T0406228

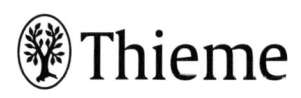

Veterinary Physiology

Edited by
Gerhard Breves
Martin Diener
Gotthold Gäbel
David Fraser

Contributors of the 6th German edition

Salah Amasheh
Walter Arnold
Jörg R. Aschenbach
Christine Aurich
Jörg-Eberhard Aurich
Heinz Breer
Cornelia Deeg
Franziska Dengler
Almuth Einspanier
Kristin Elfers
Herbert Fuhrmann
Max Gassmann

Thomas Göbel
Gerolf Gros
Melanie Hamann
Romy Monika Heilmann
Korinna Huber
Bernd Kaspers
Wolfgang Langhans
Thomas A. Lutz
Gemma Mazzuoli-Weber
Alexandra Muscher-Banse
Michael Pees
Helga Pfannkuche

Reiko Rackwitz
Susanne Reitemeier
Joachim Roth
Christoph Rummel
Hans-Peter Sallmann
Holger Sann
Axel Schöniger
Bernd Schröder
Stephan Steinlechner
Wolfgang von Engelhardt
Mirja Wilkens
Siegfried Wolffram

506 figures

Georg Thieme Verlag
Stuttgart · New York

Bibliographical data of the German National Library
(Deutsche Nationalbibliothek)
The German National Library (Deutsche Nationalbibliothek) lists this publication in the German National Bibliography; detailed bibliographic information can be found on the Internet at http://dnb.d-nb.de.

This and other books at www.shop.thieme.com.

Your opinion is important to us! Please write to us at:
www.thieme.com/en-us/contact/customer-service

© 2025. Thieme. All rights reserved.
Georg Thieme Verlag KG
Oswald-Hesse-Str. 50, 70469 Stuttgart, Germany
www.thieme.com

Printed in Germany

Translated from the German 6th edition
"Breves G, Diener M, Gäbel G. Physiologie der Haustiere.
Stuttgart: Georg Thieme Verlag; 2022"

Cover design: © Thieme
Image credits cover: picture Martin Diener; graphic:
Christiane und Michael von Solodkoff, Neckargemünd, Germany
Translation (including graphics): Prof. Dr. med. vet. Gerhard Breves,
Prof. Dr. med. Martin Diener, Prof. Dr. med. vet. Gotthold Gäbel,
Prof. Dr. med. vet. David Fraser
Copyediting: Dr. med. vet. Bianca Wiebusch, Hannover, Germany
Graphics: Christiane und Michael von Solodkoff, Neckargemünd,
Germany
Typesetting: Ziegler und Müller, Kirchentellinsfurt, Germany
Printing: Aprinta Druck GmbH, Wemding, Germany

DOI 10.1055/b000000799

ISBN 978-3-13-245170-4   1 2 3 4 5 6

Also available as eBook:
eISBN (PDF) 978-3-13-245171-1
eISBN (epub) 978-3-13-245172-8

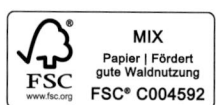

Preface

Physiology is one of the basic subjects of both veterinary and animal science. It covers knowledge of normal body functions at different levels. This includes the function of organ systems, individual organs, and detailed molecular processes of cells. A good understanding of physiology is the foundation for all clinical and para-clinical disciplines. While human physiology deals with only one species, comparative physiology of veterinary and animal science is a comprehensively demanding and challenging discipline.

This textbook is the first English version of the 6th edition (2022) of a German textbook, first published in 2000, by W. v. Engelhardt and G. Breves. Spanish, Polish and Turkish editions have been published in 2004, 2011 and 2019, respectively. Its main objective is to encompass the current state of knowledge of all aspects of physiology. In many chapters, the close relationship with pathophysiology is highlighted by including aspects of disturbed physiological functions. It is intended to offer students of veterinary medicine and related disciplines the opportunity to acquire a good understanding of physiology while at the same time indicating that physiology is not an isolated basic subject but is an indispensable basis for understanding the clinical disciplines. Thus, this book is not only addressed to veterinary and animal science students but is also intended as an aid in professional training and continued education for veterinarians working in clinics, industry or in the public health sector. In order to facilitate reading and understanding of this textbook, each chapter is introduced with "ESSENTIALS", smaller parts are summarized with "IN A NUTSHELL" and data for further in-depth knowledge is given under "MORE DETAILS". At the end of each chapter, you will find publications under "SUGGESTED READING".

The editors gratefully acknowledge the stimulating cooperation with Mrs. Anna Johne, Thieme Publisher and Dr. Bianca Wiebusch, copy editor.

Hannover, Giessen, Leipzig and Sydney, October 2024
Gerhard Breves
Martin Diener
Gotthold Gäbel
David Fraser

Vitae

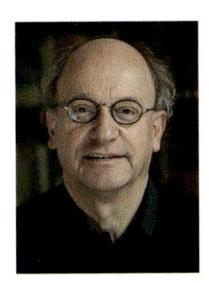

Prof. Dr. med. vet. Gerhard Breves graduated from the University of Veterinary Medicine Hannover, Germany and did his PhD (habilitation) in Physiology and Nutrition Physiology at the Institute of Physiology, Hannover. From 1987 to 1990 he was employed as a research assistant at the Institute of Animal Nutrition, Federal Agricultural Research Station, Braunschweig, Germany. In 1990 he was appointed as a Professor of Veterinary Physiology at the University of Giessen, Germany and in 1997 as a Professor of Physiology at the University of Veterinary Medicine, Hannover. His main research areas are epithelial transport processes and mechanisms and regulation of gastrointestinal metabolism.

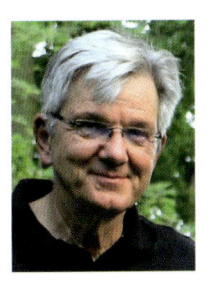

Prof. Dr. med. vet. Gotthold Gäbel studied veterinary medicine in Hannover, Germany. 1989, PhD (habilitation) in physiology at the School of Veterinary Medicine Hannover, Germany. After that, senior assistant at the Institute of Veterinary Physiology at the Free University of Berlin, Germany. Since 1993, Professor of Veterinary Physiology at the Institute of Veterinary Physiology at the University of Leipzig, Germany. Main areas of work: diarrhoea, acute and chronic rumen acidosis, regulation of intracellular pH, effect of inflammatory mediators on epithelial and neuronal processes in the gastrointestinal tract. Retired in 2021.

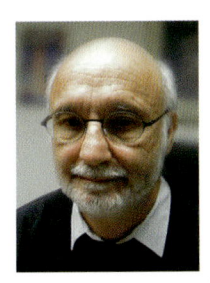

Prof. Dr. med. Martin Diener is professor of physiology at the institute of veterinary physiology and biochemistry of the Justus Liebig University Giessen, Germany. He studied human medicine and obtained his M.D. and PhD (habilitation) in pharmacology and toxicology at the University of Saarland, Homburg/Saar, Germany. After a postdoc period from 1992 to 1995 at the institute of veterinary physiology of the University of Zurich, Switzerland, he was appointed professor of veterinary physiology in Giessen in 1995. His main research interests are ion channels, epithelial transport processes and the regulation of gastrointestinal functions by the enteric nervous system.

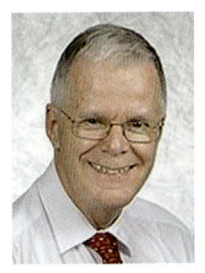

Professor David R. Fraser is Emeritus Professor of Animal Science in the Sydney School of Veterinary Science at the University of Sydney, Australia. He graduated with the Bachelor of Veterinary Science degree from that University and was then a Teaching Fellow in the Department of Biochemistry. He undertook a PhD at the University of Cambridge in the field of nutritional biochemistry. From 1967 to 1986 he was a scientific staff member of the Medical Research Council, Dunn Nutritional Laboratory, University of Cambridge, UK. He was then appointed as Professor of Animal Science in Veterinary Science at the University of Sydney and was Dean of Veterinary Science from 1994 to 1998. His main research interests are the function and metabolism of vitamin D and the special nutritional requirements of domestic animals.

Abbreviations

A

A   adult [haemoglobin]

A   area [formula]

a. (aa.)   arteria (ae) [anatomy]

AA   amino acid

AaD   alveolar arterial difference

ABC (transporter)   ATP-binding cassette (transporter)

AC   adenylate cyclase

ACE   angiotensin converting enzyme

ACh   acetylcholine

AChE   acetylcholine esterase

ACTH   adrenocorticotropic hormone

ADH   antidiuretic hormone, vasopressin, adiuretin

ADP   adenosine diphosphate

a$_{Gas}$ solubility coefficient of a gas

AgRP   Agouti-related peptide

alv   alveolar [subscript]

AMH   anti-Müllerian hormone

AMP   adenosine monophosphate

AMPA   α-amino-3-hydroxy-5-methyl-4-isoxazolpropionic acid

AMPK   adenosine monophosphate kinase

ANP   atrial natriuretic hormone, atrial natriuretic peptide, atrial natriuretic factor

AP   action potential [electrophysiology]

AP   anterior pituitary, adenohypophysis [anatomy]

AP   area postrema [anatomy]

aPPT   activated partial thromboplastin clotting time

Arc   nucleus arcuatus

ARDS   adult (acute) respiratory distress syndrome

art   arterial [subscript]

ASIC   acid-sensing ion channel

ATGL   adipose tissue triglycerol lipase

AT III   antithrombin III

ATP   adenosine triphosphate

AV   atrioventricular

Av   arteriovenous

avD   arteriovenous difference

AVT   arginine-vasotocin

B

B   total pressure or barometer reading

BAT   brown adipose tissue

BBM   brush border membrane

BCR   B-cell receptor

BE   base excess

BLM   basolateral membrane

BM   body mass

BMR   basal metabolic rate

BNP   brain natriuretic peptide

BPG   bisphosphoglycerate

2,3-BPG   2,3-bisphosphoglycerate

bST   bovine somatotropin (bovine growth hormone)

BTPS   body temperature, pressure, saturated

C

C   cholesterol [metabolism]

C   cervical segment of the spinal cord [anatomy]

C   compliance [lung]

C   concentration [formula]

CA   carbonic anhydra(ta)se

cAMP   cyclic adenosine monophosphate

cap   capillary [subscript]

CAP   compound action potential

CART   cocaine-/amphetamine-regulated transcript

CaSR   calcium sensing receptor

Ca$_v$ channel   voltage-dependent Ca^{2+}-channel

cBA   conjugated bile acid

CCK   cholecystokinin

CD   cluster of differentiation

CETP   cholesterol transfer protein

CFTR   cystic fibrosis transmembrane regulator

CFU   colony forming unit

cGMP   cyclic guanosine monophosphate

CGRP   calcitonin gene-related peptide

ch.   chapter

ChO   chiasma opticum

ChR   cholinergic receptors

CLA   conjugated linoleic acids

CLOCK   circadian locomotor output cycle kaput

CN   cranial nerve

CNS   central nervous system

CO   cardiac output

CoA(SH)   coenzyme A

COMT   catechol-O-methyltransferase

COPD   chronic obstructive pulmonary disease

COX   cyclooxygenase

Cr   creatinine

CRE   cAMP-responsive element

CRH   corticotropin-releasing hormone

CRP   C-reactive protein

CP   creatine phosphate

C segment *constant segment [immunoglobulins]*

CSF *cerebrospinal fluid [nervous system]*

CSF *colony-stimulating factor [haematology]*

CVP *central venous pressure*

CYP17A1 *steroid 17α-hydroxylase*

D

Δ *difference*

D *diffusion coefficient*

d *distance*

D *diversity [immunoglobulins]*

D_3 *vitamin D_3*

1,25-(OH)$_2$D$_3$ *1,25-dihydroxycholecalciferol, vitamin D_3, calcitriol*

25-OHD *25-vitamin D_3, calcidiol*

DA *dopamine*

DAG *diacylglycerol*

dB *decibel [unit]*

DBP *vitamin D-binding protein*

DcytB *duodenal cytochrome B*

DE *digestible energy*

dead *dead space [subscript, spirometry]*

DHPR *dihydropyridine receptor*

D$_{lung}$ *diffusion capacity of the lung*

DM *dry matter*

dm/dt *amount of substance diffusing per unit time*

DNA *desoxyribonucleic acid*

DOPA *3,4-dihydroxyphenylalanine*

dpt *dioptre*

DRA *down regulated in adenoma*

E

É *volume elasticity coefficient*

ECB *endocannabinoids*

ECF *extracellular fluid*

ECG *electrocardiogram*

eCG *equine chorionic gonadotropin*

ECL *enterochromaffin-like*

EDHF *endothelium-derived hyperpolarizing factor*

EDRF *endothelium-derived relaxing factor, nitric oxide, NO*

EDTA *ethylene diamine tetraacetate*

EDV *end-diastolic volume*

EEG *electroencephalogram*

EGF *epidermal growth factor*

ELISA *enzyme-linked immuno-sorbent assay*

EM *eminentia mediana*

EMG *electromyogram*

ENaC *epithelial Na channel*

end *end (value) [subscript]*

ENS *enteric nervous system*

EP *ejection phase [heart]*

EPO *erythropoietin*

EPP *end-plate potential*

EPSP *excitatory postsynaptic potential*

ER *endoplasmic reticulum*

ERV *expiratory reserve volume*

ESV *end-systolic volume*

ET *endothelin*

η *viscosity*

ETEC *enterotoxic Escherichia coli*

exs *expired [subscript]*

F

F *Faraday constant*

F$_{ab}$ *antigen-binding fragment*

FAD *flavin adenine dinucleotide*

FAS *fatty acid synthase*

FAT *fatty acid translocase*

F$_c$ *crystalline fragment*

FcRn *neonatal F_c receptor*

FF muscle fibre *fast, fatigable muscle fibre*

FFA *free fatty acids*

F$_{Gas}$ *fraction of gas (% volume/volume)*

FGF *fibroblast growth factor*

Fig. *figure*

FP *filling phase [heart]*

FR muscle fibre *fast, resistant to fatigue muscle fibre*

FRC *functional residual capacity*

FSH *follicle-stimulating hormone*

G

GABA *γ-aminobutyric acid*

GALT *gut-associated lymphoid tissue*

GC *guanylate cyclase*

GDP *guanosine diphosphate*

GFR *glomerular filtration rate*

ggl. *ganglion*

GH *growth hormone, somatotropic hormone (=STH)*

GH-IH *growth hormone-inhibiting hormone*

GH-RH *growth hormone-releasing hormone*

GIP *gastric inhibitory polypeptide*

G$_i$-protein *inhibitory G protein*

GIT *gastrointestinal tract*

gl. *glandula*

GLP *glucagon-like peptide*

GLUT *glucose transporter (uniporter)*

GMP *guanosine monophosphate*

GnRH *gonadotropin-releasing hormone*

G-protein *guanine nucleotide-binding protein*

GRP *gastrin-releasing peptide*

GSH *glutathione*

GSSG *glutathione disulphide*

G_t *Transducin*

GTP *guanosine triphosphate*

H

Hb *haemoglobin*

HbCO *carboxyhaemoglobin*

HbF/A *foetal/adult Hb*

HbO_2 *haemoglobin, oxygenated (oxyhaemoglobin)*

HCN channels *hyperpolarisation- and cyclic nucleotide-gated ion channels*

HCP *haem carrier protein*

HCT *haematocrit*

HDL *high density lipoproteins*

HIV *human immunodeficiency virus*

HMM *heavy meromyosin*

HR *heart rate*

HSCFA *undissociated short-chain fatty acids*

17β-HSD-2 *17β hydroxysteroid-dehydrogenase-2*

HSL *hormone-sensitive lipase*

5-HT *serotonin (5-hydroxytryptamine)*

I

I *electrical current [biophysics]*

I *volumetric flow rate [circulation]*

IBD *inflammatory bowel disease*

ICC *interstitial cells of Cajal*

ICF *intracellular fluid*

IFN *interferon*

Ig *immunoglobulin*

IGF *insulin-like growth factor, somatomedin*

IGFBP *IGF binding protein*

IH *inhibiting hormone*

IL *Interleukin*

initial *initial (value) [subscript]*

inst *interstitium/-al [subscript]*

IP_3 *inositol-1,4,5-trisphosphate*

IP_3R *inositol-1,4,5-trisphosphate receptor*

IPSP *inhibitory postsynaptic potential*

IR *insulin resistance*

IRV *inspiratory reserve volume*

IS *insulin sensitivity*

J

J *Joule*

JAK *janus kinase*

J-segment *joining segment (immunoglobulins)*

K

K_{2P} channel *two-pore domain K^+ channel*

K_a *acid dissociation constant*

kDa *kilo Dalton*

K_{ir} channel *inward rectifying K^+ channel*

K_m *Michaelis constant*

K_v channel *voltage-dependent K^+ channel*

L

L *lumbal segment of the spinal cord [anatomy]*

l *length*

LAT *L-type amino acid transporter*

lat. *latin*

LCFA *long-chain fatty acids*

LDH *lactate dehydrogenase*

LDL *low density lipoproteins*

LH *luteinising hormone*

LHA *lateral hypothalamus*

LPL *lipoproteinlipase*

LPS *lipopolysaccharides*

LRb *leptin receptor*

LT *heat-labile toxin of Escherichia coli*

lung *lung [subscript]*

M

m. (mm.) *musculus (i)*

MAG *monoacylglycerol*

MAO *monoamine oxidase*

MAP *mean arterial pressure*

MAP kinase *mitogen-activated protein kinase*

max *maximal value [subscript]*

Mb *myoglobin*

MbO_2 *oxymyoglobin*

MCH *mean corpuscular haemoglobin [haematology]*

MCH *melanin-concentrating hormone [endocrinology]*

MCHC *mean corpuscular haemoglobin concentration*

MCT *monocarboxylate transporter*

MCV *mean corpuscular volume*

MDR *multidrug-resistance-protein*

ME *metabolizable energy*

MetHb *methaemoglobin*

MGL *monoacylglycerol lipase*

MHC *major histocompatibility complex [immunology]*

MHC *myosin heavy chain [muscle]*

MIF   *Muellerian-inhibiting factor*

MMC   *migrating motor complex*

mmHg   *millimetre of mercury*

MPS   *mononuclear phagocytose system*

MR   *metabolic rate*

MRA   *moderate rapidly adapting*

M receptors   *muscarinic receptors*

MRI   *magnetic resonance imaging*

mRNA   *messenger RNA*

MSH   *melanocyte-stimulating hormone*

mTOR   *mammalian target of rapamycin*

N

n. (nn.)   *nerve (nerves)*

v   *frequency, respiratory rate*

NAc   *nucleus accumbens*

NAD   *nicotinamide adenine dinucleotide*

NADP   *nicotinamide adenine dinucleotide phosphate*

NANC   *non-adrenergic, non-cholinergic*

Na_vchannel   *voltage-dependent Na^+ channel*

ncl. (ncll.)   *nucleus (nuclei)*

NCX   *Na^+/Ca^{2+} exchanger*

NEB   *negative energy balance*

NEFA   *non-esterified fatty acid*

NEL   *net energy lactation*

NFκB   *nuclear factor kappa B*

NGF   *nerve growth factor*

NHE   *Na^+/H^+ exchanger/antiporter*

NK   *neurokinin*

NK cells   *natural killer cells*

NKCC   *Na^+-K^+-Cl^- cotransporter*

NMDA   *N-methyl-D-aspartic acid*

NPN   *non-protein nitrogen*

NPY   *neuropeptide Y*

NRDS   *neonatal respiratory distress syndrome*

NS   *nervous system*

NSP   *non-structural (glyco)protein*

NT   *neurotensin*

NTS   *nucleus tractus solitarii*

O

OBP   *odorant binding protein*

OFC   *orbifrontal cortex*

OPG   *osteoblast-derived soluble decoy receptor*

OT   *oxytocin*

P

P   *permeability [formula]*

P   *power [physics]*

p   *colloid-osmotic pressure*

p   *pressure or partial pressure [biophysics]*

$P_{50,gas}$ *half-saturation pressure*

Pa   *Pascal*

PAH   *paraaminohippuric acid*

PAR   *protease activated receptor*

PBN   *parabrachial nucleus*

PCTV   *pre-chylomicron transport vesicle*

PD   *potential difference*

PD_a, PD_b, PD_t   *potential difference at apical (a) or basolateral (b) membrane or transepithelial (t)*

PDE   *phosphodiesterase*

PDGF   *platelet derived growth factor*

$PDGFRα^+$ *platelet-derived growth factor receptor A*

P_{eff}   *effective pressure*

PEP   *phosphoenolpyruvate*

PEPCK   *phosphoenolpyruvate carboxykinase*

PET   *positron emission tomography*

PG   *prostaglandin*

PGI   *prostacyclin*

pHDL   *primary HDL reverse cholesterol transport*

Pi   *inorganic phosphate*

PI3K   *phosphoinositide 3-kinase*

PIF   *prolactin-inhibiting factor*

PIH   *prolactin-inhibiting hormone*

PIP_2   *phosphatidylinositol diphosphate*

PK   *protein kinase (PKC, PKA ...)*

pKa   *negative log base ten of the acid dissociation constant*

PL   *phospholipase (PLA, PLC)*

pleu   *pleural space [subscript]*

POMC   *proopiomelanocortin*

pp   *posterior pituitary, neurohypophysis [endocrinology]*

pp   *periportal [liver]*

Pr^{n-}   *proteinate*

PSE   *pale, soft, exsudative [meat]*

p_t   *transmural pressure*

PTH   *parathyroid hormone*

PTHrP   *parathyroid hormone-related peptide*

pul   *pulmonal [subscript]*

pv   *perivenous*

PVN   *nucleus paraventricularis*

PYY   *peptide YY*

Q

Q̇   *pulmonary perfusion*

R

R   *resistance [biophysics]*

R   *gas constant [chemistry]*

r   *radius*

ρ   *density*

RA   *rapidly adapting*

RANK   *receptor activator of NFκB*

RANKL   *receptor activator of NFκB ligand*

RBF   *renal blood flow*

Re   *Reynolds number*

REM   *rapid eye movement*

RH   *releasing hormone*

rh, Rh   *rhesus*

RIA   *radioimmunoassay*

Rm   *remnants*

RMV   *respiratory minute volume*

RNA   *ribonucleic acid*

RP   *relaxation phase [heart]*

RPF   *renal plasma flow*

RQ   *respiratory quotient*

RV   *residual volume [spirometry]*

Ry   *ryanodine*

S

S   *sacral segment of the spinal cord [anatomy]*

S muscle fibre   *slow skeletal muscle fibre*

SA   *slowly adapting*

SAA   *serum amyloid A*

SARA   *subacute rumen acidosis*

SCC   *somatic cell count*

SCF   *stem cell factor*

SCFA   *short-chain fatty acids*

SCN   *nucleus suprachiasmaticus*

SDMA   *symmetric dimethylarginine*

SERCA   *sarco-/endoplasmic reticulum Ca^{2+}-ATPase*

SGLT   *sodium dependent glucose transporter*

SID   *strong ion difference*

SLN   *sarcolipin*

SN   *substantia nigra*

SNAP   *soluble NSF attachment proteins*

SNARE   *SNAP receptors*

S_{O_2} *oxygen saturation of blood*

SP   *substance P [nervous system]*

sp   *spirometer [subscript]*

SR   *sarcoplasmic reticulum*

SRY gene   *sex-determining region of the y chromosome*

ST   *heat-stable toxin of Escherichia coli*

STAT   *signal transducer and activator of transcription*

STPD   *standard temperature, pressure, dry*

SV   *stroke volume*

T

T   *temperature*

t   *time*

T_3 *triiodothyronine*

T_4 *thyroxine, tetraiodothyronine*

TC   *total capacity*

TCR   *T-cell receptor*

TDF   *testis determining factor*

TF   *tissue factor*

TFPI   *tissue factor pathway inhibitor*

Tg   *triacylglycerol*

TGF   *transforming growth factor [immunology]*

TGF   *tubuloglomerular feedback [kidney]*

Th   *thoracic segment of the spinal cord [anatomy]*

Th   *T-helper cell [immunology]*

TJ   *tight junction*

TJMAP   *tight junction membrane associated proteins*

TLR   *toll-like receptor*

TNF   *tumour necrosis factor*

TNZ   *thermoneutral zone*

TPO   *thrombopoetin*

TPR   *total peripheral resistance*

tr.   *tractus*

TRH   *thyreotropin-releasing hormone*

TRP   *transient receptor potential (ion channel)*

TRPA   *transient receptor potential ankyrin type (ion channel)*

TRPC   *transient receptor potential classical type (ion channel)*

TRPM   *transient receptor potential melastatin type (ion channel)*

TRPV   *transient receptor potential vanilloid type (ion channel)*

TSH   *thyroid-stimulating hormone*

TV   *tidal volume*

U

U   *voltage [biophysics]*

UCP   *uncoupling protein*

UDP   *uridine diphosphate*

UGT   *UDP glucoronyl transferase*

urine   *urine [subscript]*

UT   *urea transporter*

UV   *ultraviolet*

V

V   *volume [formula]*

V   *Volt [unit]*

V̇   *volumetric volume flow*

v̄   *mean velocity [biophysics]*

V segment   *variable segment (immunoglobulins)*

v. (vv.)   *vena(ae) [Anatomy]*

VAO   *vena angularis oculi*

VC   *vital capacity*

VDN   *vena dorsalis nasi*

VDR   *vitamin D receptor*

ven   *venous [subscript]*

VF   *facial vein*

v$_{HR140}$ *running speed at a heart rate of 140 min^{-1}*

VIP   *vasoactive intestinal peptide*

v$_{La4}$ *running speed at a lactate concentration in the blood of 4 mmol · l^{-1}*

VLDL   *very low density lipoproteins*

V$_{max}$ *maximal transport velocity*

vWF   *von-Willebrand factor*

W

WHO   *World Health Organization*

Z

ZO   *zonula occludens*

ZP   *zona pellucida*

Contents

Cells and excitable tissues

Regulation of the internal milieu

Nutrition and energy balance

Endocrinology and reproduction

Addresses

Editors

Prof. Dr. Gerhard **Breves**
Stiftung Tierärztliche Hochschule Hannover
Institut für Physiologie und Zellbiologie
Bischofsholer Damm 15 /102
30173 Hannover
Germany

Prof. Dr. Martin **Diener**
Justus-Liebig-Universität Gießen
Institut für Veterinär-Physiologie und -Biochemie
Frankfurter Str. 100
35392 Gießen
Germany

Prof. Dr. Gotthold **Gäbel**
Universität Leipzig
Veterinär-Physiologisches Institut
An den Tierkliniken 7
04103 Leipzig
Germany

Prof. Dr. David **Fraser**
The University of Syndney
Sydney School of Veterinary Science
NSW 2006 Sydney
Australia

Contributors of the German edition

Prof. Dr. Salah **Amasheh**
Freie Universität Berlin
Institut für Veterinär-Physiologie (WE02)
Oertzenweg 19b
14163 Berlin
Germany

Prof. Dr. Walter **Arnold**
Veterinärmedizinische Universität Wien
Forschungsinstitut für Wildtierkunde und Ökologie
Savoyenstr. 1a
1160 Wien
Austria

Prof. Dr. Jörg R. **Aschenbach**
Institut für Veterinär-Physiologie (WE02)
Oertzenweg 19b
14163 Berlin
Germany

Prof. Dr. Christine **Aurich**
Veterinärmedizinische Universität Wien
Besamung und Embryotransfer
Veterinärplatz 1
1210 Wien
Austria

Prof. Dr. Jörg-Eberhard **Aurich**
Veterinärmedizinische Universität Wien
Klinische Abteilung für Geburtshilfe, Gynäkologie
und Andrologie
Veterinärplatz 1
1210 Wien
Austria

Prof. Dr. Heinz **Breer**
Universität Hohenheim
Institut für Physiologie
Garbenstr. 30
70599 Stuttgart
Germany

Prof. Dr. Cornelia **Deeg**
Ludwig-Maximilians-Universität München
Lehrstuhl für Physiologie
Lena-Christ-Str. 48
82152 Planegg/Martinsried
Germany

Ass.-Prof. Dr. Franziska **Dengler**
Veterinärmedizinische Universität Wien
Institut für Physiologie, Pathophysiologie und Biophysik
Veterinärplatz 1
1210 Wien
Austria

Prof. Dr. Almuth **Einspanier**
Universität Leipzig
Veterinär-Physiologisch-Chemisches Institut
An den Tierkliniken 1
04103 Leipzig
Germany

Kristin **Elfers** PhD
Stiftung Tierärztliche Hochschule Hannover
Institut für Physiologie und Zellbiologie
Bischofsholer Damm 15
30173 Hannover
Germany

Prof. Dr. Herbert **Fuhrmann**
Universität Leipzig
Veterinär-Physiologisch-Chemisches Institut
An den Tierkliniken 1
04103 Leipzig
Germany

Prof. Prof. h.c. Dr. Max **Gassmann**
Vetsuisse Fakultät Universität Zürich
Institut für Veterinärphysiologie
Winterthurerstr. 260
8057 Zürich
Switzerland

Prof. Dr. Thomas **Göbel**
Ludwig-Maximilians-Universität München
Veterinärwissenschaftliches Department Tierphysiologie
Veterinärstr. 13
80539 München
Germany

Prof. Dr. Gerolf **Gros**
Medizinische Hochschule Hannover Zentrum Physiologie
AG Vegetative Physiologie
Carl-Neuberg-Str. 1
30625 Hannover
Germany

Prof. Dr. Melanie **Hamann**
Justus-Liebig-Universität Gießen
Institut für Pharmakologie und Toxikologie
Schubertstr. 81
35392 Gießen
Germany

Prof. Dr. Romy Monika **Heilmann** PhD
Universität Leipzig
Klinik f. Kleintlastnameiere – Abt. Innere Med.
An den Tierkliniken 23
04103 Leipzig
Germany

Prof. Dr. Korinna **Huber**
Universität Hohenheim, Agrarwiss. Fakultät
Institut für Nutztierwissenschaften (460d)
Fruwirthstr. 35
70599 Stuttgart
Germany

Prof. Dr. Bernd **Kaspers**
Ludwig-Maximilians-Universität München
Veterinärwissenschaftliches Department Tierphysiologie
Lena-Christ-Str. 48
82152 Planegg/Martinsried
Germany

Prof. emeritus Dr. Wolfgang **Langhans**
Institut für Lebensmittel, Ernährung und Gesundheit
Labor für Physiologie und Verhalten
Schorenstr. 16
8603 Schwerzenbach
Switzerland

Prof. Dr. Thomas A. **Lutz**
Vetsuisse Fakultät Universität Zürich
Institut für Veterinärphysiologie
Winterthurerstr. 260
8057 Zürich
Switzerland

Prof. Dr. Gemma **Mazzuoli-Weber** PhD
Stiftung Tierärztliche Hochschule Hannover
Institut für Physiologie und Zellbiologie
Bischofsholer Damm 15/102
30173 Hannover
Germany

Dr. Alexandra **Muscher-Banse**
Stiftung Tierärztliche Hochschule Hannover
Institut für Physiologie und Zellbiologie
Bischofsholer Damm 15/102
30173 Hannover
Germany

Prof. Dr. Michael **Pees**
Stiftung Tierärztliche Hochschule Hannover
Klinik für Heimtiere, Reptilien und Vögel
Bünteweg 9
30559 Hannover
Germany

PD Dr. Helga **Pfannkuche**
Universität Leipzig
Veterinär-Physiologisches Institut
An den Tierkliniken 7
04103 Leipzig
Germany

Dr. Reiko **Rackwitz**
Universität Leipzig
Albrecht-Daniel-Thaer-Institut für Agrar- und Veterinärwissenschaften e. V.
An den Tierkliniken 29
04103 Leipzig
Germany

Dr. Susanne **Reitemeier**
Universität Leipzig
Veterinär-Physiologisch-Chemisches Institut
An den Tierkliniken 1
04103 Leipzig
Germany

Prof. Dr. Joachim **Roth**
Justus-Liebig-Universität Gießen
Institut für Veterinär-Physiologie und -Biochemie
Frankfurter Str. 100
35392 Gießen
Germany

Prof. Dr. Christoph **Rummel**
Justus-Liebig-Universität Gießen
Institut für Veterinär-Physiologie und -Biochemie
Frankfurter Str. 100
35392 Gießen
Germany

Prof. Dr. Dr. h.c. Hans-Peter **Sallmann**
Bachstr.134
31157 Sarstedt
Germany

PD Dr. Holger **Sann**
Kampstr. 52
30629 Hannover
Germany

Dr. Axel **Schöniger**
Universität Leipzig
Veterinär-Physiologisch-Chemisches Institut
An den Tierkliniken 1
04103 Leipzig
Germany

Prof. Dr. Bernd **Schröder**
Canine Science®
Bleekstraße 25
30559 Hannover
Germany

Prof. Dr. Stephan **Steinlechner**
Stiftung Tierärztliche Hochschule Hannover
Institut für Zoologie
Bünteweg 17
30559 Hannover
Germany

Prof. Dr. Dr. h.c. Wolfgang **von Engelhardt**
Auf dem Limbrinke 5
30657 Hannover
Germany

Prof. Dr. Mirja **Wilkens**
Universität Leipzig
Institut für Tierernährung, Ernährungsschäden
und Diätetik
An den Tierkliniken 9
04103 Leipzig
Germany

Prof. Dr. Siegfried **Wolffram**
Christian-Albrechts-Universität
Institut für Tierernährung und Stoffwechselphysiologie
Hermann-Rodewald-Str. 9
24118 Kiel
Germany

Editors of the former 5th German edition "Physiologie der Haustiere"

Prof. Dr. Rupert M. **Bruckmaier**

Prof. Dr. Rüdiger **Gerstberger**

Prof. Dr. Michael **Fromm**

PD Dr. Harald **Hammon**

Prof. Dr. Martin **Kaske**

Prof. Dr. Michael **Schemann**

Dr. Anne **Weißmann**

Cells and excitable tissues

1 Cell physiology

Bernd Schröder, Christoph Rummel

1.1 Basics of cell physiology

ESSENTIALS ✖

Cells represent the smallest functional unit of every living organism. Their collective functions define the physiological processes in the tissues and organs of the entire organism. The supply of energy, the transport of substances across cell membranes, the organ-specific cell anatomy and the cell-specific gene expression are basic requirements for all physiological processes in living beings.

The essential building blocks of cells are the cell nucleus, mitochondria, endoplasmic reticulum, Golgi apparatus, cytoskeleton and cell membranes. The abilities of cells to selectively absorb or release substances can vary greatly from one organ to another. The various functions of cells can also adapt to changes, or be regulated, according to their role in each organ.

1.2 The cell as the smallest functional unit of a living animal

The cell is the **smallest viable** and **reproducible functional unit** of an animal. Its ability to reproduce is one of the properties used as a criterion for life. The deoxyribonucleic acid (DNA) of the genome, as the carrier of genetic information of each cell, contains the messages defining its structures, functions and self-reproduction. The double helix of DNA in chromosomes represents the seat of the "legislative branch" in the cell, while the "executive branch" is represented by the entirety of the proteins that result from transcription and translation. The genetic information of a cell can change by **mutation**, which enables the cell to evolve according to the criteria of selection. Cells possess a **metabolic profile** that enables them not only to maintain their own structures, but also to grow and perform work. Energy-rich substances, generally ATP and NAD(P)H/H⁺, connect the energy-consuming production of substances (**anabolism**) with the energy-releasing breakdown of substrates (**catabolism**). Viable cells maintain many chemical gradients between the extracellular and intracellular spaces. Therefore, there is a constant exchange of substances and energy between the cell and its environment, so that a stable **steady state** is maintained. These processes are regulated by the structure and the permeability of the **cell membrane** (**plasma membrane**) that surrounds each cell and provides a barrier with its environment. Another decisive criterion is the **excitability** of a cell, i.e. it can receive and respond to various chemical and physical signals from outside. These processes can be mediated by specific **receptors** in the cell membrane.

IN A NUTSHELL !

The cell is the smallest viable and reproducible functional unit of an organism. The abilities of self-reproduction, metabolism and excitability are the most important criteria of a living cell.

1.3 Subcellular organisation of the cell

Although the size, shape and structure of cells are very variable, because of their wide variety of functions, all cells have a fundamentally homologous structural design. As an example, a schematic epithelial cell with its organelles is shown in **Fig. 1.1**.

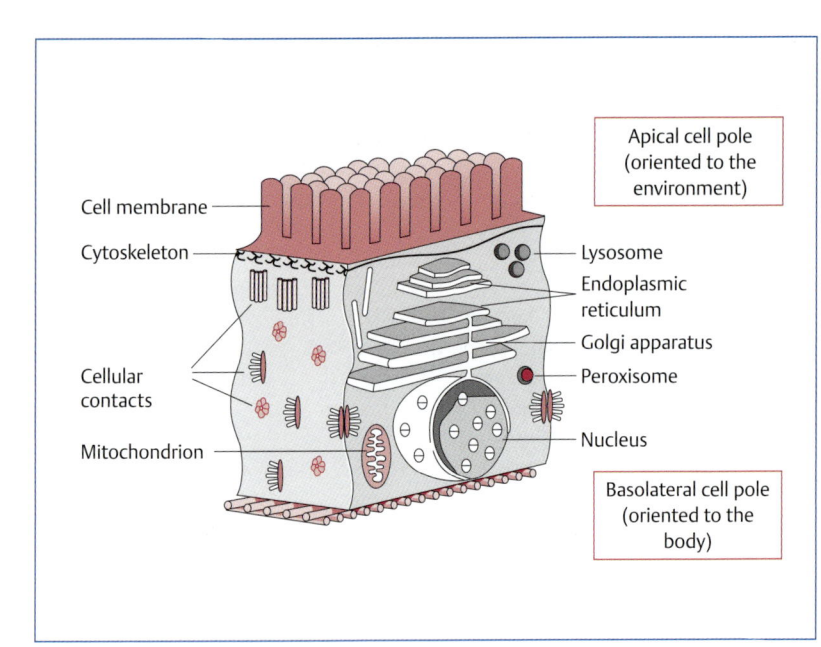

Fig. 1.1 Schematic representation of an animal cell. A **polarized epithelial cell** is shown as an example, which is connected to the environment at its **apical side** and to the inside of the body at its **basolateral side**. The nucleus is surrounded by two membranes that form the nuclear envelope. Nuclear pores penetrate through it. The intermembrane space of the nuclear envelope communicates directly with the endoplasmic reticulum (ER). The mitochondria also have an outer and inner membrane. The dictyosomes of a cell form the Golgi apparatus. Lysosomes and peroxisomes in the cell represent special vesicular functional spaces or reaction spaces (compartments). A so-called cytoskeleton (p. 29) of network-like connected protein chains stabilises the shape of individual cells. In addition, special structures for contact between cells (p. 29) in a tissue help to connect cells to one another (either mechanically and/or for communication).

Labels in figure: Cell membrane; Cytoskeleton; Cellular contacts; Mitochondrion; Apical cell pole (oriented to the environment); Lysosome; Endoplasmic reticulum; Golgi apparatus; Peroxisome; Nucleus; Basolateral cell pole (oriented to the body)

1.3.1 Intracellular organelles and the principle of compartmentalization

Animals consist of a large percentage of water (p. 331), which is an important medium for all life processes. The water in an organism is divided into functionally different reaction spaces, which are referred to as **compartments**. The intracellular body fluid can also be subdivided into a number of other compartments by subcellular structures. The complexity of the cell is expressed at the structural level by its internal organisation with biomembranes dividing the cell into numerous intracellular reaction spaces. By definition, a **membrane** is regarded as a self-contained structure, i.e. a separating layer that completely encloses a space. The term **compartment** is used to describe the sum of spaces of the same type, e.g. the entirety of mitochondria or lysosomes. The term, compartment, is not necessarily the same as the term **organelle**, which is used for different cell structures such as ribosomes or Golgi apparatus. The **cytoplasm**, which is surrounded by the cell membrane, is also a compartment in this sense. The most important compartments or organelles of the animal cell and some of their typical functions are summarised in **Table 1.1**.

Table 1.1 Division of the animal cell into compartments.

Compartment	Main functions
Cell membrane	Barrier and contact to the extracellular space, signal reception, transport of substances
Cytoplasm	Contents of a cell (other than the nucleus); general metabolism, protein synthesis, storage of glycogen, intracellular movements, cytoskeleton
Cytosol	Contents of a cell with the exception of the cell organelles and the cell nucleus
Endoplasmic reticulum (ER)	Synthesis of membrane and export proteins (mainly rough ER), lipid synthesis (mainly smooth ER); as sarcoplasmic reticulum (SR) in muscle cells, it is an important Ca^{2+} store
Golgi apparatus	Entirety of dictyosomes (= individual membrane vesicle stacks of the Golgi cisternae); oligo- and polysaccharide synthesis
Peroxisomes	Compartment for various special tasks such as oxidation of substances for detoxification; oxidases, catalase
Lysosomes	Digestion of endocytosed material; hydrolases
Cell nucleus	DNA replication, transcription, synthesis and maturation of messenger RNA, formation of ribosomal subunits in the nucleolus
Mitochondria	Respiration, ATP production

The compartmentalization of the cell is extremely **dynamic**. This applies in particular to the endoplasmic reticulum (ER) and the Golgi apparatus. Like lysosomes and the plasma membrane, they are in close contact with one another (**membrane flow)** because of the continuous release and fusion of vesicles (e.g. transport and storage vesicles). Only mitochondria have no exchange of this type with other organelles.

The purpose of compartmentalizing a cell is to separate particular metabolic pathways from one another, making them more effective, less susceptible to disruption, and easier to regulate.

> **IN A NUTSHELL** !
>
> In principle, all mammalian cells have a homologous structural design. The cell is divided into numerous compartments by intracellular membranes, each with specific functions.

1.3.2 Cell membrane

The cell or plasma membrane forms an approximately 5–6 nm thick boundary layer between the cytoplasm and the extracellular space. For each cell, it is both a barrier and a connection with the extracellular environment. It therefore has a large number of tasks, in addition to a barrier function, including control of uptake and release of substances by means of **specific transport processes**. Of particular importance are **endocytosis** and **exocytosis, cell-cell recognition**, **signal reception**, **signal processing**, **signal transmission** (signal transduction) and the formation of **cell-cell connections**.

These diverse functions of cell membranes are also reflected in their structural composition (**Fig. 1.2**). The membrane consists of a double **lipid** layer (bilayer), which is comprised partly of phospholipids (e.g. phosphatidylcholine), partly of glycolipids (e.g. ceramide group) and cholesterol. The oligosaccharide side chains of the glycolipids are located exclusively on the extracellular side of the membrane, so that the lipid bilayer is **asymmetrical**. Phospho- and glycolipids have **amphiphilic** properties, i.e. they have both **lipophilic** (**hydrophobic**) and **hydrophilic** (**lipophobic**) properties. The relative proportion of different lipids varies with the type of membrane. The amount of cholesterol in a membrane has a significant influence on its **fluidity** (**Fig. 1.4**). For example, the plasma membrane of rat liver cells contains, depending on the diet, almost 20% cholesterol as a percentage of total lipid, while intracellular membranes contain less than half this amount. **Cholesterol** plays a decisive role in the formation of so-called "lipid rafts". These are functionally and structurally important raft-like areas of the membrane that can, for example, accumulate some proteins. The characteristic arrangement of the lipid bilayer (biological unit membrane) results from the physically favourable arrangement of amphiphilic molecules in aqueous solution, in that the **non-polar fatty acid residues** (two per lipid molecule) face each other in the middle of the membrane and the **polar head groups** protrude into the extra- or intracellular space.

The cell organelles are also separated from the cytosol by membranes. In principle, the organelle membranes have the same structure as the cell membrane, but their protein content can differ significantly. The mass ratio of protein to lipid varies between e.g. 3.2 for the inner mitochondrial membrane and 0.2 in the lipid-rich myelin

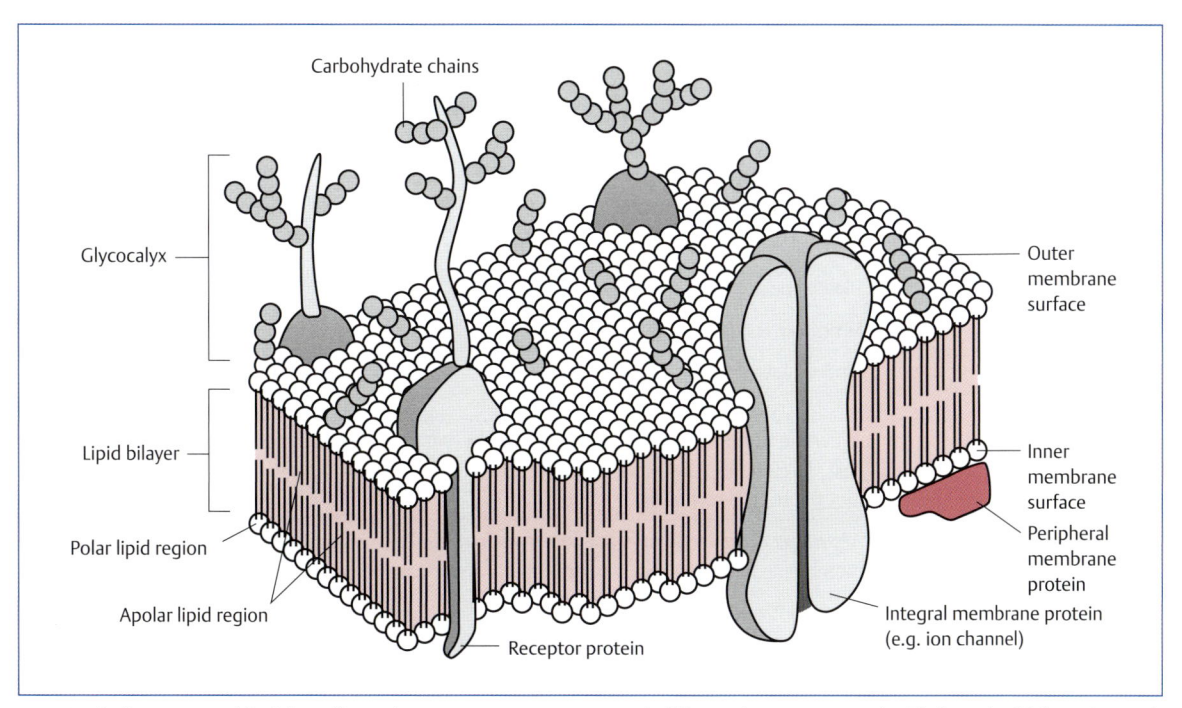

Carbohydrate chains

Glycocalyx

Outer membrane surface

Lipid bilayer

Inner membrane surface

Polar lipid region

Peripheral membrane protein

Apolar lipid region

Integral membrane protein (e.g. ion channel)

Receptor protein

Fig. 1.2 Fluid mosaic model of the cell membrane. Numerous proteins with different functions are embedded in a lipid bilayer (integral proteins, e.g. ion channels). Peripheral proteins can be bound to the membrane via specific interactions. Glycoproteins and lipids form the cell's outer layer (glycocalyx) towards the extracellular space.

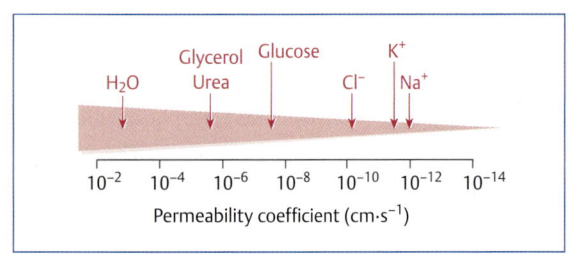

Fig. 1.3 Permeability of artificial lipid membranes for various biologically important substances. The lipid bilayer (cell membrane) has amazingly high permeability to water. Charged electrolytes are significantly less able to penetrate this "barrier". This is indicated by the permeability coefficient.

membrane, but is close to 1.0 for most membranes of mammalian cells. The **nuclear envelope** is a special case. It is folded twice and thus forms an outer and inner membrane. Mitochondria are also surrounded by two membranes, the **outer** and **inner mitochondrial membrane**. The inner membrane forms so-called cristae, invaginations into the mitochondrial matrix, which greatly increase the area. In hepatocytes, the area ratio of the inner to the outer membrane of the mitochondria is 5:1.

Due to its **hydrophobicity**, the lipid part of the plasma membrane of a mammalian cell is in principle only readily permeable to small, non-ionized molecules such as water, urea, oxygen, carbon dioxide, glycerol, and many lipid-soluble molecules. In contrast, the lipid phase of the membrane is practically impermeable to charged molecules. This applies particularly to inorganic ions such as Na^+, K^+ or Cl^- as well as non-lipid soluble substances such as glucose and fructose (**Fig. 1.3**).

In addition to lipids, the cell membrane also contains numerous proteins that can be divided into extrinsic and intrinsic proteins according to their morphological characteristics. **Peripheral** or **extrinsic proteins** can be relatively loosely attached to the hydrophilic heads of lipid molecules by electrostatic forces (e.g. the F_1 subunit of ATP synthase). In other cases, they are partially incorporated into one of the layers of the membrane (e.g. subunits of G proteins on the cytoplasmic side of the membrane). **Integral** or **intrinsic proteins** are firmly anchored in the lipid bi-

layer so that non-polar segments of the protein, which have a helix as a secondary structure, span the entire membrane once or several times (**membrane domains**). The membrane domains are connected by hydrophilic protein domains (**cytoplasmic** and **extracellular domains**) that protrude into the aqueous environment on both sides of the membrane.

In many cases, parts of non-membrane proteins, that protrude into the extracellular space, are associated with chains of carbohydrates (**glycoproteins**). Such structures on the surface of the cell membrane can form an additional envelope in many cell types. They are involved in cell-cell recognition, cell-cell adhesion, or have protective and stabilising functions. The surface of the cell membrane is so densely covered with sugar chains that a closed layer is formed, which is called the **glycocalyx** (**Fig. 1.2**). Molecules of this layer protrude up to 20 nm into the extracellular space and represent e.g. the morphological correlates of blood group and transplantation antigens (p. 241). However, these sugar residues also enable cells to specifically recognize other cells or to attach themselves to other cells. Numerous tasks and typical examples of membrane proteins are shown in **Table 1.2**.

1.3.3 Topography of membrane proteins

The topography of proteins and glycoproteins in the membrane, especially that of transmembrane proteins, is essentially determined by the amino acid sequence of their peptide chain. A prediction of the two-dimensional arrangement of the linear amino acid sequence can be given under various circumstances. For example, the occurrence of a longer series of hydrophobic amino acids in the overall sequence is interpreted as a transmembrane segment. Amino acid sequences that carry carbohydrate side chains always occur on the extracellular surface of the plasma membrane or on the luminal side of intracellular membranes. Model ideas for the spatial arrangement of a membrane protein can be derived from its two-dimensional structure. Using the well-studied voltage-dependent Na^+ channel of neurons as an example, in **Fig. 2.8** a structure-function model is shown.

Table 1.2 Functional classification of membrane proteins.

Class	Function	Examples
Receptors	Bind signalling molecules	Acetylcholine receptors, adrenergic receptors
Signalling proteins	Allow the immune system to differentiate between cancer cells, foreign cells that have entered the body, and the body's own cells	Histocompatibility antigens
Transport proteins	Allow specific polar solutes and ions to penetrate cell membranes; in some cases, such proteins also cleave ATP	Ca^{2+} channels, Na^+/K^+-ATPase
Cell-cell contact proteins	Form contacts between neighbouring cells	Gap junctions, tight junctions
Enzymes	Catalyse specific reactions of substrates in the extra- or intracellular fluid at the cell membrane	Acetylcholine esterase

1.3.4　Mobility of membrane proteins

Under physiological conditions, biomembranes are not rigid, but fluid. This means that the lipids and proteins in the bilayer are mobile and constantly moving. In principle, the molecules can either rotate around their longitudinal axis, flip over perpendicularly to the membrane plane, switch from one side of a membrane to the other (**flip-flop process**) or diffuse laterally (**Fig. 1.4**). For energetic reasons, **rotation** and **flip-flop** processes occur only very rarely (e.g. during thrombocyte activation (p. 234), the negative phospholipids of the lipid bilayer move from the inside outwards). In contrast, the lateral mobility of the membrane molecules can be relatively large depending on the cell type (**Fig. 1.4**). In addition to the mosaic-like distribution of proteins in a membrane, this property underlies the concept of the membrane as a **fluid mosaic model** (**Fig. 1.2**). Cholesterol influences these mobility properties (**fluidity**). Unsaturated fatty acids exert increased interactions via their double bonds and thereby are the primary determinants of membrane viscosity.

1.3.5　Anchoring of membrane proteins

For particular specialized cells, where a region of the membrane has a distinct function, some proteins need to be anchored and are thus firmly positioned. In **polarized** epithelial cells of the renal tubules or of the intestinal tract, the **apical** cell membrane contains different transport proteins (e.g. Na^+-dependent cotransporters) than the **basolateral** membrane (e.g. Na^+/K^+ pump) to enable directional transport, see ch. "Mechanisms of Tubular NaCl Transport" (p. 312), ch. "Absorption of minerals and trace elements" (p. 433), **Fig. 12.10**). In myelinated nerve fibres, ion channels that are involved in generation of action potential are particularly concentrated in the region of the nodes of Ranvier. In skeletal muscle cells, the receptors for acetylcholine form a non-selective cation channel (**Fig. 6.4**) and can trigger contraction. These receptors are particularly concentrated in the region of the neuromuscular junction. Elements of the **cytoskeleton** also have essential roles in anchoring membrane proteins.

1.3.6　Cytoskeleton

The cytoskeleton consists of tiny protein strands and tubes, the **filaments** and **microtubules** (**Fig. 1.1**), which span the cell and thus stabilise its shape, or are responsible for movements of the entire cell (e.g. in muscle cells with the **actin-myosin** interaction). Cytoplasmic filaments (e.g. actin) also extend into **cilia** (e.g. lung epithelium) and **microvilli** (e.g. intestinal mucosa). From studies on mammalian erythrocytes it is well known that other cytoskeletal structures such as **spectrin filaments** are linked by **actin** and **ankyrin** on the inside of the cell membrane to form a "membrane skeleton" with a hexagonal pattern. This network strengthens the cell membrane and restricts the lateral mobility of membrane proteins. Nevertheless, the membrane skeleton forms a dynamic structure that can be quickly broken down and rebuilt, particularly during growth, cell division, or differentiation. Microtubules control cytoplasmic vesicle transport and ensure that proteins are incorporated at the correct membrane position. In the meter-long nerve fibres, the neurofilaments and microtubules enable the transport of substances (e.g. neurotransmitters) or cytoplasmic cell structures (e.g. lysosomes). Special aggregations of cytoplasmic microtubules form **centrioles**, which are involved in the construction of the nuclear division spindle.

1.3.7　Cell-cell connections

Elements of the cytoskeleton support the formation of cell-to-cell connections that enable the generation and cohesion of larger cell groups. The **desmosomes** are associated with cytokeratins (**tonofilaments**, **intermediate filaments**) and the **zonulae adhaerentes** with actin filaments (**Fig. 1.5a**). Proteins that are anchored to the membrane, e.g. **zonula occludens proteins** (ZO) and the transmembrane proteins **JAM** (junctional adhesion molecule), **occludin** and the **claudins** 1–27 of epithelial cells (e.g. in intestine, liver and kidney) and endothelial cells (e.g. certain capillary endothelia) form ridge-like contact points between neighbouring cells (**occluding junction, tight junction, zonula occludens**). This allows the apical and basolateral regions of a cell to be equipped differently with proteins, so that membrane components (e.g. the cotransporter SGLT1) can be specifically incorporated into the brush border membrane of a small intestinal mucosal cell, while the Na^+/K^+ pump is located in the basolateral side of the cell (**Fig. 12.10**). In this way a functional **polarization** of the cell is achieved (e.g. **Fig. 1.1**).

Spatially, the tight junctions surround a polarized cell like a belt (0.2–0.5 µm wide) so that an epi- or endothelial cell can make many close contacts with its neighbouring cells. The distances between the contact points represent quasi pores, albeit with a very narrow diameter (e.g. 0.8 nm in the jejunum). The claudins have very different functions in terms of barrier formation. Many seal the tight junctions (e.g. claudin-1), while some others even do the opposite by creating paracellular channels (e.g. claudin-2).

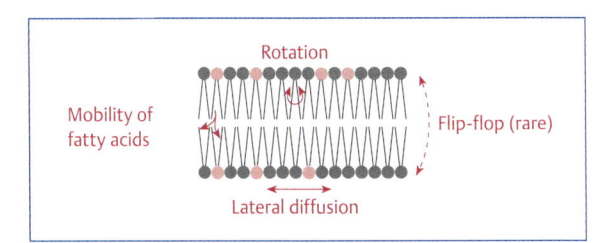

Fig. 1.4 Bilayers of lipids of cell membranes are not static structures. Rather, there are strong rotational movements, lateral diffusion and, in rare cases, a molecule switching between the inner and outer layer of the membrane (flip-flop).

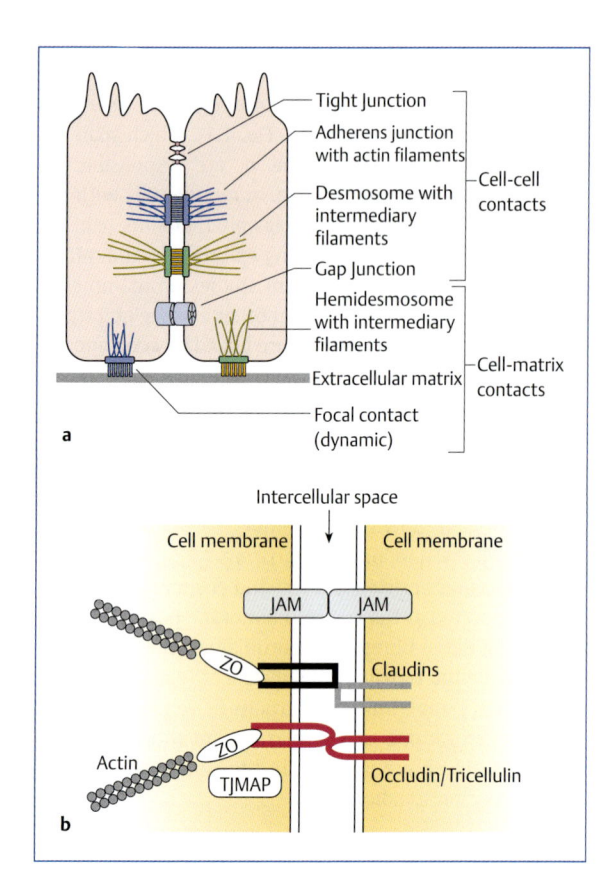

a

b

The tight junctions thus form a more or less dense barrier varying in tightness (p.311) to prevent or control disordered diffusion of molecules between cells (**paracellular transport path**). The tight junctions are regulated by a series of complex signalling pathways involving a wide range of substances, some of which are produced by the affected cells themselves. These include growth factors, cytokines, hormones, G proteins, calcium ions, protein kinases, microorganisms or products of microorganisms (e.g. in the large intestine) and xenobiotics ("foreign substances").

Fig. 1.5 Cell-cell connections

a Schematic representation of cell-cell connections, which either form belt-like barriers in epithelia or endothelia (tight junctions), attach cells to one another in a point-like manner (desmosomes and zonulae adhaerentes), or couple electrically/chemically to one another (gap junctions). The hexagonal structure of the connexons consists of six connexins each.

b Schematic representation of the basic transmembrane structures of a tight junction. The claudins have very different functions in terms of barrier formation: many seal the tight junctions (e.g. claudin-1), while some others even do the opposite by forming paracellular channels (e.g. claudin-2). The exact function of occludin is not yet known, but it probably has a barrier function.

Table 1.3 Cell-cell contacts. Contact connections are essential for tissue integrity, tissue layer organisation, and directional solute transport.

Nomenclature	Involved proteins	Main function
Tight junction (zonula occludens)	▪ Claudins ▪ Occludins	Controls the paracellular transport and the lateral diffusion of substances such as proteins in the plasma membrane and thus ensures a polar differentiation of cells, mostly sealing between the inside and outside of the body
Adhesion zone (Zonula adhaerens)	▪ Cadherins ▪ Microfilaments ▪ Actin filaments	Belt-like mechanical stabilisation of neighbouring cells, connection with the cytoskeleton
Desmosome (macula adhaerens)	▪ Cadherins ▪ Tonofilaments	Static punctiform stabilisation in the cell structure
Hemidesmosomes	▪ Integrins ▪ Attachment proteins ▪ Intermediate filaments	Fixation of cells on the basal lamina
Focal contacts	▪ Integrins ▪ Attachment proteins, actin fibres	Dynamic punctiform contacts between cells and extracellular matrix
Gap junction (nexus)	▪ Six connexins form one connexon	Protein pores for exchange of material between neighbouring cells (e.g. small intestinal epithelium) and electrical communication (e.g. smooth muscle). The connexon is the pore-forming complex of six connexin molecules. Two connexons form a gap junction channel that crosses the membranes of two adjacent cells, thus connecting the cytoplasms of those two adjacent cells.

In other cells, such as the smooth muscle cells of the gastrointestinal tract or in the cardiac muscle, the cell membranes of neighbouring cells are connected by opposing **connexons** (**gap junctions**). These hexagonal structures each consist of six identical polypeptides (**connexins**) that create a cytoplasmic connection between the cells involved, allowing both **electrical coupling** and the **passage of small molecules**. In effect, each cell forms a "half-channel" through its own cell membrane, which binds to an opposing connexon in the neighbouring cell. This creates a **channel** that connects the cytosol of both cells. Tissues such as the heart, in which a high number of gap junctions are expressed, form a functional syncytium. The permeability of the connexons can be regulated, for example, by changes in cytoplasmic Ca^{2+} concentration. **Table 1.3** provides an overview of these and other types of cell contacts between individual cells.

> **IN A NUTSHELL**   !
>
> The cell membrane consists of a lipid bilayer containing numerous proteins. This enables control of substance uptake and secretion, cell-cell recognition, and the exchange of information with the environment.

1.4 Functions of the cell membrane

1.4.1 Barrier between intra- and extracellular space

Due to its special structure, the cell membrane forms a **barrier** between the intracellular and extracellular space. As a result, different ion and protein concentrations are maintained between the inside and the outside of cells (**Table 1.4**).

In the **extracellular space**, **Na$^+$** is the most common cation and **Cl$^-$** the most common anion. In the intracellular space their concentrations are 15 and 25 times lower, respectively. This pronounced concentration gradient for Cl$^-$ ions applies to nerve and striated muscle cells. In other tissues, e.g. epithelia, it may be significantly smaller. In the **intracellular space**, **K$^+$** is more than about 40 times more concentrated than in the **extracellular space**. Adequately high concentrations of large-molecular anions, which include organic acids and proteins with different negative charges (proteinates), ensure the necessary electroneutrality in the intracellular space (**principle of electroneutrality**). The same applies to the extracellular space.

Table 1.4 also shows that there is no osmotic gradient between the extra- and intracellular space, since the total concentration of the solutes is the same in each.

Table 1.4 Typical concentrations of the most relevant ions in the extra- and intracellular space in domestic and farm animals.

Ionic species	Extracellular space Blood plasma (mmol·l^{-1})	Intracellular space Cytosol (mmol·l^{-1})	relationship outside/inside
Cations			
Sodium (Na$^+$)	142	10 (8–30)	14:1
Potassium (K$^+$)	4	155 (100–155)	1:39
Calcium (Ca^{2+})	2.5	0.1–1 µmol·l^{-1}	>2500:1 !
Other cations	2.5*	10*	–
All in all	151	175	
Anions			
Chloride (Cl$^-$)	103	4 (4–30)	26:1
Inorganic phosphate (HPO$_4^{2-}$, H$_2$PO$_4^-$)	1.5	50	1:33
Inorganic sulfate (SO$_4^{2-}$)	0.5	9	1:18
Bicarbonate (HCO$_3^-$)	27	10 (8–15)	2.7:1
Organic acids and proteinate	7	42*	1:6
All in all	139	115	
Sum of cations and anions	290	290	

*Estimate

1.4.2   Transport by diffusion

The cell membrane enables a controlled exchange of substances between the extra- and intracellular spaces. A distinction is made between non-selective and selective permeability of the membrane, depending on membrane components concerned with any particular solute transport. **Non-selective membrane permeability** allows mainly non-electrolytes such as water, O_2 and CO_2 as well as small polar (e.g. ethanol and urea) and lipophilic molecules (e.g. steroid hormones) to pass through the membrane by **diffusion**. Diffusion occurs "downhill" along a concentration gradient. The amount of substance (dm) that passes through a permeable membrane per time difference (dt) is described by **Fick's law of diffusion** (**Fig. 1.6**). Simplified, diffusion depends proportionally on the diffusion area (A) and indirectly proportionally on the diffusion distance (d). This means that a larger area contributes to an increased rate of diffusion through a membrane, and a thicker membrane has a reduced rate of diffusion. The driving force of diffusion is the concentration difference (ΔC). The diffusion coefficient (D), which is dependent on the medium and material properties, is included in the formula as a proportionality factor. The permeability for a substance is defined as the quotient of D to d and has the dimension of a velocity ($cm \cdot s^{-1}$). Diffusion is **not saturable within physiologically** occurring concentrations (**Fig. 1.6**). For example, diffusion is of great importance for pulmonary gas exchange (p. 282).

1.4.3   Transport via membrane proteins

For charged ions such as Na^+, K^+ and Cl^-, as well as hydrophilic substances such as glucose and amino acids, the lipid phase of the cell membrane represents an almost impermeable barrier, so that these substances move into or out of a cell only very slowly or not at all by simple diffusion through the lipid bilayer. Nevertheless, an exchange between the extra- and intracellular space takes place for these substances, which is made possible by membrane-bound transport proteins and/or relatively selective channels. In this way, the cell membrane possesses **selective permeability** for substances that permeate poorly.

■ Primary active transport

Active **transport** is generally defined as a process where the net flow is **"uphill"** and energy must be provided in the form of **ATP**. If the cleavage of ATP is coupled directly with the transport of the corresponding ions, this is referred to as **primary active transport**. Transport systems of this type (p. 326) that have been particularly well studied are the Na^+/K^+-ATPase, the Ca^{2+}-ATPase (e.g. in muscles) and various proton pumps (e.g. H^+/K^+-ATPase in the stomach, H^+-ATPase in the collecting duct of the kidneys). A distinction is made between electrogenic (e.g. Ca^{2+}-ATPase or H^+-ATPase) and electroneutral (e.g. H^+/K^+-ATPase) primarily active transporters (**Fig. 1.7**), which are also referred to as "**pumps**".

■ Transport through channels

Channels are membrane-spanning proteins that form a type of tunnel lined with hydrophilic amino acid residues, allowing the hydrophilic substrate (usually ions) to diffuse across the membrane. They can exist in at least two conformations, namely open (ion flow is possible) or closed (ion flow is interrupted). Channels show stochastic, i.e. random transitions from open to closed state. However, the probability with which this happens can usually be controlled by the cell, see ch. "Ionic basis of the action potential" (p. 49). Channels are named after the ion for which they are most permeable.

Channels have the highest transport rate of all transport proteins, since the interactions between ion and protein during passage are weak compared to the so-called carriers explained below. In principle, the transport of substances through open channels takes place according to the laws of diffusion in the direction of the "driving" forces. It is independent of the provision of energy (passive) and, like **diffusion, cannot be saturated** at the existing physiological concentrations (**Fig. 1.8**). As far as charged particles are concerned, the electrical potential difference across the cell membrane (**electrical gradient**) must be considered in addition to the **chemical gradient**. These two gradients

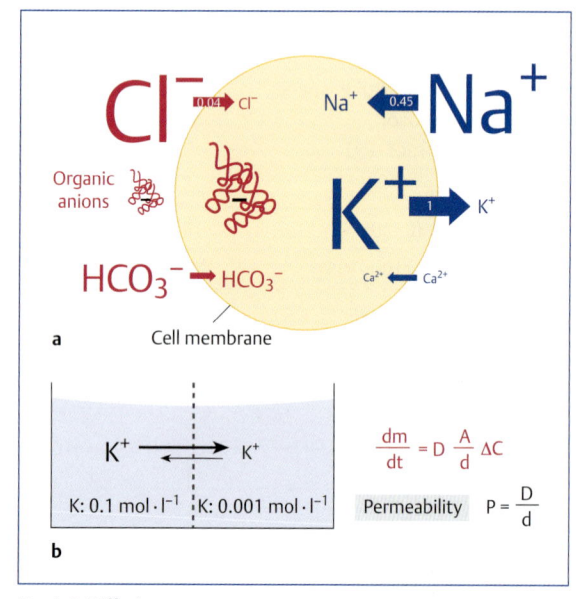

$$\frac{dm}{dt} = D \cdot \frac{A}{d} \cdot \Delta C$$

Permeability $P = \dfrac{D}{d}$

K: 0.1 mol·l⁻¹   K: 0.001 mol·l⁻¹

Fig. 1.6 Diffusion

a The distribution of anions (red) and cations (blue) between the intra- and extracellular space is crucial for understanding the functional processes of the cell. This distribution is shown here for better understanding with selected candidates roughly symbolically according to the concentrations. At rest, the conductivity for K^+ is highest in nerve cells, followed by Na^+ and Cl^- in a ratio of 1 to 0.45 to 0.04. The arrows (filled for ions for which the membrane has high permeability; dotted for ions for which the membrane has low basal permeability) indicate the direction of the chemical gradients.

b Diffusion through the cell membrane follows Fick's law of diffusion. It is non-saturable and non-selective (e.g. for O_2, CO_2, N_2 or steroids). m = amount of substance, t = time, D = diffusion coefficient, A = diffusion area , d = diffusion distance , ΔC = concentration difference.

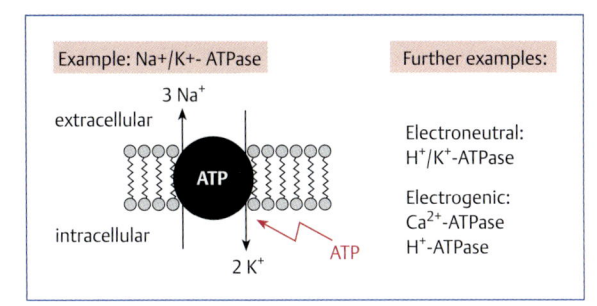

Fig. 1.7 Primary active transporters (pumps) can transport ions against a concentration gradient while consuming energy (cleavage of ATP).

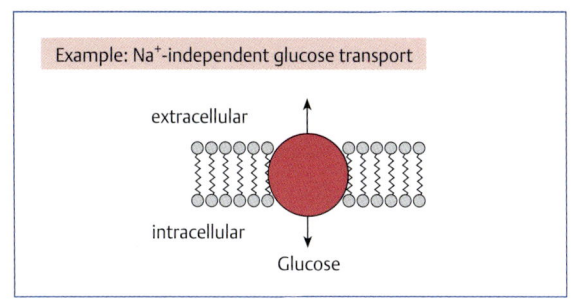

Fig. 1.9 In facilitated diffusion, substances (e.g. glucose) are transported in a saturable manner along the concentration gradient (downhill) via carriers through cell membranes

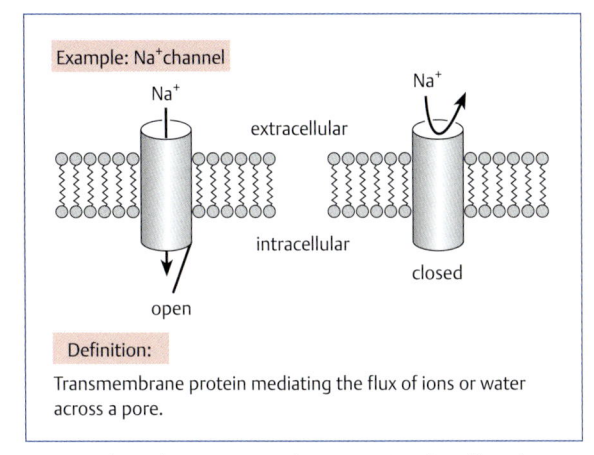

Fig. 1.8 Channels are transmembrane proteins that allow the non-saturable flow of ions (e.g. for Na^+, K^+, Ca^{2+} or Cl^-) or water (aquaporins) across the membrane through a pore.

can act on the ion flow either individually or together as an **electrochemical gradient**.

In addition to ion channels, there are also water channels (**aquaporins**), which account for the relatively high water permeability of most cell membranes (**Fig. 1.3**) or on special membranes, such as the apical membrane of the collecting duct epithelium, where the lipid phase is largely impermeable to water without aquaporins. This allows regulation of water transport in this part of the nephron through the controlled incorporation of aquaporins (p. 320).

■ Transport by carriers

The term "**carrier**" includes all membrane-bound proteins that serve to transport substances through a membrane and do not include channels or pumps. They have lower transport rates than channels because they bind their substrates more tightly and release them again more slowly. Some of the carriers transport substances for which they have the ability to bind, i.e. for which they possess an **affinity**, only in the direction of the concentration gradient, which is called a **uniport**. This means that the velocity and the direction of transport are determined by the size and direction of the concentration gradient. Other transport systems carry their substrate or several substrates only in exchange for another substance across the cell membrane,

a so-called **antiport**. Synonymously, these transporters are also referred to as **exchangers**. If two (e.g. Na^+-glucose symport in the duodenum) or even three substances (e.g. Na^+-K^+-$2Cl^-$ symport in the distal tubule of the kidney) are transported simultaneously by a carrier in the same direction, this is referred to as **symport** or **cotransport**. If substances are transported in the opposite direction, this is referred to as an antiport (e.g. Na^+/Ca^{2+} exchanger in muscle). In contrast to transport through channels, carrier-mediated transport is **saturable**, i.e. the transport velocity does not increase with increasing substrate availability. In addition, transport can be electrogenic (e.g. Na^+-glucose cotransporter), where charges are effectively transported, or it can be electroneutral (e.g. Cl^-/HCO_3^- antiporter, Na^+-HCO_3^- symporter).

Facilitated diffusion

Facilitated diffusion (**Fig. 1.9**) is the term for specific transport that occurs "downhill" in the direction of the respective "driving forces" and is saturable (**Fig. 1.11**). This designation comes from a time when little was known about the transport systems. Facilitated diffusion does not follow the laws of diffusion, but rather the principles of Michaelis-Menten kinetics. Behind these "saturation kinetics" is the fact that the transport process, in which there is physical contact between a carrier and a substrate, is characterized by an affinity between these two molecules (Michaelis constant, Km), the operating velocity and the limited number of carriers (V_{max}). Facilitated diffusion is usually mediated by uniporters (e.g. transporters for glucose, fructose or amino acids). This can be faster than simple diffusion within the range of physiological concentrations.

Secondary active transport

In the case of **secondary active transport**, an ATP-consuming step of the transport process creates a concentration gradient (e.g. primary active Na^+/K^+-ATPase, **Fig. 1.10**), which can then be the driving force for other carrier-mediated transport processes. For example, "uphill" glucose transport in renal proximal tubular epithelial cells or in small intestinal enterocytes is driven by the inward Na^+gradient, which is maintained by the activity of the basolaterally located Na^+/K^+ pump.

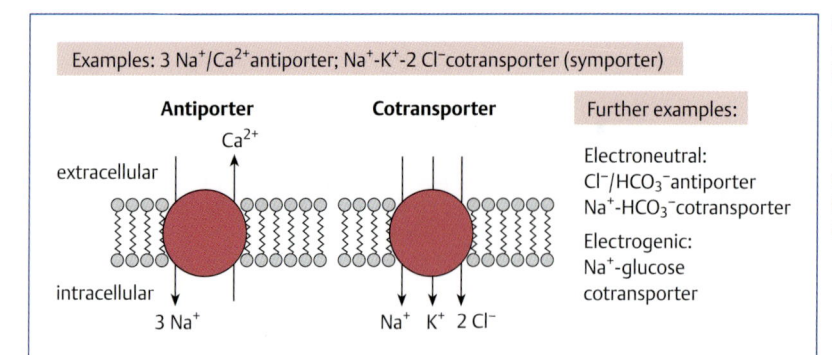

Examples: 3 Na⁺/Ca²⁺antiporter; Na⁺-K⁺-2 Cl⁻cotransporter (symporter)

Fig. 1.10 Secondary active transport processes are characterized by the fact that the driving force for transport is built up actively (energy consumption) via an electrochemical gradient (e.g. low intracellular Na⁺ and high K⁺ concentration created by the Na⁺/K⁺-ATPase). The Na⁺-K⁺-2Cl⁻ cotransporter is also referred to as the NKCC transporter (**Fig. 12.10**).

1.4.4 Transport by endo- and exocytosis

In addition to transmembrane diffusion and transport by means of transport proteins in the plasma membrane, the cell has other mechanisms available for uptake and release of substances, in which the membranes are directly involved. During **endocytosis**, particles (**phagocytosis**) or dissolved substances (**pinocytosis**) are absorbed into the cytosol by invagination and constriction of the cell membrane. Compared to phagocytosis, pinocytosis is not very specific, so it does not distinguish between different substrates very well. Conversely, during **exocytosis**, previously formed vesicles fuse with the cell membrane and the contents of the vesicle are released into the external medium. Contractile elements of the cytoskeleton are involved in these membrane fusions. There are often special receptor regions in the membrane that bind certain substances such as cholesterol, iron, insulin and some of the water-soluble vitamins or antigens and thereby trigger endocytosis (phagocytosis) in the affected area (**receptor-mediated endocytosis**). Most of the incorporated membrane vesicles are emptied inside the cell and later reused for membrane construction (**membrane recycling**), but they can also pass through the cell unchanged (**transcytosis**) and be released outside the cell at another location.

The mechanism of **exocytosis** has been well studied for some substances, such as the release of a transmitter at the presynaptic membrane, or the secretion of insulin. As a second messenger, Ca²⁺ ions are an essential factor in controlling the extent of exocytosis (**Ca²⁺-mediated exocytosis**); see ch. "Transmission of excitation, synaptic transmission" (p.59).

> **IN A NUTSHELL**   !
>
> The cell membrane forms a selectively permeable barrier between the intracellular and extracellular spaces. Lipophilic or very small substances can passively diffuse through this barrier. Lipophobic substances pass through the cell membrane via membrane transport proteins.

1.5 Membrane potential

1.5.1 Diffusion potentials and K⁺equilibrium potential

In cells, there is an electrical potential difference between the inner and the outer side of the cell membrane, which is referred to as the **membrane potential**. This voltage arises as a **diffusion potential**, which can build up on either side of the cell membrane due to the different rates of diffusion of ions through the membrane and their asymmetric distribution. For many cells, e.g. nonexcited neurons, the cell membrane is well permeable for K⁺ ions. The basis for the high K⁺ permeability are K⁺ channels. The K⁺ gradient generated by the Na⁺/K⁺-ATPase between the extra- and intracellular space is considerable (**Table 1.4**). The difference in the chemical potential (ΔW; unit: $J \cdot mol^{-1}$), which exists due to the difference in concentration between the two spaces, can be calculated according to:

$$\Delta W = R \cdot T \cdot \ln \frac{[ion]_i}{[ion]_o} \tag{1.1}$$

R stands for the gas constant ($8.314 \cdot J \cdot K^{-1} \cdot mol^{-1}$).
T is the absolute temperature (unit: K = Kelvin).
[ion] indicates the concentration inside (i) or outside (o) the cell (unit: $mol \cdot l^{-1}$).

The chemical gradient drives an efflux of K⁺ ions from the cell (**Fig. 1.11**). However, because of low anion permeability, anions cannot follow the K⁺ ions. The inside of the cell therefore has a net loss of cations so that the inner side of the membrane becomes negatively charged. This creates an electrical potential difference that corresponds to a potential electrical energy of:

$$\Delta W = z \cdot F \cdot E \tag{1.2}$$

Where z indicates the charge of the ion, F is the Faraday constant ($96485 \, C \cdot mol^{-1}$), and E is the membrane potential (unit: V).

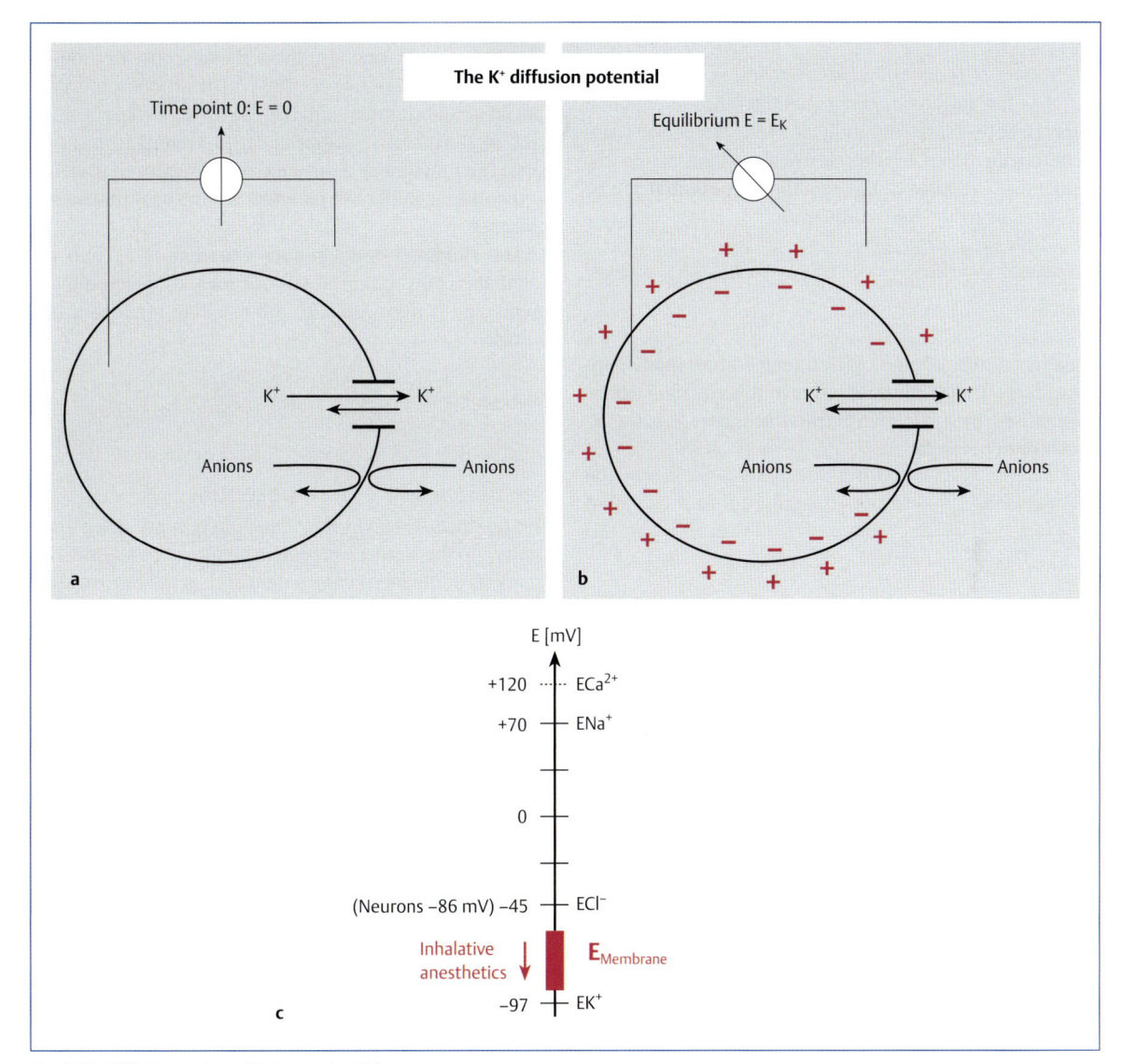

Fig. 1.11 Diffusion and equilibrium potentials

a Generation of diffusion potentials using the example of a cell where the membrane is only permeable to K^+ ions. Beginning of K^+ diffusion (**a**): Due to the K^+ concentration gradient, the diffusion out of the cell is initially greater than diffusion into the cell. The large intracellular anions, for which the membrane is impermeable, cannot follow.

b This causes the inner side of the membrane to become negatively charged. A state of equilibrium (**b**) arises between the chemically induced K^+ outflow and the electrically induced K^+ inflow. Both are exactly balanced (K^+ equilibrium potential).

c Schematic representation of the equilibrium potentials of relevant ions (black) as well as the resting membrane potential (red), which is in the negative range corresponding to the high K^+ and Cl^- conductivity under resting conditions. Depending on the cell type and ion distribution, the resting membrane potential is often between −60 and −90 mV. Volatile anaesthetics can lead to the opening of particular K^+channels (e.g. TREK-1) and reduce the ability of neurons to be activated by shifting the membrane potential to more negative values (**hyperpolarization**) and thus contribute to general anaesthesia.

The resulting **electrical potential difference** hinders the further diffusion of K^+ ions, since substances with the same electrical charge repel each other. The increasing positive charge of the membrane on the outer side impedes further outflow of K^+ from the K^+-rich intracellular space. Instead, the electrical gradient drives a flow of K^+ from the positively charged outer side to the negatively charged inner side of the membrane. A state of **equilibrium** between the two ion flows is therefore rapidly established. The efflux of K^+ from the cell interior, driven by the concentration gradient, is then equal to the influx, driven by the electrical gradient. This is referred to as **electrochemical equilibrium**, where electrical and chemical fluxes are exactly balanced. This means that the net K^+ current is zero when the K^+ **equilibrium potential** is reached.

1.5.2   Nernst equation

In the state of equilibrium, the electrical potential difference E is just large enough for the difference in chemical potential between the intracellular and extracellular space to be compensated by the electrical voltage across the membrane. The value of the **equilibrium potential** can be calculated using the **Nernst equation**:

$$E_{equilibrium} = \frac{R \cdot T}{z \cdot F} \cdot \ln \frac{[ion]_o}{[ion]_i} \qquad (1.3)$$

(Unit: V)

Under conditions of physiological temperature (body temperature 37 °C), the constant terms in this equation can be summarised by a common term which gives e.g. the **K⁺ equilibrium potential**:

$$E_K = -61 \cdot \log_{10} \frac{[K^+]_i}{[K^+]_o} \qquad (1.4)$$

(Unit: mV)

Attention: please do not confuse the two formulae! The difference lies in the use of "ln" or "$\log_{10}$". The conversion factor to go from the formula with natural logarithm (ln) to decimal logarithm ($\log_{10}$) is 2.3. In biology, the application of the "$\log_{10}$ formula" has prevailed. Swapping the numerator and denominator leads to a potential difference with a negative sign, just as the direction of the resting membrane potential is defined, which is mainly determined by K⁺.

IN A NUTSHELL   !

The Nernst equation allows the equilibrium potential of an ion on a cell membrane to be calculated, e.g. for K⁺:

$$E_K = -61 \cdot \log_{10} \frac{[K^+]_i}{[K^+]_o} \qquad (1.5)$$

with the unit mV.
With the help of this relationship, one can calculate, for example, a K⁺ equilibrium potential of −97 mV at a concentration of 4 mmol·l⁻¹ K⁺ extracellular and 155 mmol·l⁻¹ K⁺ intracellular. This means that with a potential difference of −97 mV between the inner and the outer side of the membrane, there is no net transport of K⁺ ions across that membrane.

1.5.3   Goldman-Hodgkin-Katz equation

Cell membranes are permeable to varying degrees not only to K⁺, but also to other ions, in particular Na⁺ or Cl⁻. Therefore, other ions also contribute to the resting membrane potential according to their membrane permeability, i.e. depending on the number, the conductance and the open probability of specific ion channels. All ions for which the membrane is permeable have different equilibrium potentials, which are determined by the ratio between the intra- and extracellular concentrations of the respective ion. The equilibrium potential for Na⁺ with its mirror image distri-

bution compared to K⁺ is at an extracellular concentration of 142 mmol·l⁻¹ and an intracellular concentration of 10 mmol·l⁻¹ (**Table 1.4**) at +70 mV. For Cl⁻ one can calculate an equilibrium potential of −86 mV at a concentration ratio of 103 mmol·l⁻¹ extracellular to 4 mmol·l⁻¹ intracellular. The membrane is virtually impermeable to proteins, so that their equilibrium potential is of no quantitative significance.

The **Goldman-Hodgkin-Katz equation** takes into account the contribution of **various ions**, to which the cell membrane is **permeable**, to the resulting membrane potential:

$$E_{Membrane} = \frac{R \cdot T}{F} \ln \frac{P_K \cdot [K^+]_o + P_{Na} \cdot [Na^+]_o + P_{Cl} \cdot [Cl^-]_i}{P_K \cdot [K^+]_i + P_{Na} \cdot [Na^+]_i + P_{Cl} \cdot [Cl^-]_o} \qquad (1.6)$$

(Unit: V)

The Goldman-Hodgkin-Katz equation is constructed analogously to the Nernst equation. It allows more realistic calculations of the membrane potential than the Nernst equation for many excitable cells, especially under the specific conditions of the timing of an action potential. Again, there is a proportionality factor $(R \cdot T)/F$ between the logarithm of the concentration ratios of certain ions inside and outside the cell and the resulting membrane potential $E_{Membrane}$. The charge z is missing because only monovalent ions were considered in this simplified analysis. The permeability P, which has the dimensional unit of a speed $(cm \cdot s^{-1})$, was newly introduced in comparison to the Nernst equation. P is a measure of the permeability of a membrane to an ion. The higher is P for a given ion, the better the membrane's permeability to that ion. The different ion concentrations are multiplied by the permeability of the membrane for the respective ion.

The K⁺ permeability of resting nerve or muscle cells, when measured experimentally is about 10–25 times higher than the Na⁺ permeability. As applied to nerve and muscle cells: $P_K : P_{Na} : P_{Cl} = 1 : 0.04 : 0.45$ (**Fig. 1.6a, Fig. 1.11**). Accordingly, the membrane potential is dominated by the K⁺ and Cl⁻ permeability. Since the equilibrium potentials for both ions are close to −90 mV, this means that the resting membrane potential of many neurons s is around −90 mV.

IN A NUTSHELL   !

The Goldman-Hodgkin-Katz equation (GHK equation, often also called Goldman equation for short) is:

$$E_{Membrane} = \frac{R \cdot T}{F} \ln \frac{P_K \cdot [K^+]_o + P_{Na} \cdot [Na^+]_o + P_{Cl} \cdot [Cl^-]_i}{P_K \cdot [K^+]_i + P_{Na} \cdot [Na^+]_i + P_{Cl} \cdot [Cl^-]_o} \qquad (1.7)$$

(Unit: V)
The different intra- and extracellular ion concentrations are multiplied by the permeability of the membrane for the respective ion. For example, if $P_K = 1$ and both P_{Na} and $P_{Cl} = 0$, the same results can be calculated by applying the Nernst equation.

1.6 Regulation of specialized cell functions

1.6.1 Cell volume regulation

Because the cell membrane is highly permeable to water molecules, even small differences in osmotic pressure between the cytoplasm and the extracellular fluid produce a net water movement that causes either **cell swelling** or cell **shrinkage**, depending on the direction of the gradient. As a general rule, cells are able to regulate their volume very precisely. A distinction is made between short-term and long-term mechanisms (**Fig. 1.12**).

Short-term cell volume regulation occurs spontaneously and takes place within seconds to minutes. The **Na$^+$/ K$^+$-ATPase** plays a major role in **isotonic cell volume regulation**. With an increase in the Na$^+$ influx, e.g. as a result of depolarization in a neuron or by Na$^+$-coupled cotransport systems in absorbing epithelia, the Na$^+$/K$^+$ pump will try to maintain the intracellular Na$^+$ and K$^+$ concentrations so that the intracellular fluid remains **isotonic**. A drop in intracellular osmolarity would lead to cell shrinkage and an increase would lead to cell swelling. After inhibition of the Na$^+$/K$^+$ pump (e.g. by the inhibitor ouabain), cells swell and can even burst. In the case of a **regulatory volume decrease**, the **K$^+$-Cl$^-$ cotransport system** as well as **K$^+$** and **Cl$^-$ channels** are involved in **cell volume regulation**. In response to increased osmotic pressure in the extracellular space, erythrocytes and many epithelial cell types can counteract the risk of cell shrinkage by absorbing additional, osmotically active particles, e.g. by means of the **Na$^+$-K$^+$- 2Cl$^-$ cotransporter (NKCC)** (**regulatory volume increase**). Mechanical **membrane tension** appears to play a central role in controlling cellular volume regulation. Depending on the **cell turgor**, stretch-sensitive ion channels or transporters in the cell membrane can be activated or deactivated.

Long-term cell volume regulation, e.g. with persistent hypertonicity of the extracellular space, requires hours to days, since it usually involves nucleus-mediated processes such as gene expression of specific enzymes or substrate transporters. These processes serve to increase the capacity for absorption or release of organic substrates (osmolytes) by the cell or to build up or break down macromolecules to adjust the intracellular osmolarity.

> **IN A NUTSHELL**   !
>
> The Na$^+$/K$^+$-ATPase plays a major role in short-term cellular volume regulation. When the extracellular medium is hypotonic, osmolytes can be transported out of the cell by the K$^+$-Cl$^-$ cotransporter or stretch-activated K$^+$ and Cl$^-$ channels. Conversely, under hypertonic conditions, osmolytes are taken up by Na$^+$-K$^+$-2Cl$^-$ cotransport.

1.6.2 Intracellular pH regulation

CO_2 is continuously formed in the cell during **aerobic metabolism**. In **anaerobic metabolism**, lactic acid is produced. Both aerobic and anaerobic metabolisms release **protons** (H$^+$ ions) and the intracellular pH value (pH$_i$) decreases. Intracellular pH homeostasis must be tightly regulated to maintain normal cell function because the pH value, to name just a few examples, has a direct influence on the activity of many enzymes. It affects the solubility of important electrolytes (e.g. of Ca^{2+}-, Mg^{2+}- or P$_i$-containing salts) and also exerts regulatory functions. In vitro measurements of the intracellular pH value with pH-sensitive fluorescent indicators in intact cells reveal a pH$_i$ of approximately 7.1, with a physiological pH value of 7.4 in the extracellular space.

Within a certain range, the acid equivalents can be buffered by the cell's bicarbonate-carbonic acid system. In addition, the **Na$^+$/H$^+$ antiporter** turnover rate is allosterically

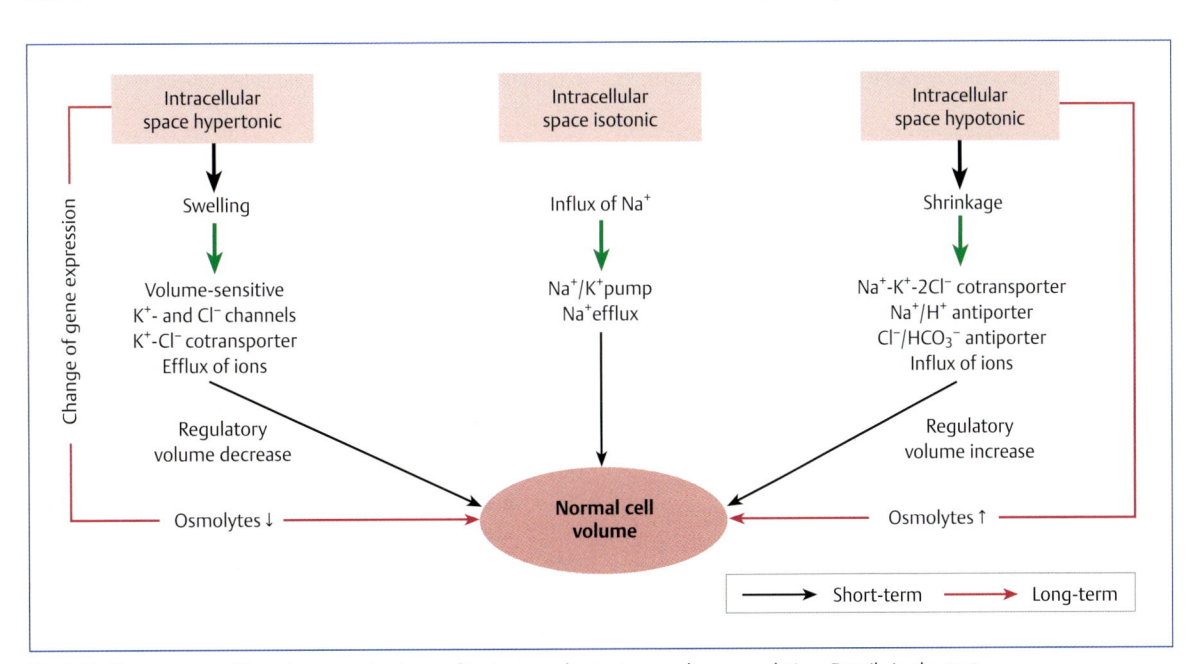

Fig. 1.12 Short-term and long-term mechanisms of isotonic and anisotonic volume regulation. Details in the text.

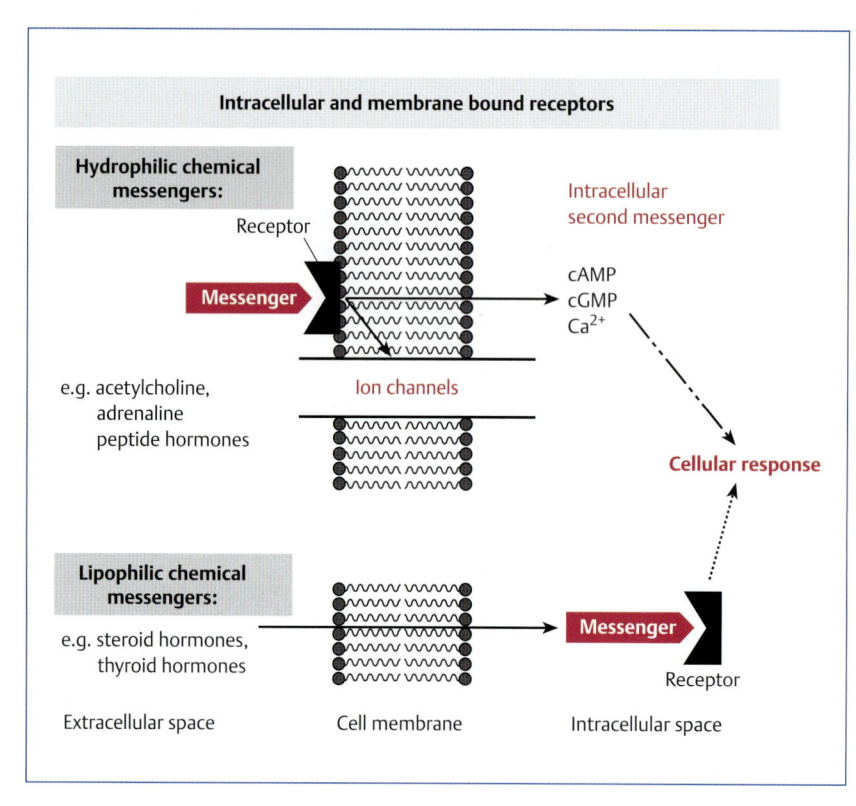

Fig. 1.13 Localisation and mechanisms of action of intra- and extracellular receptors for chemical messengers that affect the cell. Hydrophilic messengers (upper part) bind to membrane-bound receptors that act either on second messenger systems and/or on ion channels. Changes in the concentration of ions and other second messengers mediate cell responses (broken arrow), for example via activation of protein kinases. In contrast, lipophilic or gaseous chemical messengers (lower part) can diffuse through the cell membrane into the cell interior and bind to intracellular receptors. A cell response can also be mediated downstream via different mechanisms (dashed arrow). This includes the fact that lipophilic chemical messengers are transported into the cell nucleus and can induce protein biosynthesis there via transcription and translation (**genomic effect**). Such processes are slow and induce long-term changes. However, lipophilic chemical messengers can also cause non-genomic, rapid effects in the cytoplasm.

stimulated on acidification and inhibited on alkalization, leading to a correspondingly high export of protons and thus pH homeostasis (p. 351). The Na^+/H^+ antiporter is the dominant system for intracellular pH regulation in most cells and the Na^+ gradient is maintained with the utilisation of ATP (secondary active transport). What is not yet clear is the extent of the involvement of HCO_3^--dependent transport systems such as the Cl^-/HCO_3^- antiporters in cellular pH regulation.

> **IN A NUTSHELL** !
>
> pH homeostasis is predominantly regulated by the Na^+/H^+ antiporter.

1.6.3   Signal action and processing

Cells are subject to the influence of a large number of extracellular chemical messengers, such as hormones, neurotransmitters or paracrine substances. Cells can only react to the chemical messengers for which they have receptors (**Fig. 1.13**). These are proteins with binding sites with high affinity and high selectivity for their specific messengers, which then trigger a response in the cell. The receptors can be located on the cell membrane or inside the cell, either in the cytoplasm or e.g. in the nucleus. There is an important difference in the mode of action of water-soluble (hydrophilic) messengers (e.g. most neurotransmitters, peptide hormones) and fat-soluble (lipophilic, e.g. steroid hormones, thyroid hormones) or gaseous (nitric oxide: NO) messengers. While the first group of hydrophilic messengers cannot usually get into the cell interior and have

to bind to receptors on the outer side of the cell membrane, the lipophilic or gaseous messengers can easily diffuse through the lipid bilayer of the cell membrane and act on receptors inside the cell.

■ Intracellular receptors

Steroid hormones are poorly water-soluble, lipophilic extracellular chemical messengers. Because of their fat solubility, they can easily penetrate the cell membrane. After uptake in the cell, they bind to specific cytoplasmic receptors. When the hormone has bound, the receptor-hormone complex migrates to the cell nucleus, where it can trigger activation of the transcription of particular genes. The result is an increased formation of messenger RNA (mRNA), which diffuses out of the nucleus through the nuclear pores. Proteins are synthesized in the ribosomes via translation from the information contained in the mRNA. This results in a functional response in the cell, which is referred to as a **genomic effect**. It is specific to the cell affected by the hormone. As an example, the corticoid hormone aldosterone acts on the renal distal tubule to increase the formation of Na^+/K^+-ATPase, see ch. "Mechanisms of tubular NaCl transport" (p. 314). The thyroid hormones have a similar mechanism of action; however, in this case the hormone receptor is localised in the cell nucleus. Since the effect of lipophilic hormones is only established after the genetic information has been read, it may take hours or days before the maximum cell response is perceptible. On the other hand, the effect then lasts for a relatively long time. However, for a number of steroid hormones, membrane-bound receptors are now also known which mediate a rapid hormone response, i.e. they can also trigger **non-genomic effects** without inducing protein synthesis.

Nitric oxide (NO), an important neurotransmitter, behaves completely differently. NO can enter the cell as a gas (gasotransmitter) via diffusion and binds there to the enzyme guanylate cyclase, which thus serves as a receptor for NO. cGMP (p. 118) is then formed as a second messenger. The effect of NO occurs quickly and does not last long because this messenger is very unstable.

■ Membrane receptors

Hydrophilic chemical messengers bind to receptors in the cell membrane. The consequence of the binding of a hormone to its receptor is a change in the receptor conformation, which then triggers a signal in the cell, such as changing the opening behaviour of ion channels in the cell membrane. By this means, the neurotransmitter acetylcholine, after binding to the (nicotinic) acetylcholine receptor, initiates the opening of a non-selective cation channel, see ch. Path of the signal from the sensor to the effector (p. 61). The result is a depolarization of the cell, i.e. an electrical signal.

However, membrane-bound receptors can also be involved in the formation of chemical signals in Table 1.5. The change in conformation of the receptor, which occurs after the binding of the extracellular chemical messenger (**first messenger**), triggers a cascade-like reaction inside the cell and leads to the formation or release of a **second messenger**. This second, intracellular messenger "translates" the message of the first messenger, which itself cannot get inside the cell. In addition, second messengers traditionally lead to a massive **amplification of the signal**. In this way, the activation of a few receptors can affect the whole cell. These intracellular second messengers include the cyclic nucleotides, cAMP and cGMP, as well as the intracellular concentration of free Ca^{2+} ions.

■ Second messengers

The transmission of information is different for each of the three second messenger systems mentioned.

cAMP pathway

An example for agonists that have an effect via the **cAMP pathway** is the release of glucose (**Fig. 1.14**) from liver cells by the hormone adrenaline. G proteins act as a kind of amplifier between the receptor in the cell membrane and the effector protein, adenylate cyclase. The activation of a few hormone receptors is sufficient to stimulate a much larger number of **G proteins**. The consequence is an increase in the intracellular concentration of cAMP, which usually exerts its effect in the cell by activating **protein kinase A**. This is an enzyme that, under the influence of cAMP, affects other proteins, such as by phosphorylating enzymes or ion channels. The phosphorylation changes the functional state of the phosphorylated protein. Examples of this are the cAMP-dependent incorporation of aquaporins into the apical membrane of renal epithelial cells of the distal collecting duct, inhibition of glycogen synthase in liver cells, or the cAMP-dependent opening of Cl⁻ channels in intestinal epithelial cells. However, there are also receptors, such as those for the hormone somatostatin which when stimulated, via an **inhibitory G protein (G_i protein)**, leads to an inhibition of adenylate cyclase and thus to a reduction in cAMP production. In addition, cAMP can influence the transcription of genes by acting on so-called cAMP-responsive elements (CRE), which results in long-term effects of this second messenger on a cell.

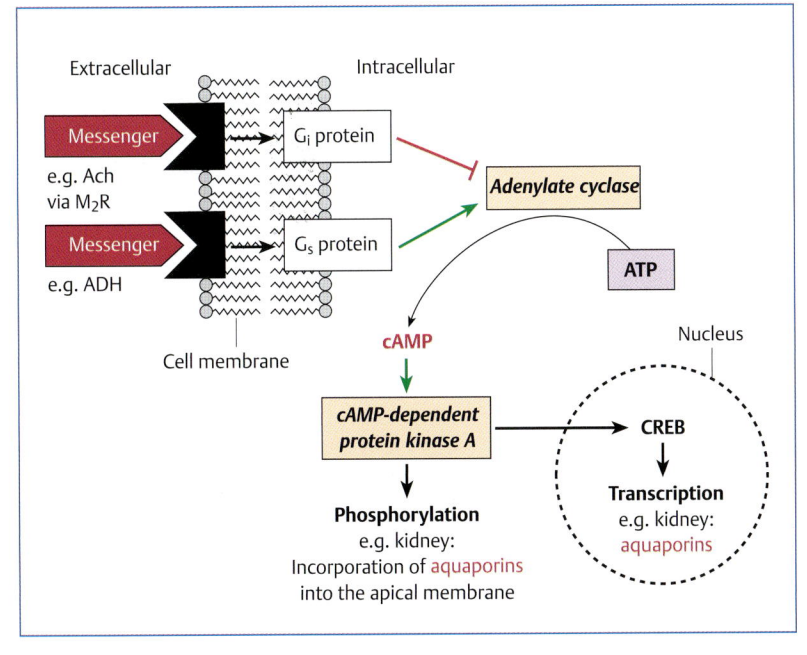

Fig. 1.14 Signalling via cAMP as an intracellular second messenger pathway. After binding to a membrane-bound receptor, adenylate cyclase (green arrow) is stimulated, mediated by G_s proteins, with subsequent formation of cAMP. The antidiuretic hormone (ADH) leads to the increased production of cAMP, which in turn activates protein kinase A and the incorporation of apical aquaporins (p. 317) stimulated into the distal collecting duct. In addition, the expression of aquaporins is increased, for example, via the transcription factor cAMP-responsive element-binding protein (CREB). In addition to G_s proteins, there are also inhibitory G proteins such as the G_i protein, which inhibits adenylate cyclase and thus the formation of cAMP (red, closed arrow). Acetylcholine (Ach), for example, binds to the muscarinic M_2 receptor and, via the G_i protein, reduces the production of cAMP in the heart with, among other things, a negative inotropic effect (e.g. inhibition of contraction force in the atrium).

Figure labels: Extracellular — Intracellular; Messenger e.g. Ach via M_2R; G_i protein; Adenylate cyclase; Messenger e.g. ADH; G_s protein; ATP; Cell membrane; cAMP; Nucleus; cAMP-dependent protein kinase A; CREB; Transcription e.g. kidney: aquaporins; Phosphorylation e.g. kidney: Incorporation of aquaporins into the apical membrane

cGMP pathway

An extracellular messenger that acts via the **cGMP pathway (Fig. 1.15)** is the hormone atrial natriuretic peptide (ANP) produced in the atria. This hormone binds to receptors in the cell membrane of renal epithelial cells of the collecting duct. The consequence of this binding is an activation of a membrane-bound guanylate cyclase. Guanylate cyclases form cGMP from GTP, which has various effects in the cell. On the one hand, like cAMP, it can activate protein kinases, which then phosphorylate certain proteins. However, it can also interfere with the degradation of cAMP by changing the activity of phosphodiesterases that break

down cAMP. Either inhibition or activation can be observed, depending on the cell type and the phosphodiesterases present. In addition, cGMP can directly influence the activity of some ion channels in the cell membrane (e.g. in olfactory or visual cells). In the case of atrial natriuretic peptide, phosphorylation of epithelial sodium channels (p. 312) favours closure of these channels and thus an increased excretion of salts and water by the kidneys.

Ca²⁺ pathway

The third way through which extracellular chemical messengers can exert intracellular effects is the **Ca^{2+} pathway**. Examples are the contraction of smooth muscle cells in vessels induced by the hormone angiotensin II, or contraction of intestinal smooth muscles evoked by acetylcholine via muscarinic $M_{1/3}$ receptors; **Fig. 1.16**). The hormone-receptor complex activates, via a GTP-binding protein, phospholipase C, which breaks down particular phospholipids in the cell membrane. This releases a sugar phosphate, **inositol-1,4,5-trisphosphate (IP_3)**. IP_3 activates Ca^{2+} channels on intracellular organelles such as the endoplasmic reticulum, which serve as Ca^{2+} stores in the cell. The result is a release of Ca^{2+} from these storage organelles and an increase in the Ca^{2+} concentration in the cytosol. The emptying of the Ca^{2+} stores represents a signal for the opening of Ca^{2+} channels in the cell membrane (capacitive Ca^{2+} influx). The concentration of Ca^{2+} ions in the cytosol is usually very low, ranging from 0.1 to 1 $\mu mol \cdot l^{-1}$, which is more than 2000 times lower than the concentration in blood plasma (**Table 1.4**). Due to the large electrochemical gradient, Ca^{2+} ions flow into the cell when the Ca^{2+} channels in the plasma membrane open. This leads to a sustained increase in the Ca^{2+} concentration in the cell.

During phospholipid cleavage, diacylglycerol, a glycerol derivative, is released. Together with Ca^{2+} ions, diacylglycerol can activate a protein kinase C, which in turn phosphorylates other enzymes. As with the cAMP and cGMP

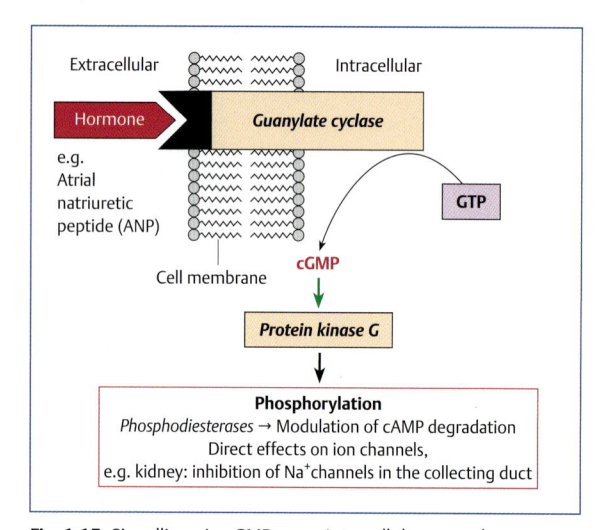

Fig. 1.15 Signalling via cGMP as an intracellular second messenger pathway. After a hormone binds to a membrane-bound receptor, a membrane-bound guanylate cyclase is activated, which forms cGMP. Thus, no G protein is involved in the cGMP pathway. When activated by the atrial natriuretic peptide (ANP), the closure of Na⁺ channels is induced by protein kinase G-mediated (green arrow) phosphorylation. However, cGMP can also activate or inhibit phosphodiesterases.

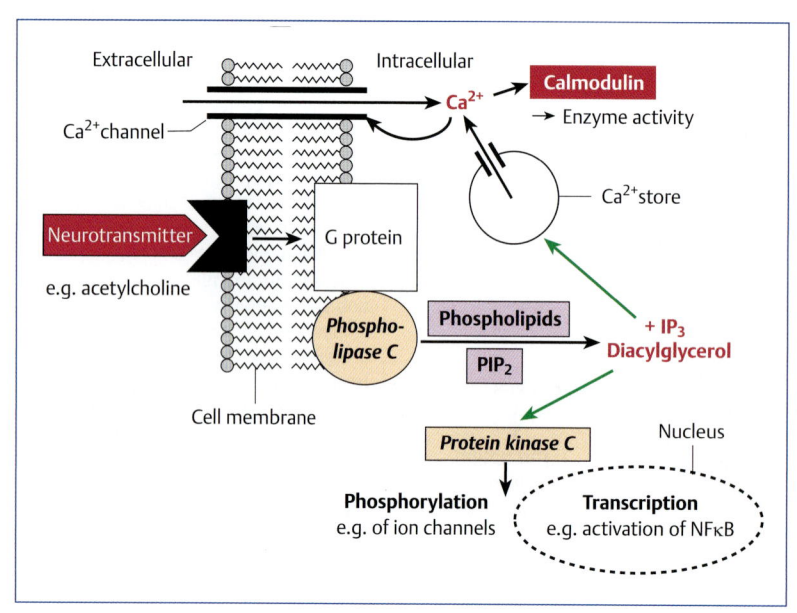

Fig. 1.16 Signalling via the intracellular Ca²⁺ second messenger pathway. After binding to a membrane-bound receptor, phospholipase C is stimulated, mediated by G proteins. This enzyme cleaves phosphatidylinositol-4,5-bisphosphate (PIP₂) into inositol-1,4,5-trisphosphate (IP₃) and diacylglycerol. IP₃ releases Ca²⁺ from intracellular stores and thereby mediates a subsequent capacitive Ca²⁺ influx from the extracellular space. Ca²⁺ has a regulatory effect on enzymes and ion channels via calmodulin, among other things. Diacylglycerol activates (green arrow) protein kinase C and thus leads to phosphorylation. Transcription can be regulated, for example, via the nuclear factor κB (NFκB).

pathway, protein phosphorylation also plays an important role in signalling within the cell in the Ca^{2+} pathway. In addition, there is an effect via the Ca^{2+}-dependent regulator protein, calmodulin, which is able to modulate the activity of many enzymes in the cell, and an effect of Ca^{2+} on some ion channels (e.g. Ca^{2+}-dependent K^+ channels). In addition, a change in the Ca^{2+} concentration in the cell nucleus can influence transcription.

Other important signalling pathways

Insulin, for example, acts via tyrosine kinases. After receptor activation, tyrosine kinases, protein kinase B, and other kinases, are activated. This in turn phosphorylates enzymes and thus regulates their activity. On the other hand, the so-called JAK-STAT pathway (janus kinase signal transducer and activator of transcription) mediates its effect mainly via the regulation of gene expression. This plays a role, for example, in the stimulation of erythropoiesis in bone marrow by the hormone erythropoietin. After binding to a receptor, STAT proteins associated with the receptor complex are phosphorylated, dissociate, dimerize, and migrate (translocate) from the cytoplasm to the nucleus. There they bind to various promoter binding sites in DNA, which regulates the expression of a wide variety of proteins. According to this special effect, activators of this signalling pathway are involved, for example, in growth processes (**Table 1.5**).

Table 1.5 Important signalling pathways and their activation.

Signalling pathways	Examples of their participation in:
cAMP	Acetylcholine (M_2 but with inhibitory G protein), ACTH, adrenaline (α_2, β_{1-3}) angiotensin II, calcitonin, prostaglandins, oxytocin, secretin, somatostatin, vasopressin (V_2)
IP_3/DAG/Ca^{2+}	Acetylcholine ($M_{1/3}$), adrenaline (α_1), antidiuretic hormone (V_1), bradykinin, cholecystokinin, gastrin, oxytocin, prostaglandins
cGMP	Atrial natriuretic peptide, nitric oxide (soluble guanylate cyclase)
Tyrosine kinase	Insulin, insulin-like growth factors (IGF-1), some growth factors
JAK STAT	Erythropoietin, growth hormone (GH), leptin, prolactin, many cytokines (e.g. interleukin-6)

IN A NUTSHELL !

The effect of hydrophilic extracellular messengers is mediated by changes in the intracellular concentration of second messengers (cAMP, cGMP, Ca^{2+}), while the effect of most lipophilic messengers is mainly mediated by a change in gene transcription.

1.6.4 Cell cycle, growth and apoptosis

The life of the cell begins with a mitotic (or meiotic) **cell division** and ends – as far as proliferating cells are concerned – with the next cell division. The timing of this **cell cycle** includes four phases (**Fig. 1.17**). The so-called **G_1 phase** (G = gap) follows immediately after the end of a mitosis (**M phase**). The now diploid cell grows and performs numerous metabolic activities such as membrane synthesis and protein assembly. The next phase of the cell cycle is called the **S phase** (S = synthesis of DNA), during which replication of DNA occurs. The cell then enters the mostly short **G_2 phase** as a tetraploid cell. This is where the preparation for the next M phase takes place. If there is an insufficient supply of the substrates required for this cell cycle, such as nutrients to maintain energy metabolism or certain growth factors, cells stop the division process and enter the so-called **G_0 phase** from the **G_1 phase**, which can last for a very long time, sometimes for the life of the cell.

The ability of tissue to regenerate, the maintenance of constant organ size and the changeability or adaptability of physiological mechanisms, presuppose that cells can be eliminated under appropriate conditions without triggering inflammatory responses or the formation of antibodies. In tissues such as the intestinal epithelium, there is a constant production of new cells from stem cells in the crypts. The mature cells at the tips of the villi in the small intestine or in the mucosa of the large intestine, perish after a few days in order to create "space" for newly formed cells. This physiological cell death (**apoptosis**; Greek "falling of the leaves") takes place according to a fixed program (**programmed cell death**). Apoptosis usually begins in the G_0 phase with the shrinking of the nucleus and ends with the dissolution of the cell membrane.

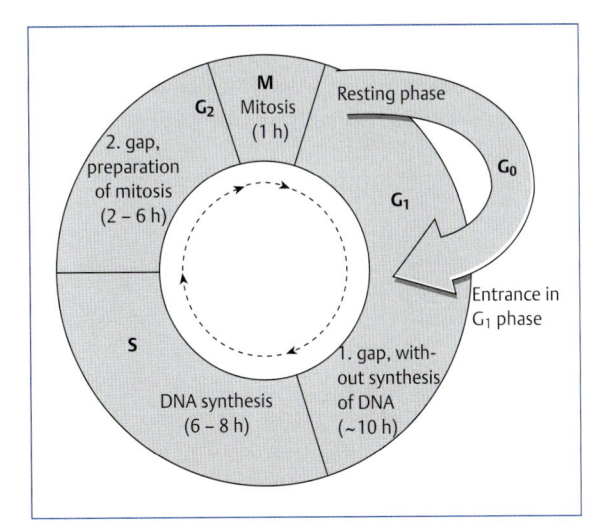

Fig. 1.17 Cell cycle of a mammalian cell with a mean generation time of 24 hours. The first three phases form the interphase: the G_1 phase, the S phase and the G_2 phase. During the shortest phase, the M phase (M = mitosis), the new chromosomes are distributed to the daughter cells in a complex process. Many non-dividing cells found in tissues exit the cell cycle and are in the G_0 state ("resting" phase).

The released DNA is rapidly degraded and phagocytosed by macrophages along with the remaining cell debris. It should be noted that only individual cells in an otherwise healthy organ are affected by apoptosis. This clearly distinguishes apoptosis from **cell necrosis**, in which multiple cells in an organ are usually damaged. It has not yet been clarified exactly how many factors and which intracellular signalling cascades are involved in triggering apoptosis. It seems to be clear that activation of a specific **endonuclease** is a key event in apoptosis. The endonuclease causes fragmentation of the chromatin.

All tissues must increase in size and cell number during the embryonic and foetal phase of growth, a process that also continues postnatally in most tissues. A distinction is made between two forms of growth. **Hypertrophy** means that the individual cells, that make up an organ, increase in size. **Hyperplasia**, on the other hand, means that the number of cells that make up an organ rises. Growth also takes place postnatally when the balance between cell formation and breakdown in a tissue is shifted in favour of the former. The prerequisite is an **anabolic metabolic state**, where there is a predominance of metabolic processes that lead to the formation of new cell substance. Individual organs differ in the way in which their growth takes place. In adipose tissue, for example, when there is increased fat storage with increased energy intake from food, there is only an enlargement of the fat-storing vacuoles of the white fat cells and thus cell hypertrophy. Other tissues such as the liver or the epidermis mediate their growth via hyperplasia. This ability ensures, for example, that the skin can regenerate quickly in the event of injury.

> **IN A NUTSHELL** !
>
> The cell cycle includes four phases: M, G_1, S and G_2 phases. Physiological cell death is called apoptosis which follows a genetically determined program.

Suggested reading

Alberts B, Johnson A, Lewis J et al. Molecular Biology of the Cell. 4th edition, New York: Garland Sicences; 2002

Cunningham JG, Klein BG. Textbook of Veterinary Physiology. Philadelphia: Saunders Elsevier; 2007

Niessen CM. Tight junctions/adherent junctions: basic structure and function. J Invest Dermatol 2007; 127:2525–2532

2 General neurophysiology

Martin Diener, Bernd Schröder

2.1 Tasks of the nervous system

ESSENTIALS ✖

While vertebrates are equipped with a variety of different neurons that differ in structure and properties, all neurons use the same basic mechanisms to process and transmit information. At its sensory end, the neuron has a zone specialised to receive signals that can then be processed and integrated in a connection zone. The third zone is responsible for propagating the integrated signals along the neuron (often very rapidly and over potentially long distances, e.g. in the order of metres in the innervation of limb muscles in large animals) to the terminal zone where the signals can be transmitted to other cells. The characteristic polarity of the neuron is important for directional conduction of excitation: signals are conducted from the sensory end of the cell to the other and not vice versa. Information transmission occurs at the sensory end through synaptic potentials, which trigger an action potential when there is suprathreshold depolarization. The most important form of signal transmission from neurons to other cells takes place via neurotransmitters, i.e. chemical messengers that change the function of the innervated cell via receptors on the postsynaptic membrane.

2.2 Neural tissue

The nervous tissue is made up of **neurons** (nerve cells) and **glia cells** that surround the neurons and fill the space between them. Neurons are excitable. This means that they are able to generate and transmit signals by rapidly changing their membrane potential. These potential changes are called **action potentials**. This refers to rapid changes in the membrane potential that terminate themselves so that the membrane potential automatically returns to its resting potential.

2.2.1 Structure and functional properties of the neuron

Neurons differ from the rest of the body's cells in several aspects. The shape and size of neurons in an animal are highly variable. These cells are able to transmit an excitation triggered by a stimulus and they can form special structures, the synapses, through which signals are transmitted either chemically or (more rarely) electrically to other nerve or effector cells.

A neuron consists of the actual cell body (**soma**), which contains the nucleus and the surrounding cytoplasm with organelles such as the Golgi apparatus and the endoplasmic reticulum etc.. Different numbers of projections emanate from the soma. As an example of the structure of a type of nerve cell commonly found in the body, in **Fig. 2.1** a motoneuron is shown schematically. Because of its star-shaped appearance, the motoneuron (p. 148) is also called a **multipolar neuron**. Usually, the neuron forms two types of projections: the axon and the dendrites. The axon conducts the electrical signals (excitations), starting from the axon hillock ("**trigger zone**"), to other neurons in the central and peripheral nervous system and to **effector cells** (**efferent excitation conduction, "output of information"**). In contrast, the dendrites, which extend from the soma like antennae (and have a large surface area), can receive the signals from the axons of other cells ("input of information") and then feed them to the soma (**afferent excitation conduction**). Often the axon splits into branches (**collaterals**) at its distal end in the periphery and can thus send its message to many different cells simultaneously. Efferents of different upstream neurons form synaptic contacts at the same nerve cell (**convergence of information transmission**). The neuron can in turn make contacts with several downstream neurons via collaterals of the axon (**divergence** of **information transmission**). Interneurons, which transmit information between neurons, are generally **bipolar** in structure, while **pseudounipolar neurons** (with one axon and only one long dendrite) usually represent sensory neurons (**Fig. 2.1**, top right).

Neurons can be functionally divided into three classes: sensory neurons, interneurons and motor neurons. Sensory neurons (p. 67) generally serve to register stimuli (in sensory physiology, these are chemical or physical events in the environment or in the body) and transmit information. **Interneurons** form by far the largest subfraction in terms of numbers; these neurons convey information between nerve cells. Motor neurons (p. 148) send commands to non-neuronal effector cells, such as muscle cells (classical motoneurons or vasomotor neurons in the case of the innervation of vascular muscles) or gland cells (secretomotor neurons), and thus influence their activity.

The junction of an axonal terminal with another cell such as a neuron or a skeletal muscle fibre is called a **synapse**. The nerve cell that transmits a signal is called the **presynaptic** neuron and the nerve cell that receives the signal is called the **postsynaptic** neuron. Depending on the localisation of the connection points between individual neurons, we speak of an **axosomatic** synapse when an axon or axon collateral ends on the soma of another neuron. Correspondingly, a synapse between an axon and a den-

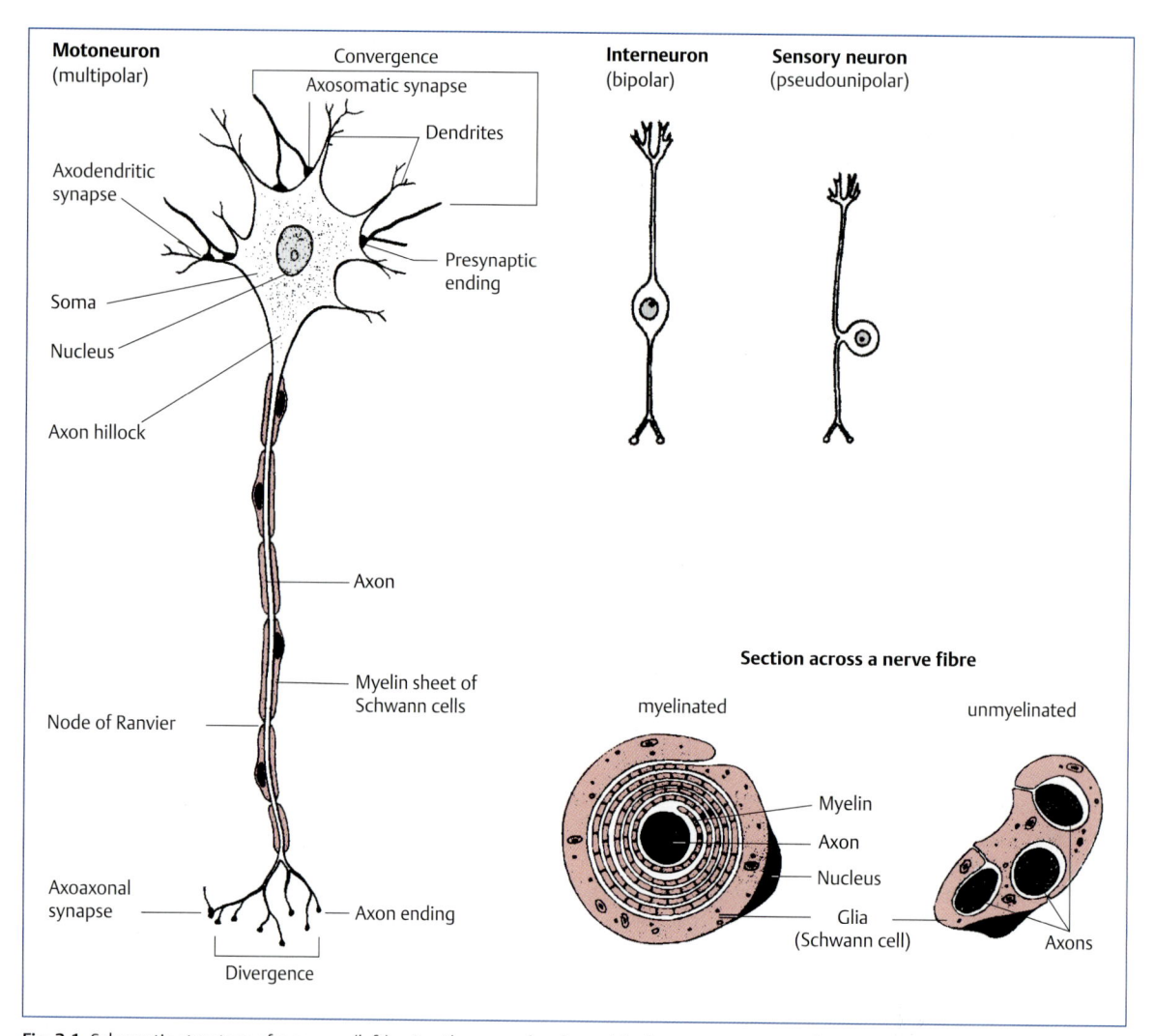

Fig. 2.1 Schematic structure of a neuron (left) using the example of a multipolar motoneuron. Further examples of neurons with different morphologies are shown on the top right. Bipolar neurons have only two processes (an axon and a dendrite) and are often sensory neurons. Pseudounipolar neurons also have only one axon and one dendrite, but they merge at their orifices to form one long process. They are found, for example, in the dorsal root ganglia. Depending on whether axons are surrounded by a myelin sheath or not, one distinguishes between myelinated and unmyelinated nerve fibres (bottom right).

drite is called an **axodendritic** synapse and between two axons an **axoaxonal** synapse (**Fig. 2.1**). Axoaxonal synapses form between the terminals of the pre- and postsynaptic cell. Therefore, they usually have no direct influence on impulse generation, but mainly modulate the transmitter release of the postsynaptic cell.

In the axon, substances that are formed in the soma, such as some neurotransmitters or their precursors, membrane vesicles, enzymes, etc., can be transported to the terminal endings with the participation of motor proteins of the cytoskeleton (p. 29) such as kinesins and dyneins (**anterograde transport**). The speed can be up to 40 cm per day. Of pathophysiological interest is the **retrograde transport** which occurs from the terminal endings of an axon in the direction of the soma, because foreign matters, such as herpes viruses or tetanus toxin, can enter the brain or spinal cord along this path.

> **IN A NUTSHELL** !
>
> The nervous tissue is made up of neurons and glial cells.

2.2.2   Functions of the glial cells

The **glial cells are non-excitable cells** of the nervous tissue that can have different functions depending on the type of glia. **Oligodendrocytes** (in the central nervous system) and **Schwann cells** (in the peripheral nervous system) have an **insulating function** (**Fig. 2.2**, **Table 2.1**). These cells surround the axons and build an insulating **myelin sheath** around them which is formed when the cell membrane of the glial cell (comparable to a roll of toilet paper) wraps itself several times around the progenitor of the nerve cell (**Fig. 2.1** bottom right). The axons of unmyelinated nerves are also surrounded by Schwann cells; however, these do not form a myelin sheath. **Astroglial cells** can build boundaries between neural tissue and blood vessels. Thus, they are involved in the formation of the **blood-brain barrier**. Glial cells also serve to nourish the neurons, since, for example, glucose must first be transported through a glial cell before it is available to a neuron, if the neuron is completely surrounded by a glial sheath.

Since, unlike neurons, glial cells retain their ability to divide throughout life, they also serve to fill neuronal cell defects (**glial scars**). Glial cells can synthesise, uptake and release various **neurotransmitters** (synaptic messengers) and **neuromodulators** (longer and/or longer range neuronal messengers). However, there is no evidence that glial cells are directly involved in information transmission, although it is now known that they can also express voltage-dependent Na^+ channels, which play a central role in the generation of action potentials (p. 49) in neurons. Another function of glial cells is to buffer excess extracellular K^+, which would otherwise accumulate in the extracellular space during intense neuronal activity. In addition to the glial cells described above, which are collectively referred to as **macroglia**, microglia (p. 128) are also found in the central nervous system, where they are capable of phagocytosis and thus perform an immune defence function.

> **IN A NUTSHELL** !
>
> Neurons are excitable cells that are generally characterised by many short cell processes, the dendrites and by a long extension, the axon. Glial cells predominantly perform support, insulation and nutritional functions in nervous tissue.

Table 2.1 The four basic types of glial cells and their main functions (CNS: central nervous system; PNS: peripheral nervous system).

Types	Functions
Microglia	Macrophage-like cells, endogenous defence and immune system in the CNS, they can eliminate cellular detritus and pathogens by phagocytosis
Astrocytes	Mechanical support of nervous tissue in the CNS, regulation of nutrient, ion and respiratory gas distribution and homeostasis, uptake and recycling of neurotransmitters, can form replacement tissue, possible role for long-term memory.
Oligodendrocytes	Supporting tissue, insulation of axons in the CNS, nutritional function
Schwann cells	Enclosing axons in the PNS with myelin sheaths (myelinated fibres) or simple sheathing or embedding by the glial cell (unmyelinated fibres), nourishing the axons, influencing axonal growth.

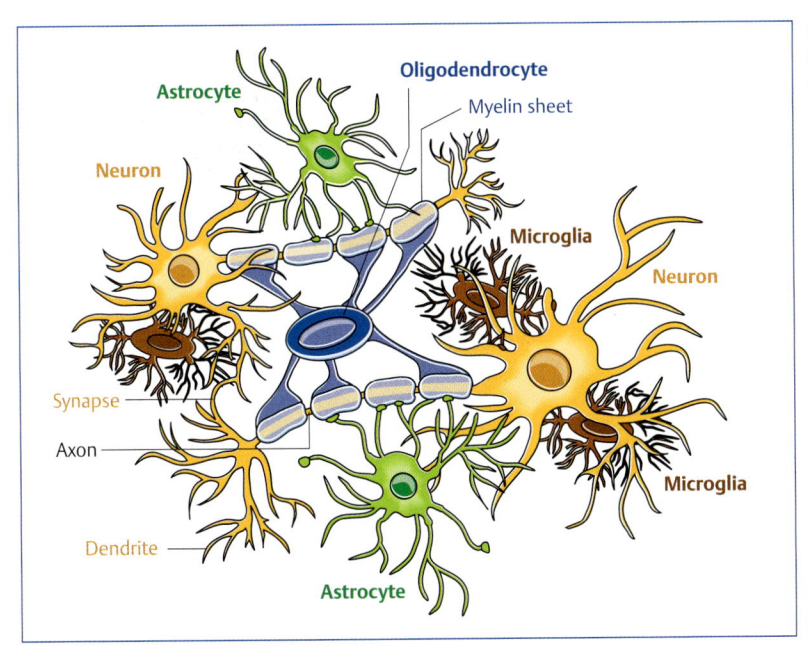

Fig. 2.2 Schematic structure of neurons and the four basic types of glial cells in the central nervous system.

2.3   Basic principles of excitation of neurons

2.3.1   Definitions

As described in ch. "Membrane potential" (p. 34), a **diffusion potential** arises at a membrane through which different ions diffuse at different velocities due to the **selective permeability** of the **cell membrane** and where a concentration gradient is present. The magnitude of this voltage can be calculated using the Goldman-Hodgkin-Katz equation. In the case of excitable cells in the resting state (i.e. without an action potential), this membrane potential is also called the **resting membrane potential**. Because of the comparatively high K^+ permeability of the neuronal membrane at rest, the resting membrane potential depends primarily on the concentration gradient for K^+ and is thus close to the K^+ equilibrium potential generated by it. By convention, this potential difference is expressed in such a way that the cell interior is negative in relation to the external environment. In most neurons, the resting membrane potential is between −70 and −90 mV. Even under resting conditions, Na^+ and K^+ ions diffuse through the cell membrane in both directions. This process, known as resting inflow or outflow, which would ultimately lead to a loss of the concentration gradients, is continuously balanced by the activity of the **Na^+/K^+ pump**. In this process, one positive charge is removed from the cell per transport step (exchange of 3 Na^+ for 2 K^+). However, this direct contribution of the pump current to the resting membrane potential is not very large. If the Na^+/K^+ pumps were blocked for a short time, the resting membrane potential would only become 2–4 mV more positive. However, the Na^+/K^+ pump is of central importance for the long-term maintenance of the Na^+ and K^+ concentration gradients between the cell interior and the external medium of cells, which is the basic prerequisite for the formation of a diffusion potential.

Changes in the resting membrane potential towards more negative or more positive membrane potentials are called **hyperpolarization or depolarization**. Such changes in membrane potential can be due to two mechanisms. First, any current flow through the membrane passively leads to a change in membrane potential according to the law of Ohm ($U = R \cdot I$), i.e. a change in voltage results when current flows across the "membrane resistor". Such changes in the membrane potential, which do not lead to the opening of voltage-controlled ion channels (**subthreshold stimuli**), represent **passive membrane responses** and are called **electrotonic potentials**. Responses of the membrane to hyperpolarization are usually passive. This also applies to responses to minor depolarizations (subthreshold stimuli). The term **stimulus** in neurophysiology refers to all causes that result in a depolarization of the membrane of an excitable cell. In the case of a sensory cell, this can be a physical or chemical event from the environment or the cell's own body; in the case of an interneuron, it can be the presence of an excitatory neurotransmitter, or experimentally, it can be the injection of a depolarizing current into a cell or the application of an external electric field. If the stimulus is so great that the membrane potential reaches the threshold value (**suprathreshold stimulus**), an action potential is triggered in an excitable cell. If the depolarization reaches a critical value, the **threshold potential**, the electrical behaviour of the neuron changes abruptly and an action potential (p. 48) is formed, which obeys the all-or-nothing principle. Action potentials are thus triggered by **suprathreshold stimuli** (i.e. suprathreshold depolarizations). The threshold value for most neurons is between −50 and −60 mV.

> **IN A NUTSHELL**   !
>
> The resting membrane potential of a neuron lies between −70 and −90 mV and is thus close to the K^+ equilibrium potential. Action potentials are triggered by suprathreshold stimuli. The threshold potential is between −50 and −60 mV.

2.3.2   Passive membrane response to subthreshold stimuli

Electrotonic potentials play an important role in neuronal excitation transmission (p. 56) and also in postsynaptic potentials (p. 61), which are generated by an electrical current at the postsynaptic membrane. They decide whether the postsynaptic potential at a dendrite ultimately leads to a subthreshold or suprathreshold depolarization at the trigger zone (**Fig. 2.10**). They also have a decisive influence on the speed with which an action potential is propagated. The passive electrical properties of a neuron, which in contrast to the active ones do not result from changes in the open probability of voltage-dependent ion channels (for further differentiation of "passive" and "active" responses see **Table 2.2**), are constant, i.e. they do not change during the stimulus or excitation conduction. A neuron has three relevant passive electrical properties: the **membrane resistance**, the **membrane capacitance** and the intracellular **series resistance** of axon and dendrites.

MORE DETAILS

The membrane resistance determines the maximum amplitude of the membrane response

According to the law of Ohm ($U = R \cdot I$), the amplitude of an electrotonic potential (ΔV), e.g. of a depolarization triggered by a prolonged stimulation current ($I_{Stimulus}$), is given by:

$$\Delta V = R_{in} \cdot I_{Stimulus} \tag{2.1}$$

The membrane resistance (R_{in}; also called input resistance, unit Ω) of the cell depends on the specific membrane resistance (R_{mem}; unit $\Omega \cdot m^2$], which is determined by the density of the ion channels in the cell membrane, their single channel conductance and their open probability. R_{in} of a cell is calculated from R_{mem}/membrane area. This means that of two neurons in which the same synaptic current is induced at a synapse by transmitter action, the respective neuron with the greater membrane resistance responds with a greater electrotonic potential. In larger neurons with dendrites and axons, the cytoplasmic resistance can also be important in addition to the membrane resistance, since passive ion movements flow not only (mediated via ion channels) through the cell membrane but also through the cytoplasm. The significance of membrane resistance for excitation conduction is discussed further in ch. Excitation propagation (p. 59).

Membrane capacitance slows down the time course of electrotonic potentials

Physically, the cell membrane behaves like a capacitor with an ohmic resistor connected in parallel (**Fig. 2.3**). The biological basis for this is that the lipid phase of the membrane can separate or store charges like a capacitor. At the same time, the membrane can also allow ions to pass through special proteins, namely ion channels, which electrically corresponds to an ohmic resistor. At the beginning of an experimentally applied current to the cell, the membrane capacitor is first charged or recharged (i.e. takes up electrical charge). This causes a time-delayed change in the voltage across the membrane. The more such a capacitor, which always has a limited capacity, is charged, the more current flows through the ohmic resistor, i.e. the ion channels, of the membrane. Accordingly, the voltage response occurs more slowly than the change in the stimulus current inducing it, such as a square-wave current pulse, and exponentially approaches its maximum amplitude, which corresponds to the voltage drop across the pure ohmic resistance of the membrane. The time in which the membrane potential has reached 63% of its final value is called the **membrane time constant τ**. This physiological parameter of the passive electrical membrane properties is 1–20 ms for various neurons. The membrane time constant τ can be calculated from the product of the membrane's resistance and capacity ($\tau = R \cdot C$). According to this, the time course of an electrotonic potential is a function of the current across the cell membrane, its duration (because this determines the amount of charge flowing into or out of the cell) and the membrane capacity. The capacity increases with the area of the cell membrane, so that a larger neuron requires more current than a smaller neuron to generate the same change in membrane potential.

The series resistance of axon and dendrites influences efficiency and speed of excitation conduction

The previous considerations regarding membrane resistance and capacitance referred to conduction of excitation within the cell body. Thus, distance effects on the propagation of the electrotonic signal could be neglected. A subthreshold membrane response such as a depolarization decreases along its travel in a dendrite, an axon or over a large cell body with increasing distance from the point of origin (**Fig. 2.4**). This is because the amplitude of the depolarization is influenced not only by the membrane resistance but also by the longitudinal resistance of the cytoplasmic interior. The longer the distance a current flows along such cytoplasmic resistance, the lower the membrane potential becomes, since the ohmic resistance of a cable increases linearly with increasing cable length. As a result, the amplitude of the electrotonic potential decreases exponentially with distance from the site of current injection (**Fig. 2.4**). Furthermore, during the passive conduction of an electrotonic potential, as is the case with the conduction of action potentials conduction of action potentials (p. 56) in the region of the internodes (this is the myelinated section of the axon between two nodes of Ranvier), mobile electrical charge is "consumed" in order to charge the capacity of the adjacent cell membrane. The distance at which the signal has finally decreased to 1/e (37%) of the initial amplitude at the point of origin is called the membrane **longitudinal constant λ**. It is greater the better the insulation of the membrane (large membrane resistance, so that less charge is consumed by ionic current through the membrane into the extracellular space) and the lower the longitudinal resistance (which in turn is in inverse propor-

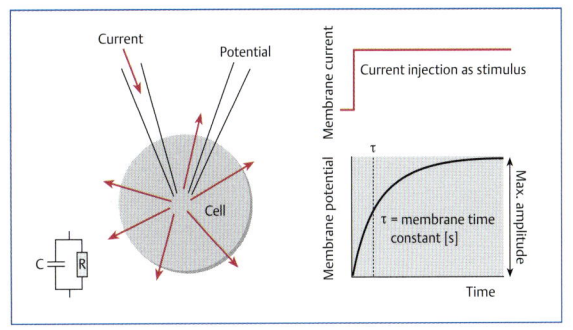

Fig. 2.3 Course of the electrotonic potential on a spherical cell. With the left microelectrode, an inward current is injected into the cell, i.e. cations flow into the cell (red arrows: current flow). With the right microelectrode, the change in the membrane potential is measured. On the right of the picture, the time course of the current into the cell (top) and the resulting electrotonic change of the membrane potential (bottom) are shown. The time that elapses until 63% of the maximum voltage change has occurred is called the membrane time constant τ . The passive behaviour of the membrane can be mimicked by an electrical "equivalent circuit" (bottom left): Physically, the cell membrane combines properties of a capacitor (C), i.e. charge can be accumulated on both sides of the membrane's lipid layer, which is impermeable to ions, and a resistor (R), i.e. current can pass the membrane through ion channels. At the beginning of the current injection into the cell, the membrane capacitor is charged first. The more such a capacitor, which always has a limited capacity is charged, (in the case of a cell membrane, a fairly constant 10^{-14} F·µm^{-2}, this means that a charge of 10^{-14} coulombs is sufficient to build up a voltage of 1 V on a membrane surface of 1 µm²), the more current flows through the ohmic resistance, i.e. the ion channels, of the membrane. At the end of the long-lasting current pulse, when the membrane capacitor is virtually completely charged and is no longer able to take up any further electrical charge, the amplitude of the resulting potential change is therefore determined purely by the ohmic resistance of the membrane. The membrane time constant τ can be calculated from the product of membrane capacitance and membrane resistance ($\tau = R \cdot C$).

tion to the axon diameter). λ thus represents an important measure for characterising the "cable properties" of nerve fibres. On various cells, the membrane length constant has values between 0.1 and 1 mm. Electrotonic potentials are therefore effective on nerve fibres for a few millimetres at most. The nerve fibre therefore has relatively poor conductive properties. The significance of the membrane time constant τ and the membrane longitudinal constant λ is discussed in connection with the spatial and temporal summation of signals (p. 64).

IN A NUTSHELL   !

The passive electrical properties of a neuron are constant, i.e. they do not change during the stimulus or the conduction of excitation. A neuron has three relevant passive electrical properties: the membrane resistance, the membrane capacitance and the intracellular series resistance of axon and dendrites.

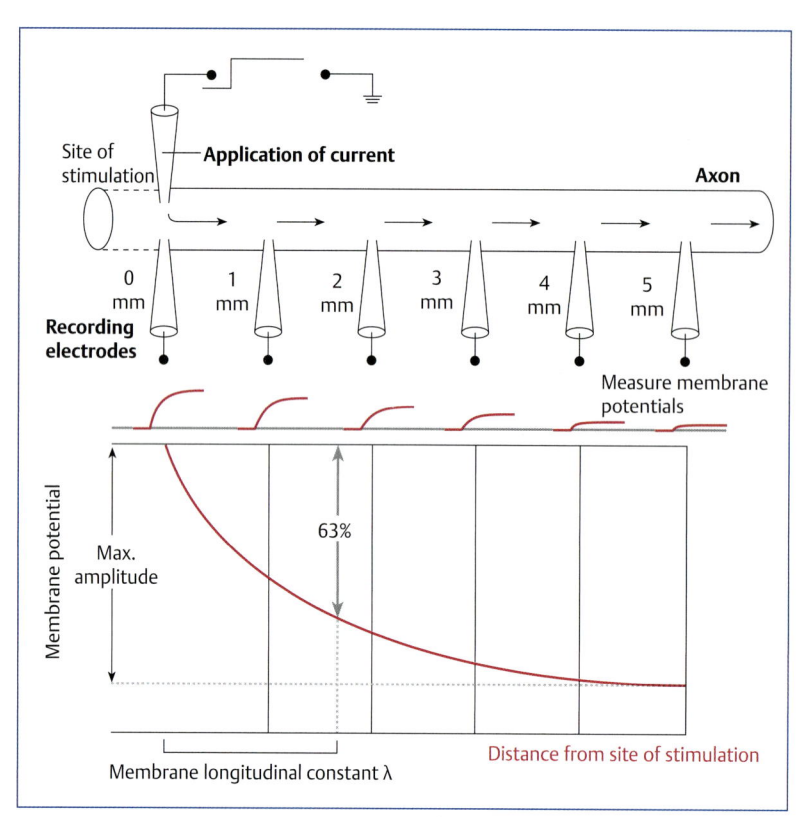

Fig. 2.4 Course of the electrotonic potential in the axon of a neuron after a subthreshold stimulus. Top: Application of a subthreshold charge of a current to an axon and resulting membrane responses at different distances (in mm) from the application site; bottom: amplitude of the respective plateau value of the membrane potential as a function of the distances from the stimulus site. The change of membrane potential decreases exponentially with increasing distance from the stimulus site. The membrane longitudinal constant λ indicates the distance from the stimulus site at which the amplitude has decreased by 63% of the initial value (measured directly at the site of current application).

2.3.3 Active membrane response to suprathreshold stimuli: the action potential

As already mentioned, the threshold potential for mammalian neurons with a resting membrane potential of −70 mV is about −50 mV. If a depolarization exceeds this threshold value, a fully developed action potential is always triggered, **regardless** of the **strength of** the **stimulus** – if one disregards the refractory phase (p.53). This constancy of the action potential is called the **all-or-nothing principle of excitation**. The action potential consists of a transient depolarization that quickly terminates itself so that the membrane potential automatically returns to the resting membrane potential. It is very short and lasts only about 1 ms in nerve cells.

The action potential differs from the passive electrotonic response (p.46) in that it depends on the opening and/ or closing of **voltage-dependent ion channels** in response to a stimulus. After a suprathreshold depolarization, the membrane potential in the **depolarization phase** ("upstroke") exceeds the value of 0 mV in less than 0.5 ms and finally reaches a peak value of maximum approx. + 30 mV (**Fig. 2.5**). The part in which the membrane has reversed its usual polarity, i.e. is positively charged on the inside, is also called the **overshoot phase**. After the reversal of the polarity of the membrane potential, **repolarization** takes place which usually restores the resting potential within 1 ms. This "normal" repolarization can be followed – to a greater or lesser extent – by a slow depolarization or **hyperpolarization**, which is referred to as a **depolarizing** or **hyperpolarizing afterpotential**.

Table 2.2 is a summary of differences between the passive membrane response and the electrical response by changing the activity of voltage-dependent ion channels, i.e. between electrotonic potentials and action potentials.

Cell, tissue

Table 2.2 Essential differences between passive and active membrane responses of neurons.

Electrotonic potentials (passive, i.e. similar to an ohmic resistor)	Action potentials (through activation of voltage-dependent ion channels)
Graded membrane response whose amplitude depends on the strength of the stimulus.	Answer according to the "all-or-nothing principle": If the membrane is suprathreshold depolarized, the amplitude is independent of the strength of the stimulus.
Summation possible.	No summation possible.
The triggering of the membrane response is not dependent on exceeding a threshold potential.	Response only after exceeding the threshold potential.
There is no refractoriness.	The membrane response shows an absolute and a relative refractory phase.
Propagated excitations weaken.	The action potential is refreshed again and again during conduction by opening voltage-dependent ion channels (in neurons these are Na^+ channels) and therefore retains its amplitude.
The duration of the membrane response depends on the level of the stimulus.	The duration is constant for a given cell type.
Depolarization or hyperpolarization.	Depolarization with "overshoot" (= reversal of the polarity of the membrane, which is positively charged on the inside during the overshoot phase).
Passive membrane response that is not dependent on the opening or closing of voltage-dependent ion channels.	Permeability change caused by the opening or closing of voltage-dependent ion channels.
Evoked by a stimulus, through neurotransmitters or also spontaneously.	Triggered by a suprathreshold membrane depolarization.

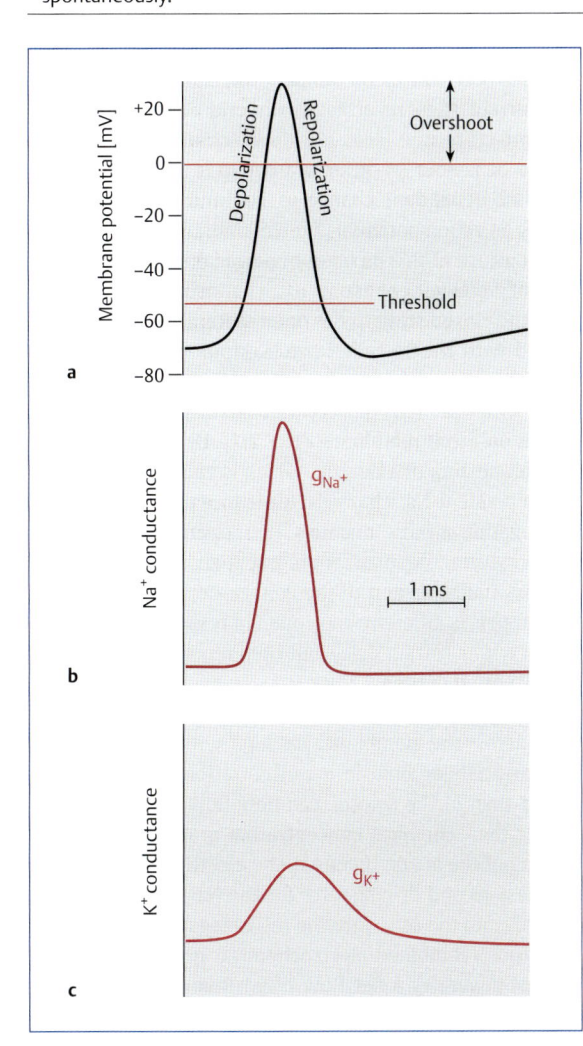

a
b
c

2.3.4 Ionic basis of the action potential

■ The Na^+ inward current and the function of the voltage-dependent Na^+ channels

The cause for the rapid change of membrane potential during the depolarization phase of the action potential is a transient **permeability increase** of the membrane for Na^+ ions (**Fig. 2.5**). Permeability is a measure of the ease of penetration through a membrane for a certain substance. It has the dimension of a velocity (unit: $cm \cdot s^{-1}$, see ch. "Transport by diffusion" (p. 32)). While the Na^+ permeability (P_{Na}; i.e. the permeability of the membrane for Na^+) in neurons under resting conditions is only about 1/25 of the K^+ permeability (P_K), P_{Na} increases to 20 times the value of P_K when the threshold is exceeded.

During the action potential, voltage- and time-dependent ionic currents flow (**Fig. 2.6**). Such membrane currents can be investigated using the voltage-clamp technique. This means that a voltage is applied to the cell with a voltage electrode and the current that flows through the membrane is measured with a current electrode. Through stepwise depolarization from a holding potential (e.g. −60 mV in **Fig. 2.6**) to different clamping potentials, voltage-dependent currents through the cell membrane can

Fig. 2.5 Time course of an action potential (**a**) and the underlying membrane conductivities (g, i.e. the ratio of the current flowing through the membrane of the respective ion in relation to the electrical voltage applied to the membrane) for Na^+ (**b**) and K^+ ions (**c**). A suprathreshold stimulation leads to depolarization (with reversal of the normal polarity of the membrane during the overshoot phase) and subsequent repolarization.

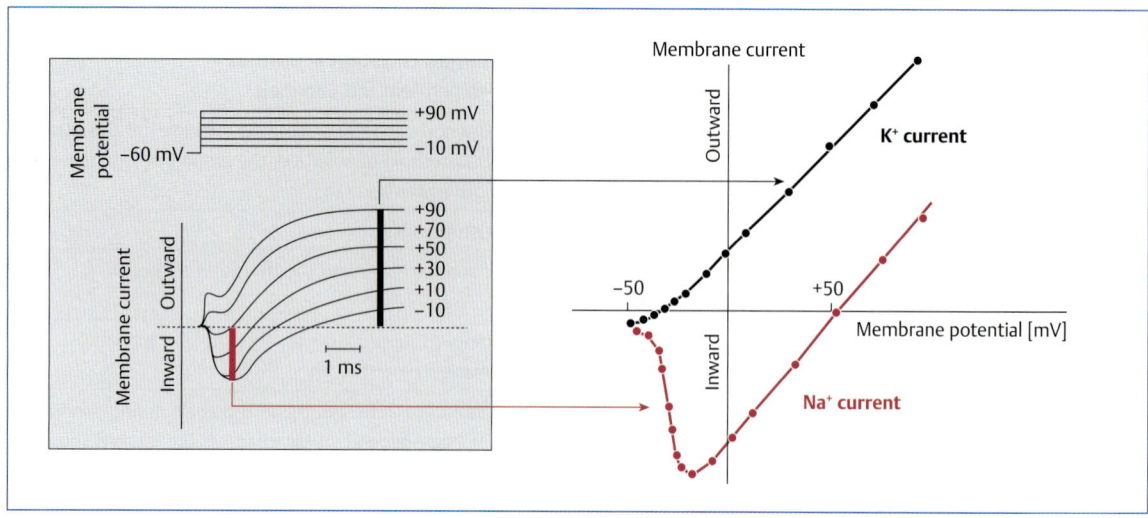

Fig. 2.6 Stepwise depolarizations of a neuron from a holding potential of −60 mV to depolarized values (−10 to +90 mV in 20 mV steps; top left) triggers time-dependent currents through the membrane (bottom left). Initially, the membrane current is dominated by a Na⁺ current (red bar), later by a K⁺ current (black bar). On the right, the maximum amplitude of the measured Na⁺ (red circles) or K⁺ current (black circles) is plotted as a current-voltage curve. The K⁺ current increases the more the membrane is depolarized. This is to be expected when the distance of the membrane potential from the K⁺ equilibrium potential and thus the driving force for the flux of potassium ions through the membrane increases. The Na⁺ current shows a more complex voltage dependence. Below a certain value, the so-called threshold value, the Na⁺ current is negligibly small. However, if the membrane is depolarized above this threshold, there is a strong influx of Na⁺ into the cell, which in this example reaches its maximum amplitude at about −30 mV. Further depolarization, however, causes the current to become smaller. At about +50 mV, which corresponds to the reversal potential of Na⁺ under the experimental conditions, the current then reverses its direction (as described by the Goldman equation) and becomes an outward current.

be measured. Depending on the potential difference, a current can flow into or out of the cell. For the technical definition of a current, an inward current is when a net positive charge flows into a cell, and an outward current is when a net positive charge flows out of a cell. Stepwise depolarization of a neuron triggers a time-dependent current, provided the depolarization is strong enough, i.e. suprathreshold. At the beginning, an inward current is induced, but this is only transient. Then the current reverses and an outward current occurs. If the membrane is depolarized more strongly, for example to +10, +30, +50, +70 or even +90 mV (**Fig. 2.6**), the inward current becomes smaller and smaller. It even disappears completely at some point. The outward current, on the other hand, which starts with a time delay, becomes larger and larger. By changing the concentration of the ions in the extracellular fluid, the ions that carry these two currents have been identified. The time- and voltage-dependent inward current is a Na⁺ current, the time- and voltage-dependent outward current is a K⁺ current.

If the amplitudes of the maximum of the Na⁺ and the K⁺ currents are plotted on a current-voltage curve, it can be seen that the K⁺ current has a relatively simple current-voltage relationship. The K⁺ current becomes larger the more the membrane is depolarized. This is to be expected when the distance of the membrane potential from the K⁺ equilibrium potential and thus the driving force for the flux of potassium ions through the membrane increases. The Na⁺ current behaves differently. It is negligibly small below the threshold value. If the membrane is depolarized above this threshold, there is a strong influx of Na⁺ into the cell. Further depolarization causes the current to de-

crease again. At about +50 mV, which corresponds to the reversal potential of Na⁺ under experimental conditions, the current then reverses its direction and becomes an outward current.

The behaviour of these two currents is responsible for the time-dependent change in Na⁺ and K⁺ conductance during an action potential (**Fig. 2.5**).

The cause of this increase in permeability is the activation of voltage-dependent ion channels, which change from the **closed state** to the **open state**. This can be investigated with the so-called patch-clamp technique, where currents can be measured through individual channel proteins with the help of very thin glass pipettes that are placed on a cell membrane (**Fig. 2.7**). Depolarization of a membrane area of a neuron, which is equipped with voltage-dependent Na⁺ channels, leads to a dramatic increase in the gating of these channels. Their open probability rises sharply during depolarization, but then drops again very quickly. The behaviour of the voltage-dependent neuronal K⁺ channels is different: they open in response to depolarization with a certain delay, but then remain activated for a longer period of time.

The opening of a Na⁺ channel leads to a charge movement across the membrane. Na⁺ ions, which are present in the extracellular fluid in a concentration about 20 times higher than in the cytosol, can now flow into the cell following their **chemical concentration gradient**. At the beginning of the action potential, the **electrical gradient** also acts as a second driving force for the Na⁺ current directed inwards into the cell, since the cell is negatively charged on the inside (combined **electrochemical gradient**). The Na⁺ current generates a net flow of positive charges into the

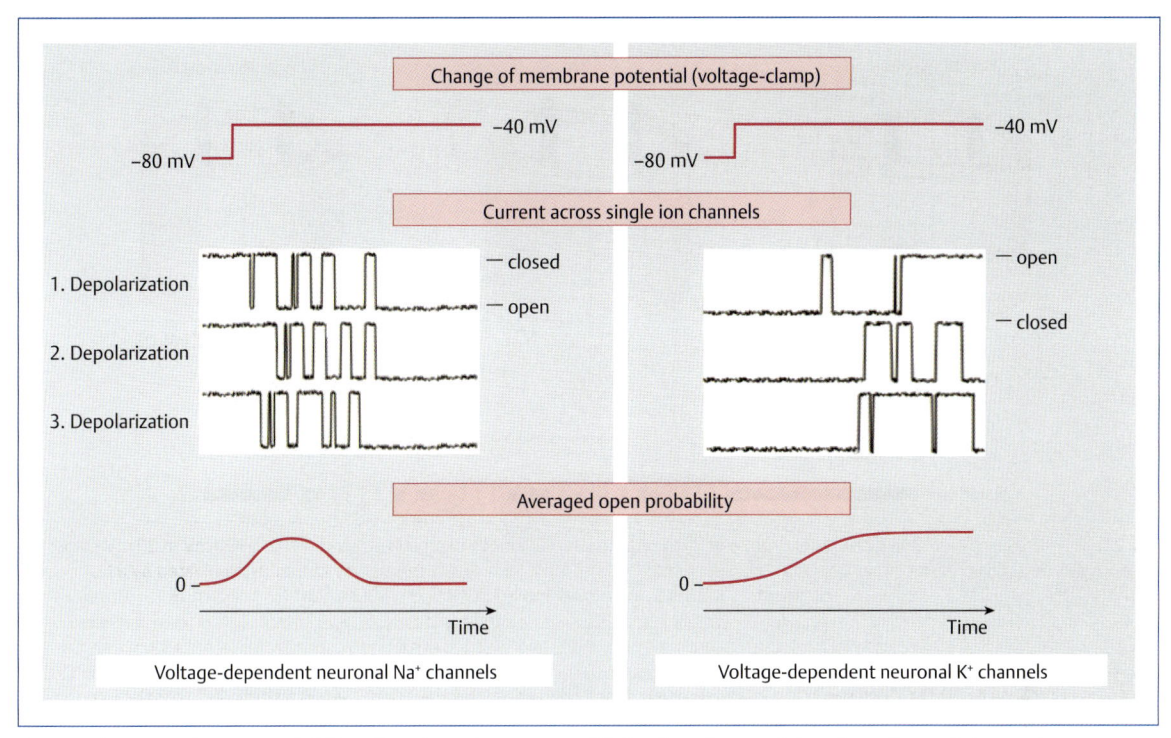

Change of membrane potential (voltage-clamp)

−40 mV   −40 mV

−80 mV   −80 mV

Current across single ion channels

1. Depolarization   — closed   — open
— open   — closed

2. Depolarization

3. Depolarization

Averaged open probability

0   0

Time   Time

Voltage-dependent neuronal Na⁺ channels   Voltage-dependent neuronal K⁺ channels

Fig. 2.7 Changes in the open probability of ion channels are responsible for the voltage and time dependence of the membrane currents during an action potential. When membrane patches containing Na⁺ channels (left) are suddenly depolarized, short-term current jumps due to the opening of an ion channel can be observed in the early phase of the depolarizing voltage step. These openings are very short (< 0.5–1 ms); the currents that flow are in the range of single-digit pA values. The opening of one and the same channel during multiple depolarizations (here: first to third depolarization) can be very different, but all responses have in common that the channel openings start relatively quickly after depolarization. When averaging this temporal profile of the probability of Na⁺ channels opening, we see that the open probability rises sharply with suprathreshold depolarization and then falls again. Neuronal voltage-dependent K⁺ channels (right), on the other hand, are only increasingly opened in the course of depolarization. They do not show any inactivation during depolarization. If one averages a larger number of such single-channel currents, one recognises the typical, time-delayed activation of the K⁺ conductance, which is responsible for repolarization.

cell. This reduces the membrane potential in terms of magnitude, i.e. shifts it in a positive direction. The depolarization additionally increases the Na⁺ permeability of the membrane, since previously unopened Na⁺ channels (provided they are in the "closed-activatable" state, **Fig. 2.8**) are opened, which finally leads to a kind of chain reaction and explains the **all-or-nothing behaviour** of the **action potential**. Finally, so much Na⁺ has flowed into the cell that positive membrane potentials are measured, i.e. the membrane has an excess of positive charge on the inside. However, before the **Na⁺ equilibrium potential** of about + 60 mV can be reached, the Na⁺ influx slows down and finally stops. Two mechanisms are responsible for this: firstly, the electrical gradient as the driving force for the inward Na⁺ current ceases to exist when the membrane is depolarized; secondly, the Na⁺ permeability quickly decreases again, i.e. the Na⁺ channels in the cell membrane inactivate very quickly (**Fig. 2.6**). By switching off the Na⁺ current, the depolarization of the membrane is terminated and the repolarization phase is initiated.

MORE DETAILS   Based on molecular biological and electrophysiological studies, the structure and function of the **neuronal Na⁺ channels** are as follows. A chain of about 1800 amino acids forms an integral protein of about 260 kDa and 8 nm in diameter from 4 × 6 subunits. It passes through the membrane several times. Various β subunits can be attached to this α subunit, which forms the actual channel. There is a whole protein family of voltage-gated Na⁺ channels (Na_v; the individual members of this protein family are designated $Na_v 1.1$, $Na_v 1.2$ etc.), which are expressed by different excitable tissues. However, each of these voltage-gated Na⁺ channels has the following properties (**Fig. 2.8**):

It contains a selectivity filter that is responsible for the channel's high selectivity for Na⁺ compared to other cations such as K⁺
– There is a voltage sensor that responds depending on the electric field applied to the membrane, i.e. depending on the membrane potential.
– An "activation gate" responds depending on the membrane potential measured by the voltage sensor so that ion flow through the channel is possible (channel open) or not (channel closed).
– Between the selectivity filter and the voltage sensor is a water-filled pore (diameter approx. 0.3–0.5 nm) through which Na⁺ ions can flow after opening.
– A cytoplasmic part of the channel (inactivation gate) can close the opening of the channel to the cytoplasm and thus inactivate the channel.

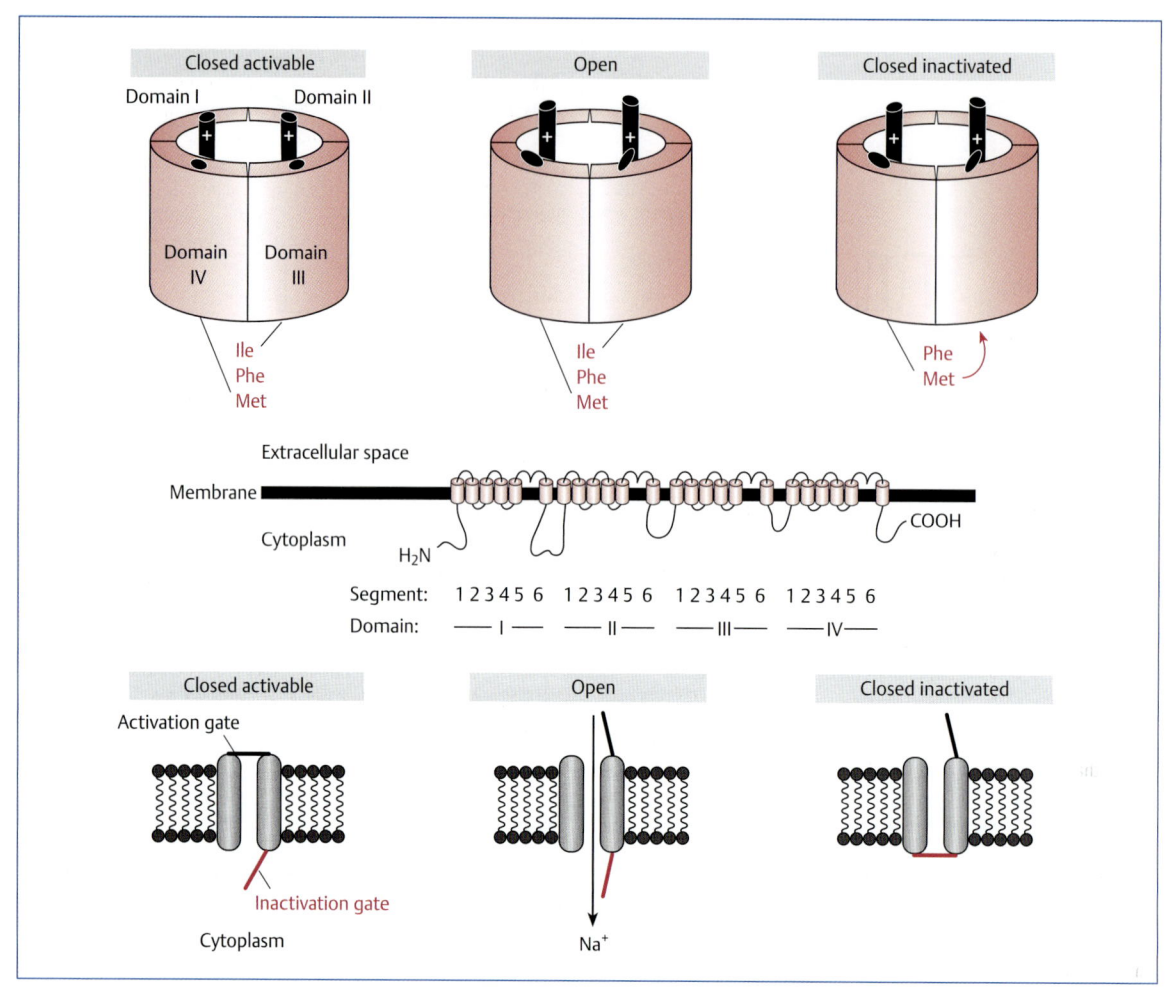

Fig. 2.8 Model representations of the activation behaviour of voltage-dependent Na⁺ channels. Neuronal Na⁺ channels consist of four domains with six segments each (top). The voltage sensors (+) are located on segment 4 (black) of the respective domains. The inactivation results from the voltage-dependent shift of a group of amino acids (red), namely isoleucine (Ile), phenylalanine (Phe) and methionine (Met) between domain III and IV on the cytoplasmic side of the channel opening. Schematically (below), the action of the movement of the activation (black) and inactivation (red) gates can be thought of as two doors in series: As soon as one (or both) of the gate structures interrupts the water-filled pore, no more ion flow is possible. In the closed-activatable state, the cytoplasmically located inactivation gate leaves the cytoplasmic channel open (bottom left). Due to a suprathreshold depolarization, which is registered by the voltage sensors, the activation gate is opened and Na⁺ flows into the cell (bottom centre). This is followed by the rapid "slamming" of the inactivation gate (bottom right). In order for the channel to be reopened by a subsequent suprathreshold depolarization, it must return to the closed-activatable state, which on the one hand takes time and on the other hand is only possible with hyperpolarized membrane potentials.

The **activation** of the Na⁺ channel is voltage-dependent. When the threshold is reached (e.g. −50 mV at a resting potential of −70 mV), the **closed** and **activatable** channel opens for a short time. In the now **open state**, it allows Na⁺ ions to pass in order to inactivate a short time after opening. This inactivation (state of the channel: **closed-inactivated**) differs from the "normal" closing of an ion channel in that the channel cannot be reopened directly from this state (as is the case in the normal "closed state"), but must first undergo a conformational change (to the **closed-activatable state**). During repolarization, the channel is in a **closed** and **inactivated** state. To return to the closed and activatable state, the channel needs time. It can only do this when the membrane potential is hyperpolarized again. If the membrane remains depolarized, this is not possible.

This behaviour of the individual voltage-dependent Na⁺ channels has important consequences for the behaviour of the entire neuron. In the case of a suprathreshold stimulus on a resting nerve cell, as shown in **Fig. 2.5** the amplitude of the action potential proves to be independent of the amplitude of the stimulus. According to the **all-or-nothing principle**, a complete, maximum action potential always occurs after the threshold is exceeded. However, this does not mean that the amplitude of the action potential must be the same under all conditions. This is because its amplitude depends on the Na⁺ influx and thus on the number of Na⁺ channels that open after the threshold is exceeded (i.e. it depends on the Na⁺ permeability of the membrane). As shown in **Fig. 2.9** the size of the Na⁺ inward current depends on the potential at the membrane just prior the start of the action potential. As a rule, this baseline mem-

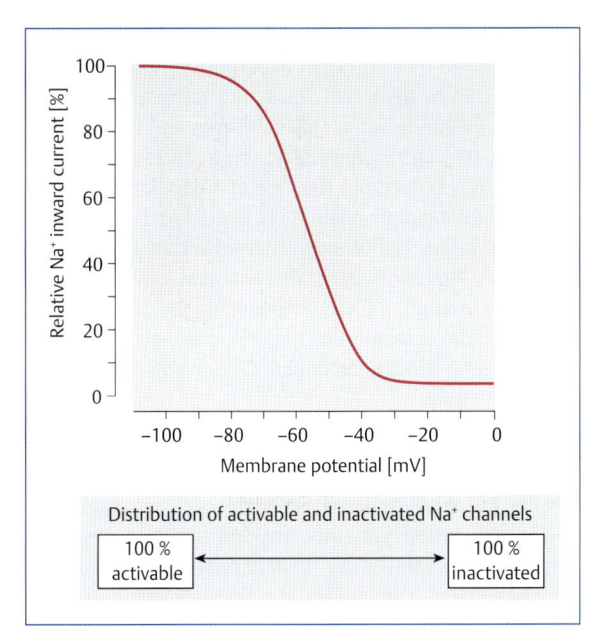

Fig. 2.9 Potential dependence of the Na$^+$ inward current triggered by suprathreshold depolarization. The artificial baseline potential from which the membrane of a neuron was suprathreshold depolarized is shown on the abscissa. For the ordinate values, the maximum triggerable Na$^+$ current was set to 100%. The reason for the fact that the Na$^+$ inward current (and thus also the amplitude of the resulting action potential) decreases when the neuron was depolarized before the stimulus is that only at strongly hyperpolarized membrane potentials are all Na$^+$ channels in the activatable state, while with increasing depolarization more and more channels are in the closed-inactivated state.

MORE DETAILS The neurotoxin **tetrodotoxin** is a toxin found in puffer fish (which makes eating "fugu" in Japan not without danger) that selectively blocks many of the known forms of voltage-gated Na$^+$ channels. Tetrodotoxin thus suppresses the axonal propagation of action potentials as well as the Na$^+$ channels present at the cell soma. The similarly acting **saxitoxin** comes from certain dinoflagellates (e.g. gonyaulax). Saxitoxin plays an important pathophysiological role in many shellfish poisonings. Other naturally occurring toxins, such as some sea anemone toxins, suppress inactivation and thus cause convulsions in animals that come into contact with the nettles of the sea anemone.

IN A NUTSHELL !

The activation and inactivation behaviour of voltage-dependent Na$^+$ channels is crucial for the course of the neuronal action potential.

---

brane potential is equal to the resting potential. Even at a membrane potential of −70 mV, which is often found in neurons, the Na$^+$ conductance cannot be activated to 100%. Maximum activation is only possible after hyperpolarization of the membrane to −80 to −100 mV. Conversely, a long-lasting depolarization to more than −40 mV leads to an almost complete abolition of excitability of the membrane, since Na$^+$ channels are inactivated at a more positive membrane potential.

If the channel is depolarized very slowly, it can go directly from the closed-activatable to the closed-inactivated state within about 1 ms. The excitation then does not reach the threshold and remains local. Such a process is also called accommodation and plays a major role e.g. at centrally excitatory synapses or sensory cells.

A pharmacological influence on the Na$^+$ channel is also of veterinary interest. Certain **local anaesthetics** (e.g. lidocaine), which are used to interrupt excitation and conduction in nerves for some time, function as Na$^+$ channel blockers. The mechanism of action is assumed to be a direct blockade of the neuronal Na$^+$ channels by local anaesthetics. For this purpose, the uncharged, basic local anaesthetic first diffuses through the nerve membrane into the cytosol. There, a hydrogen ion is attached to the amino group (protonation), creating a cation that then blocks the activated sodium channel.

■ Refractory phase

By applying long depolarizations of about 20 ms, it has been experimentally shown that the inactivation of the spontaneously closing Na$^+$ channels lasts as long as the membrane potential is kept at a depolarized value. Under natural conditions, this state corresponds to the duration of repolarization. The Na$^+$ system is now in a closed-inactivated state that lasts until the membrane potential has reached the resting value again.

If a new stimulus arrives in the closed-inactivated phase of the Na$^+$ system, the usual membrane response, i.e. the excitation, does not occur. This state, which lasts about 2 ms in nerve cells, is called the **absolute refractory phase**. In this phase, no action potential can be triggered even by very strong stimuli. The absolute refractory phase is followed by the **relative refractory phase**. During this period, some Na$^+$ channels can be reactivated by a sufficiently high stimulus. This means that the threshold during the relative refractory phase is higher than at rest and the velocity of rise as well as the amplitude of the action potential are smaller than normal.

The refractoriness limits the **maximum frequency** of action potentials of a neurons. If, for example, an action potential lasts 1 ms and is followed by a period of 2 ms in which the neuron is completely unexcitable, this results in a refractory period of 3 ms. This limits the maximum frequency with which that neuron can "fire" action potentials to 333 per second, i.e. 333 Hz. In addition, refractoriness is an essential prerequisite for the **directional** conduction of excitation (p. 56) in nerve fibres.

■ K$^+$ outward current

The basal membrane potential of nerve cells is determined by different types of K$^+$ channels, such as K$_{2P}$ channels (two-pore domain potassium channels. These are dimers of two subunits with two protein domains each, which contribute to pore formation) or inward rectifying K$^+$ channels (K$_{ir}$; these are channels that mediate a K$^+$ influx into the cell at strongly negative membrane potentials better than a K$^+$ outflow at depolarized membrane potentials). These channel types have a relatively high open probability at the resting membrane potential. Upon depolarization into the threshold range, the open probability of the inward rectifying K_{ir} channels decreases, which supports depolarization by the Na^+ inward current via Na_v channels, i.e. the generation of an action potential.

Repolarization towards the resting potential during the late phase of the action potential is accelerated by the fact that a short time after activation of the Na_v channels there is an increase in **K^+ permeability** (Fig. 2.5). This is caused by an increased open probability of voltage-dependent K^+ channels (K_v channels), of which various types are known in neurons. K^+ ions are present in the cytosol in a concentration about 30 times higher than in the extracellular fluid. This chemical gradient drives a K^+ outflow from the cell. The second driving force for the outward K^+ current during overshoot is the electrical gradient, which is directed outward from the cell for K^+ ions. The resulting **K^+ outflow** increases relatively slowly and reaches its maximum at a time when the Na^+ inflow has already decreased significantly. Therefore, there is an overall K^+-carried, outwardly directed net current of positive charges that leads to the reestablishment of the membrane potential, i.e. the **repolarization of the membrane**. Again, the K^+ outflow ceases when the membrane potential approaches the **K^+ equilibrium potential** and the K^+ permeability of the membrane decreases (by closing the voltage-dependent K_v channels).

As the slow increase in K^+ permeability shows, the activation of the K^+ channels, in contrast to the Na^+ channels, does not occur "abruptly" after reaching the threshold potential, but is strictly voltage-dependent both during and at the end of the action potential. This also implies that the K^+ channels do not close spontaneously during depolarization like the Na^+ channels, i.e. they are not inactivated, but are closed again in accordance with repolarization. This process is called **deactivation** (by removal of the activating stimulus). In contrast to the voltage-dependent Na^+ channels in neurons, which ultimately all originate from one protein family (Na_v) with more or less similar properties, there is a large number of protein families coding K^+ channels, which represent the most diverse types of ion channels.

Channels can change stochastically, i.e. randomly, from the open to the closed state (see e.g. the different opening behaviour of one and the same Na^+ or K^+ channel during a depolarization in Fig. 2.7). However, the probability with which this happens can usually be regulated by the cell. There are many different channel types with different controls: e.g. voltage-dependent (Fig. 2.7), receptor-controlled, G protein-controlled or second messenger-controlled channels. This means that there are signalling chains in the cell that regulate the open probability of particular ion channels (e.g. the activation of voltage-dependent Ca^{2+} channels in the heart (p. 178) by a cAMP-dependent protein kinase).

■ Afterpotential

In many neurons, the increase in K^+ outflow outlasts the Na^+ inflow, so that the membrane potential not only returns to the resting value after the end of the action potential, but temporarily reaches values that are closer to the K^+ equilibrium potential. This means that the action potential is followed by a so-called **hyperpolarizing afterpotential** (Fig. 2.5). As discussed above, the activatability of the voltage-dependent Na^+ channels is promoted by hyperpolarization (Fig. 2.9). Conversely, the activatability of the Na^+ system is reduced in the case of a **depolarizing afterpotential**, for example when there is a delayed inactivation of the Na^+ influx and/or only a slowed activation of the K^+ outflow. A hyperpolarizing afterpotential can also result from the opening of Ca^{2+}-dependent K^+ channels (K_{Ca} channels). The activation of these K^+ channels is due to a Ca^{2+} influx via voltage-dependent Ca^{2+} channels during the action potential.

■ Quantity of ion shifts

Despite the strong changes in membrane permeabilities during the action potential, the ion shifts through the membrane are vanishingly small in relation to the concentrations in the cytosol and in the extracellular fluid. From electrophysiological studies and physical considerations, it can be estimated that during the action potential only a few thousand Na^+ ions need to flow through a single Na^+ channel during an opening lasting 1 ms in order to shift the membrane potential in the region of the channel by 100 mV (i.e. e.g. from −70 to +30 mV). The reason for this is the very small membrane capacitance (in the case of a cell membrane, a fairly constant 10^{-14} F·μm^{-2}; this means that a charge of 10^{-14} coulombs is sufficient to build up a voltage of 1 V on a membrane surface of $1 \mu m^2$). Depending on the density of the Na^+ channels in the membrane, there would only be a change in the concentration of Na^+, which corresponds to a **change of** only one **thousandth of** the **initial concentration**. For K^+ ions, very similar values result under the same assumptions.

■ Electrolyte imbalances

MORE DETAILS The ionic currents underlying action potentials, in particular the influx of Na^+ ions, are significantly influenced by extracellular ion concentrations, as concentration gradients between intracellular and extracellular space (in addition to electrical driving forces) act as one of the driving forces for ion movements through channels. Since the triggering of an action potential depends on the opening of voltage-dependent ion channels, voltage sensors that are part of the ion channel must be able to measure potential differences across the membrane. Under resting conditions, there is a positive potential directly on the outside of the membrane and a negative potential on the inside. If a certain threshold potential difference is exceeded, the Na^+ channel opens. Changing ion concentrations in the extracellular space influences the potential dependence and the time course of the Na^+ currents. On the outer side of the membrane, there are negatively charged extensions of phospho- and glycolipids and also glycoproteins. Since the negative charges are attached to the outer membrane leaflet, the voltage sensor would measure a lower potential difference and already open the Na^+ channel at lower depolarizations. Under physiological conditions, positively charged ions, such as Ca^{2+}, Mg^{2+} and H^+, in the extracellular fluid neutralise these negative charges, so the voltage sensor measures the real potential difference present. If there is a reduction in the extracellular Ca^{2+} concentration (**hypocalcaemia**), the negative surface charge is increased, and the channel opens even at low depolarizations. High extracellular Ca^{2+} concentrations thus stabilise the membrane potential, while low Ca^{2+} concentrations lead to increased excitability of the nerves. A decrease in extracellular Ca^{2+} concentration occurs as a result of certain metabolic disorders (e.g. deficiency of parathyroid hormone, which is a hormone from the parathyroid gland that raises Ca^{2+} concentration in the blood) or Ca^{2+} deficiency in the feed. Clinical consequence of neuronal hyperexcitability can be tetanic spasms, as observed in the so-called **eclampsia** of the bitch in the parturition and post-parturition period.

Changes in the Mg^{2+} plasma level or the extracellular pH also have an influence on synaptic transmission. Magnesium ions have an inhibitory effect on transmitter release. Accordingly, magnesium deficiency can lead to the development of cramps. Such **hypomagnesaemia** sometimes occurs in connection with grass tetany in dairy cows (p. 406). Low pH, i.e. high H^+ concentrations in the blood (acidosis), have similar effects to high Ca^{2+} concentrations, while low H^+ concentrations (alkalosis) increase the excitability of cells.

With **hypokalaemia** the resting membrane potential becomes increasingly negative (e.g. from −85 mV to −95 mV). This increases the stimulus necessary for depolarization until the threshold potential is reached, i.e. the excitability of the nerve cells (and muscle tissue) decreases. In extreme cases, excitation no longer occurs. The result clinically is flaccid paralysis. In acute **hyperkalaemia** the resting membrane potential is reduced in magnitude (e.g. from −85 mV to −75 mV) and excitability increases. If the threshold potential is exceeded, the **permanent depolarization** and the resulting inactivation of voltage-dependent Na^+ channels can cause muscle **paralysis** (**hyperkalaemic paralysis**, for example, in Quarter Horses (p. 617). Clinically relevant changes in extracellular potassium concentration are, however, mainly caused by changes in the pH of blood. The different forms of acidosis or alkalosis and their development are described in ch. 15.5.

2.4 Path of the signal from the sensor to the effector

The response of a neuron to a stimulus, the generation of electrical signals, their transmission and the complex possibilities for communication between nerve cells are decisive processes in nervous systems. The cellular and molecular basis of these processes will be explained in the following.

2.4.1 Processes at the sensor and at the trigger zone: from the generator potential to the frequency-coded signal

The activation of nervous circuits is based on the activation of a sensor (receptor cell). As a polymodal sensor, it can recognise several types of stimuli or, as a monomodal sensor, it can react specifically to only one type of stimulus, see ch. "General sensory physiology" (p. 67). Special sensory cells or specialised endings of the afferent nerve fibres function as sensors. These peripheral sensors translate the actual stimulus at the **site of transduction** into an electrical potential, the **generator potential** which is also called receptor potential at sensory cells (**Fig. 2.10**). The ampli-

tude and duration of the generator potential are graded and proportional to the amplitude and duration of the stimulus. With the exception of vertebrate photosensors, which respond to light with hyperpolarization, all other sensory cells show depolarization in response to the stimulus. The cause of this generator potential in many sensory cells is the opening of **non-selective cation channels** that are permeable to both Na^+ and K^+, with the resulting Na^+ influx exceeding the K^+ outflow.

The molecular basis for depolarization can also lie in the opening of Ca^{2+} or slow Na^+ channels or the closing of K^+ channels. The generator potential propagates electrotonically to a trigger zone located in the immediate vicinity of the sensitive nerve ending. This is where it is decided whether the depolarization is sufficient to exceed the threshold for triggering an action potential. The **trigger zone** has a high density of voltage-dependent Na^+ channels, which is what makes an action potential on neurons possible. The trigger zone thus transforms the input signal, provided it is suprathreshold, into action potentials. As soon as the input signal exceeds this threshold, each further increase in its amplitude increases the frequency (**frequency modulation**) at which the action potentials are generated, but not their amplitude. The reason for the increase in frequency is that the depolarizing current acting on the axon membrane is stronger at higher generator potentials and thus the threshold can be exceeded again, sooner after an action potential. The duration of the input signals determines the number of action potentials, i.e. ultimately the duration of the time period in which a neuron fires action potentials.

For the coding of stimulus information, it is advantageous that the amplitude of the generator potential is not constant (as in the case of an action potential), since the stimulus intensity can thus be coded via the amplitude of the generator potential. However, transmission over longer distances is not possible because the electrotonic potential is only propagated over a relatively short distance due to the passive membrane properties of the nerve fibre, such as time and length constants. An electrotonic potential can only travel a relatively short distance before it "runs out" (**Fig. 2.4**). The amplitude and duration of the generator potential now decide at what frequency and over what period of time **action potentials** are propagated via the axon. The coding is therefore carried out via the number and frequency of the action potentials. Depending on the characteristics of the nerve fibre, tonic (i.e. excitation phases in which the frequency of the action potentials does not change) or phasic (excitation phases in which the frequency of the action potentials decreases over time) excitation patterns can arise. The **amplitude-encoded generator potential** is thus converted into a **frequency-encoded signal**. At the synaptic terminal the electrical signal is transformed into a **chemical signal** via neurotransmitters. The amount of transmitters released is proportional to the number of action potentials, whereby the transmitters are released in approximately constant vesicle portions ("quanta") at the synaptic terminal (p. 59).

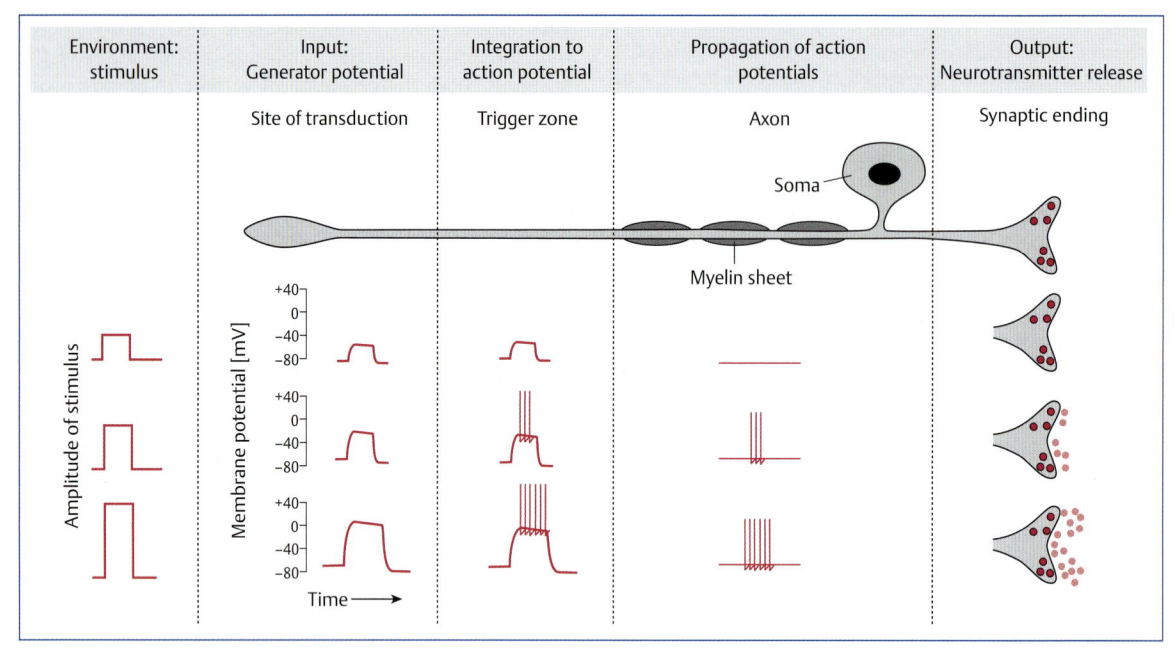

Fig. 2.10 A sensory neuron converts a stimulus (e.g. a stretch) into a generator potential. Each of the four neuronal regions (transduction site, trigger zone, axon, synaptic terminal) generates typical signals. In the first line, a subthreshold stimulus acts on the transduction site, generating only a subthreshold generator potential. In the second line, a short, stronger stimulus generates a suprathreshold generator potential, resulting in propagated action potentials with the consequence of neurotransmitter release at the synaptic terminal. In the third line, a longer lasting strong stimulus acts on the transduction zone, increasing the frequency of the triggered action potentials. Ultimately, there is a recurring characteristic sequence of the process: input, integration, conduction, output.

> **IN A NUTSHELL** !
>
> Graduated generator potentials encode the information at the sensor. Amplitude and duration of the generator potential encode the strength and duration of the stimulus. At the trigger zone, the generator potential is converted into a frequency-encoded signal, which is translated into a chemical signal at the synaptic terminal.

2.4.2 Excitation propagation: slow continuous propagation and saltatory excitation propagation

The type of excitation transmission from the trigger zone to the soma and further to the synapse depends essentially on the structure of the nerve fibre. While myelinated nerve fibres are specialised in rapid conduction, excitation propagation along unmyelinated nerve fibres is much slower (**Fig. 2.11**). In both cases, however, active transmission of the excitation occurs, i.e. sequential triggering and propagation of action potentials.

In the case of an **unmyelinated nerve fibre** (Fig. 2.11 a), a Na$^+$ influx triggers local currents, i.e. a passive ionic shift, at an excited site. Depolarization causes cations in the cytosol to be displaced from the excited site (charges of the

same type repel each other) or anions to be attracted. In other words, an electrical current flows from the excited site to the unexcited neighbouring membrane areas. The local current circuit in front of or behind the excitation front is closed by positive charges flowing on the outside of the membrane from unexcited areas to the excited area (or anions flowing in the opposite direction). These local current circuits depolarize neighbouring axon sections and can thus also excite them above threshold. Anterograde, i.e. in the conduction direction, this leads to an opening of the voltage-dependent Na$^+$ channels, which are in the closed-activatable state. In the anterograde direction, the action potential is triggered anew at each membrane site that contains a voltage-dependent Na$^+$ channel and is thus refreshed (**continuous excitation propagation**). Opposite to the direction of propagation, i.e. retrograde, the local currents meet inactivated Na$^+$ channels that cannot open in response to depolarization (the nerve is therefore refractory there).

Transmission in unmyelinated nerve fibres is relatively slow (usually only 1–3 m·s^{-1}, maximum 30 m·s^{-1}). This slow conduction is especially found in nerves that supply **the internal organs**. Relatively low conduction velocities of nociceptors are also apparent. These fibres have diameters of less than 1 μm (**Table 2.3**).

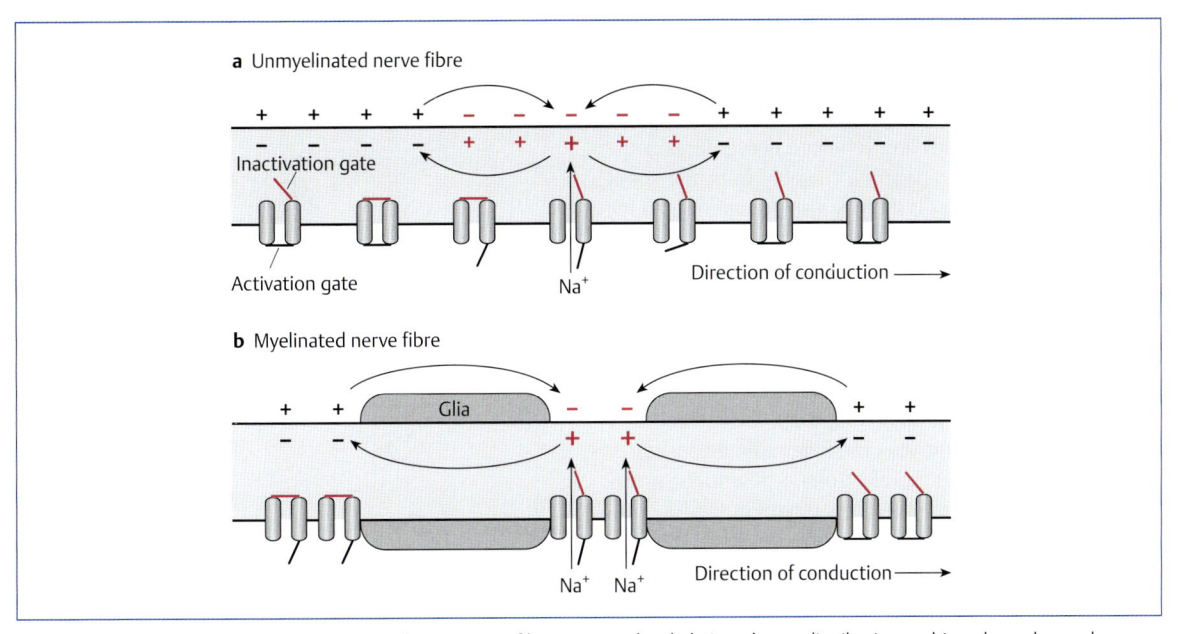

a Unmyelinated nerve fibre

Inactivation gate

Activation gate

Na⁺

Direction of conduction ⟶

b Myelinated nerve fibre

Glia

Na⁺ Na⁺

Direction of conduction ⟶

Fig. 2.11 Conduction of the action potential along a nerve fibre. For graphical clarity, charge distribution and ion channels are drawn on opposite sides of the axon.
a In an unmyelinated nerve fibre, the Na⁺ influx at an excited site (centre) triggers local circuits, i.e. passive ion shifts inside and outside the cell. These depolarize neighbouring membrane regions and lead anterogradely (i.e. in the direction of conduction) to an opening of the voltage-dependent Na⁺ channels, which are in the closed-activatable state (indicated by the position of the two "gates": Inactivation gate – red; activation gate – black). For graphical reasons, the activation gate is drawn here on the extracellular channel opening. In reality, however, it is located between the selectivity filter and the cytoplasmic channel opening. The tunnel structure of the channel at this "bottleneck" (p. 67) is widened during activation and the channel thus becomes permeable. In the anterograde direction, the action potential is refreshed at each membrane site with a voltage-dependent Na⁺ channel. Opposite to the direction of conduction, i.e. retrograde, the local currents meet inactivated Na⁺ channels, which cannot open in response to depolarization.
b In a myelinated nerve fibre, the voltage-dependent Na⁺ channels are concentrated in the region of the nodes of Ranvier. The local currents spread electrotonically in the internodes and lead to an opening of the voltage-dependent Na⁺ channels at the next anterograde node of Ranvier, whereby the action potential is "refreshed", i.e. triggered anew. Retrograde, on the other hand, the local circuits meet inactivated Na⁺ channels, whereby a direction of excitation propagation (i.e. from the soma to the synaptic terminal) is predetermined, just as in the case of the medullary nerve fibres.

Table 2.3 Classification of nerve fibres. [Data according to Erlanger/Gasser]

Fibre type	Function (example)	Fibre diameter (approx. μm)	Excitation conduction velocity (approx. $m \cdot s^{-1}$)
Aα	Primary muscle spindle afferents, motor to skeletal muscles	15	100 (70–120)
Aβ	Skin afferents (touch, pressure)	8	50 (30–70)
Aγ	Motoneuron to muscle spindles	5	20 (15–30)
Aδ	Skin afferents (temperature, nociception)	< 3	15 (12–30)
B	Sympathetic preganglionic	3	7 (3–15)
C	Sympathetic postganglionic, nociception	1, unmyelinated	1 (0.5–2)

In addition to this classification, there is also the classification of afferent nerves according to Lloyd and Hunt. These authors distinguish between four main classes of afferent nerves (fast-conducting type I to very slow-conducting type IV fibres), some of which are further subdivided. These include, for example, Ia fibres (from muscle spindles), Ib fibres (from Golgi tendon organs) and type II fibres (from touch and pressure sensors of the skin), III (temperature and fast-conducting pain fibres) and IV (slow-conducting pain fibres).

In a **myelinated nerve fibre** the myelin sheath forms an insulating layer that is interrupted at regular intervals by nodes of Ranvier (at intervals of approx. 2 mm) (**Fig. 2.11 b**). The voltage-dependent Na⁺ channels are concentrated in the region of the nodes in this type of nerve fibre. Local currents propagate electrotonically in the internodes (length about 2 mm). In this process, the amplitude of the action potential weakens slightly due to a recharging of the membrane capacitor and also to a voltage drop at the cytoplasmic resistance within the axon (series resistance (p. 46)). However, this type of conduction occurs very quickly. The distance between the nodes of Ranvier must not exceed a certain limit, because the membrane potential must still be suprathreshold at the next anterograde node in order to induce the opening of voltage-dependent Na⁺ channels. Thereby the action potential is "refreshed", i.e. retriggered. On the other hand, the local circuits encounter inactivated Na⁺ channels, making the retrograde located part of the nerve refractory. As with unmyelinated nerve fibres, a direction of excitation propagation (namely from the soma to the synaptic terminal) is thereby also predetermined for the myelinated ones. As with continuous excitation conduction, the refractory phase ensures directional excitation conduction.

In general, the speed of action potential propagation increases not only with increasing insulation (due to sheathing with myelin), but also with the diameter of the axon, since the cytoplasmic resistance opposing the current flow then becomes lower and thus the longitudinal constant λ (**Fig. 2.4**) becomes larger (i.e. electrotonic potentials spread further). It also increases with the strength of the Na⁺ current. Because of a lack of myelination, invertebrates can therefore reach high conduction velocities only through so-called giant axons, i.e. nerve fibres with a large diameter of almost 1 mm. Inhibition of the Na⁺ current by **local anaesthetics** leads to a reduction or total block of conduction.

The propagation of excitation along a nerve fibre can be measured with extracellular electrodes. If such measurements are performed on nerve bundles, the resulting signal is composed of the sum of all propagated action potentials (**Fig. 2.12**). This so-called **compound action potential** allows conclusions to be drawn about the functionality of nerves. In the case of extracellularly attached electrodes, the action potential is not monophasic as in the case of intracellular recording, in which a recording electrode is inserted into a neuron and the voltage, i.e. the difference in potential against the outside world, is measured. As a rule, the compound action potential is biphasic. Among other things, this method can also be used to measure the **nerve conduction velocity** by recording the time after which an action potential – triggered by an electrical stimulus – arrives at a recording electrode (nerve conduction velocity = distance between stimulus and recording electrode divided by the elapsed time).

MORE DETAILS How this biphasic signal develops is explained in **Fig. 2.12**. In an unexcited axon, the membrane potential is at the resting potential (cell membrane positively charged on the outside). Both extracellular electrodes are at the same potential, so no voltage is measured between the electrodes during extracellular recording. If one end (here the left end) of the nerve fibre is stimulated, this triggers an action potential. This means that the polarity of the membrane changes at the excited site. Accordingly, there is now a potential difference between the two extracellular electrodes. If the action potential now propagates along the nerve fibre, there is a period of time – assuming sufficient distance between the two recording electrodes – in which both electrodes are again over unexcited areas. Here the voltmeter, which is connected between the two extracellular electrodes, shows no deflection. Finally, the excitation arrives at the second recording electrode, resulting in a deflection of opposite polarity compared to the first deflection. When the (compound) action potential has left the range of the two electrodes, the voltmeter no longer shows a deflection.

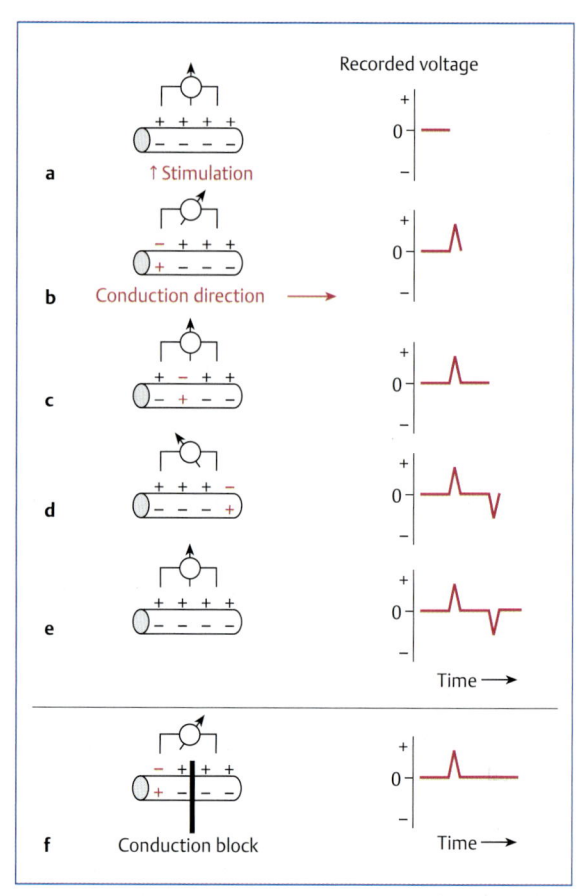

Fig. 2.12 Action potentials of nerve fibres can be recorded extracellularly and registered as compound action potentials (CAP). Two recording electrodes are placed on a nerve and connected to a voltmeter. In an unexcited axon, the membrane potential is at the resting potential (**a**): both extracellular electrodes are at the same potential, so no voltage is measured between them. If one end (here the left end) of the nerve fibre is suprathreshold stimulated, this triggers an action potential. This means that the polarity of the membrane changes at the excited site: The polarity of the membrane is reversed, resulting in a potential difference between the two electrodes (**b**). If the action potential now travels over the nerve fibre, this results in a time period in which both recording electrodes are again over unexcited regions (**c**). Finally, the excitation arrives at the second recording electrode, resulting in a deflection of opposite polarity compared to the first deflection (**d**). When the (compound) action potential has left the region of the two recording electrodes, the voltmeter no longer shows a deflection (**e**). In the case of a conduction block (**f**), a monophasic potential is produced.

With bipolar recording (**Fig. 2.12**), a biphasic potential is measured, i.e. a voltage signal that is composed of a deflection in the positive and negative direction. If the recording is monopolar (an extracellular electrode is measured against earth), a positive or negative monophasic potential is produced depending on the polarity of the electrodes. Furthermore, in the case of a conduction block, e.g. a nerve injury in the region between the two electrodes, the compound action potential is monophasic because it is not transmitted to the second recording electrode (**Fig. 2.12 f**).

IN A NUTSHELL   **!**

Saltatory excitation conduction enables the rapid axonal propagation of neural signals.

2.4.3 Transmission of excitation, synaptic transmission

Among other things, neurons have the ability to communicate with each other quickly and precisely. Nerve cells are in contact with each other or with their target **organs** via synapses. For example, a neuron can form 1000 synaptic contacts and receives around 10000 connections. The human brain contains about 10^{11} neurons and consequently about 10^{14} synapses (this is more synapses than stars in our galaxy). The excitation that reaches the synapse in the form of action potentials can be passed on to the target cell by means of **electrical** or **chemical** transmission.

■ Electrical synapses

Although most synapses use a chemical transmitter, some operate electrically via gap junctions (p.29) which allow a direct flow of ions from one neuron to the next. Gap junctions can be modulated by changes in membrane potential, cytosolic pH and cytosolic Ca^{2+} concentration. Transmission at electrical synapses corresponds to the **passive electrotonic propagation** of local, subthreshold electrical signals along an axon. Therefore, electrical synapses can conduct in both directions, whereas transmission at a chemical synapse can only occur in one direction (so-called rectifier or valve function). Since transmission at electrical synapses is based on a **direct current flow**, it is extremely fast. This type of information transmission therefore has advantages especially in triggering escape reactions. One of the classic examples is the mediation of the tail flick reaction in goldfish by a giant neuron in the brainstem (the so-called Mauthner cell), which is activated by sensory neurons via gap junctions. Electrical synapses also exist in mammals, e.g. in the brainstem and in the vestibular nuclei.

■ Chemical synapses

Morphologically, the chemical synapse consists of several components. These include the presynaptic membrane of the presynaptic terminal, the synaptic cleft (approx. 20 nm) and the postsynaptic membrane of the target cell (**Fig. 2.13 a**). In chemical synaptic transmission, transmitter release by the presynaptic neuron occurs first, followed by diffusion of the transmitter through the synaptic cleft and finally occupation of a transmitter-specific receptor on the postsynaptic neuron. The highly precise and locally very limited transmitter release often occurs through a specialised secretory apparatus in the so-called active zone in the synaptic terminals. Nerve cells of the autonomic nervous system (p.112), which innervate the smooth muscles, for example, have no synapses. They release their transmitters diffusely from so-called varicosities. Chemical synapses play a crucial role both in communication between neurons and in transmission between nerve cell and effector cell, such as in the innervation of skeletal muscles (p.148) via the neuromuscular junction.

Transmitter release at the synapse is a complex process in which various factors such as ionic currents, protein-protein interactions as well as conformational changes of the proteins and membranes are involved. Both exocytosis and endocytosis also play important roles.

The processes leading to transmitter release are timed very precisely. They begin with a Ca^{2+} influx into the presynaptic terminal (**Fig. 2.13 a**). While the action potential along the axon is essentially carried by the Na^+ influx, **Ca^{2+}** plays a crucial role in the function of the chemical synapse. Ca^{2+} influx is triggered by the incoming action potentials, which ensure the depolarization of the presynaptic membrane. Due to this depolarization, **voltage-dependent Ca^{2+} channels** (from the protein family of Ca_v channels) open, allowing Ca^{2+} to flow into the presynaptic terminal according to its chemical gradient. Within a few hundred microseconds, this leads to a thousand-fold increase in the cytosolic Ca^{2+} concentration in certain zones of the terminal from the original $0.1\,\mu mol \cdot l^{-1}$. In most neurons, voltage-dependent Ca^{2+} channels of the type $Ca_v2.1$ (also called P-type) and $Ca_v2.2$ (also called N-type), which inactivate relatively quickly, contribute to transmitter release (**Fig. 2.13 a**).

> **MORE DETAILS** The high biological importance of the voltage-dependent Ca^{2+} channels is demonstrated, among other things, by the fact that certain animals, such as cone snails, have developed highly selective toxins (in the case of cone snails, the so-called conotoxins), which inhibit various types of Ca^{2+} channels and are thus used to paralyse prey.

With increasing duration of the Na^+-carried action potential and with increasing frequency of the action potentials, the amount of Ca^{2+} flowing into the presynaptic terminal increases and thus also the transmitter release. The Ca^{2+} influx only begins towards the end of the action potential. In chemical synapses, this is one of the causes of the delay in transmission after depolarization, i.e. the time between arrival of the action potential and postsynaptic response of the target cell. Since the Ca^{2+} channels are located directly adjacent to the sites of transmitter release, they can still trigger transmitter release within approximately 0.2 ms. Other causes of the **synaptic delay time** lie in the diffusion of the transmitter from the site of release to the site of action at the postsynaptic side.

Electron microscopy shows that the presynaptic terminal contains an accumulation of small **transmitter-specific vesicles** at the specialised part of the presynaptic membrane called the **active zone**. The active zone is characterised by the presence of specific docking proteins. After a Ca^{2+} influx, the vesicles fuse with the presynaptic membrane and then release their contents by **exocytosis**. Since the content of a single vesicle is always completely released, the amount of transmitter released in a synapse is determined by the number of vesicles that fuse with the cell membrane, i.e. by the number of "vesicle quanta".

There is now relatively detailed knowledge about the intracellular processes involved in the migration of vesicles towards release sites after Ca^{2+} influx, the fusion of vesicles with the presynaptic membrane and the release of transmitter into the synaptic cleft. So far, **four groups of pro-**

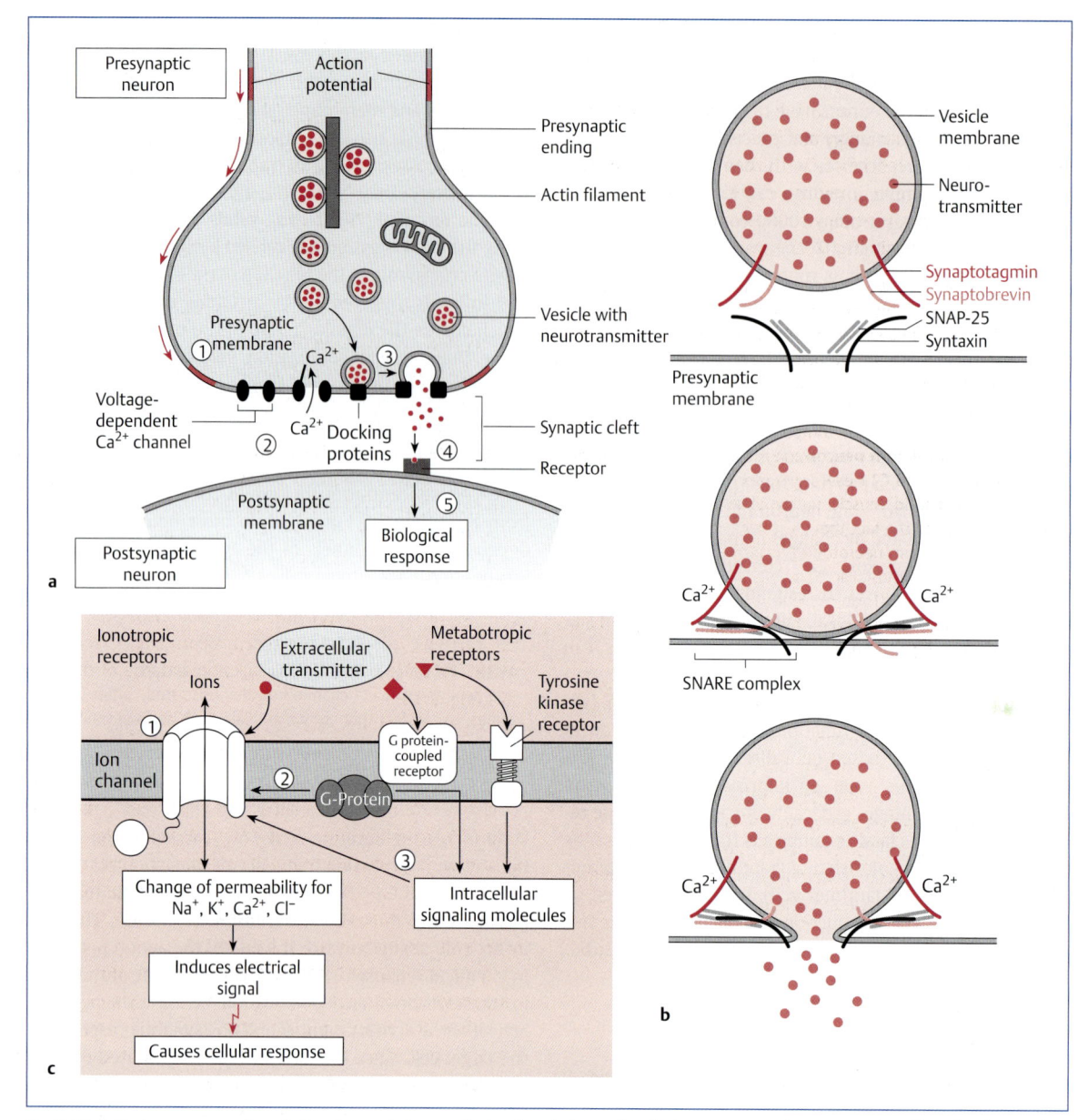

Fig. 2.13 **a** Basic processes of excitation transmission or electrochemical coupling between pre- and postsynaptic cell at the chemical synapse.
b Complex interactions of different docking proteins mediate the attachment of synaptic vesicles to the presynaptic membrane.
c Effect of transmitters via ionotropic or metabotropic receptors (using the example of a G protein-coupled receptor and a tyrosine kinase receptor).
The numbers underlined with a round circle in each part of the figure indicate the order of the respective processes.

teins have been identified that play specific roles in these processes. These **tasks** are:

- Random vesicle movements must be prevented.
- There must be a specific orientation of the vesicles towards the active zone.
- The vesicles must dock with the active zone.
- Vesicle fusion and transmitter release must occur.

Initially, only a relatively small number of vesicles are located in the immediate vicinity of the active zone; most are anchored to actin filaments of the cytoskeleton in the vicinity of the active zone and thus serve as transmitter reservoirs. The Ca^{2+} influx loosens the anchoring of the vesicles. By mobilising the vesicles, their targeted movement towards the active zones can now take place.

Attachment and fusion of synaptic vesicles to the presynaptic membrane as well as transmitter exocytosis are complex processes. They are based on the interaction of cytoplasmic proteins with binding partners in the vesicle membrane and the plasma membrane of the presynaptic terminal. These are described in more detail below, as they are important for understanding synaptic transmission under physiological and pathophysiological conditions (**Fig. 2.13 b**).

Initially, interactions occur between the vesicle protein **synaptobrevin** and the two SNARE proteins of the presynaptic membrane, **syntaxin** and **SNAP-25**. This leads to the formation of the so-called SNARE complex. SNARE stands for **soluble N-ethylmaleimide-sensitive factor attachment receptor**. The SNARE complex-independent vesicle protein **synaptotagmin** interacts with the SNARE complex in the presence of Ca^{2+}. It can bind to phospholipids of the presynaptic membrane, thus promoting vesicle fusion and transmitter exocytosis. This model idea is called the **SNARE hypothesis** (Fig. 2.13).

MORE DETAILS   Many neurotoxins interact with this process and influence different components of the synaptic fusion complex. The toxins of Clostridia bacteria in particular have a fascinating range of effects in this respect. The action of toxins produced by **tetanus toxin** and certain **botulinum neurotoxins** (botulinum neurotoxins B, D and F) is based on a cleavage of synaptobrevin. Thus, an important component of the fusion complex is inactivated. **Botulinum neurotoxin A** cleaves SNAP-25 and **botulinum neurotoxin C1** cleaves syntaxin. The different symptoms of botulism (flaccid muscle paralysis) and tetanus (muscle rigidity) are due to the fact that the toxins act on different synapses. While botulinum neurotoxin blocks the release of acetylcholine at the neuromuscular junction and thus causes flaccid paralysis, the tetanus toxin prevents the release of glycine from certain inhibitory interneurons (Renshaw cells, p. 132) in the spinal cord, resulting in cramps.

IN A NUTSHELL ❗

A prerequisite for the release of the transmitter is an increase in Ca^{2+} concentration in the presynaptic terminal after influx of Ca^{2+} via voltage-dependent Ca^{2+} channels. The release occurs via exocytosis and is based on the fusion of transmitter-filled vesicles with the presynaptic membrane. Interactions between proteins localised in the cytoplasm, in the vesicle membrane and in the plasma membrane play an important role.

2.4.4   Processes at the target cell, postsynaptic potentials

A number of chemical substances, including small molecules and peptides, serve as **neurotransmitters**. However, the effect of a transmitter depends less on its chemical structure than on the transmitter-specific receptors on the target cell and the downstream intracellular signalling cascades. For example, the transmitter acetylcholine can have an excitatory effect on some cells (e.g. smooth muscle cells of the intestine), but an inhibitory effect on other cells (e.g. pacemaker cells in the heart). Several receptor subtypes exist for most transmitters.

Transmitters are inactivated via various pathways to terminate their action at the postsynaptic membrane. As a rule, transmitters are rapidly **degraded enzymatically into ineffective cleavage products**. For example, **acetylcholine esterase** at the postsynaptic membrane cleaves acetylcholine into choline and acetate by hydrolysis. Choline can be transported back to the synaptic terminal to serve transmitter synthesis again. Diffusion of the transmitter or degradation products away from the synaptic cleft and uptake of the transmitter into neighbouring cells or into the presynaptic terminal may represent further mechanisms.

MORE DETAILS   Blocking transmitter inactivation can be of great therapeutic benefit if a reduced transmitter concentration is causally involved in a disease. Thus, acetylcholine degradation can be selectively prevented by substances that inhibit acetylcholine esterase. This is used, for example, in the therapy of myasthenia gravis in dogs. The reuptake of transmitters can also be restricted by specific "reuptake" blockers. In both cases, there is an indirect increase in transmitter concentration in the synaptic cleft. Other acetylcholine esterase inhibitors, such as malathion, which is still used in some European countries to control lice, are effective insecticides.

The transmitter-induced change in the excitability of an innervated cell is brought about by a modulation of the ionic conductance of the plasma membrane. Transmitters can directly or indirectly affect ion channels at the **postsynaptic membrane**. In both cases, membrane-spanning proteins are involved, which bind the transmitter on the extracellular side and ultimately control the opening and closing of ion channels (**Fig. 2.13c**). In direct modulation, the receptors contain both the binding site for the neurotransmitter and the ion channel in one and the same protein. Such receptors are therefore called **ionotropic receptors** or **ligand-gated ion channels**. Examples include the nicotinic acetylcholine receptors, receptors for glutamate, and glycine and GABA$_A$ (γ-aminobutyric acid) receptors (**Fig. 2.15**).

Indirect modulation takes place via receptors that do not contain an ion channel but change enzyme activities in the cell (and ultimately influence ion channels via them). Such receptors are called **metabotropic receptors** (**Fig. 2.13c**). They are often coupled (as in the case of G protein-coupled receptors) to second messenger systems with their intracellular signalling molecules (p. 38). However, they also include the receptor tyrosine kinases in which the receptor, once it has bound its ligand, acquires enzyme activity and transfers phosphate groups to tyrosine residues of target proteins, i.e. phosphorylates them.

While the ionotropic receptors induce relatively fast synaptic processes, the metabotropic receptors cause slow changes that can often last for several minutes. The metabotropic receptors therefore often serve to modulate the excitability of neurons or the sensitivity of synapses over the longer term. Such modulatory synaptic pathways are involved in learning processes, for example.

Although a nerve cell receives many inhibitory and excitatory input signals at the same time and the behaviour of the postsynaptic cell is always a result of the activity of different synapses, the individual synaptic processes will be described separately below for better understanding. Transmitters induce either excitatory or inhibitory responses (**Fig. 2.14**). Depending on which receptor types are involved, a fast (short-lasting) or slow (long-lasting) activation or inhibition occurs. Activation (by depolarization) of a postsynaptic cell occurs via **excitatory postsynaptic potentials (EPSP)**, inhibition (by hyperpolarization) via **inhibitory postsynaptic potentials (IPSP)**. Fast EPSP are in most cases mediated by the opening of ligand-gated ion channels that are permeable to both Na^+ and K^+, i.e. represent non-selective cation channels. The inward Na^+ current dominates over the outward K^+ current, resulting in depo-

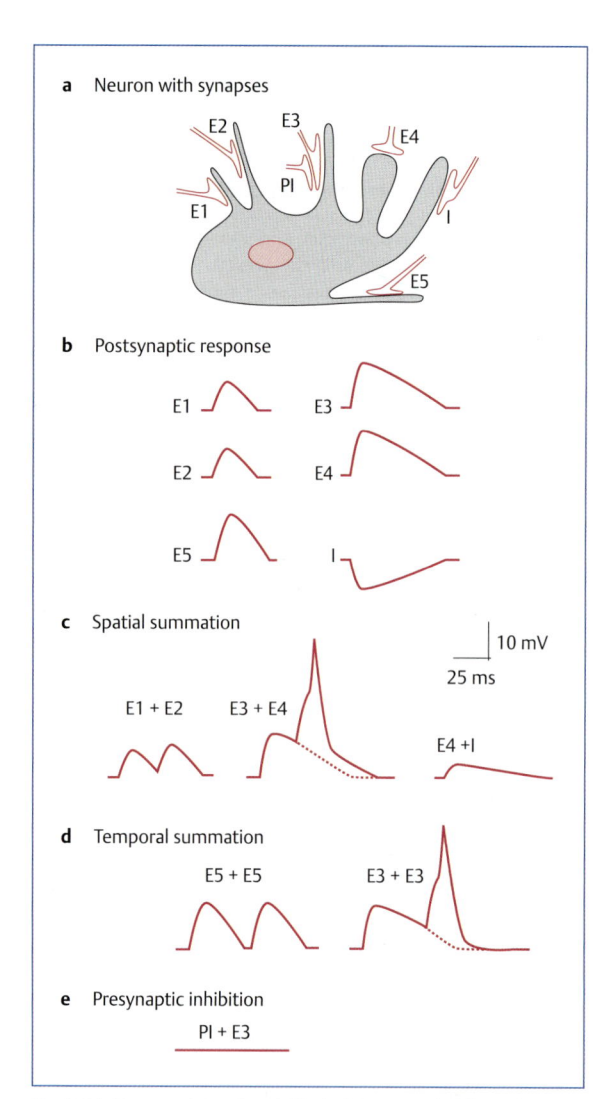

a   Neuron with synapses

E2   E3

E4

PI

E1

I

E5

b   Postsynaptic response

E1

E3

E2

E4

E5

I

c   Spatial summation

10 mV

25 ms

E1 + E2   E3 + E4

E4 + I

d   Temporal summation

E5 + E5   E3 + E3

e   Presynaptic inhibition

PI + E3

Fig. 2.14 Neurons have the ability to integrate signals as they can process multiple synaptic inputs. For simplicity, different synaptic processes are shown on a nerve cell.
a The nerve cell shown here receives several excitatory (E1–E5) and one inhibitory (I) input. In addition, an excitatory input (E3) can be presynaptically inhibited (PI).
b First, the responses of the neuron to the individual synaptic inputs are shown separately (deflection upwards = depolarization; deflection downwards = hyperpolarization). Rapid EPSP (when E1–E5 are excited) or IPSP (when I is excited) are produced. If two inputs occur at short temporal intervals at spatially separated inputs (E1 and E2 in **c**) or at the same synapse (E3 or E5 in **d**), spatial (**c**) or temporal (**d**) summation occurs. Membrane time constant and membrane resistance ultimately determine the duration and amplitude of the electrotonic signal that arrives at the trigger zone where an action potential can be initiated when the threshold is exceeded. Simultaneously occurring EPSP and IPSP are also added up (in **c** with input from E4 and I). In the example of presynaptic inhibition shown (**e**), transmitter release at an excitatory synapse (E3) is completely blocked.

larization. In some cases, excitatory potentials can also be mediated by a Ca^{2+} current.

■ Excitatory postsynaptic potentials (EPSP)

The generation of a **fast EPSP** can be illustrated by the example of the effect of the excitatory transmitter **acetylcholine** on **nicotinic receptors**. This is an **ionotropic receptor** that represents a **non-selective cation channel** (**Fig. 2.15 a**). The associated increased **Na$^+$ influx** (and K$^+$ efflux) leads to a rapid EPSP.

The EPSPs triggered by a presynaptic neuron are often too small to depolarize the postsynaptic cell to the point necessary to initiate an action potential. If several EPSPs occur in a temporally coordinated manner, they can add up and lead to an action potential. The decision is usually made at a **trigger zone**, the **axon hillock**. Here, the density of voltage-dependent Na$^+$ channels is very high, so that the threshold for the generation of an action potential is lower than in the cell body or in the dendrites. Neurons may also have additional trigger zones within the dendritic tree to amplify a weak excitatory input at distant dendrites. Sub-threshold EPSPs propagate electrotonically to the trigger zone, and so their amplitude and duration are largely determined by the passive properties of the membrane.

> **IN A NUTSHELL**   !
>
> Neurons work as "addition machines": If the sum of all signals exceeds the threshold, the excitation is transmitted in the form of an action potential; if it remains below the threshold, no excitation transmission results.

■ Inhibitory postsynaptic potentials (IPSP)

Fast IPSPs are mostly based on the opening of ligand-gated **chloride channels**. According to the chemical gradient, this leads a Cl$^-$ influx and thus induces a hyperpolarization. Typical examples are the effects of the inhibitory transmitters **GABA** (mediated via ionotropic GABA$_A$ receptors) and **glycine** (Fig. 2.15). However, due to the somewhat higher intracellular Cl$^-$ concentration, GABA and glycine lead to an excitatory effect in some non-adult neurons of the CNS (as there is then a Cl$^-$ outflow when Cl$^-$ channels open).

> **MORE DETAILS**   The GABA$_A$-mediated inhibitions in the CNS are targets for **injection narcotics** such as barbiturates, the **sedative drugs** benzodiazepines and **inhalant narcotics** such as nitrous oxide, halothane, isoflurane or sevoflurane. The effects are based on the fact that the GABA- and glycine-induced Cl$^-$ influx is increased, so that the accompanying hyperpolarization of the cell prevents the triggering of an action potential.

In some nerve cells, inhibition can also be mediated by the opening of K$^+$ channels. This stabilises the membrane potential near the K$^+$ equilibrium potential (approx. −90 mV). For example, the metabotropic GABA$_B$ receptor activates a K$^+$ channel, followed by a K$^+$ efflux.

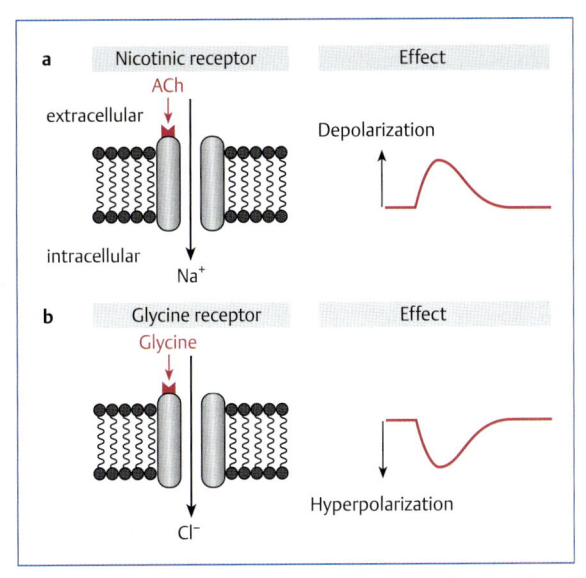

Fig. 2.15 Postsynaptic excitatory potentials (EPSP; **a**) are mediated via various ionotropic receptors, as shown here using nicotinic receptors as an example. For graphical reasons, only the influx of cations is shown, but not the K^+ movement (K^+ outflow), which also occurs through the non-selective cation channel formed by this ionotropic receptor. Postsynaptic inhibitory potentials (IPSP; **b**) are mediated via various ionotropic receptors, as shown here using glycine receptors as an example. Glycine receptors generate fast IPSP by opening ligand-gated Cl^- channels.

IN A NUTSHELL   !

After transmitter release, postsynaptic excitatory potentials (EPSP) or inhibitory potentials (IPSP) arise at the effector cell. Fast IPSP and EPSP are mediated by ionotropic receptors (ligand-gated ion channels). Long-lasting IPSP and EPSP are mediated by metabotropic receptors.

2.4.5   Integration of signals

Neurons usually receive different input signals and have to process them into a coordinated response. There are various possibilities for modulating signals at the post- and/or presynaptic level, whereby potentials can be amplified or inhibited. Some mechanisms of signal integration will be addressed in the following.

■ Principle of divergence and convergence

The stretching of a muscle can activate several hundred sensory neurons, each of which in turn contacts several hundred motoneurons. This principle of **neuronal divergence** enables a single neuron to exert a wide-ranging influence on subsequent neurons. Thus, at the input level, it is guaranteed that an input signal is distributed to several neurons. On the output level, on the other hand, there is often a connection that is referred to as **neuronal convergence**. This connection is characterised by the fact that, for example, several sensory nerve cells innervate a single motoneuron. In this way, the target cell receives the collected information of many presynaptic cells. It is often the case that the sensory information thereby comes from dif-

ferent regions or information from sensors that respond to different modalities is processed.

■ Presynaptic integration mechanisms

In addition to postsynaptic integration mechanisms, signals are also modulated at the presynaptic level. This serves to temporarily and selectively inhibit or amplify certain input signals.

Presynaptic inhibition and **amplification**: If receptors for inhibitory transmitters exist on the presynaptic membrane, this results in inhibition of transmitter release. If this is a predominantly excitatory synapse, the excitation of the postsynaptic cell is thereby suppressed. In contrast, presynaptic inhibition of a predominantly inhibitory synapse leads to reduced inhibition ("removal of the brake") of the postsynaptic cell (**Fig. 2.14**).

Presynaptic inhibitory or **excitatory modulation** may be due to the release of transmitter from one neuron being influenced by the transmitter from another nerve cell. Presynaptic inhibition or amplification can also take place through the transmitter released by the same neuron in the form of feedback modulation. This is a mechanism in all nervous systems whereby a transmitter can regulate its own release through autoinhibition, which is a protection against overexcitation. This occurs frequently in sympathetic nerves, for example, where noradrenaline inhibits its own release via presynaptic receptors.

Presynaptic inhibition is ultimately based on reduced Ca^{2+} influx or reduced Ca^{2+} sensitivity of the processes involved in transmitter release. Since intracellular Ca^{2+} is crucial for transmitter release, synaptic transmission no longer occurs without Ca^{2+} influx. Reduced Ca^{2+} influx can be caused either directly by preventing the opening of Ca^{2+} channels or indirectly through hyperpolarization of the synaptic membrane by increasing K^+ or Cl^- conductance, which results in reduced opening of the voltage-dependent Ca^{2+} channels.

MORE DETAILS   The pain-modulating effect of endogenous opioids is based, for example, on the presynaptic inhibition of the release of substance P, a transmitter that plays an important role in the conduction of excitation in the nociceptive system. Another example is the inhibitory effect of noradrenaline in the gastrointestinal tract, which is based, among other things, on a presynaptic inhibition of acetylcholine release.

A **presynaptic amplification** or activation on the other hand, is brought about by an increased Ca^{2+} influx. This can be achieved by directly increasing Ca^{2+} conductance or by closing K^+ channels. The latter would prolong the duration of the action potential and thus also the duration of depolarization, which leads to an increased Ca^{2+} influx.

IN A NUTSHELL   !

Presynaptic modulations inhibit or enhance synaptic transmission by reducing or increasing the intracellular Ca^{2+} concentration.

Cell, tissue

■ Postsynaptic integration mechanisms

Due to the high number of synaptic contacts, a nerve cell receives several input signals that can be inhibitory or excitatory. The signal produced at the trigger zone is a combination of all IPSP and EPSP (**Fig. 2.14**).

Spatial and **temporal summation: Spatial summation** of input signals becomes relevant whenever a neuron receives several input signals that occur sequentially or in parallel at several dendrites. Depending on the frequency, the sequential activation of only one synapse can cause **temporal summation** (depending on the frequency (**Fig. 2.14**). While temporal summation is based on the addition of input signals coming from one location, spatial summation involves the integration of input signals coming from different locations. The integration of the signals takes place in the soma or at the trigger zone. The passive membrane properties of the nerve cell are decisive for whether two signals combine or whether their duration is so short that they reach the trigger zone as separate EPSP.

The passive membrane properties, such as **time and longitudinal constant**, influence the propagation of synaptic potentials to the impulse-generating region, i.e. the trigger zone. This means that the **summation of synaptic potentials**, which is one of the mechanisms of neuronal integration of signals, depends essentially on the membrane properties. Neurons with a large **time constant** have longer-lasting excitatory potentials and possess a more pronounced capacity for summation than neurons with a smaller time constant. Therefore, the larger the time constant, the greater the probability that successive excitatory potentials will be additive and trigger an action potential. The time constant thus significantly influences the capacity for temporal summation. The same applies to the **longitudinal constant** of the cell. The greater the longitudinal constant, the smaller the amplitude drop of the excitatory potential on the way to the trigger zone will be. The probability that several input signals add up due to spatial summation thus increases.

To a certain extent, the time and length constants of a neuron can influence its ability to combine synaptic potentials. This changes the probability of fast EPSP adding to a slow EPSP and a concomitant increase in membrane resistance.

■ Posttetanic potentiation

Some neurons respond to high-frequency (tetanic) stimulation of the presynaptic terminal with a potentiation of their response. This potentiation is noticeable in an increased amplitude of the EPSP and persists for several minutes after the high-frequency stimulation has ended. This posttetanic potentiation is probably based on a strong increase in intracellular Ca^{2+} concentration. The resulting Ca^{2+} excess augments transmitter release and, as a consequence, the effectiveness of synaptic transmission. Thus, the information can be passed on to the postsynaptic cell via increased activation of the presynaptic cell. This process can be interpreted as a **cellular memory** since the nerve cell stores the information about the strong activation in the form of Ca^{2+} excess.

■ Long-term potentiation

A special form of postsynaptic reinforcement is long-term potentiation (**Fig. 2.16**), which is thought to play a crucial role in learning and memory. While posttetanic potentiation usually lasts only a few minutes, long-term potentiation is a process that can last several hours or days.

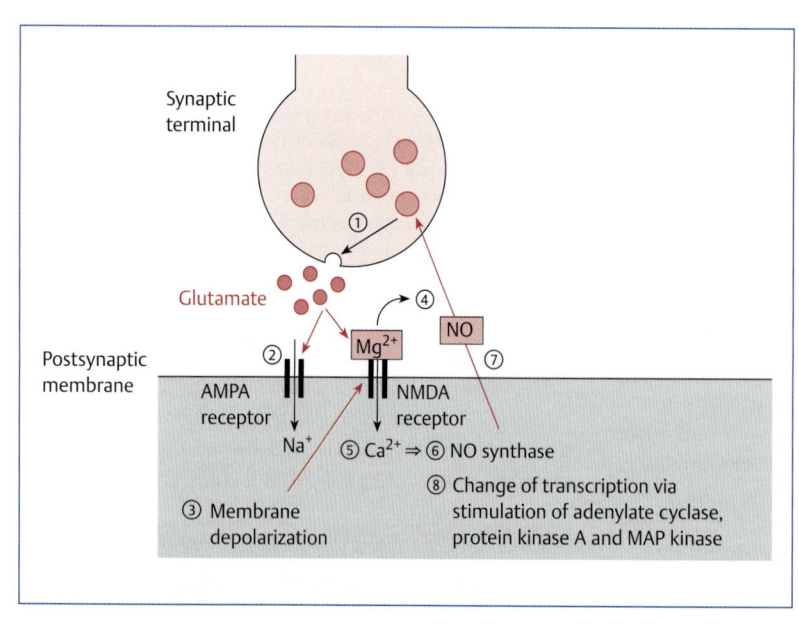

Fig. 2.16 Mechanism of long-term potentiation. Presynaptically released glutamate (1) binds under basal conditions mainly to AMPA receptors (2). The depolarization (3) triggered by the resulting Na⁺ influx leads to the detachment of inhibitory Mg²⁺ ions from NMDA receptors (4), so that glutamate can trigger an additional Ca²⁺ influx (5). This results in the stimulation of NO synthase (6). Nitric oxide diffuses into the synaptic terminal and promotes the further release of glutamate there (7). In addition, stimulation of adenylate cyclase, protein kinase A and a MAP kinase in the postsynaptic cell leads to changes in transcription and thus gene expression (8), which influence the excitability of the cell in the long term.
AMPA: α-amino-3-hydroxy-5-methyl-4-isoxazolepropionic acid
NMDA: N-methyl-D-aspartate
MAP kinase: mitogen-activated protein kinase.

Synaptic terminal

Glutamate

Postsynaptic membrane

AMPA receptor

Mg²⁺

NO

NMDA receptor

Na⁺   ⑤ Ca²⁺ ⇒ ⑥ NO synthase

⑧ Change of transcription via stimulation of adenylate cyclase, protein kinase A and MAP kinase

③ Membrane depolarization

The neurotransmitter glutamate is centrally involved in this process. There are several types of receptors for this transmitter, namely AMPA and NMDA receptors. Under basal conditions, glutamate binds mainly to AMPA receptors, which, as non-selective cation channels, allow mainly Na^+ to flow into the cell. The resulting depolarization leads to the detachment of extracellularly bound Mg^{2+} ions from NMDA receptors, which normally block these receptors. As a result, prolonged release of glutamate triggers a Ca^{2+} influx via NMDA receptors that function as ligand-gated Ca^{2+} channels. The influx of Ca^{2+} stimulates an NO synthase that converts arginine into the neurotransmitter NO. As a small gaseous molecule, NO can leave the postsynaptic cell and reaches the presynaptic axon terminal by diffusion. There, this gaso-transmitter stimulates the further release of glutamate, resulting in a long-term increase in synaptic transmission at the affected synapse.

In addition, stimulation of adenylate cyclase/protein kinase A and a MAP kinase in the postsynaptic cell leads to changes in transcription and thus gene expression, which influence the excitability of the cell in the long term.

Excessive glutamate concentrations and the associated activation of glutamate receptors have a neurotoxic effect. A dramatic increase in the intracellular Ca^{2+} concentration and the associated disruption of ion homeostasis are followed by necrosis and apoptosis. Substances that act as Ca^{2+} buffers can protect neurons from glutamate-induced excitotoxicity.

2.5 Reflexes

A reflex describes an event in which a defined stimulus causes an involuntary, neurally triggered reaction. Each reflex involves a sensor and an effector that are connected by neural pathways to form a reflex arc. Reflexes are classified according to the location of the sensor and effector in

the organism as well as the number of synapses interposed in the reflex arc. In most cases, the reflex arc is built up by several neurons, namely by an afferent (sensory) neuron coming from the sensor and an efferent neuron projecting towards the effector. Since there is only one synaptic connection in such a reflex arc, it is called a **monosynaptic reflex**, such as the patellar tendon reflex (see below). If one or more interneurons are connected between afferent and efferent, it is a **polysynaptic reflex**. If the receptor and effector are located in the same organ, they are intrinsic (mono-organ) reflexes; if they are spatially separated, i.e. the sensor and effector are located in different organs, they are called extrinsic (multi-organ) reflexes. In the language of learning theorists, a distinction is made between innate, **unconditioned reflexes** (e.g. the cough reflex) and learned, **conditioned reflexes** (e.g. "Pavlov's dog (p. 360)").

Testing reflexes is an important part of the neurological examination of an animal. For example, the patellar tendon reflex (cf. **Table 2.4**) is triggered by a blow to the patellar tendon, which pulls the kneecap (patella) slightly downwards and thereby stretches the quadriceps femoris muscle (quadriceps). The muscle spindles in the quadriceps (**Fig. 6.10**), which are also stretched by this manoeuvre, lead to the excitation of sensory cells. The excitation is conducted to the spinal cord and there passed on to motor nerve fibres, which in turn have contact with the muscle fibres of the quadriceps. The result is a contraction of the quadriceps, which manifests itself in a kicking movement of the lower leg. This reflex only works correctly if all the anatomical structures involved in the reflex arc are intact. Failures of reflexes thus allow the localisation of damage to the central or peripheral nervous system through simple clinical examinations. Other reflexes that are important for neurological-physiological examination, e.g. in dogs, are listed in **Table 2.4**.

Table 2.4 Important reflexes that are tested in certain neurological disorders or diseases as part of the examination procedure (example dog). The reflex centres, i.e. the totality of synapses and ganglion cells involved in the reflex arcs, are usually located in the developmentally older parts of the CNS, namely the medulla oblongata and the spinal cord. Reflex testing functionally examines the integrity of the structures involved in the respective reflex arc and is an important method (together with imaging techniques and others) to detect and localise lesions, especially in the spinal cord.

Reflexes	Survey of findings	Nerves involved	Involved structures in the CNS using the example of the dog
Triceps reflex (forelimb)	A reflex hammer is used to strike the tendon of the muscle above the olecranon, causing the elbow to extend.	Radial nerve	Spinal cord segments C6 – Th1
M. extensor carpi radialis reflex (forelimb)	A reflex hammer is used to strike the tendon of the muscle below the elbow, resulting in an extension of the carpus.	Radial nerve	Spinal cord segments C7 – Th1/2
Panniculus reflex	Pinching or touching the skin of the back with a pointed object causes the cutaneous trunci muscle to twitch.	Lateral thoracic nerve	Spinal cord segments C8 – Th1
Patellar tendon reflex (hindlimb)	A reflex hammer is used to strike the medial patellar ligament, resulting in extension of the knee.	Femoral nerve	Spinal cord segments L4 – L6

Table 2.4   continued

Reflexes	Survey of findings	Nerves involved	Involved structures in the CNS using the example of the dog
Tibialis reflex (hindlimb)	A reflex hammer is used to tap the anterior dorsolateral tibialis muscle in the upper third of the lower leg, resulting in flexion of the ankle joint.	Peroneal nerve	Spinal cord segments L6–S2
Flexor reflex (forelimb and hindlimb)	Pinching the toes or the interdigital space triggers a pulling away (flexion) of the corresponding limb.	Nerves involved in the forelimb: musculocutaneous nerve, axillary nerve, median nerve, radial nerve, ulnar nerve; in the hindlimb: sciatic nerve.	Spinal cord segments C6–Th1/2 for the forelimb, L4 – S2/3 for the hindlimb.
Palpebral reflex	Touching the lid margin triggers lid closure.	Afferent: ophthalmic nerve (branch of the trigeminal nerve). Efferent: facial nerve	Trigeminal nucleus areas, facialis nucleus (brainstem)
Eyelid closure reflex	Air blast or light touch to the cornea triggers eyelid closure by contraction of the orbicularis oculi muscle.	Afferent: ophthalmic nerve (branch of the trigeminal nerve). Efferent: facial nerve	Trigeminal nucleus areas, facialis nucleus (brainstem)
Pupillary reflex	Exposure of an eye triggers a miosis in the exposed eye and, depending on the species, also in the unexposed eye through contraction of the sphincter pupillae muscle (consensual light reaction).	Afferent: optic nerve. Efferent: ophthalmic nerve	Tr. opticus, colliculi craniales, ncl. parasympathicus n. oculomotorii
Swallowing reflex	Swallowing when touching the back of the throat.	Afferents: glossopharyngeal nerve, vagus nerve. Efferents: trigeminal nerve, glossopharyngeal nerve, vagus nerve, hypoglossal nerve.	"Swallowing centre" in the medulla oblongata
Anal reflex	Touching the perianal region with a clamp causes constriction of the sphincter ani and/or pinching down of the tail.	Afferents: superficial perineal nerve Efferents: caudal rectal nerve	S3 – S5

Suggested reading

Bean BP. The action potential in mammalian central neurons. Nature Rev Neurosci 2007; 8: 451–465

Catterall WA, Goldin AL, Waxman SG. International Union of Pharmacology. XLVII. Nomenclature and structure-function relationships of voltage-gated sodium channels. Pharmacol Rev 2005; 57: 397–409

Kandel ER, Schwartz JH, Jessel TM, Siegelbaum SA, Hudspeht AJ. Principles of neural science. 5th Edition. New York: McGraw-Hill Professional Publishing; 2012

3 Sensory physiology

Heinz Breer, Cornelia A. Deeg, Michael Pees, Helga Pfannkuche, Holger Sann

3.1 General sensory physiology

Heinz Breer

3.1.1 General principles of sensory physiology

■ Introduction

> **ESSENTIALS**   ✗
>
> The behaviour of animals is significantly influenced by diverse and complex information from the environment and from within the body. Accordingly, animals have distinct abilities to grasp and process information about relevant aspects of their environment and about their own status.

Reception and perception

Various physicochemical parameters (but by no means all) such as light, chemical substances or electrical fields are registered as specific stimuli (reception) by highly specialised sensors – the sensory cells (also called receptors) – and converted into electrical signals (action potentials) (**Fig. 3.1**).

In this way, the very different types of stimuli (stimulus modalities) are transferred into the uniform code language of the nervous system. Information about the actual type of stimulus is lost in this process, so it is no longer possible to tell from the electrical signal patterns whether they were triggered by physical stimuli (such as light) or chemical stimuli (such as scents). The stimulus is encoded by the neuronal "wiring" of the sensory cells with the relevant centres in the brain. Each sensory nerve always conveys "its" sensory modality, regardless of how an activation was triggered. For example, light perceptions occur even when mechanical pressure is applied to the eye, i.e. the neuronal signals contain no information about the nature of the stimulus. This direct connection between the activated sensory organ and the sensory modality (i.e. the complex sensations such as "smell", "taste", "vision" etc.) means that the afferent sensory nerves transmit the stimulus, so there is a direct connection from the sensory cells to the integration centre. This is nowadays referred to as "labelled line-coding". In the responsible areas in the central nervous system (p. 135), the subjective sensory impressions are generated by the interactions of the acute sensory information with the nervous system on the basis of the experiences of the individual. These sensations are then **perceived** as acquired experiences. The various sensory inputs not only indicate that a sensory organ has been activated, but they also pass on information about the characteristics of the stimulus. This information is called the sensory **qualities**. Such qualities for the sense of sight are, for example, the colour and brightness of the stimulus, or, for audible stimuli, the pitch and volume of the sound, and for smell, the type and strength of an odour.

Perceptions are always experiential, and represent a function of the brain, although it is uncertain which mechanisms are involved in the shaping of a subjective experience. However, it is clear that all the information contributing to an animal's "knowledge" is acquired from sensory input. These connections were already recognised by the Greek philosophers and expressed in the phrase "knowledge reaches man through the gate of the senses".

■ Sensors

Sensory organs are located on many regions of the surface and interior of the body. They function to detect and measure important physical or chemical stimuli and thus provide a continuous flow of information from the environment to the nervous system. Sensory organs usually consist of groups of sensory cells, often in association with other structures such as the lens in the eye or the auditory ossicles. They all perform the same basic operations of recoding the stimulus information into the language of the nervous system as electrical signals, representing the intensity and duration of the stimulus.

Various sensory cells are classified in different ways. Those monitoring the outside world are called exteroceptors and those registering processes and conditions inside the body are called interoceptors. Physiologically, the most important classification is determined by the type of stimulus. **Chemosensors** are those that detect taste and smell, but they are also responsible for registering components of the internal environment such as oxygen saturation and pH. **Mechanosensors** register pressure and movement stimuli, and are also the basis of the senses of hearing and balance. **Photosensors** register light and are the functional elements of vision. **Thermal sensors** detect the temperature of the body or of the environment. **Electrosensors** and **magnetic sensors** detect electric or magnetic fields.

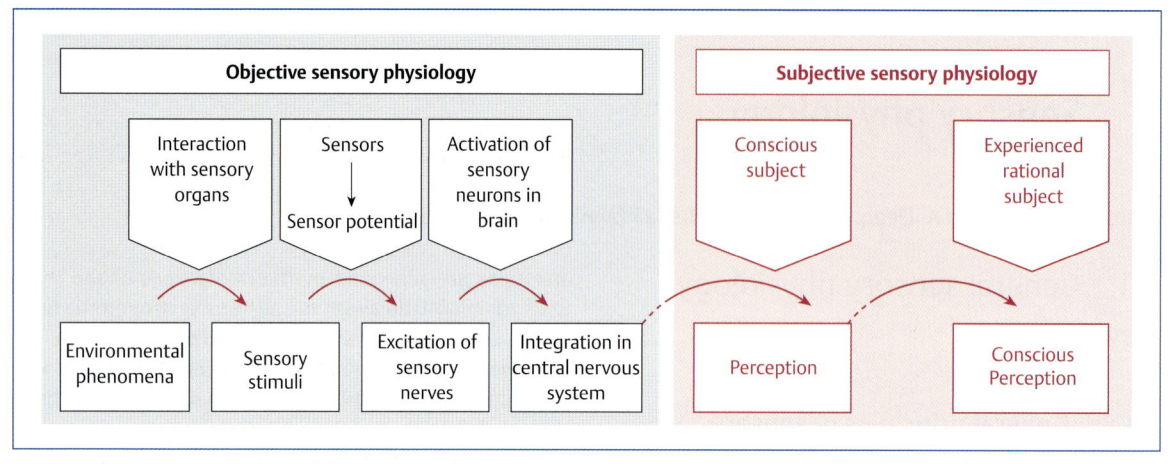

Fig. 3.1 Schematic representation of the mapping of environmental phenomena in the peripheral and central nervous system through basic sensory physiological processes. Environmental phenomena act through interaction with sensory organs as sensory stimuli (arrows), which in turn induce excitation in sensory nerves.

Sensory cells are usually extraordinarily sensitive to a very specific form of stimulus (**adequate stimulus**). In a visual cell, for example, even a single photon (energy of $3 \cdot 10^{-19}$ J) can cause a measurable electrical reaction that corresponds to an electrical potential energy of $5 \cdot 10^{-14}$ J, i.e. more than 10^5 times the energy content of the triggering photon. However, this reaction would not lead to perception. A glimmer of light needs about ten photons in order to be perceived.

The spatial area in which a stimulus can influence the electrical activity of a sensory cell is called the **receptive field** of the cell. The size of that area is determined by the peripheral branches of the afferent cell processes. The area of a single sensory cell is also called the **primary receptive field** because several sensory cells can converge on a central projection neuron so that this neuron represents the sum of many primary receptive fields. This is then called a **secondary receptive field**. The more afferent fibres that converge on a neuron, the lower is the spatial resolution.

IN A NUTSHELL   **!**

Specialisation of sensors optimises the reception of stimuli and diminishes the variety of information that is perceived.

■ Transduction and transformation

When there is a stimulus of sufficient strength to cause a change in membrane potential, this is called a **receptor potential** (generator potential) in the relevant sensory cell. This conversion of a stimulus into a change in membrane potential, by opening or closing ion channels, is called **transduction**. In some systems, this signal conversion occurs by direct action of the stimulus on the ion channels, such as in mechanosensors, but usually the signal conver-

sion is mediated through receptor-coupled transduction cascades which may be accompanied by enormous signal amplification. The amplitude of the change in membrane potential – the receptor potential – is proportional to the intensity of the stimulus. In general, it persists, albeit often in an attenuated form, as long as the stimulus continues. The receptor potential thus reflects the intensity and duration of a stimulus (**Fig. 3.2**).

The receptor potential consists of a change in the potential in a defined area, the sensory area, of the plasma membrane. It spreads electrotonically (p. 46) from its point of origin. This is accompanied by a decrease in its amplitude (decrement). For transmission to the CNS, the sensory information is converted into a sequence of action potentials (p. 48). This **transformation** into electrical impulses takes place in the spike-generating zone, which is spatially separated from the site of origin of the receptor potential (sensory zone). Stimulus conversion thus takes place in two successive steps: transduction, which is formation of a receptor potential, and transformation which is the generation and conduction of action potentials (**Table 3.1**).

This functional principle, that the sensory cell directly generates action potentials and transmits them via its axon to the CNS, applies to the "primary sensory cells". In contrast, "secondary" sensory cells generate a receptor potential that triggers the transformation into electrical impulses in the afferent nerve fibres by the release of neurotransmitters.

In all cases, the number of impulses per unit of time, i.e. the frequency of action potentials, is used to encode the stimulus intensity (**frequency modulation**). This applies to all sensory modalities in the same or similar way.

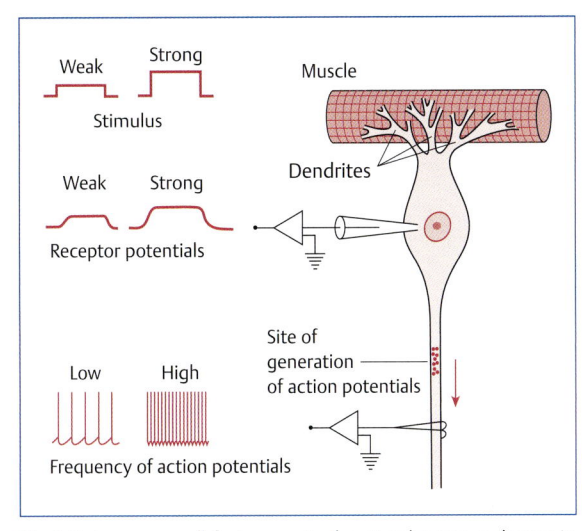

Fig. 3.2 A sensory cell first converts the stimulus into a change in membrane potential (transduction). The strength of the stimulus is reflected in the amplitude of the voltage change. For transmission to the CNS, the information is then translated into a defined frequency of action potentials (transformation). [Source: Eckert R. Tierphysiologie. 2nd ed., Stuttgart: Thieme, 1993]

Table 3.1 Sensory signal transduction.

Processes	Functional elements
Perireceptor processes ↓	Lens, ossicles, binding proteins, enzymes
Signal detection ↓	Sensors (receptors)
Signal conversion ↓	Receptor potential (generator potential)
Signal transformation ↓	Action potential
Information coding	"Wiring pattern" Pulse frequency

> **IN A NUTSHELL** ❗
>
> Amplitude frequency modulation at the beginning of the nerve fibre converts the local receptor potential into a sequence of action potentials.

■ Intensity coding

Many sensory cells are particularly sensitive. For example, some photosensors respond to a single photon and some olfactory sensory cells can detect single odour molecules. In general, sensory cells can only encode stimuli over a relatively limited intensity range, the so-called **dynamic range**. Within this intensity range, the cells respond to an increasing stimulus intensity, by increased frequency of action potential. An intensity that triggers suprathreshold excitation in 50% of all cases is called the stimulus threshold. At the upper end of the dynamic range, the sensory cell's electrical signal reaches a peak value which cannot be further increased even if the signal intensity continues to rise.

The working range and the sensitivity of the sensory cells are defined by **characteristic curves** which indicate the input-output relationships. The biophysical properties of the sensory cells mean that their electrical response increases linearly with the logarithm of the stimulus intensity. This logarithmic coding of stimuli is functionally very important. Sensory cells with a **logarithmic characteristic curve** have a very high sensitivity at low intensities and they have a very wide working range (**Fig. 3.3**). However, their ability to discriminate decreases with increasing stimulus intensity. The logarithmic input-output relationship can be seen as a compromise between high sensitivity and a wide dynamic range. The advantage of a logarithmic characteristic curve is mainly to enable a wide operating range. For example, this makes it possible for the eye to cover an intensity range of 10^9 for white light and for the human auditory system to register sounds that cover an intensity range of 10^{12}. Logarithmic characteristic curves are characteristic of exteroceptors. On the other hand, sensory cells with **linear characteristics** show a constant sensitivity to different stimulus intensities. Thus, their ability to distinguish remains the same even with increasing stimulus intensity. However, these cells only have a very narrow operating range. This makes such sensors suitable for monitoring internal stimuli, which often only fluctuate over a narrow range. Linear characteristic curves are a feature of interoceptors. Sensory cells with an **extreme value characteristic curve** show a maximum response at a particular stimulus intensity; and the response is less for both higher and lower intensity stimuli so that these cells have only a narrow working range. Extreme value characteristic curves are a feature of thermosensors.

> **IN A NUTSHELL** ❗
>
> The stimulus intensity range in which a sensory cell can perform intensity encoding with increasing energy, is called its dynamic range.

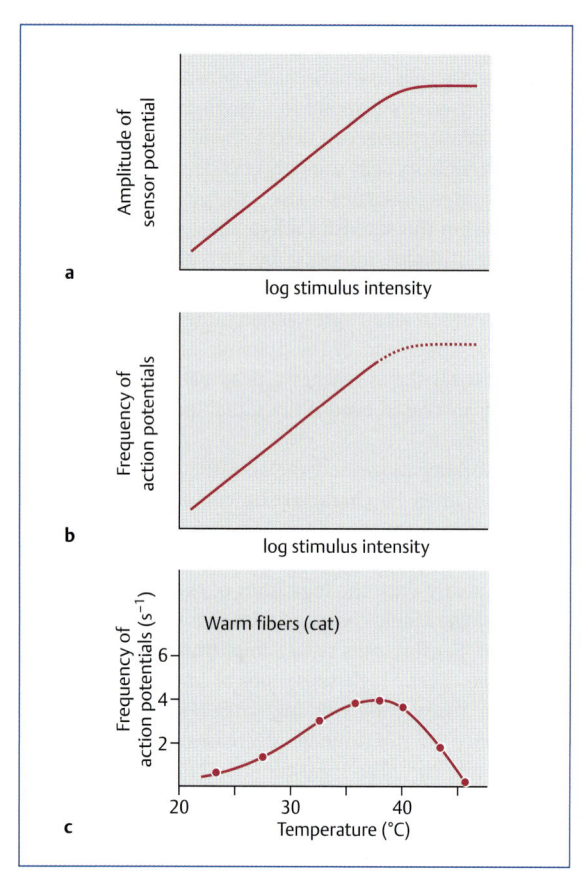

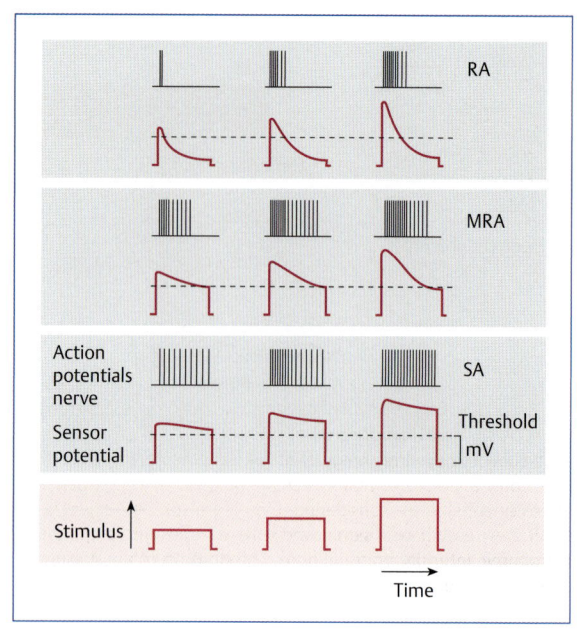

Fig. 3.4 Schematic representation of receptor potentials and action potentials of tonic and phasic receptors in response to different stimulus amplitudes. The adaptive behaviour of the action potential frequency is determined by the different rates of decrease of the receptor potential.

RA is a rapidly adapting receptor, which works as a phasic sensor; MRA is a moderate rapidly adapting receptor (phasic-tonic sensor); SA is a slowly adapting receptor (tonic sensor).

Fig. 3.3 Characteristic curves of various sensory cells. **a, b** In most sensory systems, the response is proportional to the logarithm of the stimulus intensity. There is a linear relationship over a defined range both between the amplitude of the receptor potential and the logarithm of the stimulus intensity (**a**) and between the action potential frequency and the logarithm of the stimulus intensity. **c** Thermal sensors (example cat) show an extreme value characteristic curve; based on data from Eckert R. Tierphysiologie. 2nd ed., Stuttgart: Thieme, 1993: 203 and Penzlin H, Lehrbuch der Tierphysiologie. 7th ed., Munich: Spektrum; 2005: 667

■ Adaptation

When stimuli are applied for a longer period of time, a decrease in the intensity of sensation is often observed. For example, persistent odours cease being detected after a short time of exposure. This also applies to mechanical stimuli, such as perception of the feel of clothing on our bodies. Such changes in sensation, with a constant stimulus intensity, are called sensory adaptations. These adaptations can occur at different rates and to different extents. They seem to be a feature of most senses, with the exception of pain. The causes of such adaptation can vary widely. The underlying process of adaptation can take place both in the sensory cells themselves, and also in accessory structures, as well as in the central nervous system.

Sensory cells differ in their capacity for adaptation. The tonic receptors adapt slowly and generate a relatively constant frequency of action potentials (**Fig. 3.4**). In this way, the duration of the stimulus is directly encoded. In contrast to this, the phasic receptors adapt very quickly. Action potentials are only triggered during part of the time that the stimulus lasts, possibly only at its beginning and end. The adaptation of a sensory cell can occur at different stages, ranging from the accessory structures to the transduction machinery to the generation of action potentials in the excitable membrane. Regardless of its site or its mechanism, adaptation plays an important role in expanding the dynamic range of a sensory receptor. Together with the logarithmic nature of the primary transduction process, sensory adaptation allows an animal to register changes in stimulus energy against a background noise that varies by several orders of magnitude. Occasionally, the CNS influences the reactivity of sensory organs. This efferent control allows the CNS to increase or decrease the sensitivity of the sensors depending on the situation.

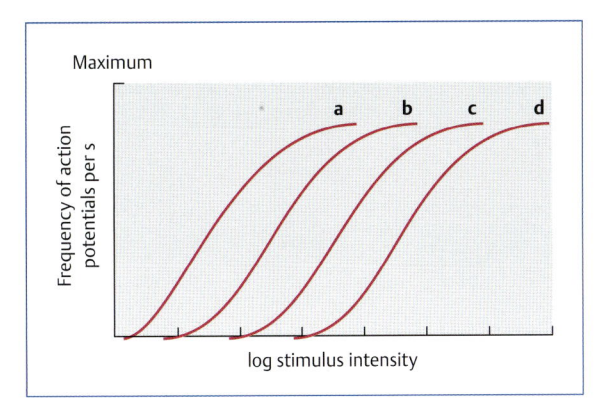

Fig. 3.5 Expanding the dynamic range of a sensory system through the recruitment of sensory cell populations. The curves labelled a–d each show the dynamic range of individual sensory afferents. They cover only a limited stimulus intensity range (3–4 logarithmic intensity units) when considering a single sensor cell. However, collectively they have a significantly greater dynamic range (seven logarithmic intensity units). [Source: Eckert R. Tierphysiologie. 2nd ed., Stuttgart: Thieme; 1993: 204]

■ Recruitment of sensory cell populations

The dynamic range of a whole sensory system is often much greater than that of a single sensory cell. This happens because individual sensory cells react with various sensitivity. In this way, as the stimulus intensity increases, those cells that are less sensitive can be recruited. The principle of recruiting sensory cell populations of different sensitivities allows for a particular stimulus to detect its intensity over a much wider range than would be possible for an individual sensory cell (**Fig. 3.5**). For example, in the two large populations of photoreceptors in the retina (p. 93), the rods are very sensitive and respond to dim light, whereas the cones respond to bright light of increasing intensity, above the maximum sensitivity range of the rods.

Suggested reading

Anson L, ed. Molecular sensing. Nature Insight 2001; 413: 185–230

Basbaum AI et al, eds. The senses: A comprehensive reference. Vol. I-VI. San Diego: Academic Press; 2008

3.2 Cutaneous senses

Helga Pfannkuche

ESSENTIALS ✖

The total body surface of domestic mammals is covered by both hairy and hairless skin. Various sensors that serve to detect the environment are integrated into the skin. The skin can thus be described as an animal's largest sensory organ. Most of the sensors found in the skin respond to specific stimuli except for the polymodal nociceptors. The skin sensors can be divided into several groups according to the types of stimuli to which they respond. Mechanosensors respond to non-noxious mechanical stimuli. Thermosensors respond to non-noxious thermal stimuli, while nociceptors and sensors for detecting itchiness respond to noxious stimuli. These sensors are either free nerve endings of pseudo-unipolar neurons in the dorsal root ganglia or they transfer their sensory potential to those nerve endings. The information obtained is then transmitted from the dorsal root ganglia via the spinal cord to the thalamus. From there, the signal is projected into both the cortex and the limbic system.

The skin sensors can collectively perceive a variety of different stimuli. The detection of these stimuli creates a direct awareness of the environment. This allows **defence against noxious agents**, and also to **forage for food** and for **social interactions**. Although most sensors are found over the whole surface of the body, their density differs markedly in different regions of the skin. A particularly high density of sensors is generally found in the facial area and particularly in those regions for **tactile detection** of the environment such as the lips, the proboscis disc of pigs, the nose of carnivores or the nasolabial plane of cattle. The **receptive fields** of the sensors in these areas are correspondingly small. A relatively low density of sensors (p. 67), with corresponding large **receptive fields**, is found in the skin over the general body trunk.

3.2.1 Mechanoreception in the skin

The reception of non-noxious mechanical stimuli occurs via sensors in both hairy and hairless skin (**Fig. 3.6**).

■ Sensors in the hairless skin

Mechanosensors of the hairless skin are Merkel cells, Ruffini corpuscles, Meissner corpuscles and Vater-Pacini lamellar corpuscles.

Merkel cells are localised in the basal epidermis. Mechanosensitive non-selective cation channels are located in their cell membrane. When the skin is mechanically deformed, these channels open and the Merkel cell depolarizes. The associated afferent nerve fibre is informed of the depolarization by the release of glutamate from the Merkel cell. An action potential then only occurs at the afferent nerve fibre. Merkel cells essentially perceive **vertical pressure on hairless skin**. They are important for the detailed perception of shapes and surface structures. Their recep-

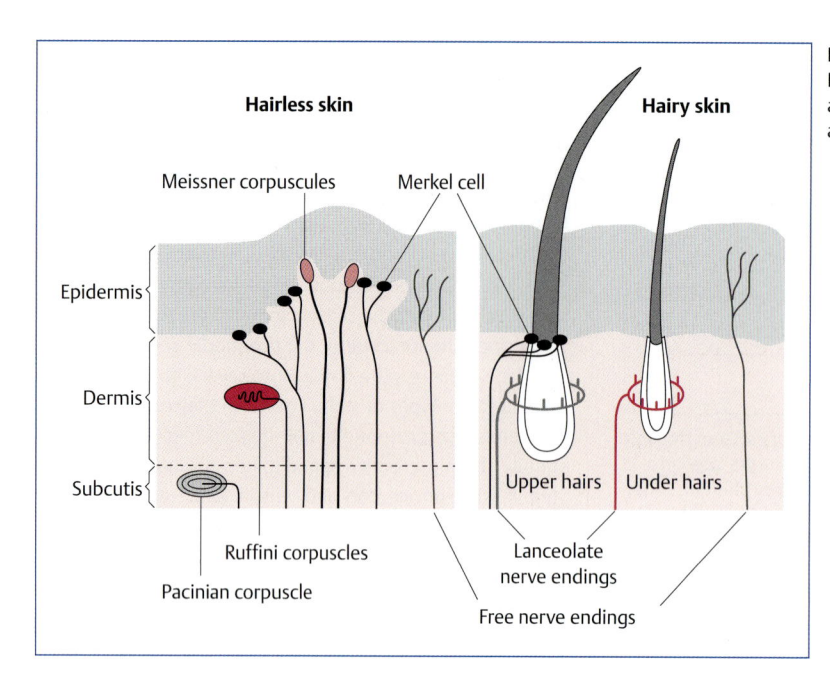

Fig. 3.6 Sensors of hairless and hairy skin. Both hairy and hairless skin contain slow and fast adapting mechanosensors as well as free nerve endings.

tive fields are small. Merkel cells are found, for example, in the paw pads of dogs and cats or in the pig proboscis. They belong to the slow adapting (SA) type of sensors, which have both a tonic and a phasic response behaviour (p. 70).

Ruffini corpuscles are localised in the dermis. They are fluid-filled capsular structures that contain the bulging ends of nerve fibres. They too, like Merkel cells, are SA sensors. However, unlike Merkel cells, they have large receptive fields. This is because they respond to **lateral tensile stress in the skin** which affects a wider skin area than a vertical pressure deformation. Dermal Ruffini corpuscles are also involved in proprioception, as the skin tenses in the corresponding areas when joints move. In addition to their localisation in the dermis, Ruffini corpuscles are also found in joint capsules and in the peridontium where they perceive tooth position and biting force.

Meissner corpuscles and **Vater-Pacini lamellar corpuscles** are rapidly adapting (RA) mechanosensors (p. 70) in hairless skin. Meissner corpuscles are located in the dermis, with very small receptive fields like those of Merkel cells. The function of Meissner's corpuscles is to register the movement of an object on the surface of the skin. They are involved in the regulation of **grip strength** and **grip control**. Vater-Pacini lamellar corpuscles are localised in the subcutis. Because of their deep location and their high sensitivity, they have very large receptive fields. Vater-Pacini lamellar corpuscles are also found in the hoof and claw corium, in the paw pads of carnivores or in the mouth of cattle.

Both types of RA sensors detect **vibrational stimuli**, but of different frequencies. Meissner corpuscles tend to cover low frequency ranges (highest sensitivity at approx. 30 Hz). Vater-Pacini lamellar corpuscles react most sensitively in high frequency ranges (highest sensitivity at approx. 250 Hz).

The rapid adaptation to mechanical stimuli in both these sensors is because of their special morphology. In both, the nerve endings are enclosed in multi-layered fluid-filled capsules. When there are mechanical stimuli, these lamellar sheaths intercept the static forces which act on the nerve endings in the middle, so that only accelerations at the beginning and end of the stimulus are mechanically transmitted to the fibre. The filter function is stronger in Vater-Pacini lamellar corpuscles than in Meissner corpuscles, so the former can adapt more rapidly than the latter. In their adaptation behaviour, the sheathed nerve endings therefore only follow the mechanical characteristics of their sheath. Without this lamellar sheath, the nerve fibre itself would show slow adaptation behaviour (p. 70).

> **IN A NUTSHELL**   !
>
> In hairless skin, there are slow adapting and fast adapting mechanosensors responsible for sensing surface structures, proprioception and grip control.

■ Sensors in the hairy skin

In mammals, the body is covered by areas of hairy skin. The hairs not only serve as protection against mechanical irritation and in thermoregulation, but they are also able to detect mechanical stimuli on the body surface according to the three types of hair: overhair (guard hair), down hair (underhair) and sinus hair.

Overhairs and down hairs are distributed over large parts of the body surface. These hairs have mechanosensitive abilities through their root innervation. **Slow** and **fast adapting sensors** are also found here, as in hairless skin. The slow-adapting sensors are complexes of Merkel cells that surround the hair root at its upper end in the transition between epidermis and dermis. **Merkel cell complexes** are mainly found around the overhair and not around the down hair.

Rapidly adapting mechanosensors are arranged in the form of **lanceolate nerve endings** around the basal root sheath of the overhairs and down hairs.

The lanceolate nerve endings can be further divided into two groups based on their receptive behaviour. One group of terminals is excited only by rapid movements of the guard hairs. The second group of lanceolate terminals is activated by movement of all hairs, but especially by those of the underhairs. These terminals respond especially to slow movement of the hairs. They have a very low threshold (p.69) and are the most sensitive mechanosensors of the skin.

According to their sensitivity and adaptation behaviour, the sensors of the hairy skin also serve to receive different stimuli. Pressure on the hairy skin leads mainly to the excitation of Merkel cell complexes. Stroking the coat most strongly excites the lanceolate terminals associated with the outer hairs, while a slight movement of the surrounding air essentially causes the sensitive lanceolate terminals on the root sheaths of the underhairs to respond (**Fig. 3.7**).

A specialised form of hairs for mechanoreception are the **sinus hairs** (vibrissae). Sinus hairs are long and stiff tactile hairs, located in places that are important for detecting orientation. In domestic mammals, this is often on the craniofacial region. Here the sinus hairs can, for example, be arranged in the form of **whiskers** and serve to investigate food, since domestic mammals do not grasp their food with hands but instead use their lips. The name sinus hair is due to the fact that the root sheath of these hairs is surrounded by **blood sinuses**, which fix the hair in its position like a water cushion. A dampening function is also discussed for these blood sinuses, which is supposed to prevent a sensory overload by only marginal mechanical stimulation of the hair. The root sheath of sinus hairs is surrounded by a wide variety of sensors, including **Merkel cell complexes**, **lanceolate terminals** and **vibration sensors**. Thus, sinus hairs are able to pick up all mechanical stimuli. **Rhythmic movements** of the sinus hairs can be seen especially in rodents where these vibrating movements optimise the tactile sensing of the environment.

MORE DETAILS Water-dwelling mammals, for example seals and sea otters, have very strong, long sinus hairs. By this means, they can detect the direction and speed of currents in water. This enables the animals to prey on fish even in murky water, as the sinus hairs detect the turbulence in the water created by passing fish.

> **IN A NUTSHELL** !
>
> In hairy skin, the mechanosensors are located near hair follicles. Overhairs, underhairs and sinus hairs have different innervation patterns that are responsible for perceiving the varying intensity of pressure and touch.

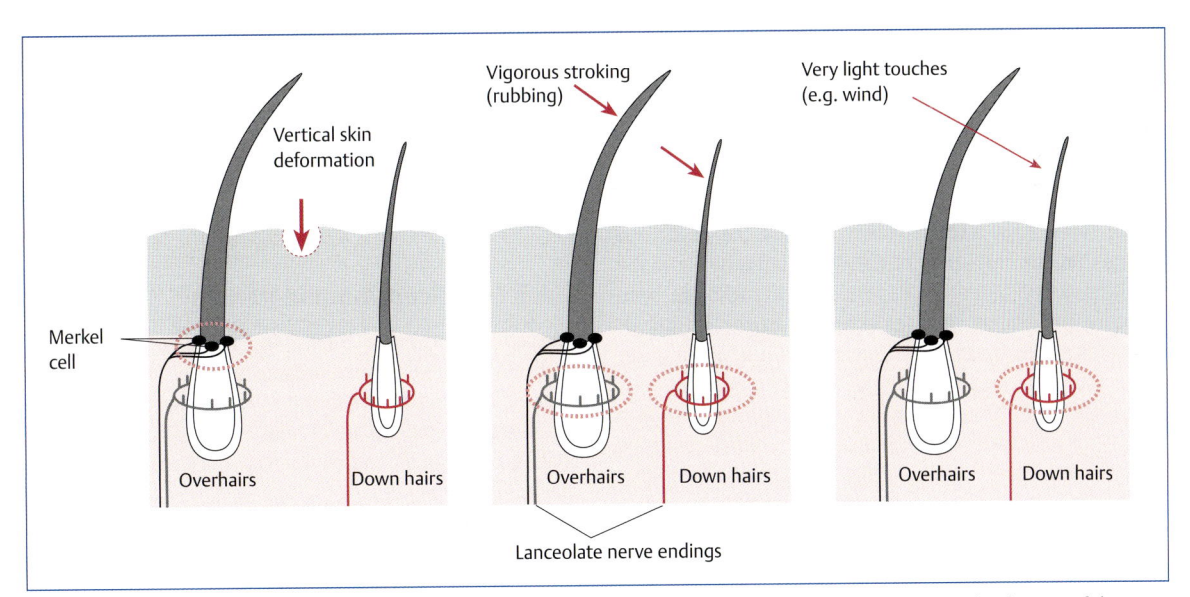

Fig. 3.7 Mechanoreception in hairy skin. In vertical skin deformation, Merkel cell complexes are mainly those excited in the area of the outer hairs. Vigorous stroking (rubbing) of the coat activates lanceolate-shaped terminals on all hair types. Very light touches are mainly received by the lanceolate-shaped terminals around the under hairs.

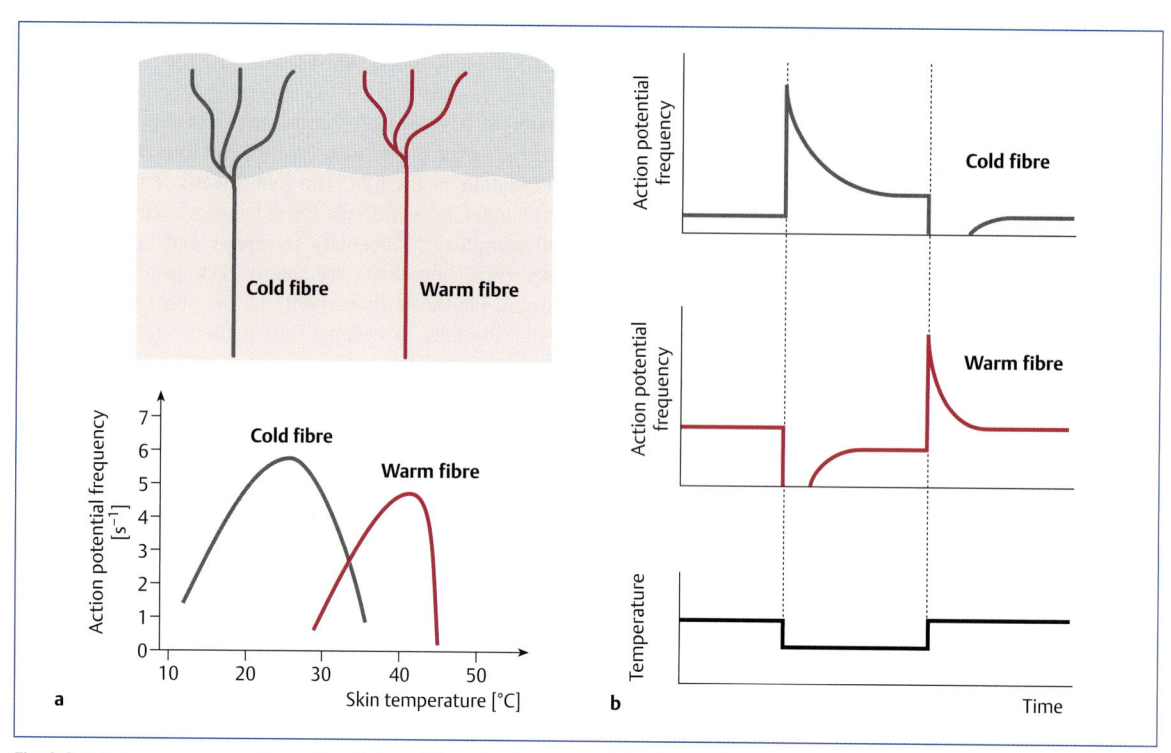

Fig. 3.8 a Temperature reception at the skin is an interaction between cold and warm fibres, which have their reception maxima in different temperature ranges.
b Cold and warm fibres react with a tonic-phasic response to temperature changes. [Source: (a) Alzheimer C, Somatovisceral Sensitivity. In: Speckmann EJ, Hescheler J, Köhling R (eds). Physiologie. 6th ed, Munich: Urban 2013: 64 and (b) Hensel H. Cutaneous Thermoreceptors. In: Iggo A (ed.). Handbook of Sensory Physiology, Vol. 2, Berlin: Springer; 1973: 79-110]

3.2.2 Thermoreception in the skin

Thermal sensors in skin are free nerve endings that respond to non-noxious thermal stimuli. They are classified as either warm fibres or cold fibres (p.506) according to the temperature at which they are maximally excited. Both sensor types show a **tonic-phasic response** (Fig. 3.8). This means that the amplitude of their depolarization and the resulting action potentials depends on the **absolute temperature** and also on **changes in temperature**. The following example illustrates this connection: If lukewarm water meets (sun-)warmed skin, the water is perceived as cold. This is because the temperature shift downwards (warm skin/"only lukewarm" water) causes the cold fibres to be excited overproportionally, while the warm fibres only generate action potentials underproportionally. If the temperature then remains the same, the action potential frequency of the cold fibres decreases again and that of the warm fibres increases, so that the "realistic" temperature of the water is then felt. This example shows that the temperature sensation on the skin depends on the response of both sensor types. The measuring ranges and maximum action potential frequencies of warm and cold fibres are shown in **Fig. 3.8**. An "overshooting" response of the thermosensors during temperature jumps also plays a role in thermoregulation during **hibernation**. The phasic response behaviour of certain thermosensors ensures that sudden increases or decreases in the external temperature which might occur during the sleep phase, are detected.

> **IN A NUTSHELL** !
>
> Thermosensors are free nerve endings in the skin that detect the temperature on the surface of the skin and, particularly, changes in temperature.

3.2.3 Nociception and itching

Nociceptors in the skin are also free nerve endings that can receive a wide variety of noxious stimuli. Of all the skin sensors, nociceptors are found in the highest density. The reception and processing of stimuli by nociceptors is described in detail in the chapter on nociception and pain (p.76).

Nociceptors not only register nociceptive stimuli but they also detect itch-inducing stimuli. The perception of pain, and of itchiness is a **protective function** which triggers appropriate reactions, such as scratching. There are no fibres that exclusively trigger a perception of itch. This sensation can be evoked by a variety of stimuli. A typical stimulus that causes itching is a release of **histamine**.

Nerve endings that perceive itch-triggering stimuli belong to the so-called **polymodal fibres**, which can be excited by different stimuli due to differently controlled receptor proteins. They are thus equally capable of detecting both pain and itch. When a polymodal nerve fibre is stimulated, it is initially not possible to deduce which type of stimulus is acting, since stimuli of different types are converted by the neurons into a comparable electrical signal. The differentiation between itching and pain as well as between different pain-triggering stimuli takes place through the integration of the signal of the polymodal fibre with other (more specific) fibres.

Thus, itching is triggered only when fibres responsible for the reception of itch-inducing stimuli are excited. If, in addition to these "itch fibres", other nerve fibres that serve to receive pain stimuli are also stimulated, the overall sensation is no longer "itch", but "pain". The nerval pathways that lead to the central nervous system and convey the sensation of "pain" simultaneously inhibit the neural pathways that convey "itch" by stimulating inhibitory interneurons. This mechanism is also the basis for the phenomenon that painful stimuli, such as intense scratching, suppress itching. Furthermore, this explains why some pain-suppressing drugs cause or enhance itching.

MORE DETAILS Nerve fibres responsible for the reception of itch-inducing stimuli can be divided into two different groups. One group of these nerve fibres is mainly stimulated by histamine and hardly at all by nociceptive stimuli. Accordingly, these nerve fibres also have histamine receptors in their cell membrane. The binding of histamine leads to the activation of an intracellular second messenger cascade. The chemical messengers produced here then cause the TRPV1 channel (TRPV1: transient receptor potential vanilloid 1) to open, see ch. "Signal transduction mechanisms at the nociceptors" (p.78). This leads to an excitation of the nerve fibre due to the resulting Na⁺ current. In the second group of "itch fibres", the TRPV1 channel is also opened by the activation of intracellular second messenger systems. Here, the stimuli are mainly proteases that are released, for example, when cells die. PAR (protease-activated receptors) are present on nerve fibres for the reception of these proteases, which are freely found in the tissue. The fibres equipped with PAR can respond not only to proteases, but their receptors are also involved in the perception of nociceptive stimuli.

Histamine not only triggers itching in different animal species. It also induces redness and swelling of the affected area because the histamine-receiving fibres not only direct their excitation towards the CNS, but also towards the skin surface. This efferent function of the afferents (p.77) leads to marked local vasodilation.

IN A NUTSHELL !

Pain and itching are registered by free nerve endings that are often polymodal, i.e. stimulated by different stimuli. The distinction between pain and itching is determined by painful stimuli also exciting those fibres that only register nociceptive stimuli.

3.2.4 Transmission and central processing of signals from the skin

Three different types of nerve fibres are involved in the afferent transmission of signals from the skin. **Table 3.2** shows the assignment of the different skin sensors to these fibre types.

Table 3.2 Leading fibres of the skin sensors.

Sensor	Afferent fibre
Merkel cells/Merkel cell complexes	Aβ
Ruffini body	Aβ
Meissner corpuscles	Aβ
Vater Pacini lamellar bodies	Aβ
Lanceolate terminals (underhair)	C, Aδ
Lanceolate terminals (over hair)	Aδ
Thermal sensors	C
Nociceptors	C, Aδ
Pruriceptors	C

The cell bodies of the fibres innervating the skin are located in the ipsilateral **spinal ganglia (dorsal root ganglia)**. Fibres innervating the craniofacial area have cell bodies in the nuclei of the trigeminal nerve. They are **pseudounipolar neurons** with a process which divides into two branches. One branch projects as a long dendritic axon into the skin area being innervated. The second branch projects as an axon via the dorsal root into the spinal cord or from the trigeminal nuclei into the brainstem.

Axons of the thermosensitive and nociceptive neurons project from the ipsilateral dorsal root to the contralateral ventral horn of the spinal cord, where they form synapses with subsequent neurons.

Axons of mechanosensitive non-nociceptive neurons do not necessarily form synapses in the spinal cord. Rather, the axon of the spinal ganglion in the ipsilateral posterior cord can extend into the medulla oblongata. However, some of the axons form synapses with subsequent neurons in the spinal cord.

Regardless of how the wiring and transmission occurs in the spinal cord, all information received in the skin is directed to the thalamus (p.135). In the case of the nociceptive and thermosensitive neurons, the neural fibres terminate in the contralateral anterior column. The downstream neuron projects up to the thalamus. The information obtained from mechanosensitive neurons is often directed to a nucleus in the medulla oblongata. The **nucleus gracilis** receives information from the caudal half of the body, while the **nucleus cuneatus** is receptive to signals from the cranial half. Within these two nuclei, there is little convergence between the incoming information. The neurons are arranged **somatotopically** and "contrast enhancement" occurs via lateral inhibition (p.137). As a result, stimuli from neighbouring skin areas can be perceived quite separately.

Projection to the thalamus then takes place from the nucleus gracilis or the nucleus cuneatus.

The contralateral thalamus receives all information coming from the skin. This is an essential relay point for information from the sensory organs on the way to the **somatosensory cortex**. In the cortex, the final processing of information, and awareness and objective evaluation takes place.

However, information is supplied not only to neurons of the lateral thalamus. The medial thalamus is also involved in processing and transmission of information. Nevertheless, the medial thalamus does not pass information to the cortex, but instead it projects to the **limbic system** where "emotional evaluation" of the stimulus takes place.

> **IN A NUTSHELL**   !
>
> The cell bodies of the fibres innervating the skin are located in the dorsal root ganglia. From there, they project via the dorsal root into the spinal cord. The information ultimately reaches the cortex and the limbic system, via the thalamus.

Suggested reading

Abraira VE. The sensory neurons of touch. Neuron 2013; 79:618–639

McGlone F, Reilly D. The cutaneous sensory system. Neurosci Biobehav Rev 2010; 34: 148–159

3.3   Nociception and pain

Holger Sann

> **ESSENTIALS**   ✖
>
> The nociceptive system serves to detect, transmit and process potentially tissue-damaging stimuli (noxae). These stimuli can trigger pain sensations in animals and humans. Mechanical, thermal or chemical noxious stimuli can be detected by specific nociceptors. Their signals are processed in the spinal cord and brain and protective reflexes are triggered as well as changes in the activity of the autonomic nervous system, motor function and affective reactions. Nociception can be modulated by inhibitory and reinforcing mechanisms (plasticity). These mechanisms often serve as targets for analgesia.

3.3.1   Pain in animals

In animals, an "early warning system" is developed to recognise possible tissue-damaging stimuli (noxae, noxious stimuli), which can help to avoid these stimuli by activating reflexes and corresponding behaviours. Recognition, transmission and processing of such noxious stimuli in the peripheral and central nervous system are called **nociception**. In humans, activation of nociception can lead to the sensation of pain. **Pain** is defined in humans as an unpleas-

ant sensory and emotional experience associated with actual or potential tissue damage. Because it is not possible to inquire about their pain sensations, this definition is not directly applicable to animals. The avoidance of pain, along with that of suffering and harm, is an elementary component of animal welfare. Therefore, a definition of pain in animals is important. In veterinary practice, one speaks of pain when the behaviour and reactions of animals to corresponding noxious stimuli show analogies to those in painful conditions in humans. Indirect conclusions about possible pain in animals are possible by examining nociception and behaviour. A sign of the activation of nociception are the so-called **pseudo-affective reactions**, characterised by changes in blood pressure, heart rate and respiration as well as by motor reflexes, protective reactions or by vocalisation. In addition, repeated noxious stimuli, such as in chronic pathological conditions, induce typical avoidance reactions. This results in the following definition for pain in animals.

> **IN A NUTSHELL**   !
>
> **Pain in animals** is an aversive sensory experience caused by actual or potential injury, triggering protective motor or autonomic responses, leading to learned avoidance of such stimuli and thus modifying behaviour.

■ Species-specific differences in pain behaviour

In veterinary practice, conclusions about pain in animals can be drawn primarily from behaviour. Species-specific differences play an important role here. In general, predators show more pronounced reactions to noxious substances than prey animals. In **Table 3.3** typical behaviours for different animal species are listed, which can be interpreted as indicators of pain. General indicators are:
- Reduced activity
- Altered group behaviour
- Reduced food and water intake
- Deterioration in appearance due to reduced self-cleaning behaviour
- Weight loss
- Vocalisation especially in acute pain
- Changed temperament (aggression, apathy)
- Altered physiological parameters (increased heart rate, respiratory rate, blood pressure)

None of these indicators is a clear expression of pain. The individual assessment of the animal based on the owner's experience should be taken into account. The distinction between stress and pain is not easy, especially since typical stress hormones (e.g. catecholamines, cortisol, endorphins) are altered in both states. As a general rule, conditions that cause pain in humans can also cause pain in pets and therefore appropriate treatment with analgesics should be given.

Table 3.3 Species-specific pain behaviour.

Animal species	Pain behaviour
Dog	Lowered head, tucked tail, tension, bent posture, avoidance of movement, restlessness (weak pain), trembling, panting, often unmotivated vocalisation (whimpering, whining, howling), apathy, aggressiveness, inappetence, disobedience.
Cat	Increased muscle tone, flight behaviour, cowering, hiding of the injured body part; less frequent vocalisations (hissing, growling), panting breathing, inappetence, greasy coat, aggression when approached.
Horse	Reduced feed intake, reluctance to be handled, removal from familiar surroundings, dull facial expression, pupil dilation, glassy eyes Colic: restlessness, lowered head, sweating, kicking the abdomen, rolling around.
Ruminants	Gloomy facial expression, hunched posture in visceral pain, removal from familiar surroundings, reluctance to be handled (sometimes aggression), inappetence, rarely vocalisations (gnashing of teeth, moaning) Colic: similar to horse, but less pronounced.
Pig	Change in social behaviour, clearer vocalisations on handling, changed gait, hiding, reluctance to move.
Laboratory rodent	Reduced food intake, unkempt coat, dirty eye rims (spectacled eyes), autotomy (biting into the painful region, e.g. toes), crying (ultrasound; in the range audible to humans on palpation).
Bird	Difficult to assess, mixed active/passive behaviour pattern, partly no reactions to noxious stimuli (learned helplessness), inappetence

Source: Hellebrekers LJ (ed). Schmerz und Schmerztherapie bei Tieren. Hanover: Schlütersche; 2000

■ Pain measurement

Visual, numerical analogue or multidimensional pain scales have been used to measure the intensity of pain. With analogue scales, the acute pain is assigned a value between no pain (0) and greatest possible pain (10). Such methods are well suited to follow changes in pain intensity after treatment but are more difficult to reach an agreed objective assessment by different observers. In multidimensional pain rating scales, different categories, such as physiological data (respiratory and heart rate, body temperature, pupil dilation, salivation), reactions to palpation, physical activity, mental status (subdued to aggressive), posture or vocalisation, are assigned corresponding values (e.g. 10). The individual values for each animal (e.g. from 0–3) are added together. For different animals such as horse, sheep, pig, cat, rabbit, ferret, rat and mouse, there are species-specific validated methods to measure pain status according to facial expression ("grimace scales"). In cats, for example, the sum of the scores (from 0–2) for the position of ears and whiskers, the tightening of the muzzle, orbital tightening and head position are used. The higher the score, the stronger the pain rating. Such pain rating scales are used especially in clinical trials to get a better comparison between different therapies.

3.3.2 Peripheral mechanisms of nociception

■ Nociceptors

The peripheral mechanisms of nociception involve activation of **nociceptors (nocisensors)** and the transmission of a signal to the central nervous system. The first step in the perception of noxious signals is the activation of nociceptors which react specifically to noxious stimuli (**Fig. 3.9**). Nociceptors in the skin can be divided into two broad groups:

- **Myelinated**, with Aδ (in the classification according to Erlanger/Gasser, **Table 2.3**; conduction velocity 2.5–30 m·s^{-1}) **fast conducting** high-threshold **mechanonociceptors**. They can only be excited by acute noxious, mechanical stimuli, such as by needle pricks, and can trigger fast, sharp pain in humans.
- **Unmyelinated** C-fibres (conduction velocity < 2.5 m·s^{-1}), which act as **polymodal nociceptors**. These react to mechanical (e.g. pinpricks, squeezing of the skin), thermal (heat, cold) and chemical noxae (e.g. high potassium ion concentrations, acid, bradykinin). In humans, activation of these nociceptors gives rise to **slow, dull** or burning pain.

Another group of nociceptors cannot be excited by physiologically occurring mechanical noxious stimuli (e.g. extreme stretching of a joint) and are therefore referred to as **dormant nociceptors**. Under pathological conditions (e.g. inflammation, overstretching of the hollow organs, ischaemia), these dormant nociceptors can be "awakened" or sensitized. They probably play an important role in pain associated with inflammation. Nociceptors are also found in muscles, joints, internal organs (viscera) and in almost all other organs of the body except the CNS. While low-threshold mechanosensors in the skin cannot encode nox-

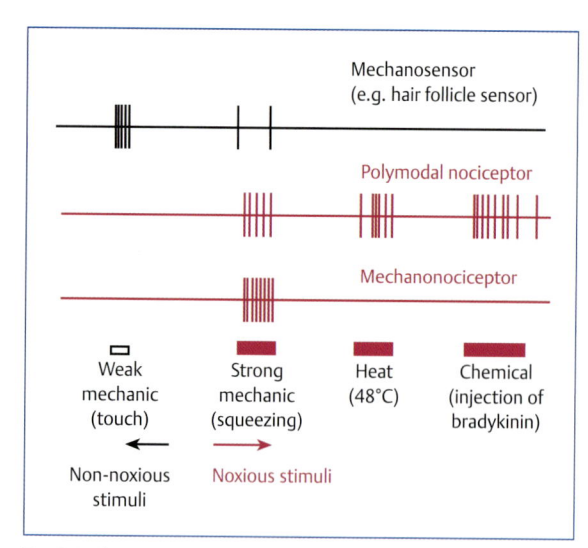

Mechanosensor
(e.g. hair follicle sensor)

Polymodal nociceptor

Mechanonociceptor

| Weak mechanic (touch) | Strong mechanic (squeezing) | Heat (48°C) | Chemical (injection of bradykinin) |

← Non-noxious stimuli   Noxious stimuli →

Fig. 3.9 Skin nociceptors and their responses to noxious stimuli. Excitation pattern of a mechanosensor (hair follicle receptor), a polymodal nociceptor and a mechanonociceptor of the skin to non-noxious (weak mechanical stimuli, white rectangle) and to noxious stimuli (red rectangles). The mechanosensor cannot encode the strength of a noxious mechanical stimulus (or chemical and thermal stimuli). The mechanonociceptor only responds to potentially tissue-damaging mechanical stimuli. The polymodal nociceptor responds to noxious mechanical, thermal and chemical stimulation.

ious stimuli (**Fig. 3.9**), low-threshold sensors in the internal organs, which respond to stretching and contractions, are able to encode noxious stimuli. Therefore, in addition to the specific nociceptors, nerve fibres responding to physiological stimuli are probably also involved in the generation of pain in the viscera.

MORE DETAILS Morphologically, the peripheral endings of the nociceptors are free nerve endings. The cell bodies of the nociceptors are located in the dorsal root ganglia and are usually smaller than those of the low-threshold mechanosensors. In addition to the classic transmitter glutamate, many nociceptors can also contain one or more neuropeptides, such as substance P or calcitonin gene-related peptide. When the nociceptors are activated, these neuropeptides can be released not only at the central synapse in the spinal cord, but also in the periphery (efferent function of the nociceptors). There they can cause, among other things, local inflammatory reactions characterised by vasodilation and plasma extravasation (neurogenic inflammation).

■ Signal transduction mechanism at the nociceptors

Different ionotropic and metabotropic receptors are involved in the reception of noxious stimuli at polymodal nociceptors (**Fig. 3.10**). So-called transient receptor potential (TRP) channel subtypes play a central role. These are non-selective cation channels which are permeable to different cations such as Ca^{2+}, Na^+ or K^+. The vanilloid receptor 1 (TRPV1), which is activated by capsaicin, the pungent ingredient of the pepper family, as well as by endogenous cannabinoids and certain fatty acid metabolites, is a sensor for noxious temperature stimuli ($> 43\,°C$). Activation with capsaicin can change the temperature sensitivity of the sensor. Thus even non-noxious temperatures can open the channel. In addition, the TRPV1 reacts to increased H^+ concentrations ($pH < 5.9$). Other TRP channels also react to temperature changes. TRPM8 responds to cold ($< 22–26\,°C$) and also to menthol. TRPA1 reacts to cold ($< 17\,°C$), chemical stimuli such as mustard oil or formalin, and also to mechanical stimuli.

In addition, there are nociceptors that are sensitive to endogenous pain-inducing substances that can be released during tissue damage. These substances include bradykinin (B_1 and B_2 receptor), adenosine triphosphate (ATP, purinergic ionotropic receptor P2X3), serotonin (5-HT; $5-HT_3$ receptor), prostaglandins (PGE_2; EP2 receptor), the nerve growth factor (NGF) (which exerts its effects via the tyrosine kinase A receptor, TrkA), and hydrogen ions ("acid-sensing ion channels", ASIC). Mechanosensitive ("stretch-activated") channels probably play a role in mechanotransduction. The activation of various protein kinases can lead to a complex modulation of the channels by phosphorylation and can thus alter the sensitivity of the nociceptors (**Fig. 3.10**).

IN A NUTSHELL

Specific mechanosensitive and polymodal nociceptors encode noxious stimuli and transmit this information to the CNS. Through various signal transduction pathways, nociceptors respond to potentially tissue-damaging signals and to mediators that are released when tissue is damaged.

Cell, tissue

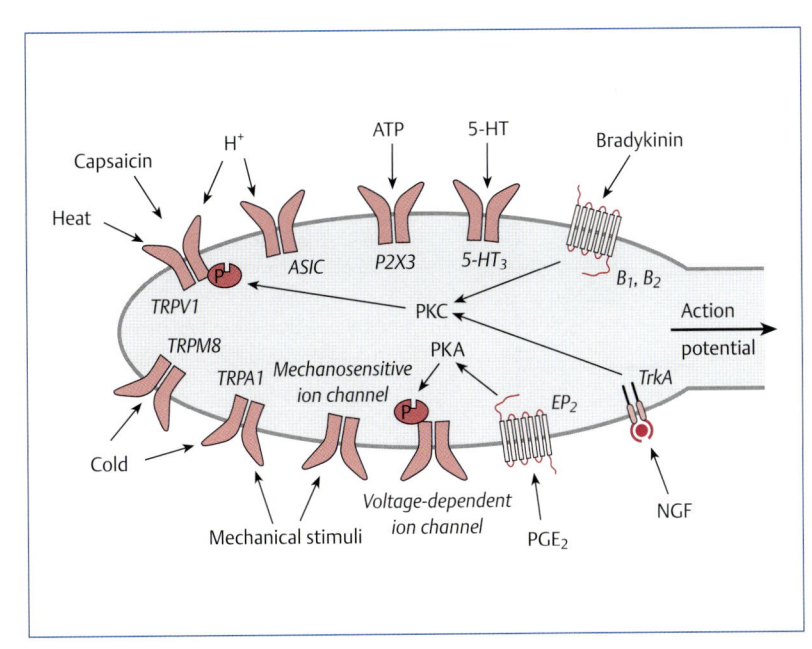

Fig. 3.10 Mechanisms of signal transduction at the nociceptive terminal. Various ionotropic and metabotropic receptors are involved in the reception of noxious chemical, thermal and mechanical stimuli. Sensitization of individual mechanisms can be modulated by various protein kinases that lead to phosphorylation (P) of the corresponding membrane proteins. B_1, B_2: bradykinin receptor subtype 1 or 2; 5-HT_3: ionotropic serotonin (5-HT) receptor type 3; ATP: adenosine triphosphate; P2X3: ionotropic purinergic receptor 3; ASIC: acid-sensing ion channel; TRPV1: vanilloid receptor 1; TRPM8: transient receptor potential channel of M (melastatin) type 8; TRPA1: transient receptor potential channel of A(ankyrin) type 1; PGE_2: prostaglandin E2; EP_2: prostaglandin E2 receptor subtype 2; NGF: nerve growth factor; TrkA: tyrosine kinase receptor A, a neuronal high-affinity receptor for nerve growth factor; PKA: protein kinase A; PKC: protein kinase C.

3.3.3 Central mechanisms of nociception

The signals from the peripheral nociceptors are further processed in the central nervous system. The first synaptic transmission of the signals from the skin nociceptors takes place in the most dorsally located layers of the dorsal horn (laminae I-II) of the spinal cord or in the corresponding regions of the brainstem for the nociceptors from the craniofacial region (trigeminal nuclei). Many neurons in these layers are most sensitive to or react exclusively to noxious stimuli.

> **MORE DETAILS** In the middle part of the dorsal horn (laminae III–IV), the afferents from low-threshold mechanosensors terminate. Most neurons located there respond best to relatively weak mechanical stimuli (touch, vibration). In the deeper layers of the dorsal horn (laminae V–VI), both nociceptive and non-nociceptive neurons are found. Primary afferent nerve fibres from muscles, joints and viscera also end in these layers as well as in lamina I.

Visceral afferent nerve fibres and sensory nerve fibres of the skin can be connected to the same spinal neurons (**viscerosomatic convergence**). Compared to skin receptors, the effectiveness of visceral sensors to excite spinal neurons is relatively low. Therefore, a strong activation of many visceral receptors is required such as the massive distension of hollow organs, traction of the mesenteries or sensitization of the visceral receptors (e.g. during inflammation) to activate spinal nociceptive neurons by visceral stimuli. Signals from visceral nociceptive sensors can be misinterpreted as noxious stimuli from the corresponding somatic regions because of viscerosomatic convergence. In humans, this is termed referred pain. The corresponding somatic regions are called Head's zones (p. 119) . An example is pain in the left arm during cardiac ischaemia or after myocardial infarction.

The nociceptive spinal neurons can act on the motor systems of the ipsi- or contralateral ventral horn in the same spinal cord segment. This triggers protective reflexes such as withdrawal reflexes or increased abdominal wall tension in peritonitis. Furthermore, the activity of the preganglionic sympathetic neurons located in the lateral horn can be modulated. This induces sympathetic reflexes such as changes in blood flow or sweating. Local spinal mechanisms thus also contribute to the motor and autonomic components of nociception and pain (Fig. 3.11).

To transmit information about noxious stimuli to the brain, the axons of the nociceptive dorsal horn neurons run to the contralateral side. They form the **tractus spinothalamicus** projecting to the thalamus, to the formatio reticularis in the brainstem (tractus spinoreticularis) and to the midbrain (tractus spinomesencephalicus). In the thalamus, the nociceptive fibres end primarily at the edge of the ventrobasal complex, but also in non-specific thalamic nuclei, i.e. thalamic areas that are not specifically linked to distinct areas of the cortex. The ventrobasal thalamic neurons then project into the somatosensory cortex (p. 135). This pathway serves to detect and localise noxious stimuli (**sensory-discriminative function**). The non-specific thalamic nuclei, the formatio reticularis and the limbic system are involved in the **affective component of nociception** such as aggression during pain. **Motoneurons** can be activated via the descending motor pathways of the CNS, in response to noxious stimulation (**motor component**). The **vegetative component** of nociception is mediated by the wiring of nociceptive signals in the brainstem, hypothalamus and descending pathways to the preganglionic neurons in the spinal cord (Fig. 3.11). This wiring can explain the vegetative reactions to strong noxious stimulation, typical of defensive behaviour, such as redistribution of blood flow (more to muscle, and less to viscera and skin), an increase in cardiac output or activation of the adrenal medulla. Pain can thus exert a direct influence on complex behavioural patterns via these various components.

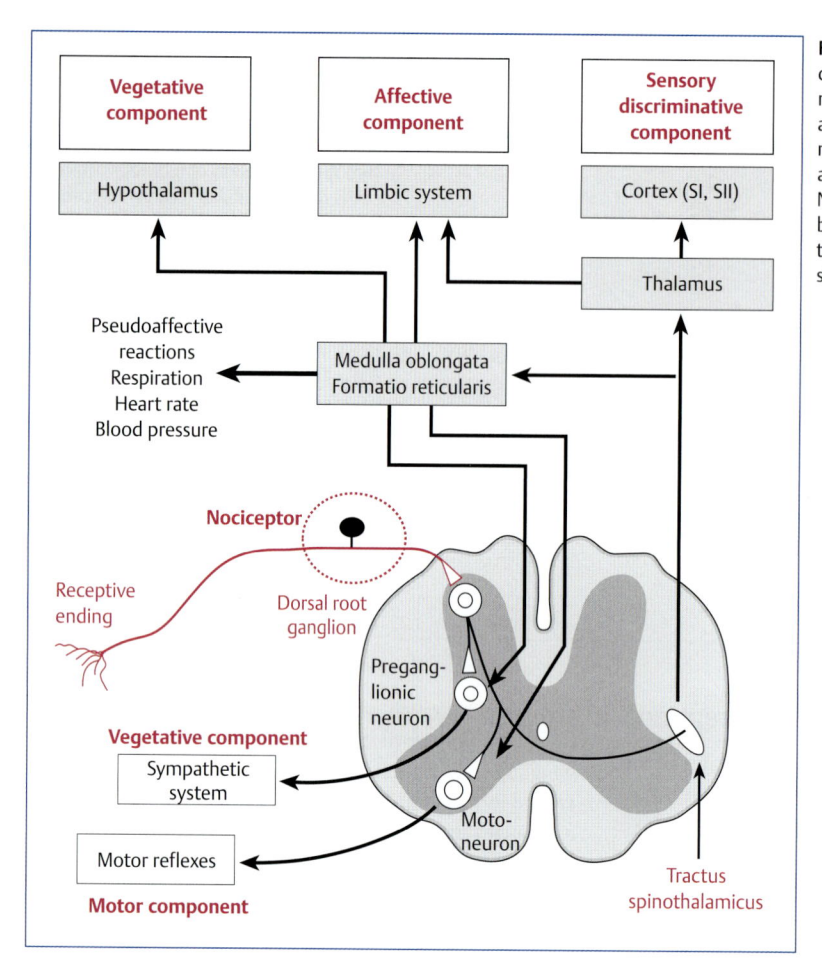

Fig. 3.11 Schematic representation of the central nociceptive pathways and the resulting main components of nociception and pain. Nociceptor activation can initiate reflex chains via stimulation of autonomic and motoneurons in the spinal cord. Nociceptive signals reach the thalamus and brainstem via the anterior column and are then processed further in the CNS (highly simplified representation).

IN A NUTSHELL   !

The processing of noxious stimuli takes place in the CNS. The resulting pain has sensory (painful yes – no), affective (displeasure), vegetative (reddening of the skin, sympathetic activation) and motor components (e.g. withdrawal reflex).

3.3.4 Plasticity of nociception

■ Sensitization of the nociception

Inflammation

One of the typical characteristics of nociception is its sensitization under pathophysiological conditions, such as inflammation. Sensitization leads to increased protection of the affected organs (e.g. in lameness or a protective posture). Elimination of noxious substances can be accelerated so that the healing process would thus be favoured.

A distinction is made between **hyperalgesia** – an increased sensitivity to noxious stimuli, and **allodynia** – where pain can be triggered by **touch stimuli**. Inflammatory processes can sensitize the peripheral nociceptors (**peripheral sensitization**) so that they react to normally non-noxious mechanical or thermal stimuli. A well-known example of this is in sunburn, where light touch stimuli

and a small increase in temperature from a warm shower cause severe pain. Local chemical factors in the inflamed tissue (**inflammatory mediators**) such as prostaglandins, bradykinin, serotonin and/or acidification, are responsible for this sensitization.

Inflammation also leads to hyperexcitability of central neurons in the spinal cord (**central sensitization**). This can lead to both hyperalgesia and allodynia. In allodynia, signals from low threshold mechanosensors are amplified in nociceptive spinal neurons, so that normally non-noxious touch stimuli can activate the nociceptive system. Sensory stimuli from regions of the skin (see "Head's zones" (p. 79)) are also amplified and the affected spinal neurons show an increase in the size of their receptive field (secondary hyperalgesia). Diseases of internal organs, such as colic, or with foreign objects in the gastrointestinal tract, can also lead to sensitization of somatic regions. Examination of the skin for hypersensitivity can help in such cases to localise the spinal segments where sensitization has occurred. An important role in central sensitization is played by the NMDA receptor (N-methyl-D-aspartate receptor), a subtype of glutamate receptor. Thus, specific NMDA antagonists such as ketamine, which is often used as an anaesthetic in veterinary medicine, can prevent central sensitization.

Neuropathic pain

In neuropathic pain, there is damage to neurons in the peripheral or central nervous system with a consequent abnormal processing of somatosensory signals. While acute pain and inflammatory pain have a protective effect on the animal as a warning mechanism, in contrast, chronic neuropathic pain, has lost this protective function. Neuropathic pain can also arise from nerve injuries or amputations, diabetes mellitus or infections (herpes zoster).

> **MORE DETAILS** Various mechanisms are involved in the pathogenesis of neuropathic pain. On the one hand, there may be inadequate neuronal activity without a corresponding noxious stimulus. On the other hand, changes in central processing can occur, for example through the sprouting of nerve endings in damaged CNS regions and a reorganisation of the wiring. The interaction of neurons with activated microglial cells (p.44) can lead to altered excitability of spinal neurons via various interleukins, chemokines and nerve growth factors. Since neuropathic pain involves mechanisms different from those of acute pain, alternative strategies for treating such pain must be implemented.

■ Endogenous antinociceptive systems

Many nociceptive neurons in the spinal cord are under the influence of inhibitory pathways, which can be regarded as the body's own "pain suppression system" (antinociceptive system). The spinal nociceptive neurons can be inhibited by local mechanisms, intersegmental spinal connections and/or descending pathways of the central nervous system (**Fig. 3.12**). By activating the descending pathways, the responses of the nociceptive spinal cord neurons to noxious stimuli are significantly reduced.

Antinociception can be triggered from the periaqueductal grey of the midbrain, the nucleus raphe magnus in the ventral medulla oblongata, the locus coeruleus in the dorsal medulla oblongata and from parts of the formatio reticularis, as well as other regions. Descending inhibition can be triggered by various physiological and pathophysiological influences such as pain, stress, anxiety, work, or high blood pressure, as well as the activation of opiate receptors e.g. by morphine, or by the body's own opioids (endomorphins, encephalins, dynorphin). The most important neurotransmitters of the descending pathways in the spinal cord are serotonin and noradrenaline (**Fig. 3.12**). In the spinal cord, local inhibition of nociception can also be achieved via encephalins or γ-aminobutyric acid (GABA)-containing neurons.

In various chronic pain syndromes and in neuropathic pain, a change in the body's own antinociception may also be observed. A central disinhibition (loss of inhibition) can lead to an imbalance between excitatory and inhibitory mechanisms, which can result in an intensification of the pain.

> **IN A NUTSHELL** !
>
> Nociception is characterised by enormous plasticity. Both endogenous amplification (sensitization) and endogenous inhibition mechanisms can be observed.

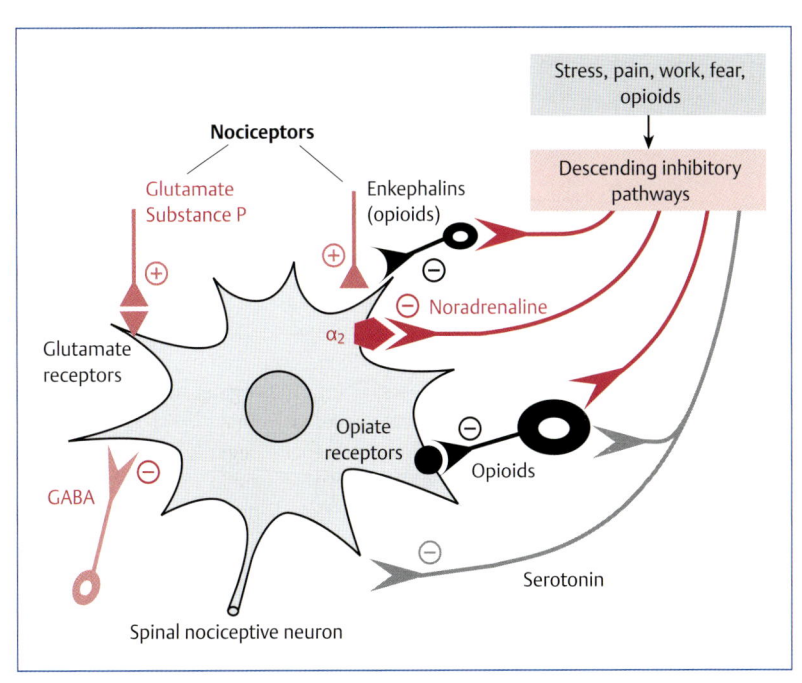

Fig. 3.12 Inhibition of spinal nociception by descending pathways from the brain and interneurons. Inhibition of the spinal nociceptive neuron can occur through noradrenaline (α$_2$ receptors), serotonin, endogenous opioids (encephalin, dynorphin) and GABA. Local enkephalinergic neurons can also presynaptically (axoaxonal synapse) reduce the release of glutamate and substance P from the central terminals of nociceptors.
+: excitatory synapse;
–: inhibitory synapse

Figure labels: Stress, pain, work, fear, opioids; Nociceptors; Glutamate Substance P; Enkephalins (opioids); Descending inhibitory pathways; Glutamate receptors; Noradrenaline; α$_2$; GABA; Opiate receptors; Opioids; Serotonin; Spinal nociceptive neuron

3.3.5   Pain management

■ Analgesics

One site of action for pain-relieving agents (analgesics) is to prevent peripheral sensitization of nociception. Thus analgesics such as acetylsalicylic acid, inhibit the formation of the sensitizing prostaglandins (**Fig. 3.13**). Furthermore, local cooling can reduce the activity of the nociceptors and slow down the process of inflammation. A short-term method of eliminating pain is to apply local anaesthesia to the affected region, the corresponding nerve or the spinal cord segments that are involved. Local anaesthetics block the voltage-dependent sodium channels that are essential for the transmission of action potentials (p.48) and thus prevent the flow of information from the periphery to the spinal cord. Since this also prevents the central sensitization of the spinal cord neurons, local anaesthesia can contribute to the reduction of postoperative pain. In the case of chronic pathological conditions, for example in the case of podotrochlosis of the horse, the corresponding nerve can be severed to eliminate pain (neurectomy). However, since neurectomies also eliminate efferent innervation and other sensory modalities, such surgical interventions are only useful after careful consideration of alternative treatments. Analgesia can be achieved in the spinal cord and brain by activating the body's own antinociceptive mechanisms. One of the oldest pharmacological pain treatments is the systemic administration of morphine, which inhibits the nociceptive system via opiate receptors. Similar analgesic effects can be obtained with α_2 adrenergic agonists, such as xylazine. Since one of the sites of action of these agents is the nociceptive spinal cord neurons, the application of morphine or α_2 agonists close to the spinal cord (epidural) also has an analgesic effect (**Fig. 3.13**). Epidural application can thus significantly attenuate any undesirable side effects.

MORE DETAILS   In neuropathic pain, there are changes in the signal processing that result in increased neuronal activity. Antiepileptic drugs, which reduce excitability by modifying calcium channels, or antidepressant agents, can limit excessive neuronal activity and thus have an analgesic effect.

■ Anaesthesia

Anaesthesia prevents the perception of noxious stimuli (**Fig. 3.13**). It has long been known that the effect of narcotics correlates well with their lipid solubility. It is assumed that narcotics exert their effect by binding to lipophilic regions of membrane proteins. This can enhance the effect of inhibitory transmitter receptors (e.g. barbiturates at the GABA$_A$ receptors), suppression of excitatory receptors (e.g. ketamine at NMDA receptors) or modification of ion channels (e.g. opening of some potassium channels). The resulting altered synaptic transmission suppresses the central processing mechanisms. As a result, complicated polysynaptic mechanisms (perception) are the first to fail during anaesthesia, depending on the dose, while simple circuits (autonomic mechanisms) or the transmission of action potentials can still be preserved and only fail with excessively high concentrations of the anaesthetic agent.

Suggested reading

Fox SM. Chronic pain in small animal medicine. London: Manson Publishing; 2013

McMahon S, Koltzenburg M, Tracey I, Turk DC. Wall & Melzack's textbook of pain. 6th Edition. Philadephia: Saunders; 2013

Self I. BSAVA Guide to pain management in small animal practice. BSAVA (British Small Animal Veterinary Association); 1st Edition; 2019

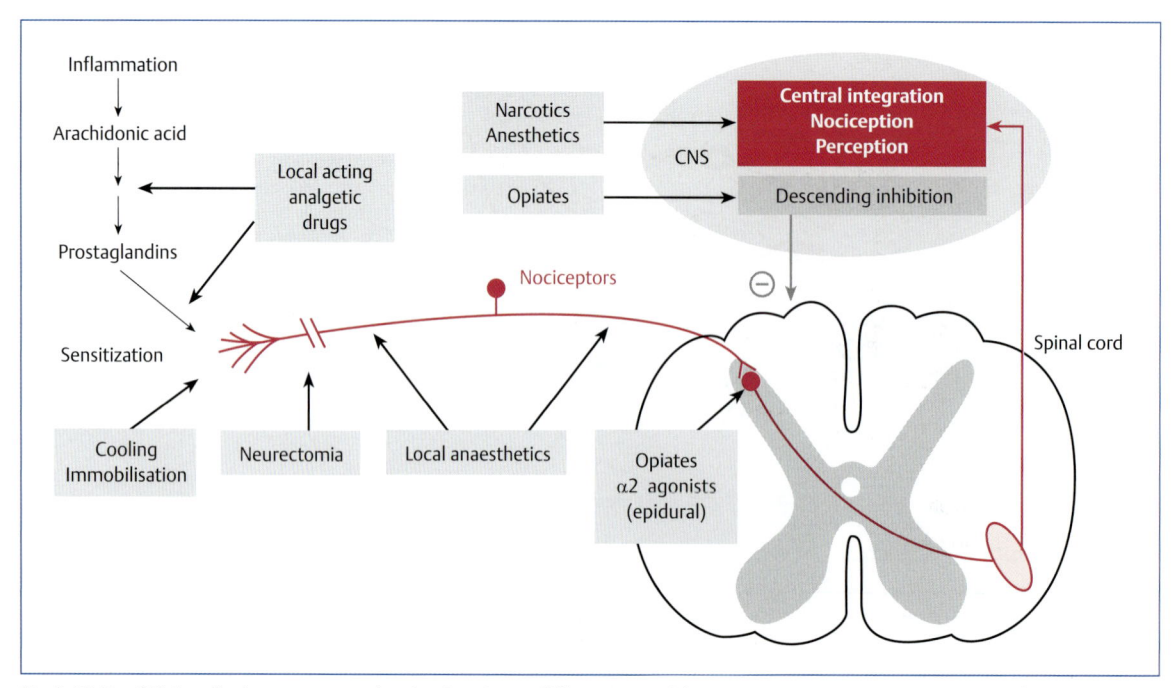

Fig. 3.13 Possibilities of pain treatment and antinociception at different sites of the nociceptive system. Arrows point to the sites of action of the respective treatment options.

3.4 Balance and hearing

Heinz Breer

> **ESSENTIALS** ✕
>
> In vertebrates, the sensory structures for both the sense of balance and the sense of hearing are located in the inner ear. While the sense of balance registers the position of the head in space and rotational movements, the sense of hearing is able to detect sound waves. In both systems, the detection of adequate stimuli occurs through highly sensitive mechanosensory cells.

3.4.1 The sensory systems of the inner ear

The sensory structures of the inner ear are located in duct-like cavities of the skull bone (petrous bone) and consist of the vestibular organ (with the semicircular canals and the otolith organs) and the cochlea (**Fig. 3.14**). This interconnected ductal structure contains a system of tubes filled with **endolymph** which, with its high K⁺ concentration, largely corresponds to an intracellular fluid. The space between the bony wall and the membranous tubular system is filled with **perilymph** (high Na⁺ concentration).

■ Sensory cells in the inner ear

The sensory cells of the inner ear are secondary sensory cells, without an axon of their own, to transmit sensory information at the synapses to afferent nerve fibres. They are called "hair cells" because the conspicuous cell processes

at the apical end appear like a shock of "hairs" under the light microscope. These consist of a larger number of smaller stereocilia arranged like organ pipes or rather **stereovilli** (stereo = stiff), which are microvillous projections with actin filaments as a cytoskeleton. In the hair cells in the organ of equilibrium, a single long cilium, the **kinocilium**, is added. All stereovilli are connected by filamentous structures, the so-called **tip links**, to each other and, if present, to the kinocilium. Tension of the tip links by deflection of the stereovilli causes mechanosensitive ion channels in the membrane to open (**Fig. 3.15**). Since the apical membrane of the hair cells with the stereocilia is surrounded by K⁺-rich endolymph, there is an influx of K⁺ ions. The driving force for this is the sum of the membrane potential of the hair cell (70 mV) and the endolymph potential (80 mV).

The resulting depolarization of the hair cells, the receptor potential of the sensory cell, causes an opening of voltage-dependent Ca²⁺ channels in the presynaptic membrane, an increased release of the transmitter glutamate, and an increased action potential frequency in the afferent nerve fibres.

There is a special situation in the organ of balance, in that not only a stimulus such as sound is registered by the hair cells, as in the organ of hearing, but also the direction of a movement must be detected. At rest, about 15% of the mechanosensitive cation channels are open, thus causing a resting potential of about –60 mV. A deflection of the stereovilli by tensing the tip link in the direction of the kinocilium, causes a depolarization of about 20 mV. This increases the synaptic activity and thus the action potential frequency in the afferent nerve fibre. Deflection of the

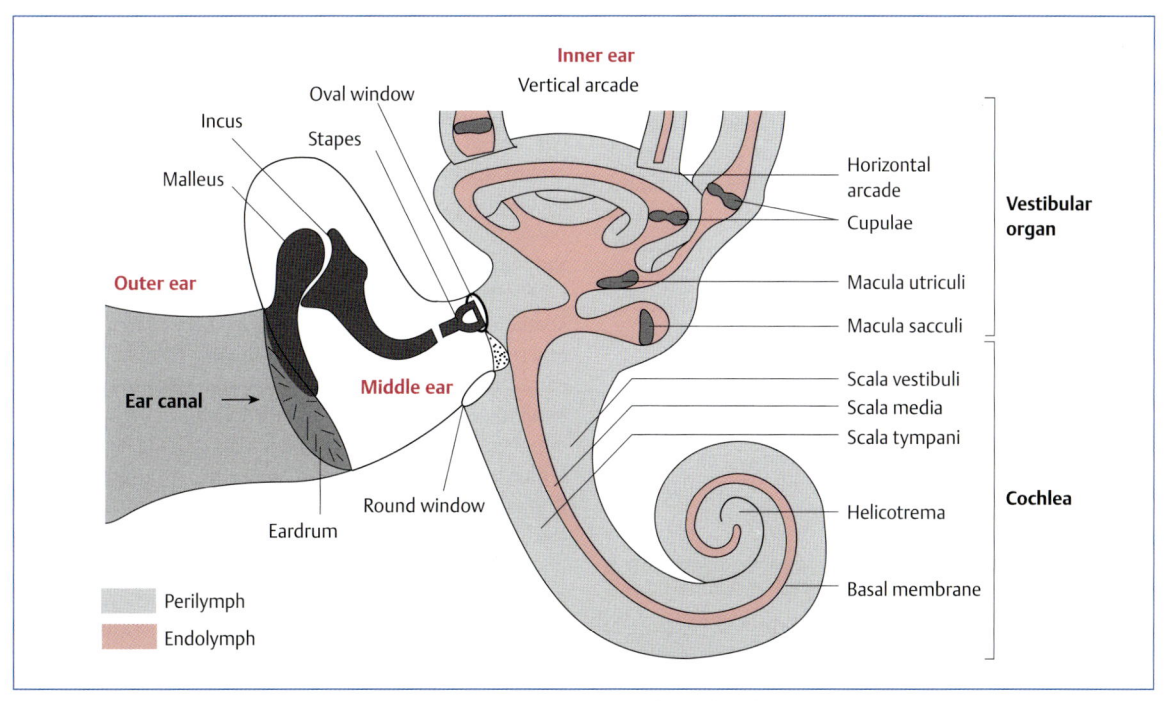

Fig. 3.14 Sensory organs of the inner ear. The auditory canal ends at the eardrum, the vibrations of which are transmitted via the ossicles (malleus, incus, stapes) to the oval window. The duct system in the petrous bone has membranous tubular structures filled with endolymph or perilymph. The sensory epithelia of the vestibular organ are located in the two otolith organs and in the ampullae of the three perpendicular canals, those of the cochlea in the organ of Corti on the basilar membrane.

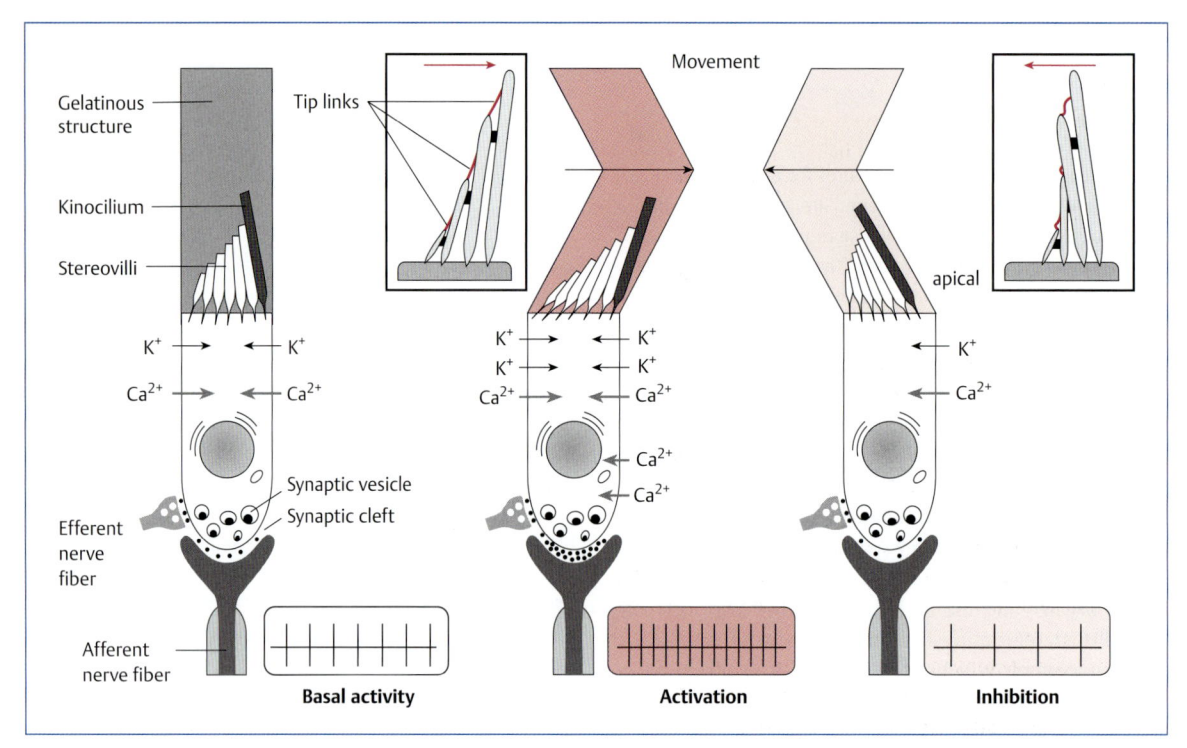

Fig. 3.15 Signal transduction of the hair cells. The hair cells are covered by gelatinous structures (cupula, otolith membrane, tectorial membrane) above their stereovilli. At rest, the afferent nerve fibres fire at medium frequency due to spontaneous transmitter release from the hair cells (resting activity). By tilting the stereovilli in the direction of the kinocilium (absent in hair cells of the organ of Corti), ion channels are opened in the hair cells by stretching the tip on the left. K^+ ions flow in from the endolymph and depolarize the hair cell. The resulting receptor potential causes activation of voltage-gated Ca^{2+} channels and an influx of Ca^{2+} ions. This causes an increased release of transmitters and thus an increased frequency of action potentials of the afferent nerve fibres (activation). A deflection of the stereovilli in the opposite direction of the kinocilium leads to a closing of the tip link-activated ion channels and thus to a hyperpolarization of the cell. This reduces transmitter release and consequently also the spike rate of the afferent nerve fibres (inhibition).

stereovilli in the other direction causes hyperpolarization of the hair cell by about 5 mV. The correspondingly reduced synaptic activity causes a decrease in the action potential frequency in the afferent axon. The hair cells and the afferent nerve fibres are therefore constantly active (**tonic activity**). Depending on the direction of inflection of the stereovilli, the synaptic activity of the hair cells and the frequency of the neuronal action potentials is increased or decreased. Therefore, the hair cells in the organ of equilibrium can register not only movement but also the direction of this movement. These hair cells are therefore asymmetrical: they respond to a mechanical stimulus either with depolarization or with hyperpolarization. In addition, the intensity of the cell response is asymmetrical for the same stimulus strength. When deflecting towards the kinocilium there is a large receptor potential, while deflection towards the small stereovilli results in a smaller receptor potential.

> **IN A NUTSHELL** !
>
> The receptor potential of the hair cells is generated by opening mechanically controlled cation channels, which modulate transmitter release and the frequency of action potentials of the afferent nerve fibres.

3.4.2　Sense of balance, vestibular organ

The organ of equilibrium or vestibular organ consists of protrusions of the membranous tube system in the duct-shaped labyrinth located in the skull bone. The labyrinth consists of the three perpendicular arcades and the two otolith organs (utriculus and sacculus; **Fig. 3.14**). The sensory epithelia with the hair cells are located in the ampoule-shaped extensions of the arcades (cristae) and in the two otolith organs (maculae).

The three semicircular **canals** are arranged in all three spatial directions, therefore their sensory systems – in interaction with the semicircular canals of the contralateral ear – are able to convert **angular accelerations (speed of head movements)** into adequate activity changes in the afferent nerve fibres. Each semicircular canal is closed in the region of the ampulla by a swivelling gelatinous cupula into which the stereocilia of the hair cells protrude. When the head rotates, the semicircular canals and the endolymph they contain move with it, but because of inertia, the fluid cannot follow this movement directly. Straight-line translational accelerations do not change the position of the endolymph or cupula, since the density (mass per volume) is the same for both. Only a relative flow in the semicircular canals, triggered by a head rotation, leads to shearing of the stereocilia, since the cupula, which is fused to the bony inner side of the arcade, moves with the head.

If this happens in the direction of the kinocilium, the afferent nerve fibres are excited. A deflection in the opposite direction causes a reduction in the frequency of the resulting action potentials.

The **otolith organs** register changes in the position of the head and linear accelerations, i.e. changes in speed along a straight line, for example when travelling in a vertical elevator. In the two otolith organs, the hair cells with kinocilia and stereocilia, are embedded in a jelly-like structure. It consists mainly of mucopolysaccharides, in which crystals of calcium carbonate (otoliths) are embedded – the **otolith membrane**. This increases its density compared to the endolymph. Changes in the position of the head cause corresponding changes in the position of the otolith membranes in the two otolith organs. This changes the shearing angle of the hair cells. With normal head posture, the constant force of gravity causes the hair cells to deflect only in the ventral saccule where the otolith membrane is vertical. In the dorsal utriculus the otolith membrane is horizontal and the stereocilia are not sheared. The non-uniform orientation of the sensory cells in the macular epithelia enables detection of different directions via modulation of the tonic activity of the hair cells. The otolith organs thus report **straight-line movements** and deviations of the head posture from the vertical.

> **IN A NUTSHELL** !
>
> The hair cells of the otolith organs and cristae in the ampullary extensions of the semicircular canals show tonic activity, the frequency of which is modulated by shearing of the hair cells.

The afferent nerve fibres from the maculae and the ampullae of the semicircular canals form the vestibular nerve projecting to the **vestibular nuclei** in the medulla oblongata. There, signals from the hair cells in the labyrinth are integrated with information from the visual system and from the proprioceptors of the muscles and joints of the neck. The convergence of these inputs enables the reflex control of body and head posture and eye movements. These vestibular reflexes are the prerequisite for positional control and other goal-directed movements. They are additionally under the control of the cerebellum and the motor cortex, so that intended movements trigger supporting reflexes, even before the movement has been executed. For the reflexive control of the compensatory eye movements when the head posture is changed, there are monosynaptic connections to the motor nuclei of the eye muscles. Compensatory eye movements serve to stabilise the visual field during active and passive body or head movements. The resulting rhythmic eye movements is called **nystagmus**.

> **IN A NUTSHELL** !
>
> The convergence of the signals from the vestibular organ, the visual system and the proprioceptors of the neck is decisively involved in the reflexive control of head and body posture as well as in spatial orientation.

3.4.3 The sense of hearing

> **ESSENTIALS** ✗
>
> The auditory system serves to register and interpret **sound waves**. Sound waves are a useful information medium. They indicate movement and they allow communication over long distances, even out of the line of sight. Sound waves are pressure fluctuations caused by a vibrating body that alternately compresses and relaxes the air (sound source).

The frequency of the pressure fluctuations is given in Hertz (Hz; oscillations per second). The maximum deviation of the **sound pressure** from the resting position is called amplitude and is measured in Pascals (Pa; $1\,N\cdot m^{-2}$). The human ear processes a sound pressure range of $2\cdot10^6$ Pa. The lowest perceptible sound pressure is $3.2\cdot10^{-5}$ Pa (**hearing threshold**), and the highest is over 100 Pa (63 Pa = pain threshold). In the range of high and low frequencies, considerably higher sound pressure levels are required to exceed the hearing threshold. By using a logarithmic scale, the values for sound pressure range are minimized to 0–120 dB. For this purpose, the logarithm of a pressure ratio to a fixed reference sound pressure (p_0,) is used with $p_0 = 2\cdot10^{-5}$ Pa. The **sound pressure level** (L) is the ratio of the effective value of the actual sound pressure to the reference sound pressure ($L = 20\cdot\log_{10} p_x /p_0$ [dB]). In acoustics, usually this sound pressure level is measured.

> **IN A NUTSHELL** !
>
> The adequate stimulus for the auditory organ is determined by the sound pressure and frequency.

In audiometry, **hearing threshold curves** are determined, taking into account physiological perception criteria. To do so, the sound pressure level is measured for frequencies from the entire hearing range at which a sound is just perceived (**Fig. 3.16**). The frequency-related hearing range is different in vertebrates (**Table 3.4**). The human ear is most sensitive in the middle frequency range between 1500–5000 Hz (human frequency range 20–20000 Hz). The frequencies generated during speech are in this range (**main speech range**). The ability of most mammals to perceive higher frequencies than humans is particularly developed in bats (upper limit 170000 Hz). Fish, which lack the cochlea, can only hear frequencies below 600–700 Hz due to a small appendage on the saccule that may be connected to sound-conducting organs.

Acoustic signals are composed of many frequencies and are called **noise**. A **tone** corresponds to a sinusoidal oscillation with a certain frequency. Loudness values are given in **phon** to express the perceived **loudness of a sound** in relation to a sine tone of 1000 Hz. For a tone of 1000 Hz, the phon and decibel values are identical.

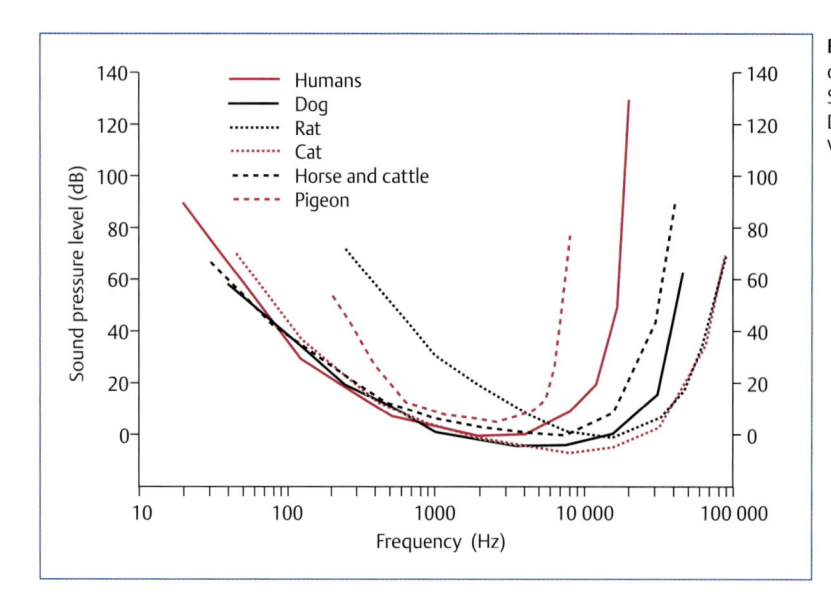

Fig. 3.16 Hearing threshold curve of various vertebrates and humans. [Source: Sjaastad ØV, Hove K, Sand O. Physiology of Domestic Animals. Oslo: Scandinavian Veterinary Press; 2007]

Table 3.4 Audible frequency ranges in animals and humans.

Species	Audible range (Hertz)
Horse	55–33000
Cattle	23–35000
Sheep	125–42000
Dog	67–45000
Cat	45–65000
Guinea pig	86–46000
Rat	250–80000
Human (juvenile)	20–20000

■ Sound conduction in the middle ear

The pressure fluctuations propagate in the air at the speed of sound. They are reflected, when they hit an object with a different sound wave impedance. **Impedance** is the product of density and sound wave velocity in a medium, for example the body of an animal. In order to register the pressure fluctuations of the air within a sensory organ in an aqueous medium, the sound energy delivered via the compressible, "sound-soft medium" of air must be transferred to the almost incompressible, "sound-hard" medium of perilymph in the inner ear. To do this, the different sound wave resistances of the two media must be adjusted. The hearing organ in land-living mammals therefore has structural specialisations for improved sound reception. The auricle acts as a funnel and concentrates the captured sound waves into the auditory canal. The most important role with regard to extensive impedance matching, i.e. improved registration of sound waves, is played by the air-filled middle ear, which is separated from the auditory canal by the eardrum and from the fluid-filled inner

ear by the oval window. When a sound wave hits the **eardrum**, a large-surface "microphone membrane" is caused to vibrate. The resulting waves are not conducted through the tympanic cavity of the middle ear by means of pressure fluctuations but instead through the lever chain of the auditory ossicles (malleus, incus, stirrup) to the small **oval window** (**Fig. 3.14**). Vibrations of the oval window transmit the sound stimulus to the fluid spaces of the inner ear. The impedance matching is thus essentially achieved by two mechanisms. On the one hand by the pressure transmission from the large-surface eardrum (approx. $50\,mm^2$ in humans) to the small-surface oval window (approx. $3\,mm^2$) and on the other hand by the leverage effect of the ossicles. The area ratio correlates with the sensitivity of the auditory system. It is approx. $15:1$ in humans, $27:1$ in dogs and $34:1$ in rats. Overall, the mechanisms in the middle ear cause approx. 60% of the sound energy to be transmitted to the inner ear. This results in an amplification of $1:50$ to $1:90$ and a gain in hearing of 10–30 dB.

Due to its transmission properties, the middle ear also serves as a **bandpass filter**. In many rodents and bats, the small and light ossicles allow transmission in the ultrasound range. In addition, the contraction of the middle ear muscles can influence and attenuate the transmission of low-frequency sounds.

> **IN A NUTSHELL**   !
>
> The auditory ossicles of the middle ear form a sound pressure amplifier system and at the same time act as a bandpass filter.

3.4.4 Cochlea

The cochlea of vertebrates is a micromechanical marvel that, on the one hand, registers movements of 0.1 nanometres and, on the other, can analyse the frequency of a sound to an accuracy of one tenth of a percent. In mammals, it is located in a winding bony duct, which is almost straight in reptiles and birds. Three superimposed membranous tubes, the scala vestibuli, scala tympani and scala media, are arranged in the bony duct (**Fig. 3.14**). The base of the cochlea adjoins the stapes of the middle ear with the oval window. Behind the oval window lies the **scala vestibuli**, which is filled with perilymph. This fluid space merges at the tip of the cochlea (**helicotrema**) into the **scala tympani**, which is also filled with perilymph and which ends at the **round window** at the base. Between the two tubes is the **scala media** filled with endolymph which houses the actual sensory organ. While the perilymph largely corresponds to the extracellular fluid with a high Na^+ concentration, the endolymph has a high K^+ concentration. The endolymph is produced by the stria vascularis.

The scala media is separated from the scala vestibularis by the Reissner's membrane, whereas the border of the scala tympani is formed by the **basilar membrane** (**Fig. 3.17**). The **organ of Corti** is located in a thickening of the basilar membrane . These sensory cells which are surrounded by supporting cells, have access to the scala media at their apical cell pole. The hair cells, which carry only stereovilli, are arranged in four rows: one row of **inner hair cells** and three rows of **outer hair cells**. In total, there are about 4000 inner and 12000 outer hair cells in humans. The sensory cells of the cochlea are innervated by nerve cells located in the **spiral ganglion**. About 90% of the nerve fibres are myelinated and lead as afferent fibres to the inner hair cells. Each cell is innervated by many fibres, each of which is unbranched and connected to only one hair cell. Only 10% of the nerve fibres project to the outer hair cells. They are not myelinated and are branched many times. These efferents are predominantly cholinergic and originate from the olivary nucleus. The axons of the 30000–40000 neurons of the spiral ganglion form the auditory nerve and project to the cochlear nucleus.

The organ of Corti is covered by the gelatinous **tectorial membrane** to the underside of which the stereovilli of the outer hair cells are attached. The villi of the inner hair cells are not attached to the tectorial membrane.

■ Formation of the travelling wave and the transduction process

The vibrations generated by sound waves at the oval window cause a shift in the volume of the perilymph in the scala vestibuli. This wave-like displacement triggers a **travelling wave towards the tip of the cochlea** and is transmitted to the walls of the endolymphatic tube. These waves generally have a very small amplitude. A maximum amplitude is reached between the oval window and the helicotrema at a characteristic point for each frequency. The basis for this differential vibration behaviour is the decreasing stiffness of the basilar membrane from the oval window to the helicotrema in a ratio of 10000 : 1. The resulting vibrations cause the tectorial membrane to deflect relative to the basilar membrane with the embedded hair cells. The relative movements of the two "membranes" against each other causes shearing of the stereovilli of outer hair cells, as only these are connected to the tectorial membrane (**Fig. 3.17**). Even tiny deflections lead to a depolarization of the cell and a reactive shortening of the cell by up to 4%. This change in length is caused by a change in the shape of the voltage-sensitive protein **prestin** in the lateral cell membrane. The shortening of the outer hair cells, which are firmly anchored to the tectorial and basilar membranes, exerts a pull on the basilar membrane and thus considerably increases its deflection. The outer hair cells are therefore not only mechanosensory cells, but at the same time electromechanical transducers.

The stimulus-synchronous contraction of the outer hair cells causes a local amplification of the basilar membrane deflection, so that the inner hair cells are stimulated at the "resonance point" as a **cochlear amplifier**. Beyond the resonance point, the vibrations are strongly damped, which further increases the **frequency selectivity of the inner ear**. The deflection of the stereovilli caused by an increased amplitude of vibration of the basilar membrane induces a depolarization of the inner hair cells. However, depolarization does not cause a change in length in inner hair cells, but rather the release of the transmitter glutamate and an activation of the afferent nerve fibres.

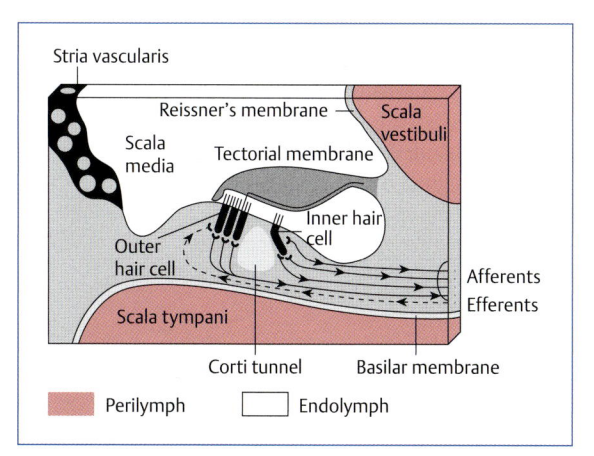

Fig. 3.17 Organ of Corti. The hair cells surrounded by supporting cells form the organ of Corti on the basilar membrane. They are arranged in one row of inner hair cells and three rows of outer hair cells. Only the stereovilli of the outer hair cells have permanent contact with the overlying tectorial membrane, the inner hair cells only during deflections of the basilar membrane. The afferent innervation of the hair cells takes place through neurons in the spiral ganglion. Here, >90% are myelinated type I fibres, all of which are in contact with the inner hair cells, while the unmyelinated type II fibres exclusively innervate the outer hair cells.

IN A NUTSHELL   !

The transduction of the sound stimulus in the inner ear is a three-stage process: 1. formation of a travelling wave, 2. amplification by outer hair cells and 3. activation of the inner hair cells.

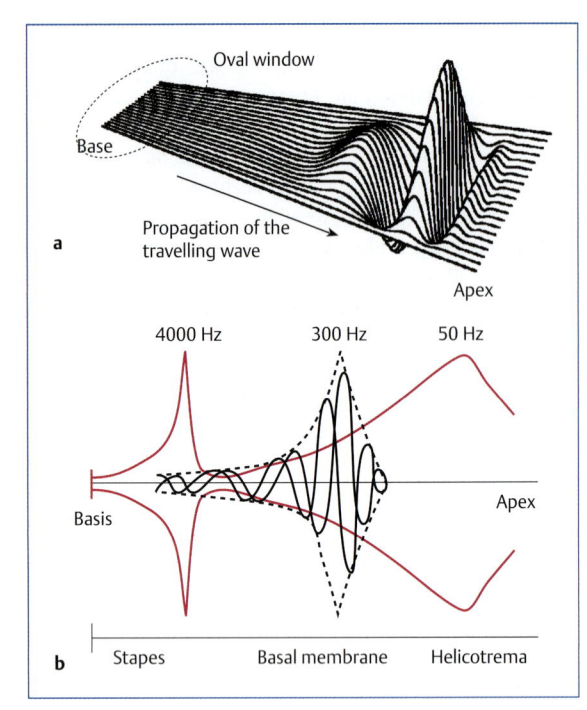

Fig. 3.18 **a** Three-dimensional representation of the travelling wave on the basilar membrane. The wavelength of the travelling wave becomes shorter and shorter along the membrane, while its amplitude increases to a maximum (envelope curve) and then dies off. **b** Travelling waves and their envelopes at different frequencies. The location of the maximum deflection corresponds to the wavelength of the sound. High-frequency travelling waves of 4000 Hz (short wavelength) have their greatest amplitude near the oval window. Low frequencies of 50 Hz (long wavelengths) reach their amplitude maximum at the helicotrema.

■ Frequency analysis of the cochlea

The frequency of a sound signal is transformed to a location of maximum response on the basilar membrane. This is due to the mechanical properties of the basilar membrane, which becomes increasingly thicker and wider from the base to the apex. In this way, a continuous gradient of decreasing stiffness is created. Each wave travels apically from the base with increasing amplitude and shorter wave periods until it reaches its maximum at the resonance point of the basilar membrane responsible for the stimulus frequency; then it rapidly decays (**Fig. 3.18 a**). For each sound frequency there is a specific point on the basilar membrane that is deflected to the maximum (= **frequency-location transformation**, Fig. 3.18 b). At the beginning of the basilar membrane the high tones and at the apex the low tones are mapped accordingly. The auditory nerve uses two strategies for frequency coding. According to this frequency-location mapping, each inner hair cell with its afferent fibres is assigned to a characteristic frequency. Thus, a spatial analysis is performed, which is basically an analysis of the frequencies of a sound. Each frequency is assigned to a specific afferent fibre and thus the pitch is encoded. In addition to the spatial analysis, the temporal pattern of action potentials in axons of the auditory nerve is used for coding. Since the times for triggering action potentials are related to the frequency of the sound stimuli, so-called phase-coupled action potentials are generated. Therefore, the sound frequency can be determined from the temporal pattern of action potentials (**periodicity analysis**).

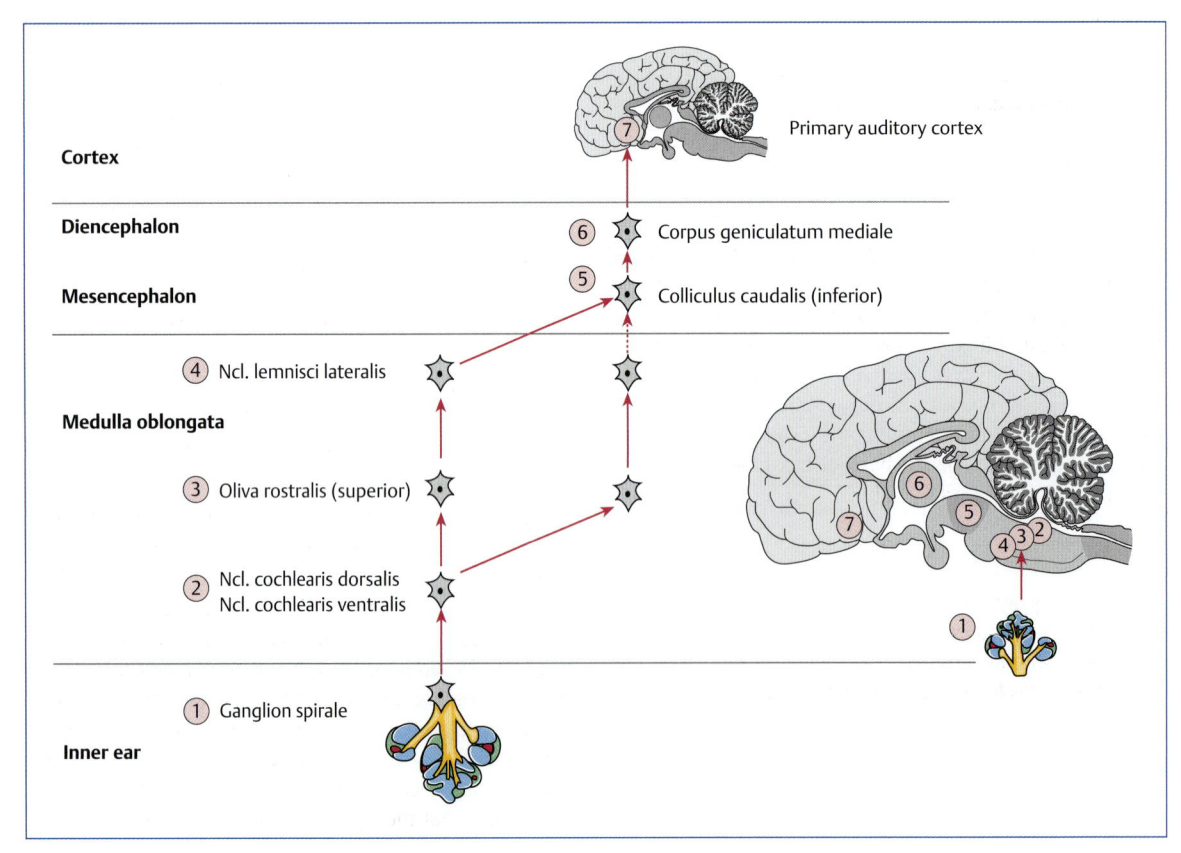

Fig. 3.19 Schematic representation of the central auditory pathway.

3.4.5 Neuronal processing of auditory signals

The neuronal activity of the afferent fibres in the VIII cranial nerve, the auditory nerve, triggered by suprathreshold stimulation of the hair cells, is processed in specialised brain regions of the auditory system. The bipolar somata of the auditory nerve in the **spiral ganglion** innervate the hair cells with the distal part of their axon and project with the proximal part to the **cochlear nuclei in the myelencephalon**. Here they form the first synapse during the processing of auditory information. Then the central ascending auditory pathway starts consisting of 5–6 neurons connected in series, which finally leads to the auditory cortex in the temporal lobe. Along this path, the fibres remain cochlea-topically ordered, i.e., throughout the course of the auditory pathway, the positions of the basilar membrane are represented in an orderly fashion. The projection of the neural pathways from the cochlear nuclei to the **superior olive** is partly contralateral and partly ipsilateral. Through the decussation of the auditory pathway, each inner ear is connected to the right and left auditory cortex. Therefore, for the first time in the course of the auditory pathway, binaural acoustic signals (recorded by both ears) can be compared in the olive complex. From here, a contralateral and ipsilateral projection to the **caudal colliculus** (ncl. olivaris rostralis, colliculus inferior) takes place in the midbrain and then to a specialised thalamic region (**corpus geniculatum mediale**). From there, the auditory pathway projects to the primary auditory cortex, where together with the surrounding secondary auditory cortex, the further processing of information takes place (**Fig. 3.19**). Overall, all central nervous stations of the auditory pathway are organised tonotopically, so that different sound frequencies (pitches) are processed in different neuron layers in the caudal colliculus. The localisation of a sound source requires binaural hearing and takes place in the cochlear nuclei, where so-called coincidence neurons play a central role. In the case of a horizontally displaced sound source, a spatial representation of the sound source is created for the two ears on the basis of the different duration and strength of a sound stimulus.

Suggested reading

Hudspeth JA. Making an effort to listen: Mechanical amplification in the ear. Neuron 2008; 59: 530–545

Moller AR. Hearing: Anatomy, physiology and disorders of the auditory system. 3rd Edition. San Diego: Plural Publishing; 2012

Phillips KR et al. How hair cells hear: the molecular basis of hair cell mechanotransduction. Curr Opin Head Neck Surg 2008; 16: 455–451

Schwander M. et al. The cell biology of hearing. J Cell Biol 2010; 190: 9–20

Sjaastad ØV, Hove K, Sand O. Physiology of Domestic Animals. Oslo: Scandinavian Veterinary Press; 2007

3.5 Vision

Cornelia A. Deeg

ESSENTIALS

How animals see the world is a fascinating topic from the human perspective, but it is also very difficult to investigate. The evolutionary development of the eye is phylogenetically of great interest, because insects and crustaceans have eyes with far better visual function than those in the otherwise more evolutionarily advanced mammals. This relates to colour perception, accommodation potency and spectral range. During evolution, these capabilities were apparently abandoned, only to be reintroduced in some mammals and humans with gene duplication of the mid-wavelength cone which allows perception of an increased range of colours. In this chapter, the general physiology of the eye is discussed, and animal-specific characteristics are highlighted.

The **organ of vision** includes the **eye**, the **optic nerves**, the accessory organs such as the lacrimal gland, eyelids and extrabulbar muscles, the central **visual pathways** and the **visual centre** of the cerebral hemispheres. The eye is a very complex sensory organ that uses a lens system to image the environment and, with the help of neuronal networks in the retina, detects and transduces light stimuli and transmits the corresponding information to the cerebrum. **Photosensors** of the retina convert the incident photons into neuronal signals, which are then processed first in the retina and later in the visual centres of the brain. The perception of an image originates in the brain and is a subjective and individually learned process.

Vision is a very important sense for most species. When we see, information about an object passes through the anterior chamber of the eye, the lens, and the vitreous body onto the **retina**. There the first information processing by neurons takes place. Information about the brightness, colour and size/orientation of the object is recorded by the **neuronal network** of the retina. It is then passed via the **optic nerves** to the **brain** where the signals are again processed and converted to a three-dimensional image. The optic nerves decussate at the optic chiasm and divide in such a way that the right hemisphere of the brain receives the information about the left side of the visual field of both eyes and vice versa for the left hemisphere.

The actual processing of the visual information in the retina varies according to the animal species. This is particularly evident in colour vision where the spectrum of visible light and the ability to detect colours differ greatly. Colours are detected by specialised **photosensors** (**cones**). Their number, distribution and specificity varies from species to species. Brightness is detected by **rods** in the retina. This information is processed in the retina by three neurons and is then passed via the optic nerve to the thalamus and the visual cortex. A perceived image is then formed in the visual cortex. The sensory impression of seeing is composed of **physical information** such as illumination, colour, contrast, form and movement, but also from **expectations** based on previous experience and **interpretations** of the brain.

3.5.1　Structure of the eye

■ Anatomical basics

The wall of the eye is anatomically and functionally divided into three layers (**Fig. 3.20**). The **outer layer** is formed by the **cornea** in the anterior part of the eye and is continued in the posterior region by the **sclera**. This layer has a mainly protective and supporting function and ensures the stable structure of the eyeball. To enable light transparency, the collagen fibres of the cornea are precisely aligned, with the lamellae of one layer lying parallel to each other at equal distances. The outer layer of collagen lamellae has a different spatial orientation, but is equally well ordered. Any damage to this structure leads to swelling of the fibres from water penetration, and thus to clouding of the cornea. A corneal transplant is a method of repair if the cornea is extensively damaged. The sclera preserves the structure of the eyeball so that the cornea and the retina retain their shape and distance. This stable framework prevents deformations that could affect visual acuity.

The **middle layer** of the eye wall is called the **uvea**. This consists of the **iris**, the **ciliary body**, and the **choroid**. The main blood vessels of the eye run through the choroid. In the anterior third of the eye, the iris bulges out to form the **ciliary muscle**, which, as a ring muscle, regulates by constriction or dilation the amount of light entering the eye. The **lens** is also attached to the ciliary muscle via the zonular fibres. Inside the posterior segment of the eye is the **vitreous body** which fills two thirds of the interior volume of the eye. The function of the vitreous body in the adult animal is largely unclear.

The **inner wall layer** of the eye is formed by the **retina**, from which axons of the retinal ganglion cells (3rd neuron) travel to the brain as the optic nerve. The retina contains the nuclei of the rod and cone photosensors in the outer granular layer, which detect light and colour respectively. In the inner granular layer are the nuclei of the horizontal, bipolar and amacrine cells (2nd neuron), which are re-

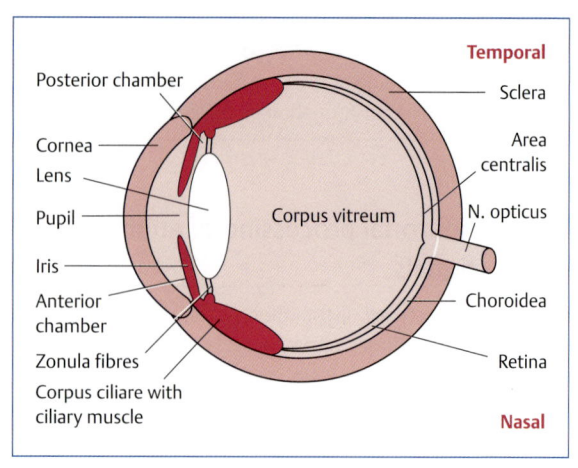

Fig. 3.20 Horizontal section through the eye.

sponsible for the further processing (lateral and horizontal connections) of the neuronal signals. These cells amplify or suppress information from the photosensors (1st neuron) and thus decide what is ultimately reported to the brain via the ganglion cells. The blood supply to the retina is partially from the choroidal vessels, but there are major differences between species, in the vascular supply of the retina. This is seen particularly in the horse retina, which is largely avascular.

■ Physical basics

An optical system is characterised by light rays being refracted when passing from one medium to another, if the optical densities of the two media are different. Where there is a spherical interface between two media, this results in a real image (**Fig. 3.21**). Incident rays are deflected at the transition from one optical medium to another and collect at the rear focal point (F_r). In a reverse optical path (which, however, plays no physiological role in the eye), rays falling perpendicularly on the rear surface of a lens would collect in the front focal point (F_f). The line connecting the front and rear focal points is called the **optical axis**. Strictly speaking, light is refracted twice when passing through a spherical lens, firstly when entering the lens and again when leaving it. However, to simplify matters, one can describe a lens as if parallel rays were refracted at a fictitious principal plane in such a way that they are deflected towards the opposite focal point. The point of intersection of the principal plane with the optical axis is called the principal point (P; **Fig. 3.21**). An optical system is characterised by the **refractive power** which is calculated from the reciprocal of the front focal length (F_f-P) in metres, and is expressed in dioptres. The refractive power of a lens depends on its curvature and essentially on the refractive indices of the media involved in the refraction. Air has a refractive index of 1.0, while liquids have a refractive index of >1.3 depending on the substances dissolved in them. The more the refractive indices vary, the stronger the refraction.

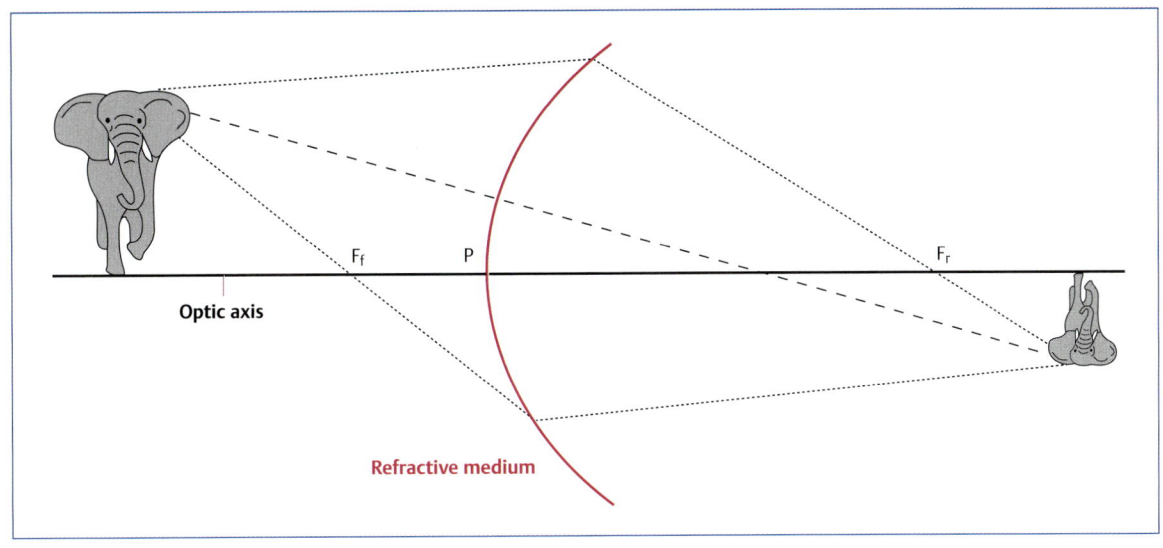

Fig. 3.21 Imaging through a simple optical system.
P = principal point, F_f = front focal point, F_r = rear focal point.

> **IN A NUTSHELL** !
>
> The refractive power of an optical system depends on the curvature of the interfaces and the refractive indices of the surrounding media.

■ Chamber fluid

The anterior chamber of the eye continuously produces **aqueous humour** which is released by the ciliary body or the posterior iris epithelium and keeps the intraocular pressure constant. In domestic animals, outflow is usually through larger vessels of the uveoscleral venous plexus and not, as in humans, through Schlemm's canal. The aqueous humour has a low protein content (about 1% that of blood plasma) with essentially the same composition as blood plasma, but also containing factors produced in the eye such as the cytokine TGF-β (transforming growth factor-β). In contrast to blood plasma, it has a higher lactate and chloride content. The proteins are released into the anterior chamber of the eye and cannot enter the posterior chamber because of the tight junctions of the iris epithelium.

On average, humans produce about 3 µl of aqueous humour per minute. A pathological increase in intraocular pressure (**glaucoma**) can be caused either by an increased production of aqueous humour or by an obstruction of its outflow. The intraocular pressure can increase from the physiological state of 20 mmHg up to 60 mmHg which can lead to secondary degeneration of the sensory cells of the retina. In domestic animals, the primary risk of glaucoma is much lower than in humans due to outflow via the venous plexus.

> **IN A NUTSHELL** !
>
> The aqueous humour essentially determines the intraocular pressure.

■ Dioptric apparatus

The eye is a composite optical system. The entirety of all light-refracting structures in the eye is summarised under the term dioptric apparatus. **Refraction** is the deviation of light rays when they pass through media of a different optical density. In the eye, light coming from the air is transmitted through the tear fluid, the cornea and the anterior chamber of the eye with aqueous humour, the lens and finally through the vitreous body onto the retina as an inverted, reduced image.

The main refraction at the eye (approx. two thirds of the total refraction) takes place at the transition from the medium air to the tear fluid, as there the refractive indices differ the most. In animals living under water or when diving, the refractive power of the eye is correspondingly significantly reduced. The cornea itself is avascular and abundantly permeated with myelin-free nerve fibres. These nerve fibres have an important protective function for the eye as part of the corneal reflex. Enzymes and secretory immunoglobulin A contained in it also protect against infections. The cornea is nourished by the tear fluid via diffusion which also protects it from drying out. The lacrimal **glands** are located dorsolateral to the eye and release tear fluid into the conjunctival sac. Outflow is via the lacrimal duct and lacrimal sac to the nasal cavity.

> **IN A NUTSHELL** !
>
> The eye is a composite optical system. The main refraction of the eye takes place at the cornea.

The active change in the refractive power of the eye is called **accommodation**. The dioptric apparatus requires a higher refractive power to produce a sharp image of near objects than for distant objects, since the focal length (f), refractive power (F), object width (g) and the image width (b), which is constant in the eye due to the fixed distance between the retina and the dioptric apparatus, are related as follows:

$$\frac{1}{f} = F = \frac{g+b}{g \cdot b} \qquad (3.1)$$

The maximum achievable change in refractive power between far and near vision is called the width of accommodation. The ciliary muscle is mainly parasympathetically innervated for near vision, but also has a small degree of sympathetic innervation. Therefore, in the absence of an accommodation target, it maintains a certain resting tone, which is determined by the dynamic balance between the two types of innervation. If the focus on an object changes, the brain registers that the image is out of focus and activates the oculomotor centres. For near vision, one needs the maximum possible **curvature of the lens**. In humans and many other mammals, this is made possible by the inherent elasticity of the lens. The maximum **near adjustment** of the lens (**Fig. 3.22** left picture) is made possible by a distinct curvature, which depends on its inherent elasticity. Contraction of the annular ciliary muscle allows the lens to change shape and thus maximise refraction of rays at the lens for near vision, by slackening the zonula fibres (lens ligaments). For distant vision, the ciliary muscle relaxes and the lens is pulled flat by the zonula fibres. The ciliary muscle is essentially parasympathetically innervated via the oculomotor nerve. Accommodation between near and distant settings takes place very quickly, the reaction being completed in 1.5 seconds.

Analysis of the properties of the ciliary muscle and lens of different animals allows conclusions to be drawn about the possible width of accommodation and thus of vision. The **width of accommodation** is sometimes significantly different in domestic mammals compared to humans. Horses, for example, have a very rigid lens and weakly developed ciliary muscles, which suggests a low capacity for accommodation. In contrast, the refractive power of the dog's lens is more than twice that of humans. In reptiles, birds and aquatic mammals, lens curvature is altered by contraction of circular muscles of the iris. In birds, accommodation often involves an additional change in corneal curvature, as they can actively lengthen or shorten the bulb axis. Amphibians and snakes, on the other hand, have another accommodation mechanism by changing the distance between the rigid lens and the retina.

> **IN A NUTSHELL**   !
>
> The change in lens refractive power (accommodation) is the prerequisite for focusing on objects at different distances.

■ Short-sightedness, far-sightedness and presbyopia

Classic short-sightedness and far-sightedness are caused by a congenital deviation of the eyeball length from the physiological length. In short-sightedness (**myopia**) light rays coming from distant objects intersect in front of the retina because the eyeball is too long for the optical system (remedied by diverging lens).

With far-sightedness (**hyperopia**) the eyeball is too short, so near accommodation is necessary when looking into the distance (remedial action with a converging lens). **Presbyopia** (aging eye condition resulting in far-sightedness) has a completely different cause. The lens epithelium is located on the front surface of the lens, under the lens capsule. These epithelial cells divide and elongate and continuously differentiate into lens fibres. The lens therefore grows throughout its life by means of the lens fibres that are deposited on it. However, no cells can be lost from the lens capsule, which is why the nucleus is constantly enlarging and condensing. Therefore, the width of accommodation also decreases with age, as the lens is no longer as elastic. This ageing process of the lens can be observed in all mammals.

3.5.2 Reflex sequences
■ Reflexes for near vision

The light waves of an approaching object are first focussed behind the retina. Information about the blurred image is then transmitted to the visual centres of the brain. The activated oculomotor centres in the midbrain then lead the accommodation reaction via the oculomotor neurons. At the same time, parasympathetic nerve fibres are activated. This leads to the contraction of the ciliary muscles which **increases the curvature of the lens**. The **pupil diameter** is also reduced to improve the depth of field.

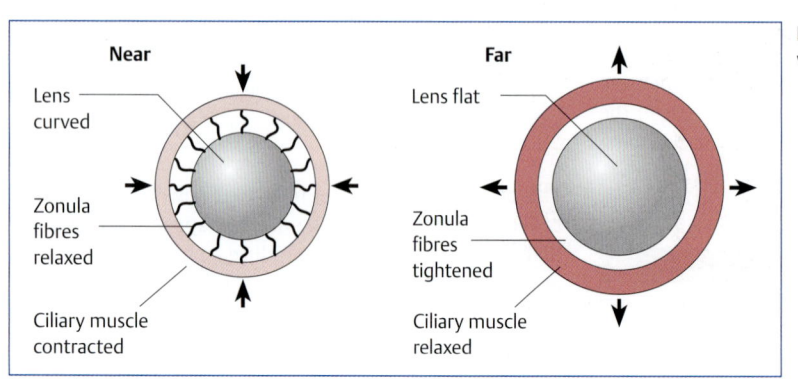

Fig. 3.22 Mechanism of near and distant vision (accommodation).

IN A NUTSHELL !

To keep the image sharp, the lens must constantly accommodate.

Pupillary reflexes

The amount of light entering the eye depends on the width of the **pupil**. Increasing the retinal luminance causes a reflex constriction of the pupil to protect the eye from glare. The **reflex arc** travels from the retinal photosensors via the optic nerves to the midbrain and from there to the oculomotor nucleus. In some animals, the pupil, which is round when open, is concentrically constricted, whereas in cats it is closed to form a vertical slit. In mammals, the exposure of one eye always leads to a constriction of the pupil in the other eye (consensual reflex). States where there is an increase in the sympathicoadrenal system (e.g. through fear) leads to a dilation of the pupils. Observation of the pupillary reaction is part of the neurological examination (cranial nerves II and III) and is used when monitoring the depth of anaesthesia.

> **MORE DETAILS** In light and very deep anaesthesia, the pupil is dilated, whereas it is constricted in the tolerance stage. In light anaesthesia, pain stimuli still have an effect, leading to dilation. In medium-depth anaesthesia, there is increased parasympathetic tone and pupil constriction. With very deep anaesthesia, the pupil is dilated again because of central paralysis of the oculomotor nerve. The pupil width cannot be used as an indication of the depth of anaesthesia with some premedications, for example, if atropine or other parasympatholytics have been given (leading to mydriasis) or if analgesia was obtained with morphine-like analgesics (miosis).

3.5.3 Signal reception and processing of light stimuli in the retina

Structure of the retina and signal processing

The **retina** contains the sensory cells of the eye. They detect light stimuli of different wavelengths and thus also enable colour vision. A total of five different cell types can be distinguished (**Fig. 3.23**) that are involved in the processing of light stimuli. The sensory cells that convert the electromagnetic energy of light into electrochemical signals are located in the outermost layer of the retina. Thus, light must first pass through the entire retina before it is registered. On the outside, the **photosensors** border the non-neuronal **pigment cells** which contain the pigment **melanin**. Melanin blackens the inside of the eye and thus prevents light reflections. A chain of three neurons is needed in the retina to process the stimuli and pass on the information. In this chain, the photosensors are the 1st neuron, which are initially connected to **bipolar cells** (2nd neuron). The bipolar cells inform **ganglion cells** (3rd neuron) about the activity of the photosensors. The axons of the ganglion cells unite to form the **optic nerve** and travel to the brain. Since there are no sensory cells in the area where the optic nerve exits (optic disc), this zone is insensitive to light (**blind spot**). Horizontal connections between the photosensors and bipolar cells are formed by **horizontal cells and amacrine cells**. Information about the state of a single photosensor cell is passed on to several ganglion cells (**divergence**), while signals of many photosensor cells are reported to one ganglion cell (**convergence**). Divergence and convergence are typical properties of neuronal networks and always occur simultaneously. This allows a high flexibility in the processing of information. The ganglion cells inform the brain about the activity in their retinal receptive field, which is composed of all subordinate cells that connect to a ganglion cell. The ratio of 1 photosensor

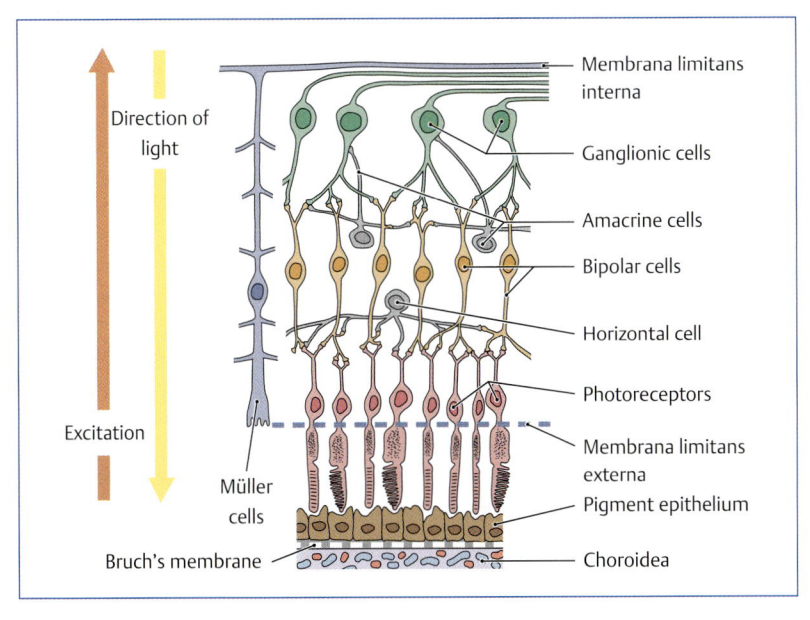

Fig. 3.23 Schematic structure of the retina. [Source: Aumüller G, Aust G, Conrad A et al. (eds.). Duale Reihe Anatomie. 4th, updated ed. Stuttgart: Thieme; 2017, Fig. M. 5.16a]

Direction of light

Excitation

Müller cells

Bruch's membrane

Membrana limitans interna

Ganglionic cells

Amacrine cells

Bipolar cells

Horizontal cell

Photoreceptors

Membrana limitans externa

Pigment epithelium

Choroidea

to 1 bipolar cell to 1 ganglion cell (at the site of sharpest vision, called the macula in humans) is the ideal ratio for sharp vision.

The photosensor cells are either **rods or cones**. Rods are so sensitive to light that they are excited by a single photon in extreme dark adaptation (p.96), but they cannot detect colour. Cones have a lower sensitivity to light but contain pigments that can absorb colours of certain wavelengths. This enables **colour vision** under daylight conditions.

MORE DETAILS In humans, there are only cones at the point of sharpest vision. In addition, the density of ganglion cells is much higher than in the periphery of the retina, so that there is an interconnection of almost one photosensor per ganglion cell. This ensures that the CNS has immediate information about the excitation state of each cone in this region. Rods are mainly found in the periphery of the retina. There, the ratio of sensory cell to ganglion cell is about 100:1 in humans. This increases the light sensitivity of the ganglion cell, but reduces the spatial resolution, which is why the periphery of the retina is unsuitable for sharp vision.

The distribution of cones and rods on the retina is species-specific and also varies from individual to individual. The density of the sensory cells determines the **spatial resolution**. For example, a high density of sensory cells helps hawks and eagles to achieve 2–6 times better distance vision compared to humans. The visual acuity of the eye depends on its spatial resolution. The decisive factor is whether two closely related points can still be perceived separately. Temporal resolution is the extent to which a rapid succession of individual stimuli can be recognised separately from one another. It has been proven that pigeons and birds of prey can perceive 150 individual images per second and are thus far superior to humans (approx. 30 individual images/second). This is likely to play an important role for manoeuvrability in flight. The higher **single-frame resolution of birds** means that the animal welfare suitability of artificial lighting needs to be considered. Neon tubes, for example, have a flicker frequency that is likely to be perceived by birds as constant flickering light. This example shows that we must not assume that animals perceive the environment in the same way as we do.

The distribution of cones and rods in the retina varies from animal to animal. Diurnal animals have many cones, which are responsible for colour vision (**photopic vision**). A majority of rods are found in cats, rabbits and owls. In these crepuscular animals, colour vision has also been demonstrated in these animals because of the presence of a few cones.

MORE DETAILS In most animals, there are also areas of the retina that are specialised for high spatial resolution. In nocturnal animals these areas are almost exclusively occupied by rods. Nocturnal animals such as rats and mice have a total of only 1–3% cones in the retina, a significant reduction in favour of the more light-sensitive rods. Birds have a favourable, low number ratio between photosensors and ganglion cells throughout the retina, which leads to a high visual acuity. Steppe animals have a horizontal strip of sharpest vision with which the horizon can be observed. This has also been demonstrated in the horse. However, horses have only a few areas within the retina that enable sharp vision. Therefore, many objects are probably perceived only dimly. Overall, in the horse retina, the ganglion cell density is very low, apart from two small specialised areas, so that a low resolving power must be assumed.

Each photosensor cell has an outer segment that is connected to the rest of the cell body via a thin cell part. In this outer segment there are numerous membrane discs or membrane folds, each with its own embedded photopigment. These are chromophores such as retinal (retinaldehyde) and various proteins. In rods, the chromophore is rhodopsin and in cones there are other opsins. These outer segments are renewed throughout life and the rejected components are removed by phagocytes in the pigment epithelial layer.

> **IN A NUTSHELL** !
>
> The eye has two different sensory cells. Rods show the lowest absolute threshold of light and are responsible for black and white vision. Cones enable colour vision.

■ Photoreception and transduction

Vertebrate photosensors are sensors that, unlike the vast majority of other sensory cells, do **not depolarize** when **stimulated**, but instead they **hyperpolarize**. In the **dark**, there is a continuous Na^+ influx across the rod membrane, the cell is thus **depolarized**. Here, cGMP as a second messenger molecule keeps the non-selective cation channels of the outer segment membrane open. The depolarizing Na^+ and Ca^{2+} influx into the photosensor cell causes a constant release of transmitter (glutamate) at the synapse. The bipolar cells activated by this, in turn have an inhibitory effect on the ganglion cell. In the state of inhibition, the ganglion cells send no information to the brain and thus indicate darkness. When light enters, the cation channels of the photosensors close so that the membrane hyperpolarizes. This reduces transmitter release. The bipolar cells no longer inhibit the ganglion cells and information is transmitted to the brain, see ch. "Sensory systems" (p.135). This means that retinal sensory cells secrete more transmitters in darkness than in brightness. **Phototransduction** is such a sensitive mechanism that in humans with extreme dark adaptation the absolute threshold of vision is 1–4 light quanta per rod per second. Cones are about 100 times less sensitive to light than rods. There are differences in these processes in various species of animals. In lizards, for example, depolarization occurs after exposure to light. No cell types other than photosensors and ganglion cells have been detected in the lizard retina.

It is the task of the photosensors to convert the incoming physical energy (light quanta) into signals that can be "read" by neurons. This process is called **transduction**. Rods and cones use a signal transduction cascade that generally consists of the same components (**Fig. 3.24**). These include opsin, 11-cis-retinal, transducin and a phosphodiesterase. The **protein opsin** and the **chromophore 11-cis-retinal** (aldehyde of retinol or vitamin A) form **rhodopsin** in the rods. 11-cis-retinal can absorb light due to a sequence of conjugated double bonds. By binding to opsin, its absorption maximum is shifted into the wavelength range of visible light. After light absorption, 11-cis-retinal changes its configuration from the 11-cis- to the all-trans-form in picoseconds due to an energy transfer (all-trans-

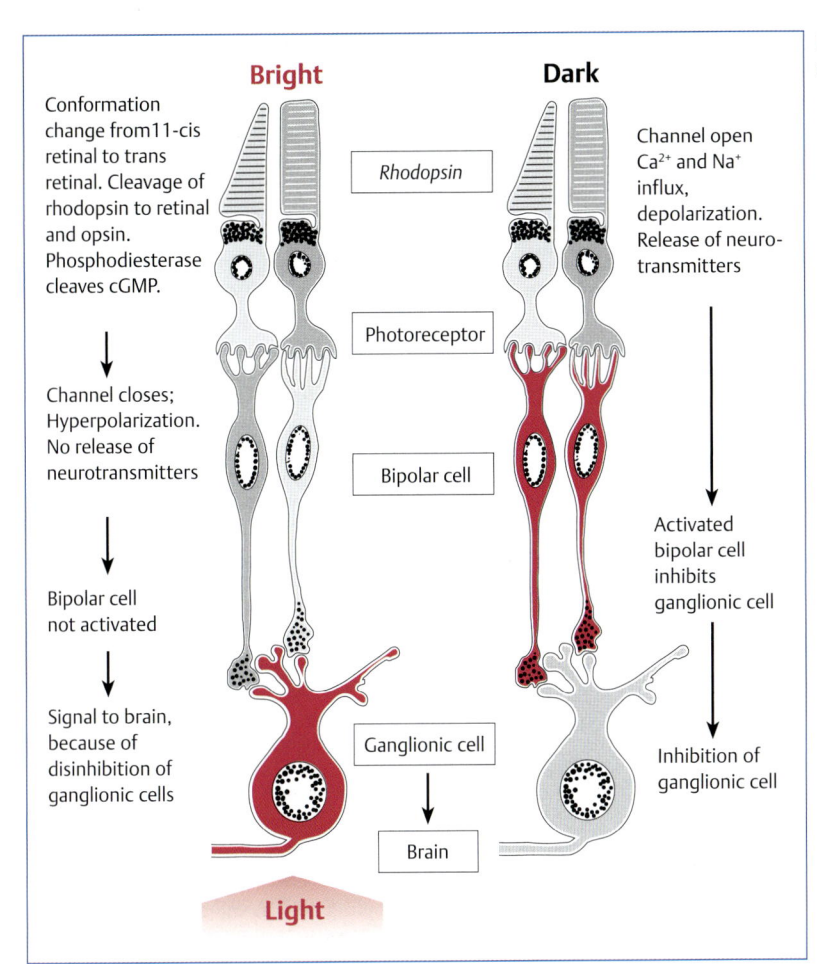

Bright

Conformation change from 11-cis retinal to trans retinal. Cleavage of rhodopsin to retinal and opsin. Phosphodiesterase cleaves cGMP.

↓

Channel closes; Hyperpolarization. No release of neurotransmitters

↓

Bipolar cell not activated

↓

Signal to brain, because of disinhibition of ganglionic cells

Rhodopsin

Photoreceptor

Bipolar cell

Ganglionic cell

Brain

Light

Dark

Channel open Ca^{2+} and Na^{+} influx, depolarization. Release of neuro-transmitters

↓

Activated bipolar cell inhibits ganglionic cell

↓

Inhibition of ganglionic cell

Fig. 3.24 Transduction process in the outer element of a photosensor.

to rods is the use of opsin isoforms (cone opsins with different colour spectra) instead of rhodopsin as in the rod. This allows the detection of a narrow range of visible light and colour vision. All other molecules of the signal transduction cascade remain the same.

> **IN A NUTSHELL** !
>
> Transduction is the conversion of a stimulus into an excitation of neuronal elements. Light stimuli lead to hyperpolarization in rods and cones.

3.5.4   Tapetum lucidum

Most domestic mammals as well as nocturnal reptiles possess a **tapetum lucidum**. Depending on the species, this has a specific localisation and structure. There is a tapetum lucidum in the choroid, which in carnivores and rodents is made up of cells or of fibrous origin in herbivores. A tapetum lucidum may be in the retina, for example in the crocodile. In histological section, this light-reflecting layer is found between the pigment epithelium and the blood vessels under the retina (choroidal tapetum lucidum). As a component, the cells of the cellular tapetum lucidum contain crystals such as zinc cysteine hydrate (dog) or riboflavin (cat). Photons that have passed through the neuronal layers of the retina are reflected by the tapetum lucidum

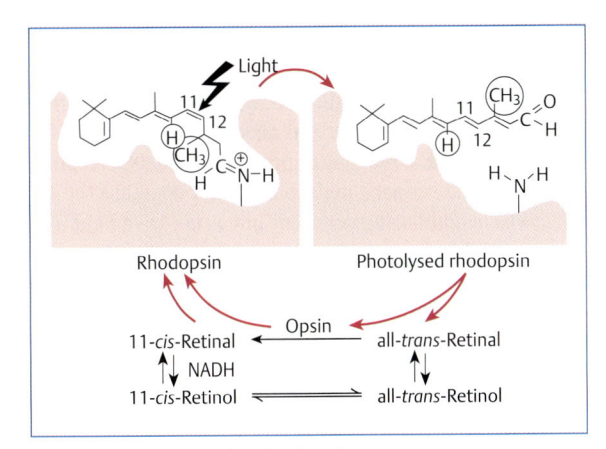

Fig. 3.25 Vitamin A in the visual cycle.

retinal; **stereoisomerisation**; **Fig. 3.25**). This rearrangement leads to the dissociation of opsin, which also changes structurally and thus becomes enzymatically active. One active opsin now activates up to 3000 transducin molecules. Transducin belongs to the family of GTP-binding proteins. It activates a phosphodiesterase, whereby cGMP molecules are hydrolytically cleaved. The decrease in concentration of the second messenger cGMP causes the cGMP-dependent cation channels to close, leading to hyperpolarization with reduced transmitter release. This cascade proceeds in the same way in the cones. The difference and can thus stimulate the receptor cells again. This enables better vision at night because the low light stimuli are better utilised. Animals with a tapetum lucidum are easily recognisable to the observer by their green to blue reflecting eyes as soon as they are illuminated by a light source in the dark.

3.5.5   Adaptation mechanisms

Adaptation is the term used to describe how the eye adapts to different levels of illuminance. In order to be able to process extreme changes in luminosity, which can vary by an order of magnitude of $1:10^{12}$ between bright day and dark night, the eye has various adaptation mechanisms. Since the eye can be exposed to very different intensities of illumination, but never bright sunshine and darkness at the same time, the eye only measures currently occurring differences in illuminance and not absolute light intensities. The retina is therefore only able to distinguish between brightness within a narrow range of luminosity and automatically adapts to the prevailing lighting conditions.

An important protective function against overexposure is the **pupil reflex**. The pigmented iris changes the amount of incident light by varying the width of the pupil. For this regulation, most animals possess two antagonistically acting smooth muscles (m. sphincter pupillae and m. dilatator pupillae), which are controlled by **parasympathetic** (sphincter muscle, **miosis**) and **sympathetic** (dilated, **mydriasis**) nerves.

Furthermore, the concentration of **visual pigments**, which are in a dynamic balance between consumption (bleaching) and regeneration, contributes significantly to adaptation. The sensitivity threshold for photoreception decreases when more photopigment is bleached than regenerated. The increased consumption of photopigments thus leads very quickly to **brightness adaptation** (in seconds, with full expression after 5 minutes). In contrast, **dark adaptation** takes 30–60 minutes and is initiated by a higher regeneration than consumption of photopigments. **Light adaptation** with the adaptation of the sensory cells to longer, stronger light irradiation proceeds very quickly because a fade is more dangerous for the neuronal network of the eye than too little exposure. Since the eye is part of the central nervous system, damage to the photoreceptors is irreversible.

The change in sensitivity of the rods takes place via transducin. With strong light incidence, transducin is shifted from the outer segment to other compartments of the rod. This reduction in transducin content correlates directly with the reduced rod response at increased illuminance. Dark adaptation occurs in two phases, an initial rapid (5–10 minutes) adaptation of the cones and a prolonged (up to 60 minutes) adaptation of the rods. It is possible that the presence of cone opsin in the dark contributes to dark adaptation because it activates the signal transduction cascade. However, the molecular mechanisms involved in light and dark adaptation are still under investigation because they have not been definitively clarified.

> **IN A NUTSHELL**   !
>
> The eye adapts to different illuminance levels (adaptation) by changing the pupil width and the ratio of bleached and regenerated visual pigment.

3.5.6   Colour vision

When sunlight (white light) is split by a prism, a coloured spectrum from violet to red is produced. This corresponds to a wavelength of 400–750 nm.

MORE DETAILS   According to the theory of trichromatic vision (von Helmholtz), light absorption in the retina in humans is provided by three different types of cones. The complementary colour theory (according to Hering) assumes that the perception of the colour pairs red-green, blue-yellow and black-white, is antagonistically connected. This means that the impression of these colours inhibits each other when the excitation originates from the same place. Counter-colour neurons have been detected at the level of the visual cortex, so that both colour vision theories can be integrated into the visual process.

In humans, the genes for the red and green opsins are located on the X chromosome; they have developed by gene duplication. These proteins are very homologous and the 30 nm difference in the spectrum is due to the exchange of only three amino acids. In humans, the gene for blue opsin is located on chromosome 7 and for rhodopsin on chromosome 3. Deficiencies in the differentiation of the colours red and green are common (2.5% of the population) and predominantly affect males. One type of cone is either completely absent or two cones have the same absorption spectrum. Lack of reception of the colour blue, on the other hand, is very rare and affects men and women equally often.

■ Colour vision of animals

The cones do not provide any information about the wavelength of the incoming stimulus, but always react in the same way when they absorb an adequate wavelength. This depends on the cone opsin present. Colour perception then arises via retinal ganglion cells that compare the response of neighbouring cones within a receptive field. The receptive field of a neuron in a sensory pathway comprises the sum of all receptive fields of all sensors (i.e. rods and cones in the case of the eye) that transmit information to this neuron. Again, convergence is found because many photosensors converge on a few ganglion cells. The proportion of signals from the different cone types are reported to the brain. In most people there are three different cone opsins, named S (short)-, M (middle)- and L (long)-opsin according to their specificity for different wavelengths. Since 2.5% of men genetically express only M- or L-opsin, they are dichromats (referred to as red-green blind).

Colour vision is more than the mere registration of the emitted wavelengths of an object. In addition to the processing of physical information, there are integrative processes in the brain that lead to **perception**. Therefore, it is difficult to determine how animals perceive colours. A first clue is the analysis of the existing sensors in the retina and their absorption maxima. In some cases, this reveals considerable differences to humans. Besides humans, only a few primates are **trichromats**. All Old-World monkeys are trichromats, while other monkey species are **dichromats**. The change occurs in the marbled monkeys, where female animals have a third cone pigment, but the males are dichromats. All other domestic mammals are also dichromats, often lacking a cone with a long-wave absorption spectrum. This is why many domestic animals cannot see colours that we perceive as corresponding to orange to red. This applies to bulls, which cannot see the red cloth at a bullfight, or dogs, which cannot recognise a red traffic light as "red".

Interestingly, spectral sensitivity is much more pronounced in many lower animals than in humans and other mammals (**Fig. 3.26**). According to current knowledge, a crustacean (mantis shrimp) has the ability to see most colours. It can distinguish up to twelve primary colours, some of which are in the UV range, and additionally it can differentiate differently polarized light. Birds and insects also often have a broader colour spectrum than mammals. They often have four colour sensors, with an additional one for the UV range. Pigeons are even pentachromats. Therefore, from a human perspective, it is difficult to imagine how these animals perceive their surroundings, because they have a much wider spectrum of colours than we do. For example, invisible to us, birds can additionally detect light with a wavelength in the **UV range**, with photosensors that have an absorption maximum of 340 nm. If you look at the plumage of birds with a UV lamp, you can see a clear sexual dimorphism between males and females that look the same colour to humans. This is why parrots, for example, can immediately recognise with their eyesight, whether another member of the same species is a male or a female.

> **MORE DETAILS** A similar UV receptor has also been found in bees, which in comparison to birds, lack the long-wave cone for the detection of red. Snakes, on the other hand, also see light in the infrared range around 800 nm. Since these completely different perceptions of animals influences their behaviour, further findings in this field are needed to understand the way their vision affects their responses to their environment.

> **IN A NUTSHELL** !
>
> Different types of cones absorb parts of the colour spectrum.

3.5.7　Central processing

■ Image perception

For images to be perceived, processing in the brain is essential. The first step of an object recognition always refers to the outer boundary of that object. This is done by measuring the differences in brightness of an object compared to its surroundings, from which the boundaries are derived. The **receptive fields** of the retinal ganglion cells are circular or ellipsoidal and each ganglion cell informs the CNS about the incidence of light on such a small area of the retina. All images are first reduced to two-dimensional information at the retina, similar to the individual pixels of a television screen. In the **visual cortex** a three-dimensional image is created from the information from both retinas. The prerequisite for this is that each point also preserves the spatial relationships to the other points in the visual field. After synaptic transmission in the thalamus, the information delivered by the axons of the optic nerves reach the **primary visual cortex** (visual cortex; **Fig. 3.27**). The projection that takes place there corresponds to a map of the retina, i.e. cells with receptive fields close to each other pass on the information to cortex cells that are also close to each other. The output of a group of different cortical cells is integrated to form an image.

■ Organisation of the visual cortex

The Nobel Prize winners Hubel and Wieser were able to show that for each point on the retina there is a set of **cortical cells** with the same spatial arrangement, which are organised in so-called columns. Only cells with the same **spatial orientation** are located in each column. These cells react optimally, for example, to short strips of light that

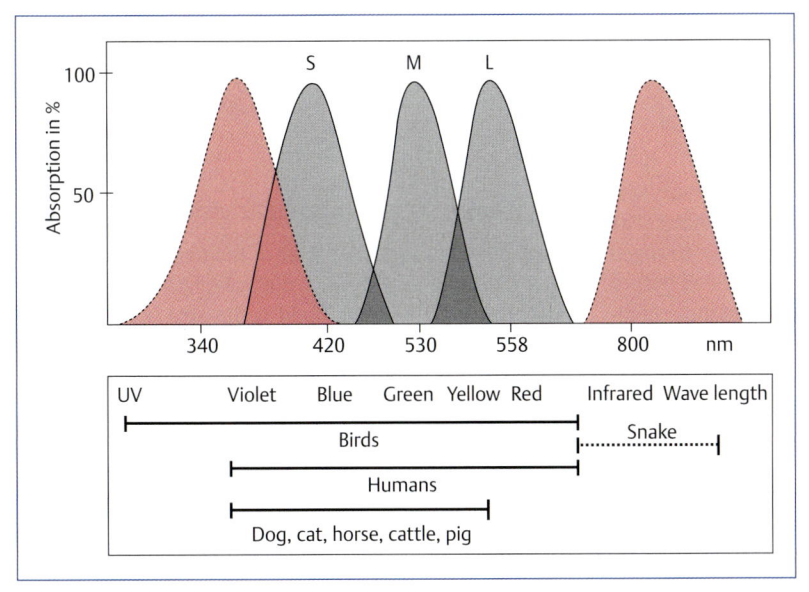

Fig. 3.26 Light absorption maxima of different cone types.

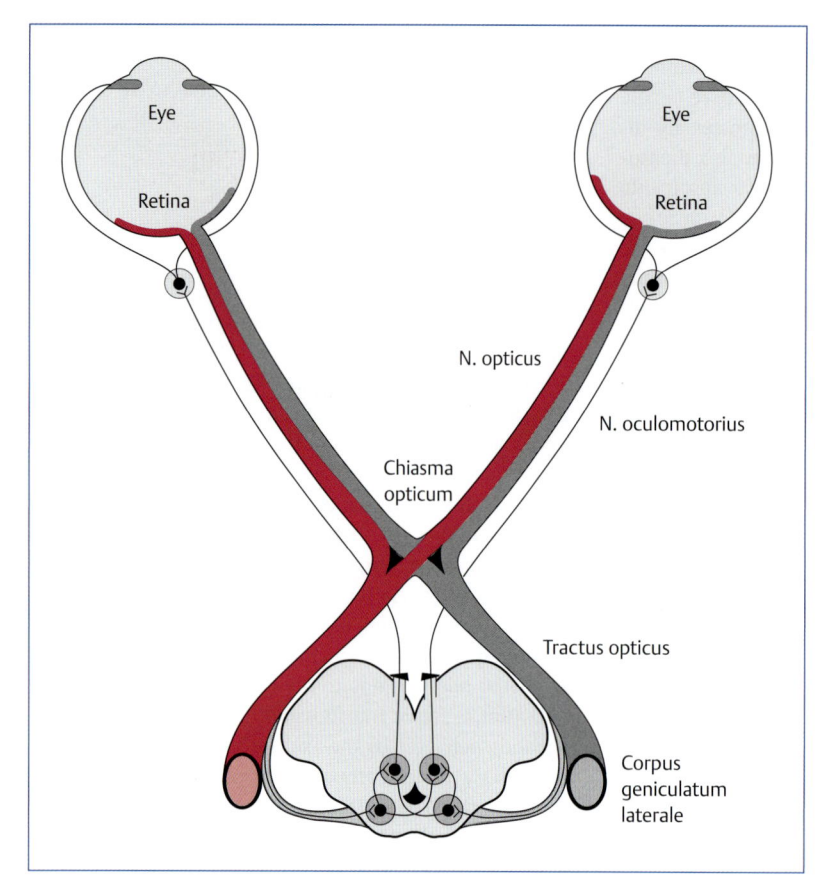

Eye

Retina

N. opticus

Chiasma opticum

N. oculomotorius

Tractus opticus

Eye

Retina

Corpus geniculatum laterale

Fig. 3.27 The visual pathway including parasympathetic innervation of the pupil. In the optic chiasm, a greater or lesser proportion of the nasal fibres of the optic nerve decussate into the contralateral optic tract and reach the lateral geniculate nucleus in the diencephalon. The radiatio optica originating there (not shown in the picture) projects to the visual cortex in the occipital lobe. A small part of the fibres of the tractus opticus does not go to the corpus geniculatum laterale, but terminates in the colliculi craniales (superiores). The consecutive neurons project to the ncl. parasympathicus n. oculomotorii (Edinger-Westphal) in the mesencephalon. The parasympathetic fibres originating there form synapses in the ciliary ganglion directly behind the eyeball and trigger miosis at the pupil.

are imaged on the retina at a very specific angle of inclination. The cells of neighbouring columns, on the other hand, react optimally to light stripes of a minimally different direction. A stimulus with a specific orientation causes the cells of the column with the same orientation to respond most strongly, whereas cells with the opposite orientation show no response. Other neurons respond maximally when the light-dark contour has not only a specific orientation but has interruptions or corners. They are particularly strongly activated by moving stimulus patterns. The totality of simple and complex cells that respond to a certain orientation of the stimulus forms an orientation column.

■ Visual association zones store individual information

Visual association zones (p. 135) surround the primary visual cortex, and these are highly developed in primates. The neurons of the association zones, which are also arranged in columns, integrate and analyse the preprocessed output of the primary visual cortex to recognise even more complex and detailed visual patterns. While lines, orientation and movement play a role in the primary cortex, neurons in the higher visual association zones of the monkey were found to respond exclusively to a complete image of a monkey face. Disfigured faces or other stimuli, on the other hand, induced no response. Cells were even found that only responded to a specific monkey face. This phenomenon has also been demonstrated in sheep. Cells in the cortex

showed a selective response to the face of certain sheep from the flock of tested animals. Information on these integrative processes has also been obtained from people who suffered damage to this cortex area after its normal development. Patients were unable to recognise people very close to them because their faces were apparently stored in these association zones. There seems to be a division into neuron populations for the **recognition** of general features of faces and individual faces. The brain achieves these immense integrative performances with few processing steps in a time of about 150 milliseconds.

> **IN A NUTSHELL** !
>
> The information from the retina is processed into an image in the visual cortex.

■ Visual field and binocular vision

The range of vision is the part of the environment that is perceived when the head is not moving but the eyes are moving freely. The **visual field** is the area perceived with the eyes in a fixed position. Due to the uneven distribution of rods and cones in the retina, the visual field varies in size depending on the colour of the object.

Parts of the field of vision are received by both eyes (= **binocular vision**). This overlapping is necessary for sharp and lifelike vision, because a single eye does not give rise to three-dimensional impressions unless there is partial overlapping with the second field of vision. **Depth** perception results when slightly different images of the same situation are displayed on our two eyes, but ultimately a single image is created from them. This is due to special cells in the visual cortex, which were first discovered in cats. **Binocular** and thus **spatial vision** is a prerequisite for a hunter like the cat to allow it to accurately judge the distances to its prey. The cat's field of vision is 180° with a binocular portion of 100°. It is in this area of overlap that depth perception is possible. While binocular vision is also predominant in humans, some animals, including the horse, hare, and snipe have predominantly monocular vision. In humans, each eye has a visual field of about 150°. The visual field of the right eye and that of the left eye overlap in the middle. This overlap is about 120°.

Depending on how the eyes are arranged (laterally or anteriorly), different numbers of optic nerve fibres also decussate at the **optic chiasm** to the contralateral side of the **visual pathway** (**Fig. 3.27**). In primates, 50% of the fibres decussate, which is the best distribution for spatial vision. In animals with side-set eyes such as ungulates, but also for example mice, 90% of the fibres decussate at the optic chiasm. The proportion of non-crossing fibres correlates directly with the size of the binocular visual field. In general, species with a large binocular visual field are hunters and at the top of the food chain, whereas animals with side-set eyes tend to be those that are hunted and are further down the food chain. For these animals of prey, it is obviously more important to have the widest possible visual field, and high spatial resolution is less important. After the optic chiasm, the fibres run as tractus opticus to the corpus geniculatum laterale in the thalamus. There, they form synapses with a consecutive neuron of the visual pathway (applies to 90% of the fibres) projecting into the primary visual cortex (occipital lobe). The remaining 10% of the fibres are not responsible for visual perceptions, but for accommodation, pupillary reflexes and circadian rhythms. So, after the optic chiasm they project either to the hypothalamus, ciliary ganglia or directly to the visual cortex.

Animals with forward-facing eyes (hunters) have good **spatial resolution** whereas animals with laterally set eyes (hunted) receive little overlapping information and therefore have little depth of field but instead have a wide field of view. In dogs, the visual field is 240° with an overlap of 60°. In hares and rabbits, the visual field is 360°, the binocular range is only 30°. Horses have a visual field of 300° with an overlapping area of 60°. A horse with a vertical head position (ridden on the reins) therefore has an area just in front of it in which it sees nothing (**Fig. 3.28**). Therefore, when jumping, it is dependent on the rider's support, as it has no spatial vision directly in front of the obstacle.

Visual field defects are called scotomas and lead to a reduced quality of perception.

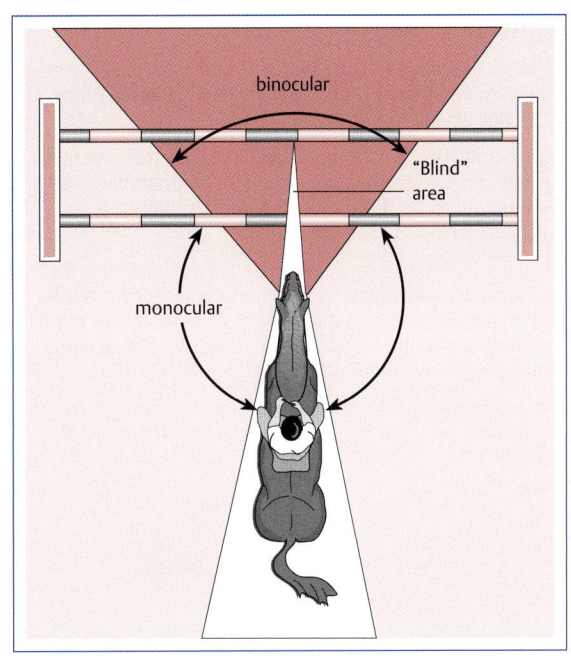

Fig. 3.28 Horse's field of vision before the obstacle.

3.5.8 Pathophysiology

Diseases of the eyes can affect vision in all animal species. Equine recurrent uveitis is a spontaneously occurring inflammation of the inner eye structures, which is very common in horses worldwide (prevalence approx. 10%). The disease occurs in inflammatory episodes that lead to destruction of the ocular tissue. This is mainly caused by **T lymphocytes**. The triggering mechanisms of this disease are still not understood. The leukocytes have a significant pathophysiological role. In a healthy state they are not able to pass through the blood-retina barrier into the interior of the eye. In equine recurrent uveitis, the blood-retina barrier breaks down. Leukocytes migrate into the iris, retina and vitreous body and are accompanied by inflammatory cytokines such as interferon-γ. The immune response is mistakenly directed against retinal proteins, which are mainly expressed in the photosensors. In the course of the disease, the retinal function is destroyed, leading to blindness in affected horses. The disease is treated with immunosuppressants. In humans, there is a comparable autoimmune uveitis, so that new findings on the disease are relevant to both horses and humans.

Suggested reading

Amann B, Hirmer S, Hauck SM et al. True blue: S-opsin is widely expressed in different animal species. J Anim Physiol Anim Nutr 2012; doi: 10.1111/jpn.12016

Degroote RL, Deeg CA. Immunological insights into equine ue-current uveitis, a spontaneous model for autoimmune uveitis. Front Immunol, Jan 8; 11: 609–855. doi: 10.3389/fim-mu.2020.609855. eCollection 2020

Lagman D, Ocampo Daza D, Widmark J et al. The vertebrate ancestral repertoire of visual opsins, transducin alpha subunits and oxytocin/vasopressin receptors was established by duplication of their shared genomic region in the two rounds of early vertebrate genome duplications. BMC Evol Biol 2013; 13: 238

Petros TJ, Rebsam A, Mason CA. Retinal axon growth at the optic chiasm: to cross or not to cross. Annu Rev Neurosci 2008; 31: 295–315

3.6 Chemical senses: sense of smell and taste

Heinz Breer

> **ESSENTIALS**
>
> All animals, even unicellular organisms, have sensory systems that allow them to detect chemical substances in their environment. In vertebrates, a distinction is made between the senses of smell and taste (**Table 3.5**). They not only have different functional roles, but also differ in the type of sensory cell and their degree of sensitivity. The primary purpose of the sense of taste is to chemically check the food to be ingested. Accordingly, the secondary taste cells are located in the oral cavity and usually only react to dissolved substances in relatively high concentrations. The sense of smell serves mainly to analyse the air we breathe. The primary sensory cells for smell are found in the nasal sensory epithelium and react to relatively small (26–300 Da) volatile compounds in sometimes extremely low concentrations. In this way, distant sources of scent can often be detected as a remote sense.

3.6.1 Sense of smell (olfactory sense)

The ability of the olfactory system to register and distinguish between an almost unlimited variety of volatile compounds in the air we breathe contributes to the fact that this sensory system plays a central role in the control of important behavioural patterns and the regulation of central vegetative functions. These include finding food sources and territories, selecting and identifying social partners, and recognising and avoiding enemies. The sense of smell is of particular importance in nocturnal animals, as well as in animals with pronounced chemical communication, especially in social animals.

Table 3.5 Characteristics of the sense of smell and taste.

	Sense of smell	Sense of taste
Sensory cells	Primary sensory cells	Secondary sensory cells
Cranial nerves	Olfactory nerve (CN I)	Facial nerve (CN VII) Glossopharyngeal nerve (CN IX) Vagus nerve (CN X)
Adequate stimulus	Mostly organic, volatile molecules	Organic or inorganic molecules, non-volatile
Biological function	Distant and close senses in the detection of food, partner and enemy recognition; orientation and communication	Near sensing, control of food intake
Distinctive qualities	Very many qualities that are difficult to delineate	Five basic qualities: sour, salty, bitter, sweet, "umami".
Sensitivity	Partly extremely high	Relatively low

Source: Lexikon der Neurowissenschaften. Heidelberg, Berlin: Spektrum Akademischer Verlag; 2000

■ Location and structure of the olfactory epithelium

The olfactory epithelium of terrestrial mammals lies protected in the posterior region of the nasal cavity. There, it covers the nasal septum and the sometimes multiple sinuous folds of the outer nasal walls in structures called turbinals which greatly increase the surface area. In species with a particularly sensitive sense of smell, the turbinal structures are sometimes very complex and provide a large surface area for the sensory epithelium. For example, the olfactory epithelium of dogs has an area of up to $150\,cm^2$, in contrast to $5\,cm^2$ in humans. Correspondingly, the number of olfactory sensory cells is extremely large (up to 250 million cells in the German shepherd dog). The olfactory epithelium (**Fig. 3.29**) is separated from the nasal lumen by a single layer of supporting cells. They have a glial cell–like function, i.e. they not only serve to delimit the nasal epithelium, but also contribute to the metabolic supply and electrical insulation of the sensory cells. At the base of the sensory epithelium, located directly on the basal lamina, there is a population of stem cells (basal cells), from which new olfactory sensory cells are generated throughout life.

The olfactory cells are chemosensory neurons that are replaced approximately every 8–10 weeks. The olfactory sensory cells are arranged as a multi-layered region in the middle area of the epithelium. They are bipolar primary sensory cells that project an unbranched axon directly into a specialised area of the forebrain, the olfactory bulb. The dendritic process of the sensory cells terminates at the luminal surface of the epithelium in a small button-like thickening with about 5–20 immobile cilia. These cilia reach a length of about 50–60 μm and thus enlarge considerably the chemosensory membrane (i.e. the sensory field) of the cells. They are embedded in a mucus layer that is produced by special glands, the Bowman's glands beneath the epithelium in the lamina propria. The mucus protects the sensitive structures from possible damaging influences in the inspired air and ensures the ionic environment for the sensory cells. Olfactory cells are the only neurons that are directly exposed to the outside world. However, the aqueous mucus also acts as a barrier to volatile and usually not very water-soluble scents.

It is assumed that the hydrophobic fragrance molecules reach the sensory cell with the help of the so-called odorant-binding proteins (OBPs) in the nasal mucus. The OBPs belong to the lipocalin family. They are relatively small proteins that bind hydrophobic molecules, such as steroids or vitamins, and thus transport them in body fluids. Whether and how OBPs transfer the scents to the chemosensory cilia membrane is still unclear. It is conceivable that OBPs contribute to the elimination of "old" fragrances. However, the inactivation of hydrophobic fragrance ligands is predominantly attributed to biotransformation enzymes (cytochrome P450; glycosyltransferases).

> **IN A NUTSHELL**   **!**
>
> The olfactory epithelium houses many millions of sensory cells specialised in the detection of odours. They are regenerated from stem cells throughout life.

■ Olfactory receptors – the molecular detectors for fragrances

In order to be able to register chemical compounds in the air we breathe, the olfactory sensory cells have receptor proteins in the cilia membrane. These odorant receptors belong to the large family of seven-transmembrane receptors, which usually couple to G proteins. This family of proteins also includes many types of receptors for transmitters and hormones. Odorant receptors are encoded by a very large gene family. The enormous diversity of odorant

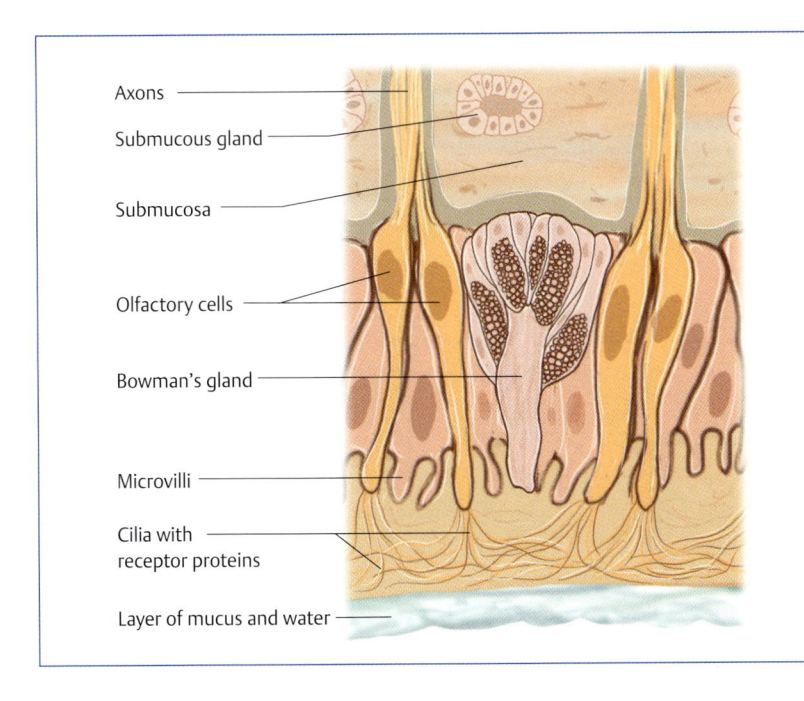

Axons

Submucous gland

Submucosa

Olfactory cells

Bowman's gland

Microvilli

Cilia with receptor proteins

Layer of mucus and water

Fig. 3.29 The olfactory epithelium is composed of three main cell types: The bipolar olfactory sensory cells project into the nasal cavity with their cilia. Their axons are bundled into nerve fibres and lead towards the olfactory bulb. The supporting cells isolate neighbouring sensory cells from each other. New sensory cells are formed from the basal cells throughout life. Below the basal membrane are the mucus-producing Bowman's glands. The supplying blood vessels and the axons of the sensory cells, which are bundled into nerves, are also located here. [Source: Schünke M, Schulte E, Schumacher U (eds.). Prometheus LernAtlas der Anatomie – Kopf, Hals und Neuroanatomie. Illustrated by K. Wesker and M. Voll. 5th ed., Stuttgart: Thieme; 2018, Fig. 13.24]

receptor genes (up to 1000 genes) allows the generation of a very large receptor repertoire. This multitude and diversity of receptors is considered to be the basis for the fact that an almost unlimited number of odorants are perceived by the olfactory system. It is of particular importance that an individual odorant receptor – in contrast to a hormone receptor, for example – does not interact specifically with "its" ligand, but reacts relatively non-specifically to a spectrum of structurally similar molecules.

The relatively broad recognition spectrum of a receptor means that a particular compound reacts with different receptor types, albeit with varying degrees of affinity. This means that each receptor is stimulated by different odorants and, conversely, each odorant also activates different receptors. This overlap allows the system, in the sense of combinatorics, an almost unlimited recognition and discrimination capacity for volatile compounds that can function as scents. In addition to the great diversity and the relatively unspecific reaction spectrum of odorant receptors, the fact that each sensory cell has only one type of receptor is of central importance for the functional principle of the sense of smell. This means that the many millions of olfactory cells can be divided into a corresponding number of receptor-specific subpopulations. The cells of a receptor-specific subpopulation are distributed over a large area in overlapping zones of the olfactory epithelium. It can there-

fore be assumed that a fragrance activates cells of different subpopulations with different intensities and thus triggers a characteristic pattern of activity in the nasal sensory epithelium.

■ Chemoelectric signal transduction

Olfactory receptors belong to the superfamily of G protein-coupled receptors (p. 39) (GPRs). Activation of the receptor in the sensory cell triggers a transduction cascade (**Fig. 3.30**). This begins with the activation of a downstream G protein – the G_{olf} – by the receptor and thus causes a stimulation of the effector enzyme, adenylate cyclase. This enzyme catalyses the formation of the intracellular second messenger cAMP and rapidly leads to an increased cAMP level. This intracellular messenger triggers the opening of cyclic nucleotide-gated, non-selective ion channels in the cilia membrane, which (in addition to a Na^+ influx) primarily lead to a Ca^{2+} influx. The influx of

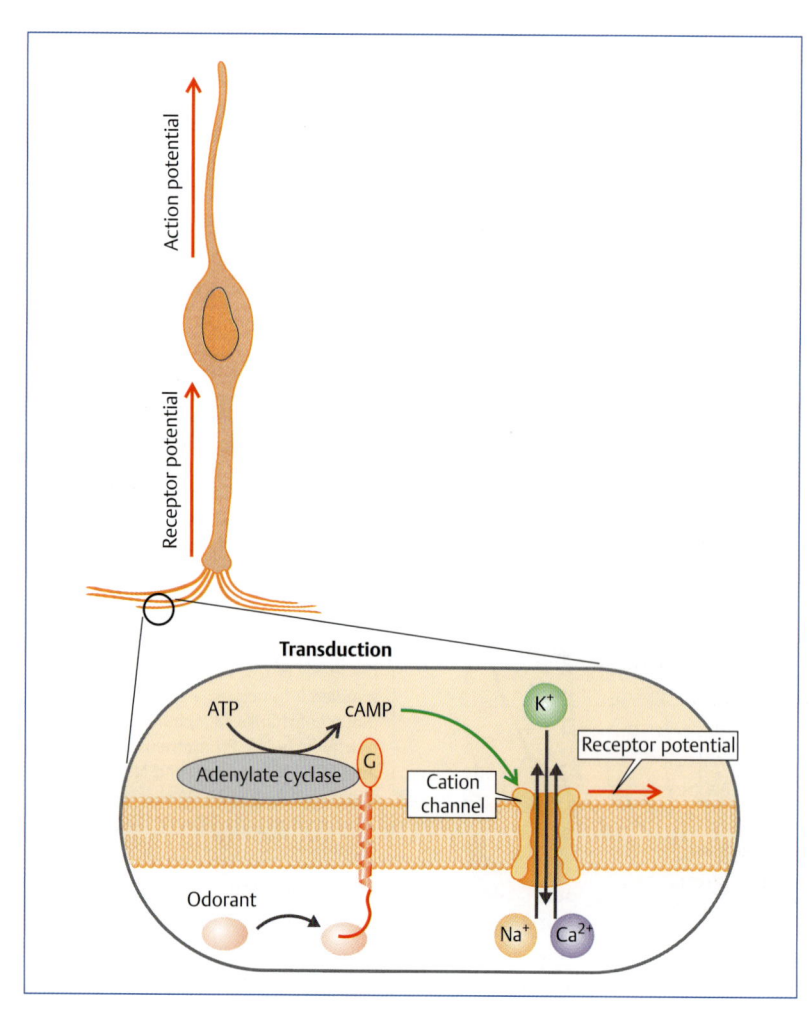

Fig. 3.30 Chemoelectric signal conversion in olfactory sensory cells.
Fragrances that bind to olfactory receptors in the cilia membrane activate the enzyme adenylate cyclase via characteristic G proteins. This leads to the production of the second messenger cAMP. The cAMP opens a cyclic nucleotide-gated ion channel that mainly allows Ca^{2+} to flow into the cell. The Ca^{2+} opens another ion channel that leads to the efflux of Cl^- and thus causes the depolarization of the cell membrane. [Source: Pape H, Kurtz A, Silbernagl S (eds.). Physiologie. 9th, fully revised ed. Stuttgart: Thieme; 2019, Fig. 21.6]

Ca²⁺ ions, however, changes the membrane potential of the sensory cell only a little, but causes the opening of Cl⁻ channels. This Ca²⁺-activated Cl⁻ conductance causes a depolarization of the cell. This atypical reaction is possible because olfactory sensory cells like secretory epithelial cells (p.453), but unlike most neurons (p.61) have an unusually high intracellular Cl⁻ concentration, which leads to the efflux of Cl⁻ ions when the Cl⁻ channels open. Through this mechanism, the sensory cells are largely independent of fluctuations in the extracellular ion concentration in the surrounding mucus. The strength of the activation is encoded in the primary sensory cell as the frequency of action potentials.

> **IN A NUTSHELL** !
>
> The binding of odorants to an olfactory receptor triggers a signal transduction cascade in the sensory cell that leads to depolarization of the cell membrane.

■ Adaptation to continuous stimulation

Olfactory cells usually react only briefly to a scent stimulus. This rapid adaptation is caused on the one hand by the fact that the Ca²⁺ ions flowing in cause a closure of non-selective cation channels in the sense of a negative feedback. They also activate a cAMP hydrolysing phosphodiesterase. In addition, the activated odorant receptors are phosphorylated and are thus "turned off". These multiple mechanisms underline the importance of adaptation for olfactory cells, which are not designed for continuous stimulation but must respond to the odorants in each breath.

> **IN A NUTSHELL** !
>
> Sustained stimulation of a sensory cell leads to the shutdown of the transduction cascade via negative feedback mechanisms.

■ Transmission of olfactory information to the brain

For the cognitive detection of odours, which initiate specific behavioural patterns, it is essential that the receptor-specific activity pattern of the olfactory epithelium is transmitted to the brain. As the primary sensory cell, each olfactory cell projects its own axonal extension directly into a specific region of the forebrain, the olfactory bulb. In this process, the axons of neighbouring sensory cells travel as axon bundles through the pores of the skull base, the ethmoid plate, to the brain. Immediately after passing through the ethmoid plate, the axons are reorganised, so that the axons of sensory cells of the same receptor type now run in common bundles and terminate together at a specific position in the bulb in a tangle-like structure – the glomerulus. In this way, the sensory cells scattered relatively widely in the nasal olfactory epithelium, but of the same receptor type, converge in a common position and thus form a receptor-specific "map" in the bulb (**Fig. 3.31**).

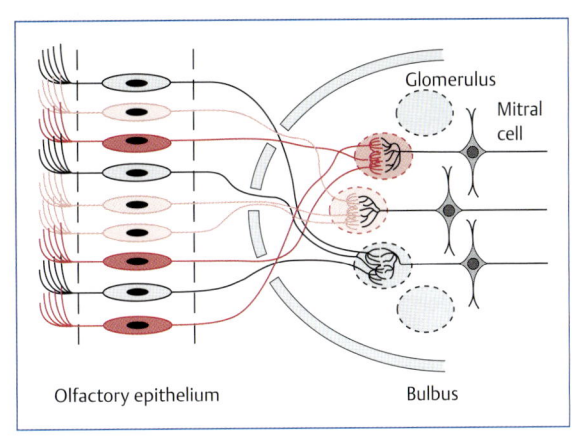

Fig. 3.31 Olfactory projection. All axons of the several thousand sensory cells in the olfactory epithelium that are equipped with the same receptor (e.g. the cells marked in red), thus having the same chemospecificity, terminate in a common glomerulus in the olfactory bulb. There, they form synaptic contacts with the dendritic projections of a few mitral cells (convergence).

The axons of sensory cells of similar receptor type, project into neighbouring glomeruli. This receptor-specific "wiring" between the olfactory epithelium and the brain is likely to result in each odorant triggering a characteristic spatial pattern of activated glomeruli in the bulb. Each odorant is therefore encoded by a specific combination of activated glomeruli.

Through this principle of **combinatorial coding** the number of different activity patterns is almost unlimited. In interaction with neuronal processing in the bulb, it allows not only the detection of complex aromas, but also the encoding of completely new chemical compounds in a foreign environment. Increasing concentrations of a fragrance often cause additional glomeruli to be activated. This is apparently because additional receptor types are being recruited and thus explains why a fragrance smells quite differently at different concentrations. For example, thioterpineol is perceived as fruity at low concentrations, but as malodorous at higher concentrations.

> **IN A NUTSHELL** !
>
> The axons of all sensory cells with the same receptor equipment converge in the bulb in common glomeruli. Specific patterns of glomerular activity are induced by specific scents.

■ Processing of olfactory information

Olfactory bulb

The glomeruli are considered structural and functional units of the bulb. A glomerulus is a complex structure enclosed by glial cells in which the branched terminals of the axons of several thousand receptor-specific olfactory cells form synaptic contacts with the highly branched dendritic projections of the downstream neurons in the bulb: the mitral cells. Initial processing of olfactory information takes place through local interneurons (periglomerular and granule cells), which establish connections between

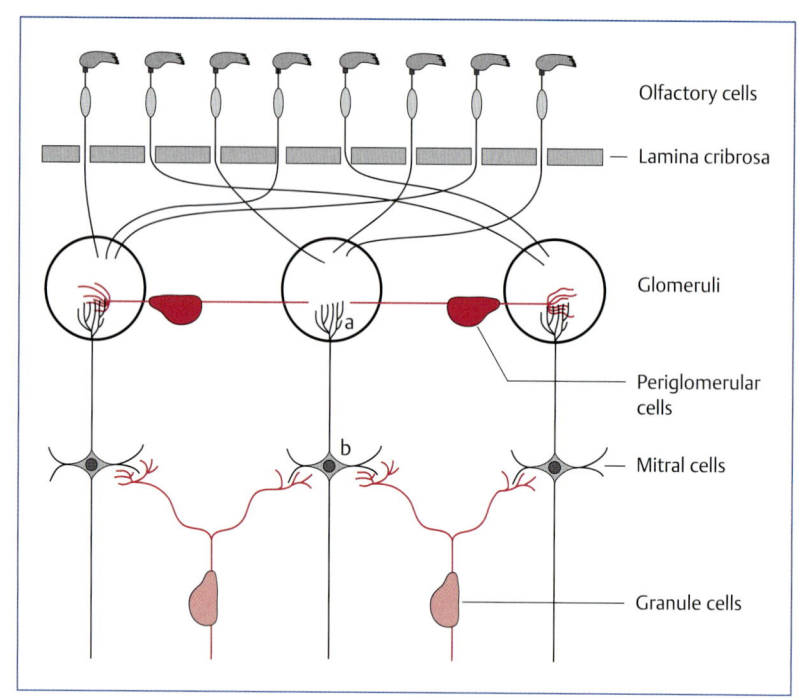

Fig. 3.32 Information processing in the olfactory bulb by local interneurons. Periglomerular cells form GABAergic, inhibitory synapses with the apical dendrites (**a**) of the mitral cells of adjacent glomeruli. The granule cells form reciprocal synapses with the basal dendrites (**b**) of the mitral cells and thus have inhibitory feedback on the activating cell. They also cause inhibition of mitral cells of adjacent glomeruli via GABAergic synapses.

neighbouring glomeruli (**Fig. 3.32**). The periglomerular cells have connections to the apical dendrites of the mitral cell and exert an inhibitory effect by means of the transmitter GABA (p. 62) on dendrites in neighbouring glomeruli. The granule cells form reciprocal synapses with the basal dendrites of the mitral cells. At the reciprocal synapse, the mitral cell releases glutamate as a transmitter, activating the interneuron. At the same synapse, the activated interneuron then releases GABA, which has an inhibitory effect on the mitral cell (**Fig. 3.32**). The interneuron also forms inhibitory synapses with mitral cells of neighbouring glomeruli and thus contributes to the contrast sharpening of the electrical activity patterns in the bulb.

This connection on two levels is reminiscent of the "wiring pattern" in the retina (p. 93) (horizontal cells, amacrine cells) and causes a pronounced **lateral inhibition**. This causes a pronounced contrast enhancement and thus improves the discriminability of scents.

interconnected convergently and divergently. It is assumed that the underlying wiring patterns are partly innate, but for the most part generated by experience. Smell information is thus obviously perceived without processing in the thalamus, a peculiarity for which the significance is still unclear.

Besides the pathways to the cortex as the basis of conscious perception, there are several connections to other brain areas. Through the interconnections to the amygdala and the hippocampus, the olfactory signals are linked to emotional aspects and affectively controlled behaviour. In addition, the connection to the hypothalamus has a direct influence on the endocrine system. This multifaceted network of the olfactory pathways in the forebrain makes it clear that the sense of smell not only serves the conscious chemical analysis of the air we breathe, but also significantly influences current emotions and contributes to the control of important bodily functions of metabolism and reproduction.

> **IN A NUTSHELL**   !
>
> The interconnection of specifically adjacent glomeruli by inhibitory interneurons leads to contrast enhancement between glomeruli with similar input signals.

> **IN A NUTSHELL**   !
>
> Olfactory information reaches the cortex bypassing the thalamus. At the same time, it is transmitted to centres responsible for processing emotions and endogenous body functions.

Higher brain centres

The information processed by the neuronal network of the bulb is transmitted to higher brain centres via the axons of the mitral cells that form the tractus olfactorius. This shows that in contrast to all other sensory modalities, the olfactory tract does not project to the thalamus, which controls access to the neocortex, but rather directly into the piriform cortex, the so-called primary olfactory cortex. Here, information from different glomeruli is apparently

■ Pheromones

Chemical components that serve the purpose of intra-species communication are called pheromones. They induce specific physiological changes in the recipient such as the production and release of hormones which can directly influence behaviour (e.g. aggression towards other members of the same species and sex). Pheromones do not represent a uniform class of substances but range from small volatile molecules to proteins with a molecular weight of up to 20 kDa. They are secreted by glands or released together with urine, sweat, saliva or tear fluid. These secretions usually contain complex "cocktails" of a variety of different components.

The composition of these mixtures can vary greatly depending on the sex, age and endocrine status of an individual. Typically, the complete mixture is necessary to trigger specific reactions, but individual components can also evoke reactions. In domestic pigs, for example, 5α-androst-16-en-3-one (androstenone) in sows in oestrus induces the so-called standing reflex. Suckling rabbits produce the substance 2-methylbut-2-enal with their milk, which triggers a stereotypic search reaction in newborn animals. Both the androstenone-induced sexual behaviour and the search behaviour for the milk source are mediated via the classical olfactory system. This also applies, for example, to trimethylamine, which occurs in the urine of male mice and exerts an attractive effect on female animal. However, the relevant olfactory sensory cells involved have a special type of receptor that belongs to the TAAR (trace amine-associated receptor) group.

In addition to the olfactory epithelium, most vertebrates have a specialised organ for registering pheromones, the vomeronasal organ, also known as Jacobson's organ. This is a blind-ended, tubular structure at the base of the nasal cavity on either side of the septum. In rodents it communicates with the nasal cavity, and in other species (e.g. even-toed ungulates) with the oral cavity via the ductus nasopalatinus. Since the vomeronasal organ ends blindly, the often non-volatile substances are brought into the oral or nasal cavity by licking or sniffing (rodents, ungulates). A "suction pump mechanism" ensures the transfer of substances into the vomeronasal organ. This is mediated by large, thin-walled vessels of the vomeronasal organ, that are rhythmically filled with blood in the manner of a venous swell body. In hoofed animals, the characteristic bleating sound ensures the transfer of pheromones into the vomeronasal organ. The chemosensory cells located there differ in several aspects from those in the olfactory epithelium. Firstly, they are not equipped with cilia, but with microvilli. The receptors of these sensory cells do not belong to the odorant receptors but represent two independent, very different protein families, which in mice have approx. 200 or 80 members, respectively. In these cells, chemoelectrical signal transduction is mediated by a G protein-activated phospholipase C and becomes operational by the activation of ion channels of the type TRPC2 (transient receptor potential canonical channel type 2). The electrically encoded information reaches a subarea of the olfactory bulb, the accessory bulb, via the axons. There, the information is processed and transmitted to special brain centres, including the hippocampus and hypothalamus, where it directly affects the endocrine system and thus social behaviour, and especially reproductive behaviour. In higher primates and various aquatic mammals, the vomeronasal organ is only rudimentary or completely absent. In Old World monkeys and in humans, the genes for most of the receptors in the vomeronasal organ and for the TRPC2 channel are also non-functional pseudogenes.

It may be that further olfactory subsystems in the nasal cavity, such as the septal organ or the Grüneberg ganglion, could also be involved in the detection of pheromones. It is also assumed that a large number of as yet unidentified chemical signalling molecules exist that serve as pheromones for communication between individuals.

IN A NUTSHELL   !

Chemical messengers that serve intra-species communication (pheromones) are detected in specialised chemosensory subsystems.

3.6.2   Sense of taste

ESSENTIALS   ✗

The sense of taste serves as a rapid and reliable assessment of food to decide whether to accept or reject it. However, the sensory impression referred to as "taste" in everyday life comes about through the integration of taste perception with olfactory information as well as tactile and thermal sensations from the oral cavity. Only the qualities sweet, bitter, sour, salty and "umami" (Japanese: "savoury", "tasty") are actually assigned as the sense of taste.

■ Taste qualities

The sweet taste is predominantly mediated by sugar molecules and serves to detect carbohydrate-rich, high-calorie food. Amino acids are responsible for the "umami" flavour taste, which facilitates the detection of proteins. In contrast, the bitter taste is triggered by a wide range of organic molecules, including compounds such as caffeine, nicotine and quinine. It generally serves as a warning of potentially toxic substances in food. As a result, there is a genetically fixed aversion to a bitter taste in many animal species. Many toxic plant constituents (alkaloids, isoprenoids, glycosides) are perceived as bitter even at extremely low concentrations and so their oral ingestion is avoided. A sour taste is caused by an increased proton concentration and probably serves to stimulate appetite (fruit acid), but also it has an aversive effect, presumably to not disturb acid-base balance from excessive acid ingestion, or also to warn against eating unripe fruit. Along with sweet taste, sour taste is also tolerated to a high intensity. A salty taste is generated by Na^+ ions in food and ensures their sufficient supply. Recent research indicates the existence of another taste quality, the taste of fat. It is assumed that the taste of fatty acids is recognised by special taste sensory cells. A high content of fatty acids in food indicates a high energy content.

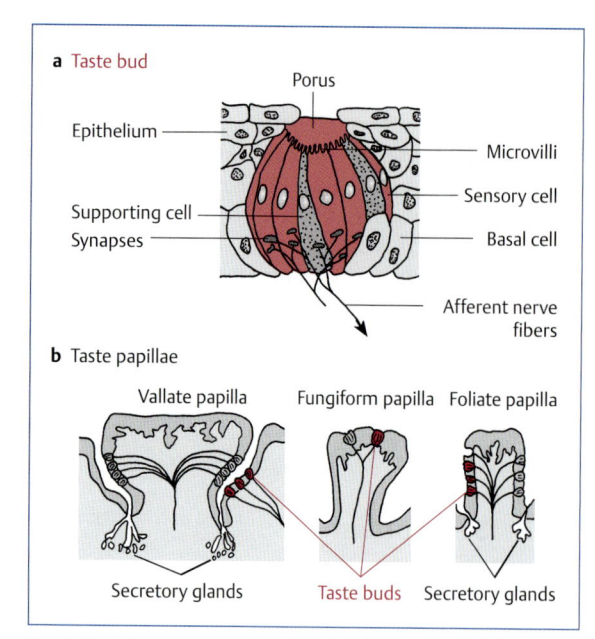

a Taste bud

- Porus
- Epithelium
- Microvilli
- Sensory cell
- Supporting cell
- Basal cell
- Synapses
- Afferent nerve fibers

b Taste papillae

Vallate papilla   Fungiform papilla   Foliate papilla

Secretory glands   Taste buds   Secretory glands

Fig. 3.33 Schematic structure of a taste bud (**a**) and of three different taste buds (**b**).

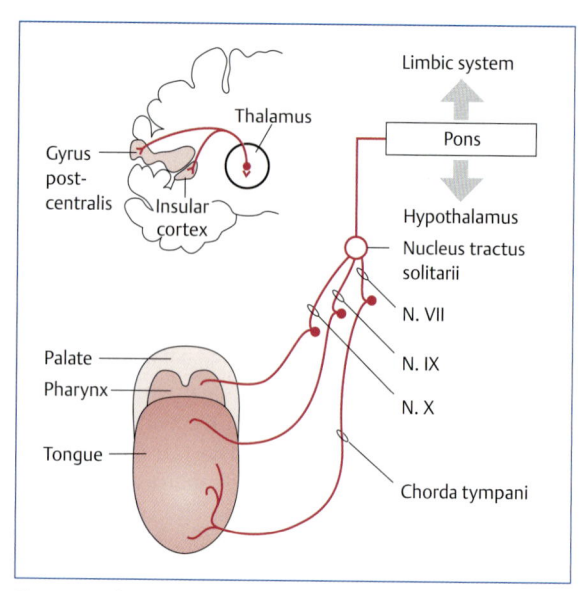

- Limbic system
- Thalamus
- Pons
- Gyrus post-centralis
- Insular cortex
- Hypothalamus
- Nucleus tractus solitarii
- N. VII
- N. IX
- Palate
- N. X
- Pharynx
- Tongue
- Chorda tympani

Fig. 3.34 Schematic representation of the afferent taste pathway. The axons of three different cranial nerves innervate the taste buds in different areas of the tongue, oral cavity and pharynx. Fibres run from the nucleus tractus solitarii via the contralateral thalamus into the neocortex, or via the pons to the hypothalamus and to various regions of the limbic system.

In general, the perception thresholds for individual taste qualities differ considerably. In humans, the thresholds for glucose are $19\,g\cdot l^{-1}$, for citric acid $0.4\,g\cdot l^{-1}$, for NaCl $0.01\,g\cdot l^{-1}$ and for the alkaloid nicotine only $0.003\,g\cdot l^{-1}$. However, it is possible that this taste perceptibility for humans has only limited applicability to other species. The sense of taste for each animal species is adapted to their evolutionary requirements for nutrients. As a result, one or more of the described taste qualities may fade into the background or be completely absent in different animal species. Chickens, for example, cannot distinguish between sweet and bitter. Domestic cats, and tigers and cheetahs, lack the ability to perceive a sweet taste. The reason for this is a deletion in the gene for the T1R2 (p. 107) receptor, so that no functional receptor protein can be generated. Furthermore, it can be assumed that there are significant differences in taste perception between the different individuals of a species.

■ Morphology

The gustatory sensory cells in the mouth act as food sensors. In fish, such cells are also found on the barbels and body skin. Taste cells have a relatively short life span of 10–14 days and are continuously generated from stem cells. In mammals and birds, the taste cells are organised in the **taste buds** (Fig. 3.33). The total number of these in domestic animal species ranges from only about a dozen to more than 30000. Humans have about 5000 taste buds. These are organised on the tongue in more complex structures called **papillae**. A distinction is made between the relatively few **vallate papillae** at the back of the tongue, which in humans have up to 1000 taste buds each, the more frequent **foliate papillae** at the back of the tongue with about 100 taste buds and the numerous **fungiform papillae** scattered over the front half of the tongue with only 3–5 taste buds. The 10–150 sensory cells in each taste

bud are spindle-shaped and arranged like orange segments. At their apical end, they have **microvilli** that serve to increase surface area and make contact with the tongue surface in a small opening, the **porus**. This allows liquid with flavours dissolved in saliva to reach the sensory taste cells. An earlier idea that each taste bud is "responsible" for one taste quality has not been confirmed, and each taste bud contains sensory cells for all gustatory qualities.

> **IN A NUTSHELL**   !
>
> 10–150 taste cells are grouped in a taste bud; the taste buds are organised in the different types of papillae on the tongue and in the oral cavity.

Innervation

The gustatory sensory cells are secondary sensory cells, as they have no axon of their own, but are innervated by afferent axons (**Fig. 3.34**). Branches of the facial nerve (cranial nerve VII) innervate the taste buds of the palate, the fungiform papillae of the anterior half of the tongue and the anterior foliate papillae. The rest of the foliate papillae and the vallate papillae are innervated by the glossopharyngeal nerve (cranial nerve IX). A branch of the vagus nerve (cranial nerve X) innervates the taste buds of the larynx.

> **IN A NUTSHELL**   !
>
> The gustatory sensory cells are innervated by different cranial nerves.

■ Receptors for sweet, "umami" and bitter substances as well as fatty acids

The basis of molecular recognition of extremely different flavours (proton: the smallest atom; bitter substances: partly very complex molecules) and the mechanisms for generation of an electrical reaction of the taste cells are very different. It can be assumed that the effect of the ions (H^+ or Na^+) is directly mediated by ion channels. In contrast, sweet and bitter substances, and also glutamate (umami), are recognised by G protein-coupled receptors that induce corresponding intracellular reaction cascades and thus trigger a response of the cell.

The receptor for "sweet" compounds, such as sugar, is a heterodimer of two G protein-coupled receptors T1R2 and T1R3. The large extracellular domain of the two subunits has multiple binding sites for diverse sweet-tasting compounds. These multiple binding sites allow the sweet receptor to respond to very different chemical substances. The receptor of "umami" cells is also a heterodimer consisting of T1R1 and T1R3. The T1R3 subunit is involved in both the sweet and the "umami" receptor.

Bitter substances are sensed by G protein-coupled receptors that belong to the so-called T2R family. In contrast to "sweet" and "umami" receptors, bitter receptors (T2R) do not have a large extracellular domain. There are relatively many T2R subtypes. The human has 25 and the mouse 36. This diversity of bitter receptor types accounts for the enormous chemical heterogeneity of bitter-tasting substances. It has been shown that the bitter cells, in contrast to olfactory cells, have many receptor types per cell. This means that even chemically very different bitter substances always activate the same sensory cell population and accordingly always generate a very similar bitter taste.

In addition to sweet, "umami" and bitter substances, fatty acids are also registered by special G protein-coupled receptors (GPRs). In cells of the gustatory system of rodents, two fatty acid receptors have recently been identified: GPR40 and GPR120. The receptor GPR120 has also been found in human taste cells. Both GPR120 and GPR40 are mainly activated by long-chain fatty acids (> 12 C atoms).

> **IN A NUTSHELL**   !
>
> Sweet, "umami" and bitter receptors are G protein-coupled receptors.

■ Signal transduction

Sweet, umami, bitter

The processes of chemoelectrical signal transduction are initiated by the interaction of taste substances with the microvilli membranes of the gustatory sensory cells. The receptor potential generated in this process causes synaptic signal transmission to the afferent nerve fibres in the secondary sensory cells. The transduction processes for the three taste qualities sweet, "umami" and bitter are largely identical. They are G protein-mediated intracellular reaction cascades (p. 38). In this process, a heterotrimeric

G protein is activated by the receptor and causes the dissociation of the α subunit from the βγ complex. The main α subunit of taste cells is called **gustducin**. The βγ complex is thought to activate a phospholipase C ($PLC\beta_2$). This catalyses the hydrolysis of the membrane phospholipid phosphatidylinositol bisphosphate (PIP_2), thus releasing the chemical messengers inositol trisphosphate (IP_3) and diacylglycerol (DAG). This activates the IP_3R3 receptor in the membrane of the endoplasmic reticulum and thus releases Ca^{2+} from intracellular stores. The increased calcium concentration in the cytoplasm then causes the activation of a non-selective cation channel (**TRPM5 channel**, transient receptor potential melastatin channel type 5) in the membrane and thus a depolarization of the cell. This depolarization then eventually leads to the release of transmitters at the presynaptic membrane of the taste cell. It is not yet clear whether other signalling pathways are activated via the α subunit of the G protein, possibly via adenylate cyclase or guanylate cyclase, and whether cyclic nucleotides (cAMP, cGMP) are involved in the transduction process.

> **IN A NUTSHELL**   !
>
> The transduction of sweet, "umami" and bitter stimuli takes place via G protein-coupled reaction cascades and the activation of TRP channels.

Fatty acids

So far, extremely little is known about the transduction mechanisms of the taste quality "fat". Since the fatty acids interact with membrane-bound G protein-coupled receptors, it can be assumed that a G protein-mediated intracellular reaction cascade is involved, similar to the transduction of sweet, "umami" and bitter stimuli.

Acid

Various mechanisms are considered for the chemoelectrical signal transduction of the taste quality "sour". Studies on taste cells of amphibians have shown that H^+ ions (actually: H_3O^+ ions) inhibit apically localised K^+ channels and thus cause a depolarization of the cell. In mammals, the so-called "acid-sensing ion channels" (ASICs) seem to be involved, i.e. Na^+ channels that open at higher H^+ concentrations. Recent research results show that the decisive stimulus does not seem to be a lowering of the extracellular pH, but rather the intracellular pH of taste cells declines. Organic acids, such as acetic or citric acid, pass through the cell membranes in an undissociated state and then dissociate in the cell according to their acid constant. The resulting H^+ lowers the intracellular pH. Inorganic acids are polar and non-permeant when dissociated. As strong acids, they are largely present in aqueous solution as H^+ ions and acid anions, whereby H^+ only enters the receptor cells in high concentrations via ion channels and thus lowers the intracellular pH value. This would explain why organic acids taste more acidic than inorganic acids at the same extracellular pH. It is assumed that H^+ ions interact with intracellular domains of membrane proteins and thus cause depolarization of the sensory cell. However, it is not yet clear which membrane proteins are involved in this mechanism.

From recent studies, other molecular elements involved in signal transduction in the "acid cells" are being proposed. In particular, the pH-sensitive non-selective cation channels PKD2L1 and PKD1L3 (polycystic kidney disease 2-like 1 and 3 protein) are thought to play a significant role.

> **IN A NUTSHELL** !
>
> The transduction of acidic stimuli has not been definitively clarified and may proceed differently in different species.

Salty

"Salt" cells express a constitutively open **epithelial sodium channel (ENaC)** in the microvilli membrane. Increased Na⁺ concentrations in saliva lead to Na⁺ influx and thus to depolarization of the cell. The ENaC channel is amiloride-sensitive, i.e. the channel is blocked by the substance amiloride, which is also used as a diuretic (p. 320). Accordingly, the addition of amiloride to salt solutions reduces sensitivity to the salt taste, which is mainly mediated by NaCl. For example, sodium chloride tastes saltier than sodium sulphate. This suggests that the anions of the sodium salts also contribute to the salt taste, especially its intensity. A possible explanation for this is the ability of the Na⁺ ions to pass through the cell-cell junctions (tight junctions) at the apical region of the taste cells. In this way the Na⁺ concentration in the interstitial space of taste buds increases. Chloride anions can follow the sodium cation through the tight junctions and thus contribute to electroneutrality. The sulphate anion cannot pass through the tight junctions, resulting in a transepithelial electrical gradient that influences the membrane potential of the taste cell.

> **IN A NUTSHELL** !
>
> Transduction of saline stimuli occurs through the influx of sodium ions through constitutively opened ion channels in the apical membrane.

■ Coding of taste qualities

Recent findings show that the processing of gustatory information already begins in the taste buds. There, morphologically distinguishable cell types are found, which apparently have different functions. Type I represents glia-like supporting cells. Proliferation of type IV basal cells ensures the constant regeneration of the short-lived sensory cells. Type II represents the sensory cells with either sweet, "umami" or bitter receptors, as well as the components of the downstream signal transduction cascade (gustducin, PLCβ₂, IP₃ R3, TRPM5). Type II cells, however, have surprisingly no synaptic contacts with the afferent nerve fibres. Only type III cells form synapses, but these cells have no receptors for taste substances. This apparent paradox posed a mystery for a long time. It is now assumed that the type II sensory

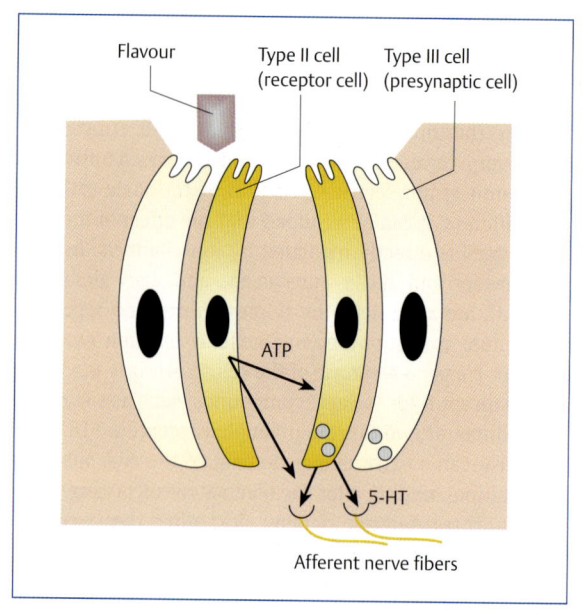

Fig. 3.35 Interactions of different cell types within a taste bud. When an adequate amount of flavourant stimulates a type II receptor cell (left), it reacts by releasing ATP. This can directly excite via purinergic receptors afferent nerve fibres or stimulate neighbouring type III cells (right) to release the transmitter substance serotonin (5-HT). Serotonin can subsequently also activate sensory afferents but may also influence neighbouring cells within the taste bud through a paracrine pathway.

cells secrete **ATP** after stimulation, which activates the type III cells via purinergic signalling. Type III cells then release the transmitter substance **serotonin** and thus stimulate the innervating fibres. Afferent fibres can also be activated directly via purinergic receptors. Acid stimuli are apparently detected by the type III cells themselves (**Fig. 3.35**). A separate cell population obviously exists for detecting a salty taste, which does not overlap with the cell populations for sweet, "umami", bitter and sour. At the sensory cell level, the taste qualities are therefore detected separately.

By integrating the activities of neighbouring cells in the type III cells, an initial processing of gustatory information already takes place in the taste bud. An individual afferent fibre reacts accordingly to several taste qualities, but with different sensitivities. The ranking of the sensitivity of an afferent fibre for the different taste qualities is called its "taste profile". Consequently, each flavour is encoded by the activity pattern of several axons. This coding principle is called "across fibre patterning".

> **IN A NUTSHELL** !
>
> A taste bud consists of different cell types that share specific functions. A sensory cell detects only one taste quality at a time; innervating nerve fibres react to several taste qualities with different sensitivities.

■ Central processing

The neuronal activity of the afferent lingual fibres in the three cranial nerves (**Fig. 3.34**) is transmitted to the nucleus gustatorius, a part of the nucleus tractus solitarii in the medulla oblongata. From there, nerve tracts project to different regions: on the one hand to various nuclei in the brainstem, where reflexive reactions related to food intake are triggered, including secretory activities such as salivation or motor processes such as chewing and swallowing. On the other hand, taste information, in terms of conscious perception, is sent to the thalamus – the "gateway" to the sensory cortex – and from there to the **primary gustatory cortex** at the base of the postcentral gyrus. Parallel to this thalamocortical projection, the gustatory information reaches areas of the lateral hypothalamus, which participate in the regulation of food intake, and the amygdala, which contributes significantly to the hedonistic component (pleasure/displeasure) of taste sensations.

At the level of the so-called **secondary gustatory cortex**, a region of the **orbitofrontal cortex** integrates taste, olfactory and visual information.

> **IN A NUTSHELL** !
>
> Gustatory information travels from the tongue to the nucleus solitarius and from there via the thalamus to the primary gustatory cortex. In the secondary gustatory cortex, taste information is integrated with olfactory and visual information; this is where the complex sensory impression for food selection is created.

■ Modulation of the peripheral gustatory system by peptide hormones

Research findings in recent years suggest that a number of peptide hormones influence the processing of taste stimuli in the taste buds. It has been shown that these are predominantly hormones secreted by endocrine cells of the gastrointestinal tract. However, they are also produced by taste cells themselves. These hormones include ghrelin, glucagon-like peptide-1 (GLP-1) and cholecystokinin (CCK). Specific receptors for these chemical messengers are found both in taste cells and in afferent nerve fibres. It is therefore assumed that these peptides act as autocrine or paracrine signals in a taste bud, and also influence the gustatory system as nutritionally relevant endocrine signals from the gastrointestinal tract. In this way, an adaptation of the reactivity of the sense of taste to the nutritional status could occur. That is, peptide hormones of the gastrointestinal tract could cause a fine regulation of the sensitivity of taste cells in a kind of "feedback reaction".

3.7 Birds and reptiles

Helga Pfannkuche, Michael Pees

> **ESSENTIALS** ✗
>
> The sense of sight is the most important sense for birds, and the bird's eye is correspondingly powerful. However, nocturnal birds of prey also have an extremely good sense of hearing, with which they are able to locate their prey. The sense of touch, smell and taste do not have a prominent role in most avian species. Migratory birds are able to orientate themselves in the earth's magnetic field with the help of a magnetic sensor.
>
> In reptiles, the most important sense depends on the species. Turtles and some lizards have a very good sense of sight. Snakes, on the other hand, have a strong sense of smell and also locate their prey through an infrared sensor.

3.7.1 Senses in birds

■ Sense of sight

The sense of sight is the most essential sense for the vast majority of avian species. Although its basic functioning mirrors that of the mammalian eye, there are some bird-specific features that give the avian eye extreme efficiency.

In most species, the bird's eye is significantly larger than eyes of mammals of comparable size. In particular the retina occupies a larger area. This area would be associated with a huge eyeball in an approximately round eye, as found in mammals. In birds, this problem is solved by a specific shape of the eyeball (**Fig. 3.36**). However, this makes it more "unstable" against deformation than a sphere. To protect against mechanical impact, the eyeball

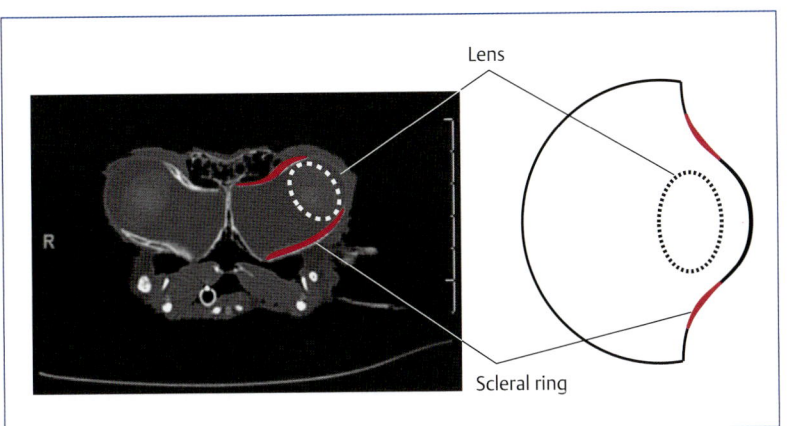

Lens

Scleral ring

Fig. 3.36 Shape and schematic structure of the bird's eye (left): Eye of an eagle owl in computer tomographic section; right: Eye of a pigeon as schematic drawing. [Source: Dr. I. Kiefer, Klinik für Kleintiere, Universität Leipzig]

is not only located in a bony orbital, as in the mammal, but a bony orbital ring is also attached. The shape of this ring differs depending on the bird species and determines the shape of the anterior part of the eye (**Fig. 3.36**). For reasons of weight and the body's centre of gravity (sitting on two uprights), they do not have a fat body as do mammals. Instead, the eye is surrounded by an infraorbital sinus which is connected to the respiratory tract and can be affected by respiratory diseases.

The large retina has no vessels, so the necessary supply of nutrients must come from another source. It is assumed that the pecten oculi plays an essential role in the self-supply of the retina and also of the vitreous body.

When considering visual characteristics, it should be borne in mind that these can differ considerably between different avian species. As an extreme adaptation, the fat martin living in dark caves has a retina in which several layers of rods are arranged on top of each other. This, together with a high convergence on downstream neurons, leads to a high light sensitivity of the retina, but at the expense of visual acuity. In addition to the sense of sight, the fat martin also orients itself by ultrasound location, similar to that of bats. The visual sense of owls is also adapted to hunting at dusk and is ideally complemented by the auditory sense.

Unlike in nocturnal and crepuscular avian species, the retina of diurnal birds is designed for colour vision with a high visual acuity. In contrast to mammals, four different cone types are found here, which can receive light in wavelengths of 320–680 nm. This means that birds are also able to perceive light in the ultraviolet range. This plays a role in hunting, for example, because mouse urine reflects light in the ultraviolet range. Tetrachromatic vision is not the only specialisation of the bird's eye. There are oil droplets in the cones. The colouration is caused by rhodopsins. A distinction is made between five different droplet colours. The light falling on the retina is filtered by the embedded oil droplets. Although this reduces the intensity, it achieves a further spread of different wavelengths.

As in the mammal, the fovea is the site of the sharpest vision. In some bird species, even two foveae have been described, where cones are stimulated either by light incident from the side or from the front. Since the mobility of the eyeball in the orbital cavity by eye muscles is less pronounced than in mammals, the entire head, and not the eye alone, is rotated to focus on an object.

Other control mechanisms are also bird-specific. For example, there is no consensual pupillary light reflex in birds, as there is complete decussation of the optic nerves in the optic chiasm. Accommodation is also different from that in mammals, as the ciliary muscle is not made up of smooth muscle cells but of striated muscle fibres. Accommodation occurs either through a change in the corneal curvature (predominant in crepuscular or nocturnal bird species) or through a change in the lens curvature (predominant in diurnal birds). In the iris, too, there is no smooth but only striated musculature. This is relevant because classical mydriatics are not effective in birds, and pupil dilation can only be achieved with muscle relaxants (curare type).

■ Hearing

Hearing plays a role in birds, especially in nocturnal birds of prey. In general, the ear has a similar structure to the mammalian ear. Instead of an auricle, there are specialised feathers around the external auditory canal. In the middle ear, of the three ossicles, only the stapes is present. The inner ear has a similar structure to that of the mammal.

Although most bird species orient themselves visually, orientation by hearing is very specialised in owls. Direction finding, for example when hunting small mammals, is not only done in two dimensions (front – back and right – left), but through a height-shifted arrangement of the ears. Sound sources can be located in three dimensions.

■ Chemical senses

The senses of smell and taste are relatively little developed in birds. However, there are some specialisations in some avian species. Vultures, for example, can detect very small amounts of ethyl mercaptan, which is used to find carrion. Some shorebirds are able to distinguish between "wormy" and "non-wormy" sand using their sense of taste. In general, birds have a high tolerance to acids and alkalis, which enables them to use partly unripe fruits as a food source.

■ Sense of touch

The sense of touch does not play a significant role in the bird's skin. Nevertheless, there are different types of feathers (filament feathers and bristle feathers) that are innervated in such a way that they have sensory functions. The beak also has a whole series of sensory endings. In the woodpecker, the tongue is an important organ that has sensitive sensors.

■ Magnetic sense

The sense of magnetism plays a role particularly in migratory birds, but also in pigeons. Two mechanisms seem to be important for orientation in the earth's magnetic field: orientation through magnetite embedded in the beak and through chryptochromes located in the retina. The former is a magnetic iron compound that aligns itself to the Earth's magnetic field. In the second case, proteins appear to convert magnetic signals into visual information in the retina.

> **IN A NUTSHELL**   !
>
> The eye is the most important sensory organ in birds. It is extremely efficient.

3.7.2 Senses in reptiles

■ Sense of sight

Unlike birds, the sense of sight is not generally the dominant sense for orientation in the environment for reptiles. Furthermore, there are major differences between the individual reptile species. While snakes are less visually oriented, the eye of some lizard species (e.g. geckos) and turtles is very efficient. Anatomically, the reptile eye is comparable to the mammalian eye, but lizards and turtles have a bony scleral ring. As in the bird's eye, the iris musculature is transversely striated and there is no consensual pupillary reflex. A special adaptation is known in the chameleon, which can align the eyes largely independently and at the same time is able to calculate distances by accommodation to objects, especially when "shooting" prey with the tongue. Thus, these animals combine all-round vision (flight animal) with three-dimensional vision (hunter). Some lizard species have a so-called parietal eye. This is equipped with a sensory epithelium, but is not used to perceive "images". Rather, the function of the parietal eye can be considered as a light sensor, which is important for various endocrinological processes.

■ Hearing

Hearing is developed in reptiles, but usually does not play a significant role in orientation. As in birds, the ossicles in the middle ear are fused into a single bone. In snakes, the inner ear in particular is developed, and an eardrum is absent. Most reptiles, but especially snakes, have their hearing in the range of low-frequency sounds. Snakes also perceive vibrations of the underground.

■ Chemical senses and sense of touch

The sense of touch and the sense of taste do not play significant roles in reptiles. The sense of smell is the most important sense in many species (especially snakes). In particular, the perception of odours by the vomeronasal organ is an important function. By licking, the odorous substances are efficiently absorbed and can be presented to the sensory cells in a side-specific manner. This even makes three-dimensional orientation possible.

■ Infrared sense

In addition to the "classical" senses, some snake species also have the possibility of perception in the infrared range. Infrared sensors are located in the so-called pit organs (**Fig. 3.37**), on the jaw between the eye and the nostril. In rattlesnakes, these pit organs are formed as singular depressions between the nasal opening and the eyes on both sides, while in pythons several pits are "threaded" in the

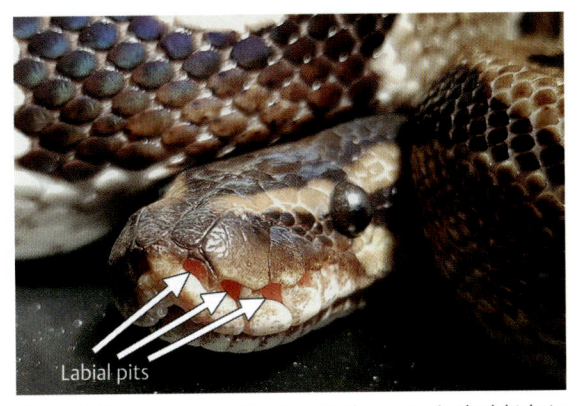

Fig. 3.37 Pit organ in a royal python (Python regius). The labial pits are clearly visible along the upper jaw. [Source: Prof. Dr. Michael Pees, Klinik für Heimtiere, Reptilien und Vögel, Stiftung TiHo Hannover]

region of the lips. The pit organs serve to locate prey by detecting heat radiation emitted by them. Free nerve endings of the trigeminal nerve, which are excited by an increase in temperature in the base of the pit, serve as sensors. This mechanism is very sensitive. Thus, mice with a body temperature of only 10 °C above the ambient temperature can be localised and struck from a distance of 60–70 cm, and rats even from a distance of 120 cm.

> **IN A NUTSHELL** !
>
> The most important senses in reptiles are the sense of sight and the sense of smell. Which sense plays the most important role depends on the species.

Suggested reading

Breer H, Fleischer J, Strotmann J. The sense of smell: multiple olfactory subsystems. Cell Mol Life Sci 2006; 63: 1465–1475

Chaudhari N, Roper SD. The cell biology of taste. J Cell Biol 2010; 190: 285–296

DeMaria S, Ngai J. The cell biology of olfaction. J Cell Biol 2010; 191: 443–452

Dotson CD, Geraedts MC, Munger SD. Peptide regulators of peripheral taste function. Semin Cell Dev Biol 2013; 24: 232–239

Lindemann B. Receptors and transduction in taste. Nature 2001; 413: 21–225

Mombaerts P. Genes and ligands for odorant, vomeronasal and taste receptors. Nat Rev Neurosci 2004; 5: 263–278

Roper SD. Taste buds as peripheral chemosensory processors. Semin Cell Dev Biol 2012; 24: 71–79

Scanes CG, Dridi S. Sturkie's Avian Physiology. Philadelphia: Elsevier; 2021

4   Autonomic nervous system

Martin Diener

4.1   Function of the autonomic nervous system

The autonomic component of the nervous system includes that part which **regulates the internal organs and metabolic processes**. Here, the role of the autonomic nervous system is closely integrated with those of the endocrine and somatic nervous systems. The **autonomic nervous system** is largely beyond voluntary control. However, there are close interactions between the autonomic and somatic nervous systems, so that processes such as micturition or defecation, which are primarily controlled by the autonomic nervous system, can also be under voluntary control.

4.2   Structure of the sympathetic and parasympathetic systems

The autonomic nervous system has different functional components: the sympathetic and the parasympathetic systems as well as the enteric nervous system (p. 361), which is described in the chapter on the Gastrointestinal Tract. The first two of these systems are the component parts of the classical autonomic nervous system. In addition, there are visceral afferents that transmit information from the internal organs to the central nervous system.

Sympathetic and parasympathetic nerves have many similarities in their structure (**Fig. 4.1**). Their cells have the basic arrangement of two-neuron chains. The central parts of the autonomic nervous system are located in the spinal cord and the brainstem, while the peripheral neurons are located outside the central nervous system in ganglia. The sympathetic ganglia are mainly located close to the central nervous system and thus distant from the organs they innervate, while those of the parasympathetic are close to the organs they innervate. The central neurons are called preganglionic neurons because they lie in front of the ganglia, while the neurons in the ganglia themselves are called postganglionic neurons by analogy. Slightly myelinated (B fibres) or unmyelinated nerve fibres (C fibres; **Table 2.3**) run from the preganglionic neurons to the postganglionic neurons. There is considerable divergence (i.e., a preganglionic neuron innervates multiple postganglionic neurons) as well as convergence (i.e., a postganglionic neuron is innervated by multiple preganglionic neurons) in synaptic connectivity within the ganglia. Thin, unmyelinated nerve fibres emanate from the postganglionic neurons and innervate the individual organs (**Table 4.1**).

The preganglionic **sympathetic neurons** are located in the spinal cord in the region of the lateral horns. Sympathetic neurons are not found in all regions of the spinal cord, but only in the thoracic and lumbar parts (Th_1 to $L_{2/3}$ in humans; in dogs, horses and cattle up to L_4 /L_6). The nerve cell bodies of these neurons send their axons to the sympathetic trunk with the **rami communicantes**. This consists of a series of paravertebral ganglia (e.g. ggl. cervicale craniale, ggl. cervicale medium and ggl. stellatum). This is where the junction with the second (postganglionic) neuron is located. In addition to the sympathetic trunk, which lies on both sides of the spine, there are a number of prevertebral ganglia of the sympathetic nervous system, which are located ventral to the spine and are unpaired (ggl. coeliacum, ggl. mesentericum craniale and ggl. mesentericum caudale). The preganglionic axons of the neurons connecting to these ganglia pass the sympathetic trunk without synaptic transmission. The fibres of the postganglionic neurons run as vegetative nerves or with the blood vessels to the organs to be innervated. The innervated targets of these nerves are the smooth muscles of all organs, the blood vessels and, in some cases, the exocrine glands as well as the heart.

The **parasympathetic preganglionic neurons** are located in the brainstem and sacral parts of the spinal cord (**Fig. 4.1.**). Parasympathetic nuclei are found in the mesencephalon, pons, and medulla oblongata. Their axons connect to cranial nerves with vegetative parts (oculomotor nerve, facial nerve, glossopharyngeal nerve, vagus nerve).

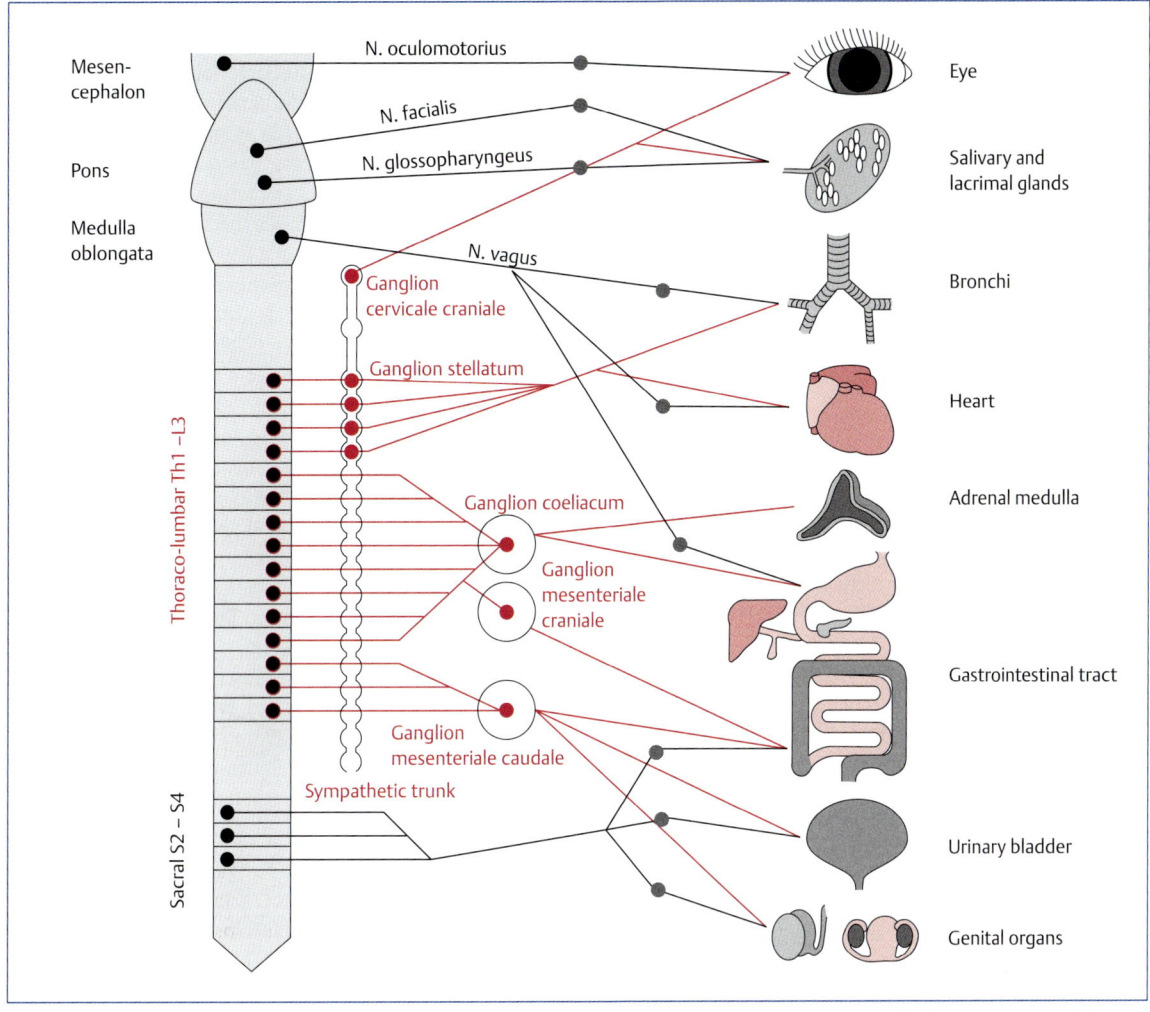

Fig. 4.1 Schematic arrangement of the sympathetic (red) and parasympathetic (grey) nervous system. In the deeper sections of the sympathetic trunk, there are neuronal junctions between pre- to postganglionic neurons, which to simplify, are not shown. The processes of these postganglionic neurons usually serve to innervate the blood vessels that run to the individual organs. The labelling of spinal cord segments with sympathetic (Th$_1$ -L$_3$) and parasympathetic parts (S$_1$ -S$_4$) refers to humans.

There are also parasympathetic preganglionic neurons in the region of the intermediate horn in the sacral segments of the spinal cord (S$_2$–S$_4$). Interconnection to the postganglionic neurons are formed in ganglia that are located close to their organs of innervation. The target organs of the parasympathetic system are smooth muscles and secretory glands. With a few exceptions (e.g. arterioles in the sexual organs), **blood vessels are not innervated parasympathetically**.

There are clear differences between the neuronal junctions in the pre- and postganglionic interconnections. The preganglionic sympathetic and parasympathetic neurons generally use acetylcholine as a transmitter for excitation at synapses with postganglionic neurons (**Fig. 4.2**). The axons of the postganglionic neurons eventually run to the organs to be innervated. In contrast to the somatic nervous system, there are no highly specialized contact points between neuron and end organ in the postganglionic junc-

tions, i.e. **no real synapses**. Instead, the autonomic nerve fibres have swellings (**varicosities**) at regular intervals, in which there are vesicles with transmitters that are released when an action potential arrives. The transmitters diffuse over a relatively long distance (up to 1 µm) through the extracellular space to the end organ, where they bind to receptors. This means that, in contrast to the innervation of skeletal muscles, no targeted activation of individual motor units is possible. While the preganglionic parasympathetic and sympathetic use the same transmitters, they differ with regard to the postganglionic transmitters. In the parasympathetic it is acetylcholine and in the sympathetic it is – with a few exceptions – noradrenaline.

IN A NUTSHELL !

Sympathetic and parasympathetic nervous systems each consist of two neuron chains.

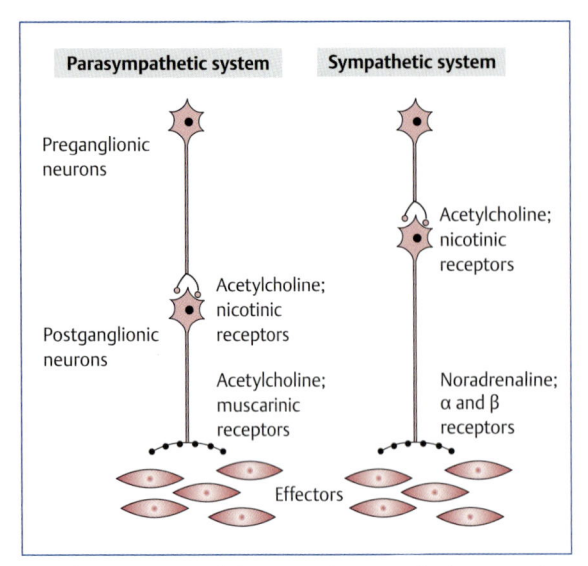

Fig. 4.2 Arrangement of the pre- and postganglionic neurons in the sympathetic and parasympathetic nervous system with the respective transmitters used and the predominant receptor types.

4.3   Sympathetic and parasympathetic effects

When the sympathetic and parasympathetic nervous systems both innervate the same organ, they often act in opposing functions and are stimulated under different conditions (**Table 4.1**). The sympathetic nervous system is increasingly activated when the body is under stress. Typical stimuli for the sympathetic nervous system are e.g. flight or fight situations. Activation of the sympathetic nervous system leads to a mobilization of performance reserves (ergotropic function) in order to adapt the animal to a **stressful** situation. The task of the **parasympathetic nervous system**, which becomes more active in resting situations and serves to maintain bodily functions (trophotropic function), is completely different.

A typical example of an **antagonism** between the sympathetic and parasympathetic nervous system is regulation of the heart rate. There is an increased rate when the sympathetic nervous system is stimulated. The parasympathetic nervous system, on the other hand, lowers the heart rate. But there are also processes in which both branches of the autonomic nervous system exert control **synergistically**. An example of this is male sexual function, where the parasympathetic nervous system produces erection through vasodilation while the sympathetic nervous system induces ejaculation. In contrast, the smooth muscle of most arterioles is an example of a tissue that is usually only innervated by the sympathetic nervous system. Stimulating the sympathetic nervous system leads to a contraction of many vessels that go to organs that are not critical, such as the arterioles of the skin or the gastrointestinal tract. There, the blood flow is reduced so that more O_2 or nutrients are available for acutely critical organs such as the heart or central nervous system. Depending on the vascular region, the sympathetic nervous system can increase or decrease blood flow in vessels that lead to skeletal muscles by triggering vasoconstriction or dilation (for the mechanism, see the section on adrenergic receptors (p. 117)). Apart from a few exceptions, the **vascular musculature is not parasympathetically innervated**. One of the few arterial vascular areas directly supplied by the parasympathetic nervous system are the penile and clitoral vessels. The veins are generally only sympathetically innervated. Stimulation of the sympathetic nervous system triggers a constriction so that blood reserves held in veins can be mobilised. A similar situation exists with the sweat glands, as they are only sympathetically innervated; the "sweat of fear" breaks out when the sympathetic nervous system is activated in a state of fear.

The muscles of the gastrointestinal tract provide an example of antagonistic regulation by the sympathetic and parasympathetic nervous system. Here the contraction of the circular and longitudinal muscles is increased by the parasympathetic nervous system, while the activity of the sphincters is reduced. The sympathetic nervous system has the opposite effect. A similar control applies to the urinary bladder: the parasympathetic nervous system promotes emptying of the bladder, whereas the sympathetic nervous system inhibits it. In the eye, the sympathetic nervous system innervates the dilatator pupillae muscle, which is why the pupil dilates when frightened, while the parasympathetic nervous system innervates the sphincter pupillae muscle and narrows the pupil.

The activity of the exocrine glands of the gastrointestinal tract, such as the pancreas, is promoted by the parasympathetic nervous system and inhibited by the sympathetic nervous system.

MORE DETAILS   With all these effects, however, one must not forget that the body does not regulate organ functions by "switching on" or "switching off" the sympathetic or parasympathetic nervous system. There is always a certain basic activity in both parts of the autonomic nervous system, which is referred to as parasympathetic tone and sympathetic tone. For both parts of the autonomic nervous system, the neurons usually exhibit spontaneous activity (0.1–4 Hz) that is organ-specific, depending on the needs of the body or the time of day. In other words, targeted changes in the activity of autonomic neural pathways lead to change in function of individual organs.

IN A NUTSHELL   !

The sympathetic becomes more active in stressful situations, the parasympathetic in resting conditions.

Table 4.1 Effects of sympathetic and parasympathetic nervous system on various organs.

Organ	Parasympathetic effects	Cholinergic receptors	Sympathetic effects	Adrenergic receptors
Heart				
Cardiac muscle	Frequency ↓	Musc. (M_2)	Frequency ↑	β_1
			Force of contraction ↑	β_1
Smooth musculature				
Vessels				
Arteries skin	–	–	Vasoconstriction	α_1
Aa. skeletal muscle	–	–	Vasoconstriction	α_1
			Vasodilation	β_2
Aa. genital organs	Vasodilation	Also NO and VIP involved	–	–
Veins	–	–	Vasoconstriction	α_1
Gastrointestinal Tract				
Longitudinal muscles	Motility ↑	Musc. (M_3)	Motility ↓	α_2 and β_2
Circular muscles	Motility ↑	Musc. (M_3)	Motility ↓	α_2 and β_2
Sphincters	Relaxation	Non-cholinergic transmitters are also involved	Constriction	α_1
Urogenital Tract				
M. detrusor vesicae	Contraction	Musc. (M_3)	Relaxation	β_2
M. sphincter vesicae int.	–	–	Contraction	α_1
Ductus deferens	–	–	Contraction	α_1
Uterus	–	–	Contraction	α_1
			Relaxation	β_2
Eye				
M. dilator pupillae	–	–	Contraction	α_1
M. sphincter pupillae	Contraction	Musc. (M_3)	–	
Further smooth muscles				
Bronchi	Contraction	Musc. (M_3)	Relaxation	β_2
Hair muscles	–	–	Contraction	α_1
Glandular cells				
Salivary glands	Serous secretion	Musc. (M_3)	Mucous secretion	α_1
Lacrimal glands	Secretion	Musc. (M_3)	–	
Digestive glands	Secretion	Musc. (M_3)	Secretion ↓	α_1
Sweat glands	–	–	Secretion ↑	Species dependent α or β, cholinergic in eccrine glands
Metabolism				
Liver	–	–	Glycogenolysis	β_2
Fat cells	–	–	Lipolysis	β_2/β_3

The functionally dominant receptor subtypes in an organ are shown. Cholinergic transmission is found at the sympathetically innervated sweat glands in humans and some primates, and at the soles of the feet in dogs and cats. The inhibition of the motility of the longitudinal and circular muscles by α_2 receptors takes place via an inhibition of acetylcholine release from enteric neurons.

4.4   Sympathetic and parasympathetic transmitters and receptors

4.4.1   Acetylcholine

The **synthesis** of acetylcholine (structure **Fig. 4.3**) requires the enzyme **choline acetyltransferase**, which combines acetate, esterified to coenzyme A, with choline. The synthesis takes place in the cytosol of the neurons. The resulting acetylcholine is stored in vesicles in the nerve endings. The basis for this transport is the acidification of the vesicles by a vesicular H^+-ATPase. An H^+/acetylcholine exchanger (vesicular acetylcholine transporter) uses the proton gradient built up by this pump to actively accumulate acetylcholine in the vesicles. Upon arrival of an action potential, the vesicles fuse with the nerve ending membrane and release acetylcholine into the extracellular space. This transmitter then diffuses to the receptors of the glandular or muscle cells.

Once stimulation of the receptors on the innervated organs has started, it must be possible to stop it again so that excitation can be controlled as required. This control is done by the degradation and diffusion of the transmitter or its cleavage products. The enzyme that inactivates acetylcholine is **acetylcholine esterase**. It is located both on the cell membrane of the end organs and on the releasing nerve endings. Acetylcholine esterase hydrolytically splits acetylcholine into acetate and choline. The acetate is "washed out" from the synaptic cleft and can then be used metabolically. Choline, on the other hand, is transported back to the nerve ending via a 2 Na^+-1 Cl^--1 choline co-transporter and can be used there for the synthesis of new acetylcholine.

> **IN A NUTSHELL**   !
>
> Acetylcholine is a transmitter at the synapse between the pre- and postganglionic neuron and at the contact point between the postganglionic parasympathetic neuron and the end organ.

4.4.2   Adrenaline and noradrenaline

Noradrenaline (norepinephrine) is the dominant neurotransmitter on the postganglionic sympathetic neurons (structure **Fig. 4.3**). Adrenaline (epinephrine), on the other hand, plays an important role as a hormone released into the blood from the adrenal medulla.

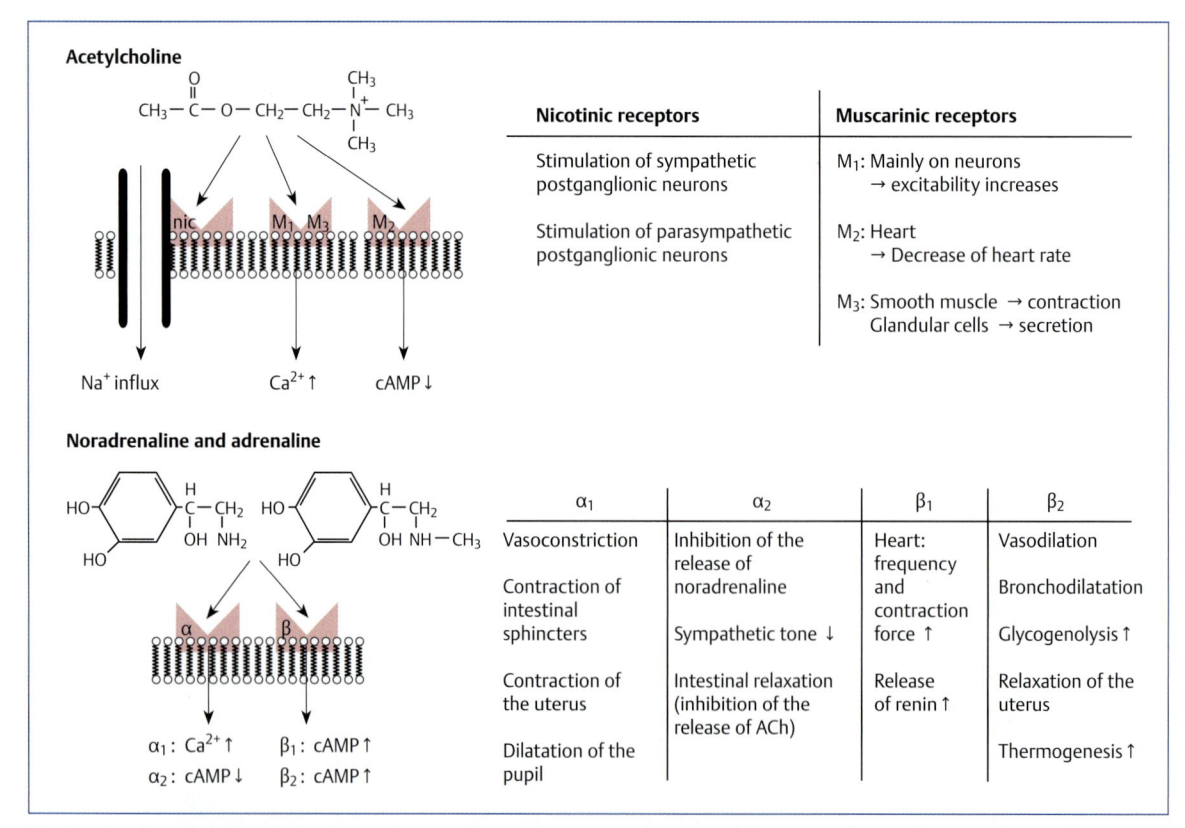

Fig. 4.3 Coupling of cholinergic (top) and adrenergic (bottom) receptor subtypes to different signalling pathways and typical locations of these subtypes (left). Acetylcholine can bind to nicotinic receptors (nic), which are ligand-gated cation channels. In addition, it can bind to G protein-coupled muscarinic receptors (M), which, depending on the subtype, lead to an increase in the cytosolic Ca^{2+} concentration (M_1, M_3) or, via inhibition of adenylate cyclase, to a decrease in the cytosolic cAMP concentration (M_2). All adrenergic receptors belong to the G protein-coupled receptors. Their main effect is an increase in cytosolic Ca^{2+} concentration (α_1), a decrease in cytosolic cAMP concentration via inhibition of adenylate cyclase (α_2), or an increase in cytosolic cAMP concentration via stimulation of adenylate cyclase (β_1–β_3).

MORE DETAILS The synthesis of both adrenergic substances begins with the amino acid tyrosine. Dopamine is produced in the cytosol of the nerve ending by hydroxylation to dopa (3,4-di-hydroxyphenylalanine) and subsequent decarboxylation. Dopamine is stored in vesicles and converted to noradrenaline by hydroxylation. Further methylation produces adrenaline from noradrenaline, in the adrenal medulla.

In contrast to the parasympathetic nerves, the diffusion of noradrenaline away from the receptor and its subsequent transport back from the extracellular space, plays the quantitatively decisive role for inactivation of transmitters in the sympathetic nervous system. Noradrenaline is transported across the membrane of the axon terminal into the cytosol by a Na^+-Cl^--noradrenaline cotransporter. There, it is taken up again into the vesicles mediated by a vesicular monoamine transporter (VMAT; acts as a monoamine/$2H^+$ exchanger) and is thus again available as a transmitter. There is also a metabolic breakdown of adrenaline and noradrenaline. Noradrenaline can be washed out of the junctions between the nerves and the innervated organ and thus enters the blood. As a result, like adrenaline, which has been released into the bloodstream by the adrenal medulla, it comes into contact with enzymes such as **monoamine oxidase** (**MAO**) and **catechol-O-methyl-transferase** (**COMT**), which are mainly localised in the lung, red blood cells and the liver. The end product of the enzymatic degradation is vanillylmandelic acid, which is excreted in urine.

> **IN A NUTSHELL** !
>
> Noradrenaline is the transmitter at the junction between a postganglionic sympathetic neuron and an end organ.

4.4.3 Cholinergic receptors

The receptors for acetylcholine on the parasympathetically innervated end organs differ significantly from the acetylcholine receptors on the autonomic ganglia. It was observed relatively early on that certain effects of acetylcholine can be mimicked by nicotine, an alkaloid in tobacco. This applies to the excitation of the postganglionic neurons by acetylcholine. Accordingly, the acetylcholine receptors in the ganglia are called **nicotinic receptors**. These are found on the postsynaptic membranes of the postganglionic neurons of the parasympathetic as well as those of the sympathetic nerves. In contrast, the acetylcholine receptors on the parasympathetically innervated end organs can be stimulated by an alkaloid of some mushrooms, muscarine. Accordingly, a distinction is made between two main types of receptors for acetylcholine, **nicotinic** and **muscarinic receptors** (**Fig. 4.2**).

The molecular structure of these different receptor types is now known (**Fig. 4.3**). Nicotinic receptors are pentamers of five subunits, which can vary significantly in their subunit composition depending on the cell type/localisation. Regardless of the respective subtype, **nicotinic receptors** usually represent **ligand-gated ion channels**. When acetylcholine binds to such a receptor, a non-selective cation channel opens and the cell membrane depolar-

izes, particularly as a result of an influx of Na^+. If the depolarization is strong enough and exceeds the threshold for the additional opening of fast, voltage-gated Na^+channels, an action potential is triggered.

The muscarinic receptors are divided into several receptor subtypes ($M_1 - M_5$; the subtypes $M_1 - M_3$ are of practical relevance) with different signal transduction. M_1 receptors are located, for example, in the central nervous system and on enteric neurons (**Fig. 4.3**). M_2 receptors are found on the pacemaker cells in the sinoatrial node and in the atrioventricular node of the heart. In contrast, the muscarinic receptors on most other end organs innervated by the parasympathetic nervous system belong to the M_3 subtype. All muscarinic receptors are **G protein-coupled receptors**. Binding of acetylcholine to a receptor triggers a conformational change in the receptor protein. This leads to a membrane-bound GTP-binding protein (G protein) being activated. In the case of muscarinic receptors of type M_1 or M_3, phospholipase C is activated after acetylcholine has bound to its receptor. This enzyme breaks down phospholipids in the cell membrane. This releases inositol-1,4,5-trisphosphate (IP_3), a chemical messenger that binds to receptors on intracellular Ca^{2+} stores, for example on the endoplasmic reticulum, and triggers the release of stored Ca^{2+} ions. Signal transmission is different for the M_2 receptors. Stimulation of these receptors leads to a decrease in the intracellular concentration of cAMP. The reason for this is that the M_2 receptor is coupled to an inhibitory G protein (G_i). This G_i protein binds to and inhibits adenylate cyclase, which converts ATP into cAMP.

> **IN A NUTSHELL** !
>
> Nicotinic and muscarinic receptors mediate the action of acetylcholine.

4.4.4 Adrenergic receptors

A similar variety of different receptor types can also be found for noradrenaline. These receptors respond not only to noradrenaline but also to adrenaline, which is why they are called adrenergic receptors. Two main forms are distinguished here, namely **α and β receptors**. For both, there are several subtypes ($\alpha_1 - \alpha_2$, $\beta_1 - \beta_3$), of which there are further variants in the case of the α receptors, which are named with letters (example: α_{1A}). The various adrenergic receptors are coupled to different signalling pathways in the cell. Stimulation of α_1 receptors leads to an increase in the cytosolic Ca^{2+}concentration. The signalling pathways involved are similar to those of the muscarinic receptors M_1 and M_3. The cAMP concentration is lowered via α_2 receptors—like the M_2 receptors—by inhibiting adenylate cyclase, while adenylate cyclase is activated via β receptors, regardless of the respective subtype.

These receptor subtypes are distributed differently in different parts of the body (**Table 4.1**). α_1 receptors are found in many organs innervated by the sympathetic nervous system. In the event of sympathetic stimulation, for example, they mediate vasoconstriction in the vessels of the skin and contraction of the sphincters in the gastrointestinal tract. An important localisation of α_2 receptors are nociceptive neurons. Their stimulation inhibits the transmission of nociceptive signals, which is exploited when analgesics are used (**Fig. 3.13**). α_2 receptors are also found on the membrane of the endings of adrenergic nerve cells. Their stimulation by noradrenaline inhibits the further release of noradrenaline.

The β receptors show a different tissue distribution (**Table 4.1**). β receptors of the type β_1 are mainly found in the heart. These are the receptors through which the sympathetic nervous system increases the heart rate via the sinus node, and the contraction force of the myocardium in stressful situations. In addition, β_1 receptors in the kidneys promote the release of the enzyme renin. In contrast, most other practically important β receptors are of the β_2 type. A third type of β receptor is known, the β_3 receptor, which in some species mediates the action of noradrenaline or adrenaline on adipose tissue.

> **IN A NUTSHELL**   !
>
> α and β receptors mediate the action of adrenaline and noradrenaline.

MORE DETAILS   In addition to their fundamental physiological significance, the variety of receptors in the autonomic nervous system is of enormous practical importance. This is because it is possible to selectively block or stimulate defined types of receptors using pharmacological agents. Since the sympathetic and parasympathetic nervous system regulate almost all functions in the body, this means that many such functions can be therapeutically modified by drugs that act in the autonomic nervous system. An example of this is **atropine**, a substance that occurs naturally in deadly nightshade. Atropine binds to muscarinic receptors without stimulating them. It thus acts as a muscarinic receptor blocker, as it prevents acetylcholine from reaching its binding site. An example of a therapeutic application is the use of atropine in anaesthesia. During anaesthesia, the parasympathetic nervous system is frequently excited, which can, for example, trigger bradycardia. This can be prevented by administering atropine before initiating anaesthesia. In the past, atropine was also used to dilate the pupil when examining the retina using an ophthalmoscope. In that system, atropine neutralizes the pupil-narrowing effect of the parasympathetic nervous system. However, atropine is no longer used for this. Instead, agents that are effective for a shorter time span due to faster degradation have replaced atropine for this purpose.

4.4.5   Cotransmitter

For a long time, it was assumed that a nerve cell only synthesizes and releases one transmitter. We now know that this is not so. There is a range of so-called cotransmitters that are released by many neurons, including those of the autonomic nervous system, in addition to the actual, classic transmitters such as acetylcholine or noradrenaline. Important cotransmitters in the autonomic nervous system are nitric oxide (NO), ATP and neuropeptides.

Nitric oxide (NO) is formed in nerve endings by NO synthase (**Fig. 4.4**). This enzyme cleaves NO from arginine, with citrulline being produced as a by-product. The form of NO synthase found in neurons is Ca^{2+}-dependent. Whenever voltage-dependent Ca^{2+} channels open after an action potential, the enzyme becomes active and forms the gas nitric oxide. Cell membranes are no obstacle for NO. It diffuses out of the nerve cell and reaches its target cell by diffusion. There, NO can pass the cell membrane almost unhindered, and then trigger a response in the cell. NO thus largely falls outside the scope of the usual neurotransmitters. It is not stored in vesicles but is synthesized and released when needed. In contrast to other neurotransmitters, nitric oxide does not act on receptors on the cell surface, but can penetrate directly into the innervated cell. In target cells, the effects of NO are mediated via cGMP as a second messenger. A cytosolic form of guanylate cyclase is activated by NO and produces more cGMP. An increase in the intracellular cGMP concentration in smooth muscle cells triggers a relaxation of the cell. Since this also applies to the smooth muscles of blood vessels, NO is an important vasodilator. The NO-induced vasodilation plays a role in penile erection, which is triggered parasympathetically by vasodilation in the corpus cavernosum, see ch. "Regulation of circulation" (p. 208).

MORE DETAILS   Another cotransmitter in the autonomic nervous system is **ATP**. As for noradrenaline or acetylcholine, certain target cells, such as smooth muscle cells, have receptors for ATP, the so-called purinergic receptors. Receptors for ATP are found, for example, on arteriolar walls and on the vas deferens, where ATP triggers a contraction. In addition, ATP has an important role in inhibiting gastrointestinal motility. The third class of cotransmitters are **neuropeptides** such as the vasoactive intestinal peptide (**VIP**) or the neuropeptide Y (**NPY**).

> **IN A NUTSHELL**   !
>
> In addition to the classic transmitters, cotransmitters are often released.

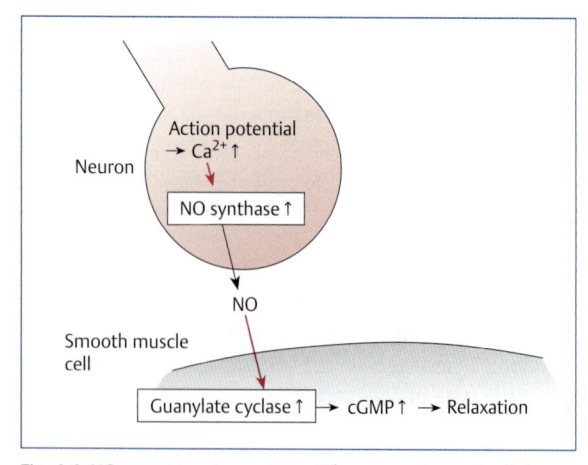

Fig. 4.4 NO as a neurotransmitter. When an action potential arrives, the opening of voltage-dependent Ca^{2+} channels at the synaptic terminals leads to an increase in the cytosolic Ca^{2+} concentration and, as a result, to a stimulation of the neuronal NO synthase, which produces NO from the amino acid arginine. This gas diffuses out of the nerve ending and binds to a cytosolic guanylate cyclase in the target cells. When it diffuses into smooth muscle cells, it stimulates the production of cGMP from GTP. This second messenger causes relaxation in smooth muscle cells.

4.5 Interaction with the endocrine system

The autonomic nervous system is closely related to the endocrine system, particularly the adrenal medulla (p. 547). In the mammalian adrenal glands, two different regions can be distinguished morphologically and functionally, the adrenal medulla and the adrenal cortex. The so-called chromaffin cells, which produce adrenaline or noradrenaline, are located in the medulla. In birds there is no separation into medulla and cortex. Adrenaline, and noradrenaline- or corticoid-producing cells are mixed here. In most species (exception: whale, chicken), the chromaffin cells produce more adrenaline than noradrenaline, the ratio is usually around 4:1. These hormones are stored in granules and released when needed through exocytosis.

MORE DETAILS Developmentally, the adrenal medulla corresponds to a large sympathetic ganglion. The chromaffin cells are descendants of sympathetic blast cells from the neural crest. Thus, they are modified "postganglionic" neurons that have lost their dendrites and axons and have become hormone-producing glandular cells. This explains the close connection between the sympathetic nervous system and the adrenal medulla. The chromaffin cells are innervated by presynaptic sympathetic neurons. The transmitter at the synapse between the preganglionic neuron and the chromaffin cell is acetylcholine. Acetylcholine triggers release of adrenaline and noradrenaline in the adrenal medulla.

Adrenaline and noradrenaline release from the adrenal medulla is induced by the same stimuli that cause sympathetic activation, such as **stress**, **fight**, **flight**, or **exposure to cold**. These adrenal messengers circulate in the blood and mobilize substrates from the liver and adipose tissue to provide metabolic energy.

> **IN A NUTSHELL**   !
>
> The autonomic nervous system and the endocrine system work closely together to control organ functions.

4.6 Vegetative afferents

Strictly speaking, the terms sympathetic and parasympathetic nervous systems only apply to the efferents in the autonomic nervous system. The reason for this is that the distinction between sympathetic and parasympathetic depends on how the efferent neurons are arranged and which transmitters they release.

However, in order to be able to do its job properly, the autonomic nervous system must receive information about the state of activity of the internal organs. This task is fulfilled by vegetative (visceral) afferents. They make up a large part of the fibres in autonomic nerves. For example, in the vagus nerve, a main nerve of the autonomic nervous system, more than 80% of the fibres that run to the abdomen are afferent, while in sympathetic nerves, such as the nervi splanchnici, their proportion is somewhat lower, at around 50%. The afferent fibres in such nerves are uniformly referred to as **visceral afferents**, regardless of

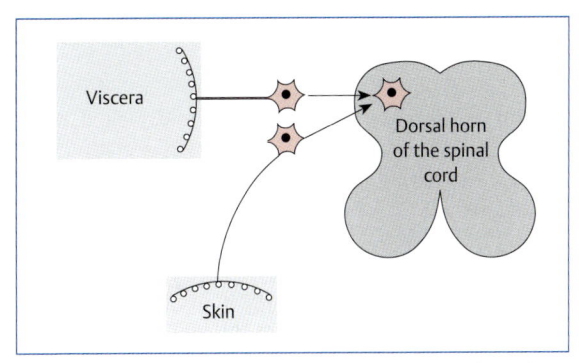

Fig. 4.5 Visceral afferents. In the dorsal horn, sensory fibres from the skin converge with afferent fibres from internal organs. As a result, pain sensation from internal organs is often wrongly perceived in areas of skin ("referred pain").

whether they join parasympathetic or sympathetic efferent nerves.

MORE DETAILS The neuronal somata of the vegetative afferents are located in the spinal ganglia or in the case of the afferents that run with the vagus nerve in the ggl. proximale (jugulare) or ggl. distale (nodosum) n. vagi. These neurons have very long extensions that branch out at the periphery. There, they are in contact with a wide variety of sensors. For example, in the gastrointestinal tract, stretch sensors provide information about the state of stretching of smooth muscles, and chemosensors provide information about the presence of particular chemical substances or the pH of the intestinal lumen. Stimulating these sensors causes action potentials to be triggered in the afferent fibres, which are transmitted in the direction of the central nervous system. There, junctions with neurons in the dorsal horn or neurons of the ncl. tractus solitarii are formed, where sensory fibres from the vagus nerve and the glossopharyngeal nerve end.

In the dorsal horn neurons, there is sometimes significant inaccuracy in the transmission of information. It appears that visceral afferents along with afferents from the skin converge on the same dorsal horn neurons (**Fig. 4.5**). Accordingly, it is often difficult for the central nervous system to distinguish where the impulse "it hurts" actually comes from, especially when it is perceived as pain. In this context one speaks of referred pain. This means that a perception of pain, which ultimately results from internal organs, is projected onto certain areas of the skin. The spinal cord is organised in segments, i.e. particular spinal cord segments are responsible for the innervation of very specific regions of the body. Pain sensation from some internal organs is therefore transmitted to certain areas of the skin, which are referred to as **Head's zones**. Since increased muscular tension very often occurs in the affected regions, it is important to know Head's zones, because these symptoms can be detected by simple clinical examinations such as observation or palpation, see ch. "Central mechanisms of nociception" (p. 79).

> **IN A NUTSHELL**   !
>
> Afferent fibres inform the autonomic nervous system about the condition of individual organs.

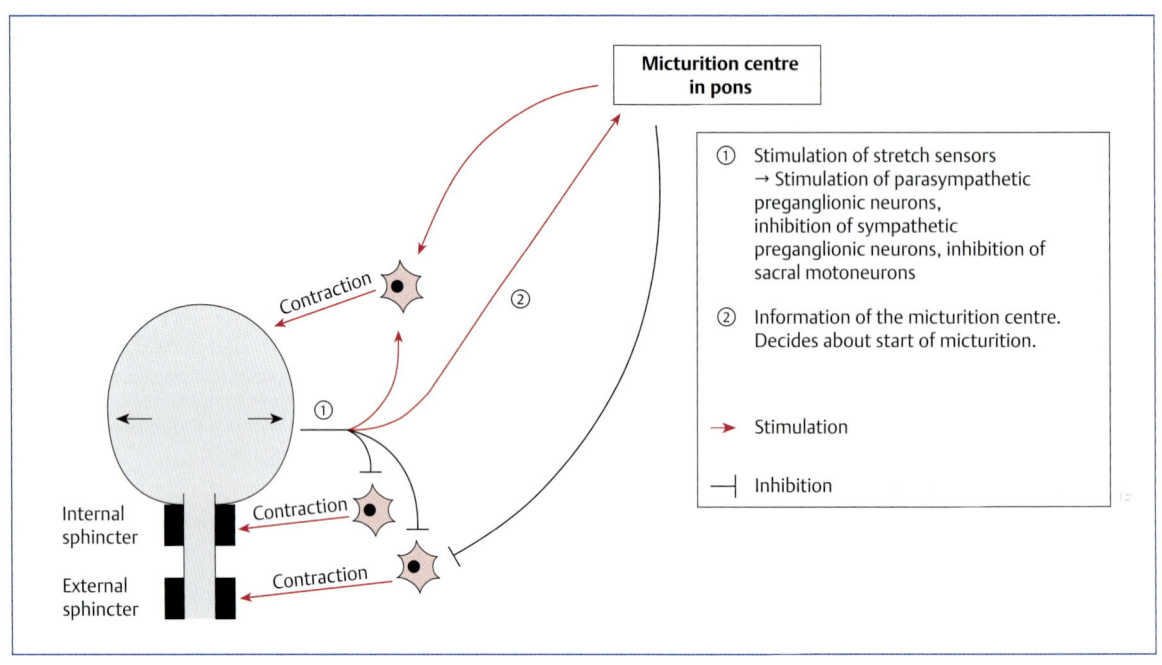

Fig. 4.6 Control of voiding of the bladder (red arrows: stimulation). Excitation of stretch sensors in the bladder results in (1) stimulation of parasympathetic preganglionic neurons (innervating the detrusor muscle), inhibition of sympathetic preganglionic neurons (innervating the internal sphincter), and inhibition of sacral motoneurons (innervating the external sphincter). As a rule, micturition only starts when (2) the micturition centre in the pons amplifies these effects. Once started, the process of voiding is self-boosting due to the pressure increase in the bladder during detrusor contraction, which causes the bladder to be completely emptied.

4.7   Vegetative reflexes

The autonomic nervous system works closely together with the central nervous system. Groups of neurons in the medulla oblongata influence many functions of the autonomic nervous system, such as in the cardiovascular system. These in turn are under the control of the hypothalamus (p. 140), which is a kind of interface between the voluntary and involuntary nervous system and the endocrine system.

> **MORE DETAILS**   The interaction between the voluntary and involuntary nervous system will be explained in more detail using as an example a reflex process, **micturition**. The bladder is innervated sympathetically and parasympathetically (**Fig. 4.6**). The parasympathetic preganglionic neurons are located in the sacral part of the spinal cord in the segments S_2–S_4. Their axons run with the pelvic splanchnic nerve to the bladder. The postganglionic neurons are located in the vesical nervous plexus in close proximity to the urinary bladder. Excitation of these parasympathetic fibres causes contraction of the detrusor and relaxation of the sphincter vesicae internus, initiating micturition. Excitation of the sympathetic nerve fibres has the opposite effect on the detrusor and sphincter. In addition, there is the m. sphincter urethrae externus, which consists of skeletal muscles and is innervated voluntarily. The corresponding motoneurons are located in the sacral part of the spinal cord.
>
> Stretch sensors in the bladder wall send the message "the bladder is full" to the spinal cord. There are connections to the preganglionic parasympathetic and sympathetic neurons: the parasympathetic neurons are activated, the sympathetic ones are inhibited. In addition, the motoneurons that innervate the skeletal muscles of the external urethral sphincter are inhibited. In order for voiding of the bladder to start, however, an additional fac-

tor must be present, namely an influence of the brain. In the pons, there are groups of neurons that control bladder emptying. Only when an activating influence of these neurons occurs does micturition begin. The pontine centres are in turn connected to other nuclei of the brainstem, the hypothalamus and the cerebrum. This ensures that there is voluntary control of micturition. Once underway, the process of micturition boosts itself due to the increase in pressure in the bladder during detrusor contraction, causing the bladder to be almost completely emptied.

> **IN A NUTSHELL**   !
>
> In many reflexes such as urination or defecation, the vegetative and somatic nervous systems work closely together.

Suggested reading

Brown DA. Acetylcholine and cholinergic receptors. Brain Neurosci Adv 2019; 3: 1–10

Browning KN, Travagli RA. Central nervous system control of gastrointestinal motility and secretion and modulation of gastrointestinal functions. Comprehen Physiol 2014, 4:1339–1368

Moncada S, Higgs EA. The discovery of nitric oxide and its role in vascular biology. Brit J Pharmacol 2006; 147/Suppl.1: S93-S201

Wehrwein EA, Orer HS, Barman SM. Overview of the anatomy, physiology, and pharmacology of the autonomic nervous system. Compr Physiol 2016; 6:1239–1278

5 Central nervous system

Martin Diener, Melanie Hamann; former collaboration: R. Gerstberger

5.1 Function of the central nervous system

ESSENTIALS ✖

The central nervous system provides the dominant control for many processes in an animal. Together with the endocrine system and local regulation by paracrine substances at tissue level, it influences the function of practically every organ in an animal. Its functions include the processing of incoming stimuli acting on sensory cells, the coordination of motor activity, the control of behaviour and (in humans) conscious thought. It is composed of grey matter (nerve cell somata) and white matter (conduction pathways). The communication of the neurons with each other or with their effector cells is characterised by a multitude of neurotransmitters and their receptors.

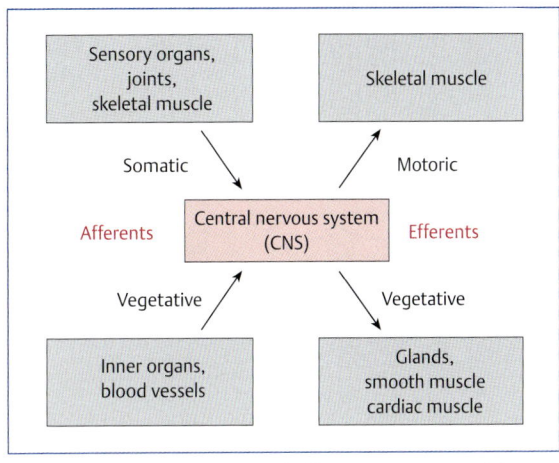

Fig. 5.1 Examples of afferent and efferent connections of the central nervous system.

5.2 Neuroanatomical structure

The term central nervous system (CNS) refers to the brain and the spinal cord. The CNS has various functions. For example, it controls muscle activity, controls the blood supply to tissues and, together with the hormone system and paracrine messengers, regulates the function of practically every single organ as well as all integrative processes of the entire animal.

The CNS needs neuronal connections to supply it with afferent information about particular parameters from specific organs or tissues (**Fig. 5.1**). Such nerve fibres can, for example, transmit signals from the locomotor system (position of a joint, stretching of a muscle), from the skin (pressure, touch, temperature) or from specialised sensory organs (eye, ear) to the CNS, which are then referred to as **somatic afferents**. If the information comes from visceral organs (e.g. gastrointestinal tract, heart, lungs), these are **vegetative afferents**.

Those nerve fibres that extend away from the CNS are called efferent pathways. They are also subdivided into **motor efferents** which travel to skeletal muscles and trigger muscle contractions, and **vegetative efferents** which serve to control internal organs. They extend to endocrine organs, to the smooth muscle cells of many organs and blood vessels or to the heart muscle, and they influence their functions.

In order for the CNS to be able to perform its diverse functions, it contains a large number of neurons. The total number of all central nerve cells is about 100 billion in humans, 10 billion in a dolphin and 0.5 billion in a cat. However, if the cognitive performance of the brain is consid-

ered, it is not only the absolute number of neurons but also their packing density and, above all, their synaptic connections with other neurons, that determine the function. These factors are most impressively pronounced in primates, elephants and birds of prey. In the human brain, depending on the anatomic localisation, there are 2000–10000 synapses per neuron. Because of this extremely dense array of interconnections, it is rather difficult to assign specific functions to individual neuronal substructures of the brain or spinal cord. There are usually groups of neurons in several substructures which are jointly responsible for any specific task.

The CNS is subdivided into seven main regions, these are – from caudal to rostral – the spinal cord, the medulla oblongata, the pons, the mesencephalon (midbrain), the diencephalon, the cerebellum, and the telencephalon (endbrain, cerebrum) (**Fig. 5.2**).

5.2.1 Structure of the spinal cord

The spinal cord is that component of the CNS located within the spinal canal (**Fig. 5.3**). The centrally located **"grey" matter** is divided bilaterally into dorsal, lateral and ventral horns. The majority of the nerve cell somata are located in the grey matter in the **ventral horn**. The myelinated axons of these motor neurons leave the spinal cord via the ventral roots into the periphery and innervate skeletal muscles. Conversely, the spinal cord receives axons from sensory neurons in the periphery via the dorsal roots, which project to neurons in the ipsilateral **dorsal horn**, among others. The action potentials transmitted by these afferents originate from sensory cells of the skin, propriosensors from muscles, tendons and joints, and the internal

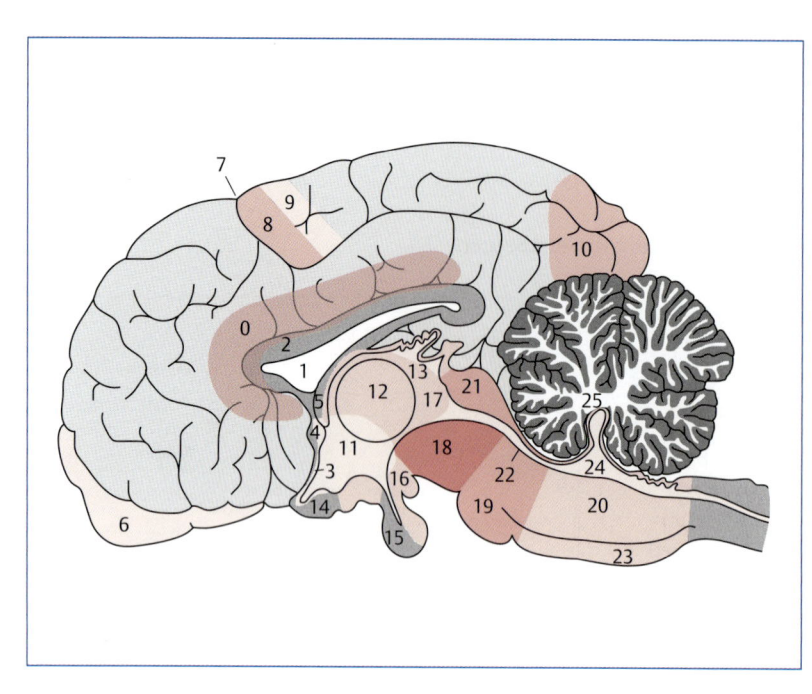

Fig. 5.2 Location of different parts of the CNS on a medial sagittal section through the brain of a dog. The position of some structures of the end brain (area motoria, sensoria and optica, basal ganglia, bulbus olfactorius), the diencephalon (hypothalamus, thalamus and epithalamus) and the brainstem (mesencephalon, pons and medulla oblongata) are projected onto the section.
Telencephalon: 0 Basal ganglia, **1** Septum pellucidum, **2** Corpus callosum, **3** Lamina terminalis, **4** Commissura rostralis, **5** Fornix, **6** Bulbus olfactorius, **7** Sulcus cruciatus, **8** Area motoria, **9** Area sensoria, **10** Area optica.
Diencephalon: 11 Hypothalamus, **12** Thalamus, **13** Epithalamus, **14** Chiasma opticum, **15** Pituitary gland, **16** Corpus mamillare, **17** III. Cerebral ventricle.
Brainstem: 18 Mesencephalon, **19** Pons, **20** Medulla oblongata, **21** Tectum, **22** Aquaeductus mesencephali, **23** Pyramis, **24** IV. Cerebral ventricle.
Cerebellum: 25 Arbor vitae.

organs. The somata of all pseudounipolar sensory neurons are localised in the ganglia (dorsal root ganglia) embedded in the dorsal roots. Preganglionic neurons of the sympathetic nervous system are located in the **lateral horn** of the thoracic medulla, and partly also in the lumbar medulla. Preganglionic neurons of the parasympathetic nervous system are localised in the sacral spinal cord (**Fig. 4.1**).

The peripherally located "**white matter**" of the spinal cord can be divided bilaterally into a ventral, a lateral and a dorsal column, in which the axons of nerve cells run. On the one hand, these are **association neurons** that connect different spinal cord segments and **commissural neurons**, the axons of which decussate to the contralateral side. On the other hand, there are **ascending or descending pathways**, the axons of which conduct information from the spinal cord to the brain or from the brain to the spinal cord. The axons of the numerous **interneurons** run within the grey matter.

> ### IN A NUTSHELL !
>
> The spinal cord contains connections to and from the brain. Motoneurons of the ventral horn innervate the skeletal muscles from here, while the dorsal horn receives somato- and viscerosensory afferents. Preganglionic neurons of the sympathetic nervous system are located in the lateral horn.

Like many other regions of the CNS, the grey matter of the spinal cord consists of ten layers according to their cytoarchitectonics, and is **somatotopically** organised (**Fig. 5.3**). This means that defined regions of the nervous system are responsible for innervation of defined regions of the body. For example, the ventral horn has a somatotopic division of motoneurons (laminae VIII and IX) for the efferent innervation of skeletal muscles. Central neuronal groups innervate the muscles of the trunk and shoulder.

Medial neurons innervate the muscles of the proximal limb regions, while lateral neurons innervate the muscles of the distal parts of the limbs. In the ventral field of the ventral horn, there are motoneurons for the extensor muscles, in the dorsal field those for the flexor muscles.

Somatotopy is also evident with the afferents arriving in the dorsal column of the spinal cord from propriosensors of the musculoskeletal system and mechanosensors of the skin. Those pathways that form the funiculus dorsalis (posterior column) conduct incoming signals towards the brainstem. They are arranged in such a way that information originating from sacral or lumbar neurons is conducted medially in the fasciculus gracilis. Information from thoracic or cervical neurons is conducted laterally in the fasciculus cuneatus. Similarly, the information from cutaneous sensors for temperature and pain, is conducted in the tractus (tr.) spinothalamicus (anterior column), and is organised in a somatotopical arrangement.

The efferent tracts such as the tr. corticospinalis or the tr. rubrospinalis, are somatotopically organised. These are connections of the motor cerebral cortex or the ncl. ruber in the brainstem with the spinal cord. They are concerned with supraspinal motor activity (p. 132) (**Fig. 5.3**).

5.2.2 Parts of the brain

The **brainstem** is the rostral continuation of the spinal cord (**Fig. 5.2**) and consists of three parts, namely the **medulla oblongata**, the **pons** and the **mesencephalon**. The medulla oblongata is the direct extension of the spinal cord into the cranial cavity and accordingly has many similarities with the spinal cord.

In all three parts of the brainstem there are collections of nerve cells of comparable function and transmitter equipment with visceromotor significance, i.e. nuclei in which **parasympathetic preganglionic neurons** are localised, see ch. "Structure of the sympathetic and parasympa-

Cell, tissue

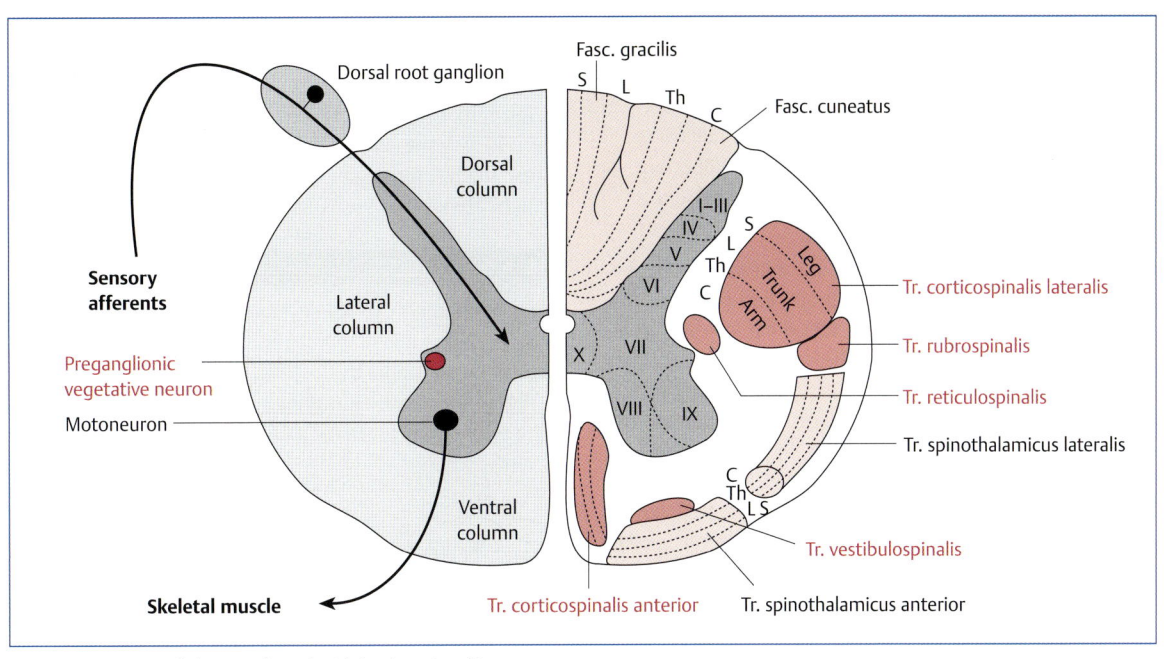

Fig. 5.3 Structure of the spinal cord with laminae I to X.
Left: Dorsal, lateral and ventral horn of the grey matter and columns of the white matter for ascending and descending tracts.
Right: Organisation of the grey matter into laminae and localisation of ascending (pink) and descending (red filled) tracts in the white matter.
S = sacral, L = lumbar, Th = thoracic, C = cervical.

thetic systems" (p. 112). These include the medullary ncl. parasympathicus n. vagi (ncl. dorsalis n. vagi), which is the autonomic nucleus of the vagus nerve for controlling the activity of numerous internal organs (lungs, heart, gastrointestinal tract), as well as the pontine ncll. parasympathici n. intermedii (ncl. salivatorius rostralis) and n. glossopharyngei (ncl. salivatorius caudalis), the axons of which run in the n. facialis and glossopharyngeus and activate salivary secretion after ganglionic transmission. In addition, neurons of the n. facialis parasympathetic nerve (lacrimal nerve) supply the lacrimal and nasal glands after forming neuronal interconnections in the pterygopalatine ganglion. Finally, in the mesencephalon is the ncl. parasympathicus n. oculomotorii (ncl. Edinger-Westphal), from which parasympathetic fibres run to the eye. Postganglionic fibres then innervate the sphincter pupillae and ciliaris muscles.

Cranial motoneurons are located in both the medulla oblongata and the pons. The nuclei of the motor cranial nerves (ncll. efferentes), which originate in the medulla oblongata, are located medially. In the medulla oblongata are the ncl. n. accessorii for the innervation of the shoulder muscles and the ncl. ambiguus, a nucleus of the vagus and glossopharyngeal nerves, for the innervation of muscles of the throat and larynx. This nucleus also contains preganglionic neurons for parasympathetic control of the heart (p. 178). In addition, there is the somatomotor nucleus of the hypoglossal nerve for the innervation of the tongue muscles. Pontine somatomotor nuclei are those of the n. abducens, the n. trochlearis and the n. oculomotorius, as well as the nuclei of the facial nerve (innervation of the facial muscles) and the motor nucleus of the trigeminal nerve (innervation of the muscles of mastication).

The **neuronal cell populations of the sensory nuclei**, which are mainly located laterally, partially extend into the medulla oblongata and the mesencephalon. These include the ncl. tractus solitarii, where sensory fibres from the vagus and glossopharyngeal nerves terminate, the nuclear region of the trigeminal nerve (ncl. principalis n. trigemini, ncl. tractus mesencephali, ncl. tractus spinalis), the ncll. vestibulares and the ncll. cochleares, in which sensory fibre connections from the vestibular and auditory organs, respectively, terminate. The pons also contains many neurons for the transmission of information between the cerebral cortex and the cerebellum.

Through the entire brainstem, i.e. from the end of the spinal cord to the beginning of the diencephalon, the so-called **formatio reticularis** runs as a net-like configuration of neurons. It consists of nuclei of mostly parvocellular nerve cells that are often difficult to distinguish from one another and diffusely merge into one another. The numerous ncll. raphes, which are involved in the descending suppression of spinal pain conduction (p. 79), and the locus coeruleus are clearly recognisable. Several "centres" of high physiological significance can be distinguished, not so much on the basis of their morphology, but rather on their functional aspects. They are located in the region of the formatio reticularis, such as the respiratory centre (p. 291), the cardiovascular centre (see ch.s on "Brainstem" (p. 139), "Regulation of circulation" (p. 208)), the "Micturition centre" (p. 120) , the vomiting centre, the eye movement centre, or the waking centre (p. 142), in which the locus coeruleus plays an important role. Substructures of the formatio reticularis are also involved in the control of muscle tone of proximal limbs and the trunk within the framework of the extrapyramidal system (p. 135).

> **IN A NUTSHELL**   !
>
> The brainstem contains preganglionic parasympathetic, motor and sensory nuclei as well as the formatio reticularis, which is composed of diffuse nuclei that are difficult to distinguish from one another and regulates important autonomic functions such as respiration or circulation.

The **diencephalon**, together with the telencephalon, belongs to the prosencephalon (forebrain) and connects rostrally to the mesencephalon (**Fig. 5.2**). It can be divided into three substructures: (1) the **epithalamus**, which essentially contains the pineal gland (syn.: epiphysis), (2) the thalamus with numerous substructures, which are important relay stations of sensory afferent pathways (p.135) – with the exception of the sense of smell – to the cortex, and (3) the hypothalamus (p.139), which is located ventral to the thalamus. The hypothalamus is the supreme coordination centre for the autonomic nervous system and thus for the homeostasis of vegetative functions as well as the neuroendocrine control of pituitary and important peripheral hormone systems (p.539).

The cerebellum (p.134) lies above the pons and midbrain. It has important functions in the coordination of movements and in motor learning. The cerebellum receives afferents from the spinal cord, the vestibular nuclei of the pons and the cerebrum, while its efferents pass through the thalamus to the cerebral cortex, the medulla oblongata and the mesencephalon. Thus, in interaction with the cortex and basal ganglia, it can take over the fine-tuning of movements.

The uppermost level of the CNS is the **cerebrum**. It consists of the **cerebral cortex** and the **basal ganglia** which are nuclear complexes of grey matter in the depths of the cerebral hemispheres. The main functions of the cerebrum are to control higher motor and sensory functions. The localisation of grey and white matter in the cerebrum is an exact mirror image of the spinal cord. On the outside is the grey matter with the neuronal somata, while on the inside is the white matter with the axons. In addition, there are the nerve cell bodies, which have been displaced into the depths in the form of the basal ganglia. The cerebral cortex is divided into different regions. The frontal lobe lies rostrally, followed by the temporal and parietal lobes; the occipital lobe is the most caudal region.

Histologically, the cerebral cortex consists of six layers (laminae). Layers I-IV have afferent functions, while layers V and VI have efferent functions. Different cortex regions can also be distinguished according to their function. Primary sensory cortex areas respond to only one sensory input, whereas the primary motor cortex has direct control of voluntary movements (see ch. on the pyramidal system (p.133). Secondary sensory or motor areas are responsible for more complex processing in the case of sensory activity or for initiating and planning voluntary motor activity. There is also the association cortex. This is where, in humans, higher functions of the brain such as conscious thought are located.

> **IN A NUTSHELL**   !
>
> The cerebrum is the highest-order control centre for the whole animal. It is supported by the diencephalon (control of sensory input by the thalamus, control of endocrine and vegetative functions by the hypothalamus) and the cerebellum (control of planned and executed movements).

5.3   Transmitters in the central nervous system

5.3.1   Transmitter diversity

The CNS expresses a large number of neurotransmitters. These originate from various classes of molecules such as **amines** (e.g. catecholamines, serotonin), **peptides** (e.g. endorphins, neuropeptide Y, substance P), **amino acids** and their derivatives (e.g. glutamate, glycine, γ-aminobutyric acid (GABA)) or even gaseous molecules (so-called **gasotransmitters** such as nitric oxide (NO)). Furthermore, since there are usually several types of receptors for each neurotransmitter, this results in a multitude of possibilities for communication between neurons via presynaptically released neurotransmitters and postsynaptically (and also presynaptically) localised receptors. **Table 5.1** gives an overview of some transmitters used in the CNS.

> **MORE DETAILS**   Often, these receptors are also sites of action for pharmaceuticals. For example, barbiturates stimulate $GABA_A$ receptors. These are ligand-gated chloride channels (ionotropic receptors). The resulting influx of Cl^- hyperpolarizses the postsynaptic membrane and thereby reduces neuronal excitability. This is the basis of the sedative (calming) and anticonvulsive (counteracting epileptic seizures) or, in higher doses, narcotic (anaesthetic) effect of barbiturates.

> **IN A NUTSHELL**   !
>
> The multitude of neurotransmitters produced by neurons in the CNS and their different receptors allow differentiated control of physiological processes, or targeted therapeutic influence of these processes by pharmaceuticals.

Table 5.1 Examples of neurotransmitters, their receptors and functions in the CNS; importance in animal and human medicine

Transmitter	Important receptors	(1) Tasks in the CNS (2) Medical significance
Acetylcholine	Muscarinic receptors (M_1-M_5; metabotropic), nicotinic receptors (with different composition of α and β subunits; ionotropic)	(1) Learning processes; drive (2) Deficiency causes dementia diseases such as Alzheimer's disease (human)
Adrenaline, noradrenaline	α receptors (α_1, α_2; metabotropic), β receptors (β_1–β_3; metabotropic)	(1) Ascending reticular activating system (ARAS); medullo-hypothalamic afferents (2) Depression, in the case of deficiency; mania, in the case of functional excess
Dopamine	D_1-D_5 (metabotropic)	(1) Movement control; control of the adenohypophysis (2) Decreased production in the substantia nigra of the brainstem as a cause of Parkinson's disease (human) Most important neurotransmitter for the reward system ("happiness hormone") and therefore important for addictive behaviour
Endorphins, enkephalins and dynorphins	μ, δ and κ receptors, etc.	(1) Endogenous inhibition of spinal pain afferents and central pain sensation (2) Activation by exogenous opiates and opioids (→ analgesia)
GABA (γ-aminobutyric acid)	$GABA_A$ and $GABA_C$ (ionotropic), $GABA_B$ (metabotropic)	(1) Most important inhibitory transmitter in the CNS (2) Stimulation of $GABA_A$ receptors by barbiturates (sedative or narcotic effect); enhancement of the effect of GABA by tranquillisers such as benzodiazepines (→ sedative effect)
Glutamate, aspartate	AMPA, kainate and NMDA receptors (ionotropic), mGluR1-mGluR8 (metabotropic)	(1) Most important excitatory transmitter in the CNS; movement control; memory (2) In case of overexcitation, death of nerve cells through apoptosis (excitotoxicity)
Glycine	Glycine receptor (ionotropic), NMDA receptor (ionotropic)	(1) Important inhibitory neurotransmitter in the spinal cord (2) Convulsions due to inhibition of glycine release by tetanus toxin at the spinal cord level
Histamine	H_1-H_3 receptors (metabotropic)	(1) Triggering vomiting; regulation of the sleep-wake rhythm (2) H_1-antihistamines as antiemetics
Neuropeptide Y	Y_1-Y_5 receptors (metabotropic)	(1) Appetite regulation
Serotonin (5-HT)	$5\text{-}HT_1$, $5\text{-}HT_2$, $5\text{-}HT_4$ to $5\text{-}HT_7$ (metabotropic), $5\text{-}HT_3$ (ionotropic)	(1) Pain; sleep-wake rhythm; depression in case of deficiency (2) $5\text{-}HT_{1B/1D}$ receptor agonists against migraine; $5\text{-}HT_3$ receptor antagonists as antiemetics

5.3.2   Neuronal projections

Often, functionally related neurons use similar neurotransmitters. Immunohistochemical labelling and neuronal tracer methods can be used to find out the site of formation of the transmitters and the projections of the neurons involved. The visualisation of such **pathways** provides important information about the communication of different regions of the CNS with each other. This is exemplified by the projection of dopaminergic neurons from their sites of formation.

Neuronal connections that use dopamine as a neurotransmitter run through the brain in relatively clearly delineated projection pathways. Three pathway systems can be distinguished (**Fig. 5.4**). The **nigrostriatal system** has its origin in neurons of the substantia nigra in the mesencephalon. It projects to the striatum, an important substructure of the basal ganglia that plays a significant role

in the execution of movements under the control of the extrapyramidal system (p. 133). A loss of dopaminergic neurons in the substantia nigra therefore causes a functional lack of dopamine in the striatum, which in humans (or experimentally in animal models after destruction of the substantia nigra) leads to Parkinson's disease with its movement disorders such as tremor, muscle stiffness (rigor) and lack of movement (akinesia).

The dopaminergic neurons of the **mesolimbocortical system** are localised in the ventral tegmental region, which is also located in the mesencephalon. From there, axons extend to structures of the limbic system (p. 138) such as the ncl. accumbens, the amygdala and the hippocampus, and also to the frontal lobe of the cerebral cortex and to parts of the olfactory system. Most of the neuronal units of the limbic system are involved in the generation and processing of emotions. Here, dopamine, among other agents, is significant, due to its positive effect in the region

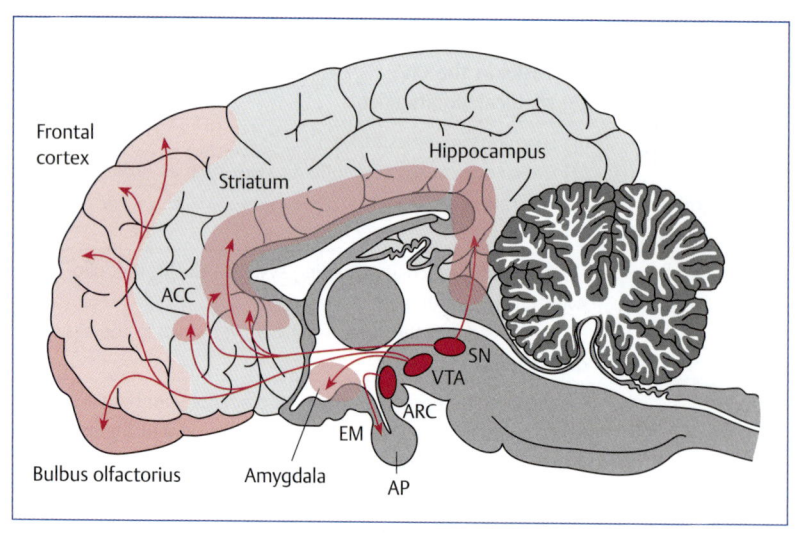

Fig. 5.4 Dopaminergic pathways in the brain, starting from nuclear regions of the mesencephalon. Dopamine production sites: Ventral region of the tegmentum (VTA) as the starting point for the meso-limbocortical pathway, substantia nigra (SN) with neurons for the nigrostriatal pathway and the arcuate nucleus (ARC), the neurosecretory neurons of which project into the eminentia mediana (EM). Pink regions represent projections with dopaminergic nerve endings, red arrows represent the projection pathways.
ACC = ncl. accumbens, AP = anterior pituitary.

of the ncl. accumbens, which has a central function in the brain's reward system. In humans, numerous euphoria-inducing drugs act by modulating this synaptic transmission.

Third, the axons of the **tuberoinfundibular pathway** project from the arcuate nucleus in the hypothalamus to the median eminence at the base of the adenohypophysis. There, dopamine is a neurosecretory product that is released into the first capillary network of the hypothalamo-adenohypophyseal system. In the anterior pituitary region, dopamine leads to inhibition of the release of prolactin, thyroid-stimulating hormone (TSH), and adrenocorticotropic (ACTH) hormone, see ch. Neuroendocrine control (p. 539).

5.4   Protective mechanisms of the brain

5.4.1   The cerebrospinal fluid space

The brain and spinal cord are soft and pressure-sensitive organs and must therefore be mechanically protected to maintain their function. This is particularly obvious when the animal is moving or when it is subjected to external shocks, such as those that occur when competing males ram each other during the rut. In addition to a bony skull-cap, the ventricular cavities of the CNS, which are filled with cerebrospinal fluid, play an important role as a mechanical "cushion".

The totality of all the cavities of the CNS that are filled with cerebrospinal fluid is called the CSF space, and is made up of inner and outer components. The **inner CSF space** consists of the four ventricles of the brain and the central canal of the spinal cord. The two crescent-shaped lateral ventricles of the cerebral hemispheres (first and second ventricles) communicate with the third ventricle at the level of the diencephalon via the foramina interventricularia (Monroi). This ventricle is ring-shaped due to the centrally located adhaesio interthalamica and is in turn connected via the aquaeductus mesencephali to the fourth ventricle in the dorsal part of the medulla oblongata

(**Fig. 5.2**). The fourth ventricle sends out long recessus laterales to both sides, which are open at their respective ends and thus form the two aperturae laterales ventriculi quarti (Luschkae). There is also another opening located medially, the apertura mediana (Magendie). The cerebrospinal fluid flows through these three openings into the **outer cerebrospinal fluid space**. This is defined by the inner two of the three meninges, i.e. the arachnoid and the pia mater, and forms the subarachnoid space. It is located as a narrow gap above the cerebral hemispheres, where in some regions it widens into cisterns, and also surrounds the spinal cord.

MORE DETAILS   Neuroimmunological, infectious or degenerative diseases of the CNS as well as tumours can be diagnosed by various analyses of cerebrospinal fluid. The CSF sample required for this is taken either from the subarachnoid space in the lumbosacral region of the spinal cord or from the cerebellomedullary cistern at the transition from the inner to the outer CSF space. Conventional and immunological CSF cytology are used to analyse the CSF sample, including detection of activated B lymphocytes, qualitative and quantitative protein diagnostics for certain activation and destruction markers, as well as microbiological diagnostic procedures.

Cerebrospinal fluid is produced primarily in the **choroid plexus** of all four ventricles. The choroid plexus consists of numerous processes, each with a central capillary lined with a fenestrated endothelium (**Fig. 8.16**) and an overlying, single-layered epithelium (**Fig. 5.5**). The epithelial cells face the ventricular cavity with their apical, microvilli-bearing membrane. They are interconnected by tight junctions and thus form the **blood-fluid barrier**. The driving force for CSF production is an active Na^+ and Cl^- transport, whereby, unusually, the Na^+/K^+-ATPase is localised in the apical cell membrane. The secretion of saline creates an osmotic gradient that allows water to flow passively, both paracellularly and transcellularly (including through membrane water channels such as aquaporin-1). In addition, some vitamins and nucleosides are taken up transcellularly.

Cell, tissue

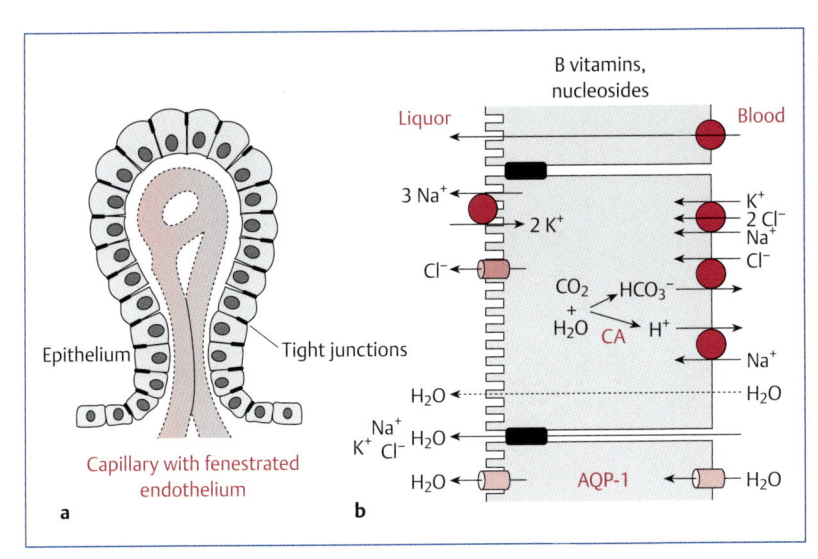

Fig. 5.5 Choroid plexus and cerebrospinal fluid.
a Structure of a "villus" of the choroid plexus consisting of a central capillary loop with fenestrated endothelium and peripheral transport epithelium with tight junctions.
b Transport mechanisms for the formation of cerebrospinal fluid via the epithelium of the choroid plexus.
AQP-1 = aquaporin-1; CA = carbonic anhydrase.

MORE DETAILS The CSF has comparable concentrations to that of blood plasma, for most of the substances dissolved in it. However, glucose, Ca^{2+} and K^+ concentrations are usually lower, while Na^+, Cl^- and Mg^{2+} are in slightly higher concentrations – but the osmolarity of both body fluids is identical. The colourless to slightly yellow CSF contains no or very few blood cells. It has a very low protein concentration in mammals, sauropsida and amphibians ($0.1–2\,mg \cdot ml^{-1}$). In contrast, fish have a much higher protein concentration ($50\,mg \cdot ml^{-1}$). Up to 400 ml (human) or 70 ml (medium-sized dog) of cerebrospinal fluid is secreted per day so that the total volume of 130 or 25 ml is thus renewed several times every 24 hours.

The **CSF** formed in this way **flows** along a pressure gradient from the site of formation to the subarachnoid space. It is collected in outpouchings of the arachnoid membrane. There pacchionian granulations drain the CSF into the venous system. Normally, regulation of CSF pressure is by the process of reabsorption. Active NaCl secretion ensures that the formation of cerebrospinal fluid occurs independently of the pressure in the CSF space and also of arterial blood pressure. However, this also means that production continues unabated in the event of drainage problems in the cerebrospinal fluid space. A hydrocephalus can thus result, if cerebrospinal fluid is prevented from venous drainage.

In addition to providing mechanical "padding" for the brain, the cerebrospinal fluid also maintains a constant extracellular environment for neurons and glial cells of the CNS, as it is in equilibrium with the extracellular fluid of the brain via the lining of the ventricular system, which consists of ependymal cells. Ultimately, the CSF space also represents a conduit system for peptide hormones and other substances.

5.4.2 The blood-brain barrier

The CNS also represents a fragile structure metabolically, as it has a very high maintenance energy metabolism. Nerve cells are almost exclusively dependent on blood glucose as an energy source. The brain also has minimal glycogen stores, which are primarily produced by the astrocytes of the CNS. However, neurons can also metabolise

ketone bodies transported in the blood of a starving animal which helps to ensure its survival. Such utilisation of ketone bodies is also found in newborn mammals during the suckling phase. Besides supplying energy, the CSF also provides amino acids and substrates for DNA/RNA synthesis, which are essential for the CNS and must be obtained from blood. On the other hand, there must be protection of the CNS against any changes, for example, in the pH or of K^+ concentration of blood, because, among other things, the membrane potential of the nerve cells would be affected. Furthermore, the CNS must be sealed off from foreign chemicals (xenobiotics) or pathogens. A strictly controlled exchange of substances between blood plasma and the extracellular fluid of the CNS is important in maintaining homeostasis of this fluid, as well as the functional integrity of the brain and spinal cord. This is referred to as the **blood-brain barrier**.

The **continuous capillary endothelium** (**Fig. 8.16**) with extremely **dense tight junctions** and basement membrane are the morphological basis of the blood-brain barrier. It can be observed in all the brain structures as the only type of endothelium (**Fig. 5.6**), apart from the so-called circumventricular organ structures of the hypothalamus and the medulla oblongata as well as the capillaries of the choroid plexus (see ch. on the cerebrospinal fluid space (p. 126)). The low passive permeability of this endothelium allows the highly selective exchange of solute molecules between the extracellular fluid of the CNS and the blood. Only substances with high lipid solubility or very small, as well as uncharged, molecules (such as water or the respiratory gases O_2 and CO_2) can diffuse through the capillary endothelium.

MORE DETAILS The endothelial cells of the brain and spinal cord capillaries contain 5 to 10 times the number of mitochondria as peripheral capillaries. There are only a small number of pinocytosis vesicles and there are numerous active enzymes that metabolise substances taken up from the blood or brain parenchyma during intracellular transport. The tight junction has 5–8 parallel strands of proteins of the claudin and the occludin family, compared to 2–3 strands in peripheral capillaries with continuous-type endothelium, such as in myocardium or skeletal muscle.

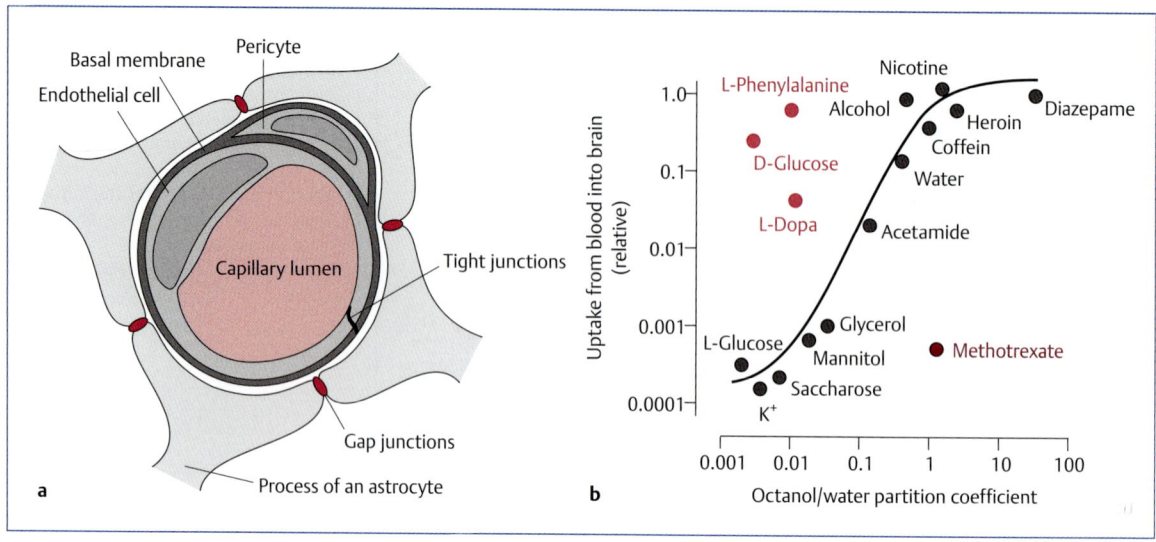

Fig. 5.6 The endothelial blood-brain barrier. **a** Representation of the cellular structures involved in the blood-brain barrier. **b** Ability of substances to pass the blood-brain barrier into the brain as a function of their lipid solubility (expressed as octanol:water partition coefficient). The permeability of most substances (grey) is grouped around a sigmoid curve in this double logarithmic representation. Larger deviations in the direction of increased uptake occur for substances (red) such as D-glucose, L-amino acids or L-dopa (precursor of dopamine), which are taken up across the blood-brain barrier by special membrane proteins. Deviations in the direction of lower uptake are found with xenobiotics such as cytostatics for tumour therapy (methotrexate, purple), which are transported back into the bloodstream by multidrug-resistance proteins; (b) based on data from Eichelbaum M, Schwab M. Wirkungen des Organismus auf Pharmaka: Allgemeine Pharmakokinetik. In: Aktories K, Förtermann U, Hofmann F, Starke K (eds.). Allgemeine und spezielle Pharmakologie und Toxikologie. 10th ed., Munich: Urban & Fischer; 2009: 36-64

Substances important for the function and survival of CNS cells, such as glucose or some amino acids, are transported by the capillary endothelium from the blood into the brain parenchyma by facilitated diffusion or active transport processes (p. 32). These substances are absorbed much better than would be expected from their relatively low lipid solubility (**Fig. 5.6**). For undesirable substances such as numerous and often lipophilic xenobiotics (like methotrexate) and important drugs, the passive protective function of the blood-brain barrier is further supported by a dense barrier of **efflux pumps** in the capillary endothelium of the brain (e.g. the multidrug resistance protein 1, MDR1). These pumps use energy to transport many foreign substances back into the capillaries after they have been absorbed into the endothelial cell.

> **MORE DETAILS**   Due to the properties of the blood-brain barrier, it is usually the lipid solubility of pharmaceuticals that determines whether they can enter the brain or not (**Fig. 5.6**). For example, stimulants or narcotics such as nicotine or heroin are highly lipophilic and thus membrane-permeant, while charged molecules such as the cytostatic drug methotrexate are practically unable to pass the blood-brain barrier. This limits the therapeutic options in the treatment of brain tumours or encephalitis.

In addition to endothelial cells, the **pericytes** and **astrocytes** are also involved in the formation and function of the blood-brain barrier. Pericytes form close cell-to-cell connections with the endothelial cells. They activate division of these endothelial cells and, because they can present antigens and perform phagocytosis (p. 248), they form an immunological barrier, for example, against neurotoxic substances. The terminals of astrocytes cover the capillaries of the CNS almost completely and are connected to each other by gap junctions. Although astrocytes are not

directly part of the blood-brain barrier, growth factors and various chemical messengers of a still largely unknown nature are released by astrocytes and cause the highly efficient tight junctions of the blood-brain barrier to form in the neighbouring endothelium.

> **MORE DETAILS**   In most domestic mammals, the endothelial blood-brain barrier is already closed at the time of birth. However, cat kittens and rat pups are born with immature blood-brain barriers. In premature births, this can also be the case in foals. The permeability of the blood-brain barrier can also increase during bacterial meningitis, cerebral circulatory disorders, tumours or in some genetic defects.

5.4.3   Microglia

The blood-brain barrier not only prevents potentially harmful substances or pathogens from passing into the brain, but also impedes the passage of components of the immune system such as antibodies. To compensate for this, the brain has its own type of immune cells, the **microglial cells**. When a noxious agent enters the brain, these highly branched microglial cells are activated. This is associated with a striking change in their shape and in the secretion of proinflammatory cytokines, oxygen radicals and nitric oxide. Activated microglial cells represent **mononuclear phagocytes** that can recognise pathogens via pathogen-associated molecular patterns. In addition, they are capable of antigen presentation to T lymphocytes that have migrated from the vascular bed (see ch. Recognition of pathogens by Toll-like receptors (p. 249). As amoeboid motile phagocytes, microglial cells constantly patrol the structures of the CNS.

> **IN A NUTSHELL** !
>
> Active protective mechanisms (microglia, efflux pumps), a passive barrier (blood-brain barrier) and a mechanical cushioning (cerebrospinal fluid space) protect the brain from potentially harmful influences.

5.5 Diagnostic methods

5.5.1 EEG and evoked potentials

The summation of numerous, simultaneously occurring excitatory (EPSP) and inhibitory (IPSP) postsynaptic potentials at the dendrites, and in some cases also axons and perikarya of the pyramidal cells in the cerebral cortex, can be determined as strongly attenuated electrical potential fluctuations at the skullcap. Electroencephalography (EEG) is therefore used in some of our domestic animals (dogs, cats, horses, birds) primarily as a diagnostic procedure that records the electrical activity of the cerebral cortex (**Fig. 5.7**). The same principle underlies the electrocardiogram, the electromyogram or the electroretinogram, which are based on electrical events in the heart, skeletal muscles or the retina.

In EEG, a distinction is made between bipolar and unipolar forms of recording. In the case of bipolar leads one electrode is placed on the left and one on the right side of the skull. A whole series of electrode pairs is used to record "brain waves" at as many points as possible. Differences in the potential between the individual electrodes of an electrode pair are measured. With unipolar recording, two electrodes are placed on the top of the skull, with one indifferent electrode serving as the reference electrode for all of them. Clinically, EEG in dogs is used in larger clinics. It is used to diagnose seizures, brain tumours or encephalitis. The voltage fluctuations that can be derived from the skin of the skull are very small and have an amplitude of 15 to a maximum of 200 μV. The frequencies of the voltage fluctuations that occur are between 2 and 30 Hz. Depending on the frequency, they are divided into different waves. α-Waves have a frequency of 8–13 Hz and, with medium-high amplitudes, represent the predominant wave form of the EEG fluctuations in humans, most mammals as well as some birds. They are found in the waking state. β-Waves have a frequency of 14–25 Hz and occur in the waking state when strong sensory stimuli from the environment affect humans or animals, as well as in sleep during dreaming. The frequency of θ-waves is in the range of 4–7 Hz; they occur in shallow sleep phases (p. 142) as well as in the awake young dog. The δ-waves with a frequency of less than 4 Hz, on the other hand, are typical for deep sleep ("slow wave sleep") and show by far the highest amplitudes.

> **IN A NUTSHELL** !
>
> With the EEG, cumulative action potentials, which primarily arise in the cortex, are derived on the surface of the skull.

In addition to the classical EEG, **evoked potentials** are registered – in humans and at least in small animals – only after specific sensory stimulation (p. 135), which can be characterised as additional waves in the EEG. Thus, for deafness diagnostics in dogs, investigations of the functionality of the auditory pathway can be carried out in sedated animals by measuring EEG changes triggered by acoustic stimuli. By superimposing several individual measurements, the "spontaneous" fluctuations in the EEG are averaged out and the reaction in the EEG response additionally caused by the sensory stimulus becomes visible.

5.5.2 MRI

In addition to EEG analysis, digital imaging techniques such as magnetic resonance imaging (MRI, **Fig. 5.8**) have made a decisive contribution to the functional analysis of cerebral structures. MRI uses strong magnetic fields to excite, for example, hydrogen nuclei in water molecules or organic substances of the body in such a way that electrical voltages can be measured in a receiver coil surrounding the head. These voltages change with the loss of excitation after the magnetic field is switched off, which is called **relaxation**. The speed of relaxation varies depending on the

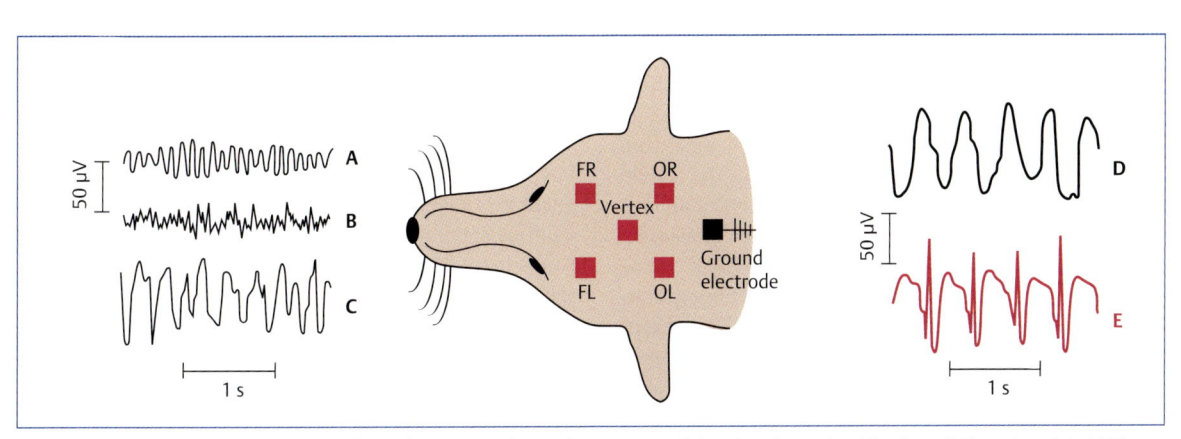

Fig. 5.7 Recording of an EEG in a dog. The red squares indicate the position of the skin electrodes. The frontal (F) and occipital (O) recording points on the right (R) and left (L) sides are shown, as well as the most important wave types, which are distinguished by their frequency: A = α-waves, B = β-waves, C = θ-waves, D = δ-waves, E = seizure waves in epilepsy.

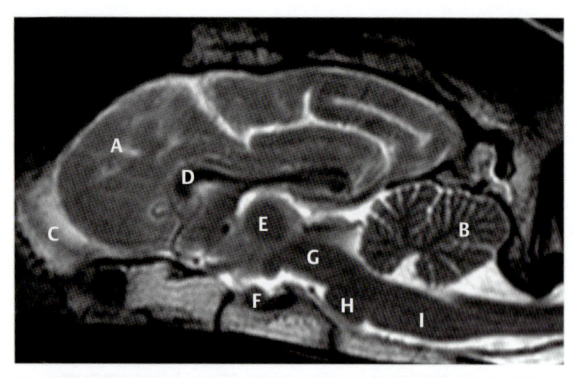

Fig. 5.8 MRI image of a dog brain. A = cerebrum, B = cerebellum, C = bulbus olfactorius, D = corpus callosum, E = adhaesio interthalamica, F = pituitary gland, G = mesencephalon, H = pons, I = medulla oblongata. [Source: Prof. Dr. M. J. Schmidt, Klinik für Kleintiere, Justus-Liebig-Universität Giessen]

type of tissue (grey brain matter, white brain matter, cerebrospinal fluid, bone). Based on this, a grey scale level can be assigned to the individual relaxation after processing by a computer in each image pixel. The final entire MRI image is composed of the individual pixels. The MRI is an excellent technique for imaging the brain and its diseases. In addition, functional magnetic resonance imaging (fMRI) can depict active areas of the brain, such as those activated during certain stimuli on the body, since such areas are reactively supplied with more blood and the magnetic properties of oxygenated and deoxygenated haemoglobin differ.

Two further imaging methods – still limited to the research sector in veterinary medicine, but already used diagnostically in human medicine – are positron emission tomography (PET) and single photon emission computed tomography (SPECT). Both procedures are examinations where metabolic processes in the brain can be visualised. For this purpose, weak radioactive substances, so-called tracers, are injected, which are distributed through the bloodstream and accumulate in particularly metabolically active regions in the brain.

5.6   Motor systems

5.6.1   Forms of movement

With the exception of the craniofacial muscles, which are innervated by motor cranial nerves, the activity of skeletal muscles is controlled by motoneurons in the spinal cord. These form the so-called spinal motor system. The activity of these neurons is in turn controlled by the brain. It is possible to distinguish between **two forms of movement**. The first are acquired, voluntary and conscious movements. Then, as a second form, there are the largely automated and thus involuntary movements, which, for example, also control posture. There are significant differences in the control of each of these types of movement. Voluntary movements are triggered by a group of higher motoneurons in the pyramidal system, which originate in the cortical region of the cerebrum. Muscle movements that

serve to control posture, on the other hand, are controlled by motoneurons of the extrapyramidal system which originate in the basal ganglia of the cerebrum. Both converge at the level of the spinal cord, i.e. at the level of the spinal motor system. In addition, both are coordinated by neurons in the cerebellum, which communicates with neurons in the motor cortex as well as neurons in the spinal cord.

5.6.2   The spinal motor system

In order to control movement or posture, the nervous system needs information about the state of the musculoskeletal system, and it does so by a process called **proprioception**. **Muscle spindles** (**Fig. 6.10**) with specialized intrafusal muscle fibres are the basis of this sense of movement. They inform the CNS about the current length of a muscle (p. 152). Excitation of the muscle spindles leads, via a **monosynaptic reflex arc**, to a contraction of the muscle in which the muscle spindle is located. They report the stretch to the spinal cord via afferent nerve fibres, which belong to the group of Ia fibres as well as II fibres. The somata of the afferent neurons that innervate the muscle spindles are located in the dorsal root ganglia. Their axons form an excitatory synapse with the α-motoneurons of the ventral horn in the spinal cord. High-frequency action potentials from these motoneurons, conducted via myelinated α-fibres, then trigger a contraction in the innervated muscle.

Intrafusal fibres of the muscle spindles are also innervated efferently by γ-motoneurons from the ventral horn. This is important, for example, in the so-called α-γ coactivation. During an active muscle contraction triggered by α-motoneurons, muscle spindles are virtually compressed and therefore initially no longer report a change in length. However, since the corresponding γ-motoneurons are also activated with a time delay, the intrafusal fibres are stretched again. In this way, the length of the muscle spindle, i.e. the sensor that is supposed to register the muscle length, is always adapted to the optimal measuring range.

Other important sensors that inform the spinal motor system about the state of the musculoskeletal system are the Golgi tendon organs. These represent connective tissue capsules traversed by tendon fibres, each surrounding the branched end of a type Ib afferent nerve fibre. They are the basis of the sense of force through which the CNS is continuously being informed about the force currently applied to a tendon. Golgi tendon organs are important for the so-called autogenous inhibition of the musculature. Their afferents end at various interneurons in the spinal cord. These are those that have an inhibitory effect on the motoneurons of the muscle where the affected Golgi tendon organ is located. The muscle tension is therefore reduced in the respective muscle. At the same time, contraction of the corresponding antagonistic muscle is increased. In addition, there are skin sensors such as the Ruffini corpuscles (p. 71), as the skin tightens at the corresponding points when joints move.

Sensors in the musculoskeletal system serve to provide the brain with as complete a picture as possible of the status of the musculoskeletal system, to be able to control motor functions. Pain pathways from the skin, muscles or periosteum are also involved. They are polysynaptically wired to excite flexor motoneurons and to inhibit extensor motoneurons, which is the basis for the flexor reflex (**Fig. 5.9**).

> **IN A NUTSHELL** !
>
> Sensors from the musculoskeletal system continuously inform the CNS about the length and strength of each muscle or the position of each joint.

Reflexes (p.65), in general, are involuntary, automatic responses to a stimulus. They are mediated by anatomically hardwired reflex arcs that include a sensor, an afferent pathway, one or several processing neurons in the CNS (or a ganglion), an efferent pathway and an effector as minimum components. Reflexes can be influenced by the CNS, so they are not stereotyped. A distinction is made between **unconditioned reflexes**, which occur in all individuals of a species (e.g. because they are innate), and **conditioned reflexes**, which have been learned by some individuals in the course of their life.

> **IN A NUTSHELL** !
>
> Reflexes serve as hardwired responses to important stimuli.

The simplest reflex – in terms of the structure of the reflex arc – is the **monosynaptic reflex arc** (**Fig. 5.9**). The stretching of a muscle, triggered for example by a blow on the tendon with the reflex hammer, is reported to the spinal cord via Ia and II fibres (p.56). The fibres entering the spinal cord via the dorsal roots form excitatory synapses with motoneurons in the ventral horn. The result is a stimulation of the motoneurons and the affected muscle shortens. Since sensors and efferent cells are located in the same organ, this is called an intrinsic (mono-organ) reflex. It is monosynaptically wired. At the same time, the antagonist of the corresponding muscle is inhibited via an inhibitory interneuron.

Polysynaptic reflexes, which are wired via several synapses, are usually extrinsic (multi-organ) reflexes, in which sensors and efferent cells are located in different organs. These include protective reflexes such as the flexor reflex (**Fig. 5.9**). The flexor reflex is triggered by pain, high-threshold pressure or temperature stimuli and ensures the removal of the limb from a danger zone by flexing the affected limb, such as quickly pulling the hand away from a hot stovetop. Here, the flexors of a limb are activated and the extensors are inhibited ipsilaterally, i.e. on the side on which the pain stimulus is received. The opposite happens on the contralateral side, for example to ensure a safe standing when pulling up a leg: The extensors contract and the flexors go limp.

Another extrinsic (multi-organ) reflex is the **panniculus reflex** which can be triggered by pinching or touching the

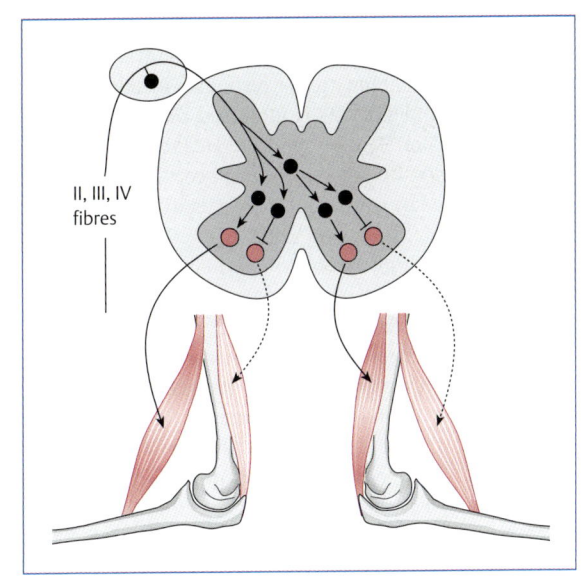

II, III, IV fibres

Fig. 5.9 The polysynaptic flexor reflex.

dorsal skin with a sharp object. The first synapses involved in this reflex are formed in the caudal cervical and cranial thoracic medulla. From there, α-motoneurons which innervate the cutaneous trunci muscle, are activated, resulting in a twitch of this muscle as a reflex response. An example of the physiological significance of this reflex is the displacement of insects that might be on the skin. This group of reflexes also includes the **corneal reflex**, which is the reflex of closing the eyelid triggered by a puff of air or a light touch on the cornea, the **eyelid reflex** (palpebral reflex), in which eyelid closure is triggered by touching the edge of the eyelid, as well as the gagging, swallowing and sucking reflex. Of great clinical importance, for example when assessing the depth of anaesthesia, is the pupillary reflex (p.93), i.e. the constriction of the pupil in response to light. It is a classic polysynaptic reflex with many synapses involved, beginning in the retina with the synapses between photosensors and bipolar cells and finally the ganglion cells, the axons of which then form the optic nerve (**Fig. 3.27**). After the decussating of the nasal fibres in the optic chiasm – which varies depending on the species – the axons run in the optic tract. The afferent fibres responsible for the light reflex do not terminate in the corpus geniculatum laterale, but run to the colliculi craniales in the midbrain and finally to the parasympathetic nucleus of the oculomotor nerve. The vegetative nerve fibres originating there form synapses with postganglionic neurons in the ggl. ciliare, the axons of which reach the sphincter pupillae muscle. Depending on the species, this results in a pronounced (e.g. human), only slight (e.g. ruminant, horse) or even no (in birds due to the total decussation of the optic nerve to the contralateral side of the brain) consensual response, i.e. a "constriction" of the pupil of the other, non-exposed eye. In addition to this parasympathetic limb of the pupillary reflex, there is also a reduction in the tone of the sympathetically innervated dilator pupillae muscle. Other reflexes that are important in the clinical neurological examination of an animal are listed in **Table 2.4**.

However, the autonomic nervous system has further modes to evoke reflex responses. It can also trigger motor responses in skeletal muscles or responses in skin or other organs. An example of this is increased muscular tension ("defensive tension") in the so-called Head's zones, i.e. the areas of the skin into which pain from certain internal organs is projected by convergence of vegetative and somatic nociceptive afferents (see ch. Vegetative reflexes (p. 120)).

In addition to motoneurons, interneurons also play an important role in the spinal control of motor function. These include the **Renshaw cells**. These are inhibitory interneurons responsible for a phenomenon called Renshaw inhibition or recurrent inhibition. Renshaw cells inhibit the activity of α- and γ-motoneurons mediated via the transmitters, glycine and GABA. They are stimulated by collaterals of the axons of α-motoneurons. Thus, if an α-motoneuron is activated excessively, the stimulation of the Renshaw cells leads to a reduction in the activity of this neuron, which acts as a kind of built-in brake and prevents excessive contraction of a muscle.

> **MORE DETAILS** However, the spinal cord is more than a simple relay station for wiring spinal reflexes or controlling skeletal muscles via the brain. In the case of a complete transection of the spinal cord (and thus the cutting of all connections to the brain), the spinal cord may even be able to control complex movement patterns (e.g. walking).

5.6.3 The supraspinal motor system

The so-called supraspinal motor system is superordinate to the spinal cord for the control of motor functions. It controls the postural and supporting motor functions. This includes involuntary muscle activities that stabilise posture and maintain balance in the gravitational field. The same applies to automated movement sequences. These are programmed movements that are either innate (breathing movements, facial expressions) or learned (walking, running, cycling). This is understood to mean arbitrary, purposeful movements that originate from an inner drive to act.

IN A NUTSHELL   !

The supraspinal motor system is superordinate to the spinal motor system.

In addition to the proprioceptors from the locomotor system, the supraspinal motor system also receives information about the position or movement of the head in space via a special sensory organ, the organ of equilibrium (p. 84). The labyrinth organ is important, for example, for righting reflexes (**Fig. 5.10**). It provides information about the absolute position of the head in space. Sensors in the neck muscles provide information about the position of the head relative to the trunk, i.e. whether the neck is held straight or is inflected ventrally or dorsally. The animal

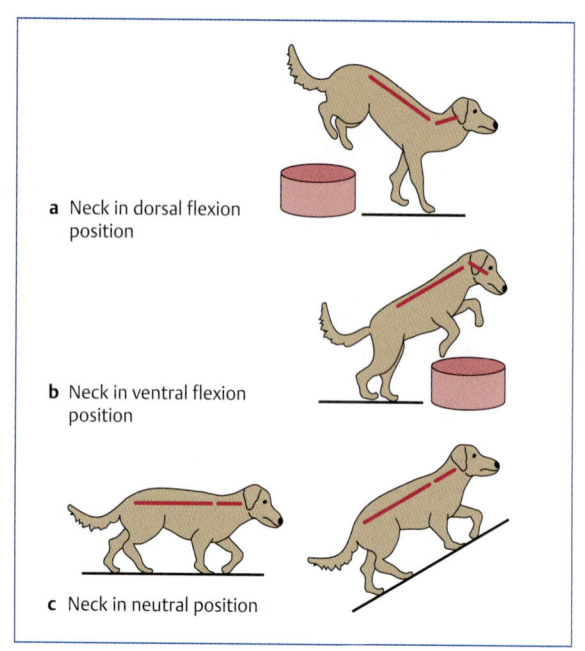

a Neck in dorsal flexion position

b Neck in ventral flexion position

c Neck in neutral position

Fig. 5.10 Vestibulocollic reflex and labyrinthine righting reflex. When the neck is flexed (**a, b**), only cervical reflexes are active because the vestibular systems are in normal position on both sides. They provide activation of the extensors of the forelimbs during dorsal (**a**) and activation of the extensors of the hindlimbs during ventral flexion (**b**) of the neck. In neutral neck position (**c**), only the labyrinthine righting reflexes become active and provide activation of the extensors in the limbs on which most of the weight force acting on the animal rests. The red lines symbolise the trunk and head axes.

needs both types of sensors to control its body and head posture. If the neck is compensatorily flexed dorsally or ventrally in an inclined trunk position, only the **vestibulocollic reflexes** are effective, because the vestibular system is in a normal position. When the head is dorsiflexed, the extensors in the forelimbs and the flexors in the hindlimbs are activated (**Fig. 5.10a**), while in ventral flexion of the head these muscle groups are activated in exactly the opposite way (**Fig. 5.10b**). In a neutral neck position (**Fig. 5.10c**) only the **labyrinthine righting reflexes** are important. They trigger activation of the extensors of the hindlimbs when the head is raised. In order to ensure a safe posture, the extensors of the forelimbs are activated when the head is lowered. These reflexes are based on interconnections between the vestibular nuclei in the brainstem and cerebellum and other parts of the brain (**Fig. 5.11**). The brainstem, in particular, is important for the automatic support of planned movements (see ch. The extrapyramidal system (p. 133). This supporting motor system network is the basis for the so-called **postural reflexes**, which regulate the normal posture of various body parts (e.g. head posture in relation to the trunk) and allow the animal to return to the normal position on two or four feet in the event of changes in body posture.

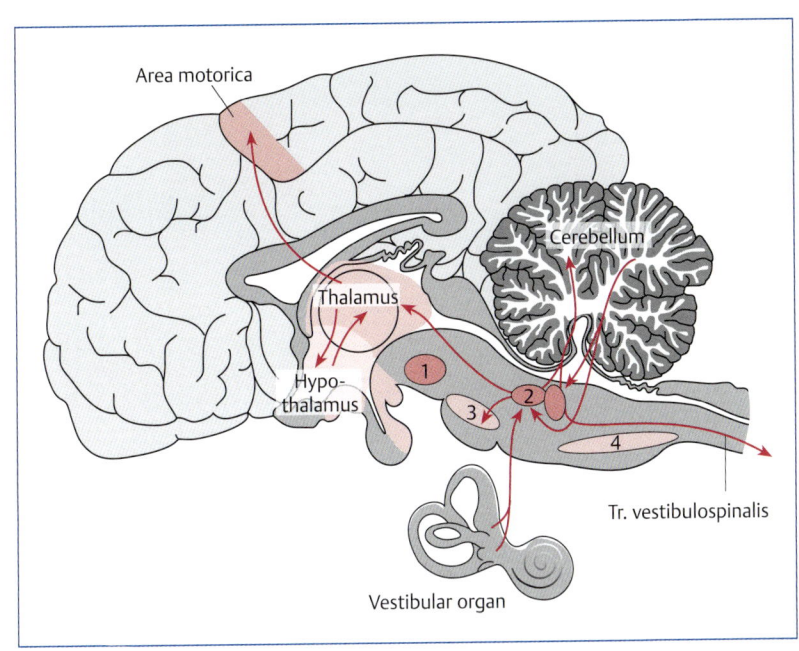

Fig. 5.11 Nuclei of the motor system network involved in involuntary motoric activity in the brainstem and pathways of the nuclei vestibulares.
1: Ncl. ruber; 2: Ncll. vestibulares,
3: Formatio reticularis in the pons,
4: Formatio reticularis in the medulla oblongata.

■ The pyramidal system

In the control of motor functions by the brain, two systems can be distinguished from each other: the pyramidal and the extrapyramidal system. All neurons within the pyramidal system arise from a specific region of the cerebral cortex, the motor cortex. These neurons are arranged somatotopically, in the form of vertical cell columns, with each innervating groups of muscles moving one joint. In a higher-order to them are neurons in the premotor cortex and in the so-called supplementary motor area, which are responsible for voluntary planning and initiation of movements.

The pyramidal cells in the motor cortex have connections to three different regions of the CNS (**Fig. 5.12**). One is to the corticospinal tract. The **tr. corticospinalis** runs from the cortex to the contralateral side of the spinal cord. A large part of its fibres decussates to the contralateral side in the **decussatio pyramidum**, from which the entire system gets its name. The fibres then run as the tr. corticospinalis lateralis in the anterior column of the spinal cord (**Fig. 5.3**). The remaining fibres run uncrossed in the tr. corticospinalis anterior, to decussate only at the level of its termination to the contralateral side of the spinal cord. More than half of the pyramidal fibres end in the cervical segments of the spinal cord to supply the upper limbs. They terminate mainly at interneurons in the spinal cord and through these, they influence the activity of the α- and γ-motoneurons, which then innervate skeletal muscles. A small part of the tr. corticospinalis reaches the motoneurons directly without mediation of interneurons.

In addition to the corticospinal trunk, motor function is influenced by the **corticonuclear tract**. It runs from the cortex to the brainstem. It is important for the control of motoneurons that innervate the cranial muscles. Thirdly, the pyramidal system consists of the **cortico-pontine-cerebellar tract**. It runs from the cerebral cortex via the pons to the contralateral cerebellar cortex. It does not directly

influence the motoneurons. Instead, it is important for the connection between the functions of the cerebral cortex and those of the cerebellum (p. 134).

Overall, the pyramidal system has the task of triggering action potentials at the motoneurons that innervate skeletal muscles. At the same time, the cerebellum is informed about these actions, which is important for the coordination of movements. For example, an animal must be prevented from simply falling over when it lifts a leg. The pyramidal system mediates complex coordinated movements, especially voluntary movements.

■ The extrapyramidal system

In domestic animals, the **extrapyramidal system**, where the pathways run outside the pyramid, is much more important for controlling locomotion. It includes motor regions of the brainstem and the basal ganglia. **Parts of the brainstem** that are important for the control of the body's posture are located in the formatio reticularis (reticular nuclei of the pons). When excited, they stimulate the α- and γ-motoneurons of extensors. The neurons of the pontine formatio reticularis are in turn stimulated by the ncll. vestibulares of the rostral medulla oblongata, so that nerve cells of the ncll. vestibulares also indirectly increase extensor tone (**Fig. 5.11**). Neurons of the formatio reticularis in the medulla oblongata trigger inhibition of the α- and γ-motoneurons of the extensors and promote the flexors. In the same way, the ncl. ruber located in the mesencephalon activates the α- and γ-motoneurons of the flexors and inhibits those of the extensors. Fibres from these nuclei travel to the spinal cord and control mainly the supporting and gait motor functions. They are in turn connected with pathways to the motor cortex and the cerebellum, so that they are continuously informed about intentional movements.

In addition to the brainstem, the **basal ganglia** also belong to the extrapyramidal system (**Fig. 5.13**). These are

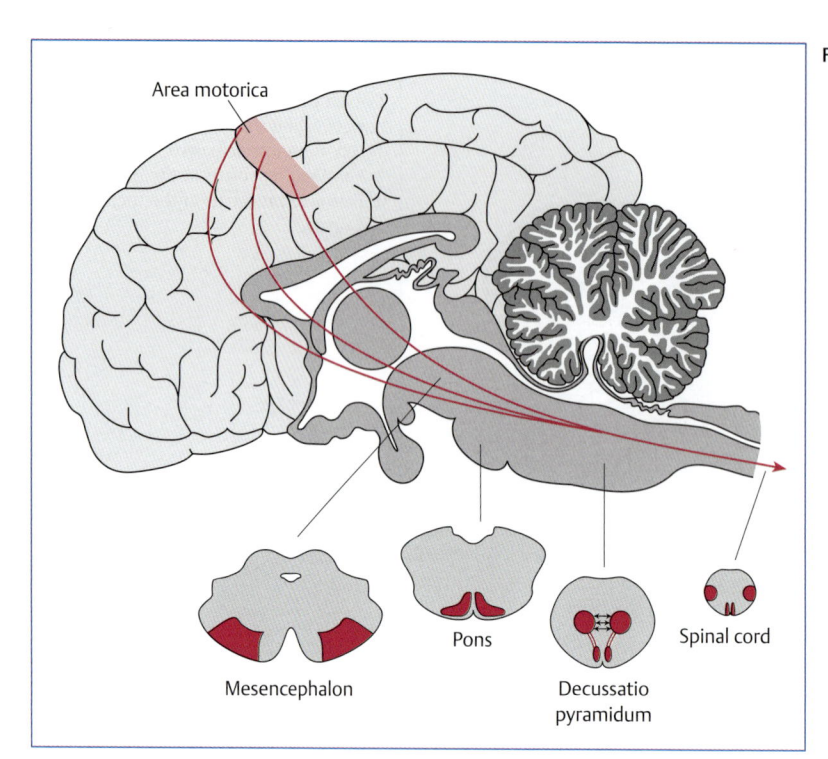

Fig. 5.12 The pyramidal tract.

Area motorica

Mesencephalon

Pons

Decussatio pyramidum

Spinal cord

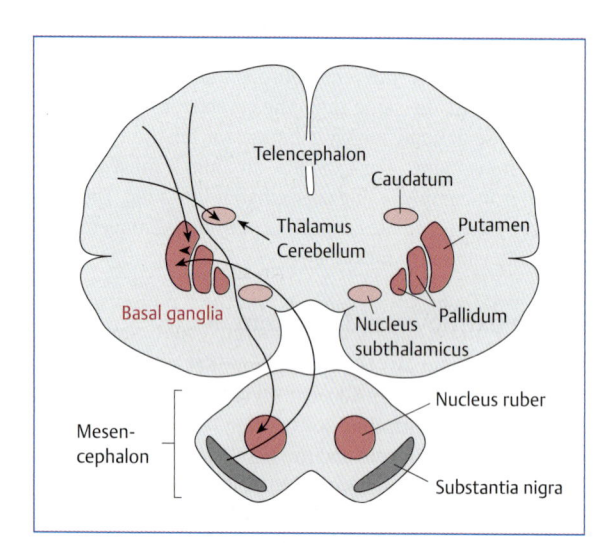

Fig. 5.13 Components of the extrapyramidal system.

Telencephalon

Caudatum

Thalamus
Cerebellum

Putamen

Basal ganglia

Nucleus subthalamicus

Pallidum

Nucleus ruber

Mesen-cephalon

Substantia nigra

the corpus striatum with its two parts, the caudate nucleus and the putamen, and the globus pallidus. Functionally, the ncl. subthalamicus, the substantia nigra, parts of the thalamus and the ncl. ruber in the mesencephalon are also part of the system.

The extrapyramidal system has a variety of tasks. It co-operates closely with the motor cortex, which is important for the smooth action of intentional movements. It is essential for the correct timing of movements and the correct amount of force by muscles involved in certain movements. It also controls learned and well-trained motor programmes, bypassing higher control centres. It mediates the involuntary adaptation of movement to sensory stimuli from the body and the environment. In animals, it is

much more important than the motor cortex. The extrapyramidal system controls numerous movements such as food uptake, copulation, following a scent, fighting, flight or even flying in birds. For birds in particular, the locomotor functions are controlled almost exclusively by the extrapyramidal system.

These central motor regions communicate with the spinal cord by **descending pathways**. They serve to control spinal reflexes and ascending somatosensory fibres. For this purpose, there are various projections to the motor neurons and interneurons in the spinal cord. They originate from the motor cortex (tr. corticospinalis), the formatio reticularis (tr. reticulospinalis), the ncl. ruber in the midbrain (tr. rubrospinalis) and the vestibular nuclei in the brainstem (tr. vestibulospinalis).

5.6.4 The cerebellum

The cerebellum also has an important role in controlling movements. In the cerebellum, a distinction is made between different types of neurons. These include Purkinje cells, basket cells, stellate cells, Golgi cells, and granule cells. The information input comes from climbing and mossy fibres. The output of information is by axons from cerebellar nucleus neurons.

The climbing fibres (tr. olivocerebellaris) are connected to cerebellar nuclei neurons and Purkinje cells, while the mossy fibres (tr. vestibulocerebellaris, tr. spinocerebellaris, tr. corticopontinocerebellaris) are connected to cerebellar nuclei neurons and, by granule cells, to the Purkinje cells. They provide information about the locomotor system as well as about the activity of spinal interneurons. Purkinje cells inhibit the activity of cerebellar nuclei neurons by releasing the transmitter GABA.

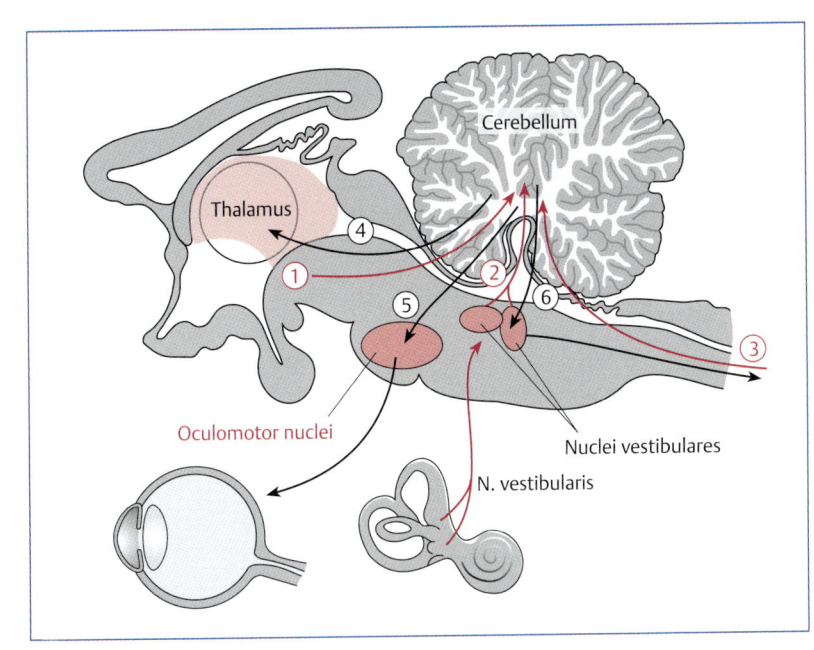

Fig. 5.14 Afferent (red) and efferent (black) connections of the cerebellum. Afferently, the cerebellum is connected to the pons via the pontocerebellar tract (1), to the vestibular nuclei via the vestibulo-cerebellar tract (2) and to the spinal cord via the spinocerebellar tract (3). Efferent connections run to the thalamus (4), the nuclei of the cranial nerves involved in ocular motor control (5), and the vestibular nuclei (6).

The cerebellum receives afferents from the cortex, which run via the pons to the cerebellum (**Fig. 5.14**). The cortex, basal ganglia and spinal cord also send information to the cerebellum through the olivary body in the medulla oblongata. It receives data from the organ of equilibrium via the vestibular nuclei. Tracts from the spinal cord travel to the cerebellum so that it receives information from muscle spindles and Golgi tendon organs. Efferent pathways from the cerebellum travel via the pons to the medulla oblongata, via the thalamus to the cortex and also to the basal ganglia.

Thanks to this "intermediate position", the cerebellum is essential for the fluidity of fast movements. It receives information from command signals starting in the cerebral cortex (**efference copy**) and information from the locomotor system about the movement that has taken place (**afference copy**). Together with information from the eye and the vestibular system, the cerebellum can create an exact picture of movements. It ensures that different motor activities that are necessary for an overall movement take place correctly one after the other or in parallel. It is also able to make corrections to motor programmes of the motor cortex and the extrapyramidal system. Symptoms of cerebellar dysfunction include **ataxia, i.e. overshooting of movements**, and, in humans, a disturbance in the rhythm of speech. Movements become jittery and transitions between individual movements are disturbed.

> **IN A NUTSHELL**   **!**
>
> The cerebellum works as a kind of "motor coprocessor" to ensure the correct sequence of complex movements.

5.7 Sensory systems

Information from sensory cells is transmitted to the CNS via hard-wired pathways. The somata of the **primary sensory neurons**, for example of the somatosensory system of the trunk and the limbs, are located in the dorsal root ganglia (**Fig. 5.15**). The first synaptic transmission occurs in the dorsal horn of the spinal cord. Tracts of mechanosensors are connected directly via the fasciculus gracilis or cuneatus (**Fig. 5.3**) to the nuclei of the same name (**secondary sensory neurons**) in the medulla oblongata. There, the **axons** decussate to the **contralateral side** and reach a **third sensory neuron** in the thalamus, via the lemniscus medialis. In contrast, afferent information about thermal or noxious stimuli – after forming junctions with secondary sensory neurons in the dorsal horn and decussation of the axons to the contralateral side – is transmitted directly to the thalamus (third sensory neuron) via the tr. spinothalamicus. For the craniofacial region, the neurons of the ggl. trigeminale, the ncl. tractus mesencephali n. trigemini and the thalamus represent the primary, secondary and tertiary sensory neurons.

The afferent pathways from the "classical" senses such as hearing (**Fig. 3.19**), vision (**Fig. 3.27**), smell (**Fig. 3.32**), taste (**Fig. 3.34**), sense of touch (p. 71) as well as the pain pathway (**Fig. 3.11**) and the afferent pathway of temperature perception (**Fig. 3.8**) are described in more detail in the corresponding chapters of sensory physiology.

The **thalamus** is located in the dorsal diencephalon (**Fig. 5.16**). The nuclei of the thalamus are divided functionally into motor, sensory, activating, and emotional nuclei. With the exception of odour-specific afferents from the olfactory bulb (p. 100), the thalamus serves as the most important relay point and filter ("gateway to consciousness") for **signal transmission** of sensory afferents to primary and secondary sensory cortex areas. The thalamus ultimately decides whether information from a sensory organ is passed on to the cerebral cortex and thus can be

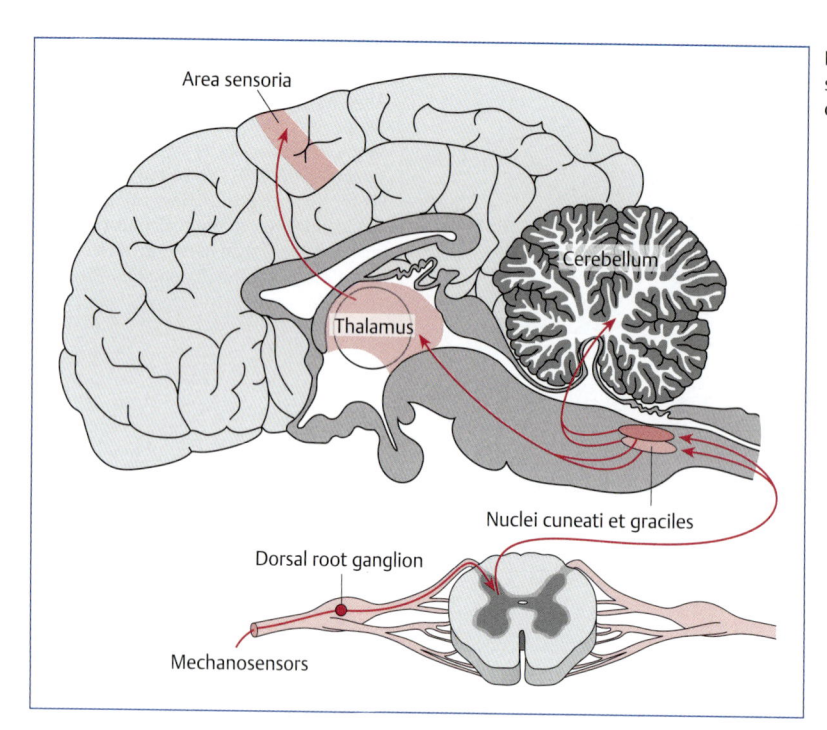

Area sensoria

Cerebellum

Thalamus

Nuclei cuneati et graciles

Dorsal root ganglion

Mechanosensors

Fig. 5.15 Lines of information from the somatosensory system to the sensory cortex.

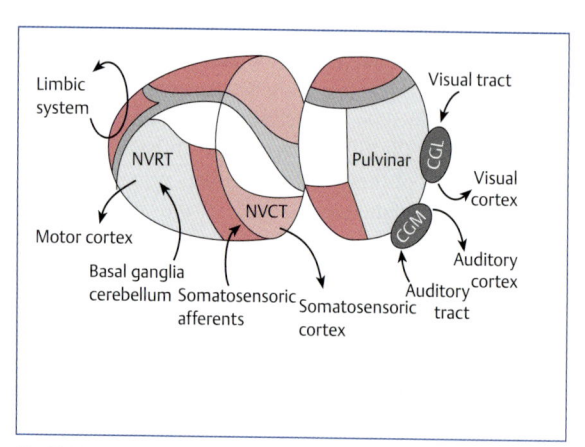

Limbic system

Visual tract

NVRT

Pulvinar

CGL

Visual cortex

NVCT

CGM

Motor cortex

Auditory cortex

Basal ganglia cerebellum   Somatosensoric afferents   Somatosensoric cortex   Auditory tract

Fig. 5.16 Structure of the thalamus. The thalamus is the most important relay station and gatekeeper of visual, auditory, gustatory and somatosensory afferents to the sensory cortex. CGL = corpus geniculatum laterale; CGM = corpus geniculatum mediale; NVCT = ncl. ventralis caudalis thalami; NVRT = ncl. ventralis rostralis thalami.

MORE DETAILS   Within the thalamus, different regions can be functionally distinguished (**Fig. 5.16**). The medial and lateral components of the ncl. ventralis caudalis thalami have inputs from proprio-, mechano-, temperature and pain sensors that reach the thalamus via the posterior column, anterior column and trigeminal pathways. They also receive afferent signals from the taste buds of the tongue (p. 105). This ventrobasal nuclear complex thus serves primarily as a "relay station" for the sensory-discriminative component of mechanosensitivity and nociception ("What happens where?"). Signals from the retina or cochlea are neurally preprocessed via the nuclei of the corpus geniculatum laterale or mediale located caudally in the thalamus and ultimately transmitted to the visual cortex in the occipital lobe or the auditory cortex in the temporal lobe. The motor ncll. ventrales rostrales thalami act as a "relay station" between the basal ganglia, cerebellum and motor cortex areas and are involved in the modulation of motor activity. Other nuclei of the thalamus enable neuronal communication with the association cortices, the formatio reticularis and the limbic system (p. 138). Because of this connection with the limbic system, the medial thalamic nuclei are more responsible for communicating affective components ("What triggers pleasure/displeasure?") of the respective stimuli.

consciously perceived. Such integration is necessary so that an accurate image of what is happening in the environment can be extracted from the information provided by individual sensory organs. For example, information that the image of an object on the retina moves from left to right can mean that the corresponding object has moved to the left or that an eye or head movement in the opposite direction has taken place. Only by integrating the information from the eye, and the organ of balance and the propriosensors, can the event "image movement on the retina" be correctly interpreted. This is partly achieved at lower levels, such as the brainstem, when the vestibular nuclei receive information not only from the labyrinth organ but also from the locomotor system in the neck region and the visual system.

The sensory projection fields of the cerebral cortex (area sensoria), where the respective sensory pathways terminate, are somatotopically structured. This means that information from certain regions of the body, for example from the trunk or the legs, is transmitted to very specific cortical areas (**Fig. 5.17**). Parts of the body that are very important in sensory perception, such as the fingertips, the head or the lips in humans, have very large sensory cortical fields, while areas that are less important, such as the legs or trunk, have very small ones. Something similar has been demonstrated in numerous other mammals and in birds.

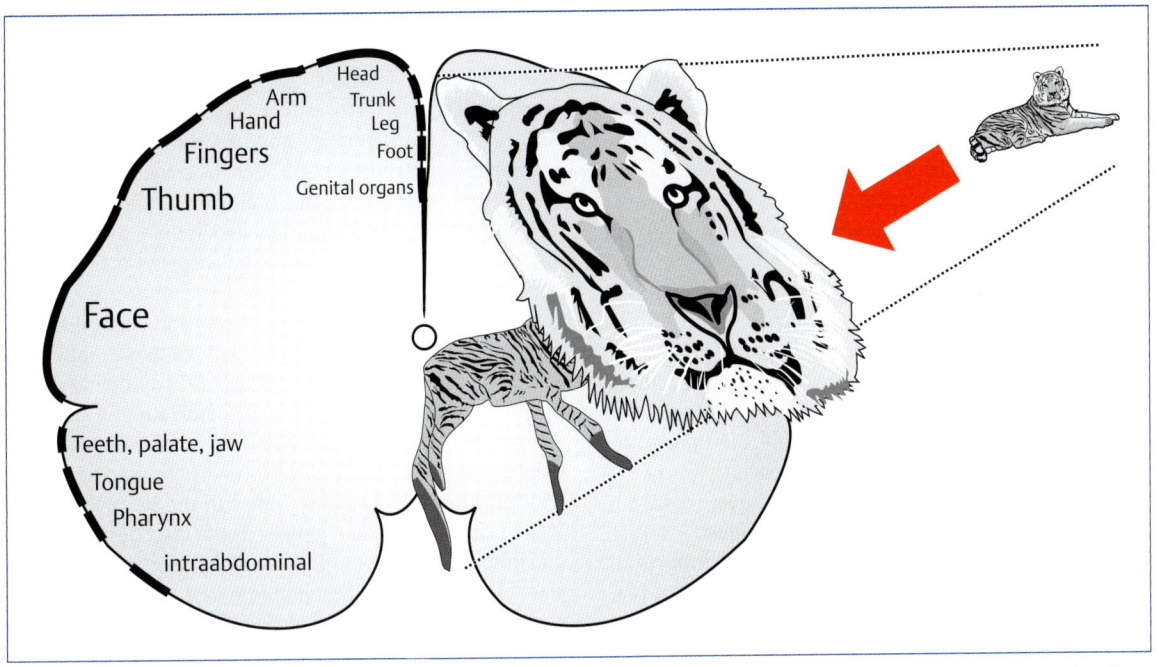

Fig. 5.17 Left: Somatotopic organisation of the sensory cortex in humans. Body regions that are disproportionately represented in the sensory cortex in relation to their size are marked with thick lines. Right: Sketch demonstrating how the somatotopic mapping of skin areas in the somatosensory cortex of felids (right) might be in comparison to body shape (top right).

MORE DETAILS   Like all other regions of the cerebral cortex, the neurons in the somatosensory cortex are arranged in six layers. Input of information from the thalamus is to neurons in lamina IV. Output of information to other cortex regions arises from laminae II and III, while the efferents of neurons in lamina V project to subcortical parts of the brain and those in lamina VI project back to the thalamus. Here, functionally related groups of neurons (which, for example, are jointly responsible for processing sensory stimuli from a body region) are arranged in the form of cell columns that run perpendicular to the brain surface. They have a diameter of several hundred micrometres and contain several thousand neurons, all of which receive information from roughly the same receptive field and a similar population of mechanosensors. Neighbouring columns receive information from other types of mechanosensors from corresponding areas of skin.

Sensory pathways do not simply conduct information from sensory organs to the CNS "like an electric cable", but they also serve to process the stimuli received by the sensory cells. Thus, it often happens that a nerve fibre connected to a secondary sensory neuron via an excitatory synapse simultaneously delivers collaterals to interneurons, which then reduce the excitability of neighbouring secondary sensory neurons via inhibitory synapses (**Fig. 5.18**). Such a circuit is called **lateral inhibition**. The result is that the activity of the neighbouring neurons is reduced. If a somewhat blurred stimulus arrives that strongly excites the receptive field of the first sensory neuron in the middle, but only weakly excites the neighbouring sensory neurons, the information that a stimulus has arrived is only transmitted via the middle secondary sensory neuron, but not via the neighbouring two. In other words, the stimulus is now much more spatially delineated. Lateral inhibition is therefore a means of enhancing contrast in the sensory system.

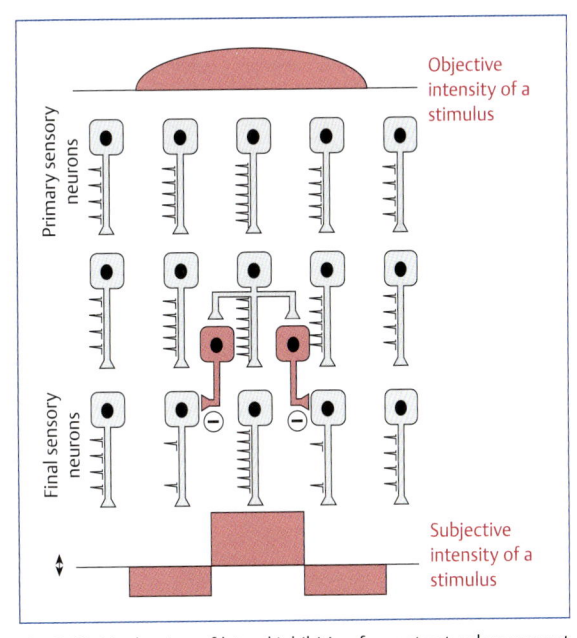

Fig. 5.18 Mechanism of lateral inhibition for contrast enhancement in sensory systems at the level of the sensors, thalamus or sensory cortex. The red neurons represent inhibitory interneurons with forward inhibition of the neighbouring target neurons.

IN A NUTSHELL !

Sensory pathways are somatotopically organised. Massive processing (processing of contrasts, suppression of information that is currently unimportant for the animal) takes place in those pathways.

Inhibitory synapses also play a role in adaptation of the sensory system to constantly present stimuli (**habituation**). Often, sensory neurons not only have an afferent connection with the CNS, but also an efferent connection, i.e. they receive commands from higher centres. These connections can also be inhibitory in nature. If a stimulus is received constantly, for example, when pressure sensors in a skin region are continuously being stimulated, this leads to reduced excitability of the sensory pathways originating from that region. Sensitivity therefore changes not only through adaptation of the sensors, but also through adaptation of the afferent neuronal pathways (p. 70).

In addition to the actual projection fields for each sensory pathway, there are also so-called sensory association fields (**Fig. 5.19**). They serve to evaluate the information provided by a sensory organ. This is important for the recognition of conspecifics, for example, on the basis of acoustic or optical stimuli. In the visual cortex, which is located in the occipital lobe and is organised retinotopically in the form of vertical cell columns, there are neurons that react particularly strongly to movements, others that react to light-dark contours in a defined spatial direction or even colour-specific patterns. There are also special neurons in the cerebral cortex for the recognition of complex structures such as features of conspecifics, competitors or predators.

> **MORE DETAILS**   In a cortical field of the primary visual cortex, there are larger areas (ocular dominance columns) that are dominated by input from either the right or the left eye. In these somewhat larger fields, one can in turn distinguish smaller neuron columns that react specifically to stimuli in a very specific spatial direction (orientation columns), for example, or groups of cells that react to very specific colours.

5.8   The limbic system

The term limbic system is used to describe a ring of brain convolutions or structures that surrounds the corpus callosum, the diencephalon and the basal ganglia (limbus = hem) and represents a kind of transition zone between the neocortex and brainstem. Anatomically, it consists of the hippocampus (located in the temporal lobe), the lobus piriformis (part of the paleocortex at the base of the brain), the gyrus cinguli (brain convolution at the median side of the cerebral hemispheres) and parts of the olfactory brain (area entorhinalis) as well as the indusium griseum (thin layer of grey matter, directly dorsal to the corpus callosum), the corpus amygdaloideum (in the temporal lobe), the corpus mamillare of the diencephalon (at the base of the brain), and the fornix (fibre tract above the roof of the third ventricle). Although the ncl. accumbens, as a nucleus of the basal ganglia, is not directly assigned to the limbic system, it has important functional relevance as part of the so-called mesolimbic system. The most important structures of the limbic system are represented by the hippocampus and the amygdala.

The limbic system plays an important role in the induction of emotions or moods. It is therefore also called the **emotional brain**. As the centre of emotions, the limbic system controls, for example, joy, fear and aggression. It also assumes important functions in the regulation of drive and motivation. It has a special significance for learning and the storage of memory content (p. 143). The limbic system also has an influence on sexual behaviour and plays an important role in the vegetative regulation of food intake, digestion and reproduction.

All in all, the limbic system can be considered as an association system that processes sensory information from the environment in the form of sensory impulses, and then coordinates them and brings them into harmony with individual physical needs. In this way, an adequate emotional response to the environmental situation is generated, for example, in such a way that fear and flight reflexes are triggered in threatening situations. The different parts of the limbic system have different functions (**Table 5.2**).

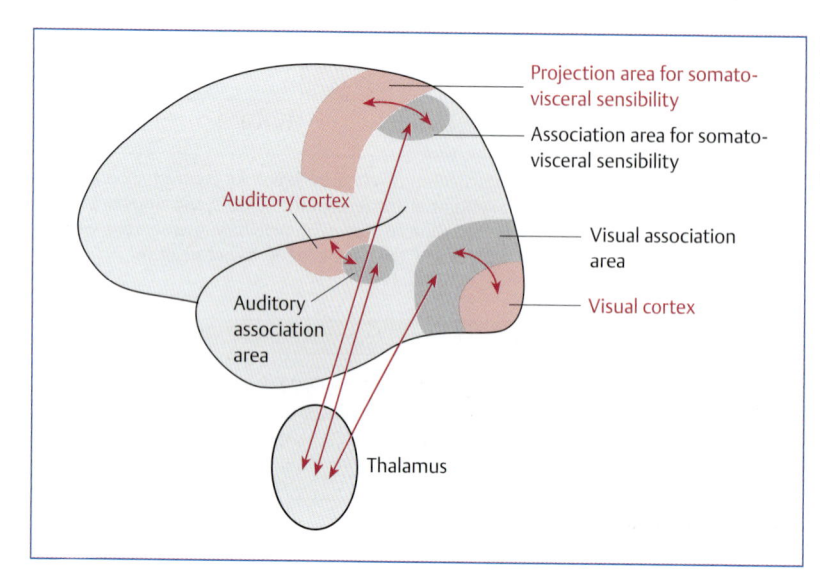

Projection area for somato-visceral sensibility

Association area for somato-visceral sensibility

Auditory cortex

Visual association area

Auditory association area

Visual cortex

Thalamus

Fig. 5.19 The thalamus and its reciprocal connection to association fields of the cortex. The association fields are located in the immediate vicinity of sensory projection fields with which they are reciprocally connected.

Table 5.2 Important structures of the limbic system and their functions.

Anatomical classification	Structure	Important functions
Cortical components	Hippocampus	• Centre for learning and memory processes • Behaviour/emotions • Vegetative control
	Cingulate gyrus	• Vegetative control • Motor drive
	Parahippocampal gyrus	• Memory formation • Input structure for sensory information and its transmission to the hippocampus
Subcortical components	Corpus amygdaloideum (amygdala)	• Centre for affective behaviour • Emotional learning • Vegetative control • Influencing sexual behaviour and functions
	Corpus mamillare	• Memory formation • Affective behaviour • Influencing sexual functions
	Nucleus accumbens (part of the meso-limbic system)	• Centre for the reward system (plays a central role in addictive behaviour) • Merging motivation and motor execution

Damage to the limbic system, for example by trauma, stroke or neoplasia, also leads to different symptoms depending on the brain structure involved. Lesions of the hippocampus often lead to loss of spatial orientation and the ability to store new memory input. Bilateral damage to the corpus mamillare leads to amnesia, i.e. memory loss. Some lesions in the limbic system can result in memories often being only evaluated without their emotional content. This results in indifference and undifferentiated social behaviour. Lesions of the amygdala can lead to changes that affect behaviour and emotions, such as exaggerated or reduced fear or aggression. Some diseases are also associated with changes within the limbic system. In humans, these include Alzheimer's dementia, depression, phobias, autism and schizophrenia.

> **IN A NUTSHELL**   !
>
> The limbic system is responsible for the formation of emotions, memory, motivation and the control of vegetative functions. It consists of various cortical and subcortical brain regions. The most important structures are the hippocampus and the amygdala.

5.9 Regulation of autonomous functions by the CNS

5.9.1 Brainstem

The brainstem contains visceromotor nuclei in the medulla oblongata, pons and mesencephalon. The axons of these preganglionic parasympathetic neurons run with the respective parasympathetic cranial nerves (see ch. Structure of the sympathetic and the parasympathetic system (p. 112)). In addition, there are also groups of neurons in the brainstem that take on more complex tasks in the autonomic regulation of organ functions (see ch. Neuroanatomical structure (p. 122)). For example, neurons of the ventrolateral medulla, of the ncl. tractus solitarii and of the ncl. ambiguus form the so-called "cardiovascular centre" (p. 210) for the short-term regulation of arterial blood pressure (**Fig. 5.20**).

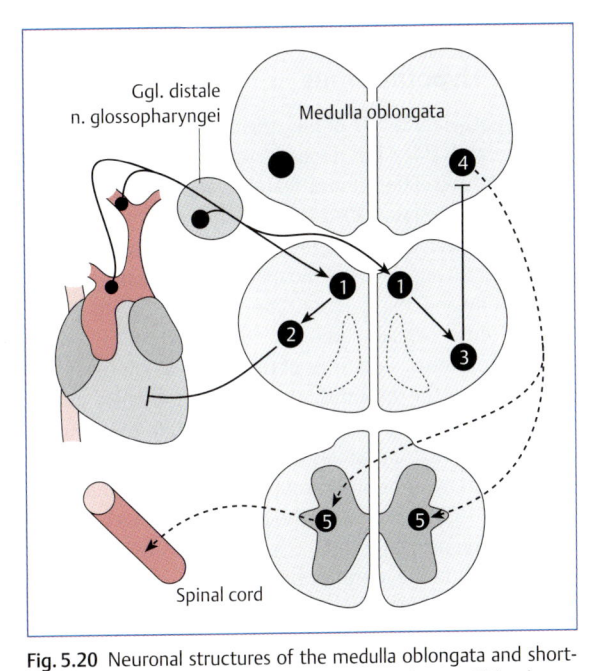

Fig. 5.20 Neuronal structures of the medulla oblongata and short-term cardiovascular regulation during elevated arterial blood pressure. The sketch shows the close connection between the "cardiovascular centre" and the vagal nuclear regions.
1: Ncl. tractus solitarii, 2: Ncl. ambiguus; 3: Caudoventrolateral medulla; 4: Rostroventrolateral medulla; 5: Intermediolateral cell column.

MORE DETAILS The neurons of the rostroventrolateral medulla oblongata are higher-ordered to the preganglionic neurons of the sympathetic nervous system in the lateral horn of the thoracolumbar spinal cord and activate them tonically. When arterial blood pressure is too high, pressure sensors located in the media and adventitia of the carotid sinus or aortic arch send their signals via sensory afferents in the vagus and glossopharyngeal nerves (ggl. distale and proximale, respectively) to the ncl. tractus solitarii in the medulla oblongata. On the one hand, this information is transmitted to neurons of the ncl. ambiguus, resulting in increased parasympathetic innervation of the heart and thus a dampening effect on cardiac activity. On the other hand, GABAergic neurons of the caudoventrolateral medulla oblongata are activated, which in turn have an inhibitory effect on the tonically active neurons of the rostroventrolateral medulla oblongata. This reduces the activity of the preganglionic sympathetic neurons in the thoracolumbar spinal cord. The consequence is a dilation of the peripheral resistance vessels due to reduced sympathetic tone and thus a fall in blood pressure. In the event of a drop in arterial blood pressure, for example as a result of hypovolaemic shock, a mirror-image response occurs (see ch. Central regulation of blood circulation) (p. 210).

Other neuronal populations of the ncl. tractus solitarii receive information from chemo- and stretch sensors from almost all parts of the gastrointestinal tract. In ruminants this is mainly from the reticulorumen. Together with the ncl. parasympathicus n. vagi and several other groups of nerve cells in the medulla oblongata, they form the "gastric centre" of the CNS (**Fig. 16.6**). It adjusts motility and secretion in the gastrointestinal tract to the overall needs of the animal. However, the term "centre" is misleading in each of these cases, as they are not anatomically delineated nuclei, but only functionally related groups of neurons.

5.9.2 Hypothalamus

The hypothalamus surrounds the third ventricle of the brain on both sides. It is divided from rostral to caudal into preoptic, anteriomedial and mammillary regions. The hypothalamus contains 20–25 nuclei that are connected to numerous other regions of the brain. Thus, some nuclei receive afferent signals from the medulla oblongata, the limbic system and the cerebral cortex. These nuclei "integrate" those signals and in turn efferently contact vegetative control structures of the medulla oblongata, the spinal cord or the thalamus. Above all, the so-called medial forebrain bundle, in which numerous axons of the involved brain structures run, serves as a "data highway". In addition, several hypothalamic groups of neurons produce hormones (p. 139) that control the anterior pituitary or produce hormones that are released into the systemic bloodstream in the posterior pituitary.

> **IN A NUTSHELL** !
>
> The hypothalamus is an important interface between the sensory nervous system, the autonomic nervous system and the endocrine system. The hypothalamus is the most relevant brain region for maintaining a constant internal environment (homeostasis) and adaptation to changing environmental conditions or stress.

Homeostasis refers to the maintenance of a state of equilibrium in an open dynamic system through internally regulating processes.

For example, the hypothalamus influences **cardiovascular regulation**. When there are changes in arterial blood pressure, or a necessary redistribution of blood flow, afferent signals are generated from the low-pressure system and arterial barosensors. These signals reach the ncl. paraventricularis of the hypothalamus via the ncl. tractus solitarii in the medulla oblongata and the locus coeruleus in the pons. Norepinephrine and dopamine serve as essential neurotransmitters in this process. Pathways that project to nuclei of the medulla oblongata (p. 139) or to preganglionic neurons of the sympathetic nervous system in the spinal cord then cause cardiac function and vascular resistance to adapt to the changed circumstances of the animal. The paraventricular nucleus and other hypothalamic nuclei in turn receive information from sensory organs, the cerebral cortex and, via hormone receptors, also from the endocrine system. The hypothalamus can therefore take on the task of reprogramming and adapting the cardiovascular system to a new situation, such as heat or cold stress, food intake, defence situations or sexual behaviour.

The hypothalamus (p. 505) also plays a central role in thermoregulation (**Fig. 5.21**). In addition to the thalamus and sensory (p. 135) cortex areas, signals from cutaneous cold sensors (and to a limited extent warm sensors) ascending in the anterior column of the spinal cord reach both the preoptic region and the ncl. medianus praeopticus. The preoptic region of the hypothalamus is the "regulator" of the feedback loop of core body temperature in homeothermic animals. In addition, numerous neurons of this nuclear region show a pronounced heat sensitivity, but only a few neurons are concerned with cold sensitivity. After integration of all "actual values" of peripheral and hypothalamic temperature signals with the "set point", an activation of thermoregulatory effector mechanisms occurs with the aim of changing heat production or heat release. Within the framework of heat production/heat conservation (muscle tremor, non-shivering thermogenesis, peripheral vasoconstriction), nerve cells of the paraventricular nucleus and the hypothalamic dorsomedial nucleus play an important role.

Within the framework of the fever reaction (p. 508) for example in inflammatory processes or in the context of infections, an adjustment of the "set point" occurs in the preoptic region.

The hypothalamus also plays an important role in the **regulation of water and electrolyte balance** (p. 334). A change in Na^+ concentration or the volume of extracellular body fluid occurs through vomiting, blood loss or diarrhoea. This leads to activation of hypothalamic and intrahepatic osmosensors or Na^+ sensors or volume sensors of the low-pressure system. Signals from the peripheral osmosensors (portal venous system of the liver) or volume sensors (vena cava and right atrium of the heart) are transmitted by vagal afferents to nerve cells of the ncl. tractus solitarii. They ultimately reach the ncl. paraventricularis as well as the ncl. medianus praeopticus of the hypothalamus

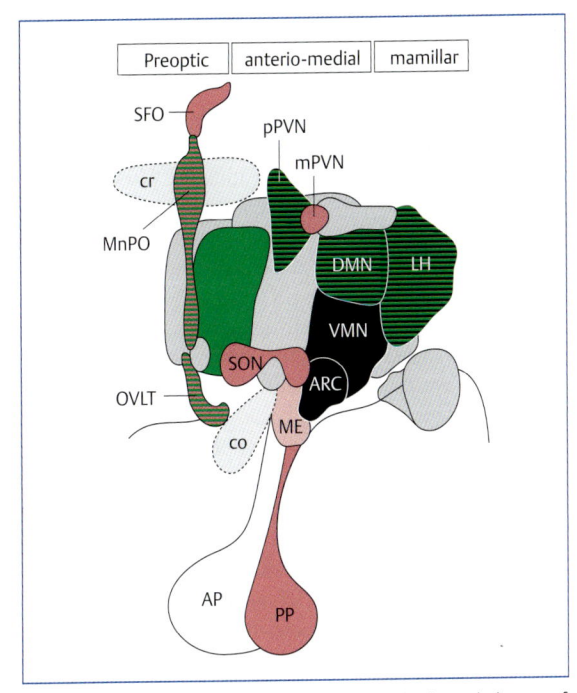

Fig. 5.21 Schematic sagittal section through the hypothalamus of a mammal. The most relevant nuclear regions involved in hypothalamic control of core body temperature (green), water and electrolyte balance (red) as well as food intake and energy balance (black) are marked. Hatching indicates regions that participate in more than one of these tasks.
AP = anterior pituitary; ARC = ncl. arcuatus; cr = commissura rostralis; co = chiasma opticum; DMN = ncl. hypothalamicus dorsomedialis; LH = lateral hypothalamus; EM = eminentia mediana; MnPO = ncl. medianus praeopticus; OVLT = organum vasculosum laminae terminalis; mPVN = magnocellular paraventricular ncl.; PP = posterior pituitary; pPVN = parvocellular paraventricular ncl.; SFO = organum subfornicale; SON = ncl. supraopticus; VMN = ncl. hypothalamicus ventromedialis.

tems are modulated. Antidiuretic hormone is produced by neurons of the paraventricular and supraoptic nuclei. It is released into blood by the posterior pituitary and stimulates reabsorption of water (p.317) from primary urine in the kidney.

Other important functions of the hypothalamus (p.539) are the control of food intake and energy balance (**Fig. 5.21**), circadian day and night rhythms (p.511) including sleep behaviour (p.142), defence behaviour or sexual behaviour.

IN A NUTSHELL   !

Brainstem and hypothalamus contain higher-order centres for the regulation of essential autonomic functions such as the adjustment of cardiovascular functions, core body temperature and salt and water balance.

In order for the brain to be able to perform such functions, which ultimately serve to **maintain the internal milieu**, it must be able to detect, for example, the Na⁺ concentration in blood or to recognise circulating chemical messengers, such as cytokines, which influence thermoregulation in the case of fever. This is the task of the **circumventricular organs** (**Fig. 5.22**). These are specific regions of the brain at the border to the third or fourth ventricle. They have a permeable blood-brain barrier. The capillaries there are usually equipped with a fenestrated endothelium. Some of these "organs" fulfil endocrine functions, such as the posterior pituitary, the eminentia mediana or the pineal organ, see ch. Special endocrinology (p.544). Others can detect substances in the circulation and therefore contain sensory neurons. These include the organum subfornicale and the organum vasculosum laminae terminalis of the hypothalamus and the area postrema in the medulla oblongata.

Close to the CSF spaces, they possess a specialized form of ependymal cells that line the inner surface of CSF spaces. These are the tanycytes, which are characterised by particularly well-developed tight junctions. They prevent substances from diffusing uncontrollably into the CSF space via the "open" blood-brain barrier around the circumventricular organs.

(**Fig. 5.21**). In mammals and birds, central osmo- or Na⁺-sensitive neurons are located in the region of the ncl. medianus praeopticus as well as the subfornical organ and the organum vasculosum laminae terminalis.

After integration of the afferent information, central (water intake, salt appetite, antidiuretic hormone) and peripheral (renal activity, sympathetic activity) effector sys-

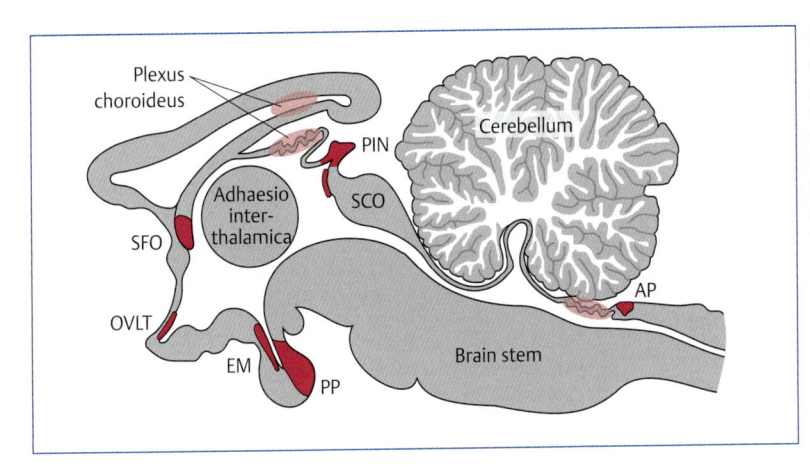

Fig. 5.22 Sensory and neuroendocrine circumventricular organs.
AP = area postrema; OVLT = organum vasculosum laminae terminalis; EM = eminentia mediana in the pituitary stalk; PP = pituitary posterior; PIN = corpus pineale (pineal gland); SCO = organum subcommissurale; SFO = organum subfornicale. The cerebrospinal fluid space is shown in white.

Cell, tissue

5.10 Sleep

In addition to information that reaches the cortex from sensory organs through the thalamus, all regions of the cortex receive additional "non-specific" excitatory input from the thalamic regions of the **formatio reticularis**. These excitatory inputs of the "**ascending reticular activation system**" (ARAS) are rhythmic and are generated in a loop-shaped conduction pathway between the thalamus and the basal ganglia. This forms the natural "**brain pacemaker**" (**Fig. 5.23**). The frequency of the oscillations changes with the degree of wakefulness (vigilance). The spectrum ranges from about 3 Hz during deep sleep and anaesthesia to about 40 Hz during high alertness, for example when reading, in the case of humans. The low frequency during sleep is a consequence of hyperpolarization of thalamic neurons and rhythmic oscillations of action potentials, which impedes the transmission of afferent information to the cerebral cortex.

Sleep is a state of unconsciousness that can be reversed by sensory stimuli. There are different stages of sleep (**Fig. 5.24**). Sleep behaviour differs in different animal species. Humans and most domestic animals show monophasic sleep, i.e. a period of sleep occurs once every 24 hours. The pig and the rabbit, on the other hand, show polyphasic sleep behaviour. Several times over a 24-hour period, they have sleep periods. Among domestic animals, felids sleep the longest, and horses and cows the least. Young animals sleep longer than adults, with high individual variation. Marine mammals such as dolphins as well as migratory birds sleep alternately with only one of the two hemispheres of the brain and thus do not run the risk of drowning or falling from the sky.

In the EEG, during normal, so-called orthodox sleep, one finds predominantly θ- and δ-waves (p. 129) as well as so-called k-complexes and sleep spindles. Muscle tone is reduced during this time. In the autonomic nervous system, the activity of the parasympathetic nervous system predominates, and the heart rate and respiratory rate are correspondingly low.

This is different in so-called paradoxical sleep. It is associated with dreaming, as we know from interviewing people who were awakened during this phase. During this time, rolling eye movements occur very frequently. This is why this form of sleep is also called REM sleep ("rapid eye movement"). In the EEG, β-waves predominate during REM sleep. The general muscle tone is reduced, but individual muscles may be activated. During REM sleep, heart rate and respiratory rate increase. In carnivores and humans, REM sleep accounts for about 20% of all sleep. In herbivores, on the other hand, it is only 5–10%, and in birds only 1%. In general, newborn animals show more REM phases than adult animals (**Fig. 5.24**).

The pacemaker for the sleep-wake rhythm is the suprachiasmatic nucleus in the hypothalamus. Serotonergic neurons in the ncl. raphe in the midline of the rostral medulla oblongata induce sleep. Noradrenergic neurons of the locus coeruleus in the pons, on the other hand, stimulate wakefulness. They belong to the ascending reticular activating system of the brainstem. We can only speculate about the function of sleep. It seems to have a restorative function for the brain. After sleep deprivation, the ability to react decreases. Immunological function is also affected and peptides released during sleep stimulate the immune system.

Fig. 5.23 Control of sleep by brainstem and forebrain. The hypothalamus is involved in the initiation of sleep through activation of the ncll. raphes in the medulla oblongata. The raphe nuclei project - mediated by the neurotransmitter serotonin - to nuclei in the pons and the ncl. tractus solitarii (NTS), inhibiting the ascending reticular activating system (ARAS). Orthodox sleep ensues. Paradoxical REM sleep is induced when the pontine nuclei inhibit the caudal reticular formation, mediated by the neurotransmitter acetylcholine.

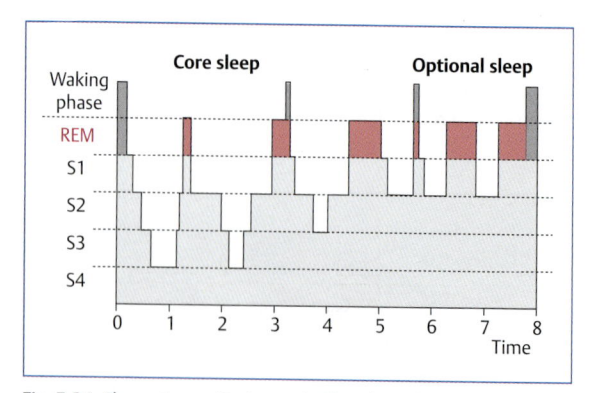

Fig. 5.24 Sleep stages. During orthodox sleep, four stages can be distinguished in the EEG (S1: primarily β-waves and a few θ-waves; S2: θ-waves with sleep spindles and k-complexes; S3: δ-waves; S4: maximum δ-waves). Core sleep describes that part of sleeping which, in the case of sleep deprivation, leads after some time to attention deficits. On the other hand, the absence of so-called optional sleep has no significant consequences. REM = rapid eye movement.

5.11 Learning and memory

Learning and memory, i.e. the uptake, storage and release of information by neuronal networks in the CNS, form the biological basis of adaptation to the environment. Without these processes, the survival of a single individual as well as that of its species would be significantly more difficult, since neither experiences of success could be repeated in a planned manner, nor failures deliberately circumvented.

Learning can be defined as the storage of information from the environment in a retrievable form in memory. It therefore enables a flexible adaptation to environmental stimuli and modifications in the environment. Memory refers to the retention of such learned changes, i.e. the ability to store what has been learned in a retrievable form. The term "memory" encompasses all aspects of memorising experiences, such as retaining, recognising and remembering those experiences.

There are several forms of memory, which are distinguished from each other. One memory form is related to the duration of the stored information, while another relates to the type of memory content. A distinction is made regarding the duration of stored information, so that there is ultra short-term memory (sensory memory), working memory and short-term memory (primary memory), as well as long-term memory (secondary memory) (**Table 5.3**).

Within long-term memory, there is also a distinction according to the type of memory content (**Fig. 5.25**).

Processes involved in the formation of memory are the reception, encoding, consolidation, storage and retrieval of stored information. In order to avoid a stimulus overload from the environment, a preselection already takes place for ultra short-term memory. Attention and emotions influence the selection and storage mechanisms. In consolidation, the "fed-in" information is embedded in already existing networks of memory units. In this process, associations are formed with existing memory units and ultimately long-term embedding in the long-term memory takes place.

Table 5.3 Forms of memory.

Memory type	Involved brain region	Duration of storage
Ultra short-term memory	Sensory areas of the cortex	Milliseconds to about 1 second
Working memory	Prefrontal cortex	Seconds to about 1 minute
Short-term memory	Limbic system, especially hippocampus	Seconds to minutes (can be extended to a few hours by repetition)
Long-term memory	Entire cortex	Hours, days, years

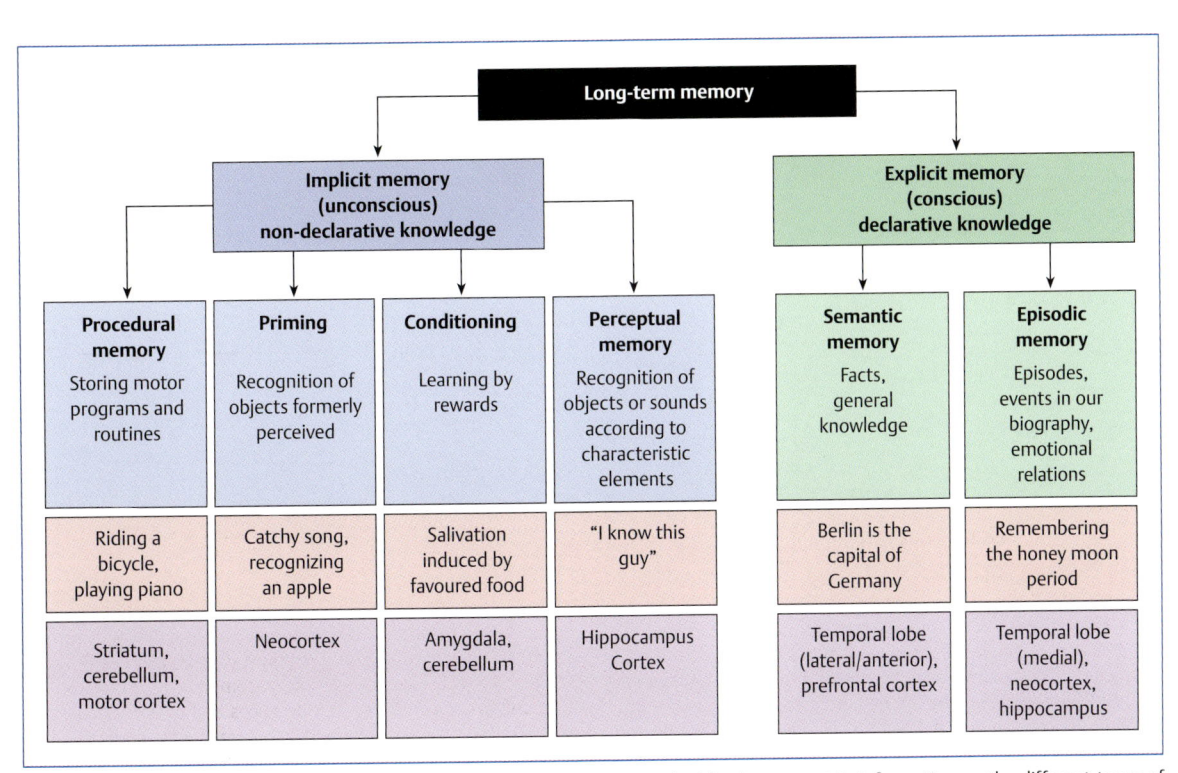

Fig. 5.25 Differentiation of long-term memory by type of memory content. The blue boxes contain information on the different types of so-called implicit memory, the green boxes on those of explicit memory. The pink boxes list examples, the purple boxes indicate the brain regions involved.

The processes that are decisive for the above-mentioned processes are a specific amplification of neuronal activity in the CNS, i.e. facilitated signal transmission by means of biochemical and structural changes at the synapses. This is referred to as synaptic facilitation or long-term potentiation or synaptic plasticity. This can be modified by different mechanisms (**Fig. 2.16**).

Information is removed from the different data memories in different ways. In sensory memory it fades away by itself, in primary memory it is overwritten by new information and in secondary memory it is displaced by subsequently learned contents.

MORE DETAILS   The highly complex system of learning and memory is susceptible to disorders. Shifts in the mineral balance, for example a calcium deficiency, can cause deficits in memory performance. **Amnesia** represents one type of disturbance in learning and memory. This is a memory disorder in which an individual can no longer access memory contents. It is not a disease in its own right, but rather a symptom of a disease or a consequence of an adverse influence on the brain. This influence can be external or internal. Amnesia can occur with brain injuries. A lesion of the hippocampus triggers anterograde amnesia. This means that no new information can be transferred into long-term memory. Consolidation is therefore disturbed. Recalling old information from the time before the hippocampal lesion, on the other hand, is unaffected. Damage to the temporal lobe or thalamus has a different effect. It leads to retrograde amnesia. Memory contents of long-term memory that originate from the time before the lesion can no longer be retrieved. However, it is possible to retrieve new memory contents.

Another type of learning and memory disorder is **dementia**, which is characterised by a progressive decline in cognitive, emotional and social abilities. The cardinal symptom here is considered to be memory impairment. At the beginning of dementia, disturbances in short-term memory and retentiveness are noticeable. This is followed by impaired orientation. As the disease progresses, patients have less and less access to long-term memory, resulting in the loss of skills, abilities and knowledge acquired during life. There are many different forms of dementia in humans. The best known is probably Alzheimer's dementia, which is also the most common form, accounting for about 60% of all dementia cases. In the meantime, neuropathological changes are also known in older dogs and cats, which are similar to those in humans suffering from Alzheimer's disease. The symptoms of cognitive dysfunction associated with these neuropathological changes are described in dogs and cats by the acronym DISHA:

- **D**isorientation/confusion: restlessness, forgetfulness, impaired learning abilities, disturbed perception, increased anxiety.
- **I**nteraction: altered pattern of interaction (increased interest or lack of interest) by the animal with humans or other pets.
- **S**leep-wake rhythm: changes – prolonged sleep phases during the day and/or restlessness at night.
- **H**ouse uncleanliness: uncontrolled urination and defecation in the house.
- **A**ctivity: reduced or increased activity of the animal.

Suggested reading

Cunningham JG. Textbook of veterinary physiology. 5th ed. Philadelphia: WB Saunders; 2012

Jaggy A, ed. Atlas and textbook of small animal neurology. Hanover: Schlütersche; 2010

Kandel ER, Schwartz JH, Jessel TM, Siegelbaum SA, Hudspeht AJ. Principles of neural science. 5th ed. New York: McGraw-Hill Professional Publishing; 2012

Lorenz MD, Coates JR, Kent M. Handbook of veterinary neurology. 5th ed. St. Louis: Elsevier; 2011

Partridge WM. Introduction to the blood-brain barrier. Cambridge: University Press; 1998

Sjaastad ØV, Hove K, Sand O. Physiology of domestic animals. Oslo: Scandinavian Veterinary Press; 2003

6 Skeletal and smooth muscles

Korinna Huber

6.1 Functions of the muscles

ESSENTIALS ✖

The most important characteristic of all muscle cells in the body is the ability to contract. This property is essential for many physiological functions.

Muscle types: Morphologically, the musculature can be divided into striated and smooth muscles. These muscle types differ in terms of excitability and the connection between the cells.

Tasks of the musculature: Transversely striated skeletal muscles are important for involuntary posture and movement control as well as for voluntary motor programmes such as running, flying or swimming. Vital processes such as breathing and blood circulation rely on the activity of the striated respiratory muscles and the heart muscle. Smooth muscles, for example in the gastrointestinal tract, uterus, urinary bladder or blood vessels, ensure the onward transport of the chyme, the expulsion of the foetus during birth, the expulsion of urine or the regulation of blood pressure and organ perfusion.

Energy metabolism of the musculature: The tasks of the different types of muscles require a very adaptable energy metabolism. In skeletal muscles, there are different cell types with specialized pathways for energy production, which explains the particularly high adaptability of these muscles to variations in performance. The metabolic heat generated during contraction can be used for thermoregulation in hypothermia (shivering in the cold).

6.2 Striated musculature

The striated muscles include the skeletal muscles and the cardiac muscle (p.166). The main function of the skeletal muscles is to maintain posture and to enable movement of the body, while the cardiac muscle is responsible for maintaining the flow of blood in the blood vessels. The cardiac musculature has morphological differences with skeletal muscle. However, in many physiological processes, the two muscle types behave similarly. Therefore, these similarities are addressed in the following chapters on skeletal muscle. The special features of the myocardium compared to skeletal muscle and smooth muscle are then described in ch. 6.4.

6.2.1 Morphology of the skeletal muscle

To enable movement of parts of the body, skeletal muscles are connected to bones (via tendons or ligaments or directly). They cause movement of one or more joints acting as a flexor or extensor during contraction. Skeletal muscle cells (synonym: muscle fibre) are long cylinders in shape and have many nuclei. **Myofibrils**, i.e. rod-like organelles arranged in parallel, are the "motors" of the muscle fibre. The muscle fibres are formed during ontogeny from the fusion of many cells, so each fibre is a **syncytium**. Several muscle fibres are combined into a fascicle and enclosed in connective tissue (perimysium). Several fascicles together form the whole muscle, which is also encased in connective tissue (epimysium) (**Fig. 6.1**). The individual skeletal muscle fibres are electrically insulated from one another by connective tissue sheaths (endomysium). Thus, they must be activated by α-motoneurons from spinal cord and brain (p.130) in order to contract. The cell surface of a muscle fibre, the **sarcolemma** (muscle cell membrane), extends deep between the myofibrils to form the **transverse tubules (T-tubules)**. They are in close spatial contact with the **longitudinal tubules (L-tubules)** (synonym: **sarcoplasmic reticulum (SR)**) and their terminal piston-shaped cisternae. This area of contact is also known as the **triad** (in cardiac muscle **diad**). These systems play a crucial role in the transmission of signals from the motoneuron to the skeletal muscle fibre and the initiation of contraction (p.150).

The ability of skeletal and cardiac muscle cells to contract is based on their myofibrils. These consist of linearly arranged small functional units. The smallest structural component of the myofibril is the **sarcomere** which contains **actin** and **myosin filaments** (**Fig. 6.2**, **Fig. 6.3**). It is connected via the **Z-line** with other sarcomeres to form long chains. The **actin filaments** are attached to the Z-lines. These are thin protein filaments, each consisting of two helically intertwined F-actins. One F-actin consists of approximately 200 globular G-actin monomers, each of which has a binding site for a myosin head (**Fig. 6.2a**). Associated with actin are **troponin** and **tropomyosin**, two regulatory proteins that are crucial for the onset of contraction. Troponin is a globular protein bound to actin with three subunits: troponin T (TnT) has a binding site to tropomyosin, troponin I (TnI) inhibits binding between actin and myosin, and troponin C (TnC) binds Ca^{2+} ions. Tropomyosin is a filamentous protein that attaches to the actin filament over a length of six G-actins. It prevents the binding of the myosin head to actin in resting muscle (**Fig. 6.2a**). Thick protein filaments, the **myosin filaments**, are located between the actin filaments. They contain

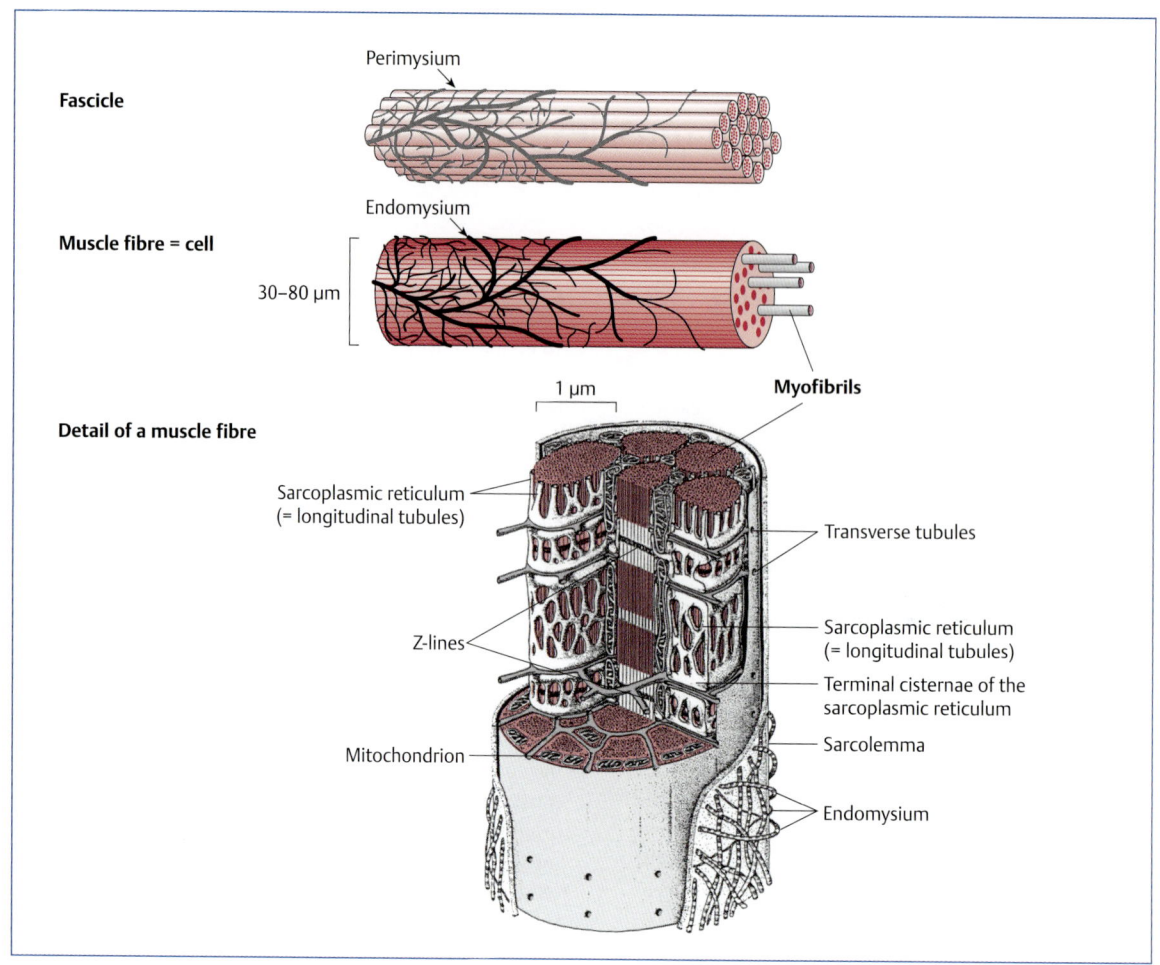

Fig. 6.1 Structure of skeletal muscle. Skeletal muscle is composed of bundles of fibres (fascicles). Muscle fibres (= muscle cells) in turn contain myofibrils, mitochondria, nuclei and L- and T-tubules. The terminal cisternae form the triads with the T-tubules. The myofibrils are composed of contractile filaments (actin and myosin; **Fig. 6.2**) and are organised in the form of sarcomeres (**Fig. 6.3**).

300–400 myosin molecules. A myosin molecule consists of two heavy chains (myosin heavy chain, **MHC**), with rod-shaped α-helical domains which wind around each other and thus form the **tail part of myosin**. The globular domains of the heavy chains form the **myosin heads**. These heads are linked in a mobile way to the myosin tail via the neck domain. An MHC isoform-specific ATPase is coupled to each myosin head. An actin-binding site is also present (**Fig. 6.2 b, c**).

In addition to contractile proteins (actin and myosin) and the regulatory proteins (troponin and tropomyosin), the muscle fibre also contains a number of structural proteins, the main representative of which is **titin**. This protein forms an elastic network and connects the myosin filaments to the Z-lines. The protein **dystrophin** connects actin filaments to the muscle cell membrane and is thus responsible for the transmission of the contraction force to the surrounding connective tissue (**Fig. 6.3**).

Skeletal muscle and cardiac muscle are both called striated muscle because of the parallel arrangement of the contractile filaments **actin** and **myosin**, and to their uniform arrangement in myofibrils in the **sarcomeric structure**.

6.2.2 Growth of skeletal muscles

The growth capacity of a muscle is determined by the metabolic type of individual muscle fibres (p. 156), and also by the number and size of the fibres. Metabolic properties are determined during intrauterine development and, depending on the species, also during early postnatal development. In part, they are genetically determined. For example, horse breeds that have been selected for endurance racing have more small muscle fibres with metabolic adaptations to enable adequate energy supply during continuous muscle activity. The different meat qualities between breeds of pigs are also likely to be based on genetically determined variations in the composition of the types of muscle fibres. The number of fibres increases during intrauterine development (**hyperplasia**), a process that is largely completed around birth in all mammals. Further muscle growth is predominantly due to an increase in fibre size (**hypertrophy**). These growth processes determine muscle mass and, in meat-producing animals, meat quality and quantity.

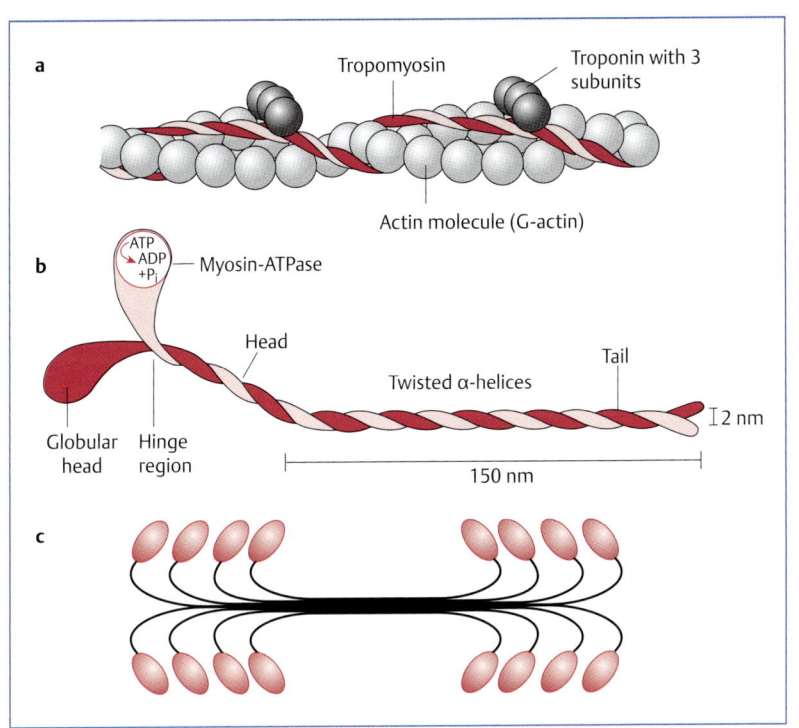

Fig. 6.2 Structure of the contractile elements of the sarcomere in skeletal and cardiac muscle. **a** Actin filaments consist of numerous globular actin molecules helically twisted in pairs together to form chains. Troponin and tropomyosin are closely linked to F-actin (consisting of G-actin monomers) as regulatory proteins. **b** The myosin molecule consists of two identical heavy chains (MHC, myosin heavy chain). In addition, there are two light chains at the myosin head. **c** A myosin filament consists of many myosin molecules twisted together at the tail. The neck regions and heads form brush-shaped ends.

Cell, tissue

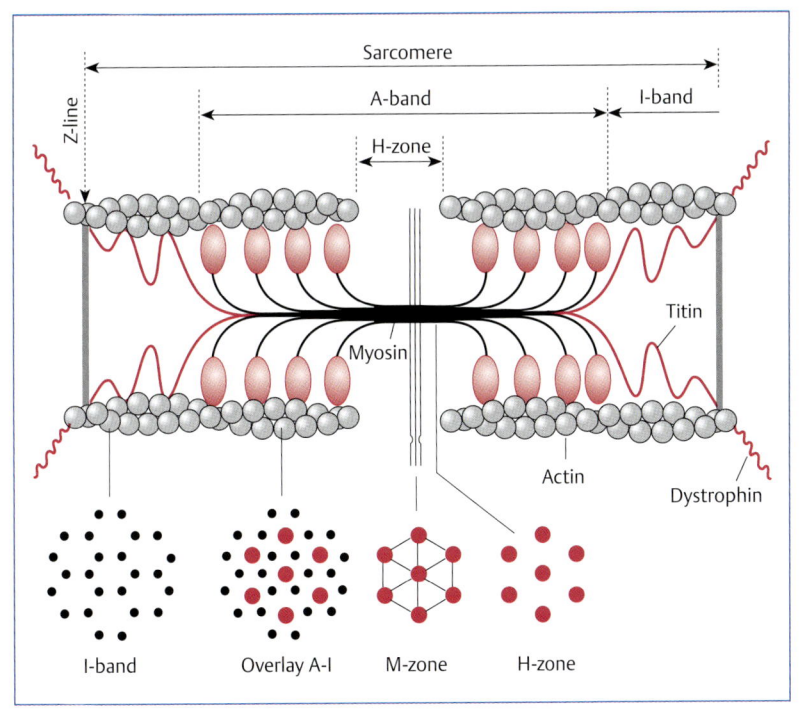

Fig. 6.3 Structure of the sarcomere in skeletal and cardiac muscle in longitudinal (top) and cross section (bottom). The sarcomere consists of myosin filaments surrounded by actin filaments. Due to its strict organisation, the sarcomere appears banded under the microscope (= cross-sectional striation of the skeletal muscle). Actin is directly anchored to the elastic Z-lines, myosin via the elastic giant protein titin. The sarcomeres themselves are linked to the sarcolemma via dystrophin, which is also elastic. The designation of the bands, overlap and zones, are taken from the histological nomenclature.

> **IN A NUTSHELL** !
>
> Muscle growth is based on an increase in the number of fibres during intrauterine development, but mainly on an increase in the size of existing fibres during postnatal development.

Postnatal muscle growth is controlled by growth hormone, insulin, insulin-like growth factor (IGF), thyroid hormones and sex hormones. All these hormones act in an **anabolic** way on protein metabolism, i.e. they increase the efficiency of protein synthesis. Muscle growth means that protein synthesis is greater than protein breakdown in the muscle. The consequence is a net protein gain. The duration of this positive muscle protein balance varies between animal species and, together with bone growth, determines the breed-specific, and also the individual-specific growth rate. Adult animals increase their body mass only through fat gain. Protein synthesis and protein degradation are therefore in balance in adults. Muscles do not continue to grow endlessly because of the action of **myostatin**, a growth factor of the **transforming growth factor (TGF-β) family**, which inhibits muscle growth and differentiation. A knock-out mutant of this gene is the **Belgian Blue** breed of cattle, which are characterised by massive hypertrophy of skeletal musculature. However, a hypertrophic increase in muscle mass can be achieved at any age through strength training. This capacity to change muscle fibre size is called **muscle plasticity**.

Old individuals usually have a negative protein balance, i.e. muscle protein breakdown is greater than protein synthesis. The onset of **senile atrophy** (**sarcopenia**) of the muscle is mainly due to a decrease in the number of muscle fibres, a change in the composition of muscle fibre type through transformation or cell death (especially of the strength-generating fibres (p. 156)), and an increasing loss of motoneuron supply. The resulting decrease in muscle strength severely limits mobility, physical performance and metabolic health. This is a phenomenon mainly studied in humans, but with advancing age of companion animals of humans (dogs, cats, horses), it is also becoming increasingly important in veterinary medicine.

Lack of exercise leads to **inactivity atrophy** in all skeletal muscles. Chronic diseases such as cancer, cardiac failure, Cushing's disease and chronic lung diseases, as well as major injuries, can cause muscle atrophy by the action of cytokines and other mediators, even in young individuals. Together with simultaneous exhaustion of all energy reserves, this leads to extreme emaciation (**cachexia**).

> **IN A NUTSHELL** !
>
> Muscle is subject to lifelong anabolic and catabolic changes and can be severely limited in its plasticity by hormones, reduced physical activity, ageing and disease.

6.2.3 Movement function of skeletal muscle

■ Muscle contraction

For a muscle fibre to contract, activation by an α-motoneuron is necessary. These neurons are located in the brainstem or spinal cord, from which **somatomotor efferent nerves** originate. Each muscle fibre is innervated by an axon terminal of a motoneuron, the point of contact being the **neuromuscular junction** or **myoneural junction**. Since a motoneuron splits into 20–1000 terminal fibres, many muscle fibres can be stimulated simultaneously. The totality of the motoneuron and all the muscle fibres it innervates is called the **motor unit**.

Neuromuscular junction

The axon of a motor neuron forms a synaptic thickening (endplate) at its end in the immediate vicinity of a muscle fibre. This thickening is surrounded by Schwann cells and is rich in mitochondria. Within this synaptic bouton, synaptic vesicles containing the transmitter **acetylcholine** (**ACh**) are stored. The actual synapse includes the **presynaptic membrane** with the **active zone** (= membrane area with high exocytosis activity), the **synaptic cleft** (approx. 50 nm) and the strongly folded **postsynaptic membrane**, which is formed by the sarcolemma, with the **basal lamina** (**Fig. 6.4 a**). If an action potential of the motor nerve (AP_{Nerve}) arrives at the neuromuscular junction, **voltage-dependent Ca^{2+} channels** open in the presynaptic membrane. The inflowing Ca^{2+} induces the translocation of the ACh-filled vesicles to the active zone of the presynaptic membrane, the fusion of the vesicles with the membrane and finally the release of the ACh into the synaptic cleft (**exocytosis**). For each action potential, 50–300 vesicles are mobilised, each releasing 5000–10000 molecules of ACh into the synaptic cleft. The empty vesicles are recycled and refilled with ACh. The released ACh diffuses through the synaptic cleft to the basal lamina and the postsynaptic membrane. The basal lamina contains many structural proteins that maintain the stability and function of the synapse. It also contains the enzyme **acetylcholine esterase** (**AChE**), which is responsible for the subsequent cleavage of ACh. At the upper end of the invaginations in the postsynaptic membrane (just opposite the active zone), about 10000 ACh receptor molecules per μm^2 are located. This **ACh receptor** is a **ligand-gated ion channel** (= ionotropic **nicotinic receptor**) that has extracellular binding sites for ACh and forms a channel for cations. After binding of ACh, there is an influx of Na^+ and thus depolarization of the postsynaptic membrane (**end-plate potential, EPP**). This EPP activates voltage-dependent Na^+ channels in the depth of the membrane invaginations. The consequence is the triggering of an action potential at the sarcolemma of the muscle fibre (AP_{Muscle}) (**Fig. 6.4 b**).

At the presynaptic membrane, the secretion of an approximately 10-fold greater amount of ACh than would be needed to evoke an action potential, and at the postsynaptic membrane, a high receptor density ensures that each AP_{Nerve} results in a contraction. The highly active AChE rap-

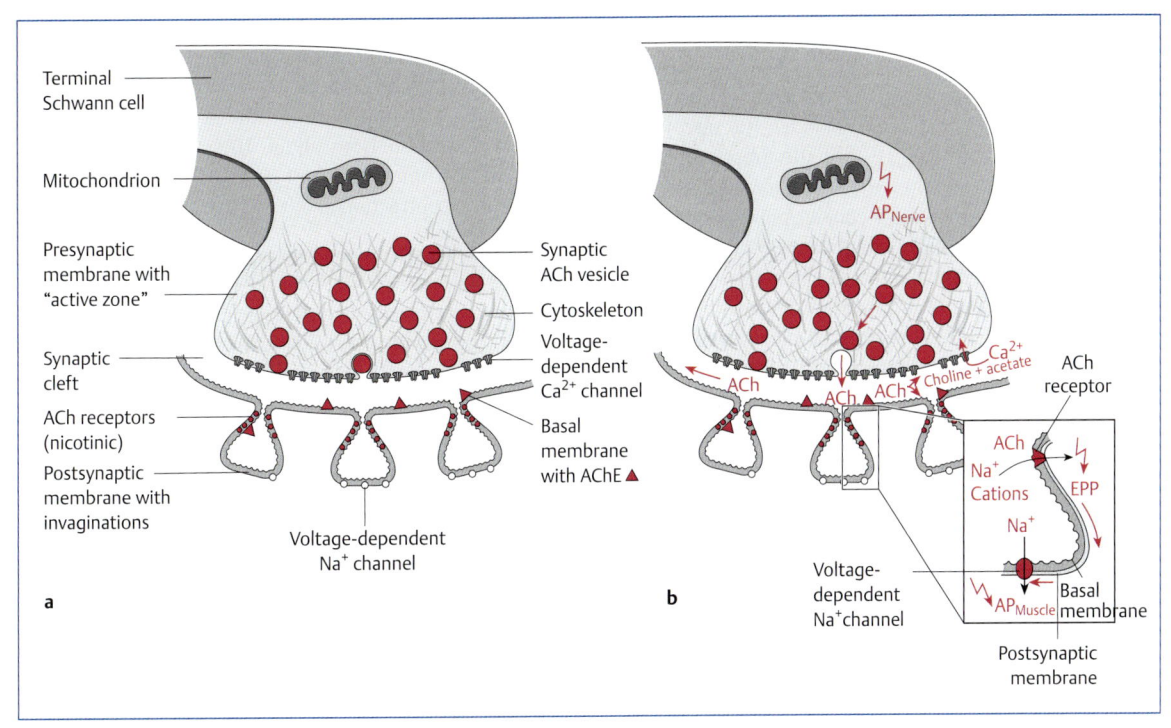

Fig. 6.4 Structure and function of a neuromuscular junction.
a The neuromuscular synapse consists of the terminal bouton of the α-motoneuron with Schwann cell sheath and acetylcholine vesicles, the presynaptic membrane with voltage-dependent Ca^{2+} channels, the synaptic cleft and the postsynaptic membrane with acetylcholine receptors (= ionotropic receptor, cation channel) and voltage-dependent Na^+ channels.
b If a neuronal action potential (AP_{Nerve}) reaches the neuromuscular junction, this leads to the release of acetylcholine (ACh) after fusion of the vesicles with the presynaptic membrane. Acetylcholine binds to its receptors at the postsynaptic membrane, Na^+ flows into the muscle cell, triggering a depolarizing end-plate potential (EPP) and thus opening voltage-dependent Na^+ channels in the depth of the postsynaptic membrane. An action potential is generated at the skeletal muscle (AP_{Muscle}).
Ach = acetylcholine; AChE = acetylcholine esterase; AP_{Muscle} = action potential muscle; AP_{Nerve} = action potential nerve; EPP = end-plate potential; ▲ = acetylcholine esterase.

idly cleaves the ACh or it diffuses out of the synaptic cleft, so that each ACh molecule can activate an ACh receptor only once on average.

MORE DETAILS   For surgical interventions, it is essential to achieve sufficient **muscle relaxation** to be able to reduce fractures or to be able to perform interventions in the abdominal or thoracic cavity. Based on knowledge of the molecular processes at the neuromuscular synapse, pharmacologically effective substances have been found that specifically block this synapse and cause the muscle to relax. For example, **D-tubocurarin** (the active ingredient in curare, muscle relaxants of the curare type) specifically blocks the ACh receptors on the skeletal muscle membrane and, as a **non-depolarizing relaxant**, ensures sustained muscle **relaxation**. **Succinylcholine** is a **depolarizing muscle relaxant** and has an activating effect on these ACh receptors, but a longer-lasting effect than ACh. There is continuous depolarization of the postsynaptic membrane and thus inactivation of the voltage-dependent Na^+ channels. In the autoimmune disease **myasthenia gravis** (severe muscle weakness), neuromuscular signal transmission is impaired by autoaggressive antibodies against ACh receptors. **Eserin** or **neostigmine** as AChE inhibitors increase the ACh concentration at the postsynaptic membrane. In this way, they improve the clinical symptoms of the disease. These substances are also used as antidotes in curare poisoning. Poisoning with **Clostridium botulinum toxin** leads to a presynaptic blockade of ACh release. The result is flaccid paralysis of striated skeletal muscles.

IN A NUTSHELL   !

The processes at the neuromuscular junction very efficiently translate nervous electrical signals (AP_{Nerve}) into muscular electrical signals (AP_{Muscle}). This translation takes place by means of a chemical transmitter via a ligand-receptor interaction (ACh/ACh receptor).

Electromechanical coupling

For conversion of an electrical signal of muscle (AP_{Muscle}) into a mechanical response, i.e. the muscle contraction, the following processes take place in skeletal muscle:
- Propagation of the electrical signal along the muscle fibre
- Conversion (coupling) of the electrical signal into a chemical signal (the Ca^{2+} switch)
- Ca^{2+}-induced muscle contraction via filament sliding and cross-bridge cycle

All these processes of electromechanical coupling also take place in a similar way in the heart muscle.

Excitation propagation and Ca²⁺ release (Ca²⁺ switch)

The muscular action potential spreads electrotonically (i.e. similar to the unmyelinated nerve) along the sarcolemma with a speed of about $5\,m\cdot s^{-1}$ over the muscle fibre. The electrical excitation reaches the triad area via the T-tubules. There, at the immediate contact point between a T- and an L-tubule (approx. 12 nm distance between the two membranes), the electrical signal is converted into a chemical signal. Two types of proteins are responsible for this coupling. In the T-tubule, these are **voltage-dependent L** (long lasting) type **Ca²⁺ channels** of the type $Ca_V1.1$ (in skeletal muscle called **1,4-dihydropyridine receptor, DHPR**). In the adjacent L-tubule, the sarcoplasmic reticulum (SR), the involved proteins are **type 1 ryanodine (and caffeine) sensitive Ca²⁺-releasing channels** (**ryanodine receptor, RyR1**) (**Fig. 6.5**). From the involvement of these Ca²⁺-selective channels, it is clear that Ca²⁺ plays a central role in electromechanical coupling. Voltage-dependent activation of the DHPR leads to the opening of the RyR in skeletal muscle via a direct, reciprocal protein-protein interaction (allosteric coupling between DHPR and RYR) or, in cardiac muscle (p. 175), to calcium-mediated opening of the RyR and a massive **release of Ca²⁺** from the **sarcoplas-** **mic reticulum** into the cytosol. Ca²⁺ is stored in large quantities in the SR of the skeletal muscle fibre. Consequently, contractions of skeletal muscle are independent of extracellular Ca²⁺. Ca²⁺ release from the SR increases cytosolic Ca²⁺ concentration from about 10^{-7} to $10^{-5}\,mol\cdot l^{-1}$ (i.e. from 10–$100\,nmol\cdot l^{-1}$ to $> 1\,\mu mol\cdot l^{-1}$). This results in muscle fibre contraction about 5–7 ms later.

> **IN A NUTSHELL**   !
>
> The propagation of excitation takes place electrotonically to the triad and triggers the release of Ca²⁺ via dihydropyridine and ryanodine receptors.

Filament sliding and cross-bridge cycle

Contraction of skeletal and cardiac muscle is based on sliding of the contractile filaments, actin and myosin into each other. In this process myosin filaments take over the active part of the **sliding** (**sliding filament theory** according to Huxley 1973). The high intracellular Ca²⁺ concentration after excitation of the muscle fibres is the switch for the start of the interactions between myosin heads and actin. The generation of force in the muscles is based on the

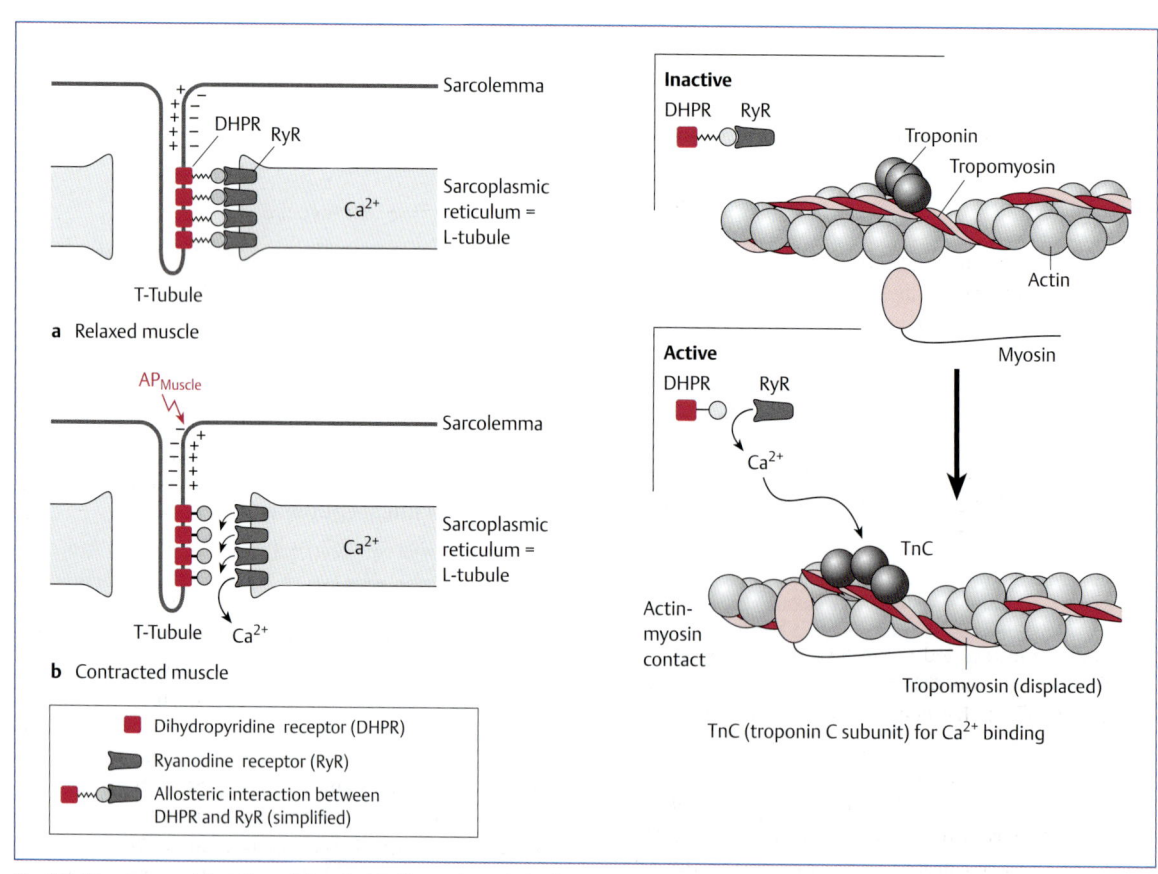

Fig. 6.5 Structure and function of the triad-Ca²⁺-switch in skeletal muscle. The close spatial connection of the T- and L-tubules (triad) enables intracellular Ca²⁺ release controlled by dihydropyridine (DHPR) and ryanodine receptors (RyR).
a Resting muscle: no AP_{Muscle} at the sarcolemma, the RyR-associated Ca²⁺ channels are closed, no contact between actin and myosin.
b Contracting muscle: AP_{Muscle} at the sarcolemma, which spreads into the T-tubules and causes intracellular Ca²⁺ release via the activation of the DHPR and RyR. Cytosolic Ca²⁺ activates troponin, removes tropomyosin from the myosin-binding site on actin and thus enables the formation of the actin-myosin contact. TnC = Ca²⁺-binding subunit of troponin.

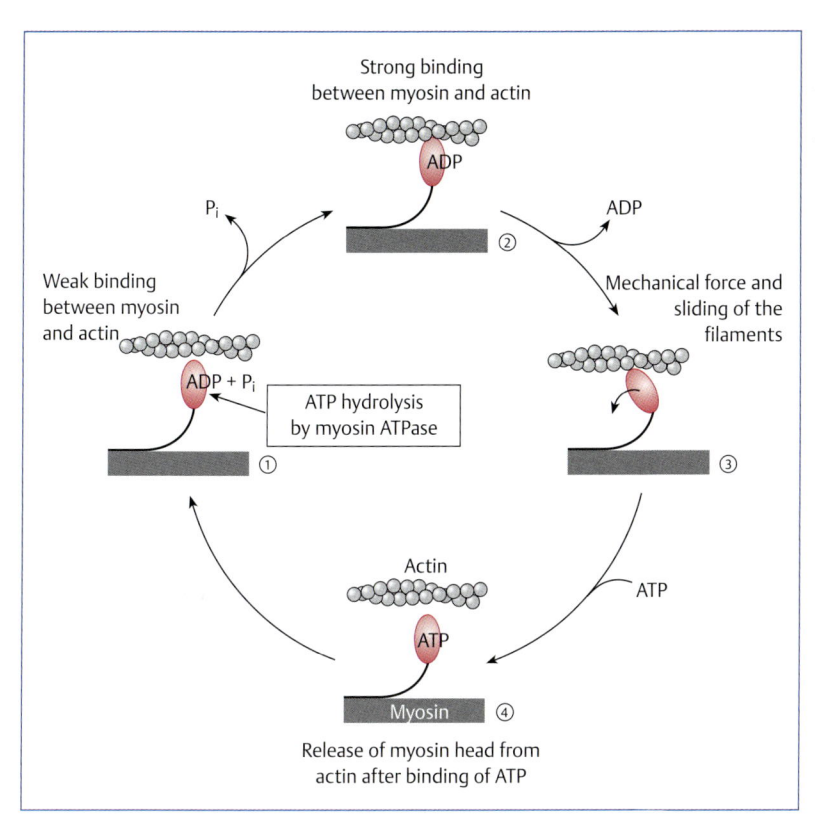

Fig. 6.6 Cross-bridge cycle in skeletal and cardiac muscle. The processes 1–4 during the cross-bridge cycle are described in detail in the text. The cyclic formation of the cross-bridges leads to force generation and length shortening of the muscle fibre.

number of contacts between actin and myosin that are established during the **cross-bridge cycle**.

To initiate contraction, Ca^{2+} binds to the TnC subunit of troponin and, through the resulting displacement of tropomyosin, makes the binding site for myosin accessible (**Fig. 6.5**). The myosin head forms a weak bond with actin, which leads to the activation of the Mg^{2+}-dependent ATPase located at the myosin head (**Fig. 6.6,1**). The ATP bound to the myosin head is hydrolysed to ADP and phosphate (P_i). With the release of the cleavage products, the weak bond changes into a strong bond (force generation) and the myosin head bends by 45° in the direction of the myosin neck ("rudder stroke", sliding of the filaments; **Fig. 6.6,2** and **3**). A single tilting movement of all myosin heads leads to a length reduction of 20 nm per sarcomere. When ATP binds again to the myosin head, the myosin releases the cross-bridge (**softening effect of ATP**; **Fig. 6.6,4**), the myosin head straightens, binds weakly to a new actin molecule, and the cycle can begin again as long as sufficient Ca^{2+} and ATP are present. The binding forces constantly oscillate between weak and strong. In this way, the myosin filaments push themselves between the actin filaments on both sides and shorten the entire **sarcomere** (**Fig. 6.7**). The force as well as the shortening of all sarcomeres is transferred to the sarcolemma by means of dystrophin and thus causes the contraction of the entire muscle fibre.

Relaxation, muscle soreness and rigor mortis of skeletal muscle

If the neurogenic excitation of a skeletal muscle fibre ceases, the muscle cell membrane repolarizes by outflow of K^+ and inflow of Cl^-. Ca^{2+} is transported back into the SR by sarco/endoplasmatic Ca^{2+}-ATPases (SERCA), which transport two Ca^{2+} ions per cleaved ATP molecule. Thus, cytosolic Ca^{2+} concentration is lowered again to 10^{-7} mol·l^{-1}. A small part of the Ca^{2+} can also be removed into the extracellular space by Ca^{2+}-ATPases and Ca^{2+}/Na^+ exchangers in the sarcolemma. Lowering intracellular Ca^{2+} concentration terminates the contraction. If the ATP concentration drops below 5 µmol·g^{-1} of working skeletal muscle, the myosin heads can no longer detach from actin when Ca^{2+} levels are high. Individual or several muscle fibres are then in a **state of rigidity** (**rigor**). If the skeletal muscle continues to move despite fibrillar rigidity, injuries of the Z-lines and muscle fibres occur due to the rigor. These injuries occur especially during eccentric movements ("braking contractions" (p. 152)) in running, ball shooting or walking downhill, but also in all movements for which the muscles are not trained. These myofibrillar injuries trigger an inflammatory process within 1–2 days, which is painful and is generally referred to as **muscle soreness**. **Rigor mortis** is also based on an ATP deficiency with a simultaneous high Ca^{2+} content of skeletal muscle cells.

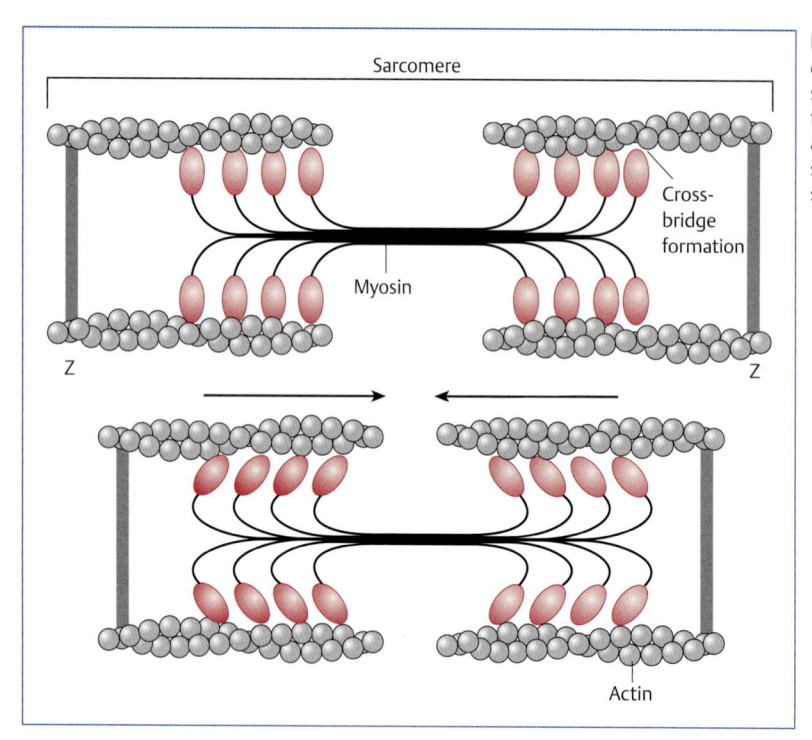

Sarcomere

Cross-bridge formation

Myosin

Z

Z

Actin

Fig. 6.7 Filament sliding in skeletal and cardiac muscle. Due to the repeated power strokes of the myosin heads, the myosin filament actively pulls itself between the actin filaments on both sides of the sarcomere, so that the whole sarcomere is shortened.

> **IN A NUTSHELL**   !
>
> The electromechanical coupling, the activation of the Ca^{2+} switch and the energy-dependent steps of the cross-bridge cycle, all lead to the generation of force and shortening of striated muscle.

■ Muscle mechanics

Muscle mechanics describes physiological relationships that define the force and mechanical action of a skeletal muscle. This includes the forms of contraction that a skeletal muscle can perform and the dependency of force generation on muscle length and excitation frequency. The regulation of muscle force is based on these biophysical relationships, the size of the muscle cross-sectional area, the composition of the muscle with different fibres types (white fibres have greater force; see also ch. Metabolic function of skeletal muscle (p.156)) and the recruitment (activation) of motor units.

Forms of contraction

If a muscle only shortens its length during contraction but does not increase its strength, such a contraction is called **isotonic**. This is the case when a muscle is only fixed at one end and shortens without an attached load. However, this is not the rule *in vivo*, as all skeletal muscles are anchored at both ends. If a muscle is fixed between two immobile attachment points, it can only increase its force when activated, but not shorten its length. This contraction is called **isometric**. In the whole animal, however, the fixation of muscles is often not rigid. Most contractions are **auxotonic**, i.e. muscle force and muscle length both change simultaneously during a contraction. In addition, there are mixed contraction forms. For example, when a heavy object is lifted, an isometric contraction is followed by an isotonic contraction, when the muscle has generated enough force to overcome the weight of the object. The opposite happens e.g. during raising the chin where an isotonic contraction is followed by an isometric contraction.

The shortening speed of a muscle is determined by the speed of the power strokes and depends on the load on the muscle. An increasing load reduces the shortening speed, with which such a load can be lifted. When the maximum lifting force is exceeded, the muscle does not shorten any more. **Concentric** contractions occur when muscle tension increases and the muscle shortens. **Eccentric** contractions are "braking contractions" when, for example, the muscle counteracts stretching by increasing its contraction activity.

Strength generation and muscle length

The force generation of a muscle is determined by its length, i.e. by its **prestretching**. If the sarcomeres are fully contracted, only a little force generation is possible because of steric hindrance (**Fig. 6.8, 1**). If the muscle is passively stretched, its active maximum force initially increases with increasing sarcomere length. At a length of 2.20–2.25 µm, the sarcomere has its **optimal length** at which all possible actin-myosin bridges can be formed and when it generates its **maximum force** (**Fig. 6.8, 2**). If the muscle is stretched further, its maximum force decreases again, as only some of the cross-bridges can be formed. When there is very strong prestretching, no more force can be generated because contact between the contractile filaments is no longer possible (**Fig. 6.8, 3**). This dependence of muscle force on muscle length can be demonstrated experimentally by measuring the isometric active

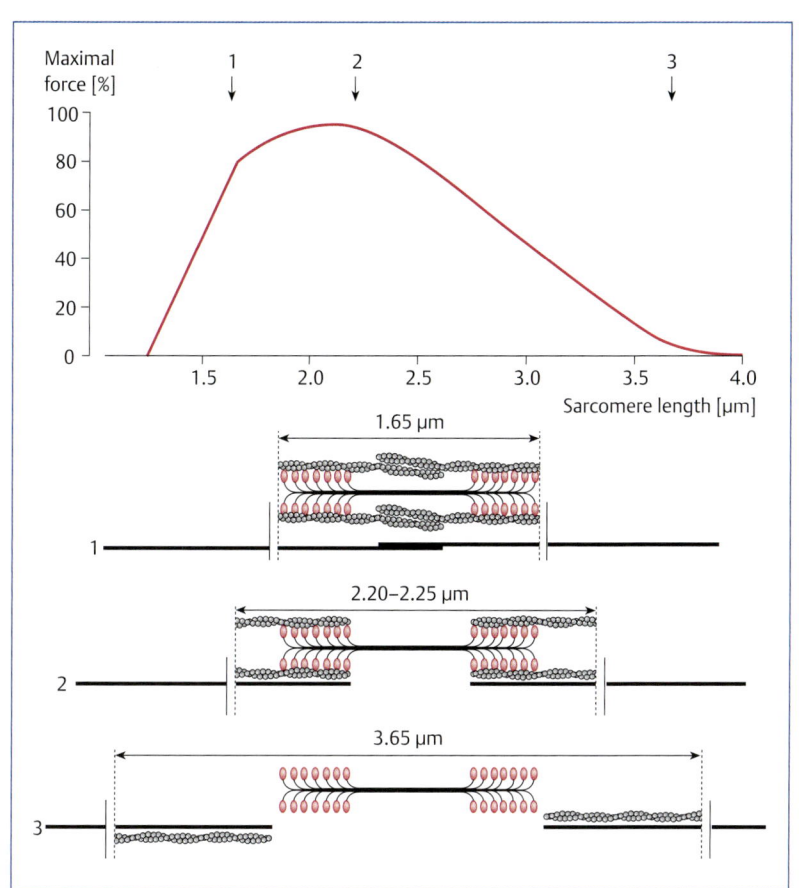

Fig. 6.8 Relationship between sarcomere length and force generation. When a muscle fibre is prestretched and the sarcomere length is increased, the active isometric muscle force increases. Maximum force (%) is reached at a sarcomere length of 2.2 μm, at which all myosin heads can form contacts with actin. Functional states 1–3 are explained in more detail in the text.

force of an increasingly prestretched muscle (**Fig. 6.9**). The optimisation of the prestretching of muscles *in vivo* is achieved by **stretch sensors** in the muscles, the **muscle spindles**. In each leg muscle, for example, 500–1000 such muscle spindles are found. Muscle spindles belong to the **phasic-tonic sensors**. These sensors react to both the absolute change in length and the speed of change in length. During an awake state, the muscle spindles are constantly active in order to coordinate by reflex arcs the postural and motor functions. Muscle spindles (**intrafusal fibres**) are muscle fibres with a nervous component. **Nuclear chain and nuclear bag fibres** are located in a spindle-shaped connective tissue sheath and lie side by side. In the thin nuclear chain fibres, the nuclei lie one behind the other in a row, while the nuclear bag fibres have a distension in the middle where several nuclei are localised. The two ends of the nuclear bag fibres are contractile, and the inner part is extensible (**Fig. 6.10**). The **tonic** chain fibres continuously monitor muscle length, while the **phasic** nuclear bag fibres measure the speed of length changes. If the muscle is stretched (e.g. during stumbling or changes in position), the change in stretch is reported via Ia (phasic) and II (tonic) afferents to the spinal cord. There, it is transmitted to α- and γ-motoneurons (efferents) in the grey matter. The axons of the α-motoneurons run to the **extrafusal** muscle fibres surrounding the **intrafusal** fibres and stimulate them to contract, thus shortening muscle length. The axons of the γ-motoneurons run to the contractile parts of the muscle spindle (= ends of the nuclear bag fi-

bres) and activate them (**Fig. 6.10**). As a result, the muscle spindle is kept taut and can react optimally to the next stimulus.

These mono- and polysynaptic reflexes are also called **postural reflexes**. In this way, overstretching of the muscle is prevented. A basal muscular tension for posture controls the fine modulation of voluntary movement sequences. In the field of medicine, checking these muscle spindle reflexes (e.g. patellar tendon reflex) is used to examine the functions of the parts of the nervous system involved (e.g. in the case of herniated discs, neuropathies).

> **IN A NUTSHELL**
>
> Muscle spindles are the sensors for reflexes in the motor system and are therefore also essential for the coordination of voluntary movements.

During passive stretching, the **plastic and elastic components** of a muscle increase in length. This increases the passive force of the muscle. The plastic components are the actin and myosin filaments. The elastic components in series are the tendons, Z-lines, the joint regions of the myosin heads, and titin. Parallel-elastic components are the endo-, epi- and perimysium. Titin plays the greatest role here for the elasticity of a muscle over its physiological range. Only when a muscle is stretched to over 170% of its initial length do the other elasticity components also come into play. If the change in length is plotted against the generation of passive force, the **passive length-tension curve** of the muscle is obtained (**Fig. 6.9 b**). The **total force** of a muscle is composed of the passive and the active force (**Fig. 6.9 b**). From a particular muscle length onwards, the contribution of the passive force in the total force predominates, because the sarcomeres are so far apart that they can no longer contribute to force generation (**Fig. 6.8**).

IN A NUTSHELL   !

The total force of a muscle is the sum of the active and passive forces. The maximum active force can only be achieved with optimal sarcomere length, which is maintained in vivo by the muscle spindles.

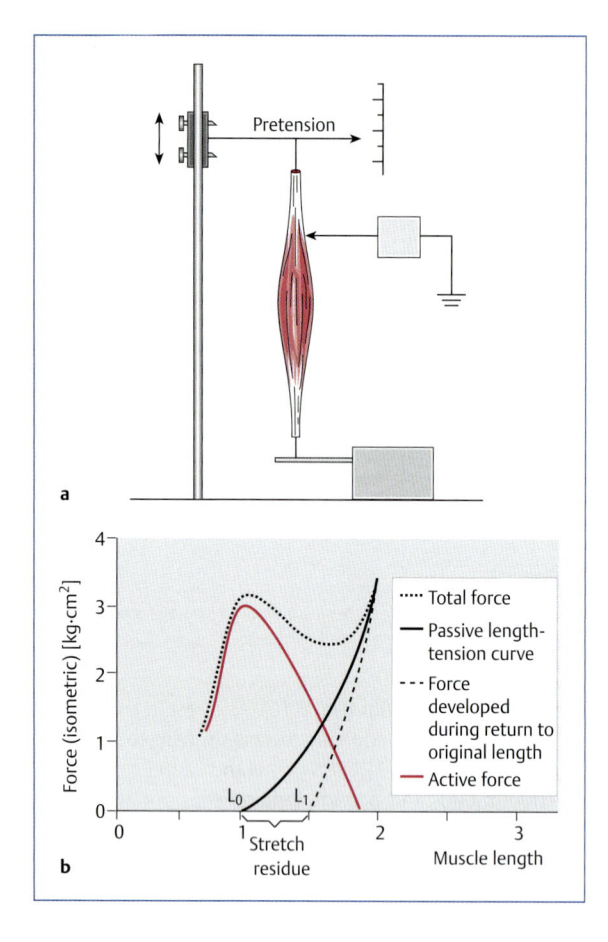

Fig. 6.9 Isometric registration of active and passive forces of a muscle.
a Measuring arrangement for recording the isometric force of a muscle. The active force is determined by stimulation with frequencies evoking single muscle twitches (**Fig. 6.11**).
b The active force increases with increasing prestretching, and reaches a maximum at the optimal length L_0 and then it drops again (red curve, **Fig. 6.8**). Passive stretching of the muscle changes its length and increases the passive force, which is based on the stretching of the plastic and elastic elements (black curve). The sum of active and passive forces gives the total force (black dotted line). If a muscle that has previously been stretched extensively (> 160–200% of its resting length) and is then relaxed (black dotted line), it does not return to its initial length (L_0) but retains a residual increase in length (L_1) due to the deformation of plastic elements in the muscle. This residue only disappears when the muscle is actively moved again.

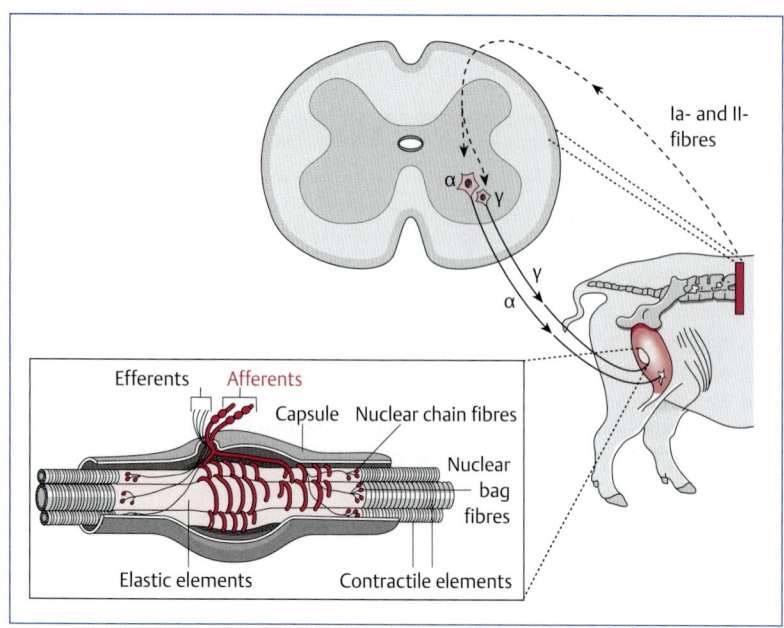

Fig. 6.10 Reflective control of muscle length via the muscle spindle apparatus. The intrafusal fibres (nuclear bag fibres and nuclear chain fibres), which are contractile as well as extensile, form the muscle spindle apparatus. The phasic Ia and tonic II nerve fibres represent the afferents that travel to the spinal cord where they are interconnected to efferent pathways, the α- and γ-motoneurons. The α-motoneurons activate the surrounding extrafusal muscle fibres, the γ-motoneurons the contractile part of the muscle spindle. Thus, the muscle becomes shorter and the spindle is synchronously adapted to this new muscle length.

Force generation and excitation frequency

Like muscle length, excitation frequency also influences muscle strength. A single stimulus triggers a **single twitch** (**Fig. 6.11,1**). Single twitches or periods of low frequency contractions allow the muscle to relax completely after each stimulus. If the stimulus frequency is increased, the contractions begin to overlap (**superposition**; Fig. 6.11,**2**), i.e. complete relaxation no longer takes place between individual contractions. Thus, the muscle begins each new contraction at a higher tension level. Above a certain frequency, the **fusion frequency**, individual contractions can no longer be distinguished from each other. This is called **tetanic contraction**, also known as a **physiologic tetanus** (**Fig. 6.11,4**). During the initial phase of the tetanic contraction, the force generation in the muscle also increases compared to the single twitch. The reason for the fusion of the contractions is that the muscular action potential occurs well before the contraction (**Table 6.1**). While the contraction associated with the first action potential is taking place, the muscle fibre is already excitable and responds to the next stimulus (refractory period completed). As a result, the contractions induced by several stimuli overlap. The reason for the increase in force is the length of time that it takes to transport Ca^{2+} back into the sarcoplasmic reticulum. With each new contraction, there is a further Ca^{2+} release, but the transport back into the sarcoplasmic reticulum does not keep pace. The cytosolic Ca^{2+} level therefore increases successively with frequent muscle stimulation. This prevents relaxation, and causes the number of active cross-bridges to increase so that muscle strength increases. Almost all contractions in physiological movement sequences are tetanic contractions.

MORE DETAILS   The tetanus described here is a physiological functional state of the muscle and has nothing to do with the clinical term "tetanus". **Tetanus** or **lockjaw** is a disease caused by the toxin of the anaerobic bacterium *Clostridium tetani*. This bacterium multiplies in deep wounds under O_2-poor conditions and produces a neurotoxin that travels along the neural pathways into the spinal cord. There the toxin blocks inhibitory synapses of interneurons. This results in hyperexcitability of the motor system, leading to violent skeletal muscle spasms. The spasm of the striated respiratory muscles eventually leads to death. Active or passive immunoprophylaxis against this tetanus toxin can be administered to animals and humans. In contrast, the term **tetany** (hypomagnesemic grass tetany in ruminants, puerperal tetany in bitches [eclampsia]) refers to states of muscular excitation that can lead to convulsions. In **grass tetany** the Mg^{2+} concentrations in plasma and cerebrospinal fluid of ruminants drop due to insufficient magnesium supply (p. 49). In the CNS, the inhibitory effect of Mg^{2+} at excitatory synapses ceases (activation of glutamatergic NMDA receptors). In addition, the release of transmitters of inhibitory synapses (blockade of glycinergic receptors at the α-motoneurons by inhibiting transmitter release) is reduced. This triggers states of excitation and muscle spasms. In **eclampsia in bitches**, a reduced plasma Ca^{2+} concentration (hypocalcaemia) leads to reduced extracellular binding of Ca^{2+}; see ch. Disorders of electrolyte balance (p. 54). The membrane potential difference is thereby lowered. This increases the excitability of neurons as the threshold potential for the initiation of action potential is reached more quickly. Increased excitability of the nerve fibres and muscle spasms are the consequence. In **parturient paresis in cows** (milk fever), blockage of the neuromuscular synapse (inhibition of acetylcholine release) due to hypocalcaemia is the main defect. The animal is immobilised because of flaccid paralysis of the musculature.

> ### IN A NUTSHELL   !
>
> Muscle strength is determined by muscle thickness, prestretch, excitation frequency, number of motor units recruited and fibre type composition.

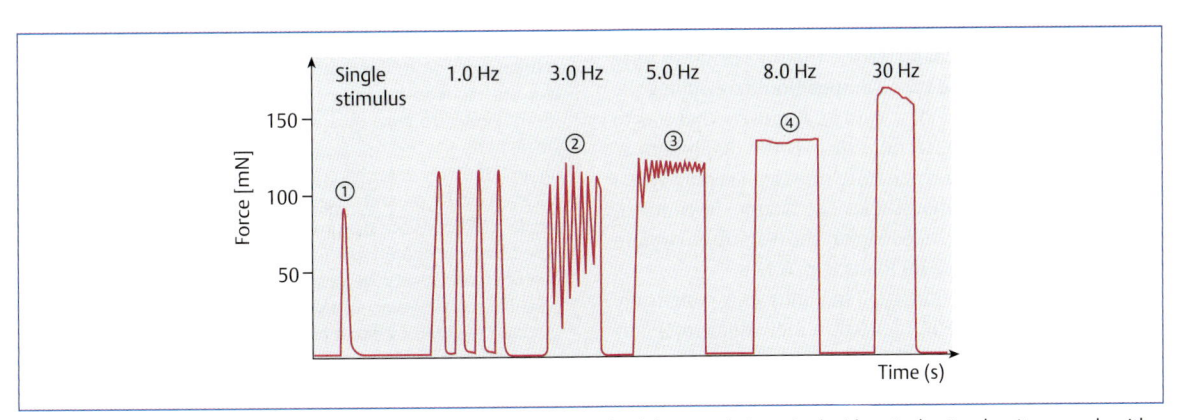

Fig. 6.11 Relationship between stimulus frequency and muscle strength. If the muscle is excited with a single stimulus, it responds with a single twitch (**1**). Excitation with a higher stimulus frequency first leads to superposition (from 3 Hz; **2**), then to incomplete tetanus (from 5 Hz; **3**) and finally to complete tetanic contraction (from 8 Hz; **4**). The force of the contraction responses increases successively from **1** to **4**, which is due to the slow increase in cytosolic Ca^{2+} concentration. At high stimulus frequency, moving back Ca^{2+} into the sarcoplasmic reticulum (SR) via the sarco/endoplasmic Ca^{2+}-ATPases (SERCA) does not match its release. Hence some Ca^{2+} remains in the cytosol, the concentration of which increases with each further stimulation.
Unit of frequency: Hz = Hertz (s^{-1}).

6.2.4 Metabolic functions of skeletal muscle

The contraction and metabolic properties can be very different in different fibres in a muscle (p.619)

■ Functional structure of the skeletal muscle

There are three main types of muscle fibres. The **type I fibre** (synonym: **S-fibre**) is red in colour due to a high capillary density, a large number of mitochondria and a high myoglobin content (haem-containing O_2 storage). This fibre slowly contracts (slow [**S**]) and generates only low but long-lasting strength. It uses predominantly aerobic, i.e. oxidative metabolic processes for energy production (p.617). Due to the good vascular supply, the storage of energy reserves in the form of glycogen in these fibres is low. They have good insulin sensitivity and therefore contribute to the maintenance of glucose homeostasis.

Type II fibres exist in two forms. The **type IIB fibre** (or **type IIX fibre** in some species; synonym: **FF fibre**) is whitish in colour due to its low capillary density, small number of mitochondria and low myoglobin content. These fibres contract rapidly (fast [**F**]) with great force, but rapidly become fatigued (low resistance to fatigue [**F**]). They have a high density of glycolytic enzymes and obtain their energy by anaerobic metabolism (glycolysis) producing lactate. These fibres use stored glycogen as the main energy substrate. The insulin sensitivity of these muscle fibres is significantly lower than that of type I fibres.

The **type IIA fibre** (**FR fibre**) is an intermediate fibre type between type I and type IIB fibres. The capillary density is greater than that of the type IIB fibre and the metabolism is predominantly aerobic. Like the type IIB fibre, it has large glycogen stores. It contracts rapidly (fast [**F**]) but generates more force than a type I fibre and does not fatigue as quickly as a type IIB fibre (resistant to fatigue [**R**]; **Fig. 6.12**).

Each muscle has a characteristic mixture of these fibre types. This **muscle fibre type composition** determines the contractile performance of a muscle. A muscle that has to provide continuous contraction, such as the diaphragm as part of its function as a respiratory muscle, has only type I and type IIA fibres so that it does not fatigue. In contrast, limb muscles that are needed for short sprints contain large proportions of type IIB fibres (**Fig. 6.12**):

The composition of fibre type in a muscle is genetically determined, but can be influenced in individuals to a certain extent, by physiological factors, and also by pharmacological intervention, within the framework of the genetic background. The different fibre types can change into each other (**fibre transformation: IIB ↔ IIA ↔ I**). In addition to their ability to hypertrophy, this phenomenon is also part of the **plasticity of muscle**. The innervation of the muscle fibre or the frequency of the incoming neural signals is one of the most important control signals for these transformation processes. By changing the composition of fibre type, the force generation of the muscle, its contraction speed and its performance can be altered. The **isoform** of **myosin**

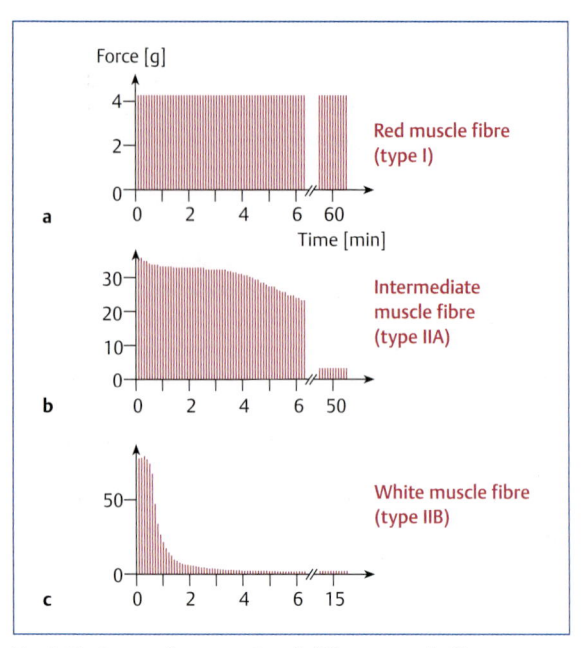

Fig. 6.12 Contractile properties of different muscle fibre types under tetanic stimulation Force given in g (note different x- and y-axis scaling).
a The red fibres can generate low-level endurance force.
b The behaviour of the intermediate fibres lies between red and white fibres in their contractile force and endurance. This is because of different metabolic requirements of the different types of muscle fibres. **c** The white fibres are able to generate great force for a short period, but then weaken.

(myosin heavy chain, MHC) (MHC I in type I fibres, MHC IIA in type IIA fibres, MHC IIB in type IIB fibres) determines the contraction speed and force generation of a fibre.

MORE DETAILS The change in fibre type is based on a change in the expression of several groups of genes. Thus, in addition to the originally present myosin isoform, further MHC are expressed in the fibres, so that initially **hybrid fibres** are formed. These can contain, for example, MHC I and IIA, MHC IIA and IIB or other combinations. With the change to a new MHC isoform, all **genes** that are required for the corresponding change in metabolism (from aerobic to anaerobic and vice versa with all intermediate stages) are also expressed at the same time. Only in the diaphragm muscles does this coupling of MHC and metabolic genes not seem to be present. Endurance and strength training for example, influence fibre type composition by shifting towards more type I fibres or more type II fibres, respectively. Loss of innervation of an oxidative slow muscle, leads to increased expression of type II fibres. However, atrophy of individual fibre types in certain (patho-)physiological situations also produces a shift in the fibre type composition. For example, in old age, the number of type I fibres increases as type II fibres die. Chronic hypoxia (lack of oxygen in the tissue, for example in patients with lung disease) shifts the fibre composition of skeletal muscles towards more type IIB fibres in order to be able to perform more glycolytic, anaerobic metabolism. Glucocorticoids (cortisone) and β_2 agonists used in the treatment of respiratory diseases shift the fibre type proportions towards type I fibres. However, age- and disease-related and pharmacologically triggered changes in the fibre type composition of muscles always result in a weakening of muscle performance.

> **IN A NUTSHELL** !
>
> Although skeletal muscles have a very uniform structure, they exhibit a high degree of plasticity in terms of their motor and metabolic performance.

◼ Energetics of skeletal muscle

Compared to other cells in the body, skeletal muscle cells exhibit the greatest change in their metabolic rate in relation to the resting state when they begin to work. This is linked to the highest fluxes of substrates in and out of the cell to convert chemical energy metabolically into mechanical energy. This proceeds with an **efficiency** of about **30%**, with the **remaining energy** being released as **heat**. When 1 mol of ATP is cleaved, 48 kJ of energy are released in the muscle, i.e. about 14 kJ for muscle work and about 34 kJ as heat generation. The heart muscle corresponds in its metabolism to that of the oxidative type I skeletal muscle fibre (p. 158).

General processes for energy production in muscle

ATP is the only energy-rich compound that can be used by the ATPases of all muscle cells (myosin ATPase, Ca^{2+}-ATPases, Na^+/K^+-ATPase). All metabolic pathways therefore aim to produce sufficient ATP so that ATP synthesis keeps pace with ATP hydrolysis, to enable adequate muscle work performance. Various metabolic pathways (p. 617) are available for the production of ATP (**Fig. 6.13**). For rapid regeneration of ATP (up to about 30 s after the onset of contraction), the reactions of **myokinase** and **creatine kinase** (CK) are required. Myokinase generates ATP and AMP by shifting a phosphate residue from one ADP to another. Creatine kinase uses creatine phosphate as a phosphate donor for the regeneration of ATP.

Skeletal muscles at rest or during very light physical activity predominantly use fatty acids from cellular stores for energy production. The oxygen (O_2) required under this condition is released from myoglobin. However, during prolonged muscle work, ATP formation is maintained by oxidation of glucose and fatty acids. Glucose is stored in muscle as glycogen and can be used in the first few minutes of muscle contraction by glycolysis to lactate in **anaerobic energy production**. In longer-lasting muscle work, the production of ATP from **aerobic metabolism** of glucose, lactate and fatty acids then becomes increasingly important. To maintain long-lasting aerobic energy supply, a corresponding increase is needed in **skeletal muscle blood flow**. This is achieved by a combination of local factors and the influence of the sympathetic nervous system (see ch. Muscle blood flow (p. 208). Only when capillary perfusion is increased and the supply of O_2 is assured, can a muscle reach its full **aerobic metabolic capacity**. In addition to the glycogen and fat stored in muscle (intra- and intercellular), glucose and fatty acids from blood can then increasingly be used for ATP production. During muscular

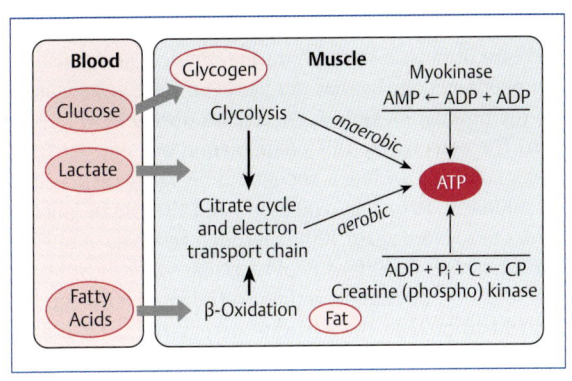

Fig. 6.13 Overview of metabolic pathways for energy production in skeletal muscle. ATP in muscle can be obtained from anaerobic and aerobic metabolic pathways. While only glucose can be used as a substrate for the anaerobic pathway, glucose, fatty acids and lactate serve as substrates for aerobic energy production. CP = creatine phosphate.

endurance exercise, glucose oxidation induced by physical activity becomes increasingly less important, whereas the contribution of fat oxidation as an energy source (p. 617) rises. The increasing availability of fatty acids in plasma, which are released from adipose tissue by catecholamines during intensive physical activity, replaces intracellular glucose oxidation, due to reduced insulin levels in blood and consequent decrease in glucose uptake by muscles. The respiratory quotient (p. 488) drops during this phase to values around 0.7. For aerobic ATP production, the **lactate** produced during anaerobic muscle metabolism can also be used as a substrate. Lactate is continuously generated during the entire time of muscle activity, even when muscle is maximally perfused and supplied with O_2. The physiological role of lactate is not yet fully understood. A large proportion of lactate enters hepatic gluconeogenesis as part of the glucose-alanine cycle. In addition, lactate has a role as a signalling molecule for the regulation of energy metabolism in muscle.

MORE DETAILS The uptake of substrates through the sarcolemma uses specific transporters. Glucose enters muscle cells by facilitated diffusion via the glucose transporter GLUT1 and the insulin-sensitive GLUT4. Fatty acid uptake from plasma or intramuscular fat is mediated by a fatty acid transport system (FAT/CD 36 and FABP). Lactate release from muscle fibres occurs via the monocarboxylate transporter (MCT) 4, and lactate uptake into muscle fibres is by MCT 1. The different muscle fibre types I, IIA and IIX/B have different functional properties with regard to their contraction speed, force and fatigability. They also have different metabolic properties. Fast fibres (IIX/B, IIA) with high force generation, have a higher rate of ATP consumption for contraction and relaxation than slow fibres (I). Accordingly, fast ATP production relies on anaerobic glycolysis, whereas slow, mitochondria- and myoglobin-rich fibres (p. 619) use oxidative metabolic processes. This is also reflected in their equipment with transporters: fast, glycolytic fibres are richer in MCT-4 transporters, while slow, oxidative fibres have more MCT-1 transporters. Slow fibres also possess fatty acid transporters, whereas the fast fibres have hardly any. GLUT4 expression is higher in fast fibres, which manage to replenish their large glycogen stores during rest because of their high glucose uptake capacity.

Skeletal muscle fatigue, the progressive, but reversible, decrease in muscle strength during physical performance, is a phenomenon that has not yet been fully investigated. Energy production from fat decreases during heavy exertion. The reasons for this phenomenon are not yet fully understood (e.g. lactate is thought to be partly responsible for inhibiting fatty acid oxidation), and the use of glucose comes to the fore again. If the **glycogen reserves** of muscle are exhausted, the intensity of muscular work must be either reduced or muscle activity terminated. Glycogen is thought to provide the pyruvate necessary for fat breakdown to maintain the citric acid cycle. If glycogen is exhausted, no further fatty acids can be used for energy. The **increase in intracellular H⁺ concentration** during **lactate production** (at physiological intracellular pH, 99% of lactate is dissociated) is also involved in muscle fatigue. The associated lowering of intracellular pH prevents the transition of actin-myosin bonds from the weak to the strong binding state. This reduces contraction speed by inhibiting myosin ATPases, inhibition of glycolysis and weakening of the binding of Ca^{2+} to troponin. The relaxation time of the muscle is prolonged because Ca^{2+} can no longer be pumped fast enough back into the sarcoplasmic reticulum. In addition, **depletion of inorganic phosphate** in muscle cells contributes to fatigue because of the decreased ability to regnerate ATP. Physical overexertion also leads to **fatigue** at a **central level** in the brain, i.e. the coordination of movements suffers. The animals become unsteady in walking, and they stumble and show ataxia.

> **IN A NUTSHELL** !
>
> Muscle work is based on a constantly dynamically adapting energy metabolism. This metabolic flexibility is the prerequisite for endurance and strength performance.

Special energetic requirements in striated musculature

Depending on the type of muscle, there are different demands on energy metabolism. Heart muscle (p. 166) and the **diaphragm** have very efficiently adapted metabolism which is necessary for their continuous contractility. The diaphragm with high oxidative capacity has a species-determined mix of slow, intermediate and fast fibres. Small animals with high respiratory rates have more fast fibres, and at the same time a higher oxidative metabolic capacity than large animals with lower respiratory rates. For respiratory work, $4.2 \, kJ \cdot min^{-1}$ energy must be expended at rest, for forced respiration up to $500 \, kJ \cdot min^{-1}$ (human). Unlike the cardiac muscle, however, the diaphragm can become fatigued.

Exogenous factors such as **nutrition, low ambient temperatures** and **training** also have an influence on the energy metabolism of muscles. Following **food intake**, glucose and fatty acids are absorbed by the muscle in an insulin-dependent manner. For this purpose, **insulin** stimulates the incorporation of GLUT4 and FAT/CD-36 transporters into the sarcolemma via a specific insulin receptor and the downstream signalling cascade involved. Glucose

is stored in resting muscle in the form of glycogen. In particularly well endurance-trained red muscle fibres, fatty acids can also be stored in the form of intracellular fat globules. An excess of dietary fat, especially saturated fat, can contribute to the development of insulin resistance in muscle, i.e. the muscle no longer responds to this hormonal signal. Hunger leads, among other things, to the stimulation of mitochondrial activity and fatty acid oxidation in muscle by activation of a central muscular metabolic switch: the AMP-activated kinase. Amino acids in the diet stimulate protein synthesis in muscle and thus ensure the replenishment of proteins that are broken down during periods of hunger or exertion. **Cold causes muscle shivering** in mammals with a regulated body temperature. This serves to generate heat. In shivering humans, intramuscular fat, glycogen (especially in extreme cold) and proteins are burnt in muscle energy metabolism, but in different relative proportions than during physical activity (different regulation of fuel selection). In the piglet, with an absence of brown adipose tissue and low body surface insulation after birth, an adaptation to this type of muscle activity develops via an increase in the number of triads, enhancement of oxidative metabolism, fat burning and mitochondrial activity in muscles. The influence of **training** on muscle energy metabolism is discussed in the chapter on performance physiology (p. 629).

> **IN A NUTSHELL** !
>
> Due to its metabolic flexibility, the musculature is capable of adapting adequately to physical performance. In addition, striated muscle is one of the main contributors to adaptation of energy nutrient homeostasis.

6.2.5   The role of skeletal muscle in health and disease

MORE DETAILS   As a storehouse for amino acids, the musculature plays a central role in overall protein metabolism of an animal. Brain, heart, liver and skin depend on amino acids present in the musculature in the postabsorptive state to maintain their specific functions. The musculature thus has the physiological function of keeping amino acid concentrations in blood plasma constant by undergoing protein degradation. In addition to supplying organs with building blocks for protein synthesis, some of these amino acids are substrates for gluconeogenesis in the liver. This is also a vital process in the postabsorptive phase and is especially essential in ruminants. After a meal, absorbed amino acids are taken up by muscles, thereby stimulating muscle protein synthesis. If the demand for amino acids in the body increases during stress, illness and injury, protein breakdown in muscle is strongly stimulated by increased cortisol secretion from the adrenal gland. For example, acute-phase proteins produced in the liver during inflammation, proteins of the immune system, and structural and functional proteins needed for wound healing, all require an increase in available amino acids. In such conditions, the daily requirement of dietary protein can increase up to 4 times the normal amount (humans). In chronic heart failure and with tumours, there is a massive loss of muscle protein, which can lead to cachexia. In old age, protein degradation often predominates due to insufficient amino acid absorption in the intestine. When feeding sick, injured or old animals, these high de-

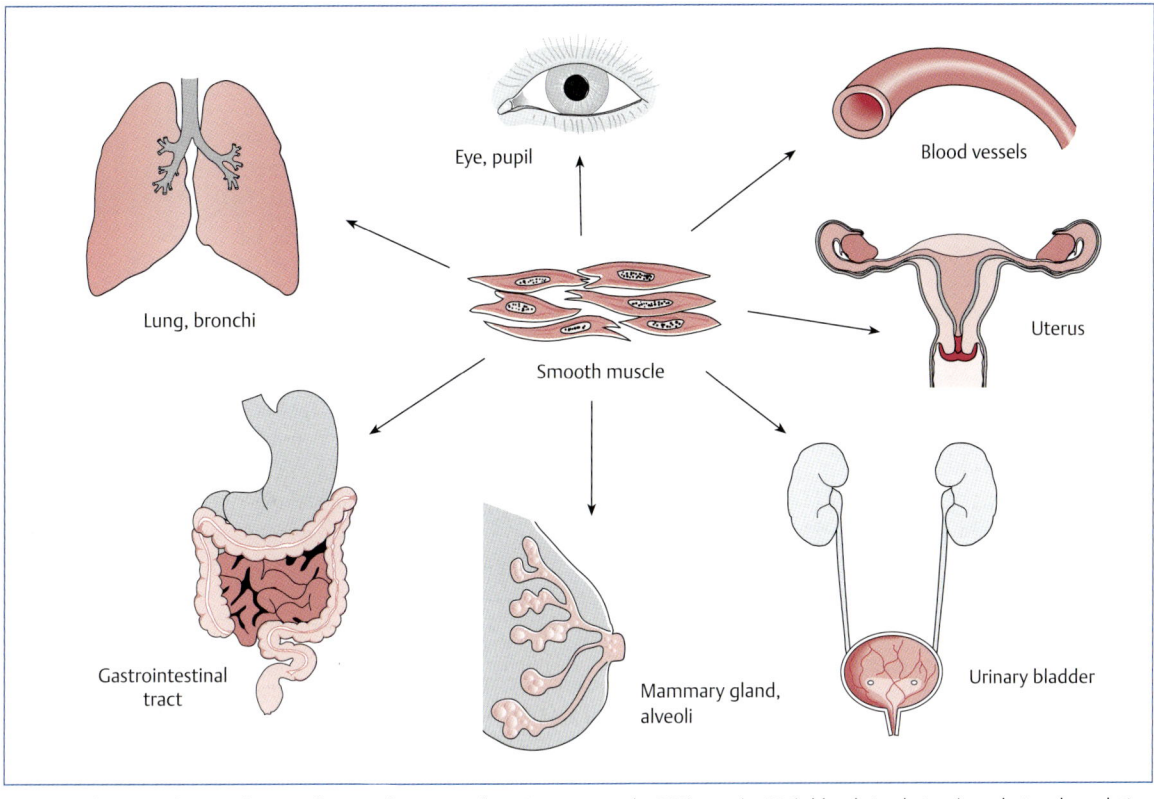

Fig. 6.14 The smooth musculature influences functions of respiratory tract (p. 273), eye (p. 114), blood circulation (see ch. Local regulation of blood flow (p. 208)), urogenital tract (p. 114), gastrointestinal tract (p. 388) and many glands (p. 114) throughout the body.

mands must therefore be met, with particular regard to the quantity and quality of dietary protein. The muscle with its metabolic capacity also seems to be involved in the development or prevention of obesity. With a good dietary protein supply and good muscling of the animal, a lot of energy is consumed in protein synthesis, and is therefore diverted from fat accumulation in adipose tissue. Since insulin-dependent glucose uptake into muscles contributes significantly to glucose clearance in plasma and thus to overall glucose homeostasis, fully functional muscle metabolism is essential for whole-body metabolic and energy homeostasis. Perturbations in muscle glucose metabolism can lead to insulin resistance and type II diabetes.

6.3 Smooth muscles

The functions of smooth muscles are very diverse and complexly regulated by neurons, hormones and paracrine chemical messengers. In contrast to skeletal muscle, activating and inhibiting influences are integrated in the functional response of smooth muscle cells. The resulting electrical responses are not always an action potential, but slow, persistent changes in membrane potential can occur that lead to a change in function. Although the total mass of smooth muscle is less than that of skeletal muscle, smooth muscle contributes significantly to the maintenance of vital bodily functions. Smooth muscle cells are found in blood vessel walls and the upper part of the respiratory tract to regulate the width of vessels and bronchi. In the gastrointestinal tract, all motor activity essential for digestive processes is based on smooth muscle activity. The

urogenital tract, the pupil in the eye and many glands are supported in their function by the work of smooth muscle cells (**Fig. 6.14**)

Influencing the function of these various smooth muscles by pharmaceuticals is of great importance in veterinary medicine. For example, the treatment of gastrointestinal motor disorders, cardiovascular and respiratory diseases and disorders of the birth process is often aimed at improving or inhibiting the contractility of the relevant smooth muscles. As a rule, the receptors for transmitters of the autonomic nervous system or for endocrine and paracrine chemical messengers on smooth muscles can be activated by appropriate drugs.

Despite the great differences in localisation and responsiveness, the main structures and functions in common are found in all smooth muscle cell types, as outlined below.

6.3.1 Smooth muscle cell morphology

Smooth muscle cells are spindle-shaped, 50–500 µm long cells with a central nucleus and irregularly arranged thin **actin** and thick **myosin filaments**. A sarcomere arrangement as in skeletal and cardiac muscle is not present. These filaments also form meshworks with **microtubules** and **intermediate filaments**. This dynamic network supports the mechanical integrity of the cell, increases contractile efficiency and is partly responsible for the increase in tone in the cells after stretching, a property that enables smooth muscles to maintain especially **long-lasting in-**

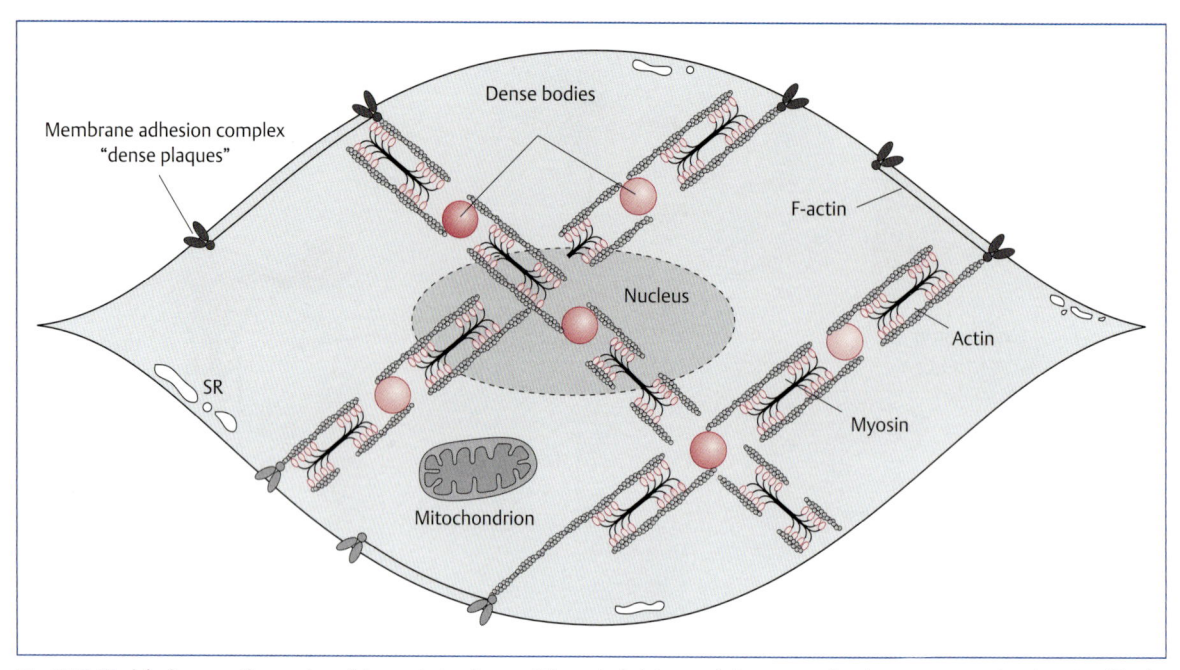

Fig. 6.15 Model of a smooth muscle cell (several structures of the cytoskeleton and the contractile elements are omitted to simplify the illustration). Components of the smooth muscle cell are irregularly arranged actin (F-actin) and myosin filaments, a weakly developed sarcoplasmic reticulum (SR), dense bodies and membrane adhesion complexes (dense plaques) for anchoring the cytoskeleton and the contractile filaments. Contraction of smooth muscle cells enables considerable reduction in volume of hollow organs because of these structural properties.

creased tension (e.g. vascular wall tension against blood pressure). In the smooth muscle cell, **dense bodies** and **membrane adhesion complexes** (dense plaques) serve to anchor this network and the contractile filaments within the cell to the cell membrane. Although much information is now available about the components of smooth muscle cells, the exact structure and arrangement of the network and anchorage points are still unclear. **Fig. 6.15** shows a possible but abstract model of smooth muscle cell morphology. In these cells, as in striated muscle cells, contraction also occurs through the interaction of actin and myosin filaments. However, the smooth muscle cell can transform from a spindle shape to a spherical shape as the contractile filaments are irregularly arranged in all three spatial directions. This leads to a pronounced reduction in volume of hollow organs, which is particularly important e.g. for emptying the uterus or the urinary bladder.

The **myosin** of smooth muscle is structurally and functionally different from the myosin types found in skeletal muscle. Smooth muscles contract much more slowly than skeletal muscles, consume much less energy during this process and can maintain long lasting contractions. Smooth muscle contraction depends on the concentration of Ca^{2+} in the cytosol, as in contraction of skeletal and cardiac muscle. The **Ca^{2+}** for contraction comes mainly from the **extracellular space** and enters the cytosol **via voltage-dependent Ca^{2+} channels** and **stretch-sensitive cation channels**. However, some smooth muscle cells also contain small intracellular Ca^{2+} stores in the form of a weakly developed sarcoplasmic reticulum. The phenotype, responsiveness and performance of smooth muscle cells (**Fig. 6.14**) are often affected by physiological or patho-

physiological status. For example, the contractile capacity of uterine muscles increases to a maximum shortly before birth, partly due to hormonal influences (adrenaline via α1 receptors, oxytocin via oxytocin receptors). The sensitivity of the bronchial musculature to bronchoconstrictors such as histamine is greatly increased in asthma.

According to the time course of the contraction, phasic and tonic contractions can be distinguished in smooth muscle. **Phasic contractions** show a certain rhythm in contraction and relaxation. This type of contraction is particularly pronounced in the smooth muscles of the **gastrointestinal tract**. The enteric nervous system and the parasympathetic nervous system intensify these contraction cycles (p.388), which are important for peristalsis (= movement of the gastrointestinal tract to transport the chyme [= food pulp]). **Tonic contractions** are long-lasting. They create wall tension in the smooth muscles of **arteries** and **arterioles**. Tonic increases in the vessel walls are produced neurogenically by noradrenaline, the transmitter of the sympathetic nervous system. Some smooth muscles also alternate between tonic tension and phasic contraction, such as in the **uterus**. As the foetus grows, the myometrium must adapt to the increasing weight of the foetus and amniotic fluid. At birth, under hormonal stimulation (oxytocin), the uterine musculature begins the process of labour, with phasic contractions to expel the foetus. Often both forms of contraction can be found in parallel in the smooth musculature of an organ, for example, the phasic-rhythmic contraction of the intestine also has a tonic component. If the smooth musculature is excited at a high frequency, the rhythmic contraction process changes into a **tetanic tone**, i.e. the smooth muscle is stimulated at a high frequency and so it contracts with maximum force. Another form of strong tonic contraction, known as a **contracture**, can be produced when the K$^+$ concentration in the extracellular space increases. This shifts the membrane potential towards the threshold potential.

IN A NUTSHELL !

The main function of smooth muscle is to adjust the luminal volume of organs (e.g. vessels, urinary bladder, uterus, bronchi) and to transport contents (e.g. chyme in the gastrointestinal tract, milk from the alveoli of the mammary gland, urine from the urinary bladder).

6.3.2 Mechanisms of smooth muscle excitation

The mechanisms of smooth muscle excitation are as diverse as the locations and functions of this type of muscle. Pacemaker cells similar to those found in the sinus node of the heart (p.172) cause a **myogenic excitation of some types of smooth muscle**. In addition, the autonomic nervous system (**neurogenic excitation**), **endo- and paracrine signalling molecules** and **electrolyte status** are the signals for smooth muscle cell excitation. In principle, smooth muscle is either a **single-unit type** or a **multi-unit type**. Like the heart muscle, smooth muscles of the single-unit type have a high degree of **intercellular coupling through gap junctions**. This type of organisation is found particularly in the gastrointestinal tract and the urogenital tract, but also in some blood vessel walls. In these cells excitation is primarily myogenic and is modulated by the autonomic nervous system (**Fig. 6.16a**). Because of their unstable membrane potential (**slow waves = spontaneous rhythmic membrane potential fluctuations**), the pacemaker cells are able to generate action potentials. These action potentials are then transmitted to associated smooth muscle cells via gap junctions and thus lead to depolarization of large groups of smooth muscle cells (as a single unit). This pacemaker activity is modulated by the autonomic nervous system. In the gastrointestinal tract, such pacemaker cells include the **interstitial cells** according to **Cajal** (**ICC**; after Ramon y Cajal 1911). They are under the modulating influence of the enteric nervous system (p.361) as well as the sympathetic and parasympathetic (p.112) nervous system. Disorders in the expression or function of these ICC can result in severe disruption of gastrointestinal motor function.

Smooth muscle cells of the **multi-unit type** have none or only very few gap junctions. Excitation occurs neurogenically through fibres of the autonomic nervous system (**Fig. 6.16b**). This type of organisation is found in muscles of the respiratory tract, blood vessels, the interior of the eyes and the hair follicles. By controlling individual or a few smooth muscle cells, a very precise fine gradation of muscle strength is possible, just as in the recruitment of activity of groups of cells in skeletal muscle. However, there are also numerous mixed forms between single-unit and multi-unit type. For example in the vascular musculature, where **neurogenic** excitation has an influence on muscle tone, this can override **myogenic** excitation or the action of hormones.

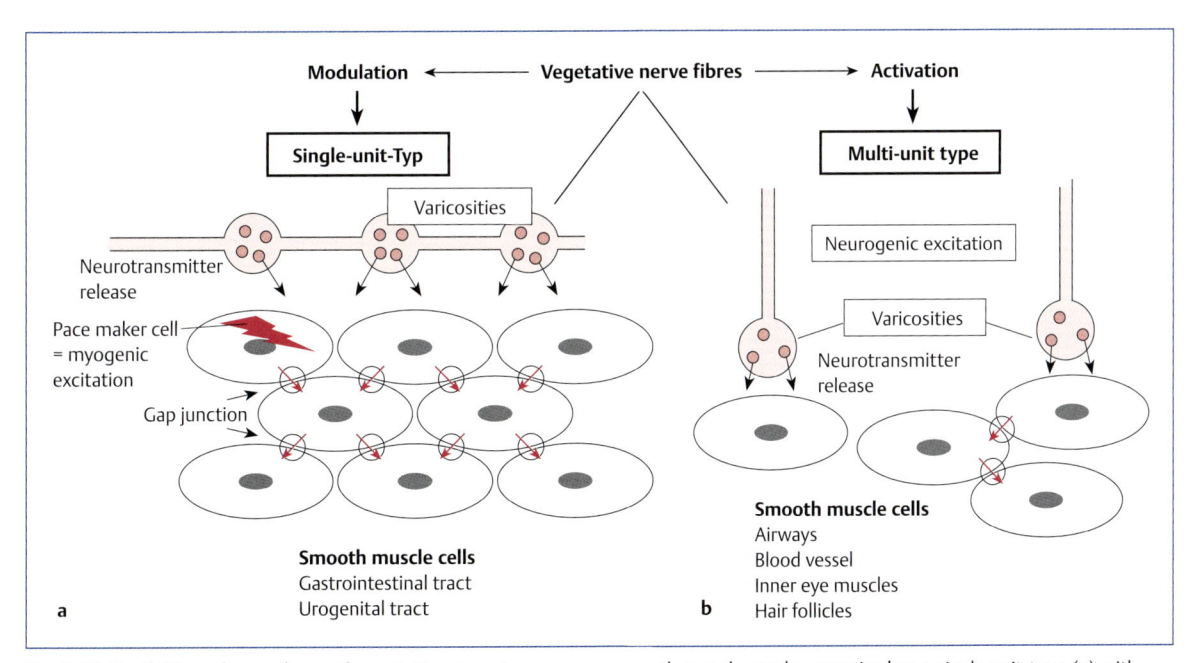

Fig. 6.16 Possibilities of smooth muscle excitation. In extreme cases, smooth muscle can be organised as a single-unit type (**a**) with myogenic excitation or as a multi-unit type (**b**) with neurogenic excitation. However, mixed forms of these types of organisation are often found in an animal.

Cell, tissue

6.3.3 Electromechanical coupling in smooth muscle

■ Electrical processes at smooth muscle cells

A prerequisite of **myogenic excitation** are the **slow waves**, i.e. rhythmic membrane potential fluctuations (from −70 to −10 mV, mouse, intestine), which are generated by the influx of Ca^{2+} ions (via cation channels) and the intracellular inositol-1,4,5-trisphosphate (IP_3)-dependent Ca^{2+} release. They also occur in relaxed musculature (**Fig. 6.17**). The **spontaneous depolarizations** (**AP, spike**) which develop during the plateau phase of slow waves, are caused by Ca^{2+} influx via voltage-dependent Ca^{2+} channels (L-type; $Ca_v1.2$ channels). While the slow waves themselves do not cause the muscle cell to contract, each spike results in a single twitch. As in skeletal muscle, high frequency action potentials can trigger a tetanic contraction. This is not possible in cardiac muscle because of the long refractory period (p. 176).

An important modulating factor of contraction activity, for example in the gastrointestinal tract, is the neurotransmitter **acetylcholine (ACh)**, which opens sarcolemmal cation channels via muscarinic receptors of type M_3 (metabotropic receptor). In contrast, smooth muscle cells of the vascular walls depolarize by the action of **noradrenaline** on α_1 adrenergic receptors, which trigger volleys of action potentials and increases the tone of the vessel wall. These mechanisms are part of **neurogenic excitation**. **Adrenaline**, a hormone from the adrenal medulla, hyperpolarizes vascular and bronchial muscles via its action at β_2 adrenergic receptors, leading to dilation, because Ca^{2+} influx has been inhibited. **Nitric oxide (NO)** is one of the most important relaxing factors on smooth muscle cells (e.g. in blood vessels and in the gastrointestinal tract). It acts by stimulating guanylate cyclase so that cGMP accumulates (as well as other mechanisms). A large number of other cellular, hormonal and neurogenic influences are involved in the electrical processes of various smooth muscle types, in activation or inhibition, by a wide variety of mechanisms.

■ Electromechanical coupling in smooth muscle cells

When smooth muscle cell membranes are depolarized, **voltage-dependent Ca^{2+} channels** open so that Ca^{2+} influx increases. At the same time, a phosphoinositol phospholipase C (PI-PLC) is activated via a G protein, which catalyses the formation of the second messenger IP_3. This signalling molecule acts on IP_3 receptors of the endoplasmic reticulum and induces Ca^{2+} release into the cytosol. Ca^{2+} binds to **calmodulin**, a regulatory protein functionally similar to troponin in skeletal muscle. The activated **Ca^{2+}-calmodulin complex** affects both myosin and actin. At the myosin head, the myosin light chain (MLC) is activated by **myosin light chain kinase by phosphorylation**. This accelerates the reaction speed of myosin ATPase by a factor of 1000. In actin, the binding site for the myosin head is protected by **caldesmon**, a protein similar to tropomyosin in skeletal muscle. Ca^{2+}-calmodulin activates a protein kinase that phosphorylates caldesmon and triggers the binding of caldesmon to the Ca^{2+}-calmodulin complex. Actin-myosin binding can then occur, i.e. the **cross-bridge cycle** and **filament sliding** start, like in these processes in skeletal muscle. At the same time as **electromechanical coupling** and the cross-bridge cycle, polymerisation of G-actin to F-actin is initiated by the increased intracellular Ca^{2+} concentration. The associated reorganisation of the cytoskeleton is an additional mechanism for the increase in strength and the reduction in organ volume observed with many smooth muscle cell types. Smooth muscle cell relaxation is mediated by the removal of Ca^{2+} by Ca^{2+} pumps and Na^+/Ca^{2+} exchangers in the plasma membrane. In addition, phosphorylation of the myosin light chains is reversed by the action of myosin phosphatase, which by itself can also lead to a reduction in muscle strength (**Fig. 6.18**). The activity of myosin phosphatase is thus a Ca^{2+}-independent pathway for regulating strength in smooth muscle.

> **IN A NUTSHELL**   !
>
> Excitation of smooth muscle cells leads to the opening of voltage-dependent Ca^{2+} channels and intracellular Ca^{2+} release into the cytosol. Depending on the type of smooth muscle, this causes phasic-rhythmic contractions and/or a prolonged increase in muscle tone.

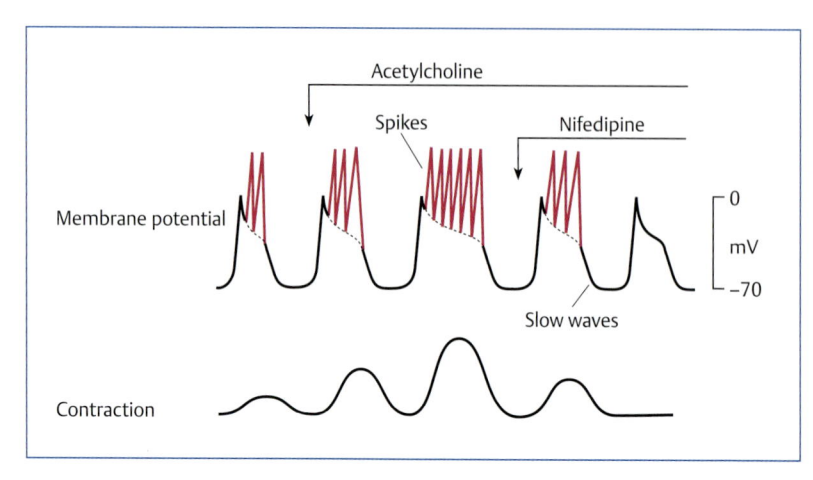

Fig. 6.17 Electrical processes and resulting phasic-rhythmic contractions in the smooth muscles of the gastrointestinal tract. Basal slow waves with spontaneously initiated spikes, lead to single twitches. If the muscles are stimulated by acetylcholine, the frequency of the spikes increases, and the contraction response becomes stronger. If the Ca^{2+} channels are inhibited by the Ca^{2+} channel blocker nifedipine, both acetylcholine-induced and spontaneous spike activity cease and the contraction response is absent.

Cell, tissue

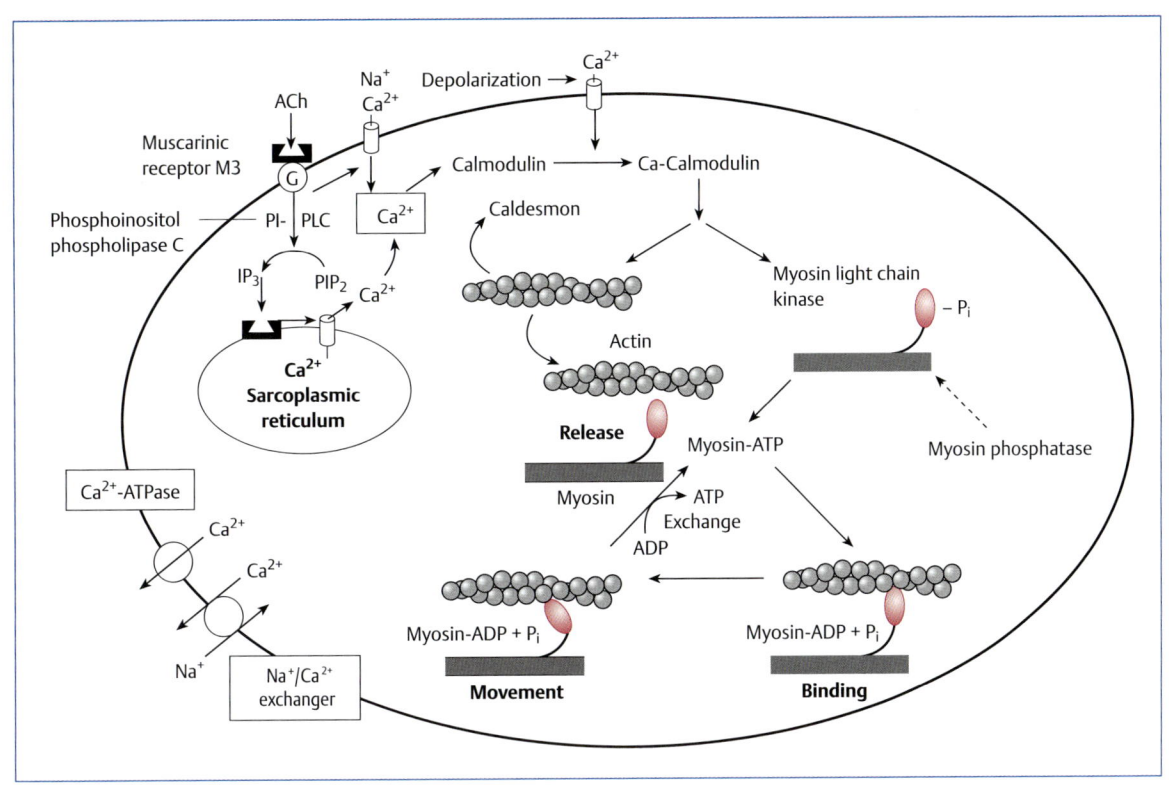

Fig. 6.18 Excitation and electromechanical coupling in a smooth muscle cell after neurogenic excitation. Acetylcholine triggers intracellular signalling cascades by binding to the M_3 receptor. This leads to the opening of non-selective cation channels which are permeable for Ca^{2+} and can also release Ca^{2+} from intracellular stores. Ca^{2+} activates calmodulin and thus initiates the processes of electromechanical coupling in the smooth muscle cell that leads to contraction (details in the text). Muscle strength is regulated by the cytosolic Ca^{2+} concentration and the activity of myosin phosphatase. In the absence of excitation, Ca^{2+} is removed from the cell via a Ca^{2+}-ATPase and a Na^+/Ca^{2+} exchanger. PI-PLC = phosphoinositol phospholipase C; IP_3 = inositol-1,4,5-trisphosphate; PIP_2 = phosphatidylinositol diphosphate.

6.3.4 Energy balance of smooth musculature

The processes of the cross-bridge cycle and filament sliding are significantly slower in smooth muscle than in skeletal or cardiac muscle. Therefore, energy consumption is lower in smooth muscle cells. In addition, stable cross-bridges between actin and myosin (latch bridges) can be formed by dephosphorylation of the myosin light chains. This makes the latch bridge more stable and allows it to hold the force for a long time without energy consumption. This is important, for example, in vascular muscles to maintain blood pressure or in the urinary bladder to hold urine as it accumulates. Both anaerobic and aerobic production of ATP are possible in smooth muscle, the former is accompanied by lactate formation. Glucose, fructose and β-hydroxybutyrate are the energy-providing substrates.

6.4 Cardiac muscle compared with skeletal muscle and smooth muscle

Cardiac muscle is a muscle tuned for endurance performance. Morphologically and functionally, it occupies an intermediate position between skeletal muscle and smooth muscle. The following briefly summarises how these three types of muscle differ (**Table 6.1**).

A detailed description of the function and control of the heart muscle can be found in ch. 7 (p. 166). The main function of the cardiac muscle as a blood pump is rhythmic contraction and relaxation, whereby the frequency and strength of contraction must adapt quickly to the needs of the animal.

Table 6.1 Overview of morphological and functional differences between the muscle types of mammals.

	Skeletal muscles	Cardiac muscle	Smooth muscles
Cell shape	Longitudinal cylindrical	Longitudinal cylindrical	Spindle-shaped
Length (µm)	up to 200 000	100–150	50–500
Number of nuclei/cell	Up to 100	1	1
Nucleus location	Marginal	Central	Central
Cross-striping through sarcomere arrangement	Yes	Yes	No
Mitochondria	Few to many (depending on fibre type)	Many	Few
Sarcoplasmic reticulum	Strongly developed	Moderately developed	Weakly developed
T-tubule system	Yes	Yes	No
Gap junctions	None	Yes	Yes (single unit)
Pacemaker cells	No	Yes (fast)	Yes (slow) (single unit)
Motor endplate	Yes	No	No
Vegetative varicosities	No	Yes	Yes
Action potential			
Duration (ms)	5	200–400	50–100
Course (mV)	-90; 10 20 ms	-85; 100 200 300 ms	-60; 50 100 150 ms
Contractions (N)	N ... ms	N ... ms	N ... ms
Refractory time (ms)	2–4	50–300	50–100
Regulatory proteins	Troponin, tropomyosin	Troponin, tropomyosin	Calmodulin, caldesmon
Tetanic contraction	Possible	Not possible	Possible

6.4.1   Morphology

In contrast to skeletal muscle cells, striated cardiac muscle cells do not have complete electrical insulation from each other. Cardiac muscle cells are conductively connected to each other by **nexus** or **gap junctions**, as is also found in smooth muscle cells of the single-unit type. Thus, the heart muscle also works as a single unit and is called a **functional syncytium**. The ability of all cells of the cardiac muscle to be excited as a unit and thus to contract as a unit is the main prerequisite for the physiological action of the heart. In contrast, the single-unit type in smooth muscle is usually limited to only parts of an organ. The cardiac muscle cell, like the smooth muscle cell, has only one central nucleus, whereas the skeletal muscle cell is a multinucleated syncytium. The high number of mitochondria in cardiac muscle cells reflects the high oxidative metabolism of this type of muscle. The sarcoplasmic reticulum is less developed in cardiac muscle cells than in skeletal muscle, but is more distinct than in smooth muscle. As in the other

muscle types, it serves as a Ca^{2+} store when the cell is excited.

> **IN A NUTSHELL**   !
>
> The cardiac muscle is a functional syncytium and therefore contracts as a unit, which is necessary for coordinated heart action.

6.4.2   Excitation

While the single cells of skeletal muscle and the multi-unit type cells of smooth muscle depend on excitation by a fibre of an α-motoneuron or a vegetative nerve fibre to contract, cardiac muscle has **autonomous** excitation generation (p. 174) similar to that found in single-unit smooth muscle. As in smooth muscle, the heart muscle contains pacemaker cells which are organised in the form of the **sinus node in the right atrium**. In contrast, in smooth muscle the pacemaker cells are diffusely distributed. The sinus node cells continuously generate action potentials that lead to a depolarization of cardiac muscle cells with a long-lasting **plateau phase**, resulting from Ca^{2+} influx from the extracellular space. The resulting action potential of heart muscle, with a duration of 200–400 ms, lasts much longer than that of the skeletal muscle cell with 5 ms or a nerve cell with 1 ms. The smooth muscle cell, on the other hand, can have action potential lengths of 1–100 ms, depending on the type of muscle. As in single-unit-type or multi-unit-type smooth muscle, the autonomic nervous system (p. 114) plays an important role in **regulating** the **contraction processes** of the heart. The Ca^{2+} influx during the plateau phase is not only responsible for the maintenance of the action potential, but also induces a release of Ca^{2+} stored intracellularly in the sarcoplasmic reticulum (**Ca^{2+}-induced Ca^{2+} release**).

> **IN A NUTSHELL !**
>
> The cardiac muscle is autonomously excited by pacemaker cells. The autonomic nervous system regulates the actions of the heart in a superordinate way.

6.4.3 Electromechanical coupling and contraction

While Ca^{2+}-troponin in striated muscle enables the contacts between actin and myosin, in smooth muscle this is controlled by the Ca^{2+}-dependent activation of calmodulin. In cardiac muscle, the contraction lasts 200–400 ms and occurs almost simultaneously with the action potential. In skeletal muscles, the duration of contraction depends on the composition of the fibre types of the muscle. In type IIB fibre-rich muscles, contraction lasts 10–30 ms, in type I fibre-rich muscles 40–70 ms. The contraction duration in smooth muscles can range from 200 ms to 3000 ms depending on the type, but continuous contractions are also possible. However, the contractions in both skeletal and smooth muscles always occur after the action potential has expired. In the case of high-frequency stimulation of skeletal muscles and smooth muscles, a tetanic contraction occurs in both these muscle types, i.e. individual twitches merge into a single, more powerful contraction. This is due to the fact that the contraction starts **after** the action potential and thus during the time of electrical re-excitability of the muscle cells. With the continuous accumulation of free Ca^{2+} in the cell during frequent excitation, relaxation does not occur, and the muscle force rises. This is different in cardiac muscle, where action potential and contraction occur almost simultaneously. The cell can only be excited again when the contraction has also ended. The heart muscle is therefore not tetanisable, which is a prerequisite for the change between diastole and systole.

> **IN A NUTSHELL !**
>
> The cardiac muscle cannot be tetanised by high-frequency stimulation like skeletal muscle and certain smooth muscles.

Suggested reading

Allen DG, Lamb GD, Westerblad H. Skeletal muscle fatigue: cellular mechanisms. Physiol Rev 2008; 88: 287–332

Berchtold MW, Brinkmeier H, Müntener M. Calcium ion in skeletal muscle: its crucial role for muscle function, plasticity, and disease. Physiol Rev 2000; 80: 1215–1265

Gladden LB. Lactate metabolism: a new paradigm for the third millennium. J Physiol 2004; 558: 5–30

Hirsch NP. Neuromuscular junction in health and disease. Br J Anaesth 2007; 99: 132–138

Te Pas MFW, Everts ME, Haagsman HP. Muscle development of lifestock animals – Physiology, genetics and meat quality. UK-Cambridge, USA: CABI Publishing Oxfordshire; 2004

Circulatory and respiratory system

7 Heart

Gerhard Breves

7.1 Functions of the heart

ESSENTIALS ✖

The **heart** is an **autonomous organ**, the function of which is made possible by specialised muscle cells, for generation and conduction of excitation, along with other cells of the myocardium.

– The **cardiac cycle** consists of **systole** (isovolumetric contraction phase and ejection phase) and **diastole** (relaxation and filling phase). At the beginning of systole, the first heart sound is produced, with the second heart sound following at the beginning of diastole.

– The **work of the heart** is adapted to changing loads by the extent of mechanical muscle prestretching (**Frank-Starling mechanism**) and the influence of the autonomic nervous system. The heart works as a **pressure-suction pump** and consists of two atria and two ventricles, each connected in series. The direction of blood flow is controlled by inlet valves (atrioventricular valves) and outlet valves (aortic and pulmonary valves). The right heart drives the pulmonary circulation, the left heart the systemic circulation. Cardiac output is the product of heart rate (HR) and stroke volume (SV).

– The basis for the **contraction of myocardial cells** is the ability to generate action potentials. Muscle contraction is controlled by an influx of Ca^{2+} into the myocardial cell from the extracellular space and an intracellular release of Ca^{2+} from the sarcoplasmic reticulum.

– **The autorhythmia of** the **heart** is initiated when an action potential arises in the primary pacemaker (sinus node, sinoatrial node) through spontaneous depolarization which propagates via the conduction system to the myocardium. The sympathetic nervous system can increase the heart rate (positive chronotropic action), the conduction velocity in the AV node (positive dromotropic action) and the force of contraction (positive inotropic action). The parasympathetic nervous system decreases the heart rate (negative chronotropic action).

– The rhythmically changing **electrical activity of** the **myocardium** generates an electrical field that is conducted via the extracellular fluid to the surface of the body. There, the time-dependent potential differences can be registered as an electrocardiogram (**ECG**) by means of electrocardiography with electrodes. The standard recording points are on the limbs (limb leads according to Einthoven or Goldberger) or on the chest wall (Wilson's leads).

7.2 Heart as a pump

The cardiovascular system forms a self-contained system in which blood is constantly transported through the systemic and pulmonary circulations to all regions of the body. These circulations are vascular transport systems composed of arteries, arterioles, capillaries, venules and veins (**Fig. 8.1**). At the centre of these transport systems is the heart as a combined **pressure-suction pump** which drives the continuous outflow and return of blood to the heart. The heart is surrounded by a connective tissue sac, the **pericardium**. It consists of an outer layer (parietal pericardium) and an inner layer (visceral pericardium, **epicardium**). A thin, liquid-filled space is present between the two sheets. The epicardium is the outer layer of the heart wall with the **cardiac muscle** as the contractile element. The innermost of the three layers of the heart wall is the **endocardium**. It lines the chambers of the heart and the valves. Functionally, the muscular hollow organ heart is divided into two parts, the left and right heart, which are separated by the interatrial and interventricular septum. Both parts of the heart consist of an **atrium** and a **ventricle**. Between them, are the two **atrioventricular valves** (right heart **tricuspid valve**, left heart **bicuspid valve**, Fig. 7.1 a). The cranial and caudal **vena cava** directs blood flow into the right atrium, as does a large cardiac vein, which carries venous blood from the heart muscle into the right atrium (**coronary sinus**). These three veins transport oxygen-poor blood to the heart. Four veins arising from the lungs lead arterial, oxygen-rich blood into the left atrium. The blood supply to the cardiac muscle is provided by the coronary vascular system (right and left **coronary artery**). The coronary arteries originate from the aorta just above the **aortic valve**.

The four heart valves are located in the **atrioventricular valve plane** (Fig. 7.1 b). Their function is to partially separate the cardiac chambers and to serve as inlet and outlet valves. Thus, a directed flow of blood through the heart is achieved. The inlet valve between the right atrium and the right ventricle is the **tricuspid valve**. The **bicuspid valve** (also called the mitral valve from Latin: mitre, bishop's mitre) is the inlet valve between the left atrium and the left ventricle. The **pulmonary artery** arises from the right ventricle, while from the left ventricle the main artery is the **aorta**. The **pulmonary valve** is located between the right ventricle and the pulmonary artery; the **aortic valve** is between the left ventricle and the aorta. Both act as outlet valves. Whereas the aortic and pulmonary valves each consist of three semilunar cusps (**semilunar valves**), the tricuspid and bicuspid valves form the **atrioventricular valves**. The first consists of three leaflets (= tricuspid) and the second has two leaflets (= bicuspid). The leaflets are limited in their range of movement by **chordae tendineae** (tendinous cords, heart strings). The chordae tendineae are connective tissue–like, delicate structures between the leaflets and the protrusions of the ventricular muscles, the **papillary muscles**. The chordae tendineae maintain the position of the atrioventricular valves and their tension; they prevent a reflux of blood into the atria during ventricular systole.

> **IN A NUTSHELL** !
>
> The heart is the pump that generates pressure and thereby provides the energy to move blood. The heart valves act as inlet and outlet valves to ensure that the blood flow is directed.

7.2.1 Heart action in four-quarter-beat

The structure of the heart is that of two functional pumps, running in parallel and simultaneously (right and left heart), each with an atrium and a ventricle. Each ventricular pump works separately in a four-quarter mechanical cycle. The cycle begins with the **isovolumetric contraction phase** (first beat, Fig. 7.2 a), followed by the **ejection phase** (ejection, second beat) and the **isovolumetric relaxation phase** (relaxation, third beat). The cycle concludes with the **filling phase** (fourth beat). During each **cardiac cycle** ("heartbeat"), the isovolumetric contraction phase and the ejection phase constitute the **systole**, while the isovolumetric relaxation phase and the filling phase are called **diastole**. In the **electrocardiogram** (ECG), which will be discussed in detail later, the electrical activity of the heart from the R wave to the end of the T wave corresponds to the mechanical ventricular activity of systole. The interval from the end of the T wave to the R wave corresponds to diastole (Fig. 7.2 b). During the isovolumetric contraction

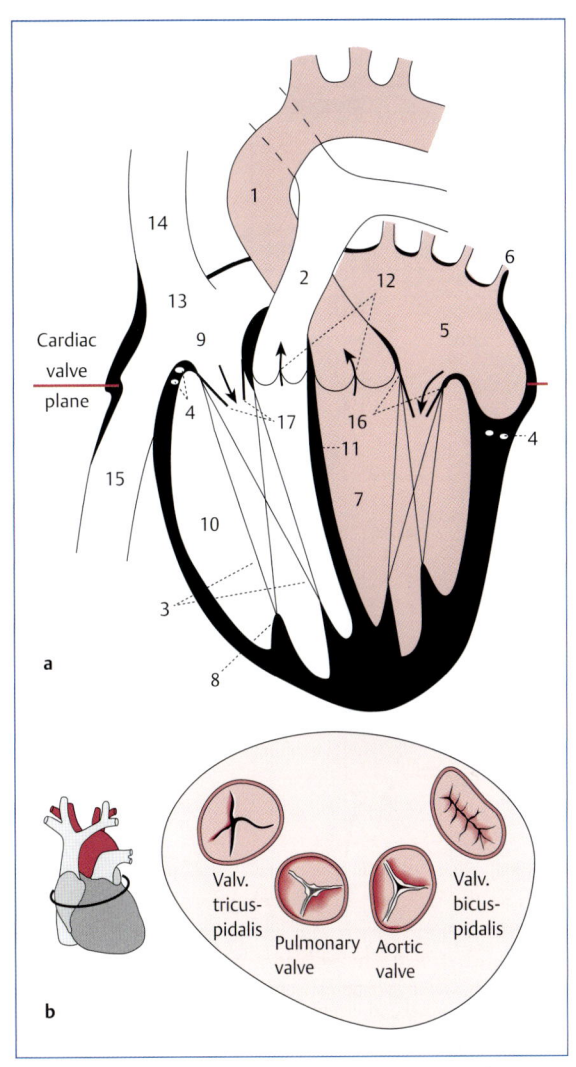

Fig. 7.1 a Schematic of the mammalian heart showing the two atria (9 right atrium, 5 left atrium) and the two ventricles (10 right ventricle, 7 left ventricle). The ventricles are separated by the interventricular septum (11). The interatrial septum is connected to the aorta (1) and the pulmonary artery (2). Between the atrium and the ventricle are the valvula tricuspidalis (17) and valvula bicuspidalis (16). The inlet valves are also commonly called atrioventricular (AV) valves. The leaflets are connected to papillary muscles (8) by chordae tendineae (3). This mechanism prevents the valves from opening during ventricular systole. During diastole blood flows from the cranial (14) and caudal (15) veins through the right atrium into the right ventricle. In the left heart, arterial blood (pink) from the pulmonary veins (6) enters the left atrium. During the following systole, the stroke volume (SV) of the right ventricle is ejected via the pulmonary valve into the pulmonary artery ((2), pulmonary circulation). The SV of the left ventricle is pumped into the aorta via the aortic valve ((1), systemic circulation). The outlet valves are also called semilunar valves (12).
b Cross section through the heart showing the atrioventricular valve plane schematically from above. It is formed by inlet and outlet valves. Note: The ventricular myocardium of the left ventricle is much thicker than that of the right ventricle because a higher systolic ventricular pressure must be generated in the systemic circulation than in the pulmonary circulation. The sinus node (13) in the venous sinus of the right atrium is the primary pacemaker of the heart. The blood supply to the heart is via coronary vessels (4).

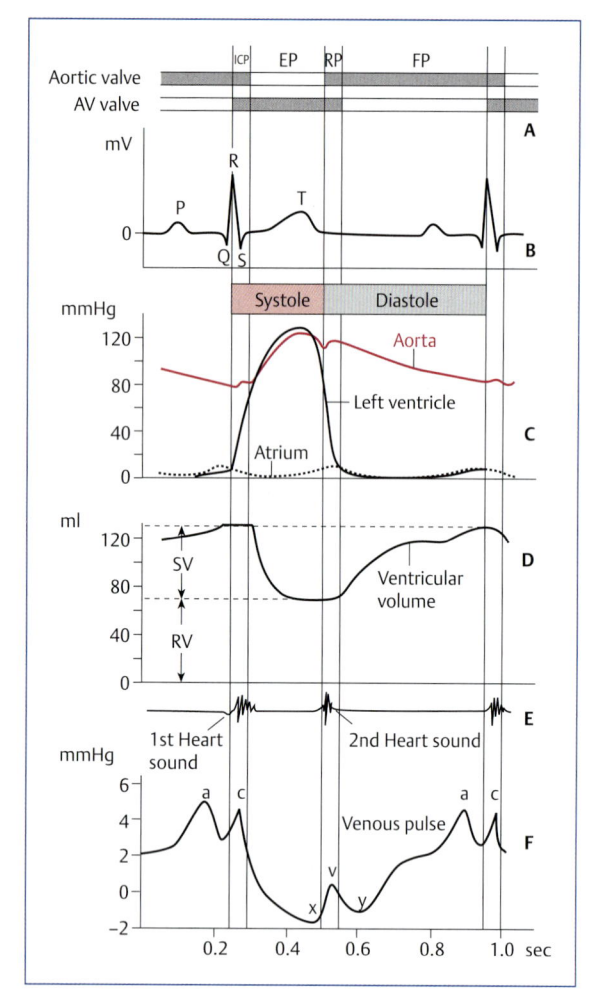

Fig. 7.2 Mechanical and electrical activity of the heart action in individual phases of a pig weighing about 70 kg.
A The four phases of the cardiac cycle: **Systole** (ICP: isovolumetric contraction phase, and EP: ejection phase), **diastole** (RP: isovolumetric relaxation phase, and FP; filling phase). The aortic valve (left heart as an example) is open (white) during EP, otherwise always closed (grey). The atrioventricular valves are open (white) during filling, otherwise always closed (grey).
B Associated **electrocardiogram** (ECG, schematic) showing the propagation of the electrical activity during the cardiac cycle. The meaning of the characteristic waves (P, Q, R, S, T) will be explained later, see ch. ECG analysis (p. 185).
C Pressure curve during systole and diastole in the left atrium and **left ventricle** and in the **aorta**. Note: The pressure amplitude in the aorta is considerably attenuated by distensibility of the vessels ("Windkessel function" (p. 196), Fig. 8.7, Fig. 8.19).
D During systole, the ventricles are never fully emptied. At rest, the **stroke volume** (SV) is even smaller than the remaining **reserve volume** (RV).
E The heart's action in four phases produces two main heart sounds (p. 169), which can be visualised in a phonocardiogram. The first heart sound is associated with the closing of the AV valves. The second heart sound is produced by the vibration of the blood column in the vessels immediately after closure of the semilunar valves. Note the incision (p. 197) (notch in the pressure curve) during the R phase.
F Pressure curve in the cranial vena cava (venous pulse). The deflections are generated by: a = atrial contraction, c = tightening phase of the right ventricle, protrusion of the AV valve, x = lowering of the cardiac valve plane, v = raising of the cardiac valve plane with the AV valve still closed, y = filling of the right ventricle.

and the isovolumetric relaxation phases, when no blood flows in the ventricles, all valves are closed. During **ejection**, the **pulmonary** and **aortic valves** (semilunar valves) are open, while the **atrioventricular valves** (bicuspid and tricuspid valves, AV valves) are closed. During the **filling phase**, the process is reversed, the AV valves are open, and the pulmonary and aortic valves are closed. These **heart valves** regulate blood flow by passive closing and opening, depending on changes in pressure. This process is supported by the anatomical arrangement of the valves in the so-called **atrioventricular valve plane** (Fig. 7.1 a, b). This is a stiffened plate of connective tissue which, due to fixation of the pericardium to the diaphragm at the cardiac apex (apex cordis), shifts depending on the state of contraction. In this way, it has a decisive influence on haemodynamics (**atrioventricular plane displacement**). By the shortening of the ventricular myocardium during systole, the cardiac valve plane moves towards the apex of the heart and causes the relaxed atria to dilate. This results in suction which, at the beginning of diastole, causes the rapid **inflow** of blood from the **atria** into the **ventricles**. During diastole, the increase in length of the ventricular myocardium shifts the cardiac valve plane back towards the base of the heart. The AV valves open and the blood is redistributed from the atria to the ventricles. Together with atrial contractions, the ventricles fill rapidly with blood.

> ### IN A NUTSHELL !
>
> – **Isovolumetric contraction phase**: All valves are closed.
> – **Ejection phase**: The outlet valves are open.
> – **Isovolumetric relaxation phase**: All valves are closed.
> – **Filling phase**: The AV valves are open.
>
> The **atrioventricular plane displacement** is responsible for the rapid **early diastolic filling of the ventricles**.

7.2.2   The ventricles are never completely empty

During a cardiac cycle the ventricles never empty completely. As shown in **Fig. 7.2 d**, each ventricle contains approximately 130 ml of blood at the end of **diastole** (**end-diastolic volume**, EDV; example of a 70 kg pig). During systole, under resting conditions, approximately 60 ml is ejected (**stroke volume**, SV), but 70 ml remains (**end-systolic volume**, ESV). The ratio of stroke volume to end-diastolic volume gives the **ejection fraction**, a measure of cardiac function. As can be seen in **Fig. 7.2 c**, **the left ventricular pressure** is very low at the beginning of systole. It is close to 5 mmHg in this phase. Because of the forceful contraction of the ventricular myocardium, the pressure increases very rapidly until it exceeds the aortic pressure (**isovolumetric contraction phase**). Then the aortic valve opens and the stroke volume leaves the ventricle (**ejection phase**). Because at the beginning of **systole** the ventricular volume initially remains the same (**Fig. 7.2 d**), this phase is called **isovolumetric contraction phase**. The ejection of the stroke volume is initially rapid and then slows down when the **ventricular** and **aortic** pressures fall after reaching their maxima. When the ventricular pressure drops even further, ejection is stopped and there is a brief reflux of blood in the region of the aortic valve. The aortic valve then closes. The transition from systole to diastole produces the so-called **incisura** in the pulse pressure curve in the arteries near the heart, so that the pressure curve appears as a **dicrotic** (two-peaked) **notch** (aorta in **Fig. 7.2 c**, **Fig. 8.7**, **Fig. 8.8 a**). In **diastole**, the ventricular myocardium relaxes and the left ventricular pressure drops back to a value of about 5 mmHg (ventricular **preload**; the preload of the right ventricle is about 3 mmHg). In **Fig. 7.2 c** the pressure amplitude in the left ventricle is about 120 mmHg. The mitral valve remains closed until the ventricular pressure falls below that in the left atrium (relaxation of the myocardium). The first phase of ventricular **diastole** is called the **isovolumetric relaxation phase**. Ventricular filling is initially rapid (atrioventricular plane displacement (p. 167)) and then slows until an action potential is initiated by the pacemaker cells of the sinoatrial node (onset of the P-wave in ECG), triggering **atrial contractions**. As can be seen in **Fig. 7.2 d**, during diastole 80–90 % of **ventricular filling** is completed before atrial contraction begins. The atrial contraction ultimately causes only the final residual filling of the ventricle (end of the **filling phase**). At the onset of ventricular systole, the atrial muscle cells begin to relax again. The processes described here for the left heart also apply to the right heart in terms of timing and blood flow rates, although the pressure conditions there are different. The maximum systolic pressure in the right ventricle is only about 20–30 mmHg.

> **IN A NUTSHELL** !
>
> The maximum pressure in the left ventricle is about 120 mmHg, while that in the right ventricle is only about 20–30 mmHg.

7.2.3 Heart sounds

The physiological heart action causes characteristic sounds (first and second heart sound, **Fig. 7.2 e**). They can easily be recorded and documented phonocardiographically. The **first heart sound** is a low-frequency, muffled sound that occurs during the isovolumetric contraction phase. It is caused by the ventricle rapidly tightening around the non-compressible blood, causing it to vibrate together with the AV valves. The **second heart sound** is produced when the valves of the aorta and the pulmonary artery close. It is a bright, loud, shorter tone. Occasionally, a **third heart sound** can also be detected as a very quiet sound, shortly after the second heart sound. It cannot be heard with a stethoscope in healthy animals. This third heart sound is produced during early ventricular filling by the inflowing blood.

MORE DETAILS If the heart sounds are accompanied by murmurs, these usually indicate pathological changes in the heart valves or stenoses. These are not referred to as heart sounds, but instead are called heart murmurs.

> **IN A NUTSHELL** !
>
> The first heart sound is produced by the isovolumetric contraction of the ventricles, and the second heart sound comes from the closure of the aortic and pulmonary valves.

7.2.4 Pumping capacity at rest

The processes depicted in **Fig. 7.2** repeat with each heartbeat. They pump a new **stroke volume** (SV) into the pulmonary artery and the aorta with each subsequent cycle. The number of heart beats per minute is called the **heart rate** (HR). The **resting heart rate** varies widely in animals, decreasing significantly with increasing body mass (**Fig. 7.3 a**). An elephant with a body mass of about 4000 kg has a resting heart rate of 24 per minute, an Etruscan shrew with a body weight of 2.4 g has a resting heart rate of 800–1200 per minute.

Cardiac output (CO) is the total ejection volume pumped out by each ventricle in one minute. It is the product of SV and HR and correlates positively with body mass (**Fig. 7.3 b**).

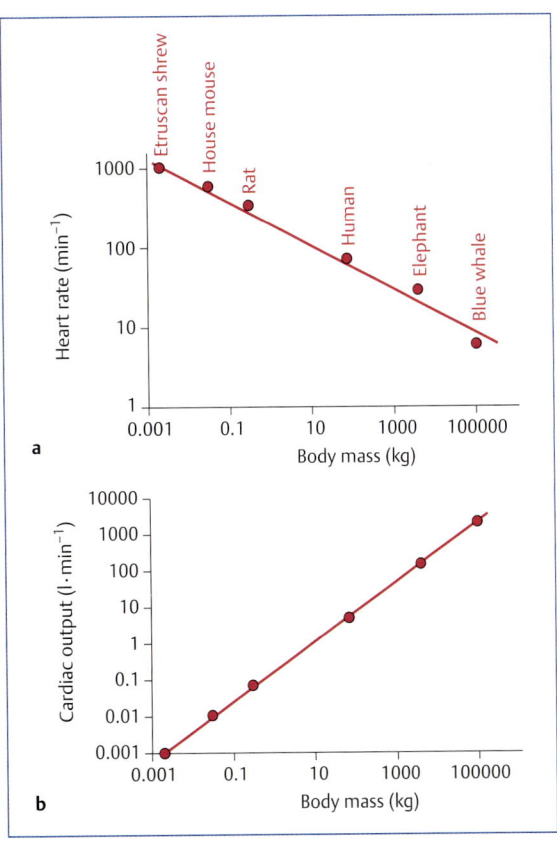

Fig. 7.3 Relationship between resting heart rate (**a**), resting cardiac output (**b**) and body mass in different mammals.

For a pig (70 kg) with a resting HR of 85 beats·min⁻¹ and a SV of approx. 60 ml (**Fig. 7.2 d**), the result is 5.1 l·min⁻¹. A rough estimate of the total blood volume (p. 212) of an adult animal is obtained by multiplying the body weight by a factor of 0.07: e.g. 70 kg·0.07 = 4.9 kg or about 4.9 litres of blood. This means that even under resting conditions the entire blood volume is transported through the lungs or heart once per minute.

IN A NUTSHELL   !

The resting heart rate varies widely in different animal species, and decreases with increasing body mass. At rest, the entire blood volume is transported through the lungs or heart once per minute.

7.2.5   Adjustment of cardiac power during physical work

As already mentioned in ch. 7.2.2, the **stroke volume (SV)** is the **end-diastolic volume (EDV)** minus the **end-systolic volume (ESV)**. The SV can be increased by (1) an increase in end-diastolic volume (e.g. by increased filling during diastole) or by (2) a decrease in end-systolic volume or by both processes simultaneously. The effects of increasing end-diastolic volume on SV are shown in **Fig. 7.4 a**. The physiological mechanisms underlying this relationship are based on the fact that stretching the ventricular musculature (prestretch (p. 152), **Fig. 6.8**) increases the force of the next contraction, and that stretching the muscles during diastole leads to increased release of Ca^{2+} from the sarcoplasmic reticulum in myocardial cells. The latter triggers the beating force, i.e. the **prestretch has a positive inotropic** effect. This effect is comparable to the so-called Bayliss effect on smooth muscle cells (see ch. Autoregulation, myogenic tone (p. 208). **Fig. 7.4 a** shows the interdependence of the end-diastolic ventricular volume and the stroke volume in a large dog. **Resting conditions** are shown approximately in the middle of the curve (dashed lines). It is clear that the SV can be proportionally adjusted upwards or downwards within a certain range of EDV changes. This raises the question of what the end-diastolic volume ultimately depends on.

7.2.6   Frank-Starling mechanism

The **wall tension** caused by the end-diastolic ventricular volume and the resulting end-diastolic **ventricular pressure** is called the **ventricular preload of the heart**). End-diastolic ventricular pressure is identical to atrial pressure because the AV valves are open during diastole. Thus, ultimately ventricular preload is also influenced by processes that act on **atrial pressure** such as the pressure in the pulmonary veins. **Fig. 7.4 b** shows that, for example, an increase in preload to 5 mmHg leads to a proportional increase in EDV. Physiologically, this effect means that preload-induced increases in EDV lead to an increase in stroke volume (**Fig. 7.4 c**). Conversely, a decrease in preload

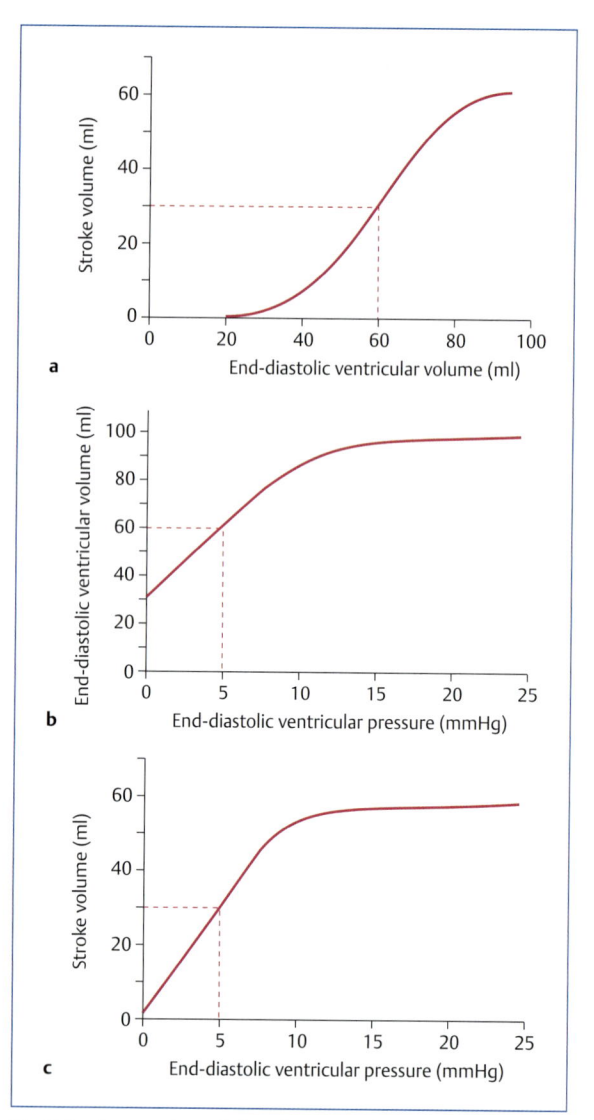

Fig. 7.4 a Increase in end-diastolic ventricular volume (EDV) augments stroke volume; **b** Increase in end-diastolic ventricular pressure (preload) augments EDV; **c** Combination of the functional relationships in a and b: Increase in ventricular preload augments stroke volume. In all functional relationships a maximum is reached (a–c, examples for the left ventricle of a larger dog, dashed lines indicate values at rest). With increasing EDV, the ventricular wall is stretched until it reaches the limit of its elasticity; based on data from Klein BG (ed.). Cunningham's Textbook of Veterinary Physiology Philadelphia: Elsevier; 2013

can decrease stroke volume, for example, in **haemorrhagia** (bleeding).

The **autoregulation of stroke volume** as a function of the end-diastolic volume was first studied by the scientists Otto Frank and Ernest Henry Starling and is known as the **Frank-Starling mechanism**. The Frank-Starling mechanism also achieves, above all, that the **right** and **left heart** adapt to **equal ejection volumes**. If, for example, the right heart were to pump only 1 ml more blood per beat than the left, the difference would already correspond to approx. 60 ml after one minute and would lead to pulmonary oedema within a very short time. These effects of the end-diastolic ventricular volume on the stroke volume of the right and left ventricle ensure an autoregulatory adjustment of the stroke volumes at a constant heart rate. This also allows rapid coordination of the pumping of both ventricles to rapid fluctuations in blood pressure, such as when an animal lies down or stands up.

> **IN A NUTSHELL** !
>
> Frank-Starling mechanism: autoregulation of stroke volume ensures that the stroke volumes of both ventricles remain equal.

In addition to preload, end-diastolic volume is also influenced by ventricular **compliance**. Compliance is a measure of the distensibility of a body structure such as the vessels (p. 196) or the lungs (p. 270). Ventricular compliance describes the increase in volume with increasing filling pressure. **Fig. 7.5** (upper curve) shows that with normal ventricular compliance there is no problem for end-diastolic filling at a preload up to approx. 5 mmHg. At a preload of 10 mmHg, the EDV would be significantly higher. With reduced compliance due to inelastic connective tissue in the ventricular wall, the EDV is significantly lower (**Fig. 7.5** lower curve). The normal EDV is reached under these conditions only with a preload of 10 mmHg (dashed line).

> **IN A NUTSHELL** !
>
> Compliance is a measure of the distensibility of a body structure, such as the vessels or lungs. The compliance of the ventricles describes the ventricular volume increase with increasing filling pressure.

In addition to preload and compliance, **filling time plays a role as a third factor in controlling end-diastolic volume**. The filling time is determined by the heart rate. An in-

crease in heart rate is usually accompanied by an increase in contractility (p. 170). Under resting conditions there is sufficient time for filling. Ventricular filling is virtually complete when atrial systole begins (**Fig. 7.2d**). However, if the heart rate rises sharply during heavy physical work, the duration of the diastole and thus the filling time decrease significantly (**Fig. 26.14**). Ch. 7.2.8 discusses why cardiac output does not decrease significantly with heavy work and thus with increasing heart rates.

> **IN A NUTSHELL** !
>
> An increase in heart rate is at the expense of diastolic filling time.

7.2.7 Ventricular contractility

Contractility is the force and velocity of myocardial contraction exerted by the cardiac muscle itself without the influence of preload or afterload. With increasing contractility, the stroke volume increases, and with decreasing contractility it decreases (**Fig. 7.6**). The contractility of the myocardium is fully influenced by the hormonal action of noradrenaline (p. 116) in control by the sympathetic nervous system (p. 178). The effect of **adrenaline**, released from the **adrenal medulla**, is comparable (**Fig. 7.13**). The ventricular wall then contracts more forcefully, faster and in a shorter time. Stroke volume (**Fig. 7.6**) and thus also cardiac output increase accordingly, which can lead to a rise in blood pressure (**Fig. 8.23**, **Fig. 8.24**).

MORE DETAILS The stimulating effect of noradrenaline and adrenaline on contractility occurs via the excitation of adrenergic $\beta 1$ receptors (p. 117) in the heart (**Table 4.1**; **Fig. 4.3**). Hypertension can be treated by inhibiting the adrenergic signalling pathway with β_1 receptor blockers such as propranolol.

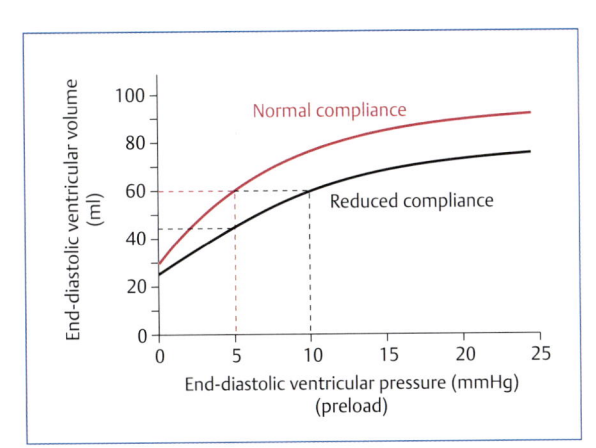

Fig. 7.5 End-diastolic ventricular volume and end-diastolic ventricular pressure. Ventricles with reduced distensibility (compliance) require a greater filling pressure (preload, e.g. 10 mmHg versus 5 mmHg) to achieve a normal end-diastolic volume (e.g. 60 ml for a dog, 30 kg); based on data from Klein BG (ed.). Cunningham's Textbook of Veterinary Physiology Philadelphia: Elsevier; 2013

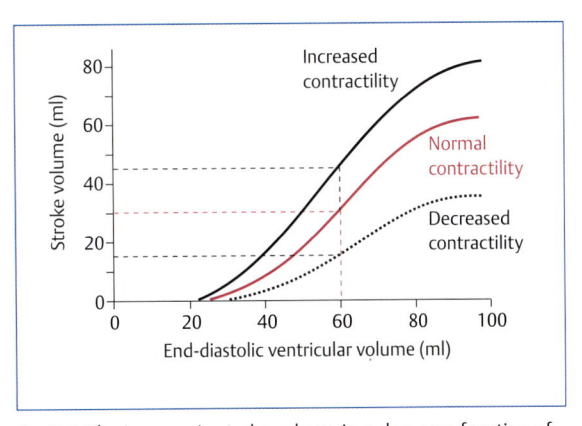

Fig. 7.6 The increase in stroke volume in a dog, as a function of end-diastolic ventricular volume (EDV) at normal (**Fig. 7.4a**), decreased, and increased contractility. Increased ventricular contractility is shown graphically as an upward shift, decreased contractility as a downward shift of the functional curve. With normal contractility and normal EDV of 60 ml, in this example of a dog (30 kg), the stroke volume is about 30 ml. If the contractility increases with unchanged EDV, the stroke volume is increased to 45 ml. If the contractility decreases, the stroke volume is only 18 ml; based on data from Klein BG (ed.). Cunningham's Textbook of Veterinary Physiology Philadelphia: Elsevier; 2013

Ventricular contractility is the main factor in regulating end-systolic ventricular volume. In addition, arterial blood pressure influences the pumping capacity of the heart. A significant elevation of arterial blood pressure makes it difficult to eject stroke volume because left ventricular pressure must exceed aortic pressure during systole for blood to be pumped out. This aortic pressure determines the **afterload**, i.e. the wall tension that the myocardium must exert to open the aortic valve. It is mainly determined by two factors – the pressure in the aorta, which must be overcome with every systole, and the compliance of the arteries, see ch. 8.3.4 (p. 196).

7.2.8 Adjustment of cardiac output at work

Since cardiac output is the product of stroke volume and heart rate, it is to be expected that cardiac output doubles with a doubling of heart rate (**Fig. 7.7** black line; **Table 7.1**). With increasing physical exercise and the associated increase in heart rate, the ejection rate increases beyond even the expected values (**Fig. 7.7** red line). This increase occurs through a combination of increased preload (increased stroke volume) and an increase in heart rate. Crucial to these changes is the activation of the sympathetic nervous system, which increases heart rate, augments the force of contraction and causes contraction and relaxation to occur more rapidly (**Fig. 7.13**). At very high heart rates, the stroke volume decreases due to the then very short filling phase, the increase in cardiac output thus becomes smaller as the heart rate (p. 624) continues to rise, see ch. Frank-Starling mechanism (p. 170).

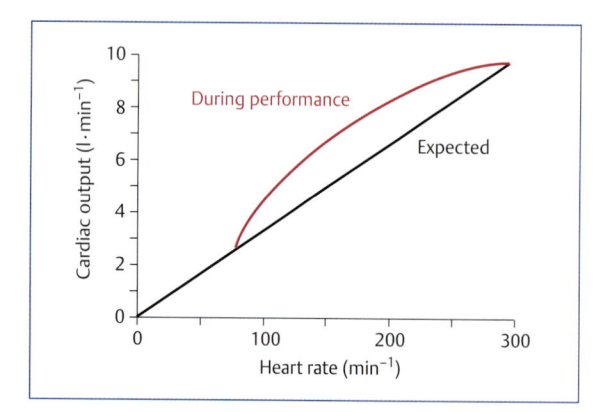

Fig. 7.7 Assuming that stroke volume remains constant, then cardiac output (CO) increases linearly with increasing heart rate (expected dependency as black line). The red line shows the increase in CO for a dog running alongside a bicycle. This increase in CO with increasing heart rate is greater than the expected linear relationship due to sympathetic influence; based on data from Klein BG (ed.). Cunningham's Textbook of Veterinary Physiology Philadelphia: Elsevier; 2013

Table 7.1 Typical adjustments of cardiac parameters in a large dog (30 kg) during physical exercise.

Parameter	Resting state	Physical exercise
Ventricular end-diastolic volume (ml)	60	55
Ventricular end-systolic volume (ml)	30	15
Stroke volume (ml)	30	40
Ejection fraction (%)	50	73
Heart rate (beats · min^{-1})	80	240
Cardiac output (l · min^{-1})	2.4	9.6

Based on data from Klein BG (ed.). Cunningham's Textbook of Veterinary Physiology. Philadelphia: Elsevier; 2013

7.3 Electrical activity of the heart

The heart muscle, like skeletal muscle, is a striated muscle, but as well as this similarity there are also important differences (**Table 6.1**). The electrical processes in the heart are mediated by cells of the **cardiac conduction system** (**Fig. 7.9a**). The contraction of the myocardium is triggered by action potentials initiated by spontaneous depolarizations in specialised cardiac muscle cells. The **primary pacemaker** is the sinoatrial node. If the sinus node fails, then the **atrioventricular node** (**AV node**) can take over this function, but at a much lower frequency (**secondary pacemaker**). The AV node has the capacity for spontaneous electrical depolarization. This does, however, not normally come into play because the sinus node "imposes" its higher frequency on the AV node. The cardiac muscle forms a functional **syncytium** via **gap junctions** (**Fig. 7.8**), through which the pacemaker potential quickly spreads to every muscle cell. The cardiac action potential is very long, thus guaranteeing relaxation and refilling between heartbeats. **Noradrenaline**, released from sympathetic nerve endings at the sinus node, stimulates heart rate (positive **chronotropic effect**). Parasympathetic nerve endings reduce heart rate by the action of **acetylcholine** (negative chronotropic effect). Noradrenaline causes faster and more powerful contractions in all heart muscle cells (positive **dromotropic, inotropic** and **lusitropic**). The effect of the parasympathetic nervous system is limited to the sinoatrial node, the atria (negative inotropic) and the AV node (negative dromotropic).

> **IN A NUTSHELL** !
>
> The electrical activity of the heart is controlled by the cardiac conduction system. Dominant pacemakers are the cells with the fastest depolarization, usually the sinoatrial node cells. In principle, however, every cell of the cardiac musculature can trigger an action potential.

7.3.1 Comparison of contractile elements in cardiac muscle and skeletal muscle

The structural units of the heart are the cardiac muscle fibres (**cardiac muscle cells – cardiomyocytes**). Each cardiomyocyte contains a few hundred **myofibrils** similar to those of skeletal muscles (p.145). In cardiac and **skeletal muscles**, each myofibril consists of many **sarcomeres** arranged in series. They form the smallest functional unit of muscle. The contractile elements of the sarcomere are **actin** and **myosin**. They are responsible for contraction and also relaxation through their interaction with ATP (**cross-bridge cycle**, **sliding filament theory**). This leads to shortening and force generation of the skeletal and cardiac muscle (p.150) (**Fig. 6.6**; **Fig. 6.7**). Cardiomyocytes have a central nucleus and are much shorter than skeletal muscle fibres. Desmosomal end-to-end linkages (**intercalated discs**) give rise to long cell chains that function like a long muscle fibre (**Fig. 7.8 a**). The cardiomyocytes branch and connect to other parallel cell strands through these branches, forming an interconnected plexus. Between the cell strands run collagen fibrous septa with small blood vessels and capillaries. Capillary density in cardiac muscle is very high (pig: 1000–1500 capillaries per mm^2, skeletal muscle 100–300 capillaries per mm^2). The end-to-end connections appear as bright lines under the light microscope and are called **disci intercalares**. They contain three types of cell junctions: 1. **desmosomes**, which closely anchor neighbouring cells to each other by means of the intermediate filaments; 2. **zonulae adhaerentes**, which fix the actin filaments of the sarcomeres to the two ends of the cells (equivalent to the Z-lines of skeletal muscles); 3. **gap junctions**, which allow the passage of excitatory electrical currents (**Fig. 7.8 b**). A **stem cell population** analogous to the **satellite cells** of the skeletal muscle is only weakly developed in the cardiac muscles of mammals, so that the capacity of heart muscle to be able to regenerate is not strong.

7.3.2 Two types of cardiac muscle cells

Most **cardiomyocytes** do not generate their own, spontaneous action potential. Some cardiomyocytes, however, are specialised and can spontaneously depolarize to threshold. Thus, they initiate action potentials that can then trigger a heartbeat. Such myocytes are called **pacemaker cells**. A population of such cells is localised in the **sinus node** of the right atrial wall. Under physiological conditions, these cells depolarize in a regular rhythm. Their action potentials reach the ventricular myocardium via the electrical conduction system. The sinus node thus functions as the primary pacemaker. Consequently, the heart is able to generate through these pacemaker cells, its own muscle action potentials followed by contractions (**autorhythmia of the heart**). The heart's pumping capacity is adjusted mainly by changes in heart rate, by sympathetic and parasympathetic innervation of the sinoatrial node.

7.3.3 Cardiac muscles as a functional syncytium

An important difference between cardiac and skeletal muscles are the electrical **gap junctions** (**Fig. 7.8 b**; **Fig. 6.16**, smooth muscle cell; **Fig. 1.5a**, cell-cell contacts) between cardiac muscle cells. Action potentials propagate in the longitudinal direction of a cell, through gap junctions at the end of the cell to a neighbouring cell, or through cell branches to a neighbouring cell strand. As the action potentials propagate from cell to cell through the cardiac tissue, neighbouring cells contract synchronously, quasi as one unit. They also relax simultaneously. As a result, the heart muscle behaves largely like a single cell and is referred to as a **functional syncytium**. The gap junctions are formed by special channel proteins called connexons (**Fig. 1.5a**); see ch. on cell-cell connections (p.29)). Like cardiac muscle cells, smooth muscle cells (p.161) also form gap junctions, but skeletal muscle does not. The T-tubules of cardiac muscle cells are larger than those of skeletal muscles, and they are often branched. The Ca^{2+}-storing **sarcoplasmic reticulum** is moderately developed in heart muscle (**Table 6.1**). Heart muscle cells also require extracellular Ca^{2+} for contraction. One third of a cardiomyocyte is composed of mitochondria. This indicates the high metabolic activity of cardiac muscle, see ch. Energetics of the Heart (p.180).

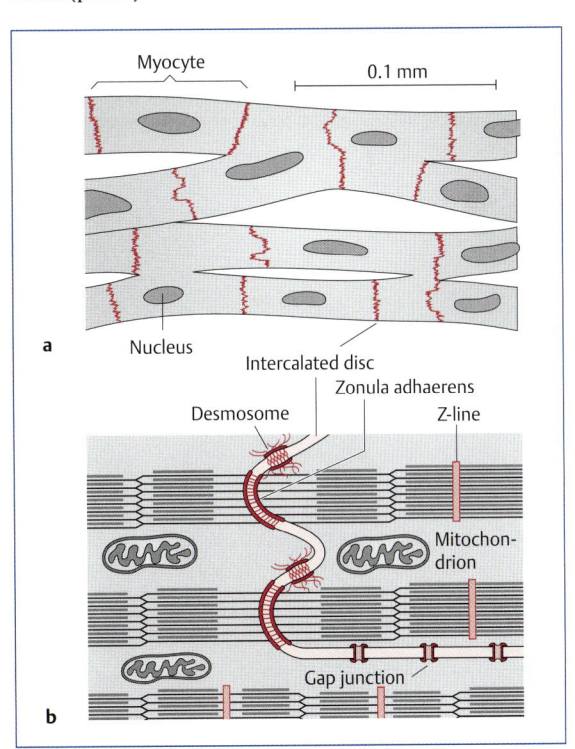

Fig. 7.8 **a** Basic structure of the myocardium with the branched transverse connections, central nucleus and striation (schematic). The muscle cells adhere to each other at the intercalated discs (disci intercalares).
b Enlarged area of an intercalated disc. There are three types of cell contacts: (1) **desmosomes**, which attach the cell membrane of adjacent fibres to each other, (2) **zonulae adhaerentes**, which are not only cell-cell connections but also bind to the actin filaments, and (3) the electrically conducting **gap junctions**. The cardiomyocyte contains numerous mitochondria.

7.3.4 Generation and conduction of electrical impulses

The **cardiac conduction system** is formed by the **sinus node**, the **atrioventricular node** (AV node, Aschoff-Tawara node), the **His bundle** (AV bundle), the **Tawara branches** (bundle branches) and the **Purkinje fibres** (Fig. 7.9 a). Each heartbeat begins with a spontaneous action potential from one of the pacemaker cells in the sinoatrial node (Fig. 7.9 a). It then propagates from cell to cell in the atrial muscles of the right and left atrium (**internodal pathways**). This is followed by contraction of the atria. The **action potential** then travels to the atrioventricular node and then to the start of the His bundle at the septum. The AV node is the only way for the action potential to propagate from the atria to the ventricles because without this connection the atria are separated from the ventricles by a non-excitable layer of connective tissue within the **atrioventricular plane**. The conduction of excitation from the beginning of the AV node to the beginning of the His bundle is slow in comparison with the ventricular conduction of excitation ("**snail path**"). This slow conduction creates the necessary delay between atrial and ventricular contractions (**Fig. 7.9 b**). After the slow conduction from the AV node and the subsequent first part of the His bundle, the action potential then continues rapidly towards the cardiac apex ("**racetrack**"). The second part of the His bundle consists of specialised muscle cells that can conduct excitation very quickly. The action potential is distributed to the two Tawara bundles, which run in the septum, up to the apex of the heart. There, the bundles branch into a network of **Purkinje fibres** that conduct the action potentials to the inner sides of both ventricles. Thus, the action potentials are first distributed to the subendocardial muscle cells. From there, they propagate very rapidly from cell to cell through the cardiac wall towards the pericardium. Since the action potential spreads extremely quickly in the millisecond range from the distal part of the His bundle to the outer part of the ventricular myocardium, there is an almost synchronous **contraction of cardiac muscle cells in both ventricles**. With the subsequent atrial and ventricular relaxation and the filling phase, the cardiac cycle is completed.

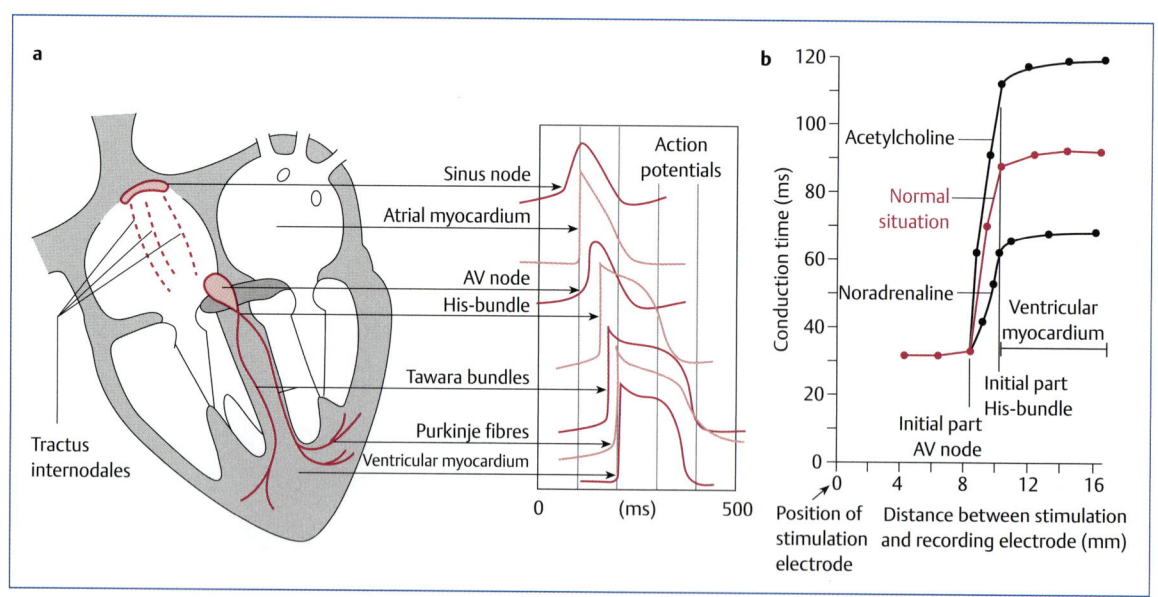

Fig. 7.9 a Shape of a characteristic action potential in different regions of the heart. Action potentials of the **pacemakers** (primary pacemaker (sinus node), secondary pacemaker (AV node)) as well as the other parts of the **cardiac conduction system** (His bundle, Tawara bundle, Purkinje fibres) appear as solid red lines. The action potentials of the atrial myocardium and the ventricular myocardium are dashed in red. The temporal shift corresponds to the sequence of excitation during cardiac action.
b Dependence of conduction time on the distance between the stimulus site and the recording electrode under control conditions and under the influence of acetylcholine and noradrenaline. The neurotransmitters only influence the conduction time in the region of the AV node. An increase in conduction time means a decrease in conduction velocity.

7.3.5 Long-lasting cardiac action potentials

Depolarization of the membrane of cardiomyocytes leads to mechanical **contraction of heart muscle**. This process of **electromechanical coupling** is analogous to the corresponding process in skeletal (p. 149) muscle and smooth muscle cells (p. 162). However, the **action potential** (AP) of skeletal muscles is short and lasts only up to 5 ms (**Table 6.1**). In contrast, the APs of heart muscle last considerably longer (200–400 ms; **Fig. 7.9 a; Table 6.1**). This is the result of coordinated **changes in ionic conductances** of the cardiomyocyte membrane for Na^+, K^+ and Ca^{2+} ions. The **Ca^{2+} channel type** of the **sarcolemma** (voltage-dependent Ca^{2+} channel of the type Ca_v 1.2) of cardiac muscle cells, is also known as the **dihydropyridine receptor** (**Fig. 6.5**). It corresponds functionally to the **L-type Ca^{2+} channel** of a **pacemaker cell** (L = long lasting, long-lasting current or slowly inactivating). Its **threshold potential** is –40 mV. Different types of K^+ channels, such as voltage-dependent K^+ channels (K_v) and "inward rectifying" K^+ channels (K_{ir}), which have a high conductance only at negative membrane potential (close to the resting membrane potential), also contribute significantly to the cardiac action potential.

Fig. 7.10 shows the action potential of a cardiomyocyte and the sequence of conductivity changes of the cell membrane for the **ions** mentioned. The action potential starts from a **resting membrane potential** of about –90 mV. In this phase, many **K^+ channels** are open and most **Na^+ and Ca^{2+} channels** are closed. When the myocardial cell is depolarized to the **threshold potential**, the closed activatable **voltage-dependent Na^+ channels** open abruptly. This al-

lows a rapid influx of extracellular Na^+ causing a charge reversal at the membrane (**phase 0**). The Na^+ channels inactivate very quickly and the membrane begins to repolarize. K^+ channels are activated by depolarization. They open for a short time, allowing a K^+ outward current (rapidly activatable voltage-dependent K^+ channels, e.g. of the type K_v 12.2 . This generates a "transient outward" current) (**phase 1, initial peak**). It is a peculiarity of cardiac muscle cells that repolarization is interrupted after a short time, resulting in a slightly descending **plateau** of long duration (approx. 200 ms, **phase 2**). The plateau is the result of many K^+ channels being closed and thus K^+ conductivity of the membrane decreases (by reducing the current through inwardly rectifying K^+ channels of the type K_{ir} 2.1). In addition, many of the **Ca^{2+} channels** are open, so that Ca^{2+} conductivity is high. The Ca^{2+} channels are voltage-dependent and are located in the **sarcolemma** and in the **T-tubules**. These T-tubules are located on one side along segments of the **sarcoplasmic reticulum** (**Fig. 6.5**) and thus form **diad structures** in the myocardium. In contrast, in skeletal muscle (p. 148), the T-tubules face the sarcoplasmic reticulum on two sides (triads (p. 150), **Fig. 6.5**). Since Ca^{2+} concentration in extracellular fluid is higher than in the cytosol, rapid Ca^{2+} influx occurs. The combination of a reduced K^+ outflow and a Ca^{2+} influx causes the long depolarization of the membrane. After about 200 ms, a population of K^+ channels (slowly activatable voltage-dependent K^+ channels, e.g. of the type K_v7.1) opens again (**reopening**) and the Ca^{2+} channels then become inactivated. This combination eventually leads to repolarization (**phase 3**) and allows the resting membrane potential to be reached again (**phase 4**). Ca^{2+}, which flows into the cardiomyocyte during

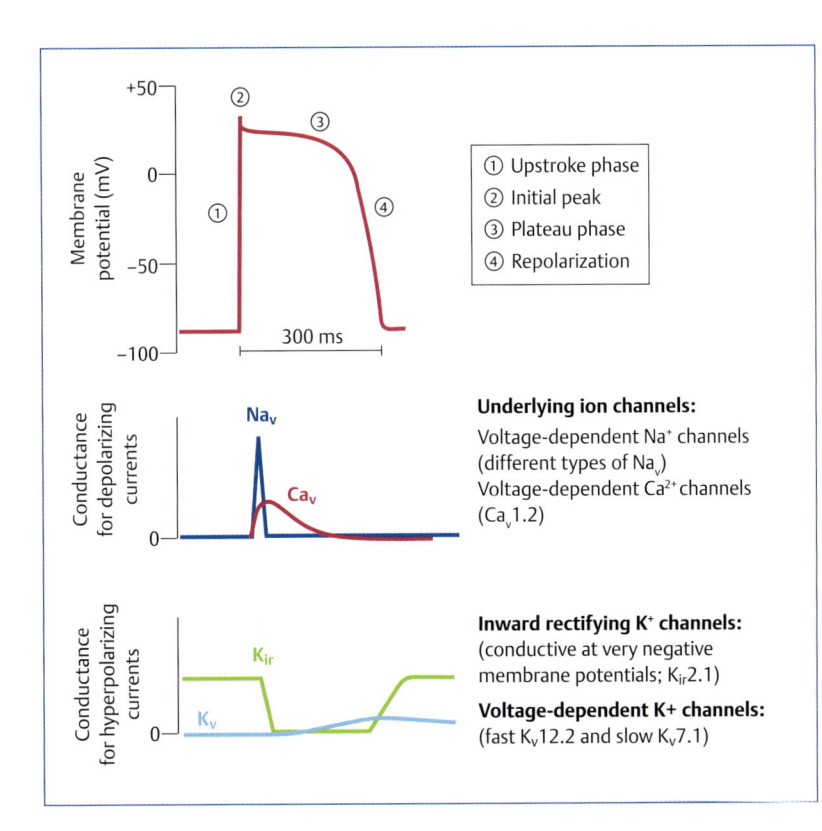

Fig. 7.10 ① Upstroke phase ② Initial peak ③ Plateau phase ④ Repolarization

Underlying ion channels:
Voltage-dependent Na^+ channels (different types of Na_v)
Voltage-dependent Ca^{2+} channels (Ca_v1.2)

Inward rectifying K^+ channels: (conductive at very negative membrane potentials; K_{ir}2.1)

Voltage-dependent K+ channels: (fast K_v12.2 and slow K_v7.1)

Fig. 7.10 The action potential of myocardial cells arises from changes in conductivities of the cell membrane for K^+, Na^+ and Ca^{2+}. In the resting state (resting membrane potential), the cell membrane is most permeable to K^+ due to a high conductance of inwardly rectifying K^+ channels (K_{ir}). The action potential is generated by the characteristic sequence of transient conductance changes for Na^+ (Na_v), K^+ (K_{ir}, K_v) and Ca^{2+} (Ca_v) (phase 1, upstroke; phase 2, initial peak; phase 3, plateau; phase 4, repolarization); the numbers 1–4 mark the different phases.

the plateau phase (replenishing effect of Ca^{2+}), initiates a massive **release of Ca^{2+}** from sarcoplasmic reticulum through ryanodine receptors (p.150), which act as intracellular Ca^{2+} channels, (**trigger effect** of Ca^{2+}). It is estimated that 90% of the Ca^{2+} required for contraction originates from the sarcoplasmic reticulum. In less than 100 ms, the concentration of Ca^{2+} increases 100-fold from about 10^{-7} $mol \cdot l^{-1}$ to 10^{-5} $mol \cdot l^{-1}$, initiating a contraction, as in skeletal muscle, by binding to **troponin C** (Fig. 6.5). The contraction is actively terminated by pumping Ca^{2+} out of the cytosol, either across the cell membrane into the extracellular fluid, or back into the sarcoplasmic reticulum. Another way for the muscle cell to export Ca^{2+} from the cytosol is through the **Na^+/Ca^{2+} antiport system** (**NCX**, **Na^+/Ca^{2+} exchanger**).

> **IN A NUTSHELL** !
>
> The action potential of cardiomyocytes begins with depolarization from −90 mV to approx. + 30 mV (initial peak), followed by a plateau and subsequent repolarization to the resting membrane potential. Depending on the heart rate, the total duration of the action potential is 200–400 ms.
> The rapid release of Ca^{2+} ions causes contraction of the myocardial cells (electromechanical coupling).

7.3.6   Heart is not tetanisable

The fast Na^+ channels are inactivated at the peak of the myocardial action potential (initial peak). As long as the **Na^+ channels** are not **reactivated**, no new action potential can be initiated. Only when the resting membrane potential is almost reached again, the inactivated closed state of this type of channel can change to the **closed activatable state**. Until then, the **cardiac muscle cell is refractory**. The closed non-activatable Na^+ channel configuration guarantees that no second action potential can occur before the previous one is completed. This in turn allows relaxation and filling between contractions. The contraction of the ventricular muscle cells is almost complete when the Na^+ system can be reactivated after the **relative refractory period** (see ch. Ionic basis of the action potential (p.49)). The cytosolic Ca^{2+} concentration has already returned to the resting level at this time point. The long action potential and the resulting long refractory period ensure that the heart only performs single contractions. **Superposition** or **tetanus**, as in skeletal muscle, cannot take place (see ch. Force generation and excitation frequency (p.155) and cardiac arrhythmias (p.188). During most of the time of an action potential, cardiomyocytes cannot be excited by a second stimulus (**absolute refractory period**; Fig. 7.19c). The Na^+ channels are closed and inactivated until the membrane potential falls below −40 mV. Then the **relative refractory period** (Fig. 7.19c) begins, during which some of the Na^+ channels of cardiomyocytes are still inactivated. Therefore, greater than normal stimulus strengths are required to initiate action potentials during this relative re-

fractory period. The resulting action potential has a smaller amplitude and duration than a normal response. After this abnormal action potential has elapsed, normal excitation is possible again. The action potentials of **atrial cardiomyocytes** are similar to those of ventricular cardiomyocytes, but they are shorter. This is because the voltage-dependent Ca^{2+} channels are open for a shorter time, while at the same time the K^+ channels are closed for a shorter period. This does not result in a clear plateau (**Fig. 7.9 a**). As a consequence, the refractory period of **atrial myocytes** is significantly shorter than that of the **ventricular musculature**. The atria can therefore potentially "beat" faster than the ventricles.

> **IN A NUTSHELL** !
>
> During the absolute refractory period, the myocardium cannot be excited by an additional stimulus. During the relative refractory period, some cardiomyocytes can be activated by greater stimulus intensities. The contraction of the ventricular muscles is almost complete when the Na^+ system responsible for depolarization can be activated again after the relative refractory period. Due to the long refractory period, the heart muscle is not tetanisable.

7.3.7   Autorhythmia of the heart

Pacemaker cells of the sinus node depolarize spontaneously up to a threshold potential and then initiate action potentials. This spontaneous depolarization is called the **prepotential** (Fig. 7.11 phase 4). It is a special feature of the sinoatrial node. Pacemaker cells therefore do not have a constant resting membrane potential, they function **autorhythmically**. The action potential of pacemaker cells does not have the steep upstroke of the myocardial cells carried by the Na^+ current. The voltage-dependent fast Na^+ channels are replaced in these cells by pacemaker HCN ion channels (formerly called "funny" channels generating a "funny" current I_f, Fig. 7.11). Of the **HCN channels** ("hyperpolarization- and cyclic nucleotide-gated channels"), four isoforms are known so far (HCN 1–4, in the heart predominantly HCN4). They are **non-selective cation channels** that generate the prepotential of the autorhythmic pacemaker cells through **Na^+ influx**. During the action potential, when membrane potential rises rapidly, they are closed. They only reopen spontaneously through hyperpolarization after a maximal repolarization has been accomplished. The maximum potential (end of phase 0) is reached while the atrioventricular muscles are still relaxed. It then triggers an atrioventricular contraction. In pacemaker cells, there are various types of K^+ channels that are also involved in spontaneous depolarization. At the maximum of the action potential, K^+ conductance is comparatively high (I_K, Fig. 7.11, phase 3), and most **K^+ channels** are then open. Afterwards, the K^+ channels begin to close, K^+ conductance decreases, and the pacemaker cells repolarize down to about −60 mV. The Ca^{2+} channels also contribute to the action potential. In the late phase of the prepotential, shortly

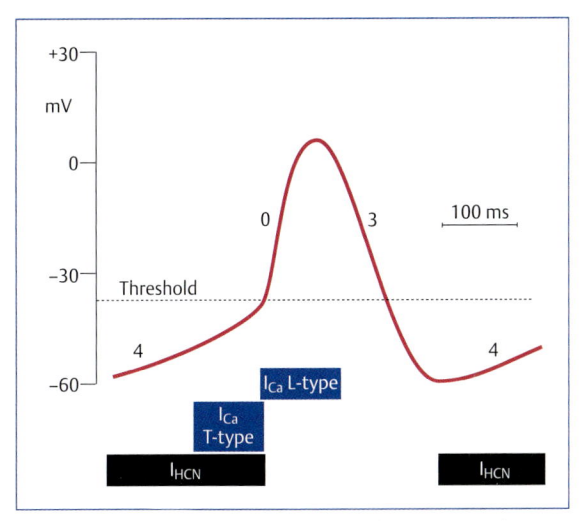

Fig. 7.11 A pacemaker cell of the sinus node spontaneously depolarizes to threshold, thus initiating its own action potential. The prepotential arises from an increase in Na+ influx through the HCN4 channel. An increase in Ca²⁺ influx through Ca²⁺ channels of the T-type (I_{Ca} T-type) finally accelerates establishment of the threshold. When the threshold is exceeded, there is a steep rise of membrane potential, which is primarily carried by a strong increase in Ca²⁺ influx (Ca²⁺ channels of the L-type, I_{Ca} L-type). The absence of fast Na+ channels in pacemaker cells is reflected by the much slower rise of the action potential in pacemaker cells of the sinus node compared to the rate of increase in myocardial cells (**Fig. 7.10**). Phases 0, 3 and 4 (marked with these numbers in the figure) correspond to those in myocardial cells. Phases 1 (initial peak) and 2 (plateau) are absent in pacemaker cells.

before the threshold is reached, some **T-type Ca²⁺ channels open** (**Fig. 7.11** T = transient current (I_{CaT}) carried by Ca_v3 channels, which are fast inactivating channels with a threshold potential of about −55 mV). Consequently, Ca²⁺ influx supports the reaching of the threshold. If the threshold is exceeded, many more of these Ca²⁺ channels open, this time of the **L-type** ($Ca_v1.2$). Thus, the rising phase of the action potential in the pacemaker cells, in contrast to the processes in myocardial cells, is carried by Ca²⁺ influx (**Fig. 7.11**, phase 0; I_{CaL}). After the peak of the action potential has been reached, the Ca²⁺ channels close spontaneously.

The cells of the AV node behave similarly to pacemaker cells in the sinoatrial node. They also show pacemaker activity and a slowly developing action potential. This is also initiated with a prepotential, but this prepotential is less steep compared to that of the sinus node cells (**Fig. 7.9a**). The action potentials of the **sinus node** propagate from cell to cell through the atria to the AV node, before the action potential of the AV node can be initiated. The sinus node therefore "imposes" its rhythm on the AV node.

However, under certain pathophysiological conditions, the pacing activity of the AV node can be critical in maintaining life. For example, if the sinus node is dysfunctional and does not initiate action potentials, the **AV node** can act as a **secondary pacemaker**, i.e. it can trigger ventricular contractions from its spontaneous rhythm. However, excitation in the AV node is much slower and thus the heart rate is reduced (frequency about only half of that of the sinus node). Without this excitation generation in the AV node, cardiac arrest would occur if sinus activity failed. This is why the AV node is also called an **escape pacemaker**.

Another important characteristic of cells in the AV node is their prolonged conduction time compared to atrial cells (**Fig. 7.9b**). This protects the ventricles from being stimulated from the atrium at a very high rate which would make efficient pumping impossible, as for example, in **atrial flutter**. In a condition called **AV block**, where conduction to the AV node is partially or completely disrupted, the AV node can also act as a pacemaker for the ventricles. The long conduction time and long refractory period of the AV node is also important under physiological conditions. Thus, during ventricular excitation, this refractory period prevents reactivation of the atria by action potentials running back from the ventricular myocardium.

The functions of cells in the AV node, like those in the sinus node, are affected by the **autonomic nervous system** (**Fig. 7.12**). Under the influence of the **sympathetic nervous system**, **the conduction velocity** is increased (**positive dromotropic**), the **refractory period is shortened** (adaptation to increased heart rate) and depolarization is faster, so that the frequency of the secondary **pacemaker** can be increased. The **parasympathetic nervous system** has exactly the opposite effect (**negative dromotropic**)

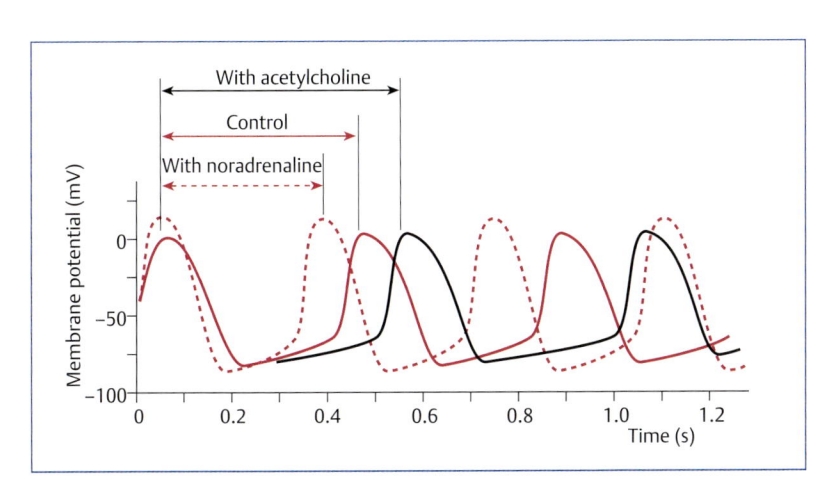

Fig. 7.12 Without any influence of neurotransmitters, a spontaneous rhythm of action potentials is established in the pacemaker cells of the sinus node (control, red line). Acetylcholine reduces the number of depolarizations by prolonging the prepotential (black line), while noradrenaline has the opposite effect (dashed line); based on data from Klein BG (ed.). Cunningham's Textbook of Veterinary Physiology Philadelphia: Elsevier; 2013

with a prolonged refractory period and reduction in the frequency of the secondary pacemaker.

The **His bundle** also has its own rhythm, but it can only initialise about one third of the excitations per minute compared to the sinus node. Thus, the His bundle, as the **tertiary pacemaker** of the heart can act as a backup function for the AV node. In principle, every heart muscle cell has the ability to generate excitation (**automatism**).

> **IN A NUTSHELL**   !
>
> Pacemaker cells do not have a constant resting membrane potential, they function autorhythmically. The lowest membrane potential after completed repolarization is at about −60 mV. The prepotential of varying length runs from there, triggering an action potential at −40 mV. Depolarization occurs through Ca^{2+} influx, repolarization through K^+ outflow.

7.3.8 Sympathetic and parasympathetic nervous system regulate heart rate

The heart is innervated by afferent and efferent nerve fibres of the autonomic nervous system. The **efferents** of the **sympathetic** and parasympathetic (p. 114) have the primary function of mediating **chronotropic, dromotropic** and **inotropic effects** on cardiac action. Chronotropic effects affect the heart rate. Dromotropy refers to the influence on the conduction velocity and inotropy describes effects on the contraction force. In addition, there are **bathmotropic effects** of the autonomic nervous system. Bathmotropy is the influence on the threshold of stimulation and thus the excitability of the heart. Positive bathmotropy means that the stimulus threshold is lowered. Negative bathmotropy means an elevation of the stimulus threshold.

> **MORE DETAILS** Positive bathmotropic drugs that lower the stimulus threshold include **adrenaline, noradrenaline** and **cardiac glycosides**. Negative bathmotropic drugs elevate the threshold, for example **acetylcholine** or **lidocaine**. By definition, the fifth parameter used to classify effect of the autonomic nervous system on the heart is **lusitropy**, which is the effect on the ability of the heart muscles to relax rapidly and completely. Positive lusitropy means an increase in relaxation capacity. Negative lusitropy refers to a decrease in relaxation capacity.

The neurotransmitters noradrenaline from the sympathetic nervous system (nervi cardiaci, nervi accelerantes) and acetylcholine from the parasympathetic nervous system, increase or decrease the **heart rate** (positive or negative chronotropic effect; **Fig. 7.12**). Sympathetic nerve fibres which run to the sinoatrial node, activate β adrenergic **receptors** via noradrenaline. These are predominantly $β_1$ type receptors as the $β_2$ type plays only a subordinate role in the heart (**Table 4.1**). This activates downstream signal transduction pathways (G_s-protein → adenylate cyclase→ cAMP (p. 39) → protein kinase), and accelerate Na^+ influx through **HCN channels** during the prepotential (p. 176). Thus, the heart rate rises (positive chronotropic effect). The humoral chemical messenger

adrenaline from the adrenal medulla has the same effect. Parasympathetic nerve fibres of the vagus nerve, which terminate at pacemaker cells of the sinus node, lead to a decrease in heart rate via acetylcholine. This negative chronotropic effect is triggered by **muscarinic receptors (M type)** (M_2 type, **Fig. 4.3**). When the Na^+ influx via the HCN channels is reduced, the Ca^{2+} influx via T-type Ca^{2+} channels is slowed down (G_i protein-mediated) and the K^+ outward current is increased (G_s protein-mediated). The rise in the prepotential is now flatter and the threshold is reached later (**Fig. 7.12**).

The autonomic nervous system can regulate cardiac activity over a wide range. At rest, the **vagal tone** is predominant. For example, the mean heart rate in a large dog is 60 beats·min^{-1} during sleep, 90 beats·min^{-1} during a waking state at rest, and approximately 175 beats·min^{-1} during physical exercise, when the sympathetic nervous system is the main regulator (**Fig. 26.13**).

> **IN A NUTSHELL**   !
>
> The sympathetic nervous system has a positive chrono-, dromo- and inotropic effect on cardiac action. The parasympathetic nervous system acts as an antagonist to these actions.

7.3.9 The sympathetic nervous system has a positive inotropic and lusitropic effect on cardiac muscle cells

Sympathetic nerve endings secrete **noradrenaline** in all parts of the heart tissue, not just in the sinoatrial or the atrioventricular node. All **cardiac muscle cells** express β adrenergic **receptors**. Circulating noradrenaline and adrenaline released from the adrenal medulla can also stimulate these receptors. This leads to action potentials with higher amplitude and shorter duration in the myocardial cells, resulting in more powerful and faster contractions (**Fig. 7.13**). Activation of $β_1$ receptors in particular (**Table 4.1**), causes more **Ca^{2+} channels** to open during the **plateau phase** (phase 2, **Fig. 7.10**) of the action potential, so that more Ca^{2+} can flow into cells from the extracellular space. Because **Ca^{2+} influx** is the primary depolarizing event during plateau, this process elevates the plateau. The increased depolarization, in turn, causes a faster **reopening of the K^+ channels**, which accelerates repolarization and shortens the action potential; see ch. on cardiac autorhythmia (p. 176). The greater the amplitude of the action potential, the faster it propagates from cell to cell. Thus, conduction velocity increases.

The augmented Ca^{2+} influx after β receptor activation promotes Ca^{2+}-induced Ca^{2+} release (p. 149) from the **sarcoplasmic reticulum** (SR) via the **ryanodine receptor (Ca^{2+} channel**). Therefore, the cytosolic Ca^{2+} concentration increases to such an extent that contraction is more powerful and has a faster onset. This contraction is terminated sooner because β receptor activation promotes the activity of the Ca^{2+} pumps, which then work faster to move Ca^{2+}

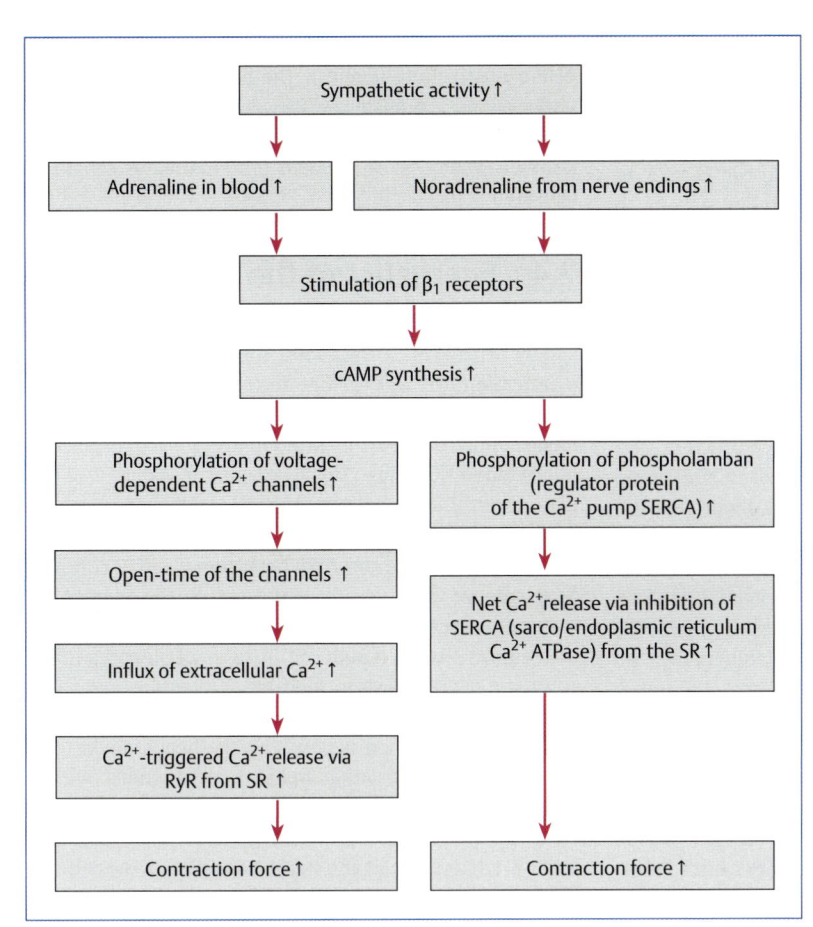

Fig. 7.13 Effect of the sympathetic nervous system on cardiac muscle cells. SR: sarcoplasmic reticulum, RyR: ryanodine receptor = Ca^{2+} channel, cf. **Fig. 6.5**, ↑ increase, ↓ decrease.

Circulation, respiration

back into the sarcoplasmic reticulum. This effect is mediated by the SR membrane protein **phospholamban**, which controls uptake of Ca^{2+} into the sarcoplasmic reticulum. In the dephosphorylated state, it inhibits the pump (**SERCA**, sarco/endoplasmic reticulum **Ca^{2+}-ATPase**). After β adrenergic stimulation, phospholamban is phosphorylated by protein kinase A and its action as an inhibitor is thus prevented. Consequently, more Ca^{2+} is taken up into the sarcoplasmic reticulum and cardiac muscle cells can relax more quickly. In the phosphorylated state, phospholamban has a positive lusitropic effect (**Fig. 7.13**). More Ca^{2+} ions are transported across the cell membrane into the extracellular space by **Ca^{2+} pumps** and **Na^+/Ca^{2+} exchangers** (**NCX**, stoichiometry 3:1). The proportion of total Ca^{2+} transported across the sarcoplasmic reticulum and across the cell membrane are 90% and 10%, respectively.

7.3.10 The parasympathetic nervous system acts on the sinus node, AV node and atrial musculature

Qualitatively, the cardiac actions of the **parasympathetic nervous system** are exactly opposite to those of the sympathetic nervous system. Because the sympathetic nervous system has **positive** chronotropic, dromotropic and ino-

tropic effects, the parasympathetic nervous system has corresponding **negative** chronotropic, dromotropic and inotropic effects. These contrasting effects are essential in adjusting the functions of the sinoatrial and AV nodes, and in the action of muscle cells of the atria. As already described, **acetylcholine** is released at parasympathetic varicosities. It acts on **muscarinic receptors** of the M_2 type (**Fig. 4.3**). In the ventricles, the acetylcholine effect is of very minor importance because, in comparison to the number of sympathetic nerves, only very few nerve fibres of the vagus nerve innervate the ventricles. Acetylcholine reduces the heart rate at the **sinus node**, slows down conduction at the **AV node**, and reduces the contractile force of the atrial muscles. The few parasympathetic nerve fibres in the ventricular musculature end in association with sympathetic nerve fibres, which express **M_2 receptors**. When these M_2 receptors are activated, the release of noradrenaline can be inhibited (presynaptic inhibition; (p.63) **Fig. 4.3; Table 4.1**).

IN A NUTSHELL   !

The sympathetic nervous system acts on all parts of the heart via noradrenaline, the parasympathetic nervous system acts through acetylcholine mainly on the sinoatrial and atrioventricular nodes as well as in the atria.

7.3.11　Afferent fibres of the sympathetic and parasympathetic nervous system

Afferent sensory fibres of the vagus nerve run parallel to the efferent fibres of the autonomic nervous system, to neurons of the nucleus tractus solitarii and other regions of the CNS (p.122) involved in cardiovascular regulation, see ch. Regulation of autonomic functions by the CNS (p.139). These afferent fibres pick up activity from atrial receptors, which are essentially involved in the regulation of blood volume (p.212). There are two types of functional volume receptors (stretch receptors). These are the **A receptors** which are activated during atrial contraction, and the **B receptors** which are activated during the filling phase of the atria. This is how information about pressure and volume reaches the CNS. The activity of the volume receptors (especially the B receptors) directly influences two systems on the efferent side. On the one hand, increased excitation of the volume receptors inhibits sympathetic neuronal activity, especially the part that innervates the kidneys. This leads to reduced activity of the renin-angiotensin-aldosterone system (p.307) (**Fig. 12.7**). On the other hand, afferent impulses from the B receptors reach osmoregulatory regions in the hypothalamus, which are involved in the control of ADH secretion. Thus, with an increase in intravascular volume, an increased action potential frequency of the **volume receptors** causes an inhibition of **ADH secretion**, leading to increased diuresis. This volume regulatory reflex to acute changes in intravascular volume is known as **Gauer-Henry reflex**. The ventricles also contain stretch receptors with vagal afferents, but these are of comparatively low density. They are only excited during the **isovolumetric contraction** and under physiological conditions act only to maintain the negative chronotropic vagus effects.

> **MORE DETAILS**　If the ventricles are extremely dilated, this mechanism can trigger reflex **bradycardia (reduced heart rate) and vasodilation**. In addition, subendocardial sensory nerve fibres project to the central nervous system, by which a thoracic pain sensation is conveyed in certain heart diseases (e.g. circulatory disorders) (**angina pectoris**).

7.3.12　Atrial natriuretic peptide

In addition to the ability of **muscle cells of** the **right atrium** to affect cardiac action through neuronal and hormonal regulators, they themselves also have **endocrine functions**. Thus, the acute or chronic stretching of the atria caused by volume load is an adequate stimulus for the secretion of **atrial natriuretic peptide** (ANP). This hormone belongs to the group of natriuretic hormones along with the "brain natriuretic peptide" (BNP) and the "C type natriuretic peptide" (CNP) found in the CNS. Atrial natriuretic peptide is a 28 amino acid peptide hormone. Its most important actions are (1) **attenuation** of **sympathetic tone**, (2) **inhibition of** the **renin-angiotensin-aldosterone system** and (3) **reduction of renal Na⁺ reabsorption** (see ch. Regulation of sodium transport (p.312), volume regulation (p.334)).

Through its suppressing action on renal Na^+ reabsorption, ANP exerts a diuretic effect. The hormone acts on membrane-bound guanylate cyclase which stimulates intracellular cGMP synthesis, so that phosphodiesterases, ion channels and cGMP-dependent protein kinases can all be activated.

7.4　Energetics of the heart

Cardiac muscle depends on a continuous and adequate supply of oxygen. If the **blood supply** is insufficient, the contractile force will rapidly decrease. Cardiac arrest can occur just a few minutes after a heart attack. Without a blood supply, the heart muscle soon begins to die. The **coronary blood flow rate** (**Fig. 8.1**) at rest is about 5% of cardiac output. During exercise, the blood flow rate may well be increased by a factor of 4 to 6. The difference between maximum and basal **coronary perfusion** is called **coronary flow reserve**. It is usually expressed as the quotient of maximum stress and resting volumetric flow rate. The coronary flow reserve is reduced in cases of stenoses in the coronary arteries, also in high blood pressure and many other heart diseases.

Coronary perfusion depends on the heart rate, arterial pressure, neural regulation and particularly metabolic factors. These include **local** (H^+, K^+, CO_2) and **endothelial chemical messengers** (NO, PGI_2), **hormones** (catecholamines, angiotensin II) and **neurotransmitters** (noradrenaline, acetylcholine). A decrease in oxygen partial pressure leads to the production of mediators (especially adenosine), which then cause vasodilation and thus improve coronary perfusion. The cardiac muscle thus adjusts its own blood flow to demand (autoregulation (p.208)). A particular situation applies to the left ventricle, where the high pressure during systole compresses the submyocardial vessels. Only during diastole, when the arterial pressure is higher than the ventricular pressure, will sufficient blood flow reach the myocardium through the coronary vessels (p.201).

The **oxygen demand** of the heart at rest is about 10–15% of total resting oxygen utilisation. During heavy work, the demand increases about 5-fold. The extent of capillarisation of cardiac muscle (p.173) is considerable. The O_2 extraction capability in the **coronary circulation** is remarkably high (about 70%). This is more than twice as high as that of the whole animal at rest, which amounts only to about 25%. Thus, O_2 extraction in the coronary circulation cannot be substantially increased. Therefore, when cardiac output increases, the augmented demand for oxygen must largely be met by an increase in blood flow rate.

Energy metabolism of the **myocardium** is almost exclusively aerobic (**Fig. 26.2**). A large part of the energy requirement is for contractions (60–70%). The rest is for structure maintenance and electrophysiological activities connected with ion pumps (Ca^{2+}-ATPase, Na^+/K^+-ATPase). As a rough estimate, 40% of the substrates for ATP production during physical rest are **fatty acids** and **triacylglycerols**, 30% **glucose**, 20% **lactate** and 10% **ketone bodies**, **pyruvate** and **amino acids** (**Fig. 7.14**). Efficient energy me-

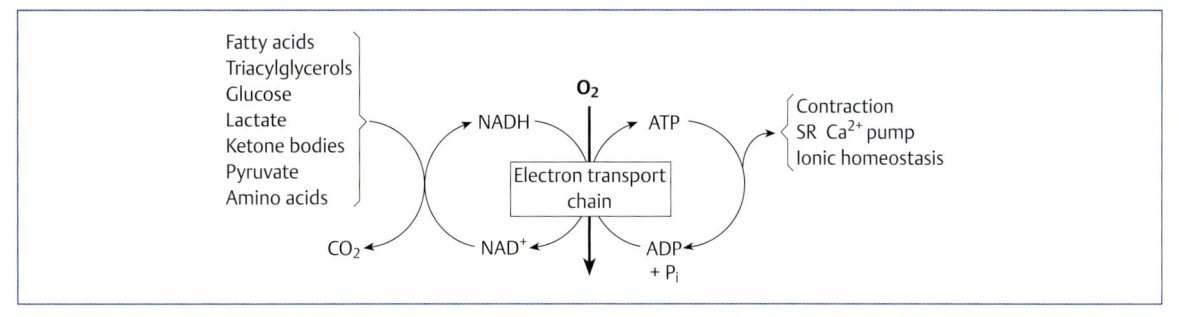

Fig. 7.14 Coupling of contraction force, ATP hydrolysis, oxidative phosphorylation and NADH production by dehydrogenases in the metabolism of the cardiac muscle. The heart is an "omnivore". The cardiomyocytes are mainly dependent on oxidative phosphorylation for energy production. As substrates, the heart normally burns free fatty acids and triacylglycerols, followed by glucose and lactate. If the supply delivered by the coronary arteries changes, the heart may also switch to other substrates such as ketone bodies, pyruvate and amino acids. SR = sarcoplasmic reticulum.

tabolism is needed to produce sufficient ATP for the continuous work of the myocardium. The myocardium cannot store a lot of ATP ($5\,\mu mol \cdot g^{-1}$). However, it has a high ATP utilisation rate (about $0.5\,\mu mol \cdot g^{-1} \cdot s^{-1}$ at physical rest). This means that ATP stores would be depleted within about ten seconds after a block in oxidative phosphorylation. The supply of another important energy store, namely **creatine phosphate** (ATP formation by the creatine kinase reaction), is also not much larger at $7{-}10\,\mu mol \cdot g^{-1}$. Its use fades into the background under normal conditions. The ATP required for cardiac work comes predominantly from **oxidative phosphorylation** (under physiological conditions > 95% **glycolysis** and GTP formation in the **citrate cycle**) (see ch. Energetics of skeletal muscle (p. 157); Metabolism of erythrocytes (p. 232). The heart can therefore be described as an "**omnivore**" with regard to energy metabolism (**Fig. 7.14**). During physical exertion, the proportion of lactate for energy production increases up to 60%. During exertion, more lactic acid is produced by skeletal muscles, because part of their energy metabolism is anaerobic. Hence, during exercise, there is a decrease in the relative proportion of other energy substrates for myocardial metabolism.

MORE DETAILS If the oxygen supply to the myocardium decreases (**ischaemia**), then lactate is formed from pyruvate and the myocardium releases lactic acid instead of consuming it. Therefore, an increase in coronary venous lactate concentration (more precisely: a decrease in the arteriovenous lactate quotient) is a clinical indicator of myocardial hypoxia.

> **IN A NUTSHELL** !
>
> Substrates for oxidative cardiac metabolism at rest and during physical work are mainly free fatty acids, glucose and lactate. The heart is an energy substrate "omnivore".

7.5 ECG – basics

7.5.1 Physical principle

An **electrocardiogram** (**ECG**) is a recording of the sum of the electrical activities of all cardiomyocytes. At rest, the individual heart muscle fibres have a negative membrane potential with respect to the extracellular space. When an action potential is initiated, a membrane recharge occurs, which is caused by a rapid sodium influx (**Fig. 7.10**). After excitation of a cardiomyocyte, neighbouring fibres are depolarized very quickly so that an action potential (p. 175) is also initiated in them. There are differences in potential between the currently excited and unexcited regions of the heart, which can be interpreted as small electrical dipoles that are surrounded by an **electric field (Fig. 7.15 a)**. Each point of the electric field has a specific potential. Points of the same potential can be represented by so-called **isopotential lines** (**Fig. 7.15 a**). The voltage differences between outside and inside of the cells (**intracellular recording** registering a monophasic change in potential difference, **Fig. 7.15 b**), are not taken into account in the **extracellular ECG recording**. Here both electrodes are located outside the cell measuring a biphasic change in potential difference. In this case, potential differences between different isopotential lines are recorded. At each time point of the propagation of depolarizing or repolarizing events, a large number of individual dipoles (elementary dipoles) are found in the heart. They can also be represented as **vectors** which are directed from minus to plus, i.e. from the excited to the unexcited tissue (**Fig. 7.15 a**). By definition, deflections of the vectors from minus to plus are upwards (positive potential differences using the example of the atria, **Fig. 7.16 a**). The individual vectors of excited myocytes can be combined. This results in a spatial **integral vector**. This vector changes constantly in size and direction and symbolises an electric field that propagates in the body via the extracellular fluid. It can also be registered on the surface of the body, albeit in a greatly attenuated form. Since the fibres in the heart run mainly from the base of the heart to the apex, the integral vector reaches its greatest extension on this line, which is also called the **electrical axis** of the heart. The integral vector is represented as an arrow with changing length and direc-

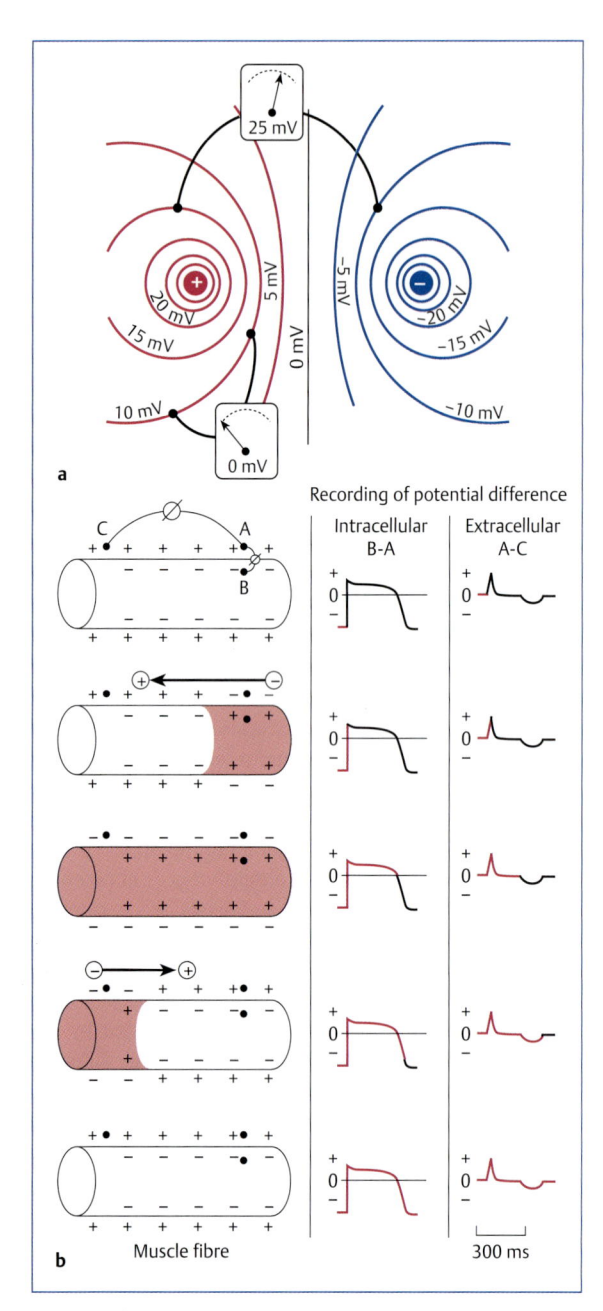

a

Recording of potential difference

	Intracellular B-A	Extracellular A-C

b Muscle fibre

300 ms

Fig. 7.15 a Schematic representation of a dipole of the excited cardiac muscle fibre with the electric field represented by the isopotential lines. There is a potential difference between the isopotential lines which can be measured with a voltmeter if the cell is in an electrolyte solution. If the recording electrodes are on the same isopotential lines, the voltmeter would read 0 mV, because there is no potential difference between these points. The magnitude and direction of the electric field can be represented by a vector. If many muscle cells are excited at the same time, as in atrial and ventricular excitation, an integral vector results. **b** Fluctuations in potential during depolarization and repolarization along a heart muscle fibre from right to left. The middle column shows the time course recorded with a typical extra/intracellular recording (monophasic recording, between points A and B). This time course corresponds to the representation explained in **Fig. 7.10**. In the non-invasive form of extracellular recording (resulting in a biphasic signal), as already described for the compound action potential in nerve fibres (**Fig. 2.12**), both electrodes are located on the cell surface. Now the potential difference prevailing between points A and C in the case of an action potential is measured (also **Fig. 7.16 a**). The results of the extracellular recording are shown in the right column. In electrocardiography, the electrical activity of the heart is recorded with an extra/extracellular electrode on the surface of the body. Red colouring = depolarization.

T wave. The ECG is an expression of the electrical, but not the mechanical activity (contraction), of the heart. It therefore does not provide any direct information about the pumping activity of the heart.

> **IN A NUTSHELL**
>
> The electrocardiogram records the temporal sequence of electrical potential differences on the surface of the body caused by the action of the heart, which result from depolarization and repolarization of cardiac muscle. The deflections shown in the ECG correspond to potential differences in the order of 1 mV.
>
> The vector points from minus to plus, i.e. from excited to unexcited tissue. By definition, a vector from minus to plus in the ECG causes a deflection upwards.

tion in space. If its negative base as in **Fig. 7.16 b** is virtually fixed in the centre of the heart, its positive tip performs three oval vector loops during a heartbeat. This is shown in **Fig. 7.16 b** as a snapshot of the maximum integral vector in which the R wave is recorded in the ECG. First, the **atrial loop** is formed. It represents excitation of the atria and appears in the ECG as a **P wave** (**Fig. 7.19**). This is followed by the **ventricular loop**. It represents ventricular excitation which appears in the ECG as a **QRS complex**. The movement of the integral vector during cardiac action concludes with the **repolarization loop**. This appears in the ECG as a

7.5.2 Standard recording procedure

For clinical electrocardiography, lead systems have become established which, with the aid of particular recording points, provide the most comprehensive spatial recording possible of the electrical processes in the heart. With the aid of the bipolar **limb leads** according to **Einthoven** (**Fig. 7.17 a**), the unipolar limb leads according to **Goldberger** (**Fig. 7.17 b**), the adaptations of the limb leads for the horse (**Fig. 7.17 c**) and the **chest wall leads** according to **Wilson** (**Fig. 7.17 d**), an extensive spatial recording can be carried out.

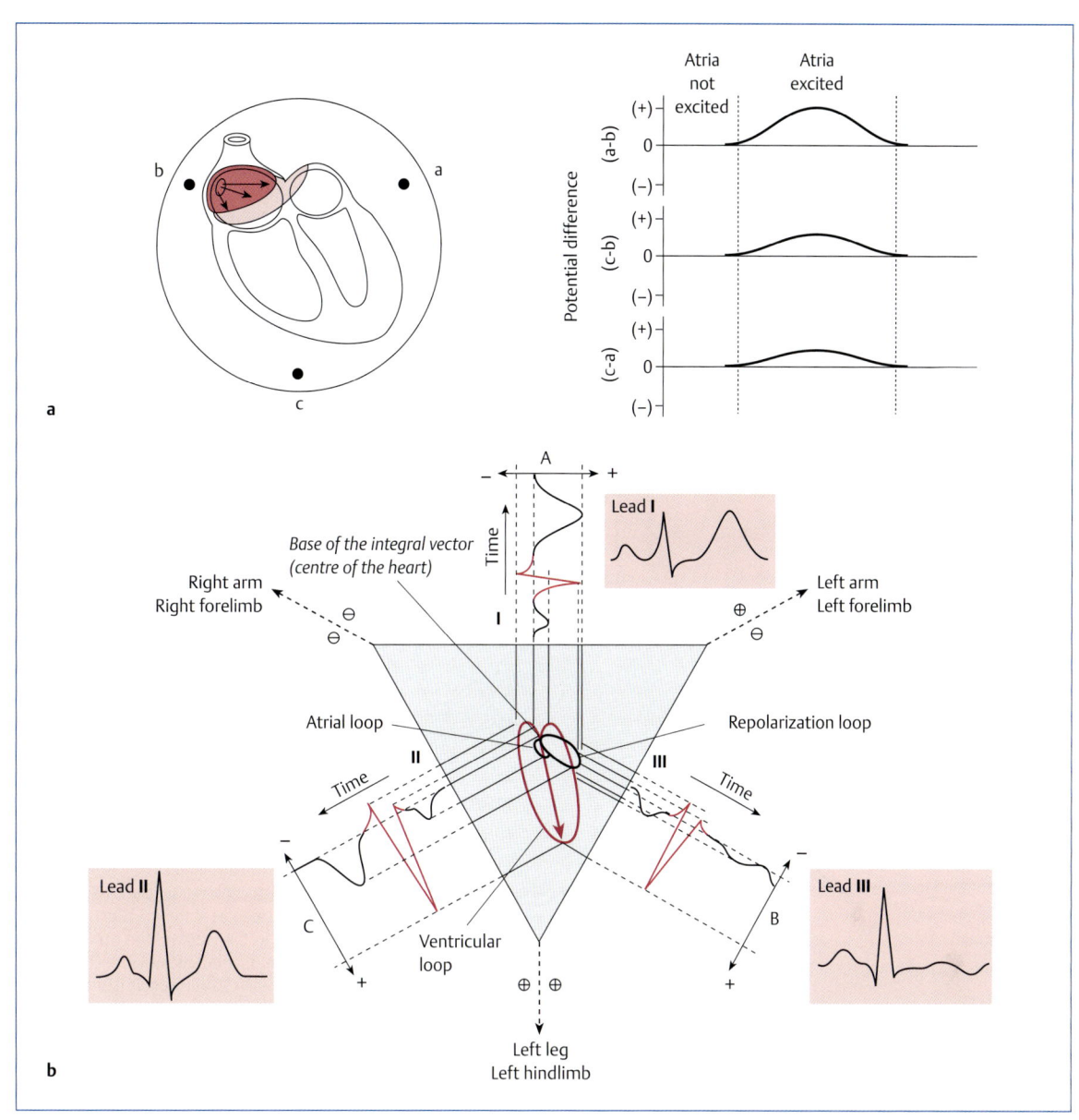

Fig. 7.16 Origin of the ECG.
a An unexcited heart would not show any potential differences (P_D) other than 0 mV between the recording electrodes a, b and c. When the depolarization wave propagates from the sinus node towards the AV node (arrows in the right atrium), point a is initially positive compared to point b. When the atria are fully excited, the P_D = 0 mV. Because parts of the left atrium are also already excited, there is also a difference in charge between cardiac apex c and point b. Between c and a, this difference is only small.
b Position of Einthoven leads (p. 182) I, II and III and projections of the electrical integral vector. At each time point of the propagation of depolarization or repolarization waves, an integral vector emanates from the heart, the direction and size of which varies in the three-dimensional space of the body. In this snapshot, the time point with the maximum integral vector (resulting in the R wave in the ECG) is shown. The temporal first loop is the atrial loop, which is caused by atrial excitation. The second and usually largest loop (red) is the ventricular loop produced by ventricular excitation. The repolarization loop corresponds to the return of membrane potential in the ventricles to resting values. The direction of the electrical axis of the heart (p. 186) can be determined with the help of the respective largest integral vector generated in the individual loops.

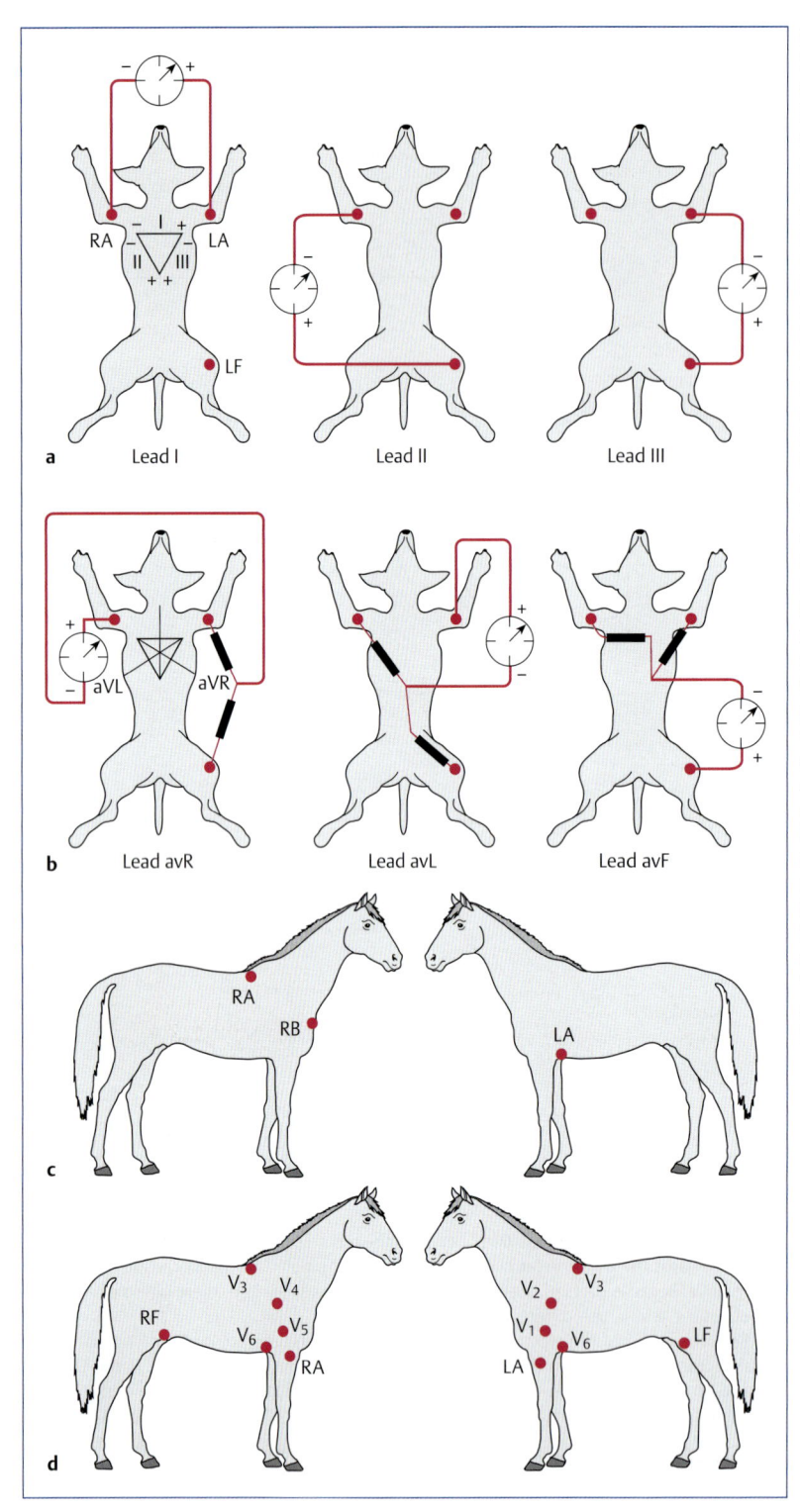

Fig. 7.17 Standardised ECG leads according to Einthoven, Goldberger and Wilson.
a The leads according to **Einthoven** are bipolar limb leads that are routinely recorded via three electrodes plus a grounding electrode. In this example, the electrodes are placed on the dog according to the traffic light scheme as follows: Lead I between the right (RA) and left front leg (LA), lead II between the RA and left hind leg (LF) and finally lead III between the LA and LF.
b The **Goldberger** leads are also limb leads, but they are unipolar. Three leads are used and the potential changes are measured between a different and an indifferent electrode. The indifferent electrode is created by connecting two recording points together via a resistor as a "zero point": Lead aVR (augmented voltage right, RA against LA and LF), lead aVL (augmented voltage left, LA against RA and LF) and lead aVF (augmented voltage foot, LF against LA and RA). By interconnecting two of the electrodes against the third electrode according to Goldberger, three additional leads are obtained compared to the Einthoven measurement, which, plotted as vectors, also form an equilateral triangle and are rotated by 30° compared to the Einthoven triangle.
c Standard ECG lead in the horse between base and apex.
d Chest wall leads according to **Wilson**, adapted for the horse (RA right front leg, LA left front leg, RF right hind leg, LF left hind leg). In the unipolar measurement according to Wilson, six electrodes (V1–V6) are placed as standard. Electrode V3 is attached to the withers, the other electrodes are distributed over the thorax.

7.5.3 Spatiotemporal analysis of the ECG

In the ECG, a distinction is made between (1) **waves** (= deflections from the isoelectric line upwards or downwards), (2) **segments** (region between two waves) and (3) **intervals** (sums of waves + segments). Segments are represented by the **isoelectric line**. The isoelectric line is the line in the ECG that is horizontal. It occurs when there are no excitation wavefronts along the fibres. This is the case during complete excitation of the atrial and ventricular muscles and after complete repolarization of the ventricular muscles until the onset of the next atrioventricular excitation. The deflections are designated consecutively in alphabetical order with capital letters beginning with the letter "P".

The **P wave** represents the atrial excitation starting from the sinoatrial node. The corresponding integral vector describes the atrial loop (**Fig. 7.18 a, b**). The P wave is directed upwards because at this point in time in lead II the left hindlimb is positive in relation to the right forelimb. The repolarization of the atria produces only a weak signal, which is largely covered by the **QRS complex**. Consequently, this repolarization is not visible in the ECG. During the PQ segment, the atria are fully excited. The evaluation of the PQ segment is not particularly clinically relevant. The **PQ interval** indicates how fast an action potential is transmitted from the sinus node in the atria via the AV node in the direction of the cardiac apex to the Purkinje fibres (**Fig. 7.18 c**). Due to the slow conduction in the AV node, the PQ interval is essentially an expression of the atrioventricular conduction time.

The **QRS complex** is formed by Q, R and S waves of different amplitude and direction, which altogether reflect the excitation propagation in the ventricular musculature (**Fig. 7.18 d, e, f; Fig. 7.19 b**). The excitation of the ventricles begins on the left side (towards the left ventricle) and initially spreads towards the base of the heart. In the ECG, this corresponds to the **Q wave** (**Fig. 7.18 c**). When most of the base of the heart is excited, the direction of propagation of the excitation wave now turns to the apex of the heart (**R wave, Fig. 7.18 d**). The last part of the ventricular muscles to be excited is near the atrial septum of the right ventricle. The ventricular wall there begins to depolarize on the inside (minus), the outer tissue is still in the unexcited state (plus), so that the integral vector changes direction again (**S wave, Fig. 7.18 e**). At the end of the S wave, the ventricles are fully excited.

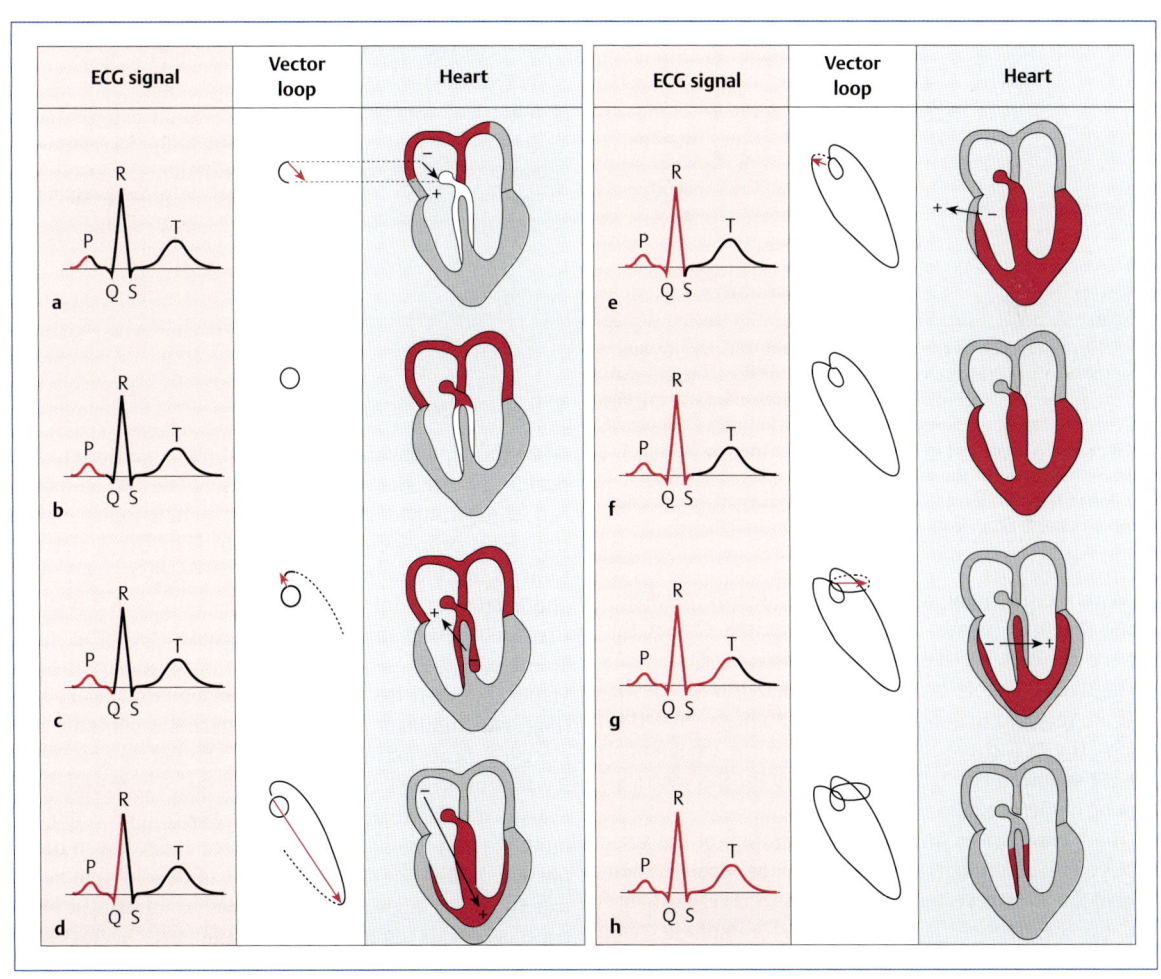

Fig. 7.18 Typical waves in the ECG signal during a cardiac cycle. By definition, the waves are listed from P to T and correspond to specific phases of the cardiac electrical activity (from **a-h**, the excitations are marked in red). The vector diagram shows the time course of the three vector loops.

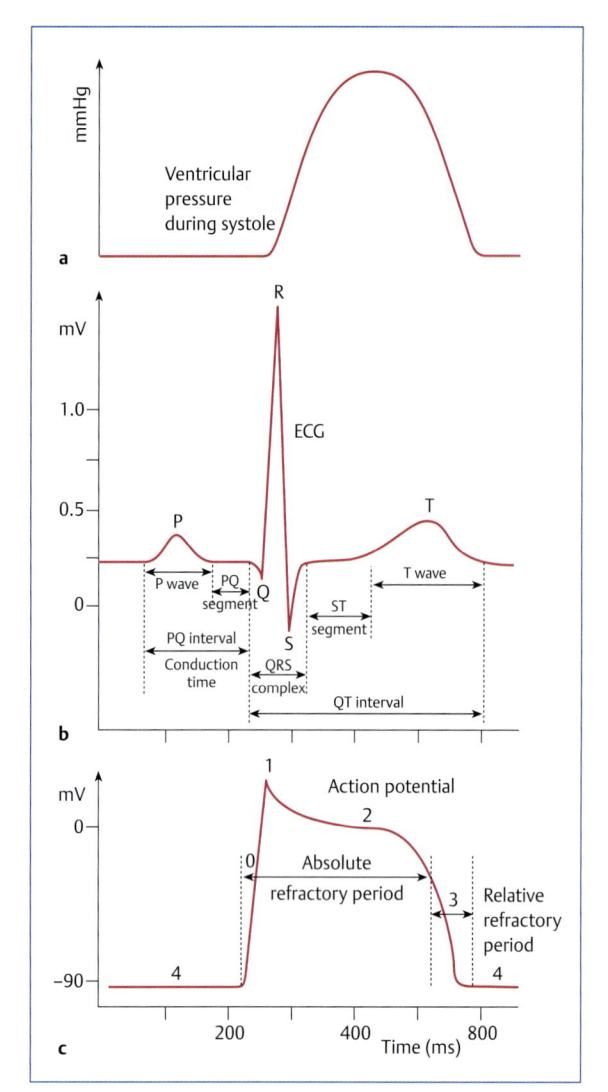

is usually not the case, or only occasionally so, if repolarization occurs at different rates in different myocardial regions. In Einthoven lead II, for example, the T wave is directed upwards in humans and primates (**Fig. 7.18**; **Fig. 7.19 b**), because the action potentials at the base of the heart and subendocardially last longer than at the apex of the heart and subepicardially. The base is thus still depolarized when the apex is already repolarized.

Until the beginning of the next atrial excitation, the **TP segment** follows. Comparing the electrical heart signals (ECG) with the mechanics of the cardiac cycle, the beginning of the TP segment corresponds to the beginning of the isovolumetric relaxation phase of diastole. It lasts until about halfway through the filling phase (FP, **Fig. 7.2 a, b**). By definition, diastole in the ECG extends from the end of the T wave to the R wave (actually to the Q wave, but this is often not as easy to measure as the R wave, sometimes the Q wave is not visible). Systole lasts accordingly from the R wave to the end of the T wave (**Fig. 7.2 a, b**).

> **IN A NUTSHELL**   !
>
> The P wave corresponds to the spread of excitation across the atria. The PQ segment shows the sustained excitation of the atria up to the AV node.
> The Q wave of the QRS complex indicates the onset of ventricular excitation, the R wave shows the spread of excitation of the large myocardial mass towards the apex of the heart (electrical cardiac axis).
> The S wave is formed at the end of the complete excitation of the left ventricle.
> The ST segment shows the complete excitation of the ventricles.
> The T wave is generated by the repolarization of the ventricles.

Fig. 7.19 Comparison of the time course of the ECG of a cardiac cycle (**b**) with the pressure course in the left or right ventricle (**a**) and the action potential of a myocardial cell intracellular recording (**c**). The assignment of the letter identification in the ECG proposed by Einthoven is explained in detail in the text. The numbers 0–4 indicate the phases of the action potential (cf. **Fig. 7.10**). The function of the absolute and relative refractory periods is discussed in more detail in ch. "Heart is not tetanisable" (p. 176).

With the beginning of the repolarization of the membrane potential (phase 1, **Fig. 7.19 c**) at the end of the Q wave, the muscle cell enters the plateau phase (phase 2) during which systole occurs (**Fig. 7.19 a**). Now all muscle cells are reversed in polarity, there are no more excitation fronts. The ECG curve therefore runs on the isopotential line (**ST segment**, **Fig. 7.18 f** and **Fig. 7.19 b**). The ventricular loop of the integral vector has ended.

The **T wave** arises from the repolarization of the ventricles and is accordingly represented by the repolarization loop of the integral vector (**Fig. 7.18 g, h**). It is very variable and can be positive, jagged, negative or biphasic (e.g. horse, Einthoven lead II), depending on the type of lead and the animal species. If the repolarization occurs in the same order as the excitation propagation, then a negative T wave results, as is often observed in dogs. However, this

7.5.4   Electrical heart axis

From the bipolar limb leads according to Einthoven, the position of the **electrical heart axis of the QRS complex** can be determined. It shows the main direction of excitation wave propagation in the ventricles. This is not the same as the **anatomical heart axis**. Although the electrical and anatomical cardiac axes can be identical in direction, they often deviate from each other, even in a healthy heart. The steeper the heart lies in the thorax, the greater the deviation between the anatomical and electrical heart axis (dog, cat, ruminant, horse). To determine clinically the electrical heart axis from the ECG, the net height of the R waves of at least two QRS complexes of corresponding leads is measured and the position determined is plotted on the corresponding side of the isosceles **Einthoven triangle** (Fig. 7.20 a). For the classification of the different **heart axis types**, the angle α forms the basis, as it takes the electrical heart axis (direction of the maximum R vector) with the horizontal. It largely corresponds to the anatomical longitudinal axis of the heart. The line connecting the vector peaks represents the resulting vector loop for excita-

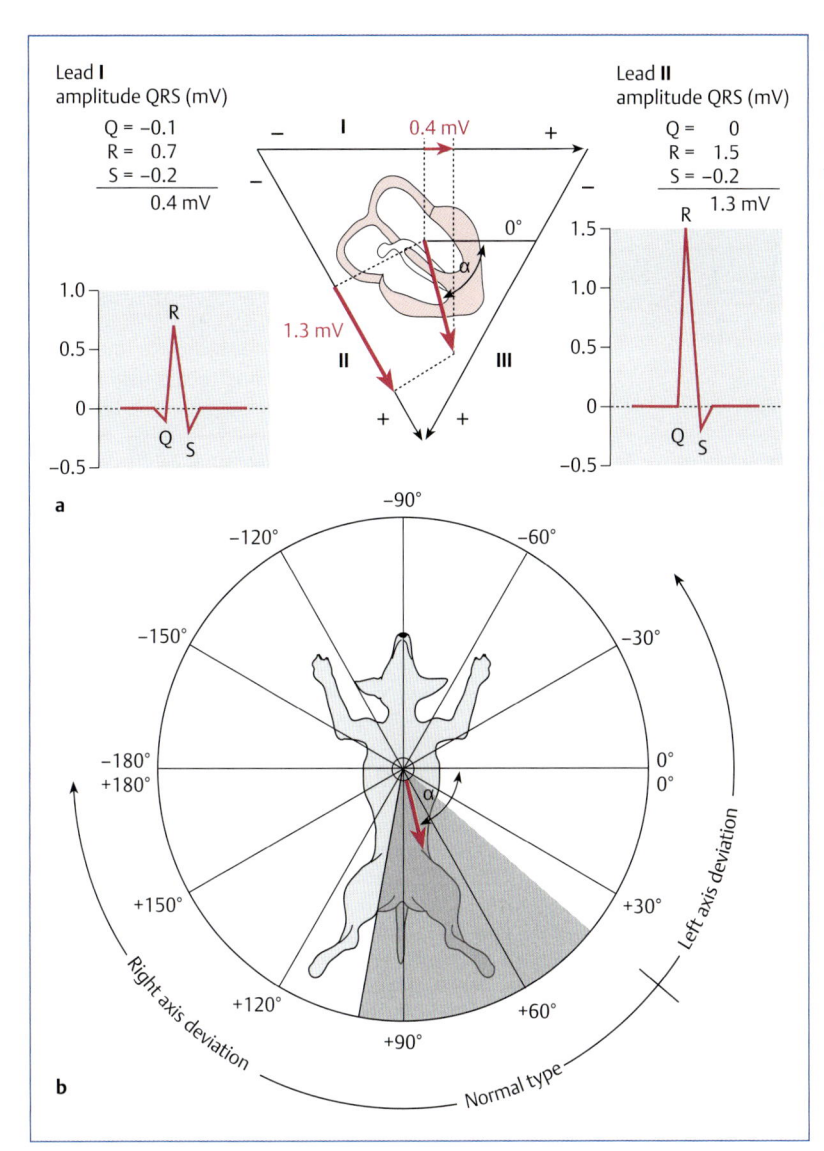

Lead **I**
amplitude QRS (mV)

Q = –0.1
R = 0.7
S = –0.2
––––––––
0.4 mV

Lead **II**
amplitude QRS (mV)

Q =   0
R = 1.5
S = –0.2
––––––––
1.3 mV

Fig. 7.20 Estimation of the position of the electrical cardiac axis in a dog.
a The net ECG deflections of the QRS complex of two Einthoven leads (here I and II) are plotted on the corresponding side of the isosceles Einthoven triangle (starting from the side bisector in the minus to plus direction). The intersection of the perpendiculars starting from the respective vector base forms the starting point of the integral vector. The intersection of the perpendiculars starting from the vector tips determines the length and position of the integral vector (electrical heart axis). For the classification of different position types of the heart, the angle α (here 75°) between the heart axis and the horizontal line (0°) forms the Einthoven triangle.
b Scheme for determining the position type in dogs using the angle α determined in **a**. In the given example, the electrical heart axis is in the normal range (= dark grey area).

tion propagation in the ventricles. In the dog, the normal range of the electrical cardiac axis is between 40° and 100° (**Fig. 7.20 b**). In the cat it varies physiologically between 0° and 160°. Deviations should be interpreted as an indication of altered excitation propagation across the ventricles. For example, a rightward deviation may be due to right ventricular hypertrophy, and a leftward deviation may be due to left ventricular hypertrophy.

IN A NUTSHELL   !

The electrical heart axis can be determined as the angular deviation from the horizontal line in the Einthoven triangle.

7.6 Cardiac disorders

Primary cardiac dysfunction occurs mainly as a reduced pumping capacity (**cardiac insufficiency, heart failure**). This is usually because of altered cardiac muscle function, as a result of **arrhythmias** or **valvular heart diseases**. Secondary cardiac malfunction is predominantly caused by disorders in the upstream or downstream vascular regions. The term cardiac insufficiency refers to a state where an adequate blood supply to the periphery cannot be guaranteed, because of exhaustion of functional and morphological compensatory mechanisms. The compensatory mechanisms include the Frank-Starling mechanism (p.170) (stronger contraction through preload increase), the **sympathetic tone** (HR ↑, preload ↑, afterload ↑, O_2 consumption ↑, **Fig. 7.13**), **hypertrophy** of the ventricles (in chronic pressure and/or volume stress) and an increase in **aldosterone concentration** resulting from a drop in blood pressure and subsequent reduced renal perfusion, renal sodium and water reabsorption ↑, blood volume ↑, preload ↑, (see ch. Distribution and regulation of blood volume (p.212); renin-angiotensin system (p.307).

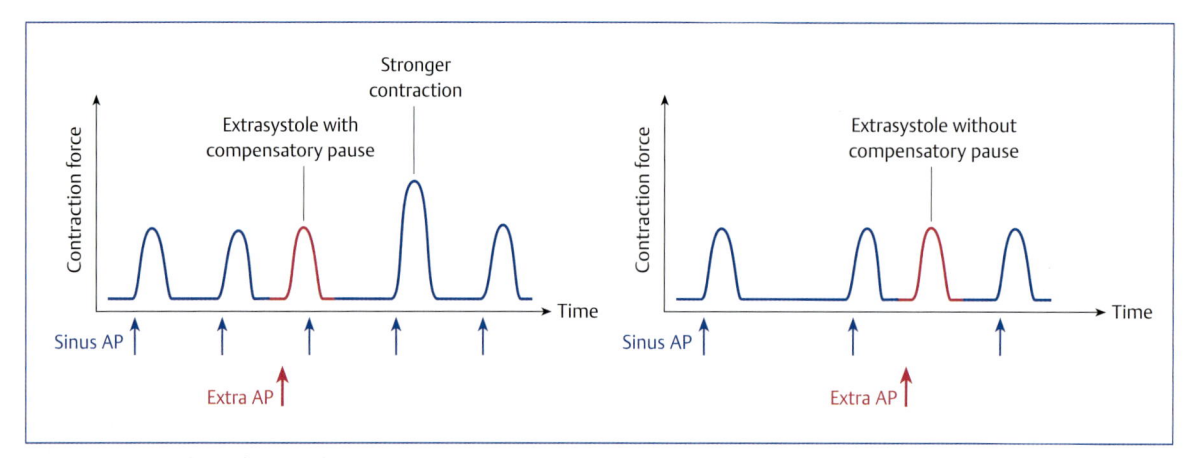

Fig. 7.21 Extrasystoles with and without a compensatory pause. An additional stimulus from an ectopic centre causes an extrasystole. The subsequent regular ventricular excitation fails if the excitation from the sinus node falls within the absolute refractory period of the extrasystole, resulting in a compensatory pause. Only the next excitation of the sinus node produces a response. Since the ventricles now contain more blood than normal, the contraction is stronger than normal (left). Extrasystoles can also be embedded in the heart rhythm without a compensatory pause (right), especially at lower heart rates.

7.6.1 Cardiac arrhythmias

Extrasystoles: Contractions outside the physiological sinus rhythm are called **extrasystoles** ("heart stumbles"). Extrasystoles most often arise in the AV node (supraventricular extrasystoles), the His bundle and Purkinje fibres. **Ectopic centres** can also be located in the atrial (**supraventricular extrasystoles**) or ventricular muscle (**ventricular extrasystoles**). If, with a slow basic rhythm, the extrasystole falls between two normal sinus action potentials (**interposed extrasystole, Fig. 7.22 a**), the basic frequency remains unaffected. However, less or no blood may be pumped if the ventricles are not sufficiently filled again. With a higher heart rate, an extrasystole is usually followed by a **compensatory pause**. The subsequent regular ventricular excitation is omitted because the excitation originating from the sinoatrial node falls within the absolute refractory period of the extrasystole. Only the next excitation of the sinus node can then evoke ventricular excitation again. As the ventricles now contain more blood than normal, the contraction is stronger than usual (**Fig. 7.21**). In the case of a ventricular extrasystole, the propagation of excitation can be retrograde via the AV node to the atria, as the AV node and atrial muscles are not refractory in this case (see ch. Heart not tetanisable (p.176). A negative P wave then appears in the ECG.

> **MORE DETAILS Arrhythmias:** In an ECG, **cardiac arrhythmias** and **conduction disorders** (heart blocks) can be easily recognised. An **arrhythmia** is generally understood to be a disorder of the normal heartbeat sequence, caused by irregular processes in the initiation and conduction of excitation in the heart. Changes in heart rate observed in **respiratory sinus arrhythmia** represent **physiological frequency variability** (Fig. 7.22 b). During inspiration, the heart rate increases. During expiration, it decreases again. There are various explanations for this. During inspiration, the intrathoracic pressure (p.203) leads to an increased return of blood flowing into the large veins close to the heart. The increased blood supply is supposed to lead to a reflex increase in heart rate, via receptors in the right atrium. Another explanation of respiratory arrhythmia lies in the close connection of the neuronal centres in the CNS that control breathing and

heart activity. During inspiration, stretch receptors are activated in the airways and thorax. These are linked to the motor nucleus areas of the vagus nerve via inhibitory interneurons in the medulla oblongata. The stimulation of the stretch receptors should lead to an inhibition of the cardiac vagus fibres.

Cardiac arrhythmias are usually sudden disorders in the initiation and/or conduction of excitation. Causes include mechanical overload, O_2 deficiency and noxious stimuli such as toxins, pharmaceuticals, inflammation, or cell death. Perturbations of the intra- and extracellular milieu, influence on membrane transport systems (e.g. Na^+/K^+-ATPase) or reduction of cell metabolism (ATP ↓) can lead to changes of the resting and action potential and thus to disorders of the normal electrical action of the heart. This can originate from the **sinus node** itself (**nomotop** = "located at the physiological site": sinus tachycardia, sinus bradycardia, sinus arrhythmia) or from **ectopic centres** (= "not located at the physiological site", i.e. heterotopic). Sinus **tachycardia** is usually caused by increased activity of the sympathetic nerve endings at the sinus node. For example, when a dog suffers circulatory shock (p.214) due to severe blood loss, the heart rate is reflexively upregulated by a factor of 2 to 3 via barosensors and the cardiovascular centre, so that the animal quickly gets a heart rate of 200 beats · min⁻¹. **Sinus bradycardia** as a result of increased vagal tone, is not uncommon in athletes and animals that do a lot of performance training. Bradycardia can also be caused by medication, for example by β receptor blockers. In contrast to **sinus tachycardia, paroxysmal tachycardia** occurs suddenly and ends abruptly (**Fig. 7.22 c**). This sometimes lasts only a few seconds, but it may be present for several days. Tachycardia can occur supraventricularly or ventricularly when muscle cells there become more excitable than the sinoid pacemaker cells. Only when the abnormal situation stops can sinus rhythm regain control of the heart's action. Supraventricular paroxysmal tachycardias are thought to be caused by action potentials that retrogradely excite atrial muscles from the AV node. Ventricular paroxysmal **tachycardias** are particularly dangerous because with this form there is basically a risk of life-threatening ventricular fibrillation or cardiogenic shock. This is often accompanied by a pronounced O_2 deficiency of the ventricular muscles.

Atrial flutter or fibrillation are special forms of tachyarrhythmias. This can occur transient (paroxysmal) or continuous (permanent). In contrast to paroxysmal tachycardia, these arrhythmias are almost always caused by an organic, life-threatening heart disease. These include inflammatory heart diseases (**myocarditis, pericarditis, endocarditis**), pressure and volume load

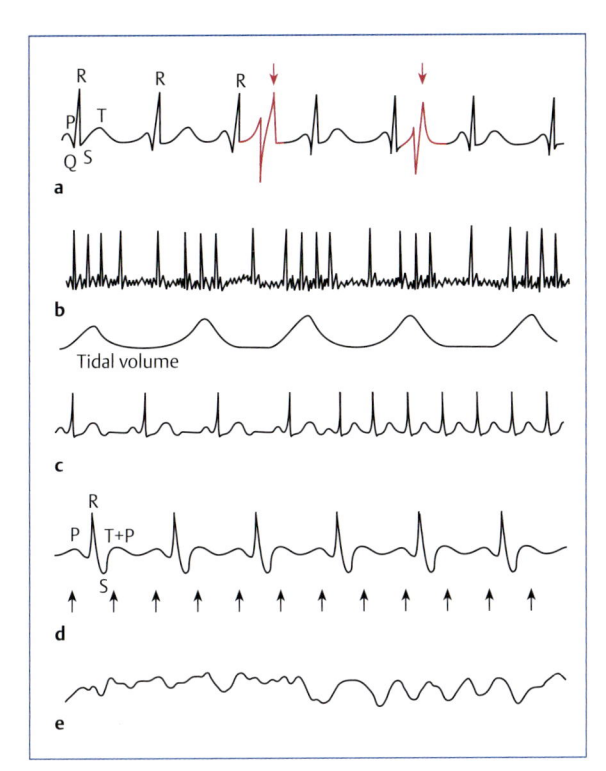

Fig. 7.22 Various ECG curves.
a Two extrasystoles (arrows) which do not disturb the basic rhythm
b Respiratory sinus arrhythmia ECG: top line. Curve of the associated respiratory volumes, bottom line. Inspiration causes tachycardia.
c Paroxysmal arrhythmia. Sudden onset of tachycardia (right half of figure).
d Atrial flutter 2:1 rhythm.
e Ventricular fibrillation.

on the atria and ventricles (e.g. **cor pulmonale**, pressure increase in the pulmonary circulation), infectious, toxic and ischaemic myocardial damage as well as **hyperkalaemia** and **hypocalcaemia**. Atrial flutter in dogs usually drives atrial contractions with a frequency of 300–500 per minute. Only every second atrial excitation is transmitted to the ventricles in the AV node because of the long refractory period (2:1 rhythm, **Fig. 7.22 d**). When there are more than approx. 200 action potentials per minute, these cannot be transmitted in the AV node in dogs. In atrial fibrillation, the depolarizations appear in a very rapid, irregular and uncoordinated sequence. P waves are not seen in the ECG, or are only recognised with difficulty. The pumping function of the atria effectively stops due to lack of coordination. However, since most of ventricular filling (p. 167) is passive and the AV node functions as a low-pass frequency filter, this does not initially have any dramatic consequences for overall pumping capacity of the heart. Nevertheless, the pumping capacity decreases due to a reduction in the heart rate. In humans, the ventricular rate usually increases to 140–150 beats·min^{-1} during atrial fibrillation. Activation of the AV node during atrial fibrillation (e.g. under positive dromotropic action of the sympathetic nervous system) can lead to irregular ventricular tachycardia and negatively affect pumping performance. The transitions to ventricular flutter and fibrillation are flowing. Especially with ventricular flutter, the pumping capacity is greatly reduced. Ventricular fibrillation, for example as a result of a heart attack, is a life-threatening situation. If left untreated, ventricular fibrillation leads directly to death because of the heart's lack of pumping power. In the ECG, you can see fibrillatory waves with a frequency of about 300–800 beats min^{-1} (hu-

man, **Fig. 7.22 e**). In ventricular fibrillation, local disorders in the conduction or course of excitation cause so-called **circulating excitations** in parts of the myocardium (**"re-entry effect"**), so that the cardiac muscle no longer works in a coordinated manner. The pumping capacity of the heart drops abruptly to zero and blood circulation stops. Circulating excitations can occur when the spread of the depolarization is partially delayed in certain regions of the heart muscle, so that after passing through those regions it encounters tissue that is already excitable again. At the beginning of the T wave, the refractoriness of many cardiomyocytes is terminated, and if an extra impulse encounters activatable cells during this time, circulating excitations and ventricular fibrillation can be particularly easily triggered (**vulnerable phase**). Ventricular fibrillation can occur, for example, in an electrical power accident, when the alternating current has a chance to fall in the vulnerable phase of the myocardium (dependent on the electrical system of the country) 50 or 60 times per second. When an electrical current flows through the heart in a lightning strike, cardiac arrest follows. Compared to an electrical accident with an alternating current, ventricular fibrillation occurs less frequently from lightning strike, and **asystole** usually occurs immediately.

Heart blocks: These are arrhythmias caused by disorders in the conduction of excitation. Causes include coronary heart disease, myocardial infarction, side effects of medication, myocarditis, injuries, electrolyte imbalances (especially strongly increased K$^+$ levels). Depending on the localisation of the disorder, a distinction is made:

1. **Sinoatrial block**: disturbed conduction from the sinus node to the atrial muscles.
2. **Atrioventricular block** (AV block): disturbed conduction of excitation from the atria to the ventricles.
3. **Intraventricular block** (thigh block): disturbed conduction of excitation in the ventricles.

The bundle branch block is divided into right bundle branch block or left bundle branch block according to the respective ECG findings. The AV blocks occur in the AV node and His bundle, the degree of severity can be diagnosed with electrocardiography.

In **1st degree AV block**, the conduction of excitation is delayed (prolonged PQ segment) and there is a delayed onset of contraction of the ventricles. This disorder can be recognised by a prolongation of the PQ interval in the ECG. It often remains subclinical and thus not recognised, and usually requires no treatment.

In **2nd degree AV block**, there is partial failure of conduction (**Fig. 7.23 a**). Several possibilities can explain this:
– The PQ interval becomes longer and longer. Eventually it becomes so long that an atrial excitation is no longer transmitted to the ventricles, and a single ventricular contraction fails. The next ventricular excitation is then transmitted normally again. Then the prolongation of the PQ time starts again (**Wenckebach periodic cycle**), **Fig. 7.23 c**.
– Sudden absence of a ventricular action in response to atrial excitation, without the PQ interval being prolonged beforehand. In this case, only every 2nd, 3rd or 4th atrial action can be transmitted to the ventricle (2:1 or 3:1 or 4:1 block). This type of block, which is usually localised in the His bundle, is known as **Mobitz block**. The prognosis is less favourable compared to Wenckebach block, as there is a risk of the rhythm turning into **total AV block** (3rd degree AV block) (**Fig. 7.23 b**).

In **3rd degree AV block**, there is a complete loss of conduction between the atrial muscles and the ventricles. In an emergency, the ventricles stop contracting or continue to beat in a slow **escape rhythm asynchronously to the atria**. This originates from the secondary (AV node) or the tertiary pacemakers (His bundle, Tawara's bundle and Purkinje fibres). The frequency of these pacemaker cells is between 20 and 40 beats min^{-1} (pig). A 3rd degree AV block is a typical indication for implantation of a pacemaker.

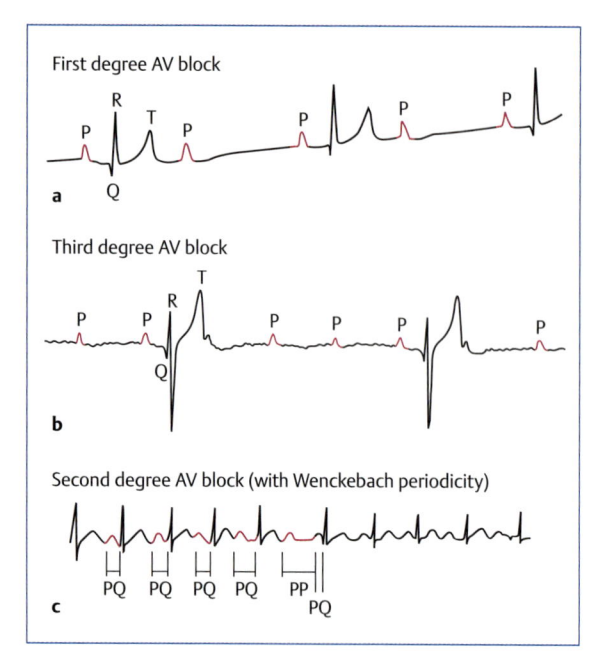

a First degree AV block

b Third degree AV block

c Second degree AV block (with Wenckebach periodicity)

PQ   PQ   PQ   PQ   PP
PQ

Fig. 7.23 Different AV blocks. **a** 2nd degree AV block, some sinus impulses are not transmitted. **b** 3rd degree AV block, sinus rhythm and ventricular rhythm are uncoupled. **c** 2nd degree AV block with Wenckebach periodicity: The PQ segment is continuously prolonged until a QRS complex fails. Then the whole sequence starts again.

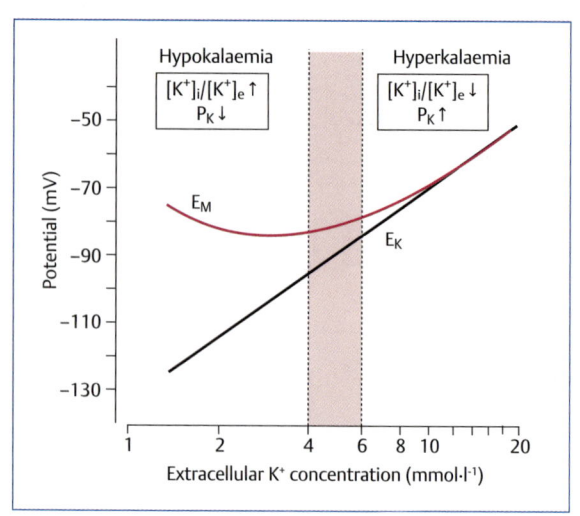

Fig. 7.24 Dependence of the membrane potential (E_M) of a cardiomyocyte on the extracellular K^+ concentration ($[K^+]_e$). E_K is the potassium equilibrium potential calculated on the basis of the Nernst equation (assuming intracellular K^+ concentration $[K^+]_i = 150\,mmol \cdot l^{-1}$). **Normokalaemia** lies between 4 and 6 mmol $\cdot$ l^{-1} K^+ in blood plasma. Above and below this, the membrane changes its K^+ permeability (P_K). As a result, E_M approaches the potassium equilibrium potential in **hyperkalaemia**, i.e. E_M becomes more positive. With **hypokalaemia**, P_K decreases, the influence of K^+ on the membrane potential decreases and E_M again becomes more positive. This means that the cardiomyocyte becomes more excitable in both hypokalaemia and hyperkalaemia, as the threshold can be reached more easily.

7.6.2 Electrolytes

Of all the ions in the extracellular fluid that can affect cardiac action, K^+ is of the greatest practical significance. An increase in extracellular K^+ concentration has two effects on the myocardium. First, the resting membrane potential is decreased because the transmembrane K^+ gradient is reduced. Second, **hyperkalaemia** ($K^+ > 6\,mmol \cdot l^{-1}$) causes an increase in the K^+ conductivity of the cell membrane. This is due to an abnormal closing behaviour of particular K^+ channels (**Fig. 7.24**). Experiments have shown that the resting membrane potentials of cell membranes of atrial muscle fibres, the Purkinje fibres and the ventricular cells in diastole correspond approximately to the K^+ equilibrium potential. With the help of the Nernst equation (p. 36) in **normokalaemia**, with 150 mmol $\cdot$ l^{-1} K^+ intracellular (**Table 1.4**) and 4 mmol $\cdot$ l^{-1} K^+ in blood, a theoretical resting membrane potential of –96 mV can be calculated. A doubling of K^+ concentration in the blood during hyperkalaemia (from 4 to 8 mmol $\cdot$ l^{-1} K^+) increases excitability of the cardiac muscles, as the heart cells depolarize towards the threshold potential (according to the Nernst equation to theoretically –78 mV). Thus, cardiac cells can be more easily excited. If the extracellular K^+ concentration increases further, the membrane potential is depolarized to such an extent that the cells no longer repolarize sufficiently after a single action potential. Consequently, the activatability of the voltage-dependent sodium channels is reduced further and further (**Fig. 2.9**). The heart is thus arrested in diastole (**diastolic cardiac arrest**). This is used in cardiac surgery. During certain surgical interventions, the heart is treated with a so-called **cardioplegic solution**

($K^+ > 15\,mmol \cdot l^{-1}$) so that it is immobilised for a time. With normal blood flow, it usually starts beating again without complications. When the extracellular K^+ concentration in **hypokalaemia** falls below 4 mmol $\cdot$ l^{-1}, the resting membrane potential, according to Nernst, should theoretically increase and thus the cells should be less excitable. However, since K^+ conductivity of the cell membrane decreases at the same time, the influence of K^+ on the resting membrane potential is reduced and, contrary to expectations, the cells can even depolarize more easily. Because of the abnormal behaviour of K^+ conductivity of the cell membrane, both hyperkalaemia and hypokalaemia can increase excitability in the heart, which often leads to cardiac arrhythmias.

Suggested reading

Dobson GP. On being the right size: Heart design, mitochondrial efficiency and lifespan potential. Clin Exper Pharmacol Physiol 2003; 30: 590–597

Dobson GP, Faggian G, Onorati F et al. Hyperkalemic cardioplegia for adult and pediatric surgery: end of an era? Front Physiol 2013; 4, Article 228: 1–28

Eisner D, Bode E, Venetucci L et al. Calcium flux balance in the heart. J Mol Cell Cardiol 2013; 58: 110–117

Fenske S, Hennis K, Rötzer RD et al. cAMP-dependent regulation of HCN4 controls the tonic entrainment process in sinoatrial node pacemaker cells. Nat Commun 2020; 11: 5555

Ferrantini C, Crocini C, Coppini R et al. The transverse-axial tubular system of cardiomyocytes. Cell Mol Life Sci 2013; 70: 4695–4710

Greger R, Windhorst U. Comprehensive Human Physiology. Berlin, Heidelberg: Springer; 1996

Klein BG. Cunningham's Textbook of Veterinary Physiology. Philadelphia: Elsevier; 2013

Scicchitano P, Carbonara S, Ricci G et al. HCN channels and heart rate. Molecules 2012; 17: 4225–4235

Sjaastad ØV, Sand O, Hove K. Physiology of Domestic Animals. Oslo: Scandinavian Veterinary Press; 2012

Stanley WC, Recchia FA, Lopaschuk GD. Myocardial substrate metabolism in the normal and failing heart. Physiol Rev 2005; 85: 1093–1129

8   The circulatory system

Michael Pees, Helga Pfannkuche, Wolfgang von Engelhardt

8.1   Tasks of the cardiovascular system

Wolfgang von Engelhardt

ESSENTIALS ✗

- **Sufficient blood flow** to all tissues and organs is necessary to maintain their functions.
- The cardiovascular system must be able to **adapt quickly** to changing requirements. For example, during physical exercise there is a rapid increase in cardiac output and an increase in blood flow to the working muscles. Despite this significantly increased blood flow to muscles, the blood flow to some organs, such as the kidneys and brain, must remain constant.
- **The tasks** of the cardiovascular system are to transport nutrients, gases, metabolic products, immunoglobulins, hormones, enzymes and electrolytes. In addition, the circulatory system is involved in thermoregulation.
- Essential basic principles of transport in the circulatory system are (1) **convective transport** of blood along a hydrostatic pressure gradient generated by the heart and (2) the **diffusive exchange of gases and other solutes** between blood and tissue.
  - **Convection** enables rapid transport over **long distances**. Components of blood are moved quickly through the systemic and pulmonary circulation. Oxygen can thus be transported from the lungs to distant parts of the body within a few seconds.
  - **Diffusion** is the main transport mechanism over **short distances** (in the range of μm), whereby the transport of a substance always takes place from a site of higher concentration to a region of lower concentration. The transport of substances by diffusion over long distances is very slow. The time required for diffusion increases with the square of the diffusion distance. A glucose molecule takes 0.5 ms to diffuse through a 1 μm thick capillary wall, but many hours through a 1 cm thick boundary layer.
- The hydrostatic pressure required for filtration in the capillaries and glomeruli of the kidney must be maintained in the circulation.

8.2   Circulatory systems and vessel walls

Wolfgang von Engelhardt

The circulatory system consists of a self-contained system of parallel and also serially arranged blood vessels. There are two pumps connected in series. The right and the left heart generate directed blood flows (**Fig. 8.1**). The **systemic circulation** (or "systemic circuit") with the so-called **high-pressure system** is the volume between the left ventricle and the right atrium. The blood volume between the right ventricle and the left atrium is the **pulmonary circulation** (or "pulmonary circuit"), the so-called **low-pressure system**. In both vascular sections, a functional and morphological distinction is made between arteries, arterioles, capillaries, venules and veins. The link between **two capillary regions, connected in series** and originating from a vein, are called **portal vessels**. Examples are the blood flow in the vessels between the intestine and the liver and in the vessels between the hypothalamus and the anterior pituitary. Parallel to these blood vessels, there is a **lymphatic vascular system** in which fluid from the interstitial space is collected and returned to the venous system via the **thoracic duct**.

The structure and composition of the vessel walls vary in different regions of the vascular system (**Fig. 8.2**). All vessel walls are lined with **endothelium**, which is an effective **selective barrier** between the intravascular space and the vessel wall or interstitial space. There is only very limited passage across this barrier of water-soluble, large-molecular substances. The **vascular walls of capillaries** consist only of endothelium and basement membrane. Many **smooth muscle cells** are present, especially in those vessels in which flow rate and blood pressure can change rapidly and where stored blood can be released quickly (see ch. Local blood flow regulation (p.208); Central regulation of blood flow (p.210)). This applies to the **arterioles** and to a lesser extent also to the arteries, but is a very minor property of venules and small veins. In the vessel walls of the large veins (**Fig. 8.13**), there are considerably fewer smooth muscle cells than in arterioles, relative to the cross section of the vessel walls. However, the total size of the large vein vascular bed is extensive. Consequently, when

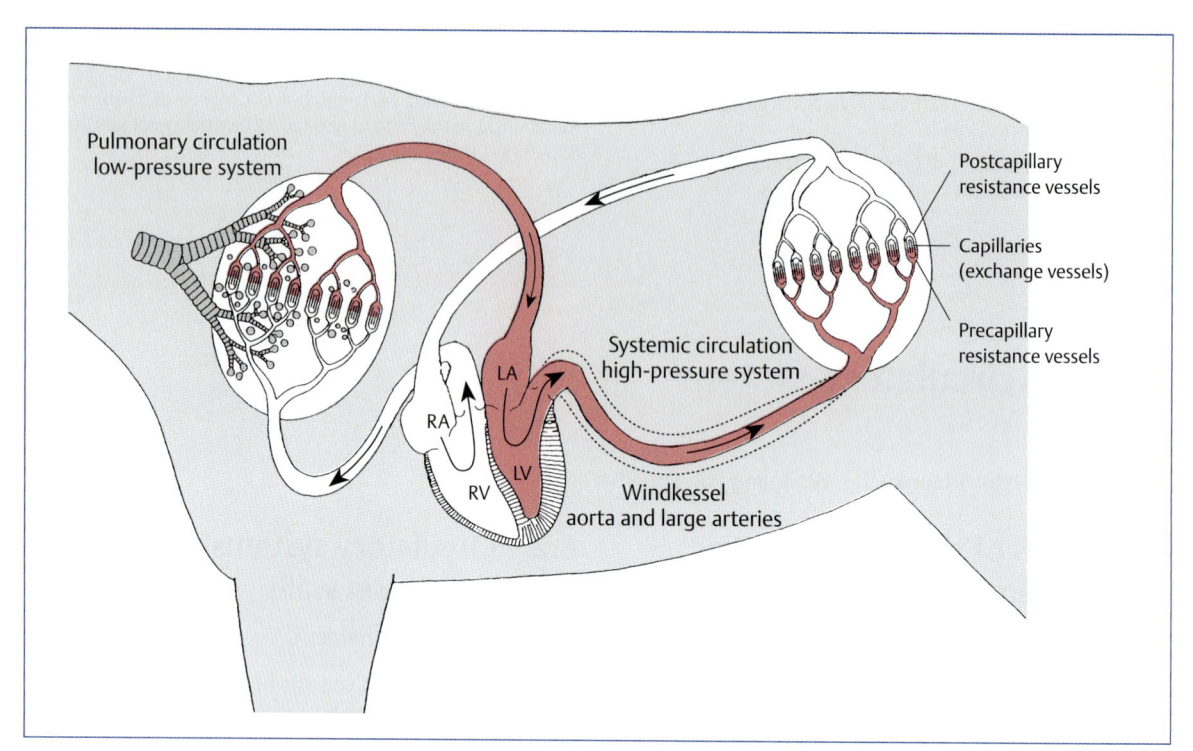

Fig. 8.1 Systemic circulation (with the high-pressure system) and pulmonary circulation (low-pressure system). The function of the aorta and the large arteries is shown schematically.
RA = right atrium; LA = left atrium; RV = right ventricle; LV = left ventricle; arterial blood: red.

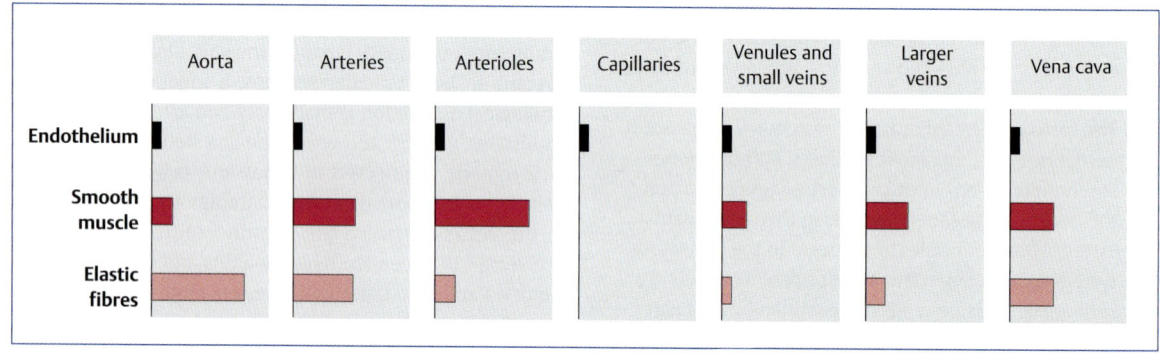

Fig. 8.2 Relative data on blood vessel wall composition in different vascular regions (the length of the bars indicates the proportion of the respective tissue in the vessel wall). It should be noted, when comparing the proportions of the different tissues in vascular walls, that the walls of arteries are significantly thicker than those of veins.

there is blood loss, the blood volume in the large veins can be rapidly decreased by contractions of those smooth muscles in the vein walls, so that enough blood can flow to the heart to maintain circulation (see ch. Distribution and regulation of the blood volume (p. 212). The proportion of **elastic fibres** is greatest in the aorta, but many elastic fibres are also found in the larger and medium-sized arteries (p. 196).

Because of the frequent branching of blood vessels, their **total cross-sectional area increases** approximately 750-fold from the aorta to the capillaries. This cross-sectional area then decreases substantially again approaching the vena cava. Consequently, the **average flow velocity** of blood in an average-sized dog decreases from the aorta ($20\,cm \cdot s^{-1}$) to the capillaries ($0.07\,cm \cdot s^{-1}$). In the venous system, the flow velocity increases again, so that in the vena cava, blood flow velocity is $15\,cm \cdot s^{-1}$. Flow velocities and cross-sectional areas in the vessels in different parts of the circulatory system are summarised in **Table 8.1**.

Table 8.1 Number of blood vessels in the systemic circulation, mean diameter and total cross-sectional area of the vessels, mean blood pressure and mean flow velocities in the different sections of the systemic circulation in a medium-sized dog.

	Aorta	Large arteries	Arterioles	Capillaries	Venules	Large veins	Vena cava
Number of vessels[*1]	1	40	$4 \cdot 10^7$	$1.2 \cdot 10^9$	$8 \cdot 10^7$	40	1
Diameter (mm)[*1]	10	3	0.02	0.008	0.03	6	12.5
Total cross- sectional area (relative to aorta, aorta = 1)[*1]	1	3.8	160	750	710	14	1.5
Mean pressure (mmHg)	100	95	30	15–30	15	10	0–4
Mean flow velocity (cm · s⁻¹)[*2]	20	10–15	0.75	0.07	0.35	3	15

Source: Values from: [*1] Swenson MJ, Reece WO. Duke's Physiology of Domestic Animals. 11th ed, Ithaca, London: Cornell University Press; 1993; [*2] Caro CG, Pedley TJ, Schroter RC et al. The Mechanics of the Circulation. Cambridge: University Press; 2012

8.3 Biophysical basis of haemodynamics

Wolfgang von Engelhardt

ESSENTIALS ✖

Blood flow follows a pressure gradient. The **volumetric flow rate** is the volume of blood that flows per unit of time, and is determined by the **blood pressure** and the **flow resistance** of the vessels. Regulation of flow resistance occurs mainly in the arterioles. The average **flow velocity** of blood in different sections of the vascular system is inversely proportional to the total cross-sectional area of the vessels, so that flow velocity in the widely ramified capillary network is very low. To understand these interrelationships, the law of Ohm, the continuity principle, the Kirchhoff rules and the Hagen-Poiseuille law are all important.

In the vessels, there is usually a **laminar flow** of blood with a parabolic velocity profile. However, **turbulence** can occur at high flow **velocities** in the large vessels. This is seen mainly in pathophysiological conditions, such as vascular stenoses and valvular heart diseases.

The state of expansion of a blood vessel is expressed by its **wall tension**, while its expansion capacity is indicated by its **compliance**. The reciprocal of compliance is the **volume elasticity coefficient**. The distensibility of veins is greater than that of arteries.

8.3.1 Flow rate, pressure, resistance

Blood, like any fluid, has an internal fluid friction that creates resistance to flow. To overcome this flow resistance, a pressure difference is required in the blood vessels.

The relationship between driving pressure difference (Δp), resistance (R) and volumetric flow rate (I) can be defined analogously to the **law of Ohm**.

The **flow rate** (volumetric flow rate) is the volume of blood that flows through an organ per unit of time (e.g. ml · min⁻¹).

$$I = \frac{\Delta p}{R} \tag{8.1}$$

This general law also applies to the amount of blood ejected from the heart, the **cardiac output** (CO). The mechanical activity of the left ventricle produces a mean **blood pressure** in the aorta at rest (MAP) of about 100 mmHg (= 13.3 kPa; **Table 8.1**). This pressure overcomes the **flow resistance** of the vascular circuit (**total peripheral resistance**, TPR). Blood returns into the right atrium under a very low pressure (**central venous pressure**, CVP) of 0 – 4 mmHg (= 0 – 0.5 kPa). The pressure difference for the systemic circulation is thus about 98 mmHg (= 13.0 kPa).

For a complete cycle, cardiac output is defined by:

$$CO = \frac{P_{art} - P_{ven}}{TPR} \tag{8.2}$$

CO = cardiac output, MAP = mean arterial blood pressure, CVP = central venous pressure and TPR = total peripheral resistance.

According to the **continuity principle**, the volumetric flow rate is the same in every region of the vascular system.

$$I = A_{CrossSection} \cdot \bar{v} \tag{8.3}$$

with $A_{CrossSection}$ = vessel cross-section area,
$\bar{v}$ = mean flow velocity

Flow resistance (R) can be determined according to the law of Ohm, as the quotient of pressure difference (Δp) and flow rate (I):

$$R = \frac{\Delta p}{I} \tag{8.4}$$

The **total resistance** (R_{total}) for **resistors connected in series** is equal to the sum of the respective individual resistances (**1st rule of Kirchhoff**):

$$R_{total} = R_1 + R_2 + R_3 + \text{etc.} \tag{8.5}$$

The total flow resistance of a group of **blood vessels connected in parallel** is always smaller than the resistance of each individual vessel, since the total cross-sectional area of the circuit increases. In the case of vessels connected in parallel, such as within organs or when divided into various organ circuits, the reciprocal **value of the total resistance** is equal to the sum of the **reciprocal values of the partial resistances** or the sum of the **conductivities** (since the reciprocal value of a resistance is the conductivity; **2nd rule of Kirchhoff**):

$$\frac{1}{R_{total}} = \frac{1}{R_1} + \frac{1}{R_2} + \frac{1}{R_3} \text{ etc.} \tag{8.6}$$

or

$$R_{total} = \frac{1}{\frac{1}{R_1} + \frac{1}{R_2} + \frac{1}{R_3} \text{ etc.}} \tag{8.7}$$

The **Hagen-Poiseuille law** is a specification of the resistance in the law of Ohm to the conditions in a tube through which liquid flows:

$$I = \frac{r^4 \pi \Delta p}{8 \eta L} \tag{8.8}$$

r = radius of the vessels, Δp = pressure difference, η (eta) = viscosity, L = length of the vessel.

If $\Delta p/R$ (law of Ohm) is substituted for I in this equation, then

$$R = \frac{8 \eta L}{r^4 \pi} \tag{8.9}$$

Since the **radius** takes effect in its **4th power**, this means that for changes in flow rate, **small changes in the radius produce significant changes in resistance**. If the radius increases by 20 %, this will cause an increase in flow rate to more than double the initial value. These radius changes occur mainly in the region of the arterioles.

However, the application of the Hagen-Poiseuille law to blood circulation and to haemodynamics has some restrictions, as this law applies to **rigid tubes**. Blood vessels, however, are flexible. This law applies also only to **uniform** and **laminar flow**, whereas blood flows in arteries in a pulsating manner and turbulence can occur.

> **IN A NUTSHELL** !
>
> The total resistance of a blood vessel changes to the 4th power of the vessel radius. Therefore, very small changes in the radius have very large effects on the total resistance, and thus on blood pressure and/or on flow rate, analogous to the law of Ohm.

8.3.2   Characteristics of blood flow

Blood moves through a blood vessel at an average flow velocity. The **flow velocity** (measured e.g. in $cm \cdot s^{-1}$) depends on the flow rate and the cross-sectional area of the vessels through which the blood is moving. The following equation describes the relationship between mean flow velocity ($\bar{v}$), flow rate (I) and the cross-sectional area ($A_{Cross\,Section}$) of the tube. The average flow velocity in a tube corresponds to the quotient of the flow rate and the cross-sectional area of the tube:

$$\bar{v} = \frac{I}{A_{CrossSection}} \tag{8.10}$$

From this it follows for vessels with a circular cross-section that

$$I = \bar{v} \cdot A_{CrossSection} = \bar{v} \cdot r^2 \cdot \pi \tag{8.11}$$

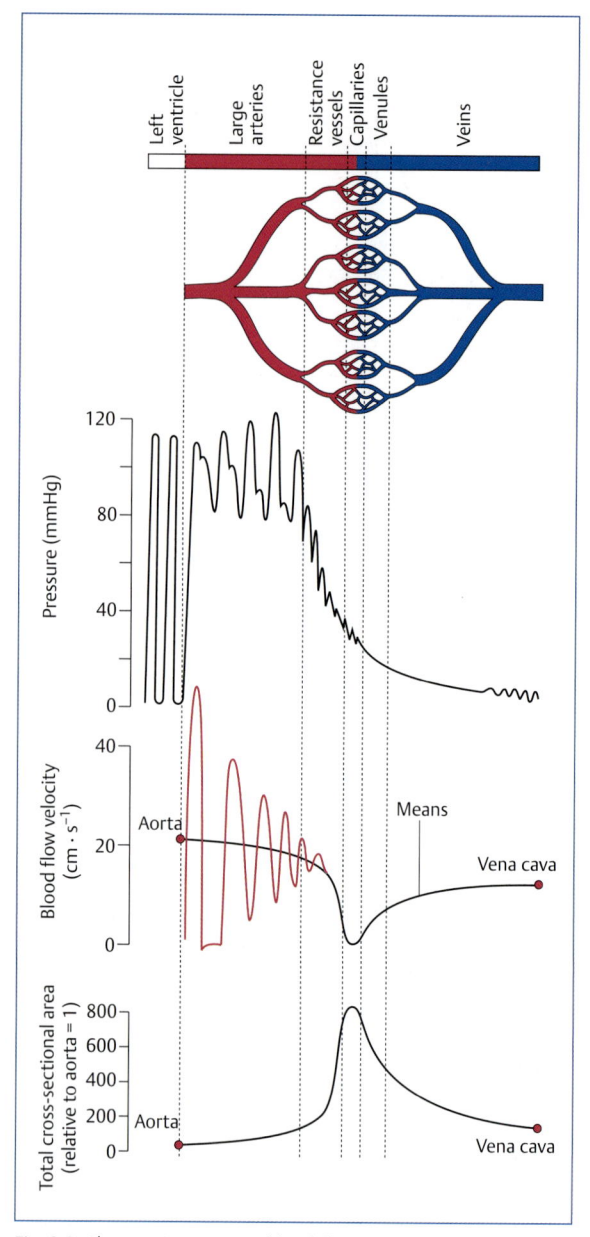

Fig. 8.3 Changes in pressure, blood flow velocity and total cross-sectional area of the vessels in the different sections of the systemic circulation. The flow velocity is inversely proportional to the total cross-sectional area of the vessels. The flow velocity of blood is highest in the arteries and veins and lowest in the capillaries. The total cross-sectional area is highest in the capillaries.

If the total cross-sectional area in individual vessel sections changes, with blood flowing at a constant flow rate, the flow velocity changes with these changes in cross-sectional area. With frequent branching in the capillary beds, the total cross-sectional area increases considerably, and thus the flow velocity in the capillaries is very low (**Fig. 8.3**). The average flow velocity in the aorta is about 300 times greater than in the capillaries (**Table 8.1**).

> **IN A NUTSHELL** !
>
> Blood flows more slowly in vessel regions with larger total cross-sectional areas.

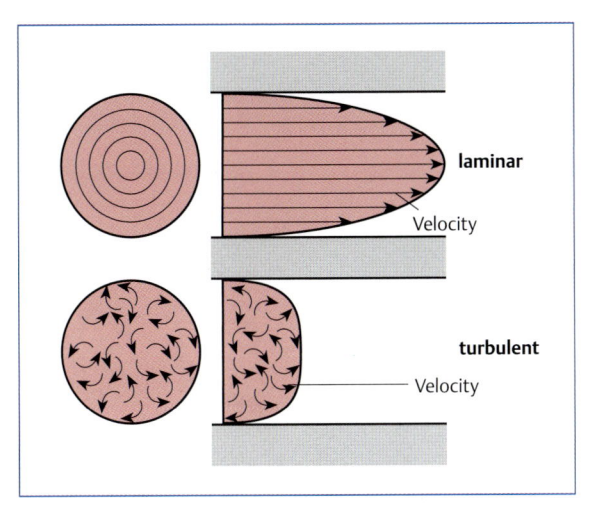

Fig. 8.4 Velocity profiles in laminar and turbulent flow.

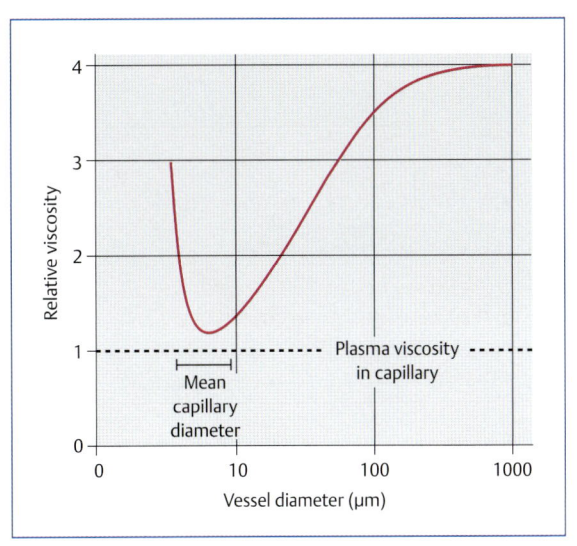

Fig. 8.5 Dependence of the relative viscosity of blood (plasma viscosity = 1) on vessel diameter. In small blood vessels, the viscosity of blood decreases with decreasing vessel diameter and reaches a minimum at a diameter of 4–10 μm (Fåhraeus-Lindquist-Effect). [Source: Klinke R, Pape HC, Silbernagl S. Physiologie. 5th ed., Stuttgart: Thieme; 2005: 191]

Laminar flow: In blood vessels further away from the heart, all particles in a fluid move parallel to the vessel axis. Axial flow in the centre has the highest flow velocity. The fluid immediately adjacent to the wall does not move at all. The result is a parabolic velocity profile (**Fig. 8.4**). This also means that the **shear stress** is not the same across the cross-section area of the vessel. Shear stress has the dimension of a pressure, it is a force per unit area with the force acting along the area. In blood vessels, it is the force that is necessary in laminar flow to move the individual imaginary fluid layers (**Fig. 8.4**) against each other. In the centre of the vessel, shear stress is close to zero, at the vessel wall it is very high. Shear stress leads to the displacement of the individual liquid layers against each other. The viscosity of the liquid determines the speed of the displacement.

In **turbulent flow**, the average fluid movement is slower for the same pressure difference. Vortices are generated and thus energy is lost. Fluid and blood corpuscles no longer move only parallel to the vessel axis, but also transversely to that axis (**Fig. 8.4**). Only in laminar flow is there a linear relationship between volumetric flow rate and pressure difference for a vessel with a constant cross-sectional area (law of Ohm). This law no longer applies in **turbulent flow** because vortices form with a consequent additional loss of energy. The transition from laminar to turbulent flow depends on the diameter of the vessels ($2r$), the mean flow velocity ($\bar{v}$), the density (ρ) and the viscosity (η) of the fluid. The dimensionless **Reynolds number** (Re) combines these quantities:

$$Re = \frac{2r\bar{v}\rho}{\eta} \qquad (8.12)$$

If the Reynolds number in a bloodstream exceeds a critical value of 2000–2200, laminar flow changes into a turbulent flow. The Reynolds number in the aorta, and also in the pulmonary artery, during the ejection phase are considerably greater than this critical value, especially in large mammals. This means that turbulent flow occurs in these vessels for a short time, even under physiological conditions. However, increased flow velocities occur mainly in

conditions of vascular stenoses and valvular insufficiencies. The turbulence that then occurs gives rise to murmurs on auscultation, which are important for diagnosis of these conditions.

8.3.3 Viscosity of the blood

The Hagen-Poiseuille law (p. 194) is only valid for so-called **Newtonian fluids** (e.g. water, oil), where their viscosity depends only on temperature. **Blood**, however, is a **non-homogeneous suspension of blood cells in blood plasma**. The non-homogeneous non-Newtonian fluid, blood, has a variable viscosity, which is referred to as its **apparent viscosity**. For example, with decreasing **flow velocity** and thus decreasing shear stress, the apparent blood viscosity increases significantly. This is due, among other things, to the formation of **erythrocyte aggregates ("rouleaux")** in small blood vessels.

Furthermore, the viscosity of blood depends on the **diameter of the vessels through which it flows** (Fig. 8.5). For small vessels with a diameter of less than 300 μm, the apparent viscosity of blood decreases with decreasing vessel diameter (**Fåhraeus-Lindquist effect**). This can be explained by the deformability of erythrocytes. A relatively cell-poor marginal zone is formed, which serves as a low-viscosity sliding layer for the locomotion of the central cell column (see ch. Erythrocytes (p. 227)).

Circulation, respiration

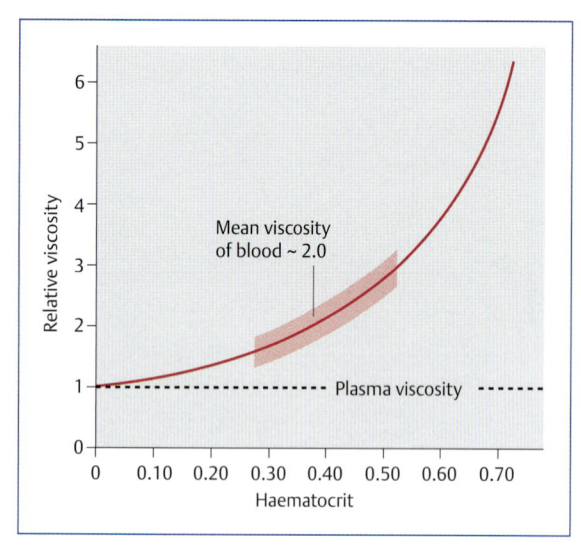

Fig. 8.6 Dependence of the relative viscosity of blood on haematocrit (plasma viscosity=1). Reference values for haematocrit in domestic animals see **Table 9.5**.

The apparent blood viscosity depends on the **haematocrit** (**Fig. 8.6**). The higher the haematocrit and the higher the plasma protein concentration, the more viscous the blood. Unlike blood, however, blood plasma is a Newtonian fluid with viscosity dependent on temperature. In discussions about the flow behaviour of blood, we therefore often speak of the **relative viscosity**, which is the apparent blood viscosity divided by the plasma viscosity.

> **MORE DETAILS**   By releasing locally stored erythrocytes, the spleen of horses (and also llamas) can augment the haematocrit in blood by up to 60% of the resting values (p.626). In domestic ruminants, and dogs and cats, this change in haematocrit is lower after release of erythrocytes from the spleen. The rise in haematocrit, and thus the increase in haemoglobin concentration, has the advantage for horses in that O_2 supply to the working muscles can be considerably increased. Likewise, llamas can avoid hypoxia in their tissues through increased haemoglobin concentrations even at the low O_2 partial pressures at high altitudes. On the other hand, these increased haematocrit levels have the disadvantage that they augment both the viscosity of blood and also the peripheral resistance. As a result, the demands on the heart are high. Nevertheless, the well-trained heart of racing horses can cope with this considerable additional load.

> **IN A NUTSHELL**   !
>
> The viscosity of blood is not a constant. It increases with increasing haematocrit and decreasing flow velocity, and it decreases with decreasing vessel diameter in the very small blood vessels.

8.3.4   Compliance of the blood vessels

Considering the passive mechanical behaviour of the vessel walls, the quantity and structural arrangement of the smooth musculature is only one of the relevant factors. The **compliance** of the elastic and the collagenous fibres in the media and the adventitia is also of great importance (**Fig. 8.2**). In the large arteries close to the heart, elasticity

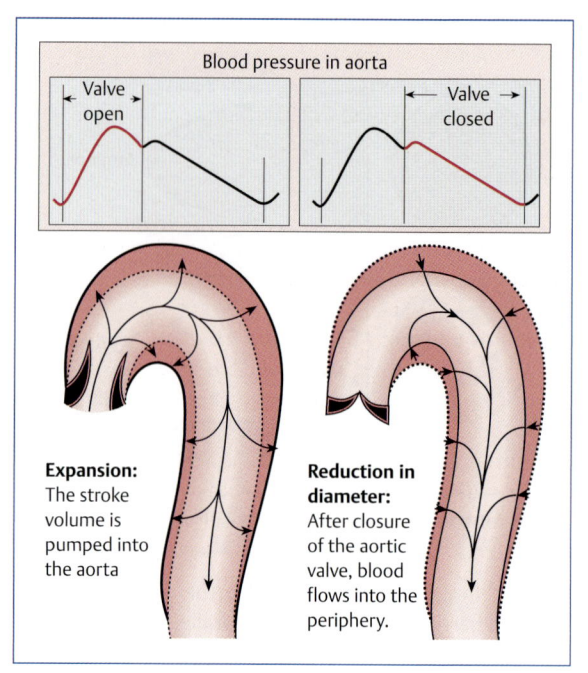

Fig. 8.7 Windkessel effect of the aorta. The increasing pressure during the expulsion of the stroke volume leads to passive (exaggeratedly drawn) dilation of the aorta (left side of the picture). The stored blood volume continues to flow into the periphery of the circulation after the aortic valve closes (right side of the picture). The Windkessel function extends over the entire aorta and the large arteries in which there are also many elastic fibres. [Source: Klinke R, Pape HC, Silbernagl S. Physiologie. 5th ed., Stuttgart: Thieme; 2005]

in the vessel walls is well developed. This elasticity decreases with increasing distance from the heart. Due to the rise in pressure generated by the heart during systole, the lumen diameter of blood vessels close to the heart is increased and their wall is stretched (**Windkessel function**; **Fig. 8.1**; **Fig. 8.7**; **Fig. 8.19**). Part of the stroke volume is retained by this **vascular expansion**, and a part of the kinetic energy is converted into potential energy by stretching of elastic fibres in the vessel walls of the aorta and large arteries (**Fig. 8.7**, left side). After closure of the aortic valve, the elastic fibres shorten again during diastole. The kinetic energy is converted to mechanical work so that the stored volume flows further into the periphery of the circulation (**Fig. 8.7** right-hand side). The Windkessel function results in a **low blood pressure amplitude** and a **more continuous flow** of blood. The more rigid the wall of the large arteries, the lower is the Windkessel effect, and the greater are both blood pressure amplitude and mechanical stress on the heart, which has to perform greater acceleration work.

> **MORE DETAILS**
>
> **Windkessel (function)** A Windkessel is a gas-filled container that is required for storage of fluid and to compensate for pressure fluctuations. Every piston pump at a water well, used to have such an air vessel. The gas in the air chamber is compressed with each piston stroke. Between the piston strokes, the air expands again, so that there is a continuous flow of water from the pipe despite the intermittent increase in pressure. The diaphragm pressure tanks of heating systems also have such a Windkessel function.

The state of distension of a vessel is determined by its **distensibility** and by the transmural pressure. The difference between intravascular and extravascular pressure is the **transmural pressure** (p_t). Since the extravascular pressure (tissue pressure) is very low, the intravascular pressure in the arteries is usually approximately that of the transmural pressure. Exceptions are the vascular systems in the myocardium of the left ventricle and to some extent also in skeletal muscle, where considerable tissue pressures occur during muscle contractions. The result is that during systole, and also during contraction of skeletal muscle, a decrease in the vessel diameter and even a complete vessel collapse can occur (see ch. Energetics of the heart (p. 180) and Flow velocity pulse in the arteries (p. 201)). There is also considerable extravascular pressure fluctuations in the veins (p. 202) of the thoracic region, and thus altered filling of the vessels (p. 212) can occur during the respiratory cycle (see ch. elastic respiratory resistances (p. 270)). The greater the transmural pressure, the greater the strain on the vessel walls. To quantify these stresses, the term wall tension is used. Wall tension (T) is defined as the force per unit area. In addition to the transmural pressure (p_t), the wall tension also depends on the radius (r) of the vessel and the thickness of the vessel wall (d). The modified **Laplace's law** reads:

$$T = \frac{p_t \cdot r}{2d} \tag{8.13}$$

MORE DETAILS For example, the vessel diameter increases in the case of a pathological vascular dilation (**aneurysm**). When the vessel wall does not become thicker, vascular ruptures can occur. Since systolic blood pressure rises during hard physical work, racehorses with an existing thin-walled aneurysm occasionally suffer sudden vascular ruptures during a race, and thus bleed to death quickly.

The passive distension properties of individual vascular sections are described by their **compliance** (C) (distensibility, elastic distensibility). It is defined as the ratio of a change in volume (ΔV) to the corresponding change in transmural pressure (Δp):

$$C = \frac{\Delta V}{\Delta p} = \frac{1}{\acute{E}} \tag{8.14}$$

In a similar way to pulmonary compliance, vascular compliance (C) is also measured by pressure-induced volume

changes. The **volume elasticity coefficient (É), which is the reciprocal value of compliance**, is also frequently used in the assessment of distensibility (É). É is small for large distensibility and vice versa:

$$\acute{E} = \frac{\Delta p}{\Delta V} \tag{8.15}$$

8.4 Haemodynamics in the individual vascular systems

Wolfgang von Engelhardt

8.4.1 The arterial system

■ Pulse pressure (pulse wave) and blood pressure

The rhythmic pumping action of the heart resulting in a rise in blood pressure in the downstream vessels, generates a wave of pressure change, the **pulse pressure** or **pulse wave**. This is accompanied by a pulsatile change in volumetric flow rate. This wave propagates in the direction of the capillaries. The pulse wave travels much faster than the blood volume itself.

Parallel to the increase in pressure during systole, there is an expansion of the vessel. The resulting changes in cross-sectional area of an artery largely correspond to the course of the pressure curve. This expansion of the vascular wall is palpated as a **pulse** during clinical examination.

The **pulse pressure** is caused by the stroke volume being pumped into the blood-filled aorta. Due to inertia, blood in the aorta resists acceleration. There is an increase in pressure that remains localised. Due to the rapid rise in pressure during systole, the elastic fibres (p. 196) in the wall of the aorta and in the large arteries near the heart are stretched. This **Windkessel function** in the aorta and the large arteries leads, in accordance with the elasticity of the vessel walls, to a dampening of the pulsation of blood pressure and to a more continuous flow of blood along the aorta and the large and medium-sized arteries (**Fig. 8.8**).

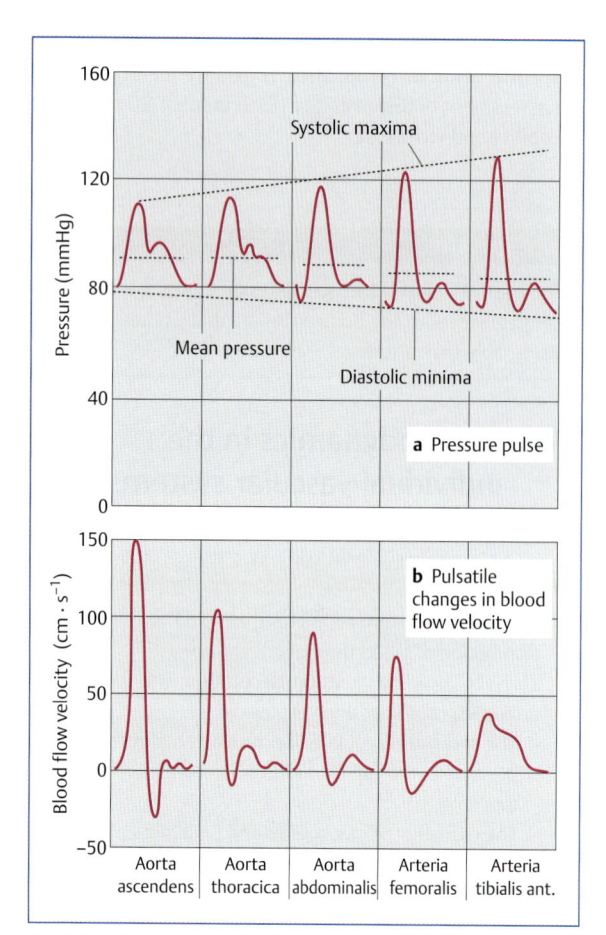

Fig. 8.8 Pulse pressure and pulsative changes in blood flow velocity along the aorta and the great and middle-sized arteries. The increase in pressure amplitude (**a**, upper drawing) is a result of the increase in systolic pressure and the small decrease in diastolic pressure. The mean pressure drops only slightly along these arteries. The strong pulsatile behaviour of flow velocity in the ascending aorta decreases with increasing distance from the aortic valve (**b**, lower drawing). [Source: Klinke R, Pape HC, Silbernagl S. Physiologie. 5th ed., Stuttgart: Thieme; 2005]

As a wave, this pulse pressure travels along the arterial walls away from the heart towards the periphery. Its velocity of propagation is the **pulse wave velocity**. It amounts to **$5–6\,m \cdot s^{-1}$** in the **vessels near the heart** and increases to over **$30\,m \cdot s^{-1}$** in the **peripheral arteries**. This increase in pulse wave velocity towards the periphery can be explained by the decreasing elasticity of the peripheral arteries.

> **IN A NUTSHELL**   !
>
> Pulse wave velocities must not be confused with the much slower pulsating changes in flow velocity (p. 201).

MORE DETAILS Due to the lower elasticity of the aorta and arteries in **older animals** as well as in older people, less of the kinetic energy expended by the heart can be stored there during systole. The difference between systolic and diastolic blood pressure (blood pressure amplitude) and also the pulse wave velocity are therefore usually higher. Consequently, the flow velocity is also greater in older animals.

In different arterial regions, the **pulse pressure** differs depending on the anatomical location (**Fig. 8.8 a**). In the arteries close to the heart, such as the ascending aorta, an **incisura** is present. This is because shortly before and during the closing of the aortic valves, there is a brief backflow of blood before the aortic valves close completely. This causes a momentary drop in pressure, followed by a rise. This incisura is not apparent in vessels far from the heart. It should be noted that the **pulse pressure maximum**, and also the amplitude of the **pulse pressure** in the arteries, both increase with increasing distance from the heart. There are two reasons for this phenomenon:

- Because of the decreasing elasticity of the arterial walls towards the peripheral circulation, less of the kinetic energy produced by the heart is able to be stored there.
- The pressure waves are **reflected** in the peripheral branches so that forward and backward pressures are combined.

> **IN A NUTSHELL**   !
>
> Pressure and volumetric flow rate in the arterial system show characteristic pulsations, the shape and amplitude of which are determined by the distensibility (Windkessel effect) of the vessel walls.

Arterial blood pressure in the systemic circulation

In systole, a maximum arterial pressure of 120–140 mmHg, called the systolic pressure, is produced in the circulation of most domestic animals (**Table 8.2**). The minimum pulse pressure before the start of the next systolic rise is the **diastolic pressure**. The difference between the two is the **blood pressure amplitude**. Superimposed on these rhythmic pressure changes between systolic maximum and diastolic minimum are higher-ordered rhythmic changes in blood pressure (see ch. Blood pressure fluctuations at rest (p. 201)).

MORE DETAILS Blood pressure amplitude can increase above normal values, when there is reduced compliance (distensibility of the arterial walls), in old age, when there is arteriosclerosis, and in aortic valve insufficiency, because of backflow of blood into the heart. It is lower in aortic valve stenosis. Blood pressure amplitude, and also mean blood pressure, can both increase, without a change in heart rate, if either stroke volume or total peripheral resistance are increased.

Mean arterial blood pressure is determined by integrating the pulse pressure curve over time. It is not exactly the arithmetic mean of the systolic and diastolic blood pressures, but is somewhat lower due to the shape of the pressure curve. The resting blood pressure is about the same in the various domestic mammals. In laboratory animals, however, the resting blood pressures are usually somewhat lower (**Table 8.2**). It is interesting to note that arterial pressure is significantly higher in birds. Very old domestic animals, in a similar way to older humans, have higher mean and higher systolic blood pressures than younger animals because of reduced elasticity of the arterial walls.

Table 8.2 Mean resting blood pressure in the arteries of the systemic circulation at heart level in domestic animals, laboratory animals, birds and giraffe (averaged values).

	Systolic blood pressure (mmHg)	Diastolic blood pressure (mmHg)	Mean blood pressure (mmHg)
Domestic mammals	120–140	80–95	95–107
Rabbit, guinea Pig, rat, mouse	100–110	60–70	80–90
Birds	175–250	145–170	160–190
Giraffe	260	160	219

Source: Swenson MJ, Reece WO. Duke's Physiology of Domestic Animals. 11th ed., Ithaca, London: Cornell University Press; 1993
1 mmHg = 133.3 Pa

> **IN A NUTSHELL** !
>
> Mean arterial blood pressure at rest in the large and medium-sized arteries in domestic and laboratory animals is similar to that in humans.

When comparing blood pressure data, it is important that the arterial blood pressure is measured at the level of the heart. In the legs and in the raised head, the respective hydrostatic pressure caused by gravity must be added or subtracted. For example, with a mean blood pressure at heart level of 95 mmHg, the upright person has a pressure of about 180 mmHg in the arteries of the feet and 70 mmHg in the arteries of the head.

MORE DETAILS One explanation for the higher blood pressure in birds could be the nucleated erythrocytes, which are on average larger than in mammals Table 9.5) and perhaps also the nucleated thrombocytes. Therefore, deformability of these cells in birds could be lower, so that comparatively higher blood pressure is required to enable blood to flow through capillaries.

A special situation applies to giraffes (**Fig. 8.9**). Mean blood pressure at heart level of the giraffe is about 215 mmHg. This high pressure is necessary so that a mean blood pressure of 65 mmHg can still be achieved in the head of a 4.5 m high animal.

Arterial walls in giraffes are unusually thick to withstand this high pressure. If giraffes suddenly lower their heads to drink water, pressure in the cranial arteries would be expected to rise to very high levels. However, valves in the large neck veins prevent venous blood from flowing back into the head when the head is lowered. This prevents excessive hydrostatic pressure in brain capillaries. In addition, it is assumed that a network of elastic blood vessels, close to the brain, can retain blood when pressure rises, and this contributes to relieving the pressure.

Arterial pressure in the pulmonary circulation

The systolic pressure in the pulmonary arteries varies between 20 and 40 mmHg (hence the so-called **low-pressure system** when pressure is < 30 mmHg). The diastolic pressure is between 10 and 20 mmHg (**Fig. 8.10**). In cattle, horses and pigs, slightly higher values have usually been found (on average about 26 mmHg) than in humans, dogs, cats and small ruminants. The resistance in the pulmonary arterioles is low. The flow velocity of the blood in the pulmonary capillaries is high and the contact time in these capillaries is short, especially when cardiac output increases during physical work (**Fig. 11.25**).

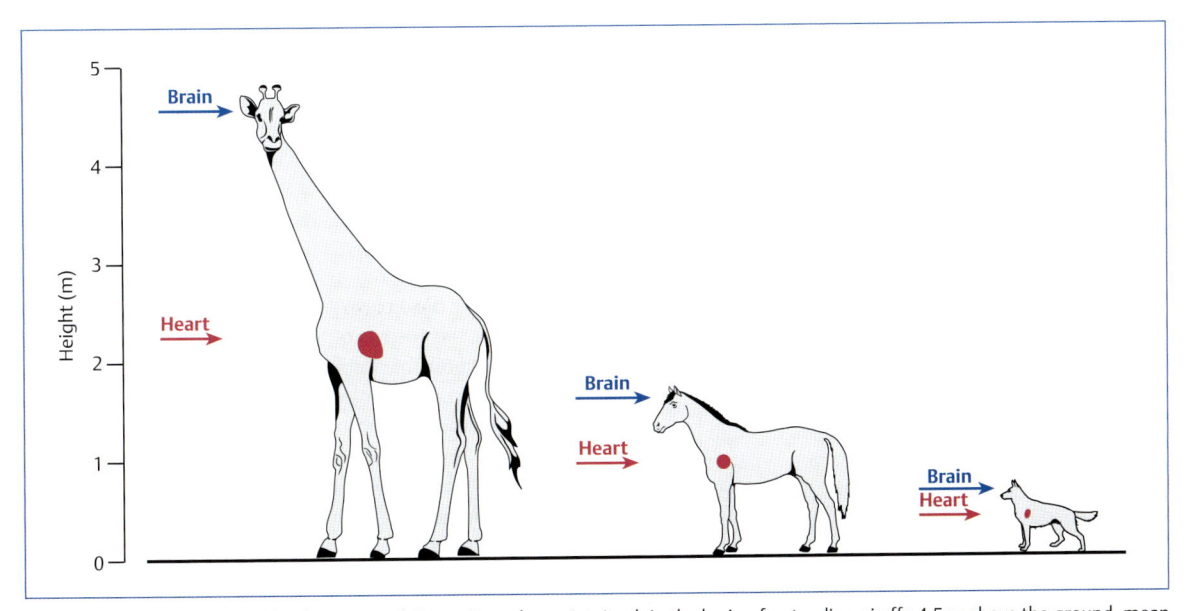

Fig. 8.9 In order for a mean blood pressure of 60 mmHg to be maintained, in the brain of a standing giraffe 4.5 m above the ground, mean blood pressure, at heart level, must be about 220 mmHg. For a horse or dog, a mean blood pressure at heart level of about 100 mmHg is sufficient to ensure cerebral perfusion.

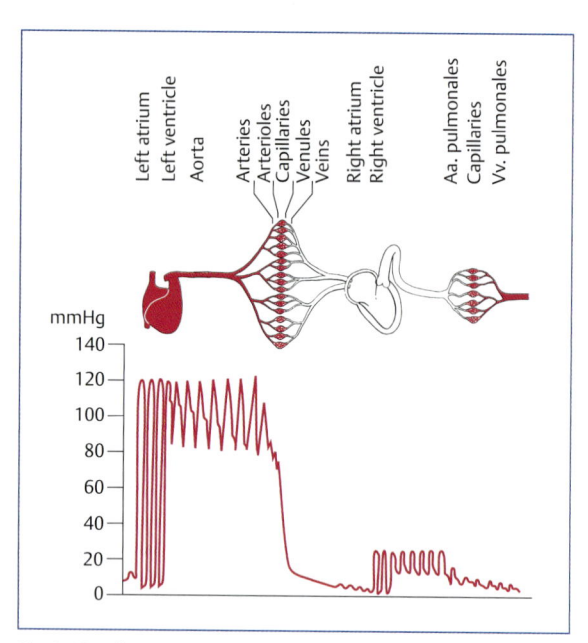

Fig. 8.10 Schematic representation of blood pressure in the systemic and pulmonary circulation of a domestic animal.

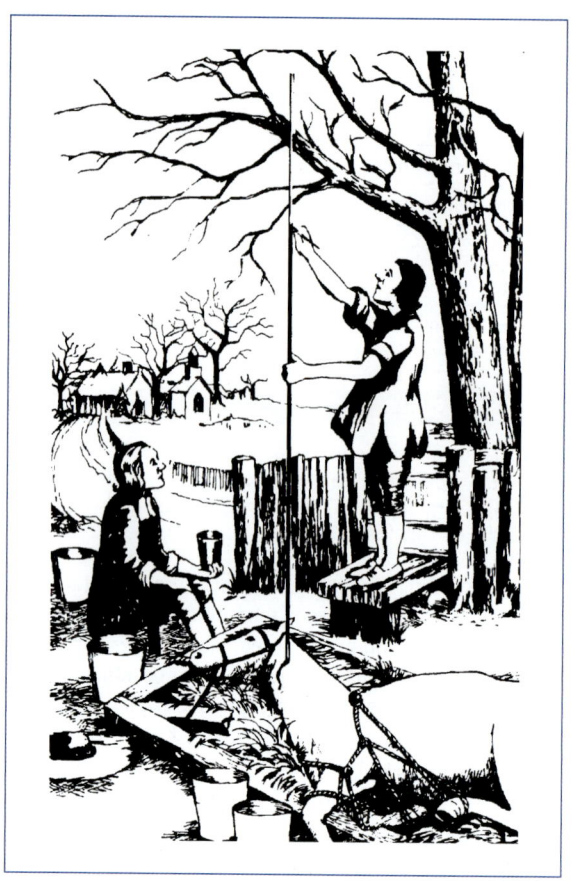

Fig. 8.11 Stephen Hales (1677–1761) made the first direct measurement of blood pressure in animals in 1728. He measured the height of the blood column in a vertical glass tube. [Source: Hall WD. Stephen Hales: Theologist, Botanist, Physiologist, Discoverer of Hemodynamics. Clin Cardiol 1987; 10: 487-489]

> **IN A NUTSHELL**   !
>
> The blood pressure in the pulmonary artery is much lower than in the aorta. The resistance in the pulmonary arterioles is low.

Blood pressure measurement

After inserting a cannula into an artery, systolic and diastolic pressure can be measured with a pressure gauge (**direct method**). This invasive method is very accurate. However, it is reserved for special situations, such as monitoring animals under anaesthesia.

> **MORE DETAILS**   Historically, it is interesting to note that the first blood pressure measurement was carried out on a horse by Stephen Hales in 1728. The height of the blood column was measured in a glass tube connected to the carotid artery (**Fig. 8.11**).

In humans, blood pressure is generally recorded using the clinically common **indirect method** (according to **Riva-Rocci**). A cuff placed around the upper arm is inflated until the cuff pressure exceeds the expected systolic pressure. The pressure is then slowly released. At a cuff pressure between the systolic and the diastolic pressure, characteristic sounds (**Korotkoff sounds**) are heard when the artery distal to the cuff is auscultated at the same time. These sounds are caused by **turbulent blood flow**. When the cuff pressure is high, initially no blood flows through the compressed artery. The turbulence occurs when the blood flows very quickly through the still partially compressed vessel for a short time when the cuff pressure is released. The first occurrence of the **sound marks the time when the systolic blood pressure can be read on the manometer**. As the cuff pressure continues to decrease, the Korotkoff sounds initially become louder. Eventually they be-

come duller and quieter, and then they disappear. This is the sign that the turbulent flow through the periodically constricted vessel is now changing into the laminar flow of the permanently open vessel. The pressure read at the time when the Korotkoff sounds disappear, is the **diastolic blood pressure** (Fig. 8.12).

Indirect blood pressure measurements are less satisfactory in domestic animals than in humans. Because of anatomical limitations, Korotkoff sounds cannot always be reliably perceived during a blood pressure measurement in domestic animals. Hypertension and hypotension are increasingly encountered as diseases in small animal practice. For the diagnosis of cardiovascular diseases, when monitoring the success of therapy and during anaesthesia, a simple and reliable indirect blood pressure measurement would be of considerable help. Various methods of indirect blood pressure measurement have therefore been repeatedly tested in animals. The most frequently used (but unfortunately not always with satisfactory results) is the **oscillatory method**. Here the cuff is applied to the forelimb (dog, cat, rabbit, pig) or to the hindlimb (dog) and also to the root of the tail (horse, pig, dog). The cuff is inflated. The cuff pressure is then slowly released. When the systolic pressure is reached, the arteries under the cuff fill increasingly and some blood begins to flow through the artery

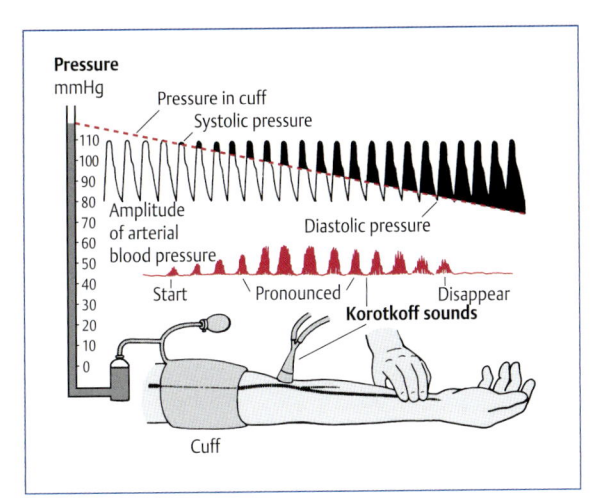

Fig. 8.12 Indirect blood pressure measurement according to Riva-Rocci. Murmurs (Korotkoff sounds) occur when the cuff pressure falls below the systolic blood pressure. They disappear when the blood pressure falls below the diastolic blood pressure.

that is still closed during most time of the pressure wave. The resulting pressure fluctuations at the arterial wall are registered by the cuff as oscillations. The cuff pressure at the beginning of this oscillation is considered the **systolic blood pressure**. The oscillations then increase as the cuff pressure continues to decrease. Finally, the oscillations disappear when the cuff pressure no longer compresses the arteries under the cuff, which is the **diastolic blood pressure**. However, variation in these measurements is usually large. It is therefore recommended to determine an average value from several measurements.

Occasionally, **Doppler sonography** is also used when measuring blood pressure. Here the detector is fixed distally to the cuff. This makes it possible to record the resumption of blood flow when the pressure is slowly released from the cuff. This is then the **systolic blood pressure**. Diastolic pressure cannot be measured with this method.

Blood pressure fluctuations at rest

The characteristic time-dependent changes in the **pulse pressure** caused by cardiac activity (**Fig. 8.7**) and the spatial differences in different arterial sites (**Fig. 8.8 a**) have already been pointed out. These periodic fluctuations between the systolic maximum and the diastolic minimum are finally caused by the heart, i.e. the rhythmic change between systole and diastole.

In addition, there are **Traube-Hering waves** that are caused by respiration. They are, therefore, synchronous with respiratory movement. Only a brief explanation is given here, as it is discussed in more detail in the chapters on respiration, venous return and blood pressure (p.203) and special features of the pulmonary circulation (p.213). During deep **inspiration**, the pressure in the thoracic cavity is reduced (**Fig. 11.15**). As a result, more blood is drawn from the veins of the abdominal cavity into the right atrium and the right ventricle. Due to the increased end-diastolic filling of the right ventricle, the **stroke volume of**

the right heart increases via the Frank-Starling mechanism (p. 170). Consequently, the blood pressure in the pulmonary artery rises during inspiration. This is different in the **systemic circulation**. During deep inspiration, blood is retained in the pulmonary vessels. The **backflow of blood** to the **left heart** and the resulting wall tension of the myocardium (preload) is reduced. This results in a lower end-diastolic filling of the left ventricle. Consequently, there is a slight fall in the systolic blood pressure and also the mean blood pressure in the systemic circulation. At the peripheral arteries, these changes are recorded as Traube-Hering waves. During the subsequent **expiration**, the conditions are reversed.

In addition, **Mayer waves** are observed at rest. These are periodic fluctuations of blood pressure occurring at intervals of about 20–40 seconds. They are due to **vegetative tonus changes**. The activities of the sympathetic and parasympathetic nervous system, via the **control circuit** for short-term blood pressure regulation (**Fig. 8.22**), are continuously adjusted within the setpoint values with a certain time delay. Thus, there is a slight, rhythmic change in blood pressure.

In addition, there are diurnal **fluctuations**, whereby the arterial blood pressure of diurnal animals is lower at night than during the day.

Blood pressure at work

With increasing workload, **systolic blood pressure** rises, but diastolic pressure changes little or not at all compared to its resting values. The strong vasodilation and the resulting decrease in peripheral resistance in the working muscles, is the reason why the **diastolic pressure** remains relatively constant. With increasing fatigue, and also with increasing thermoregulatory heat production, the diastolic pressure can then often fall due to increased dilation. The blood pressure amplitude increases with exertion, since with rising cardiac output proportionally less energy can be stored in the vessels of the lungs. **Fig. 26.15** shows the blood pressure changes with increasing running speeds of sport horses.

Blood pressure increases also during fight or flight, mating, or feeding.

■ Pulsation of flow velocity (pulsating blood flow) in arteries

In the discussion of pulse pressure (p.197), the arterial **blood flow velocity pulse**, i.e. rhythmic changes in blood flow velocity caused by volume displacement, has already been mentioned. The velocity pulses (or flow waves) result from the passage of blood into the ascending aorta during the ejection phase of the left ventricle. The flow rate and thus also the blood flow velocity reach their maximum in the first third of systole and then drop sharply (**Fig. 8.8 b**). The area above the zero line of the flow velocity pulse in the aorta corresponds to the stroke volume of the heart. At the end of systole, there is a brief reverse flow in the aorta towards the closing aortic valve (area below the zero line). As already mentioned, this is the cause of the incisura in the pulse pressure (**Fig. 8.8 a**). During the subsequent diastole, no blood flows in the ascending aorta and the flow velocity is approximately zero until the beginning of the next ejection phase.

It has also already been pointed out that the discontinuous pumping action of the heart in the large and middle arteries is increasingly dampened by the Windkessel function from central to peripheral. The amplitude of the flow pulse thus decreases towards the periphery (**Fig. 8.8 b**). In the capillaries, the flow is then practically continuous. The **flow velocity** of the blood in the individual vessels depends on the **total cross-section area** in each vascular bed (see ch. Flow, pressure, resistance (p. 193) – extended law of Ohm). In the large arteries, the **average flow velocity** in a medium-sized dog at rest is 10–20 cm·s^{-1}, in the medium and smaller arteries less than 10 cm·s^{-1}. Due to the large increase of the cross-sectional area in the capillary bed, the flow velocity drops to very low values (about 0.07 cm·s^{-1}; **Table 8.1**).

> ### IN A NUTSHELL   !
> The flow velocity of blood (velocity pulse) is much lower than that of the pulse wave (pulse wave velocity) which propagates at a higher speed. The flow velocity is only about 1/20 of the pulse wave velocity.

A special feature is the shape of the **flow velocity pulse** in the **coronary arteries** and the **blood flow rate in the myocardium**. During systole, the blood flow to the myocardium in the left ventricle drops to very low values, as the vessels in the myocardium of the left ventricle are compressed from the outside by the rising interstitial myocardial pressure during contraction. Even the capillaries are closed for a short time. The major part of the **blood flow** to the **left ventricular myocardium** occurs during **diastole** (!). Blood flow to the right ventricular myocardium is largely continuous because the pressure in the right ventricle is low.

> ### IN A NUTSHELL   !
> The myocardium of the left ventricle is mainly supplied with blood during diastole.

8.4.2 The venous system

The two main tasks of veins are the return flow of blood to the heart and the **storage** of a large **volume of blood** (**Fig. 8.13**). The **veins** are therefore also referred to as **capacity vessels** (**Fig. 8.19**).

> ### IN A NUTSHELL   !
> About 70% of total blood volume is in the veins.

It is important that a considerable part of this blood volume (p. 212) can be quickly made available to the circulation when needed (see ch. Special features of the pulmonary circulation (p. 213)). The venous pressure at the level

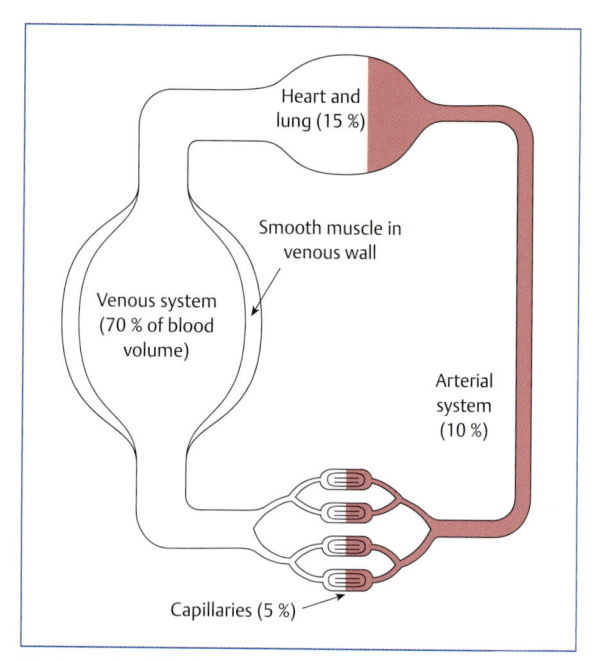

Fig. 8.13 Blood distribution in the systemic and pulmonary circulation. By far the largest proportion of total blood volume is in the veins. The veins are therefore the most important blood reservoirs.

of the heart is close to 0 mmHg. Due to gravity, the pressure values above the heart are even less than 0 mmHg. When the jugular vein is punctured with the head stretched upwards, air can therefore be aspirated through the cannula! 1.20 m below the heart, a venous pressure of 90 mmHg could be expected in standing cattle due to gravity. The **muscle pump**, the **respiratory pump** and the **atrioventricular plane displacement** drive venous **return to the right heart**. As a result, venous pressures in the limbs are usually lower than calculated on the basis of gravitational influence.

■ Muscle pump

The muscle pump makes an important contribution to venous return from the limbs. In most of the small and medium-sized veins of the body, **venous valves** are present at regular intervals. These valves prevent backflow of blood in the veins. In a standing animal or human, the venous valves subdivide the blood column segmentally. The resulting hydrostatic pressure in the veins of a limb may actually be much lower than the hydrostatic pressure calculated from the height of the blood column due to these valves. The veins are compressed by **contraction of** the **skeletal muscles**. Because of the valves, the blood thus flows towards the heart (**Fig. 8.14**).

> ### IN A NUTSHELL   !
> During physical activity, the muscle pump transports blood in the veins from segment to segment towards the heart through contractions of the skeletal muscles.

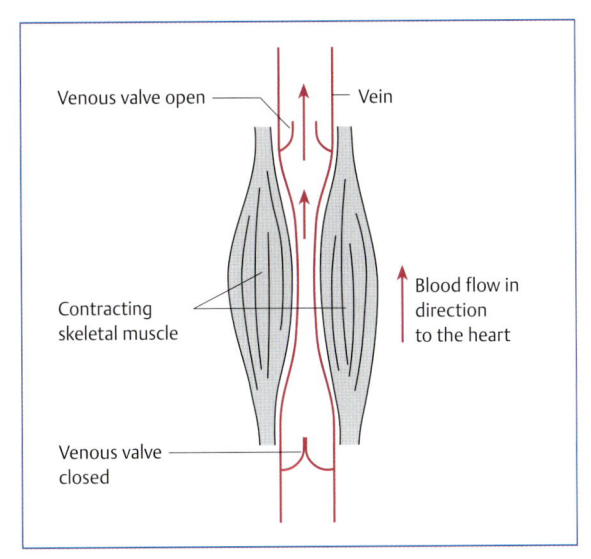

Fig. 8.14 Muscle pump. During contraction of skeletal muscle, the diameter of the veins is reduced; the venous pressure increases in this section of the vein. The venous valves cause blood to flow towards the heart.

In a very sedentary animal, however, there may be increased filling of the veins and thus a progressive opening of the venous valves. As a result, a continuous column of blood may eventually be produced, and the blood pressure in the lower part of the limbs then corresponds to the force of gravity. Due to this increased venous pressure, the pressure in the capillaries (p.204) is increased. Thus, the balance between capillary filtration and reabsorption is shifted towards increased filtration (Fig. 8.18). This is partly responsible for the formation of **oedema** in the lower parts of the limbs during prolonged standing. This is observed especially in stabled horses, when they have had insufficient exercise.

■ Respiration, venous return, and blood pressure

During **inspiration** the intrathoracic pressure falls. This dilates the intrathoracic veins and also the atria. The consequence is an increase in blood flow from the extrathoracic veins into the intrathoracic veins and into the right atrium. In addition, during inspiration, a contraction of the diaphragm increases abdominal pressure. This also results in increased **venous inflow** into the **thoracic veins**. During expiration, venous valves prevent blood from flowing back into the extrathoracic veins. The increased venous return during inspiration (**respiratory pump**) **improves** end-diastolic **filling** of the **right ventricle**. This increases the stroke volume of the right ventricle via the Frank-Starling mechanism (p.170) (Fig. 7.4). The augmented stroke volume **raises** the **pressure** in the **pulmonary artery**.

The effect of respiration on filling of the **left ventricle** is approximately **opposite** to that of the right heart. During inspiration, blood is retained in the lungs due to low thoracic pressure. As a result, the filling of the left ventricle is reduced and the arterial pressure in the systemic circulation decreases somewhat. During **expiration**, the filling in-

creases so that stroke volume and arterial blood pressure rise. These fluctuations in blood pressure (p.201) caused by breathing are called **Traube-Hering waves**.

■ Atrioventricular plane displacement

The rhythmic shifting of the atrioventricular valve plane (p.167) causes a reduction in pressure in the right atrium and adjacent vena cava during each ejection phase. This has a suction effect on the venous blood. At the onset of diastole, the atrioventricular valve plane shifts towards the blood-filled atria. Thus, the open AV valves dip rapidly into the atrial blood. This explains the rapid filling of the ventricles at the onset of diastole.

■ Venous pulse

The small pressure and diameter fluctuations in the veins close to the heart, which are characteristic of resting animals, are called the venous pulse (**Fig. 7.2f**). The **a-wave** is caused by atrial contraction. The **c-wave** that follows shortly after, is mainly a result of the tricuspid valve protruding into the right atrium during the isovolumetric contraction of the ventricles. The subsequent depression to a **minimum (x)** is caused by the shift of the atrioventricular valve plane during the ejection phase. During the isovolumetric relaxation of the ventricles, the pressure in the atrium and in the vena cava initially rises as long as the atrioventricular valve is still closed. When this valve opens, the pressure falls again because of blood inflow into the ventricle. Consequently, a positive wave, the **v-wave**, with a subsequent **depression (y)** occurs. As the ventricle continues to fill, the pressure gradually rises again until the next **a-wave**.

8.4.3 The microcirculation in the terminal vascular bed

The terminal vascular bed comprises the **arterioles**, the **capillaries** and the **venules** (Fig. 8.10; Fig. 8.15) as well as the drainage system of the lymphatic capillaries (p.207), ending blindly in the tissues. In individual organs, the structure of the terminal vascular bed is adapted to the specific needs of each organ.

■ Arterioles

Significant changes in resistance, which are essential for the regulation of organ perfusion in the systemic circulation, take place in the **arterioles** (**precapillary resistance vessels and sphincter vessels**) (Fig. 8.15; Fig. 8.19). In the vascular walls of arterioles, there are many circular layers of smooth muscle cells responsible for the resistance changes (p.208) (Fig. 8.2). The relative proportion of smooth muscle is greater in the wall of arterioles than in all other vessels (Fig. 8.2). In the pulmonary circulation (p.213), changes in resistance and also the possibilities for regulation are smaller and much less developed than in the systemic circulation.

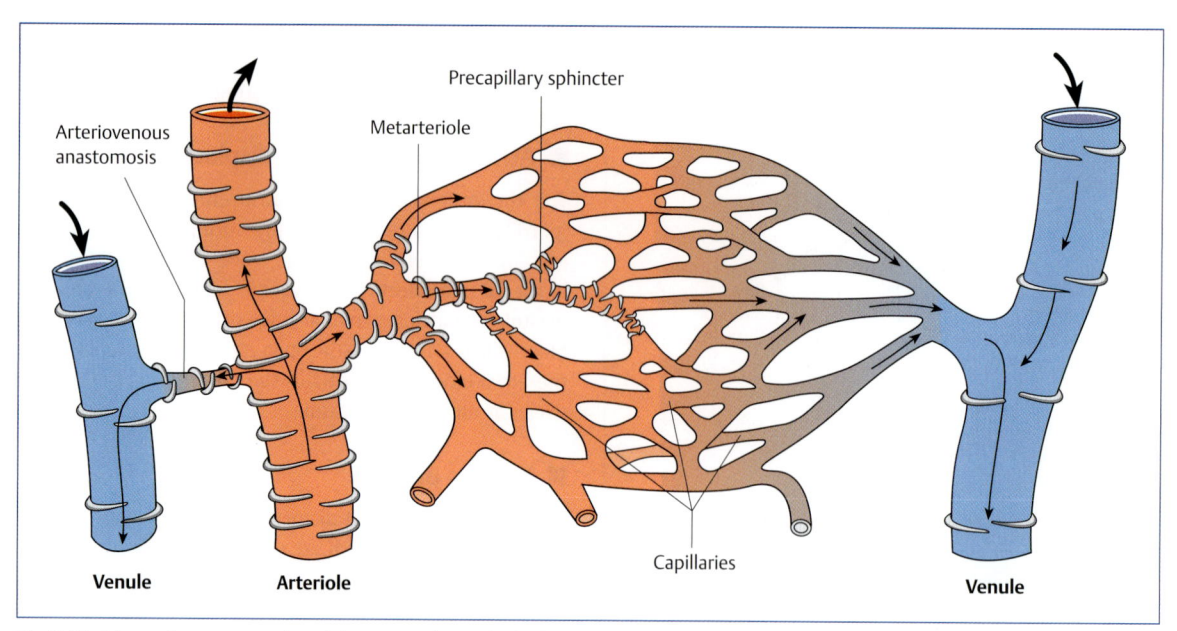

Fig. 8.15 Schematic representation of the terminal vascular bed with arterioles, capillaries and venules. The smooth musculature is shown by grey circles on the vascular walls. An example of an arteriovenous anastomosis (direct connection between arteriole and venule) is shown.

The **sphincter vessels** are blood vessels that have a closure mechanism consisting of smooth muscle cells arranged in a ring. By opening or closing sphincter vessels in the terminal region of the precapillary resistance vessels, the number of capillaries supplied with blood, and therefore the size of the capillary exchange surface, is regulated (**Fig. 8.15**; **Fig. 8.19**).

> **IN A NUTSHELL !**
>
> The arterioles are precapillary resistance vessels through which flow rate and blood pressure are tightly regulated.

■ Capillaries

The exchange of substances between blood and tissues takes place in the capillary bed of every organ. The wall of capillaries consists only of endothelial cells with a basement membrane (**Fig. 8.2**). In most organs, capillaries of the **continuous type** are present (**Fig. 8.16**). Small molecules (up to almost the size of plasma proteins) and especially lipid-soluble substances, can pass easily through the capillary endothelium. In the **brain capillaries** well-developed **tight junctions (zonulae occludentes)** are found between the endothelial cells. The **permeability of the brain capillaries** is therefore **low** (blood-brain barrier (p. 127)). In the glomeruli of the kidney (**Fig. 12.5**), but also in the intestinal mucosa and in some exocrine and endocrine glands, the **capillaries** are **fenestrated** (**Fig. 8.16**) containing passageways through the endothelium such as transendothelial cellular channels, pores or gaps. However, the basement membrane is still completely intact in this type of endothelium. The permeability of these fenestrated

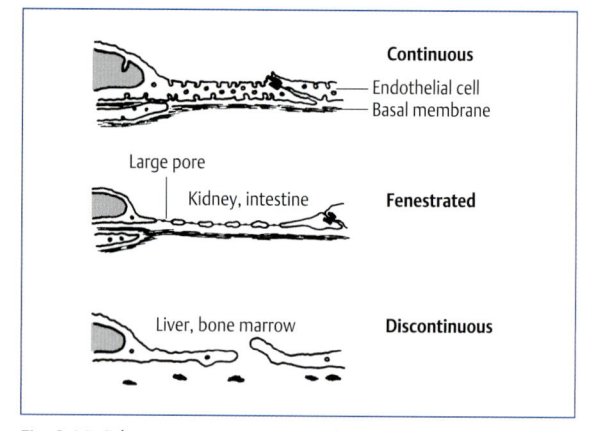

Fig. 8.16 Schematic representation of the three most important types of capillary endothelium.

capillaries is 100- to 1000-fold higher for small molecules than in continuous-type capillaries. In liver, spleen, and also in the bone marrow, the capillaries are discontinuous. In these **discontinuous capillaries** (**Fig. 8.16**), there are large inter- and intracellular gaps that also include the basement membrane. These capillaries allow the passage of proteins, other macromolecules and also corpuscular substances.

> **IN A NUTSHELL !**
>
> The most important barrier for the exchange of substances between the intra- and extravascular space is the vascular endothelium.

Solute exchange between blood and interstitial space

Exchange of solutes by diffusion

The exchange of solutes by diffusion is by far the main mechanism of transport across capillary walls. Very small, uncharged substances, which include the respiratory gases CO_2 and O_2, as well as lipid-soluble substances, can pass freely through the entire endothelial layer of the **capillary wall** and also in the **postcapillary venules**. For larger substances the **permeability** is considerably lower. Plasma proteins cannot leave the blood vessels, or only to a small extent. The exchange processes by diffusion can be extensive in the capillaries. This is demonstrated by the following estimate for humans, where, for all capillaries of the body, a diffusion exchange of 80000 litres of water and 20 kg of glucose takes place over 24 hours.

> **IN A NUTSHELL** !
>
> The exchange of solutes between blood and the interstitium takes place mainly by diffusion.

Distribution of fluid between blood and interstitium

Although the exchange of fluid through the capillary wall between blood and interstitial fluid is based mainly by diffusion, filtration and reabsorption processes are crucial for the **net movement of water**. **Filtration** and **reabsorption** in the capillaries depend on the **hydrostatic (Δp)** and **colloid-osmotic (oncotic) (Δπ) pressure differences**. The net outward movement is called **filtration**, the net inward movement is called **reabsorption**.

Effective filtration pressure

The net fluid transport through the capillary wall is determined by the **effective filtration pressure** (p_{eff}) between blood and the interstitial space. The effective filtration pressure results from the pressure differences between hydrostatic (Δp) and colloid-osmotic (Δπ) pressures taking into account the pressures in the capillary (p_{cap}) and those in the interstitial space (p_{inst}):

$$p_{eff} = \Delta p - \Delta \pi = \left(p_{cap} - p_{inst}\right) - \left(\pi_{cap} - \pi_{inst}\right) \tag{8.16}$$

Since the intravascular **hydrostatic pressure** is usually higher than the extravascular pressure in the interstitium, fluid would be constantly lost from blood through the capillary wall into the interstitium. The **colloid-osmotic pressure**, which is generated by proteins (p. 220) that are unable to pass through the capillary wall (or only pass to a very small extent), opposes this outward hydrostatic pressure, and thus water is retained.

The **colloid-osmotic pressure** does not change significantly throughout the capillary bed (mean values for $\pi_{cap} \approx$ 24 mmHg). However, the **hydrostatic pressure** falls from about 30 mmHg at the beginning of the capillary to about 19 mmHg at the end. Therefore, the effective filtration pressure along the capillary decreases. The hydrostatic pressure in the tissue is normally very low. Data reported

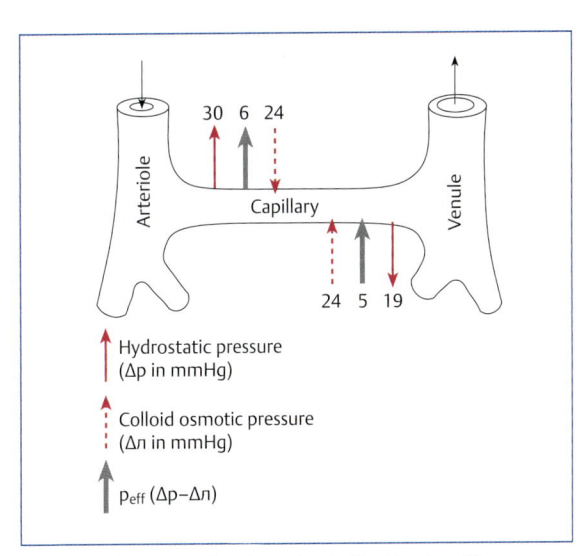

Fig. 8.17 Filtration and reabsorption in the blood capillary. The hydrostatic and colloid-osmotic pressures and the resulting effective filtration (p_{eff}) are indicated by arrows for the arterial beginning and end of the capillary. Pressure data are given in mmHg.

in textbooks varies because of the difficulty in measuring this pressure accurately. The mean pressure in the interstitium might be 1 mmHg. The **colloid-osmotic pressure** in the **interstitium** (π_{inst}) is close to zero in most organs because there is very little protein in the interstitial fluid. However, in the liver and to a limited extent in the gastrointestinal tract, smaller protein molecules can partially diffuse through the wall of capillaries forming a less dense barrier. In these organs, the colloid-osmotic pressure in the interstitial fluid is therefore somewhat higher.

At the beginning of the capillary, the effective filtration pressure directed outwards is greater (+6 mmHg) (**filtration**). At the **end of the capillary**, the **effective filtration pressure** is then directed inwards (−5 mmHg) due to the low hydrostatic pressure in the lumen of the capillary. This allows water from the interstitium to re-enter into the capillary (**reabsorption**). The effective filtration pressures at the beginning and end of the capillary show that under normal conditions the net fluid transport out of the capillary is greater than the inward transport (**Fig. 8.17**). The **outward forces** are slightly **greater** than the inward forces. Overall, this difference results in **greater net filtration** into the tissue (**Fig. 8.18** – normal). This difference, also called net filtration, amounts to about $21 \cdot d^{-1}$ in a healthy animal weighing 50–80 kg. This fluid is transported out of the interstitial space as **lymph** via the lymph vessels (p. 207).

> **IN A NUTSHELL** !
>
> The hydrostatic and colloid-osmotic pressures in the vessels and in the tissues are critical for net fluid exchange through the capillary wall.

In comparison to the extensive diffusion processes just discussed, it is important for quantitative consideration that only about 0.5% of the plasma fluid flowing through the

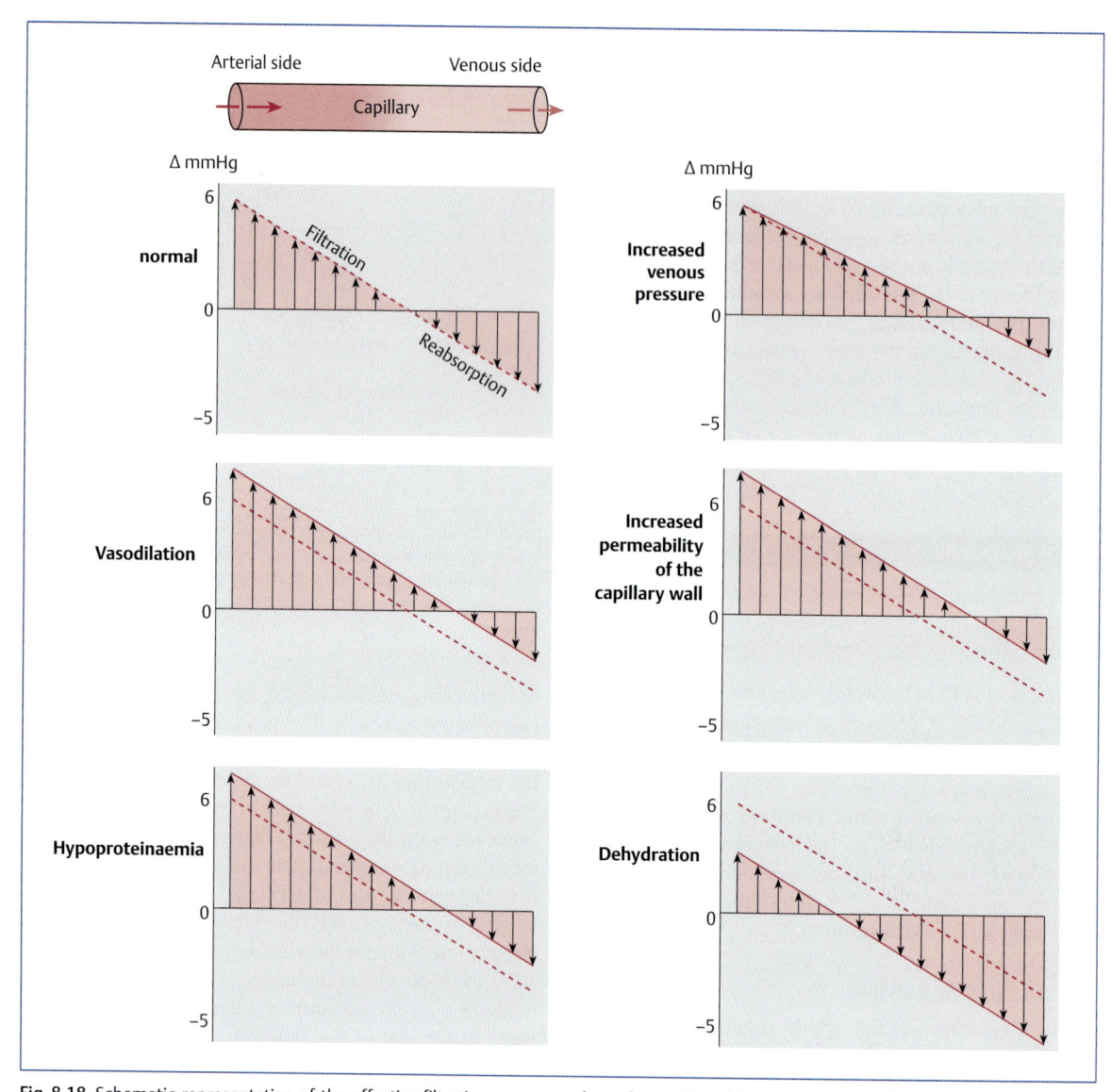

Fig. 8.18 Schematic representation of the effective filtration pressures along the capillary (given as pressure differences in mmHg). If the outward forces of the capillary (increased hydrostatic pressures, decreased colloid-osmotic pressures or elevated vascular permeability) are increased, oedema develops. If the reabsorption forces predominate (dehydration), exsiccosis occurs. Filtration and reabsorption under normal conditions are each indicated as a red dashed line.

capillary is filtered out in the arterial section of the capillary. Thus, about $20 \cdot l \cdot d^{-1}$ is filtered into the interstitium at the beginning of the capillary in a medium-sized animal of about 70 kg.

With vasodilation of the arterioles, and with increased permeability of the capillary wall, and also in hypoproteinaemia, the pressures responsible for filtration are increased, compared to those responsible for reabsorption. However, the **causes** of these increased forces driving fluid transport out of the capillary are very **different**. In vasodilation the hydrostatic pressure is increased on the arterial side of the capillary. When there is increased permeability of the capillary wall to proteins, the colloid-osmotic pressure in the interstitium is increased. In hypoproteinaemia the colloid-osmotic pressure in the blood plasma is reduced. All these different factors result in increased effective filtration pressure at the beginning of a capillary. This can lead to oedema.

Oedema

Oedema can have very different causes (**Fig. 8.18**):

- Due to **increased venous pressure** (e.g. venous congestion in cardiac insufficiency), the hydrostatic pressure in the venous part of the capillary is increased. The pressures in the capillary responsible for reabsorption are thus reduced.

- With **vasodilation** of arterioles, the hydrostatic pressure in capillaries is also augmented. Thus, the pressures leading to filtration are higher than those for reabsorption.

- When there is **increased permeability of the capillary wall** (as with insect bites, burns, local inflammations and allergic reactions), plasma proteins can leave the capillaries and enter the interstitium. This reduces the colloid-osmotic pressure differences between blood and interstitial fluid. Filtration is then increased, and reabsorption reduced. Local mediators for such changes in permeability include histamine and cytokines.

- In the case of **hypoproteinaemia** (e.g. in starvation, renal leakage of protein into urine, hepatic parenchymal damage, and exudative enteropathies), the colloid-osmotic pressure in the plasma is reduced and thus filtration into the interstitium overwhelms reabsorption.
- When **lymphatic drainage is disturbed**, the hydrostatic pressures in the tissue increase. This reduces the forces responsible for filtration. The pressures necessary for reabsorption are not sufficient to transport the fluid accumulated in the interstitium into the capillaries.

Dehydration and exsiccosis

When **dehydration** (**Fig. 8.18**) leads to plasma fluid loss, the plasma protein concentration rises with consequent increased colloid-osmotic pressure. This reduces filtration and increases reabsorption. This increased reabsorption can lead to fluid loss from the interstitium and to exsiccosis.

> **IN A NUTSHELL** !
>
> When the hydrostatic and/or colloid-osmotic pressures in the capillary beds change, oedema or exsiccosis develop.

■ Venules

The **postcapillary venules** (internal diameter 8–13 µm) are formed by the union of several venous capillaries. Their wall consists of endothelium, basement membrane, some collagenous fibres and an envelope of pericytes (Rouget cells), which contain contractile elements. As in capillaries, there is still some exchange of substances across the walls of postcapillary venules. With **venule** inner diameters of 30–50 µm, the number of smooth muscle cells in the wall increases (**Fig. 8.2**). When the tone of these smooth muscle cells rises, the venules are known as postcapillary resistance vessels (**Fig. 8.19**). These venules can then change the effective filtration pressure in the capillaries.

8.4.4 Lymphatic system

Fluid from the interstitium enters the lymphatic vessels through gaps in the lymphatic capillaries. The muscle cells in the wall of the lymph vessels contract rhythmically. Numerous valves similar to venous valves cause a directed flow. In a similar manner to the effect of the muscle pump (**Fig. 8.14**) on venous blood flow, alternating pressure on the outside of lymph vessels is also relevant for lymphatic flow. The lymph capillaries lead into large lymph vessels. Before lymph from large lymph vessels reaches a vein, it flows through numerous **lymph nodes**. In the lymph nodes, lymph composition can change so that the **postnodal lymph** often has a higher protein concentration than the **prenodal lymph**. The postnodal lymph is therefore not representative of the composition of the interstitial fluid, nor of the rate of formation of the lymph.

> **IN A NUTSHELL** !
>
> Excess interstitial fluid is removed as lymph.

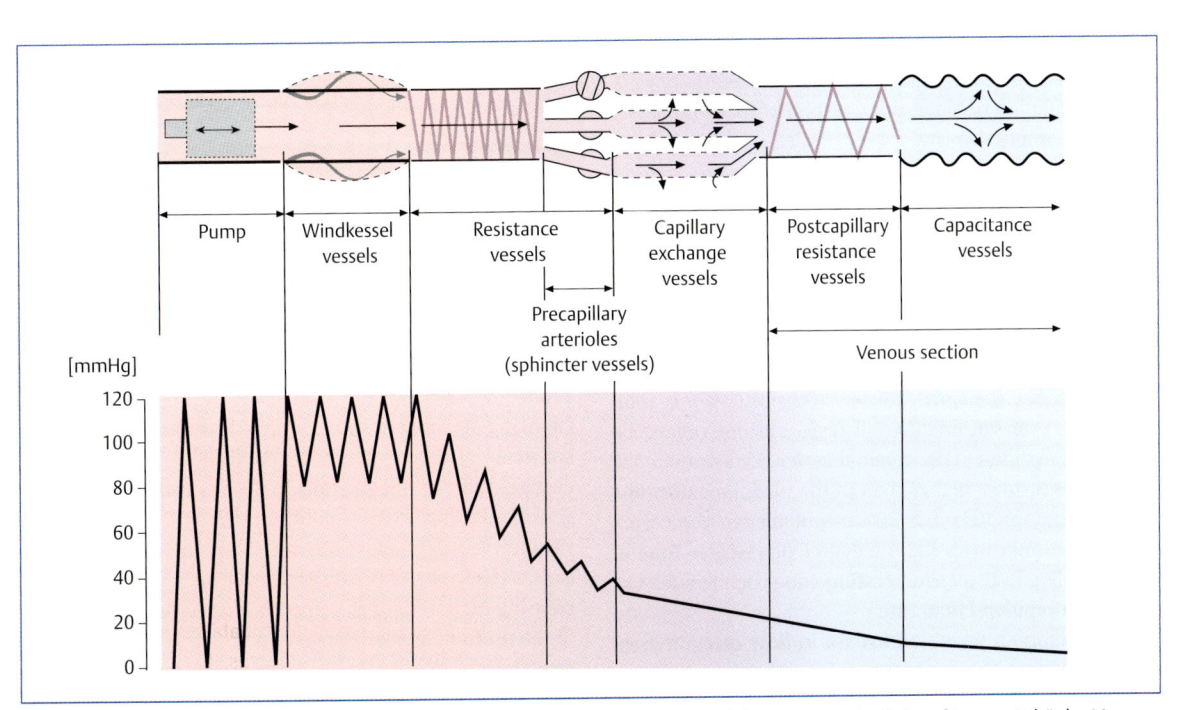

Fig. 8.19 Schematic representation of functional differences in vascular segments of the systemic circulation. [Source: Schünke M, Schulte E, Schumacher U. 2.1 Übersicht und prinzipieller Wandaufbau. In: Schünke M, Schulte E, Schumacher U (eds.). Prometheus LernAtlas der Anatomie – Innere Organe. Illustrated by K. Wesker and M. Voll. 5th ed., Stuttgart: Thieme; 2018]

8.5   Regulation of blood circulation

Wolfgang von Engelhardt

ESSENTIALS   ✗

– At rest and under changing workload, all organs must be sufficiently supplied with oxygen and metabolic substrates, and there must also be adequate removal of metabolic wastes. This requires **finely tuned regulation** of **blood circulation**. Cardiovascular regulation can be short-, medium- or long-term. A distinction is made between local and central regulatory processes.
– While in most organs the blood flow rate adapts to a change in demand, in individual organs – even when the arterial blood pressure in the body changes – a constant flow rate is maintained by autoregulation.

8.5.1   Local blood flow regulation

Blood flow is regulated by numerous, sometimes competing, influences on the smooth musculature (p. 159) in the arterioles, the **precapillary resistance vessels** and the **sphincter vessels** (**Fig. 8.15**; **Fig. 8.19**; multi-unit type, **Fig. 6.16**). The tone of the smooth muscle cells in the vascular walls can be altered by several, very different processes. It is particularly important that **smooth muscles** in these vascular segments can adjust their tension largely by **autoregulation**. Through these changes in **vascular tone**, the vessel width can be made narrower or wider as blood pressure rises or falls. Thus, autoregulatory vascular resistance can change in such a way that a **constant blood flow rate** is maintained. Besides these **myogenic** changes in muscle tone, **neurogenic**, **humoral** and **endothelium-mediated** mechanisms (p. 208) are also involved in flow rate regulation. In most situations where there is physiological regulation of blood flow, several of these processes are acting simultaneously.

■ Resting blood flow and maximum blood flow increase in tissues

The level of **resting blood flow rate** is different in the various organs (**Fig. 8.20**). In tissues with a high resting metabolism (heart, skeletal muscle, or brain) and also in organs in which flow rate does not only serve the supply of the tissue (kidney), the flow rate per 100 g of tissue is relatively high. Even within different regions of one organ, the flow rate can differ. In the cerebral cortex, for example, the flow rate is 3 times higher than in the medulla oblongata. In the kidney (p. 305) it is 20 times higher in the cortex than in the inner medulla. The degree of **vascular tone** of the **vessel** wall (also called **resting tone**) determines the rate of **resting blood flow rate**.

The maximum possible **increase in flow rate** varies in different tissues. The greatest possible rise occurs in vascular regions where there can be greatly increased demand, such as in skeletal muscles and skin. During heavy work, the rise in flow rate in these tissues can exceed 70 times the resting blood flow (**Fig. 26.16**). In most other tissues,

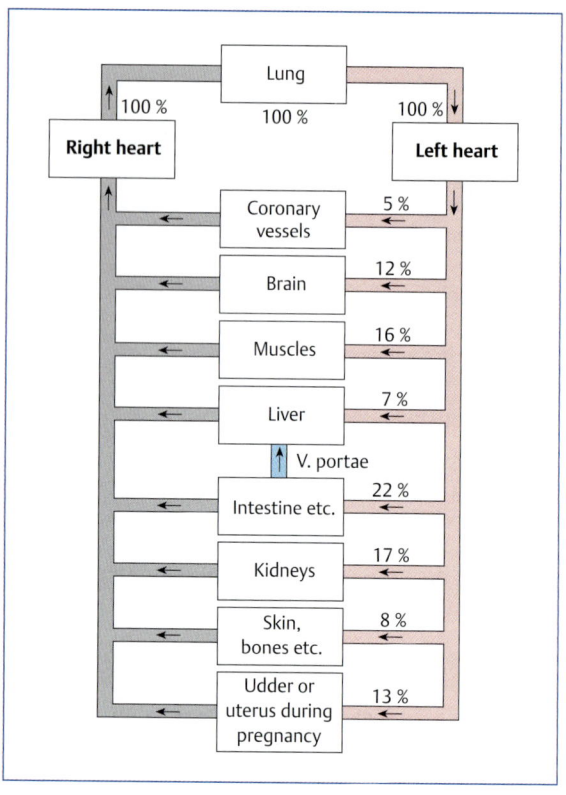

Fig. 8.20 Diagram of the blood circulation and the resting blood flow rate. Systemic and pulmonary circulation are connected in series. The blood flow to the individual vessels takes place in parallel. The percentage values indicate what proportion of cardiac output flows through the different organs at rest. Blood flow direction is indicated by arrows.

flow rate increases to about a 5-fold maximum. In the **kidneys** and, to a lesser extent, in the **brain**, perfusion is largely **constant** and **independent** of the regulatory processes in the rest of the body (**autoregulation**).

IN A NUTSHELL   !

Resting blood flow rate is related to the resting tone of the vascular walls.

■ Control of local blood circulation

Autoregulation, myogenic tone

While in most organs blood flow adjusts according to changing demand, in some organs flow rate is kept largely constant by autoregulation even when arterial pressure changes. This autoregulation (p. 306) is achieved by myogenic excitation of the smooth muscles (p. 161) in the resistance vessels (**Bayliss effect**). The rising blood pressure causes stretching of the walls of arterioles. This leads to increasing excitation of the smooth muscle cells in the walls of the precapillary resistance vessels. The consequence is a **stretch-induced contraction** keeping **flow rate** in these organs **largely constant during changes in blood pressure**. These autoregulatory reactions are mainly found in vessels of the kidney (p. 305), to a lesser extent also in **brain** and **heart**, and to a much lesser extent in skeletal muscles, liv-

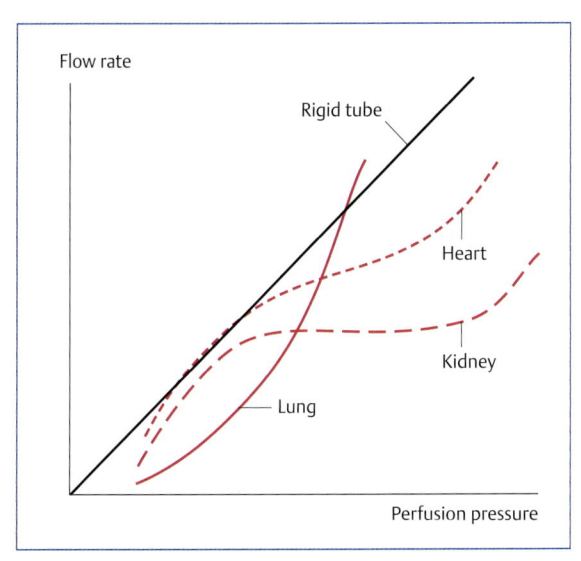

Fig. 8.21 Relationship between perfusion pressure and flow rate for a rigid tube, an organ with strong autoregulation (kidney), an organ in which autoregulation plays a moderate role (heart), an organ without autoregulation (lung).

er, and the gastrointestinal tract. Such autoregulation is **not present in** the vessels of the pulmonary circulation (p. 213). There, passive dilation occurs when perfusion pressure increases and the flow rate even increases disproportionately (**Fig. 8.21**).

The molecular mechanism of myogenic autoregulation in the organs in which the Bayliss effect applies, lies in the opening of mechanosensitive cation channels in the membranes of the smooth muscle cells of the resistance vessels. Ca^{2+} flows into the smooth muscle cells of the resistance vessels and, as shown in **Fig. 6.18**, binds to calmodulin. The myosin light chain is activated and, after phosphorylation, the smooth muscle cells contracts. With the reduction of the diameter of the blood vessel, the vascular resistance increases significantly. Since the radius is effective in its 4th power, small changes in the radius are decisive in altering the flow resistance (Hagen-Poiseuille law (p. 194)).

As soon as intravascular pressure returns to initial values, the organs with pronounced autoregulation are adjusted back to the approximate original vascular tone by myogenic regulation. In this way, a largely constant flow rate with only slight changes can be maintained in these organs even when blood pressure shows stronger fluctuations.

> **IN A NUTSHELL** !
>
> In organs with pronounced autoregulation, flow rate changes little or not at all when arterial blood pressure rises.

Increased flow rate due to tissue metabolites

As the metabolic activity of a tissue rises, so does the metabolically induced dilation of the blood vessels. Elevated CO_2 **partial pressure**, rising **lactate** and H^+ **concentrations**, **adenosine** and **inorganic phosphate** formed during ATP breakdown, increased **extracellular K^+ concentrations** as a result of, for example, increased muscle activity cause **local vasodilation and thus an increase in flow rate**. This metabolic regulation is mainly responsible for the pronounced increase in blood flow of working skeletal muscle. Vascular dilation occurs mainly by inhibition of the voltage-dependent Ca^{2+} channels in the smooth muscle cells (p. 162) of the arterioles and through inhibition of the secretion of noradrenaline (p. 117).

Neural regulation

Vasoconstriction is achieved primarily through **sympathetic noradrenergic control**. The basic processes involved in this regulation are discussed in ch. 4 (p. 112) and in central regulation of blood circulation. Only a few details about the local control of flow rate are considered here.

The arterioles and small arteries, and to a lesser extent the veins, are innervated by postganglionic noradrenergic nerve fibres. By releasing noradrenaline from varicosities, and its binding to α_1 receptors, the tone of vascular smooth muscle cells is increased, and thus flow rate decreases. Any circulating catecholamines (adrenaline and noradrenaline) will also influence blood flow in a concentration-dependent manner. At low adrenaline concentrations, the activation of β_2 receptors causes vasodilation, and thus an increase in flow rate. At high adrenaline concentrations, there is an α_1 effect as with noradrenaline. The physiological effect of catecholamines in a particular tissue depends on the local density of α_1 and β_2 receptors. In the skin vessels, the α_1 receptors predominate. In the vessels of the gastrointestinal tract and the muscles, both α_1 and β_2 receptors are present. In the coronary vessels, β_2 receptors (p. 117) predominate (**Table 4.1**).

MORE DETAILS

Sympathetic cholinergic control

Sympathetic cholinergic vasodilation has so far only been demonstrated in skeletal muscle of dogs, cats and goats. It is not known whether it is also present in other animals. This control seems to be particularly important in the start-up phase of muscle work.

Parasympathetic cholinergic control

Parasympathetic cholinergic vasodilation plays a minor role, compared to sympathetic innervation. A parasympathetic cholinergic innervation of blood vessels has so far been shown mainly in the genitals, in the coronary vessels and in the brain. Vasodilation in the genitals leads to blood filling of erectile tissues and simultaneous relaxation of muscles surrounding the cavernous tissue.

Humoral regulation

Even at extremely low concentrations, **angiotensin II** causes strong vasoconstriction. The renin-angiotensin-aldosterone system (p. 307) is discussed in the kidney chapter. The effects of **antidiuretic hormone** (ADH, also called vasopressin because of its effect on blood vessels (p. 212)) and **atrial natriuretic peptide** are discussed in the chapter on blood volume regulation (p. 212).

Locally limited changes in perfusion can also occur with mechanical stimuli, change in temperature, and in inflammatory and allergic conditions. Several paracrine signalling molecules play a role in this dilation. These include **prostaglandins**, **bradykinin** and **histamine**. Bradykinin and histamine also increase the permeability of the capillary walls and thus promote the development of local oedema (**Fig. 8.18**). **Serotonin (5-hydroxytryptamine, 5-HT)** has vasodilatory and vasoconstrictive effects, depending on the various **5-HT receptors**, and also strong bronchoconstrictive effects (**Fig. 8.25**).

The role of endothelium in the regulation of vascular tone

The endothelial cells release numerous substances affecting vascular muscles. These include **nitric oxide (NO**, identical to endothelium-derived relaxing factor, EDRF), **prostacyclin (PGI$_2$)**, **endothelium-derived hyperpolarizing factor (EDHF)** with a **vasodilatory effect** as well as the strongly vasoconstrictive peptides, the endothelins (p. 328) (ET).

> **IN A NUTSHELL**　　　　　　　　　　!
>
> The endothelium is an essential modulator of vascular functions.

MORE DETAILS　The **NO-induced vasodilation** plays a decisive role in penile **erection**. An essential part of the physiological process of erection is triggered by the release of NO in the corpus cavernosum. This activates the enzyme guanylate cyclase, which catalyses the formation of cyclic guanosine monophosphate (cGMP) (**Fig. 4.4**). This triggers a slight muscle relaxation in the corpus cavernosum, which allows the inflow of blood and thus erection. The action of cGMP is terminated by the enzyme phosphodiesterase type 5 (PDE5), which cleaves cGMP. In erectile dysfunction, sildenafil (company name **Viagra®**), which is a potent **inhibitor of PDE5**, can be used to reduce the amount of cGMP broken down in the corpus cavernosum. A higher concentration of cGMP in the corpus cavernosum can lead to a stronger erection.

> **IN A NUTSHELL**　　　　　　　　　　!
>
> The blood flow to the organs is regulated by many competing influences on the resistance vessels.

8.5.2　Central regulation of blood circulation

In order for different cardiovascular requirements to be met within physiological limits under resting conditions and during exertion, control processes and higher-level co-ordination (p. 139) are needed (**Fig. 8.22**, **Fig. 8.23**, **Fig. 8.24**, **Fig. 8.25**). These coordinated processes consist mainly of adjusting **arterial blood pressure**, **cardiac output** and controlling **blood volume**. Important aspects in the adjustment of heart rate and cardiac output (p. 169) have already been discussed. In general, for cardiovascular regulation, **regulation of arterial blood pressure** is of central importance. **Fig. 8.25** summarises the major factors that influence mean arterial blood pressure. Many of these have already been discussed.

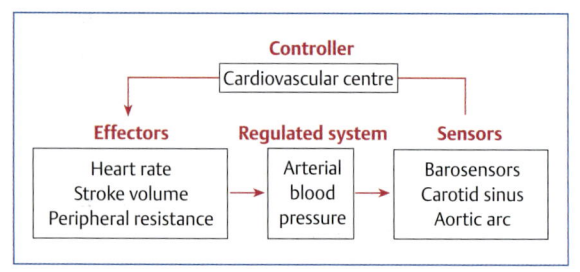

Fig. 8.22 Control circuit for short-term regulation of arterial mean pressure.

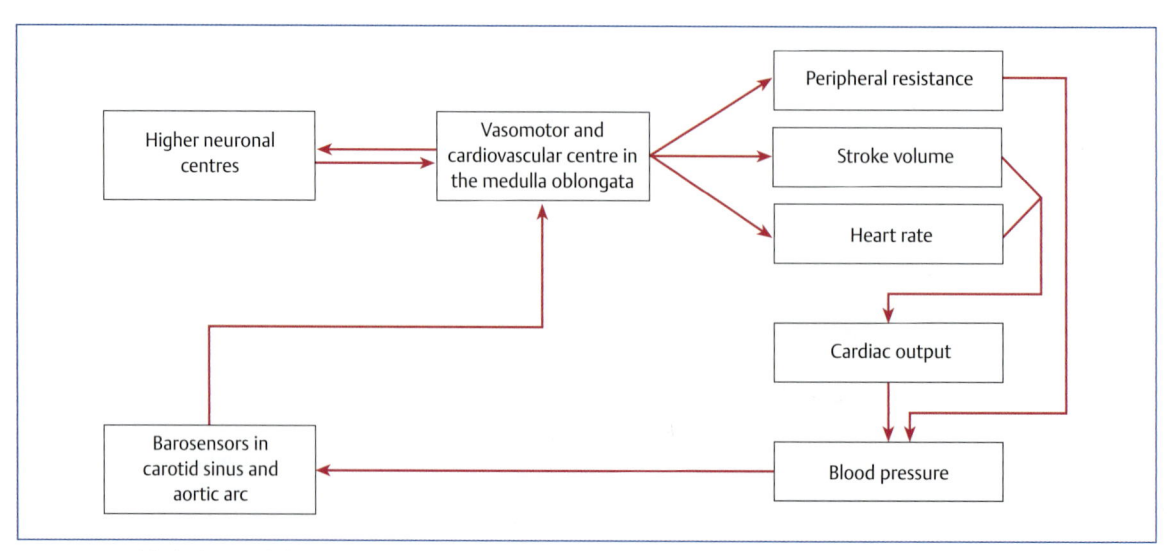

Fig. 8.23 Simplified scheme of short-term blood pressure regulation.

Short-term blood pressure regulation

Cardiovascular reflexes are used to maintain adequate blood pressure in the short term, according to the principle of a control circuit (feedback loop) with a regulator, effectors, and sensors (**Fig. 8.22**). Pressosensors (p.140) that detect pressure changes (often also called **pressoreceptors** or **barosensors**) are stretch-sensitive end organs in the **carotid sinus** where it divides into external and internal carotid artery. Pressosensors are found also in the vascular wall of the **aortic arch** (**Fig. 8.24**, right). These receptors have a phasic-tonic sensitivity where the mean action potential rate is higher at higher mean pressure than at low mean pressure. In order to understand the regulatory circuit, it is important to recognise that the afferents leading to the **cardiovascular centre** in the medulla oblongata (p.139) exert a constant **inhibitory** influence on the autonomic nuclear regions of the brainstem. This means that when the arterial pressure drops, the **sympathetic tone** rises, while the **parasympathetic tone** falls. This leads to an increase in heart rate (p.178) and cardiac **stroke volume** and also to an increase in **peripheral resistance**. The **pressoreceptor reflex** thus enables rapid, controlled counter-regulation in the event of short-term changes in pressure in the large arteries (**Fig. 8.23**).

The short-term regulation of mean arterial pressure after a major **blood loss** is shown in **Fig. 8.24**. With re-duced excitation of the **pressosensors**, there is **reduced inhibition** of the **cardiovascular centre**. As a result, the **cardiac output** and the **resistance** in the **peripheral vessels** are increased (p.209). This leads to a rise in mean arterial pressure.

During the transition from lying to standing (**orthostasis**), there may be a short-term **increase in blood volume** in the capacitance vessels of the **limbs**. This causes a temporary fall in venous return to the heart, in central venous pressure, in stroke volume and in systolic blood pressure. This leads to rapid adaptation via the barosensors. If there are orthostatic regulation disorders, circulatory **collapse** may occur.

However, regulation of arterial blood pressure is not only from effectors of the cardiovascular system described here. Further influences (**Fig. 8.25**) arise from chemosensors (p.291), nociceptors (p.76) and afferents from the limbic system (p.138) as well as the cerebral cortex (p.121).

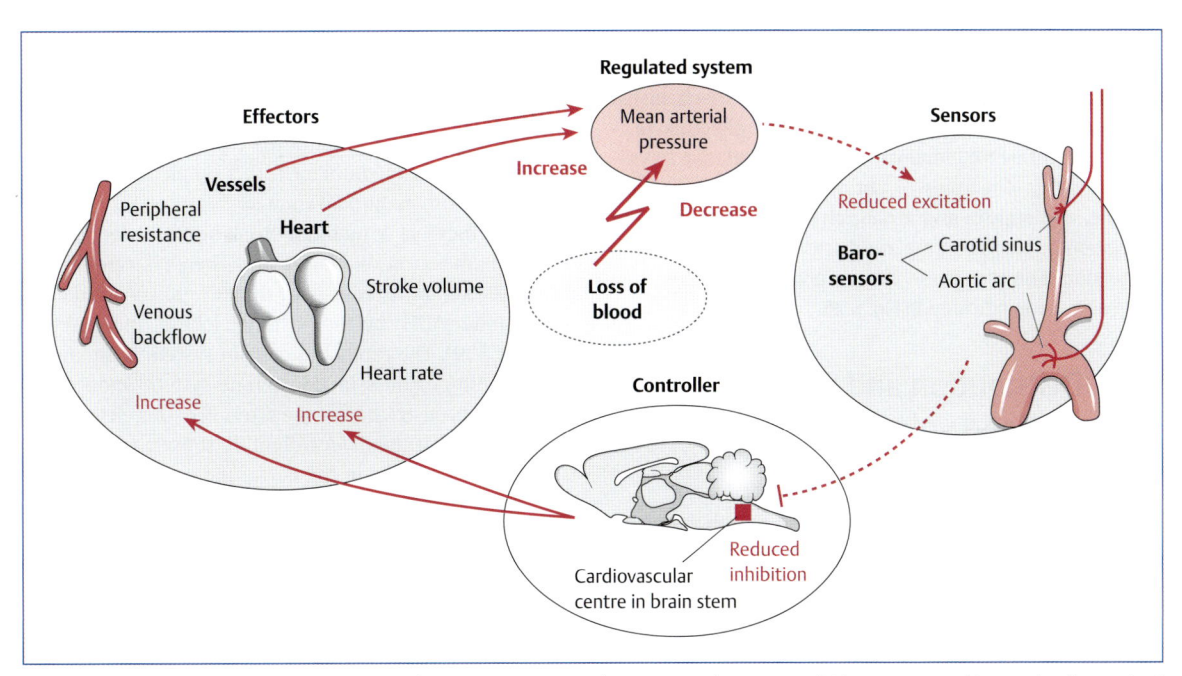

Fig. 8.24 Short-term regulation of mean arterial pressure. A primary drop in arterial pressure, which was assumed here to be the result of blood loss, initiates a chain of regulatory processes that lead to sympathetic activation via the barosensors. Thus, cardiac activity and vascular constriction are induced. [Source: Klinke R, Pape HC, Silbernagl S. Physiologie. 5th ed., Stuttgart: Thieme; 2005: 198]

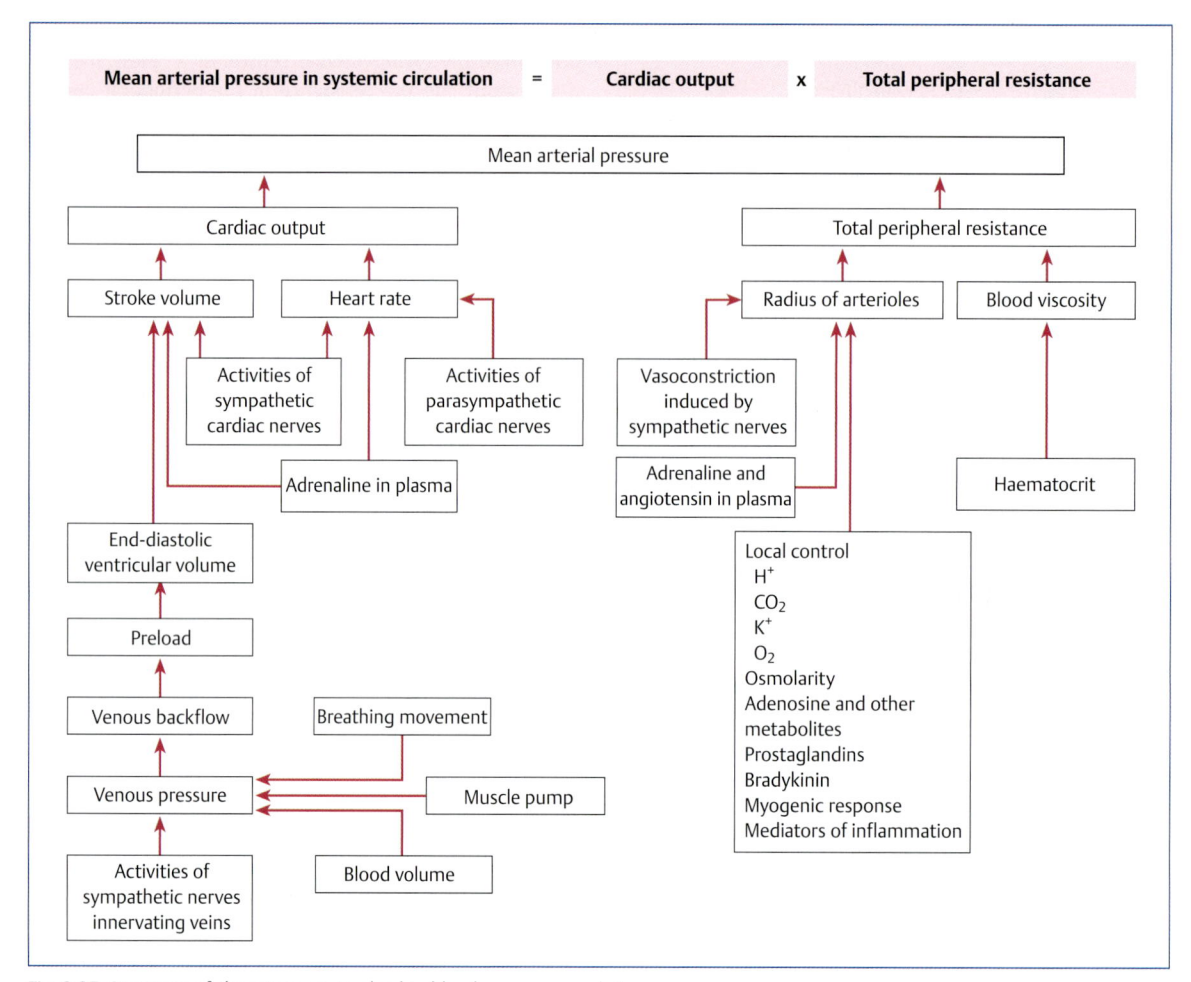

Fig. 8.25 Summary of the processes involved in blood pressure regulation.

■ Medium- and long-term cardiovascular regulation

The renin-angiotensin system is mainly involved in **medium-** and **long-term** regulation. **Long-term mechanisms** of cardiovascular regulation are primarily affecting processes that influence blood volume (p.212) relative to vascular capacity. The roles of **antidiuretic hormone, aldosterone, angiotensin** and **atrial natriuretic peptide** in the regulation of blood volume are discussed in the following subsection. Some of these factors and the changes they bring about are indicated in **Fig. 8.25**.

8.6   Distribution and regulation of blood volume

Wolfgang von Engelhardt

Blood volume in monogastric animals is usually between **70 and 80 ml · kg⁻¹ body weight**. In fat pigs and in ruminants, blood volume is usually lower (about 55–75 ml · kg⁻¹ body weight) due to the low blood supply to adipose tissue in pigs, or the large volume and weight of the forestomach in ruminants. Young animals have a higher blood volume per kg body weight than adult animals.

In the event of blood loss, there may be a **short-term** increase in **venous tone**. This allows sufficient extra blood to flow to the heart. Sympathetic activation also causes a rise in **resistance of** the **arterioles**. This leads to a decrease in the effective filtration pressure and an increase in reabsorption in the venous part of the capillaries (**Fig. 8.18** dehydration). In the medium term, this supplements the vascular space with additional volume.

When there is a **medium- to long-term** decrease in blood volume, atria dilation is low. Thereby, water excretion in the kidney is reduced by the secretion of **antidiuretic hormone** (ADH) by the posterior lobe of the pituitary gland (p.539). The **renin-angiotensin system** (also known as the renin-angiotensin-aldosterone system) induces increased vasoconstriction of the arterioles. This elevates the wall tension that the myocardium must exert to overcome the diastolic pressure in the aorta, and to open the aortic valve (afterload). The secretion of **aldosterone** leads to increased reabsorption of Na⁺ and thus also of water. In addition, the sensation of thirst (p.335) is triggered by these hormones. Volume deficiency causes a reduction in perfusion of the kidney (p.306) by the action of sympathetic stimulation. The system starts with the release of the enzyme **renin** from cells of the juxtaglomerular apparatus. This peptidase forms angiotensin I from **angiotensinogen** (an α_2 globulin in blood plasma). Angiotensin I is then cleaved by angiotensin-converting enzyme (ACE) present in the plasma and in endothelial cells (especially in the lungs). This results in the formation of **angiotensin II** (**Fig. 12.7**). In addition to the strong vasoconstrictor effect already mentioned, angiotensin II promotes ADH secretion and, above all, the release of **aldosterone** from the adrenal cortex. This enhances renal reabsorption of Na^+ and water in the collecting tube (p.313) and also their absorption in the colon (p.440).

Atrial natriuretic peptide is produced and stored in the wall of the atria. When the atria are dilated, the release of atrial natriuretic peptide is stimulated due to an increase in volume. Sodium reabsorption in the collecting tube is thus reduced, more water is excreted and this counteracts the increase in blood volume, which consequently then decreases.

8.7 Special features of the pulmonary circulation

Wolfgang von Engelhardt

The **pulmonary circuit** is part of the **low-pressure system**. The total flow resistance and thus the pressure are considerably less in the pulmonary vascular system than in the systemic circulation. The vascular resistance in the pulmonary circulation is only about one tenth of the resistance in the systemic circulation.

> **IN A NUTSHELL** !
>
> In the pulmonary vascular system, the total flow resistance, and thus the pressure, is considerably less than in the systemic circulation.

Flow resistance in the pulmonary vascular system is mainly due to **passive pressure** from the high **elastic distensibility** of the pulmonary vessels. Their **vascular tone** is low, unlike in the systemic circulation. An increase in perfusion pressure causes passive dilation of the vessels and the flow rate increases disproportionately (**Fig. 8.21**). The pulmonary vessels have only a thin layer of smooth muscle cells. The typical arterioles of the systemic circulation are absent in the pulmonary circuit. Although the pulmonary vessels are abundantly innervated by sympathetic vasoconstrictor fibres, under physiological conditions there is **no significant** neuronally controlled **regulation of blood flow**. Rather, the physiological significance of this innervation is that sympathetic stimulation can increase the filling of the left ventricle with blood stored in the pulmonary vessels.

> **IN A NUTSHELL** !
>
> In the pulmonary circuit, the magnitude of flow resistance is largely determined by passive pressure changes in vessel diameter. There is no significant neural regulation of the pulmonary circulation.

However, at low alveolar O_2 partial pressures, local **vasoconstriction** occurs in the pulmonary vessels (Euler-Liljestrand mechanism (p.282)). Hence, when there is **alveolar hypoxia**, local flow rate in the pulmonary vessels is reduced. At low alveolar O_2 partial pressures, there is therefore less O_2 in the alveoli on the one hand and less blood in the alveolar capillaries on the other. Because of this lower capillary flow rate, although less O_2 diffuses into the capillaries, O_2 saturation of the blood can increase. During transient hypoxia, this is a useful physiological adaptation.

However, if hypoxia and thus also vasoconstriction in the entire lung continue for a long time, blood pressure in the pulmonary arteries rises significantly (**pulmonary hypertension**). This then often leads to **hypertrophy of the right ventricle**.

Pulmonary hypertension is much more frequently caused by mitral valve insufficiency (**Fig. 7.1**) than by vasoconstriction. The blood then flows back through the incompletely closing mitral valve into the left atrium and into the pulmonary veins during systole.

> **MORE DETAILS** The amount of backflow in mitral valve insufficiency depends on how leaky the closed mitral valve is. Depending on the degree of insufficiency, pulmonary hypertension results. Pulmonary hypertension leads to a massive right ventricular strain and usually has a very poor prognosis.
>
> When cattle are kept at altitudes above 2000 m for long periods of time in the Rocky Mountains, irreversible pulmonary hypertension may develop, as a result of the low O_2 partial pressure. These animals become seriously ill (High-mountain Disease or Brisket disease). In this disease, the number of smooth muscle cells in the pulmonary arteries is increased, vasoconstriction is considerable, pulmonary hypertension results and ultimately right heart failure occurs.

Pulmonary flow resistance is strongly dependent on ventilation. During **inspiration**, pleural pressure decreases. This augments transmural pressure (difference between intravascular and extravascular pressure). Thus, blood volume in the intrathoracic low-pressure system rises (**Fig. 11.14**, **Fig. 11.15**). During diastole, the filling of the right atrium and the right ventricle is also increased, and with it the stroke volume of the right ventricle. During **expiration**, the opposite effects occur (see Traube-Hering waves (p.203)).

When there is low intravascular pressure, blood supply to the lungs is much more dependent on **hydrostatic influences** than is the blood supply to the systemic circulation. The upper regions of the lung, depending on the position of the body, are much less supplied with blood than the lower regions. The flow rate increases from top to bottom in accordance with the increasing intravascular pressure. Flow rate is very low in the upper sections and flow in the pulmonary arteries occurs mainly during systolic pressure peaks.

In addition to blood inflow through the pulmonary artery, there is a small nutritive supply of arterial blood to the bronchi through small bronchial vessels branching from the aorta.

IN A NUTSHELL   !

The regional blood supply to the lungs is not homogeneous and varies from upper to lower anatomical regions.

During **physical work**, despite the strong rise in cardiac output, there is only a relatively small increase in pressure in the pulmonary artery because of the high elastic distensibility of the pulmonary vessels. However, this rise in pressure is sufficient to allow adequate perfusion of the upper lung sections.

Since the colloid-osmotic pressure of plasma is much greater than blood pressure in the pulmonary capillaries (**Fig. 8.10**), **outward filtration** does not normally occur. The inward effective filtration pressure predominates, as do the forces of reabsorption.

> **MORE DETAILS**   A large increase in pulmonary capillary pressure is mostly of cardiac origin, e.g. with left heart failure. When the colloid-osmotic pressure falls below the hydrostatic pressure in the pulmonary capillaries, such as when plasma protein concentration declines during starvation, or when there is excessive fluid intake, an outward filtration can occur, where fluid leaks into the alveoli. Despite increased lymphatic drainage, **pulmonary oedema** can then result.

The short distance for pulmonary diffusion enables very effective gas exchange.

8.8   Circulatory failure, shock

Wolfgang von Engelhardt

During circulatory failure, cardiac output is not high enough to ensure sufficient flow rate to the various organs. Causes are hypovolaemia, heart failure or considerably increased peripheral vasodilation.

> **MORE DETAILS**   During **hypovolaemia**, the heart is not filled with enough blood during diastole. Therefore, the atrial pressure drops. Stroke volume decreases and thus cardiac output is reduced. Hypovolaemia can occur with blood loss and also with loss of other body fluids, through the kidneys, from diarrhoea, vomiting, burns, excessive sweating, ileus or from ascites. Shock usually occurs when blood loss exceeds 25% of total blood volume.
>
> **Cardiac failure** leading to shock may have its origin primarily in the heart itself (valvular defect, heart insufficiency, heart attack), or secondarily it may be triggered by pulmonary embolism, hypothyroidism or hyperparathyroidism.
>
> A sudden **dilation of peripheral vessels** can occur with allergies, anaphylaxis, sepsis, fever, intense pain, and shock. If cardiovascular regulation is no longer adequate, the CNS is no longer supplied with sufficient blood and unconsciousness follows.

8.9   Foetal circulation and circulatory changes during and after birth

Wolfgang von Engelhardt

Gas exchange in the foetal circulation takes place via the placenta. Oxygen-rich blood (only about 80% saturated with O_2) flows through the umbilical vein (v. umbilicalis) to the foetus. A small amount of this blood reaches the liver. This blood coming from the placenta then **mixes** with desaturated blood from the lower half of the foetal body. This **mixed blood**, which flows via the inferior vena cava into the right atrium, has an O_2 saturation of only 60–65%. Most of the blood passes into the left atrium through the **foramen ovale** in the atrial septum. The remaining blood is pumped from the right ventricle into the pulmonary artery. Resistance in the collapsed pulmonary vessels is high. About 75% of the blood passes from the pulmonary **artery** through the **ductus arteriosus (Botalli)** into the aorta due to the existing pressure gradient. Therefore, the amount of blood that flows back through the capillary regions of the lung via the pulmonary veins to the left atrium is quite small before birth. The foetal organs are supplied with mixed blood via the aorta. Some of the blood returns via the umbilical artery back to the placenta (**Fig. 8.26**). Because of the foramen ovale and the ductus arteriosus, both ventricles are largely connected in parallel in the foetal circulation.

During **birth** there is a major change in the cardiovascular system:

1. The **increase in tone** and compression of the uterine arteries by contraction of the **uterine musculature** during labour, lead to a **decrease in uterine flow rate**.

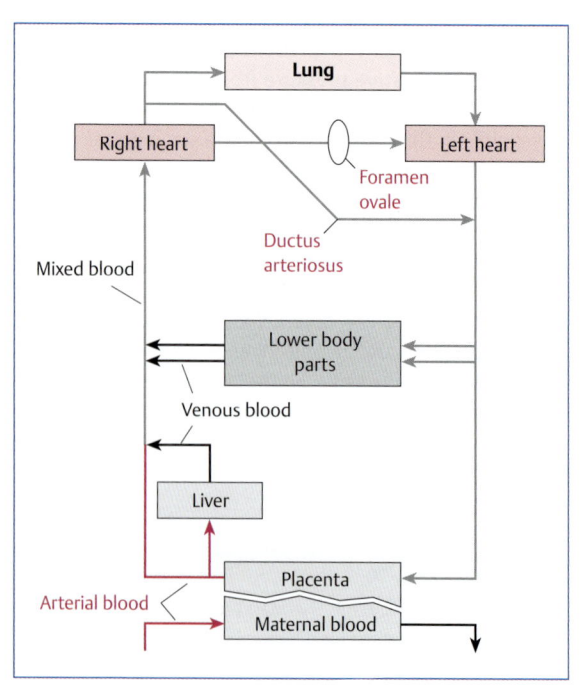

Fig. 8.26 Schematic representation of the foetal circulation. Red = arterial blood, black = venous blood, grey = mixed blood.

Circulation, respiration

2. The increase in peripheral resistance in the foetal placenta **increases foetal aortic pressure**.

3. As placental perfusion falls, the **partial pressure of CO_2** in the foetal blood increases. **Lung respiration is stimulated** bychemosensors in the foetus.

4. As the **lungs inflate**, flow resistance in the pulmonary circulation decreases. This leads to a reversal of the pressure gradient between the aorta and the pulmonary artery. **Initially**, this causes a reversal of **flow** in the **ductus arteriosus**. Blood flows from the left heart through the initial portion of the aorta into the **pulmonary artery**.

5. The pressure gradient between the right and left atrium is also reversed, as the **pressure in** the **right atrium decreases** due to the absence of blood returning from the placenta. At the same time, **pressure in** the **left atrium increases**, due to the greater inflow of blood from the lungs. This compresses the valve in the left atrium against the **foramen ovale**. At first, the foramen is **functionally** closed, but in the following days the valve grows and the **foramen ovale** becomes permanently **closed**.

6. In the **ductus arteriosus**, contraction of the smooth muscle causes a slow narrowing and thus a functional **closure** within 1–2 days after birth. Complete anatomical closure of the ductus arteriosus and the foramen ovale can occasionally take several weeks.

Suggested reading

Anwaruddin S, Martin JM and Askari AT. Cardiovascular Hemodynamics: An Introductory Guide. New York, Heidelberg, Dordrecht, London: Springer; 2013

Caro CG, Pedley TJ, Schroter RC, Seed WA. The Mechanics of the Circulation. Cambridge: University Press; 2012

Klabunde RE. Cardiovascular Physiology Concepts. Baltimore, Philadelphia: Lippinott Williams & Wilkins, Wolters Kluwer; 2012

Klein BG. Cunningham's Textbook of Veterinary Physiology. St. Louis: Elsevier; 2013

Levick JR. An Introduction to Cardiovascular Physiology. 4th ed. Oxford: University Press; 2003

Nichols WW, O'Rourke MF, Vlachopoulos C. McDonald's Blood Flow in Arteries. Theoretical, experimental and clinical principles. 6th ed. Boca Raton: CRP; 2011

Renkin EM, Michel CC. Handbook of Physiology, Section 2: The Cardiovascular System. Bethesda: American Physiological Society; 1984

Scanes CG, Dridi S. Sturkie's Avian Physiology. Philadelphia: Elsevier; 2021

8.10   Cardiovascular system in birds and reptiles

Helga Pfannkuche, Michael Pees

> **ESSENTIALS**   ✖
>
> The cardiovascular system of sauropsida shows both parallels and differences to that of mammals. While homeothermic birds have a mainly similar structure and function of the cardiovascular system to that of mammals, the cardiovascular systems of poikilothermic reptiles is markedly different from that of mammals and birds. In most reptile species, the heart has only one ventricle. However, there is no mixing of the blood. Instead, various mechanisms enable targeted control of the intracardiac flow rate, and thus of the demand-dependent blood supply to the pulmonary or the systemic circulation. Pressure shunting and washout shunting are the most important mechanisms for this.

8.10.1   Cardiovascular system in birds

In general, the avian cardiovascular system is very similar to that of mammals. The heart has four chambers and there are two completely separate circuits to the lungs and to the rest of the body.

As for the other avian organ systems, the cardiovascular system is adapted to the demands of flying. Although the flying mode of locomotion enables birds to live in widely differing habitats, there is also a high energy requirement and thus high demands on the cardiovascular system. At the same time, the lowest possible body weight is needed. The avian heart is therefore larger compared to that of mammals, and stroke volume is also higher. Likewise, heart rate in birds is generally relatively higher. Also, of clinical importance, are the high blood pressure values that can be measured in birds. In turkeys, for example, this can be over 300 mmHg. These pressures are also a reason for stress susceptibility and acute circulatory failure in birds. It also explains the frequently described aortic rupture in turkeys.

A special feature compared to the mammalian heart is the muscular right atrioventricular valve, which has no chordae tendineae and is regulated by an additional **nodus truncobulbaris**. This valve can become defective in diseases of the right heart because, like the myocardium, it can also become severely hypertrophied, observed diagnostically by ultrasound.

Like reptiles, birds have not only a hepatic, but also a **renal portal system**. This means that blood flowing from the back half of the body towards the heart can be directed to the kidney. The physiological significance of this system in birds is not yet clear. However, it could play a role in control of salt balance and the even distribution of perfusion of the kidney.

8.10.2   Cardiovascular system in reptiles

The heart of reptiles is very different from that of mammals and birds. Most reptiles have a three-chambered heart. This consists of two atria and one ventricle. Only crocodiles have two separate ventricles, similar to mammals and birds.

The presence of only one ventricle poses special challenges to the function of the heart. In diastole, both the oxygen-poor venous blood from the systemic circulation (p. 191) and the oxygen-rich blood from the pulmonary veins, flow via the two atria into the common ventricle. Thus, there is at least some mixing. However, mechanisms in the reptilesn heart ensure that this mixing is not "at random" and that blood from the atria within the ventricle is selectively directed into the afferent arteries. The advantage of this selective blood distribution is particularly evident in the snake heart. It has been demonstrated that after ingestion of a prey animal, twice the amount of blood is directed into the pulmonary circuit (p. 191) to obtain the oxygen necessary for the digestive process to start. Conversely, reptiles can also use a "pulmonary bypass" and pump blood directly back into systemic circulation without a lung passage when oxygen demand is low.

Two mechanisms have been developed to regulate blood flow in reptiles, pressure shunting and washout shunting. These are not strictly separated from each other but differ according to species.

■ Pressure shunting

Pressure shunting is found especially in the heart of turtles and snakes (**Fig. 8.27**). The principle of pressure shunting is that most of the blood from the ventricle during systole flows into the draining vessel which has the largest diameter and thus the smallest flow resistance. During systole, blood can be pumped either into the pulmonary artery or into the aortic arches. At first glance, such a mechanism does not seem very efficient. However, it also has great advantages for reptiles, which do not have such a tightly regulated respiratory cycle as mammals and birds. For example, with right-left shunt, the lungs are completely bypassed, and blood circulates only in the systemic circulation. This benefits aquatic turtles when diving, for example, as no oxygen is "wasted" by blood passing through the lungs. When the animal comes to the water surface, blood can then pass through the lungs several times via a left-right shunt and thus be optimally saturated with oxygen. Right-left shunting is also useful for snakes that swallow large prey and can hardly breathe during swallowing.

Control of shunting is by contraction or relaxation of the vascular musculature. For a right-to-left shunt, the pulmonary artery and other pulmonary vessels are constricted by activation of parasympathetic fibres. Dilation of the arteries of the systemic circulation occurs through NO-mediated relaxation of the vascular musculature (p. 118). The left-right shunt is accompanied (p. 209) by sympathetically mediated constriction of the arteries of the systemic circulation. In parallel, the parasympathetic tone of the pulmonary vessels decreases, resulting in vasodilation.

■ Washout shunting

Washout shunting is found mainly in lizards and turtles. The ventricle is partially divided. This enables blood from the left and right atria to be pumped out separately. For this purpose, two strong muscle ridges are formed in the ventricle, which divide it into three compartments: the cavum pulmonale, the cavum venosum and the cavum arteriosum (**Fig. 8.28a**). This division also leads to the reptile heart being described by some authors as having five compartments. The muscle ridges, which serve to separate the three compartments, do not completely close them off from neighbouring compartments. Nevertheless, they modify the direction of blood flow coming from the two atria and thus lead to the separation of oxygenated and deoxygenated blood.

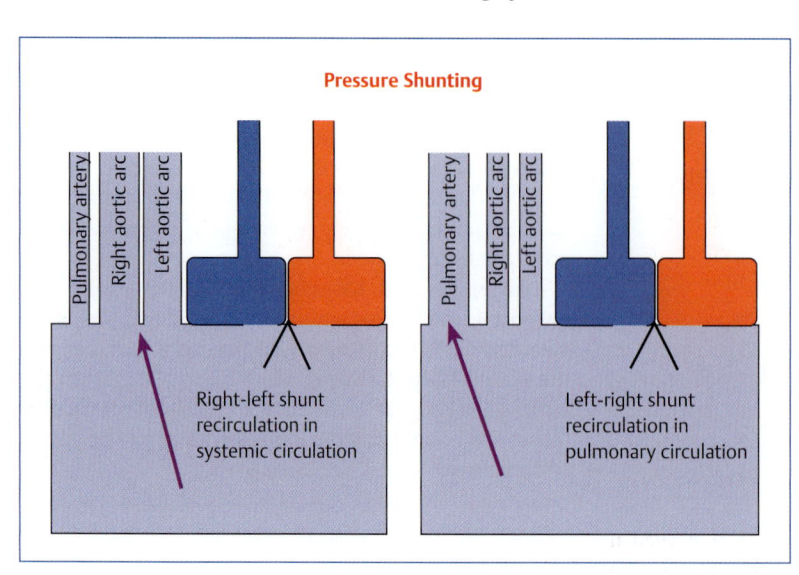

Pressure Shunting

Pulmonary artery | Right aortic arc | Left aortic arc

Right-left shunt recirculation in systemic circulation

Pulmonary artery | Right aortic arc | Left aortic arc

Left-right shunt recirculation in pulmonary circulation

Fig. 8.27 Pressure shunting in the reptile heart. Blood flow is controlled by dilating or constricting the efferent vessels – either into the systemic circulation when the arteries of the systemic circulation are dilated (left) or into the pulmonary circulation when the arteries of the pulmonary circulation are dilated (right). Further explanations are given in the text.

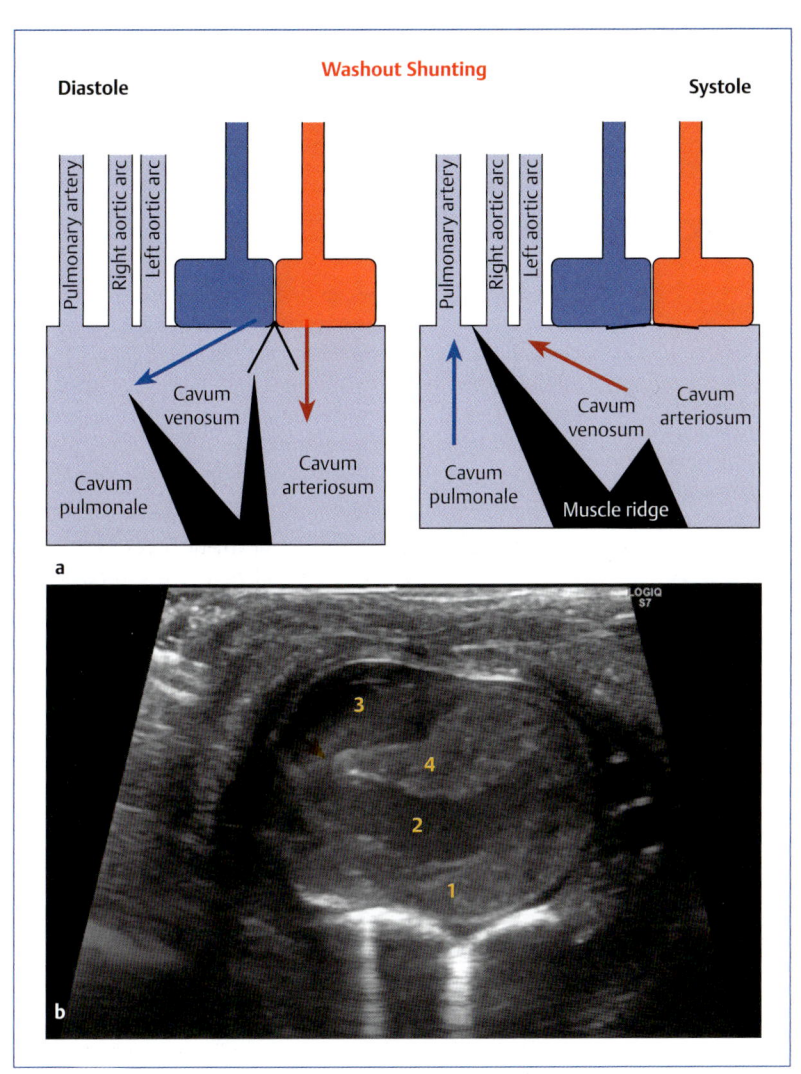

Washout Shunting

Diastole

Systole

Pulmonary artery · Right aortic arc · Left aortic arc

Cavum venosum
Cavum arteriosum
Cavum pulmonale

Cavum venosum
Cavum arteriosum
Cavum pulmonale
Muscle ridge

a

b

Fig. 8.28 Washout shunting in the reptile heart.

a Blood flow is controlled by muscle ridges and by the position of the AV valves during diastole (left) and systole (right). Further explanations are given in the text.

b Echocardiographic image of the muscular ridge in the ventricle of a royal python (python regius): The selective contractility of the muscular ridge allows blood flow to be controlled between the two major subdivisions of the ventricle (2) (arrow).
1 = ventricular wall, 2 = cavum pulmonale, 3 = cavum arteriosum/venosum, 4 = muscular ridge. [Source: Prof. Dr. Michael Pees, Klinik für Heimtiere, Reptilien und Vögel, Stiftung TiHo Hannover]

Circulation, respiration

Fig. 8.28b schematically shows the change in flow direction during a cardiac cycle. In diastole, the musculature of the ventricle and thus also that of the muscular ridges is relaxed. The muscular separation between the cavum arteriosum and cavum venosum, together with the open AV valves protruding into the ventricle, results in the oxygen-rich blood from the left atrium being directed for the most part into the cavum arteriosum. Deoxygenated blood from the right atrium, on the other hand, flows towards the cavum pulmonale. During the subsequent systole, ventricular geometry changes in such a way that the cavum pulmonale is separated from the rest of the ventricle by the muscle ridges. Blood contained here is pumped into the pulmonary artery towards the lungs. The two aortic arches receive the oxygen-rich blood from the cavum arteriosum and the mixed blood from the cavum venosum.

■ Special features of the circulatory system

In reptiles, two aortic arches arise from the ventricle of the heart. They unite caudally to the heart.

Like birds, reptiles have a **renal portal system** which directs blood from the hindlimbs to the kidneys. The advantage of this system for reptiles is probably that even if blood supply to the kidneys is reduced, blood from the

portal venous system supports renal perfusion. However, the portal vein system is not necessarily used all the time. Under stress, blood flow to the kidney can probably also be prevented by means of valves.

> **IN A NUTSHELL** !
>
> The reptiles heart has only one ventricle in most species. The blood flow within the heart is controlled by different mechanisms.

MORE DETAILS Interestingly, in crocodiles one aortic arch arises from the left ventricle and one from the right ventricle. The two aortic arches are connected via the **foramen of Panizza** near their point of origin, so that right-left shunts are possible for crocodiles with diversion of blood from the right ventricle into the systemic circulation. This plays a role, especially when diving underwater. The reduction in perfusion of the lungs is further assisted by a narrowing of the pulmonary artery, which is equipped with nodule-like structures in its wall for this purpose. In crocodiles that are on land and breathing air, blood from the right ventricle is directed to the left aorta at rest, and blood from the left ventricle is directed to the right aorta. With increasing activity, systolic pressure in the left ventricle increases, thus oxygen-rich blood is also forced through the foramen of Panizza into the left aorta as it is expelled.

9 Blood

Max Gassmann, Thomas Göbel, Bernd Kaspers, Thomas A. Lutz

9.1 Functions of blood

Max Gassmann, Thomas A. Lutz

> **ESSENTIALS** ✖
>
> Blood (sanguis) is a highly complex transport medium. It is a suspension of various cells in a protein-containing, buffered electrolyte solution. The blood volume in mammals amounts to approx. $\frac{1}{13}$ of the fat-free body mass (e.g. in a 20 kg dog, blood volume is approx. 1.5 l). Blood transports oxygen from the lungs to the tissues and carbon dioxide in the reverse direction. Nutrients are transported in blood from the intestine to the tissues and corresponding waste products are transported to the excretory organs. In addition, hormones, micronutrients, molecules involved in humoral immunity, and body heat are transported by blood (**Table 9.1**). The blood thus has a central homeostatic role.

The **transport functions** include various solutes derived from the respiratory and gastrointestinal tracts. Blood also transports metabolic intermediates between organs such as adipose tissue, muscles and liver. It also delivers metabolic end products to excreting organs such as kidneys, liver, gall bladder, intestines or even the sweat glands. In addition, blood serves to transport hormones, vitamins, trace elements and other micronutrients as well as heat. As a circulating part of the extracellular fluid, blood plasma thus ensures the maintenance of **homeostatic conditions** with regard to volume, solute concentrations, electrolyte distribution, osmotic pressure, H⁺ ion concentration and temperature.

To maintain homeostasis, both blood volume and concentrations of blood constituents are constantly monitored by control processes, and if necessary, corrected via appropriate feedback mechanisms. Two examples are: (1) blood sugar concentration is regulated by insulin and glucagon, among other factors, and (2) blood pressure (p. 208) is adjusted by angiotensin, aldosterone and the autonomic nervous system. The most strictly controlled property of blood is the osmolarity of extracellular fluid. The functions of the blood in cellular and humoral immune defence and mechanisms for protection against blood loss are described in detail in ch. 9.4 (p. 234) and ch. 10 (p. 244).

Table 9.1 The functions of blood.

	Function
1.	Maintenance of homeostasis in the tissue fluid (defined, among others, as isotonicity, ion composition, isohydria, isovolaemia and isothermia; according to Claude Bernard [1813–1878]).
2.	Gas transport (oxygen and carbon dioxide) between lungs and tissues.
3.	Transport of nutrients from the digestive tract to the liver.
4.	Transport of nutrients and metabolic intermediates between tissues (e.g. lactate after work, from muscle to liver).
5.	Transport of metabolic waste products to the excreting organs (e.g. urea from the liver to the kidney).
6.	Transport of hormones (e.g. erythropoietin from the kidney to the bone marrow), vitamins and micronutrients (e.g. trace elements).
7.	Heat transport, e.g. transfer of excess heat from internal organs (p. 500).
8.	Defence function: transport of leukocytes, immunoglobulins (e.g. IgG) and other components of humoral immunity, e.g. complement system (p. 247).
9.	Haemostasis and coagulation (p. 234); protection against blood loss.
10.	Maintenance of blood volume (p. 212) and thus blood pressure (e.g. for kidney filtration).

9.2 Non-cellular components of the blood

Max Gassmann, Thomas A. Lutz

> **ESSENTIALS**   ✖
>
> The non-cellular components of blood are water, electrolytes, proteins (incl. fibrin), non-protein nitrogen compounds, carbohydrates, lipids, vitamins and other micronutrients. Maintaining the appropriate plasma concentrations is vital, and the levels of many of these components are efficiently regulated.

9.2.1 Blood plasma

By centrifuging blood, heavier cellular blood components (red and white blood cells and platelets) can be separated from blood fluid. Blood clotting (p. 236) is inhibited by the addition of anticoagulants such as heparin, sodium EDTA or sodium citrate. In blood that has been rendered **uncoagulable**, centrifugation leads to separation into **blood plasma** and **blood cells**. If, however, blood is allowed to **coagulate** before centrifugation, it is separated into **blood serum** and a **blood clot**, which contains all blood cells. Blood serum thus corresponds to the plasma fraction without fibrin that leads to clotting.

In terms of weight, water is the largest component with approx. 900–910 g per litre of plasma. The next largest fraction comprises blood proteins, with approx. 65–80 g per litre. Electrolytes, glucose and non-protein nitrogen compounds (NPN) are present in a true solution, whereas blood proteins are in colloidal solution. Proteins also bind blood lipids, iron and especially some of the divalent cations, Ca^{2+} and Mg^{2+}.

Water requirements for most animal species considered in veterinary medicine are met primarily from drinking water and the fluid content of their feed. However, species living in desert conditions, such as the kangaroo rat, have to derive most of the water they require through oxidative metabolism. Since water loss, unlike water intake, is a continuous process, there is a constant potential risk of dehydration for an animal. For example, in a medium-sized dog, 5-days of dehydration, under otherwise "normal" environmental conditions, leads to about 10% loss of body weight. This loss of water affects both the intracellular and the extracellular space. In such severe dehydration, most animals refuse to eat. An exception to this are camels. In these animals, water loss is mainly from intracellular and intercellular fluids and not, as in most domestic animals, from blood plasma. Further aspects of blood plasma isohydria are discussed in ch. 12.9.2 and ch. 13.8.

> **IN A NUTSHELL**   !
>
> **Blood plasma** is an aqueous liquid in which all non-cellular blood components are dissolved or emulsified.

9.2.2 Electrolytes of plasma

A high extracellular sodium concentration is critical for maintaining extracellular fluid volume (**Table 9.2**). Besides inorganic ions such as Na^+ and Cl^-, K^+, Ca^{2+}, Mg^{2+} and HCO_3^-, $H_2PO_4^-/HPO_4^{2-}$, SO_4^{2-}, various plasma proteins (p. 220) are also important in maintaining fluid volume. Inorganic electrolytes are the main determinants of the **osmotic pressure of blood plasma**. Over 95% of total osmotic pressure is determined by the **quantities of dissolved inorganic electrolytes** (approx. 5000 mmHg).

> **IN A NUTSHELL**   !
>
> Na^+ and Cl^- together account for about 85% of the osmotically active particles in the plasma.

Table 9.2 Approximate average concentration of constituents present in mammalian plasma.

Ion/substance	g · l⁻¹	mmol · l⁻¹
Na^+	3.25	140
K^+	0.18	5
Ca^{2+}	0.10	3
Mg^{2+}	0.02	1
Cl^-	3.60	101
HCO_3^-	0.6	24
$H_2PO_4^-/HPO_4^{2-}$	0.04	2
SO_4^{2-}	0.02	1
Protein	63–80	1
Glucose	0.8 (0.35–2.00)	4.4 (2.0–11.0)
Lipids	5.0	-
Urea	0.15	-
Total NPN	0.3	-

Osmolality is practically the same in all body compartments, at about 290 mosmol · kg⁻¹. The main difference between blood plasma and interstitial fluid is the protein concentration. Although plasma proteins generate an osmotic pressure of only approx. 25 mmHg, this so-called **colloid-osmotic** or **oncotic** pressure is of utmost importance for the distribution of water between intravascular and extravascular spaces (see ch. Microcirculation in the terminal vascular bed (p. 203))

Isotonicity, the maintenance of osmotic pressure in the extracellular space, is one of the basic requirements for the function and for the communication of all cells of the body. Thus, an increase of osmotic pressure in the extracellular space leads to shrinkage of cells. A reduction of extracellular osmotic pressure causes cell swelling and, in extreme cases, cell bursting (e.g. haemolysis of erythrocytes in pure water). Saline solution infusions usually have the same osmotic pressure as plasma (isotonicity). Hypertonic infusions lead to water flow from cells into the extracellular space and hence into blood. Occasionally, hypertonic infusions are used in the therapy of hypovolaemic shock. In contrast, with hypotonic infusions, water flows into the cells.

Another important prerequisite for homeostatic cell function is **ion composition**. This means that both the total number of osmotically active substances, and also their relative proportions, must be in a physiological range. The basic ionic composition of extracellular and intracellular spaces determines the membrane potential and thus is important for all bioelectrical processes in and between the cells, as well as for membrane transport (see ch. Functions of the cell membrane (p. 31)). It should also be noted that slight differences between the interstitium and the intravascular fluids are caused, among other things, by the so-called Donnan effect. Because negatively charged plasma proteins bind some of the circulating cations, the total cation concentration in blood is somewhat higher than in the interstitium.

9.2.3   Plasma proteins

The **functions of plasma proteins** include: specific and non-specific **transport** of a wide variety of substances, **pH buffering**, regulation of **colloid-osmotic** (oncotic) **pressure**, effects on **blood viscosity**, **blood coagulation**, and specific or non-specific **defence against infection**. In addition, many plasma proteins have enzymatic functions (see ch. on blood coagulation (p. 236)). Apart from immunoglobulins, produced in lymphatic organs, and lipoproteins, derived from the intestine and other organs, most plasma proteins are synthesised by the liver. This also explains the multitude of defects, like coagulation disorders and oedema, observed in liver diseases, such as cirrhosis.

Individual plasma proteins can be isolated by various methods. **Electrophoresis** is used to separate the plasma proteins in a gel according to their charge and mass (**Fig. 9.1**). The relatively small, strongly negatively charged prealbumin in the globulin fraction (not present in all species) migrates rapidly towards the anode in the electric field. Proteins with a relatively large molecular mass and low net charge (e.g. IgG) remain almost at the application site. As shown in **Fig. 9.1** the sequence on a gel is: prealbumin/albumin, $\alpha_{1,2}$, $\beta_{1,2}$, γ globulins. The division into α and β globulins and their subgroups is not function-specific. γ Globulins are mainly **immunoglobulins** (IgA, IgG, IgM), which serve the body's immune defence (see ch. Opsonisation and phagocytosis (p. 248)). In many diseases, specific changes occur in the protein electrophoretic pattern. For example, acute-phase proteins appear in the course of an inflammation (**Table 9.3**). With refined techniques (e.g. immunoelectrophoresis), it is now possible to distinguish between more than 100 individual plasma proteins, some of which are used for precise diagnosis of disease.

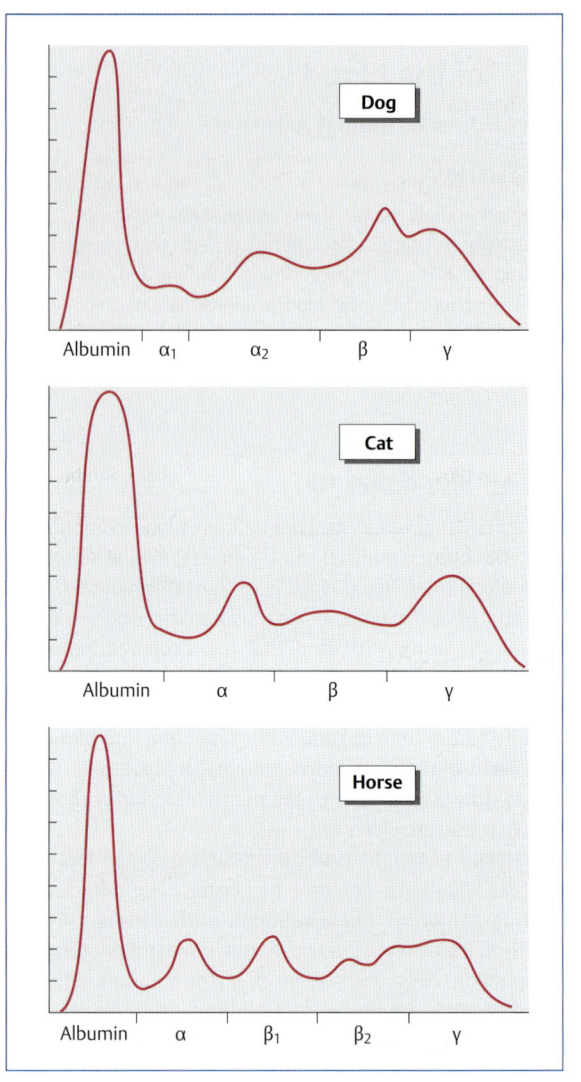

Fig. 9.1 Electrophoretic separation of plasma proteins of dogs, cats and horses (also **Table 9.3**).

IN A NUTSHELL   !

The proteins **albumin**, **fibrinogen** and various **globulins**, comprise about 7% by weight of the plasma. Other proteins, such as enzymes or hormones, are present in smaller but physiologically important quantities.

MORE DETAILS   The **concentration of proteins in plasma** depends above all on water balance. Thus, in dehydration, with an unchanged amount of plasma protein, the concentration of protein is increased (**Fig. 8.18**). Physiological fluctuations in plasma protein concentrations are seen, for example, as different age-dependent patterns. Albumin and globulin concentrations are often lower in young animals than in adults. Older animals sometimes have an increased total protein concentration, because of a relative increase in the proportion of globulins. During pregnancy and lactation, plasma protein concentration is sometimes reduced.

Table 9.3 Functions of some globulins and causes for their changes in animals.

Proteins	Function	Changes and associated disorders
α Globulins		
α₁ Fraction		
α_1-Proteinase inhibitor	Protease inhibitor	• Increase: inflammation, hepatitis • Decrease: Cirrhosis
α_1-Acidic glycoprotein	Immune regulation	• Increase: inflammation, tissue trauma, neoplasia, acute or chronic hepatitis
α_1-Antichymotrypsin	Enzyme inhibitor	• Increase: inflammation
High-density lipoprotein (HDL) (α_1 -lipoprotein)	Cholesterol transport	• Increase: hypothyroidism
α₂ Fraction		
α_2-Macroglobulin	Protease inhibitor	• Increase: inflammation, acute or chronic hepatitis
Coeruloplasmin	Copper transport	• Increase: inflammation, tissue trauma
Haptoglobulin	Binding of dimeric haemoglobin, immune regulation	• Increase: inflammation, tissue trauma, use of corticosteroids, pregnancy/birth • Decrease: acute haemolysis, haematoma formation
Serum amyloid A (SAA)	Immune regulation, lipoprotein metabolism	• Increase: inflammation, tissue trauma, birth, familial amyloidosis in Abyssinian cats
β Globulins		
β₁ Fraction		
Low-density lipoprotein (LDL)	Lipid transport	• Increase: nephrotic syndrome, hypothyroidism, cholestatic liver disease
Transferrin	Iron transport	• Increase: chronic iron deficiency, blood loss • Decrease: inflammation
Ferritin	Iron deposition, storage	• Increase: inflammation, iron overload, acute haemolysis • Decrease: iron deficiency, chronic blood loss
C-reactive protein (CRP)	Modulation of the immune response	• Increase: inflammation, tissue trauma, neoplasia, administration of corticosteroids, birth.
Fibrinogen	Haemostasis, scaffold for tissue repair	• Increase: inflammation, pregnancy/birth • Decrease: disseminated intravascular coagulation
Factors of the complement system (C 1,2,3b,4,5)	Complement system	• Increase: inflammation
β₂ Fraction		
Factors of the complement system (C 3,6,7)	Complement system	• Increase: inflammation
γ Globulins		
Immunoglobulins of the type IgA, IgE, IgG, IgM	Immune defence	• Increase: chronic inflammation, chronic infection, neoplasia, immune-mediated disease, liver disease • Decrease: inherited or acquired immunodeficiency syndrome

Albumin is mainly responsible for **non-specific transport** of other molecules. Albumin (molecular weight: 66 kDa), makes up approx. 60% of total plasma proteins. Albumin is a homogeneous class of protein. It contains no prosthetic groups. Plasma albumin has a half-life of about 10–15 days. It transports bilirubin and fatty acids as well as divalent cations. Many exogenous substances such as drugs can also bind to albumin. Only the non-protein bound propor-

tion of cations in blood is biologically active. This proportion is significantly influenced by plasma pH, which affects the degree of ionisation of plasma proteins. This is clinically relevant, especially for Ca^{2+} (hyperventilation → alkalosis → stronger negative charge of the plasma proteins → increased binding of Ca^{2+} to plasma proteins → decrease in free Ca^{2+} → increase risk of tetanic spasms). When measuring electrolyte concentrations in plasma, the unbound, i.e.

ionised fraction should therefore always be determined separately.

Globulins are a very heterogeneous protein fraction consisting of various glycoproteins, lipoproteins and metalloproteins. The half-life of globulins in plasma is on average five days. The molecular weight of plasma proteins varies considerably between approx. 40 and 1300 kDa. In contrast to albumin, globulins are often involved in the **specific transport** of a wide variety of substances, such as lipids, hormones, trace elements (Fe, Cu), and vitamins (**Table 9.3**). In most cases, proteins help to solubilise water-insoluble substances. The α_1 globulins include, for example, the vitamin B_{12}-binding transcobalamin or the steroid hormone-binding transcortin. The Cu transporting protein coeruloplasmin (p. 436) is located in the α_2 globulin fraction. Many lipoproteins, and the iron binding transferrin, are β globulins.

Plasma proteins (approx. $65–80\,g\cdot l^{-1}$) are an ever present, readily available **nutrient supply for an animal**. In starvation, these proteins can be used as a source of energy for cells. In addition, plasma proteins serve as an "amino acid buffer" for the turnover and synthesis of various cellular proteins. An important function of plasma proteins is maintenance of **colloid-osmotic (= oncotic) pressure**, resulting mainly from the unequal distribution of proteins between intravascular and extravascular space, where protein concentration is low. Although the contribution of proteins to total osmotic pressure is small, only these macromolecular proteins maintain colloid-osmotic pressure, since they cannot diffuse through the vascular endothelium, unlike the small-molecule components. Quantitatively, albumin is again the most important, accounting for about 80% of the colloid-osmotic pressure. The functional significance of the colloid-osmotic pressure lies in the regulation of fluid exchange (**Fig. 8.17**) between capillaries and interstitium. Plasma proteins represent a counterforce to the hydrostatic pressure. If there is an imbalance between the colloid-osmotic and hydrostatic forces, oedema may result as a pathological accumulation of fluid in the interstitium. One important cause of oedema is hypoproteinaemia (**Fig. 8.18**), which can result from severe liver, kidney or intestinal diseases, or from malnutrition (e.g. swollen bellies in severely malnourished children in developing countries). Oedema also occurs when there is an increase in hydrostatic pressure (e.g. in cardiac insufficiencies); (see ch. Microcirculation in the termimal vascular bed (p. 203)).

Plasma proteins are **amphoteric molecules**, i.e. they behave like bases towards stronger acids and like acids towards stronger bases. Thus, in addition to bicarbonate (HCO_3^-) and phosphate ($H_2PO_4^-/HPO_4^{2-}$) buffers, they play an important role in pH regulation (for the **buffering function** of plasma proteins see ch. Buffer systems (p. 346)). In addition, plasma proteins determine the viscosity of the blood plasma (p. 195), which is about twice that of water.

Enzymes are also found among the plasma proteins, of which the transaminases are of particular diagnostic importance (see textbooks of clinical chemistry). An increase in the activity of these transaminases in blood can provide diagnostic criteria for specific organ damage, since the enzymes leak from damaged cells into blood in larger quantities. See also the importance of plasma proteins as specific clotting substances (p. 236) as well as antigen-specific and -nonspecific components of humoral immunity (p. 244).

■ Erythrocyte sedimentation rate

Erythrocyte sedimentation rate is a non-specific parameter that is still occasionally measured for diagnosis in horses. It indicates changes in the composition of blood plasma. The erythrocyte sedimentation rate is increased in inflammatory diseases. Although it is very non-specific, it is an indicator of inflammatory processes, and is very easy to perform.

Blood cells suspended in blood plasma have a higher specific gravity than plasma. Therefore, they have a tendency to sediment. In the living animal, blood cells are kept in suspension by the flow of blood. However, in stagnant blood with an anticoagulant such as Na citrate, sedimentation occurs, with **erythrocytes settling** more rapidly than that of the leukocytes because of their **higher specific gravity**. Only the sedimentation **rate** of erythrocytes is of practical diagnostic relevance.

The causes of increased or decreased aggregation are not yet fully understood. Cell count per volume unit also has a considerable influence on the erythrocyte sedimentation rate, which is why the red blood cell count (or the haematocrit) must be taken into account. The lower the red blood cell count, the higher the rate of sedimentation. In anaemia therefore, erythrocyte sedimentation rate may not be a valid diagnostic criterion.

9.2.4　Non-protein nitrogen compounds

> **IN A NUTSHELL**　　　　　　　　　　　　　　　!
>
> Non-protein nitrogen substances are summarised under the term NPN (non-protein nitrogen) or residual nitrogen.

The nitrogen content of the NPN fraction is on average $500\,mg\cdot l^{-1}$ plasma. **Urea**, the end product of protein and amino acid metabolism in mammals, represents the largest proportion of NPN compounds. Urea is formed in the urea cycle in the liver during the detoxification of ammonia (NH_3), which is released by oxidative deamination of glutamate in practically all body cells. $NH_3 + H^+$ forms NH_4^+. Urea is produced from $NH_4^+ + HCO_3^-$.

In herbivores, **hippuric acid** is the second largest component of NPN. This is a detoxification product of benzoic acid from the gastrointestinal tract. The next is **creatinine**, a breakdown product of creatine. Thus its concentration in plasma is a measure of catabolic processes in muscle. Other NPN components are amino acids, oligo- and polypeptides (including peptide hormones such as insulin or glucagon), purine and pyrimidine derivatives, allantoin and uric acid (p. 325). **Allantoin** or **uric acid** are degradation products of purine bases. In birds (p. 337), they are also the degradation products of amino acid metabolism.

Circulation, respiration

MORE DETAILS   In mammals, **uric acid** is largely produced in the peroxisomes and then converted by uricase to allantoin. Primates are an exception, as this uricase step is not present. Birds also do not convert uric acid to allantoin so that uric acid can crystallise in organs (especially the kidneys) and in joints. This formation of crystals is also known as gout in humans. In **Dalmatian dogs**, the conversion of **uric acid into allantoin** is disturbed, because of a defect in the transport of uric acid into peroxisomes. Because of this, Dalmatians have higher uric acid concentration in (p. 325) blood and urine compared to other dog breeds. Uric acid containing bladder stones are therefore found more frequently in this dog breed.

NPN compounds are mostly **excreted in urine**. The term azotaemia is used when the NPN fraction in plasma rises, usually as a result of renal dysfunction. **Uraemia** is a serious syndrome, although the exact cause of the accompanying severe disorder of general health is unclear. The increase in the concentration of those solutes in blood that are typically used for diagnosis, is probably not directly responsible for the disturbed general health status.

9.2.5   Carbohydrates

The portal vein collects blood coming from abdominal organs, which is loaded with nutrients from the intestine, as well as hormones and metabolic products. Depending on the composition of food, blood of the portal vein contains different monosaccharides. After passing through the liver, however, blood of the hepatic vein contains only **glucose**. Since glucose is the most important source of energy for the CNS and various other organs, blood glucose level is very well maintained by hormonal control systems (p. 546). It is kept as constant as possible within a relatively narrow range. Apart from minor species differences, fasting glucose values of about $4–7\,\text{mmol}\cdot\text{l}^{-1}$ are generally found in monogastric mammals and about $2–4\,\text{mmol}\cdot\text{l}^{-1}$ in ruminants. Birds generally have higher blood glucose values (around $10\,\text{mmol}\cdot\text{l}^{-1}$).

MORE DETAILS   **Monogastric animals** absorb large amounts of glucose from the intestine, whereas in **ruminants** the short-chain fatty acids formed by microbial fermentation in the forestomachs are the main end product of carbohydrate digestion. Glucose is subsequently synthesised by gluconeogenesis (p. 469) in the liver from these short-chain fatty acids, mainly from propionate. Gluconeogenesis is also the most important source of glucose for cats, using amino acids as substrates, as cats consume very little carbohydrates in their natural diet. For this reason, in ruminants and in cats, unlike other monogastric animals, the activity of gluconeogenesis is related to food intake (p. 546).

The blood sugar concentration (p. 546) is mainly regulated by the pancreatic hormones, insulin and glucagon. In most monogastric animals, food intake increases blood glucose concentration, and this is counter-regulated by insulin, secreted from the pancreatic β-cells.

9.2.6   Lipids and fatty acids

> **IN A NUTSHELL**   !
>
> The concentration of lipids in blood fluctuates widely, depending mainly on food or fat intake.

After digestion of triacylglycerols (formerly called: triglycerides), the long-chain fatty acids and also monoacylglycerols are absorbed in the small intestine. They are relinked as triacylglycerols in the intestinal epithelial cells (**Fig. 16.59**) (see ch. Digestion and absorption of fats (p. 429). The triacylglycerols then associate with apolipoproteins to form **chylomicrons**, along with small amounts of cholesterol and fat-soluble vitamins and phospholipids. Chylomicrons enter the blood via the lymph vessels (**Fig. 16.60**) (see ch. Digestion and absorption of fats (p. 429). After a high-fat meal, blood serum contains up to $20\,\text{g}\cdot\text{l}^{-1}$ lipids in emulsified form and therefore has a milky turbid appearance; this is the so-called lipaemic serum or plasma. Removal of chylomicron lipid from blood occurs partly under the influence of insulin, which activates lipoprotein lipase, thus enabling the uptake of lipids by various cells.

MORE DETAILS   Lipids are mainly **transported in blood bound to plasma protein**. The fat and protein content of lipoproteins (p. 467) (**Fig. 17.4**) varies widely. Lipoproteins are classified according to their density into **VLDL** (very low density lipoproteins), **LDL** (low density lipoproteins) and **HDL** (high density lipoproteins) (**Fig. 17.4**). The HDL consist of 50% lipids, while VLDL have a lipid content of about 90%. VLDL are cleaved by endothelial lipoprotein lipase to produce LDL. The LDLs are very rich in cholesterol and, when there is a low level of HDL in humans, this probably leads to deposition of **cholesterol and its derivatives in the vascular wall**. This could result in vascular occlusion (atherosclerosis), especially of the coronary vessels. It should be noted that not only HDL concentration, but also its functionality (e.g. antioxidant properties and cholesterol absorption capacity) and the size of HDL subtypes are of pathophysiological significance.

Long-chain fatty acids are mainly transported bound to albumin. Their concentration in blood increases in response to stress, thus providing the body with an additional energy substrate. **Short-** and **medium-chain fatty acids** are absorbed by the intestinal epithelium. They reach the liver via the portal vein. Short-chain fatty acids, the end product of microbial carbohydrate fermentation in the ruminant forestomachs (and in the monogastric large intestine), are therefore found in greater concentrations in the blood of ruminants.

9.2.7   Other blood constituents

The concentration of **ketone bodies** resulting from the breakdown of fat is particularly high in states of **starvation, diabetes mellitus**, or in **ketosis** of **cattle**. Ketone bodies can be used as source of energy in tissues including the CNS. **Lactic acid** is produced as an important metabolic product in anaerobic muscle metabolism (p. 627) (**Fig. 26.2**). In the liver, it can be converted to glucose via the so-called **Cori cycle**. Blood lactate level is used as an indicator of performance when measuring training status (p. 630) (**Fig. 26.19**). An increase in lactate level also occurs in states of shock, when there is a local increase in anaerobic metabolism because of a temporary decline in blood perfusion of tissues (tissue hypoxia).

Various **pigments** affect the colour of blood plasma. Besides carotenoids (e.g. from carrot consumption) and other pigments, colour is also determined by **bilirubin** content (see ch. on erythropoiesis and erythrocyte degradation (p. 230)). Equids have a relatively high concentration of bilirubin in blood under physiological conditions, but it is elevated in all animal species in various disease processes (prehepatic, hepatic and posthepatic icterus). Accordingly, in severe chronic liver disease, the mucous membranes, and also the sclera of the eye, take on a yellow colour (jaundice = icterus).

Vitamins belong to the large number of micronutrients which are transported in blood. Water-soluble vitamins such as the B vitamins are dissolved in blood, while those not soluble in water are transported in a bound form (e.g. vitamin E is transported in lipoproteins). The role of **vitamin B_{12} (cobalamin)**, of particular importance for blood, is explained in more detail in the section below.

MORE DETAILS   Cobalamin is an organometallic compound with a central one-, two- or threefold positively charged cobalt ion. Cobalamin is the only known biologically active compound containing cobalt. It can only be synthesised by bacteria. Cobalamin must therefore either be ingested in the diet or, in ruminants, can be produced by microbial fermentation in the rumen and can be subsequently absorbed by the small intestine. Ruminants therefore need sufficient amounts of cobalt in their diet to meet this requirement for cobalamin. Cobalamin absorption in small intestine only occurs when bound with intrinsic factor (p. 415), secreted by gastric gland cells. Cobalamin is a coenzyme of methionine synthetase, methylmalonyl-CoA mutase, and leucine mutase. Among other things, cobalamin is important for the formation of precursors of DNA synthesis. Therefore, tissues with high mitotic rates have a high requirement for cobalamin. Hence, cobalamin is important for haematopoiesis in bone marrow (see pernicious anaemia in the chapter on haemoglobin and oxygen transport (p. 229)).

Suggested reading

Vogel J, Kiessling I, Heinicke K et al. Transgenic mice overexpressing erythropoietin adapt to excessive erythrocytosis by regulating blood viscosity. Blood 2003; 15: 2278–2284

Weiss DJ, Wardrop KJ. Schalm's Veterinary Hematology, 6th ed. Iowa: Blackwell Publishing; 2010

9.3   Cellular components

Max Gassmann, Thomas A. Lutz

> **ESSENTIALS**
>
> **Erythrocytes** make up more than **99%** of the cellular blood components. The main function of red blood cells is the transport of oxygen throughout the body. For this process, oxygen binds reversibly (oxygenation) to the red blood pigment, **haemoglobin**, in erythrocytes. The other cell components in blood are white blood cells (**leukocytes**) and platelets (**thrombocytes**). These two cell types have important roles either in the body's immune defence against infections (**leukocytes**), or in haemostasis and blood clotting (**thrombocytes**). The production rate of erythrocytes is mainly determined by the demand for oxygen, while the production rate of leukocytes is related to the state of the immune system.

9.3.1   Haematopoiesis

> **IN A NUTSHELL**   !
>
> Haematopoiesis refers to the production of the various blood cells in the blood-forming tissue.

Postnatal haematopoiesis takes place mainly in the **marrow** of flat bones and in the **lymphatic system**. After birth, haematopoiesis that previously took place in the liver and spleen during embryonic and foetal life, becomes insignificant. The **haematopoietic system** is characterised by four basic features:

1. It is one of the **most active tissues for cell division** in the body. This explains the susceptibility of haematopoiesis to chemo- and radiation therapy in tumour diseases, which target rapidly dividing cancer cells.
2. Compared to erythrocytes (life span in mammals between 60 and 160 days), **white blood cells**, with the exception of certain lymphocytes (memory cells), have a relatively **short life span** of only a few days.
3. All blood cells (erythrocytes, granulocytes, monocytes, thrombocytes and lymphocytes) are derived from a small population of **pluripotent haematopoietic stem cells**, also known as a colony-forming unit (CFU).
4. The haematopoietic system is **regulated** very **efficiently** and can adapt quickly to changing needs (e.g. lack of oxygen or infection).

The haematopoietic stem cells have a great regenerative capacity. The number of blood cells being continuously formed is enormous. In mammals, for example, about 50 billion erythrocytes are produced per litre of blood each day. The **pluripotent stem cells**, are capable of self-renewal, and are central to the production of all the blood cells. It is apparent that the number of these stem cells, which do not exhibit characteristic morphological properties, is extremely low. In animal experiments, for example, in a mouse, the entire haematopoietic system, previously de-

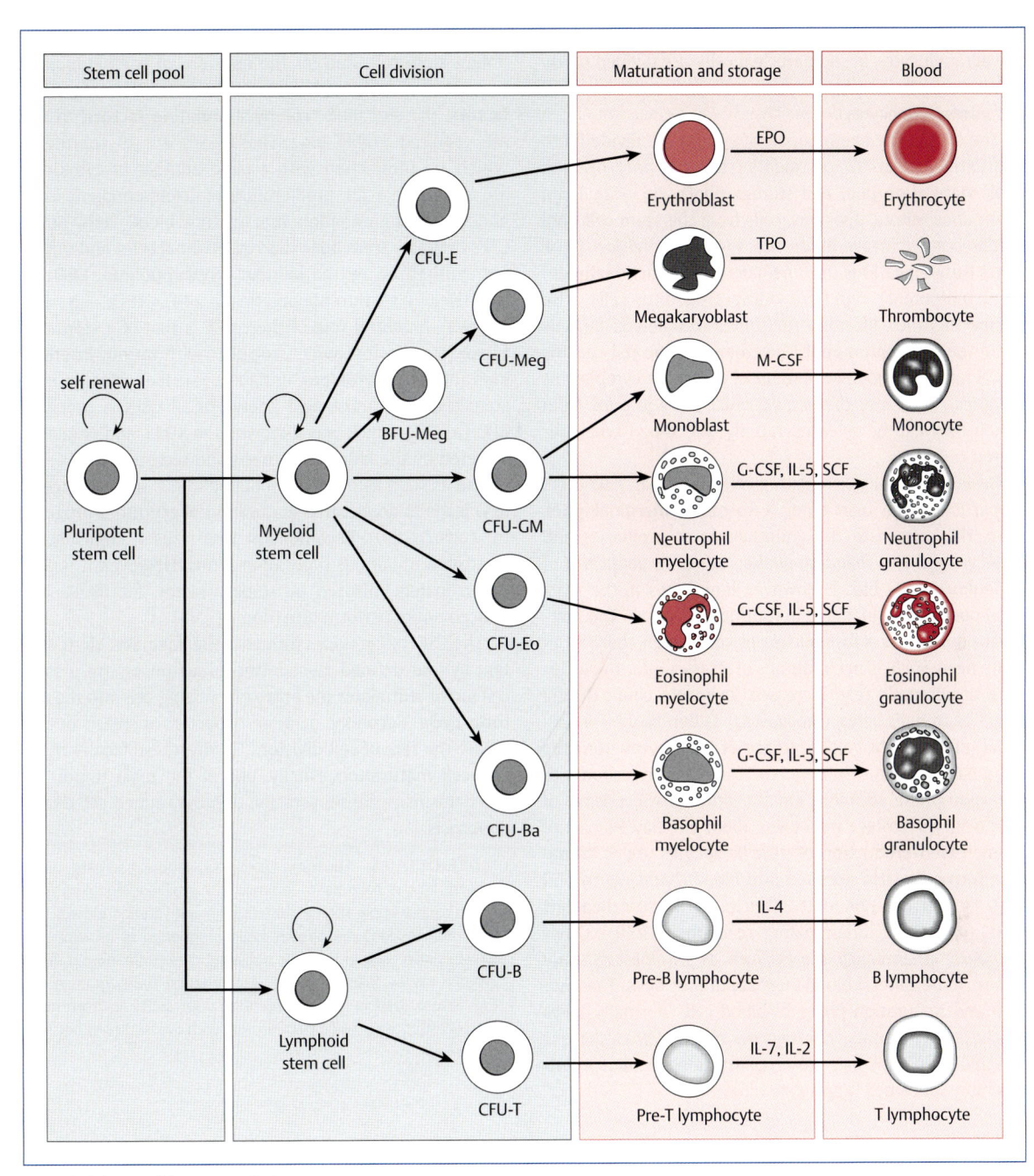

Fig. 9.2 Scheme of haematopoiesis.
The pluripotent stem cells as well as the myeloid and lymphoid stem cells are capable of self-renewal. Further explanations are given in the text.
BFU-Meg = burst-forming unit megakaryocytes, CFU-E = colony-forming unit erythrocytes, CFU-Meg = colony-forming unit megakaryocytes, CFU-GM = colony-forming unit-granulocytes/monocytes, CFU-Eo = colony-forming unit eosinophil granulocytes, CFU-Ba = colony-forming unit basophil granulocyte, CFU-B = colony-forming unit B lymphocyte, CFU-T = colony-forming unit T lymphocyte; EPO = erythropoietin, TPO = thrombopoietin, M-CSF = macrophage colony-stimulating factor, G-CSF = granulocyte colony-stimulating factor, SCF = stem cell factor (steel factor), IL = interleukin.

stroyed by cytotoxic radiation, could be restored by the introduction of just 30 isolated stem cells.

Multipotent progenitor cells are the first to differentiate from the stem cells. Two main differentiation lineages from these progenitor cells can be distinguished: the **lymphoid** (lymphatic stem cell) and the **myeloid** (myeloid stem cell) cell lineages (**Fig. 9.2**). Subsequently, **unipotent progenitor cells** are generated where the direction of their

differentiation is now irreversibly determined. These committed cells (erythropoietic, granulo-/monocytopoietic, thrombopoietic) are designated as CFU-E, CFU-GM, CFU-Meg (**Fig. 9.2**). The three main types of **mature cells** are **erythrocytes** (red blood cells), **leukocytes** (white blood cells) and **thrombocytes** (platelets). It should be noted that the classifications of leukocytes are different according to their origin and to their morphological characteristics. All so-called granulocytes belong to the myeloid cell series. The agranulocytes, or mononuclear cells, are divided partly into the lymphoid (lymphocytes) and partly to the myeloid cell series (monocytes).

The cells of the haematopoietic system are divided into four extravascular compartments (stem cell pool, division pool, maturation pool and storage pool) (Fig. 9.2). From continuous mitotic divisions, cells from the **stem cell pool** of the bone marrow enter the so-called **division pool**. Then, through various intermediate steps, functionally defined (unipotent), rapidly dividing progenitor cells arise for specific roles. After cell division is completed, the cells are in the **maturation pool**. They then develop cell-specific characteristics (e.g. development of particular cytoplasmic granules), and enter the extravascular **storage pool**, from which they can be released rapidly into blood when required.

Besides becoming circulating cells in blood, leukocytes in particular can also enter a so-called **marginal pool**. Here, they attach to the endothelium of capillaries and small vessels. This marginal pool accounts for about **half** of all **leukocytes** in blood. However, leukocytes in the marginal pool are not included in routine cell counts. The marginal pool allows a fast release of cells when there is an acute need, such as in conditions of stress, under the influence of adrenalin (e.g. increased leukocyte count during stress of animals being transported). When there is a bacterial infection, the initial **release of leukocytes** from the marginal pool occurs in only 20–30 minutes in response to the appropriate stimulus. On the other hand, release of cells from the storage pool takes about one day. As part of an increased production of new leukocytes, more **immature forms** are also released into blood (band neutrophil with curved but not lobular nucleus: the so-called **left shift**) (see ch. on inflammatory reactions (p.250)). Other immature preliminary stages, such as myeloblasts, only appear in peripheral blood after about four days. The division and maturation phase of blood cells normally takes 10–12 days (just under six days per phase). When there is a high demand, the maturation phase, in particular, is considerably shortened (approx. two days).

For the development of different blood cells from pluripotent stem cells and for the response of haematopoietic tissue to an increased demand, haematopoietic **growth factors**, the so-called **"colony-stimulating factors" (CSF)**, are required (**Table 9.4**). These CSFs are glycoproteins which, on interaction with a large number of cytokines, are responsible for proliferation of haematopoietic cells and their differentiation into mature blood cells. Some CSFs originate from bone marrow stromal cells, and others are synthesised by the kidneys (**erythropoietin, EPO**) or the liver (e.g. thrombopoietin (p.234), **TPO; Fig. 9.2, Fig. 9.3**). A central role of these CSF is that of a **stem cell factor** (steel factor), which, together with various **interleukins** and other **cytokines**, initiates the cell division cycle of stem cells. The most well known of all CSFs is probably EPO (p.328), which was discovered in 1948, and is mainly secreted by the kidney. Synthesis and secretion of EPO increase as soon as oxygen demand exceeds oxygen supply. EPO leads to accelerated maturation of erythroid progenitor cells (p.230). Recombinant EPO is used clinically, in treatment of various types of anaemia. However, it is also unfortunately misused by some athletes, for illegal enhancement of performance (doping).

The CSFs or cytokines influence the haematopoietic system by four defined mechanisms of action. Firstly, a stem cell factor stimulates the **entry** of a resting cell into the **mitotic cycle**. Secondly, a range of factors increase or decrease the rate of **cell division**. Thirdly, these factors regulate **cell maturation**. Finally, one of the most important mechanisms is the suppression of programmed cell death, **apoptosis**.

MORE DETAILS   For some years now, various haematopoietic growth factors have been commercially available, enabling their broad clinical application in both human and veterinary medicine. Recombinant EPO has already been mentioned as an example, which is also used in anaemic dogs and cats (suffering e.g. from chronic kidney failure). On an experimental basis, granulocyte CSF is also used in the treatment of dogs suffering from bone marrow suppression due to treatment with cytostatics or because of parvovirosis.

Table 9.4 Haematopoietic stem cell biology.

Haematopoietic growth factors	Synonyms	Size (kD)	Origin
Stem cell factor	Steel factor, mast cell growth factor	37–42	Bone marrow cells, foetal tissue
Granulocyte macrophage colony-stimulating factor (GM-CSF)	CSF α	18–30	T lymphocytes, monocytes, endothelial cells, fibroblasts, macrophages
Granulocyte colony-stimulating factor (G-CSF)	CSF β	19.6	Monocytes, macrophages, endothelial cells, fibroblasts, neutrophils
Macrophage colony-stimulating factor (M-CSF)	CSF-1	90	Monocytes, macrophages, endothelial cells, placenta
Erythropoietin (EPO)	–	38	Kidney, foetal liver and many other organs
Thrombopoietin (TPO)	–	35–70	Liver, kidney

9.3.2　Erythrocytes

The haematocrit, which is mainly determined by the number and size of erythrocytes, averages about $0.41 \cdot l^{-1}$ in mammals. The viscosity of the blood is significantly affected by the number of erythrocytes and their deformability as well as by the concentration of plasma proteins.

■ Physiological properties and reference values

> **IN A NUTSHELL**　　!
>
> Mature **red blood cells** (**erythrocytes**) are blood cells highly specialised for **oxygen transport**.

In the great majority of mammals, erythrocytes have a **biconcave disc shape** in cross-section. Because of this shape, erythrocytes possess a very large surface-to-volume ratio. This large cell surface area contributes significantly to rapid and efficient diffusion of oxygen and carbon dioxide across the cell membrane.

Mammalian erythrocytes are devoid of a **nucleus**. Yet they are able to maintain a range of complex metabolic functions (p. 232) over their **life span of 60–160 days** (which varies between species). In contrast to mammals, all other vertebrates, i.e. **birds**, **reptiles, amphibians** and **fish**, possess large, **nucleated** erythrocytes, which usually have a biconvex shape. The advantages and disadvantages of non-nucleated compared to nucleated erythrocytes are unclear.

The **diameter** of mammalian erythrocytes varies between species. In domestic animals, diameter is approximately between 5 and 7 µm (**Table 9.5**). While most mammals have round erythrocytes, in **camelids** they are spindle-shaped. Erythrocytes can pass through capillaries with a diameter smaller than the erythrocytes themselves. This passage through capillaries is possible by the high deformability (p. 195) of a red cell's membrane. However, this deformability decreases as the erythrocytes age, at which point they are eliminated in the spleen.

Circulation, respiration

Table 9.5　Reference values of haematocrit, haemoglobin concentration in blood, red blood cell count, and diameter in different species.

Animal species[1]	Haematocrit ($l \cdot l^{-1}$)	Haemoglobin concentration ($g \cdot l^{-1}$)	Red blood cell count ($\times 10^{12} \cdot l^{-1}$)	Erythrocyte diameter (µm)
Cattle	0.21–0.30	84–120	4.9–7.5	5.7
Sheep	0.27–0.45	90–150	9.0–15.0	4.5
Goat	0.22–0.38	80–120	8.0–18.0	3.2
Pig	0.32–0.50	100–160	5.0–8.0	6.0
Horse[2]	0.24–0.53	80–190	5.5–12.9	5.5
Dog	0.37–0.55	120–180	5.5–8.5	7.3
Cat	0.24–0.46	82–153	5.9–11.2	5.7
Rabbit	0.30–0.50	80–150	4.0–7.0	7.0
Guinea pig	0.32–0.50	110–170	3.4–8.7	7.0
Llama[3]	0.25–0.45	100–190	9.6–17.7	2.8–7.8
Bactrian camel[3]	0.25–0.42	70–160	6.2–15.5	3.5–6.8
Chicken[4]	0.22–0.35	70–130	2.5–3.5	7.5–12.0
Goose[4]	0.44	109	2.6–3.3	7.2–12.2
Duck[4]	0.40	115	3.0–4.5	6.2–12.1
Frog[4]	0.30	78	0.2–0.6	15.0–25.0

[1] Values vary considerably between different breeds or lines of the same species.
[2] Values from cold-blooded to warm-blooded and thoroughbred horses increasingly
[3] Spindle-shaped
[4] Nucleated
Reference
for mammals and chicken: Weiss DJ, Wardrop K. Schalm's Veterinary Hematology, 6th ed., Iowa: Blackwell Publishing; 2010

MORE DETAILS   There is obviously no correlation between the body size of mammals and the cell volume of their erythrocytes. Thus, the size of mouse erythrocytes roughly corresponds to those of an elephant. Extreme environmental conditions have led to erythrocyte adaptations in different animal species. For example, the spindle shape of the erythrocytes in camelids could improve blood flow properties through the capillaries of llamas, vicuñas, alpacas and guanacos. These New World camelids live at high altitudes (5000 m above sea level) in the Andes, where oxygen partial pressure is low. Camels have adapted to survive in hot, dry deserts, and can go for up to two weeks without consuming water. When drinking, they can absorb a considerable amount of water in a very short time (up to ⅓ of their body weight). Such a large and rapid water intake would be fatal for the majority of mammals. In camels, however, there is no haemolysis although the blood plasma gets hypotonic. The erythrocyte membranes of camelids have many scaffolding proteins (especially the spectrins). These maintain structural integrity of the ellipsoid-biconcave erythrocytes. Other adaptive mechanisms are also known. **Mountain goats**, for example, have very small erythrocytes, but their number is correspondingly increased. This augments the total erythrocyte surface area, to compensate for the low oxygen partial pressure at high altitude and to ensure efficient oxygen exchange and transport. Marine mammals may use their large, thick erythrocytes as oxygen stores during prolonged periods of diving (p. 289).

Within individuals of a species, the cell sizes within an erythrocyte population show a Gaussian distribution. **Normocytes** are erythrocytes whose size lies within the normal range. The term **microcytes** describes those cells where the size tends to be smaller, whereas **macrocytes** refers to erythrocytes which tend to be larger. Where there are marked differences in size between erythrocytes, as happens in some diseases, this is described as **anisocytosis**.

The **number of erythrocytes** in the blood (red blood cell count) differs between species, with a negative correlation between erythrocyte size and number in mammals, as already mentioned (**Table 9.5**). Therefore, total volume of all blood cells, the so-called **haematocrit**, is relatively similar between mammalian species. Factors that affect the red blood cell count, which in domestic mammals averages 5–$14 \cdot 110^{12} \cdot l^{-1}$ (5–14 million·µl^{-1}) blood, are the sex, the degree of physical training, breed (e.g. thoroughbred horse vs. cold-blooded horse) and also age (**Table 9.5**). It should be noted that in newborn dogs and cats, the number of erythrocytes per unit volume is only about half that of the adult animals.

Haematocrit is the proportion of cellular components in the total blood volume. Since erythrocytes greatly outnumber leukocytes and thrombocytes, the haematocrit is essentially determined by the **number and size of erythrocytes**, as well as the distribution of body fluids. Reference values, in large animal species, lie between 0.28 and $0.52 l \cdot l^{-1}$ (**Table 9.5**; formerly described as a percentage, i.e. 28–52%). Physically trained animals tend to have higher values. In those animal species with a so-called storage spleen (p. 195) (horses, camelids and seals, and to a lesser extent also dogs and cats), haematocrit rises sharply during physical exercise, during which the erythrocyte depot in the spleen is released by activation of the sympathetic nervous system (so-called work erythrocytosis). In horses,

oxygen transport capacity (p. 626) can be increased in this way by up to 60% in the short term, and in some breeds of dog by about 20%. When there is a relative deficiency of oxygen, e.g. when living at high altitude, there is acclimatisation with a physiological increase in haematocrit by stimulation of erythropoiesis by EPO.

MORE DETAILS   How high can the haematocrit rise? Recent studies on Peruvian coastal dwellers doing their work at over 5400 m above sea level revealed the highest value ever measured in a human of 0.91! Values between 0.8 and 0.92 were also found in genetically modified, transgenic mice overexpressing the human EPO gene. When there is excessive erythrocytosis, normal blood flow to the tissues seems to be possible only through generalised (nitric oxide-induced) vasodilation and increased deformability of the erythrocytes.

The **total resistance of the arterioles** is mainly determined by the **vessel diameter** and the flow properties (**viscosity**) of the blood (see ch. Flow rate, pressure, resistance (p. 193) and Central regulation of blood flow (p. 210)). About ⅔ of the total viscosity of blood is determined by the relative number of erythrocytes, and about ⅓ by plasma proteins (**Fig. 8.6**). Because of the great influence of the **proportion of erythrocytes** on **blood viscosity**, any change in their number has a marked effect on the **flow properties** of blood (**Fig. 8.5**). If the number of erythrocytes is reduced (anaemia), blood viscosity also declines. If the number increases (polyglobulia, erythrocytosis), viscosity also increases. Other cell components, such as the platelets and leukocytes, have a minor effect on viscosity. Blood is not a homogeneous, so-called Newtonian fluid. This means that the viscosity of blood decreases with increasing shear stress due to the aggregation and deformability of erythrocytes. The faster the blood flows, the lower is the **relative** viscosity (p. 195). Precondition for changes in shape of erythrocytes in the blood stream is the considerable flexibility of the cell membrane and its submembranous cytoskeleton, formed by a meshwork of different proteins. It should be noted that young erythrocytes are more deformable than older ones.

MORE DETAILS   Viscosity (p. 195) is relatively high at slow flow velocity and consequently low shear stress, because at slow flow speed erythrocytes aggregate into larger conglomerates. However, especially in smaller vessels (diameter < 300 µm), a low-cell marginal flow with reduced internal friction results, as erythrocytes are then predominantly in the axial blood flow (laminar flow, **Fig. 8.4**). The thickness of the cell-poor boundary layer increases (relative to the vessel diameter) the smaller the vessel becomes. However, in very narrow capillaries (diameter < 5–10 µm), where deformability of individual erythrocytes is the limiting factor, the conditions are reversed and viscosity increases sharply (**Fig. 8.6**). Finally, as in any fluid, blood viscosity in a vessel also depends essentially on temperature, which can also be important in appendages of the body (e.g. legs, nose) of homeothermic animals (warm-blooded animals).

Pathological increases and decreases in haematocrit can have various causes. A **pathological increase** of **haematocrit** can occur when there is considerable and prolonged loss of fluid. This is the case e.g. in diarrhoeal diseases or heavy sweating. Because of the accompanying reduction in plasma volume, the relative number of cells per unit of (blood) volume increases and thus also does the haematocrit. **Polyglobulia**, i.e. a marked increase in the number of erythrocytes, can also result, e.g. in reaction to oxygen deficiency. A distinction is made between **polyglobulia vera**, in which the EPO concentration in the serum is normally increased, **pseudopolyglobulia** because of reduced plasma volume, and other forms of polycythaemia (various genetic, partly unknown causes of the disease).

Disorders in haematopoiesis, or chronic blood loss with a secondary shift of fluid to intravascular compartment, and a corresponding **reduction** in the number of erythrocytes, can cause a **pathological reduction in haematocrit**. Immediately after acute haemorrhage, the haematocrit at first usually remains constant, as there is a loss of both blood cells and plasma in the same proportion as in whole blood. Only when there is partial compensation of the missing blood volume by fluid influx from the interstitium, does a temporary decrease in haematocrit subsequently occur. A low haematocrit (e.g. in anaemia), leads to turbulence of the blood flow because of reduced blood viscosity. This can lead to heart murmurs (p. 169) even in animals with healthy hearts.

■ Haemoglobin and oxygen transport

> **IN A NUTSHELL** !
>
> The main function of erythrocytes in blood is to transport oxygen reversibly bound to intracellular haemoglobin.

The main function of erythrocytes is transport of oxygen (p. 275) from the lungs to the various body tissues. In this process, **haemoglobin**, the red blood pigment, plays a major role. In contrast, only about 10% of carbon dioxide (p. 280) in blood is bound to haemoglobin as carbamino-haemoglobin. The rest is transported from tissues to the lungs in the form of dissolved HCO_3^-. Species differences in haemoglobin (Hb) concentrations are listed in **Table 9.5**.

MORE DETAILS Many invertebrates can transport **oxygen physically dissolved in blood** or in haemolymph. In the animal kingdom, there are other blood pigments besides haemoglobin that can bind and transport oxygen. One example is **haemocyanin**, a copper-containing blood pigment found in arthropods and molluscs, which, unlike haemoglobin, is **freely** dissolved in the **plasma**. In this way, oxygen can be bound directly at the surface and transported to inner parts of the body. However, since such an oxygen transport system relies strictly on diffusion, it can only be used by small organisms or those with a low energy expenditure. More highly developed vertebrates need more oxygen for their high metabolic activity. Consequently, they need more blood pigment to transport oxygen. The required **increase** in the amount of haemoglobin dissolved **freely in the plasma** would lead to greatly **increased blood viscosity** and consequently poor blood flow. Nature has solved this by packaging **haemoglobin** in **erythrocytes** in a very high concentration (5 mol·l^{-1} or about 95% of the dry matter of an erythrocyte). Viscosity of total blood thus remains relatively low.

The **building blocks of haemoglobin** consist of an oxygen-carrying **prosthetic group** (**haem**) and a species-specific **protein moiety** (**globin**). The muscle pigment, myoglobin, has the same structure, as well as other globins (e.g. neuroglobin and androglobin), where only the protein differs from that of haemoglobin. The **haem molecule**, which is responsible for the red colour of blood, consists of a divalent **central iron atom** (Fe^{2+}) and four substituted pyrrole rings which form a protoporphyrin ring around the iron

(**Fig. 11.18**). The central Fe^{2+} has six coordination sites, four of which are linked to the protoporphyrin system, one is linked to a side chain of the globin molecule, and the last one links to oxygen. Oxygen binds to this Fe^{2+} atom, via a loose coordinated bond. In contrast to monomeric myoglobin, haemoglobin is composed of four subunits (tetramers), two of which are identical. The complete haemoglobin therefore consists of **four haem molecules**, each with two α or β polypeptide chains. Animal haemoglobins are structured analogously to human haemoglobins. Each haemoglobin molecule can therefore bind reversibly and transport a maximum of four oxygen molecules.

The ability of haemoglobin to **bind oxygen** is linked to the presence of polypeptide chains. The haemoglobin of embryos, foetuses or infants differs in its protein content (embryonic and foetal **haemoglobin** (**Fig. 11.22**), see ch. CO_2 transport (p. 280)). Oxygen-carrying haemoglobin is called **oxyhaemoglobin** and the process itself is called **oxygenation**. The divalent iron atom remains unaffected, i.e. there is **no oxidation** of the Fe^{2+} atom. For **deoxygenation**, release of oxygen depends on oxygen partial pressure. Under physiological conditions, oxidation of divalent iron (Fe^{2+}) to trivalent iron (Fe^{3+}), which results in formation of methaemoglobin, occurs only to a small extent. Oxygen cannot bind to Fe^{3+}. Therefore, methaemoglobin is inactive for O_2 transport. Because of a reducing system (methaemoglobin reductase), methaemoglobin concentration in circulating erythrocytes is limited to 1–2% of total haemoglobin. Oxygen loading of haemoglobin is dependent on parameters such as oxygen and carbon dioxide partial pressure, temperature, pH value, content of 2,3-bisphosphoglycerate (2,3-BPG) and the number of oxygen molecules already bound (**Fig. 11.20, Fig. 11.2**).

MORE DETAILS Impaired oxygen transport capacity of blood is generally described by the term **anaemia**. This can be caused by a reduction in number or mass of erythrocytes, a decrease in haemoglobin content of whole blood or of individual erythrocytes (hypochromic anaemia), or an impairment of oxygen transport capacity of erythrocytes. The causes of anaemia are very diverse and range from simple blood loss to diseases associated with an impaired synthesis of new erythrocytes or of haemoglobin (e.g. due to iron deficiency, drugs that damage bone marrow, or radiation therapy) or an augmented degradation of erythrocytes (e.g. haemolysis caused by toxins or parasites).

Haemorrhagic anaemia occurs, for example, in trauma with penetrating wounds, in bleeding lesions triggered by ulcerations of the gastrointestinal tract (e.g. after chronic use of anti-inflammatory drugs), by intestinal neoplasms or intestinal parasites (e.g. Uncinaria, hookworms). The most important deficiency anaemias are blood formation disorders due to iron or cobalamin deficiencies. **Iron deficiency** is common in piglets, because sow's milk cannot meet the iron requirements of fast-growing piglets. Prophylactic iron supplements are therefore often administered parenterally to piglets. Vitamin B_{12} (**cobalamin**) deficiency in ruminants may be because of an insufficient supply of cobalt, or of cobalamin itself in monogastric animals (see ch. Digestion in the forestomachs, vitamins (p. 405)). Vitamin B_{12} deficiency can also arise from insufficient absorption from the intestine because of the absence of intrinsic factor (p. 415) produced by gastric mucosal cells. Bone marrow with its high mitotic rate is particularly dependent on cobalamin, which is necessary for the formation of precursors of DNA synthesis. Cobalamin deficiency therefore leads to what is known as **pernicious anaemia**, characterised by a hyperchromic macrocytic megaloblastic anaemia. As well as cobalamin deficiency, an inadequate supply of folic acid can also lead to similar anaemia symptoms.

Haemostatic anaemia results from inadequate haemostasis or blood clotting (p. 236) in thrombocytopenias, thrombopathies or in acquired disorders of the coagulation system e.g. poisoning with the vitamin K antagonist warfarin, or from hereditary conditions, e.g. von Willebrand disease (p. 234) found in Doberman Pinscher and German Wirehaired Pointer dogs.

Haemolytic anaemia results from a destruction of existing erythrocytes. Haemolysis can be triggered by immune reactions such as in viral equine infectious anaemia, by various blood parasites such as anaplasma or babesia (piroplasmosis) or by certain bacteria such as leptospires. Haemolyses, with typical Heinz bodies in blood count, are triggered, for example, by poisoning with plant toxins (e.g. brassica spp.) or by certain drugs. Also, excess zinc and copper can lead to toxic haemolysis. Postpartum haemoglobinuria is associated with hypophosphataemia.

Finally, various hereditary **enzymatic defects** can cause a deficiency of erythrocytes, such as a reduced activity of pyruvate kinase (West Highland White Terrier), phosphofructokinase (quail dog) or glucose-6-phosphate dehydrogenase.

■ Erythrocyte indices

MORE DETAILS For a more detailed diagnosis of anaemia, so-called **erythrocyte indices** are used. These parameters can be calculated from simple determination of red blood cell count (RBC, expressed in number $\cdot l^{-1}$), haemoglobin content ([Hb] in $g \cdot l^{-1}$) and haematocrit (HCT):

- **MCV (fl):** mean corpuscular volume. Average erythrocyte volume calculated from the quotient HCT/RBC.
- **MCH (pg):** mean corpuscular haemoglobin. Average haemoglobin content of a single erythrocyte, calculated from the quotient [Hb]/RBC.
- **MCHC (g $\cdot l^{-1}$):** mean corpuscular haemoglobin concentration. Mean haemoglobin concentration in erythrocytes, calculated from the quotients [Hb]/HCT or MCH/MCV.

A decrease in MCV is called microcytosis and an increase is called macrocytosis. The mean haemoglobin concentration in erythrocytes (MCHC) is reduced in extreme iron deficiency or augmented in some forms of haemolytic anaemia. The reference values for some animal species are given in **Table 9.6**.

■ Erythropoiesis and erythrocyte degradation

> **IN A NUTSHELL**   !
>
> Erythropoiesis is regulated by the hormone erythropoietin (EPO). The local oxygen partial pressure in the kidney is the main factor regulating the secretion of EPO. Erythrocytes are formed in the bone marrow, and aged erythrocytes are destroyed, mainly in the spleen. Bilirubin is formed from haemoglobin released during erythrocyte destruction through several intermediate steps.

Like all blood cells, erythrocytes have a mesodermal origin. During **early embryonic development**, the first **erythroid precursor cells**, the so-called **erythroblasts**, are formed. They contain embryonic haemoglobin. In the developing foetus, erythropoiesis occurs predominantly in the **liver** and to a smaller extent also in the **spleen**. From about the middle of gestation, erythropoiesis is **permanently** transferred to **bone marrow**, and continues there throughout life.

Erythrocytes are derived from a **pluripotent stem cell** which has the capacity for self-renewal, differentiation and proliferation (**Fig. 9.2**). During development into a mature erythrocyte in mammals, the differentiating cell becomes smaller and loses the nucleus and nucleoli. The **erythroid progenitor cells** in **bone marrow** can be recognized by their size, nuclear-cytoplasmic ratio, nuclear structure, and stainability of the cytoplasm (**Table 9.7**). With increasing **age**, the main site of formation shifts from the bone marrow of large tubular bones to that of the **ribs**, later to that of the **sternum** and finally to that of the **vertebral** and **pelvic bones**. This age dependency must be taken into account in diagnostic bone marrow punctures.

Formation of new erythrocytes in healthy animals matches the rate of removal of old red blood cells. Erythropoiesis is regulated by the hormone **erythropoietin** (EPO (p. 328)), which is mainly synthesised and secreted by the **kidneys**, and, depending on the species, to a lesser extent in the liver.

Table 9.6 Reference ranges for MCV, MCH and MCHC.

Animal species	MCV (fl)	MCH (pg)	MCHC (g $\cdot l^{-1}$)
Cattle	36–50	14–19	380–430
Sheep	28–40	8–12	310–340
Goat	16–25	5–8	300–360
Pig	50–68	17–21	300–340
Horse	37–59	12–20	310–390
Dog	60–77	17–23	320–360
Cat	37–55	13–17	260–360

Source: Weiss DJ, Wardrop KJ. Schalm's Veterinary Hematology, 6th ed. Iowa: Blackwell Publishing; 2010

Table 9.7 Cell shapes observed during erythropoiesis in mammals.

Cell shapes	Characteristics
Proerythroblast	Young, immature, large, round cell; nucleated, sharply defined nucleoli; cytoplasm strongly basophilic
Erythroblast	Smaller, round cell; no nucleoli; smaller nucleus; cytoplasm from basophilic to polychromatic; increasing haemoglobin content
Normoblast	Cell becomes even smaller; denser nucleus; haemoglobin content complete; cytoplasm polychromatic to orthochromatic
Reticulocyte	Without nucleus; fine, net-like framework (lat. rete=net; precipitation of ribonucleoproteins in reticulocyte staining); no longer able to divide; still moderate RNA, protein and haem synthesis; appears in blood
Normocyte (mature erythrocyte)	Small, round cell with a central depression (biconcave shape, except in camelids – where it is spindle-shaped), without nucleus

EPO is a glycoprotein with a molecular weight of about 34 kDa. After binding to **EPO receptors** on **erythroid progenitor cells**, it prevents their programmed cell death (apoptosis). As a result, they can mature into **reticulocytes** and enter bloodstream. Regulation of EPO expression is **oxygen-dependent**. Erythropoiesis can be stimulated by living at high altitude, or when there is a severe blood loss, or with carbon monoxide poisoning. In all of these examples, partial pressure of oxygen in blood is reduced.

The winners of the Nobel Prize in Physiology or Medicine (2019) succeeded in identifying the so-called prolyl hydroxylase 2 (PHD2) as a cellular oxygen sensor, which is found in all cells. PHD2 mutations cause Tibetans to show a reduced response to oxygen deficiency. At normal oxygen partial pressure and sufficient iron supply, PHD2 is active and induces the degradation of the α subunit of hypoxia-inducible transcription factor 2 (HIF-2α). As soon as certain kidney cells register a local reduction in oxygen partial pressure, PHD2 is inactivated. Thus, HIF-2α, which is continuously synthesised in the cell, is instantly stabilised and forms the heterodimer HIF-2. Subsequently, HIF-2 binds to an enhancer sequence of the EPO gene (hypoxia-response element, HRE), thereby increasing its transcription rate. EPO not only stimulates erythrocyte maturation, but also production of erythroferrone (ERFE) in erythroblasts. Erythroferrone is the link to iron metabolism. It acts by inhibiting production of hepcidin in the liver. In the absence of hepcidin, the iron transporter ferroportin (Fpn) is not degraded in intestinal cells and macrophages, so that iron is absorbed in the intestine or is recycled from macrophages and enters the bloodstream, where it is transported bound to transferrin (**Fig. 9.3**).

MORE DETAILS Severe and especially chronic kidney diseases can lead to reduced EPO production and thus to impaired erythrocyte formation resulting in anaemia. To be effective, when recombinant EPO is administered therapeutically, iron, vitamin B_{12} and folic acid must also be available in sufficient quantities to stimulate erythropoiesis.

In recent years, it has been shown that EPO performs other functions that have nothing to do with blood formation. The EPO receptor is also found in neuronal cells. Both stimulation of endogenous EPO production and application of recombinant EPO led to a clear improvement in patients after a cerebral infarction (stroke), but only if EPO was not applied together with tissue plasminogen activator. Further protective effects of EPO after oxygen deprivation have been observed in cells of the retina, spinal cord and heart muscle.

While erythrocytes of humans, horses and cattle remain functional for an average of 120, 145 and 160 days, respectively, erythrocytes of pigs and cats have an average lifespan of only 62 and 70 days, respectively. There is a direct relationship here to mammalian metabolism: A relatively high number of reticulocytes is normal in smaller animals because of their higher rate of red blood cell production. **Reticulocytes** represent the direct precursor cells of erythrocytes, which mature into adult erythrocytes within 2–4 days in blood (**Table 9.7**). In horses and other odd-toed ungulates, reticulocytes are not normally found in peripheral blood. This is due to their delayed release from bone marrow. Detection of reticulocytes in birds is difficult because the progenitor cells have a ring of particles surrounding the nucleus. These particles are distributed in the cytoplasm during maturation and remain in the mature erythrocyte. In dogs, approximately 1% of erythrocytes are renewed each day, which corresponds to a **new formation rate** of approx. 1 million erythrocytes per second in a 20 kg dog!

Older erythrocytes are characterised by reduced metabolic activity, membrane deterioration coupled with water loss, and decreasing deformability. Erythrocytes are predominantly **degraded in the spleen**, where cells of the mononuclear phagocyte system phagocytose old erythrocytes. The polypeptide chains of haemoglobin undergo almost complete proteolysis and degradation products are transferred into the amino acid pool. Iron is almost completely recycled and made available to the bone marrow for utilisation in further erythropoiesis. The protoporphyrin ring of haemoglobin is converted into bilirubin via several intermediate stages (verdoglobulin, biliverdin). The lipophilic, toxic unconjugated bilirubin is transported bound to albumin and, after esterification with glucuronic acid in hepatocytes, conjugated bilirubin is excreted into the intestine in **bile** (**Fig. 17.7**) (see ch. Formation of the

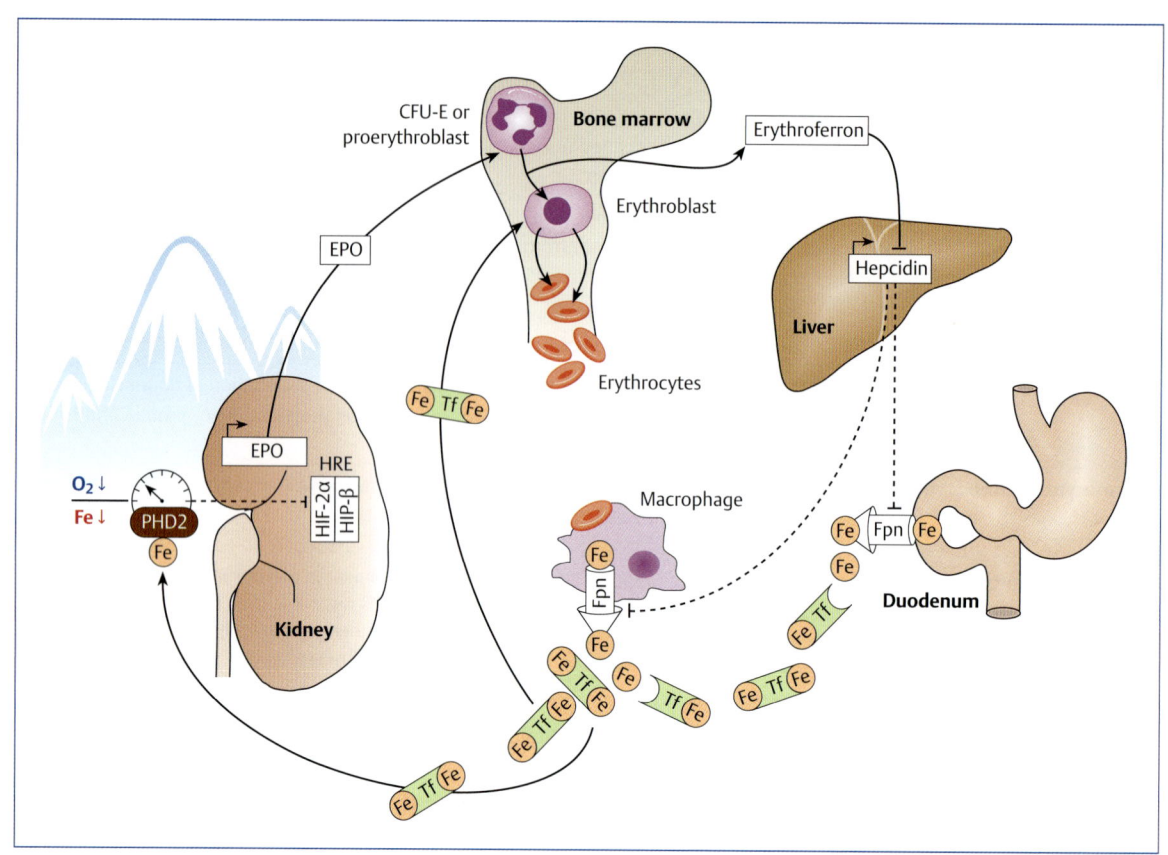

Fig. 9.3 The cellular oxygen sensor and the link between EPO (regulation of hypoxia) and hepcidin (iron regulation).
The cellular oxygen sensor is prolyl hydroxylase 2 (PHD2), which requires sufficient oxygen and iron to initiate the degradation of the α subunit of hypoxia-inducible factor 2 (HIF-2α). In states of oxygen deficiency (e.g. severe blood loss, anaemia or living at high altitudes), PHD2 activity is severely restricted, so that HIF-2α is stabilised and forms the HIF-2 complex together with its constitutively expressed heterodimerisation partner HIF-β. This binds the enhancer sequence HRE (hypoxia-response element) located at 3' of the EPO gene and thus increases transcription of EPO mRNA. As a result, more EPO reaches the bone marrow in blood, where it accelerates the maturation of differentiating CFUs and erythroblasts into mature erythrocytes. It also induces secretion of erythroferrone by these precursor cells.
Erythroferrone in blood is taken up by the liver and inhibits production of hepcidin. Hepcidin in the membrane of intestinal cells and of macrophages binds the cellular iron transporter ferroportin (Fpn), and promotes its degradation. Because erythroferrone inhibits formation of hepcidin, Fpn degradation does not occur. Thus, iron, from intestinal absorption and from macrophages, can enter bloodstream where it binds to transferrin (Tf). In this way, iron is available for the formation of haemoglobin, myoglobin or for use in other factors and molecules such as PHD2.

bile pigments (p. 475)). In the intestine, conjugated bilirubin is degraded to form colourless urobilinogen which is partially reabsorbed and, after being metabolised in the liver, can be excreted in urine (enterohepatic circulation) (**Fig. 16.61**).

■ Erythrocyte metabolism

IN A NUTSHELL !

The erythrocyte, which is highly specialised for oxygen transport, obtains energy for ion transport processes from anaerobic glycolysis. Erythrocytes possess an efficient protection system against oxidative damage.

Mature, circulating mammalian erythrocytes have **neither nucleus nor mitochondria** and are therefore not capable of cell division or synthesis of DNA, RNA, proteins, lipids or haem. Erythrocytes are therefore **metabolically limited**, but are highly specialised cells for oxygen transport. They are no longer able to metabolise substrates aerobically and use **anaerobic glycolysis** for energy metabolism. Glucose, and in smaller quantities fructose, or in some species inosine, are the most important substrates. Glucose uptake in erythrocytes occurs passively by glucose uniporters, i.e. via facilitated diffusion.

A large part of the energy gained is required for active ion transport processes, in which mainly the Na^+/K^+ pump and an Mg^{2+}-dependent Ca^{2+} pump are involved. The Ca^{2+} pump is responsible for keeping the concentration of free Ca^{2+} in erythrocytes as low as possible. In addition to these ion transport processes, ATP is primarily needed for maintaining the shape of erythrocytes as well as for synthesis of the tripeptide **glutathione (GSH)** (GSH). Formation of **glutathione** is an important **protection against oxidation** for erythrocytes. There is a great oxidative damage potential (p. 290) in erythrocytes because of their high oxygen content. This promotes the formation of superoxides and peroxides. **Oxygen radicals** are destroyed by superoxide dismutase. In addition, the selenium-containing glutathione peroxidase serves to break down organic peroxides. In this reaction, GSH is converted by a redox system to diglutathione (GSSG), which contributes significantly to the degradation of lipid peroxides. Apart from this, free SH groups are protected from oxidation. Such SH groups, that are susceptible to oxidation, are mainly found in enzymes of the erythrocyte membrane and in haemoglobin. The pentose phosphate cycle of the erythrocyte is important for regeneration of GSH from GSSG. This reaction is catalysed by the enzyme glutathione reductase. With increasing age, the erythrocytes lose this capability for synthesis of glutathione. This, along with other factors, leads to destruction of old erythrocytes. For example, haemolysis can be provoked or enhanced in vitro, by blocking the SH groups. As a further oxidation protection mechanism, erythrocytes possess a high catalase activity, by which peroxides are degraded to water and oxygen. Here, NADPH serves as an oxidation protection for the catalase enzyme itself.

Glycolysis also produces reduced nicotinamide dinucleotide (**NADH$_2$**) which in turn is an important cofactor for **haemoglobin reductase** (or methaemoglobin reductase). As already mentioned, this enzyme catalyses **reduction** of **methaemoglobin** to **haemoglobin**. Methaemoglobin is continuously produced in small quantities in erythrocytes. As a by-product of glycolysis, 2,3-bisphosphoglycerate (2,3-BPG (p.278)), is also produced in erythrocytes. It regulates release of oxygen and diminishes oxygen affinity of haemoglobin (**Fig. 11.21**). 2,3-BPG is found in relatively high concentrations in erythrocytes of dogs, horses, pigs and humans, whereas it is significantly lower in cats and in ruminants.

9.3.3 Leukocytes

> **IN A NUTSHELL** !
>
> On the basis of their morphology and characteristic staining, the **leukocytes** or **white blood cells** (Greek: leukos = white) are divided into **lymphocytes**, **monocytes** as well as **neutrophil, eosinophil** and **basophil granulocytes**.

The classification of leukocytes differs according to their origin and morphological characteristics. All so-called granulocytes belong to the myeloid cell line, whereas agranulocytes (or mononuclear cells) belong partly to the lymphoid (lymphocytes) and partly to the myeloid cell line (monocytes). The leukocytes are functionally part of the immune system (p.244) and are discussed in that section.

The leukocytes that can be detected in blood represent only a very small proportion (approx. 5%) of the total number of leukocytes in the body. The importance of the marginal pool has already been pointed out. The majority of total leukocytes are distributed throughout various organs of the body. After formation in bone marrow, granulocytes and monocytes are transported in blood and distributed to their target location. They then stay in their target tissue, while lymphocytes are constantly circulating. Accordingly, examination of leukocytes in blood reflects the reaction state of the immune system (p.244). The total number of leukocytes varies greatly from animal to animal, with values of approx. $3-30 \cdot 10^9 \cdot l^{-1}$, i.e. 3000–30000 cells per µl blood (**Table 9.8**). The term **leukocytosis** applies if total leukocyte count exceeds the upper limit of the reference range, characteristic of each animal species. A reduction below the lower limit is called **leukocytopenia or leukopenia**.

MORE DETAILS Analysis of different leukocyte types in the so-called **leukocyte differential count** provides additional information on the percentage of the respective cell types in the total white blood cell (WBC) count (**Table 9.8**). Thus, it is helpful for various diagnoses. It is determined by counting the different leukocytes in specially stained blood smears. In some species, the granulocytes make up more than 50% of the leukocytes (human, horse, dog, cat). In contrast, in ruminants, pigs, chickens, rats, mice and rabbits the lymphocytes dominate the white blood cell count. Also found in the blood smear are the small **platelets** (thrombocytes (p.234)), which are of great importance in haemostasis.

Table 9.8 White blood cell count (cells per µl) and leukocyte differential blood count.

Animal species[1]	White blood cell count (per µl)	Neutrophils	Lymphocytes	Monocytes	Eosinophils	Basophils
		(% of total leukocytes)				
Cattle	5100–13300	20–50	45–65	2–6	2–6	0–2
Sheep	4000–8000	10–50	40–55	0–6	0–10	0–3
Goat	4000–13000	30–48	50–70	0–4	1–8	0–1
Pig	11000–22000	28–47	39–62	2–10	0–11	0–2
Horse	5400–14300	22–72	17–68	0–14	0–10	0–4
Dog	6000–17000	50–70	16–28	0–4	0–4	0–1
Cat	10000–15000	60–78	15–35	0–4	0–4	0–1
Rat	6000–20500	20–25	70–75	2–3	2–3	0–1
Mouse	4000–12000	20–30	40–60	3–5	3–5	0–1
Rabbit	5200–12000	8–50	20–90	1–4	1–3	1–10
Chicken	12000–30000	25–50	40–60	2–5	2–5	2–3
Human	3000–11000	57–70	20–30	5–7	2–4	0–1

[1] Values may vary between different breeds or lines of the same species.
Reference for leukocyte counts: Weiss DJ, Wardrop KJ. Schalm's Veterinary Hematology, 6th ed. Iowa: Blackwell Publishing; 2010

Suggested reading

Franke K, Gassmann M, Wielockx B. Erythrocytosis: the HIF pathway in control. Blood 2013; 122: 1122–1128

Gassmann M, Mairbäurl H, Livshits L et al. The increase in hemoglobin concentration with altitude varies among human populations. Ann N Y Acad Sci 2019; 1450: 204–220

Gassmann M, Muckenthaler MU. Adaptation of iron requirement in hypoxia conditions at high altitude. J Appl Physiol 2015; 119 (12): 1432–1440. Doi: 10.1152/japplphysiol.00248.2015

Gassmann M, van Tissot Patot M. Hypoxia: adapting to high altitude by mutating EPAS-1, the gene encoding HIF-2α. High Alt Med Biol 2011; 12(2): 157–167

Goetze O, Schmidt J, Spliethoff K et al. Adaptation of iron transport and metabolism to acute high-altitude hypoxia in mountaineers. Hepatology 2013; 58: 2153–2162

Grimm C, Wenzel A, Groszer M et al. HIF-1-induced erythropoietin in the hypoxic retina protects against light-induced retinal degeneration. Nature Medicine 2002; 8: 718–724

Jefferson JA, Escudero E, Hurtado ME et al. Excessive erythrocytosis, chronic mountain sickness and serum cobalt levels. Lancet 2002; 359: 407–408

Jewell UR, Kvietikova I, Scheid A et al. Induction of HIF-1α in response to hypoxia is instantaneous. FASEB J 2001; 15: 1312–1314

Sargin D, Friedrichs H, El-Kordi A et al. Erythropoietin as neuroprotective and neuroregenerative treatment strategy: comprehensive overview of 12 years of preclinical and clinical research. Best Pract Res Clin Anaesthesiol 2010; 24(4): 573–594

Staub K, Haeusler M, Bender N et al. Hemoglobin concentration of young men at residential altitudes between 200 and 2000 m mirrors Switzerland's topography. Blood 2020; 135: 1066–1069

Vogel J, Gassmann M. Erythropoietic and non-erythropoietic functions of erythropoietin (Epo) in mouse models. J Physiol (London) 2011; 15; 589 (Pt 6): 1259–1264

Weiss DJ, Wardrop KJ. Schalm's Veterinary Hematology, 6th ed. Iowa: Blackwell Publishing; 2010

9.4   Haemostasis and blood clotting

Bernd Kaspers, Thomas Göbel

> **ESSENTIALS**
>
> Damage to a blood vessel leads to loss of blood from the vascular system. Even under physiological conditions, small, imperceptible vascular injuries and bleeding occur constantly in an animal. In order to keep blood loss as low as possible, vascular injuries activate complex and very strictly regulated processes. These lead ultimately to cessation of bleeding (haemostasis: Greek haem = blood, stasis = stasis) and repair of the damaged vessel. Four mechanisms can be identified in the process of haemostasis:
> - **Vasoconstriction**
> - **Formation of a thrombocyte aggregate** (haemostasis)
> - **Blood clotting**
> - **Formation of connective tissue** (final wound closure)
>
> While the first three of these processes occur within seconds to minutes, and thus very quickly stop the bleeding, the process of connective tissue formation begins only after hours to days. It leads to the final closure of the injury and to extensive restoration of the original tissue structure. There are numerous interactions between these individual mechanisms.

9.4.1   Vasoconstriction

Immediately after an injury, there is a **vasoconstriction** and thus a significant reduction in blood flow rate. This reaction of the vessel is triggered firstly by neuronal reflexes, secondly by local myogenic spasms and thirdly by local humoral factors (e.g. thromboxane A_2). The degree of vasoconstriction depends on the type and extent of an injury. A sharp cut will bleed much more than a blunt trauma such as a contusion. Vasoconstriction can last for many minutes to hours, allowing time for the subsequent processes of haemostasis.

9.4.2   Formation of a thrombocyte aggregate

In the region of an injured vessel wall, thrombocytes (platelets) accumulate very quickly, to form **thrombocyte aggregates**. This closes the constantly occurring, very small vascular lesions without the need to activate the system of plasmatic coagulation (p. 236). The relevance of the formation of a platelet plug to stop bleeding is seen in the majority of haemostasis disorders in dogs, which can be attributed to low platelet counts, or malfunctions of platelet aggregation (e.g. von Willebrand disease).

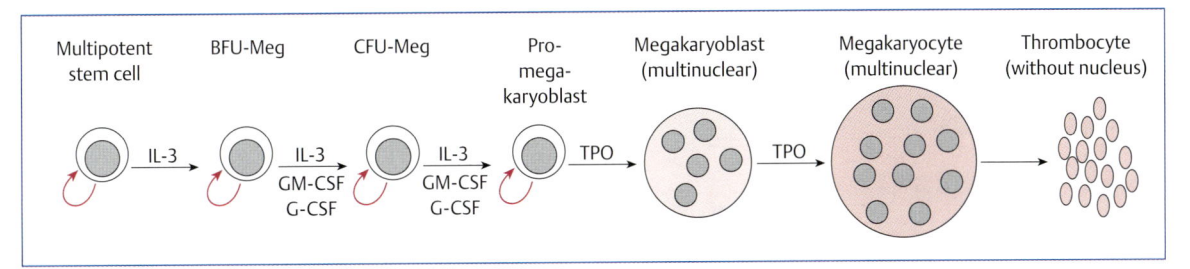

Fig. 9.4 Formation of thrombocytes. In bone marrow, megakaryocytes mature from multipotent haematopoietic stem cells via several precursor stages. Differentiation (→) and proliferation (↺, self-renewal) processes are regulated by numerous growth factors. Megakaryocytes disintegrate into up to 1000 thrombocytes when they leave the bone marrow.
BFU-Meg = burst-forming unit-megakaryocytes, CFU-Meg = colony-forming unit-megakaryocytes, GM-CSF = granulocyte/macrophage colony-stimulating factor, G-CSF = granulocyte colony-stimulating factor, TPO = thrombopoietin, IL-3 = interleukin-3.

■ Production and degradation of thrombocytes

Thrombocytes originate in **bone marrow** from myeloid stem cells (**Fig. 9.2**). At first, the **megakaryocytes** mature (megakaryocytopoiesis; **Fig. 9.4**) under the influence of numerous haematopoietic growth factors, including colony-stimulating factors and thrombopoietin.

The mature megakaryocytes leave bone marrow and then enter the blood stream. During this process and during the passage of the megakaryocytes through pulmonary arteries, the cells disintegrate into **thrombocytes**, with up to 1000 platelets being produced per megakaryocyte. In **mammals**, these thrombocytes are **non-nucleated** and have a size of 2–4 μm. In sauropsida (**birds** and **reptiles**), they are **nucleated** and somewhat larger (e.g. 4–8 μm in chicken). The number of thrombocytes in blood varies greatly from animal to animal, with values of $2.5 \cdot 10^4$ (chicken), $2 \cdot 10^5$ (horse) to $1 \cdot 10^6$ (rat) cells per μl of blood. Their **lifespan** is about 3–10 days. Accordingly, 2–5 million platelets have to be newly formed per second. During ageing of thrombocytes, significant changes occur in the carbohydrate pattern of their cell membrane. These changes are recognised by cells of the mononuclear phagocyte system of the **spleen** and **liver**, which eventually leads to phagocytosis and **degradation** of old **thrombocytes**.

■ Morphology and metabolism of thrombocytes

Thrombocytes, although they do not have a nucleus in mammals and can no longer proliferate, have many of the **characteristics of complete cells**. They have mitochondria, a smooth endoplasmic reticulum and a Golgi apparatus as well as numerous granules. Morphologically, electron-dense granules can be distinguished from so-called α-granules and lysosomes. The electron-dense granules contain various adenine nucleotides, serotonin, inorganic phosphates and calcium. In the α-granules, numerous proteins are stored, including platelet factor-4, β-thromboglobulin, growth factors, fibrinogen, coagulation factor V and VIII, fibronectin, von Willebrand factor, and thrombospondin. The lysosomes contain various acid hydrolases. During platelet aggregation, the content of the granules is released and thus becomes available for haemostasis.

■ Thrombocyte function

In the region of a vascular injury, platelets adhere to exposed connective tissue structures within seconds. This **thrombocyte adhesion is triggered** by the **von Willebrand factor** (**vWF**; **Fig. 9.5**). This factor is the largest plasma protein and has a molecular weight of up to $20 \cdot 10^6$ kDa. It consists of numerous, identical subunits. Its plasma concentration is only $10 \, \mu g \cdot ml^{-1}$. vWF is produced by vascular endothelium and by megakaryocytes which store the factor in Weibel-Palade bodies and in α-granules. Endothelial cells release vWF into blood and into the subendothelial matrix. If injury to the endothelium occurs, vWF binds to exposed collagen structures of the subendothelial matrix. This binding is made possible by the fact that shear forces increase in the region of the vessel injury, which leads to unfolding of the previously globular vWF and formation of vWF strands and networks. Consequently, binding sites for collagen and adhesion molecules on the platelets are exposed. This allows binding of vWF to the subendothelial matrix and to a membrane receptor complex (GPIb/IX complex) on thrombocytes. The result is an initial **adhesion of platelets** to the subendothelial matrix (**Fig. 9.5**). This is an important regulatory mechanism, as vWF in the folded form is unable to bind to the GPIb/IX complex, thus preventing platelet aggregation in an intact vessel. In vessels where shear forces are low (e.g. veins), fibrinogen-mediated adhesion of thrombocytes also occurs after vascular injury. At high shear forces (arterioles, microcirculation), thrombocyte adhesion is mediated almost exclusively via the vWF. The adhesion of the thrombocytes leads to their **activation**, whereby the shape of thrombocytes changes and their granules are released (**Fig. 9.5**). Some of the released substances such as ADP, serotonin (see ch. Humoral regulation (p. 209); Inflammatory reaction (p. 250)) and thromboxane A_2, activate further thrombocytes. The **activation of thrombocytes** leads to a conformational change in another receptor complex, the GPIIb/IIIa complex, which enables its binding to fibrinogen. **Fibrinogen bridges** are formed between activated **thrombocytes** (**Fig. 9.5**) leading to a **thrombocyte aggregate**, thus achieving an initial closure of the vascular injury.

The inhibition of thromboxane A_2 formation by acetylsalicylic acid (**Table 9.9**) leads to an inhibition of platelet function and to a reduction of thrombocyte aggregates in the body, an effect that is also used therapeutically.

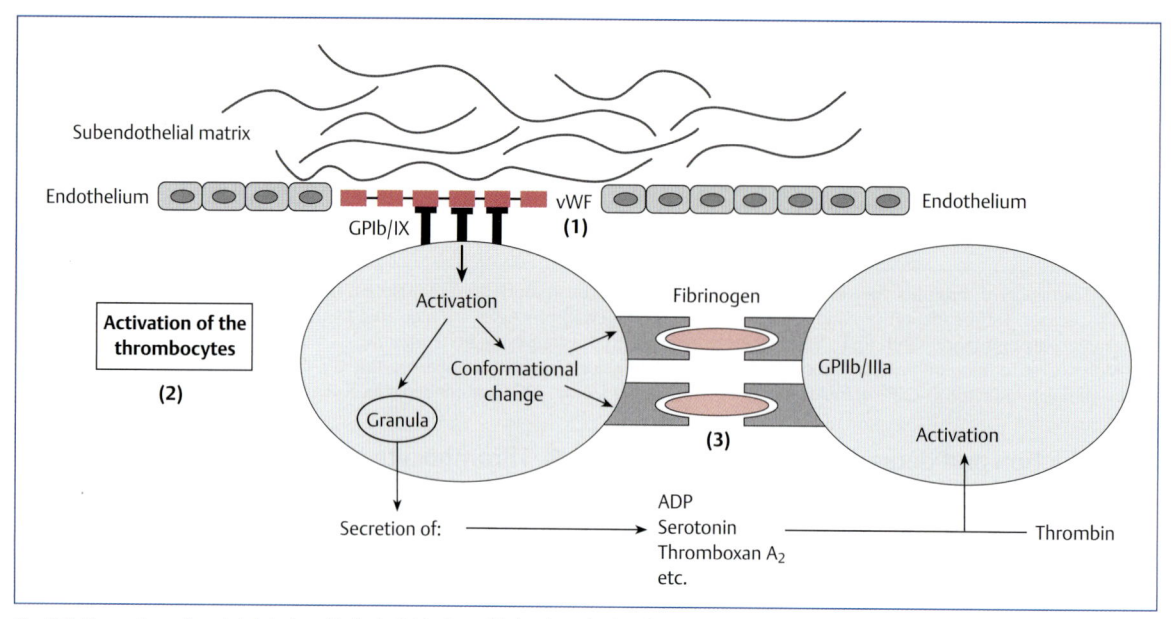

Fig. 9.5 Formation of a platelet plug. Endothelial lesions (1) lead to the binding of von Willebrand factor (vWF) to collagen fibres of connective tissue and subsequent adhesion of thrombocytes to the immobilised vWF, via the adhesion molecules GPIb/IX. The adhesion process triggers platelet activation and secretion of numerous factors from the granules (ADP, serotonin, thromboxane A_2) (2). Neighbouring thrombocytes are activated by these factors and by thrombin from plasmatic coagulation, which leads to the formation of fibrinogen bridges between the adhesion molecules GPIIb/IIIa (3). This causes a thrombocyte plug to form at the site of the lesion.

> **IN A NUTSHELL** !
>
> Thrombocytes adhere to the subendothelial matrix in the region of vascular injuries. This adhesion is mediated by von Willebrand factor.

The **thrombocyte plug** is called a **white thrombus**. It cannot be dissolved in vivo. However, it can be detached by flowing blood. Formation of fibrin (coagulation), which begins shortly after thrombocyte aggregation, and the associated cross-linking of the thrombocyte aggregate, lead to a stabilisation of the thrombocyte clot. Erythrocytes are also deposited in the fibrin clot, so that a **red thrombus** is formed. Finally, **retraction of the clot** occurs, resulting in further stabilisation, collapse of vessel walls and cessation of bleeding. Retraction is caused by contraction of filaments of the thrombocyte's cytoskeleton.

> **IN A NUTSHELL** !
>
> Thrombocyte adhesion and aggregation lead to temporary occlusion of a vascular lesion.

9.4.3 Coagulation

■ Fibrin formation

More than 50 factors are involved in the formation and dissolution of a blood clot. These are referred to as **procoagulants or anticoagulants**, respectively. Whether clotting occurs depends on the balance between these two groups of factors. When there is vascular damage, the procoagulants predominate and cause the formation of a fibrin clot. The factors involved are internationally designated with Roman numerals (e.g. prothrombin is factor II), their activated form is marked with an "a" (e.g. thrombin is factor IIa). Active factors are formed by a proteolytic cleavage of a peptide from the inactive precursors. The activated factors are often themselves proteases, i.e. protein-cleaving enzymes, which can then activate downstream factors. In the course of the **coagulation cascade**, there is a clear amplification of the reaction from stage to stage, a principle that can be found again in the complement cascade (p. 247).

Plasmatic coagulation is only triggered when there is **injury to the endothelium**. The **intact endothelium** separates factor III (tissue thromboplastin or "tissue factor"), which is localised in tissues, from its binding partner factor VIIa, which is dissolved in blood, and thus **prevents clotting** (Fig. 9.6 a). Factor III is a membrane-bound protein expressed on numerous cell types (smooth muscle cells, pericytes) in the vascular wall and in the subendothelial matrix (fibroblasts). Only when vascular injuries occur does factor III come into contact with factor VIIa circulating in the plasma, and thus activates fibrin formation (Fig. 9.6 b). VIIa is always present in small quantities in blood, but how it is activated from factor VII is not yet clear. The binding of factor VIIa to factor III leads to a large increase in the proteolytic activity of factor VIIa (about 10^5-fold). This cleaves factor X to factor Xa and thus causes the formation of another complex, that of factor Xa and cofactor Va. The factor Xa/Va complex (prothrombin activator) now causes activation of **prothrombin** (factor II) to **thrombin** (factor IIa), the most important protease in the coagulation cascade. Thrombin finally cleaves four small peptides from the fibrinogen molecule, exposing the binding sites for polymerisation of fibrin monomers into **fibrin strands**. At the same time, thrombin also activates factor

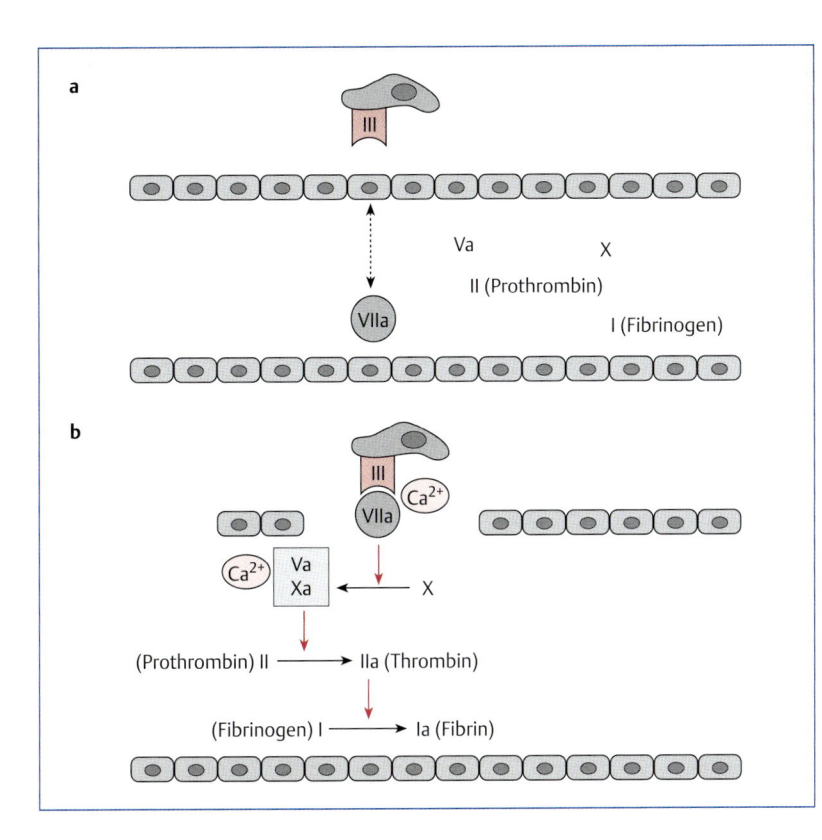

Fig. 9.6 Activation of plasmatic coagulation.
a An intact endothelium prevents clotting by physically separating factor III (in tissue) and factor VIIa (in the blood). **b** If an endothelial lesion occurs, factor VIIa binds to factor III and starts the clotting cascade. As a result of the factor III/factor VIIa interaction, factors X and II (prothrombin) are activated and finally fibrin is formed. Factor Va plays an important role as a cofactor, as it increases 1000-fold, the enzymatic activity of factor X.

XIII to XIIIa, which catalyses cross-linking of fibrin strands to form a **fibrin network** (**Fig. 9.10**).

> **IN A NUTSHELL** !
>
> Plasmatic coagulation leads to the formation of a fibrin network and thus to a stable vessel occlusion.

The pathway described here is called the **extrinsic pathway of blood coagulation**. It is the **in vivo** pathway of **fibrin formation**, as demonstrated by numerous clinical studies and experimental models in mice with experimentally induced factor deficiency. However, shortly after activation of this pathway, inhibition occurs by the tissue factor pathway inhibitor (TFPI) present in plasma. This inhibitor prevents the formation of factor Xa.

To achieve the effective formation of a fibrin clot, further factors must be activated (**Fig. 9.7**). In recent years it has become clear that the factor III/VIIa complex not only converts factor X to Xa, but also causes the activation of factor IX to IXa. Factor IXa forms an enzyme complex with cofactor VIIIa that also activates factor X to Xa. Thus, there is not only a continuation of fibrin formation, but a considerable intensification of the process.

All the processes described take place at **cell membranes** of endothelial cells, and of thrombocytes in the developing thrombus and of subendothelial cells. In this way, fibrin formation is limited to the region of vascular injury. The cofactors V (**Fig. 9.8 a**) and VIII (**Fig. 9.8 b**) are plasma proteins that are activated by thrombin to form cofactors Va and VIIIa and bind to membrane phospholipids (**Fig. 9.8, (1)**). The membrane-bound factors Va and VIIIa have a high affinity for factors Xa and IXa, respectively, and

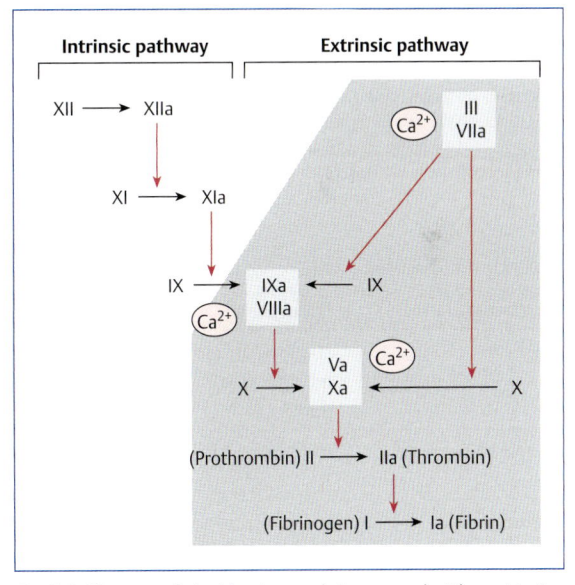

Fig. 9.7 Diagram of the blood coagulation cascade. The extrinsic pathway of blood coagulation (light grey background) is activated by factor III/factor VIIa interaction (**Fig. 9.6 b**). Initially, this leads to direct activation of factor X (but with a time delay), and also to activation of factor IX. This results in an intensification of the coagulation process.
In vitro, coagulation can also be induced by autocatalytic activation of factor XII on negatively charged surfaces (e.g. glass) (intrinsic pathway of blood coagulation). Activation of this pathway is used for functional testing of factors IXa, VIIIa, Xa and IIa in laboratory diagnostics.

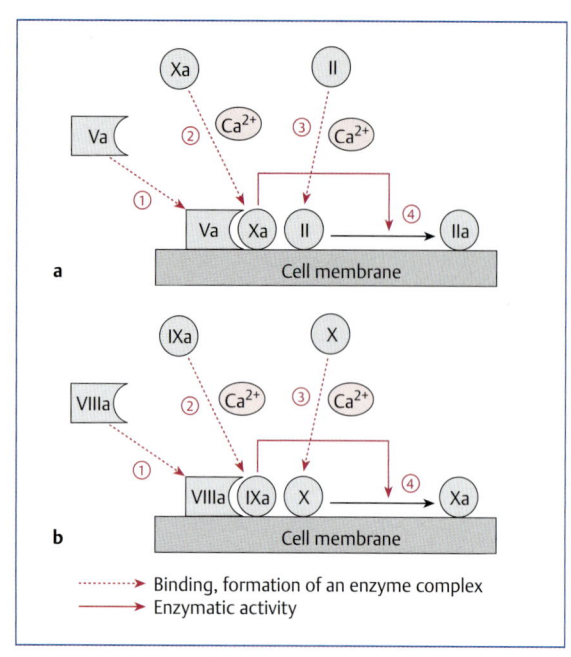

Binding, formation of an enzyme complex ┈┈┈▶
Enzymatic activity ────▶

Fig. 9.8 Formation of the prothrombin activator complex. The coagulation processes described all take place in a strictly membrane-associated manner. This process is shown here for the prothrombin activator complex (**a**) and for factor X (**b**).
a Factor Va binds to cell membranes (1) of subendothelial cells, thrombocytes and endothelial cells in the region of a vascular injury, and then associates with factor Xa (2). Only in this complex is factor Xa proteolytically highly active and cleaves factor II (prothrombin, (3)) to IIa (thrombin, (4)). Ca²⁺ ions are essential for binding to the membranes.
b Binding of factor VIIIa (functionally homologous to Va, (1)) and IXa (functionally homologous to Xa, (2)), which together activate factor X (3) to Xa (4), is similar. Ca²⁺ ions are also necessary for formation of these complexes.

thus mediate their binding to the cell membrane (**Fig. 9.8**, (2)). In addition, formation of complexes from factors Xa and Va or IXa and VIIIa cause an up to 1000-fold increase in enzymatic activity of the proteases (factor Xa or IXa). Without binding to the respective cofactor (Va or VIIIa), these proteases are functionally inactive and binding (**Fig. 9.8** (3)) and activation (**Fig. 9.8** (4)) of factors II and X would not take place. This becomes clear in **haemophilia A** in which a factor VIII deficiency leads to severe coagulation disorders and bleeding. Such coagulation disorders are also found in domestic animals, especially in dogs.

In addition to the factors mentioned so far, **Ca²⁺ ions are also essential factors** in the coagulation process (**Fig. 9.8**). Coagulation can be prevented by removing Ca²⁺ ions from blood. In practice, substances such as citrate, oxalate or ethylenediamine tetraacetic acid (EDTA), which bind Ca²⁺ ions tightly, are therefore often used to prevent blood clotting in vitro (**Table 9.9**).

Phospholipid membranes have many fixed negative charges on their surface. Since many coagulation factors also have strongly negatively charged domains, their binding to phospholipid membranes is not readily achieved. Divalent Ca²⁺ ions can on the one hand bind to negatively charged components of coagulation factors and on the other hand interact with phospholipid membranes. Ca²⁺ ions thus mediate the binding of coagulation factors to membranes. Ca²⁺ deprivation prevents this process and thus, among other things, prevents formation of the prothrombin activator complex, since both factor Xa and prothrombin (factor II) only bind to phospholipid membranes in a Ca²⁺-dependent manner (**Fig. 9.8**).

Table 9.9 Anticoagulants.

Anticoagulant	Occurrence	Mechanism of action	Relevance
Heparin	Endothelial cells, basophil granulocytes, mast cells	Binding to AT III, heparin-AT-III complex binds thrombin	Application as anticoagulant in vivo and in vitro (heparin plasma)
Heparan sulphate	Endothelial surfaces	Like heparin	Physiological anticoagulation at the intact endothelium
Hirudin	Isolated from the leech	Binds thrombin directly	–
Coumarin derivatives	E.g. in lazy clover	Vitamin K antagonist Inhibition of γ-carboxylation of factors II, VII, IX, X	Poisoning in domestic animals due to ingestion of rat poison baits, oral anticoagulant therapy
EDTA, citrate, oxalate	Synthetic	Complex formation with Ca²⁺ by removing the Ca²⁺ ions, numerous reaction processes in the coagulation cascade are inhibited	Obtaining plasma samples for laboratory diagnostics
Acetylsalicylic acid	Synthetic	Cyclooxygenase inhibition, inhibition of thrombocyte activation through inhibition of thromboxane A₂ formation	Inhibition of platelet aggregation in vivo

The proteins that are bound to membranes through Ca^{2+} ions are all proenzymes. Synthesis of these proteins (factor II, VII, IX and X) in the liver is vitamin K-dependent. **Vitamin K** is a component of an enzyme complex that converts glutamate residues in the region of the N-terminus of the coagulation factors mentioned to γ-carboxyglutamate. This results in an increase in negative charge in this molecular region. Vitamin K deficiency thus leads to an absence of γ-carboxylation which is why the Ca^{2+}-mediated binding of coagulation factors to phospholipid membranes does not occur.

Vitamin K belongs to the fat-soluble group of vitamins and is found as phylloquinone (vitamin K1) in green plants. Furthermore, it is produced as menaquinone (vitamin K2) by microorganisms in the ruminant forestomachs (p.405) and in the large intestine (p.440). While (microbial) vitamin K synthesized in the rumen is absorbed during passage through the small intestine, vitamin K produced in the large intestine cannot be absorbed. This is only available to those animals that ingest their faeces (coprophagy/caecotrophy, **Fig. 16.81**). If the intake of faeces is prevented due to the housing conditions (e.g. cage housing of chickens), vitamin K deficiency symptoms, with bleeding, can occur.

> **MORE DETAILS** Vitamin K deficiency causes severe coagulation disorders. Vitamin K analogues, such as **coumarin derivatives** (dicumarol or warfarin), are used therapeutically to inhibit coagulation. However, they are also used as **rodenticides** in the control of rats and mice, where the ingestion of these substances also leads to coagulation disorders and thus **bleeding to death** (**Table 9.9**). Dicumarol is also found in sweet clover and in some herbs.

The concept of coagulation in vivo described here differs in parts from the "classical" concept of the coagulation cascade, in which two independent pathways lead to the formation of the prothrombin activator (factor Xa/Va) (**Fig. 9.7**). Besides the extrinsic pathway of blood coagulation already described, there is an **intrinsic pathway**. This begins with the **autocatalytic activation** of factor XII to XIIa on negatively charged surfaces and leads via factors XI/XIa and IX/IXa to the activation of X to Xa. This system has been intensively investigated in vitro by adding blood samples to negatively charged surfaces such as glass, kaolin or dextrans. Since patients with factor VIII or factor IX deficiency are prone to life-threatening bleeding (haemophilia A and B), the intrinsic pathway was also long considered the crucial pathway in vivo. However, the relatively commonly seen factor XII deficiency does not lead to blood clotting disorders.

Only when it became clear that the initial complex of the extrinsic pathway of blood coagulation (factor III/VIIa) also activates factor IX of the intrinsic pathway (**Fig. 9.7**), this "dilemma" was solved. In contrast to factor XII deficiency, factor XI deficiency leads to bleeding in vivo, as has been observed in humans and dogs. Factor XI can be activated not only by factor XIIa, but also by thrombin. Here, a positive feedback activation obviously exists, which is important in case of severe bleeding.

Under physiological conditions, therefore, there is no autocatalytic activation of factor XII to XIIa. Nevertheless, this process plays an important role. On the one hand, it initiates the coagulation of blood when it is introduced into so-called serum tubes after activation at the negatively charged surfaces in the tube. Thus, after centrifugation of clotted blood, serum can be obtained for laboratory diagnostics. On the other hand, the activation of the intrinsic pathway is used to determine the activated partial thromboplastin time.

In vivo, however, the system is only activated under pathophysiological conditions. If negatively charged molecules such as RNA, DNA or polyphosphates are released from cells or if the system comes into contact with surfaces of bacteria and misfolded proteins, factor XII can bind there, be activated and induce formation of thrombin. An amplification mechanism also exists in this system. After autocatalytic activation of factor XII to XIIa, the latter can convert the plasma protein prekallikrein to the protease kallikrein, which then converts more factor XII to XIIa in a positive feedback. Another plasma protein, the high-molecular-weight kininogen, further enhances the formation of factor XIIa.

An additional in vivo function of factor XII activation is the formation of bradykinin. This is formed by partial proteolysis of high-molecular-weight kininogen by kallikrein. After binding to its receptor, bradykinin leads, among other things, to vasodilation, increase in vascular permeability and induction of pain (p.78) (**Fig. 3.10**). Finally, the factor XIIa-kallikrein system is also involved in fibrinolysis (**Fig. 9.10**).

■ Coagulation testing

> **MORE DETAILS** In the diagnosis of coagulation disorders, so-called **global tests** (global coagulation assays) are usually used first. These tests measure the time that elapses between activation of the coagulation system and formation of a visible or measurable fibrin strand. To examine the extrinsic pathway of blood coagulation (factors VII, X, V, II), a plasma sample (e.g. citrate plasma) is mixed with Ca^{2+} ions and factor III and the sample is stirred with an eyelet. Depending on species, a fibrin strand should then form after 7–15 seconds (Quick test). Similarly, the function of the factors of the intrinsic pathway of blood coagulation (XI, IX, VIII, X and V as well as II) is tested by adding negative charged surfaces (e.g. kaolin, dextran) and Ca^{2+} to citrated plasma and also measuring, while stirring, the time until fibrin formation (activated partial thromboplastin time, aPPT). If a plasma sample shows a prolonged clotting time, the cause can be found by testing the function of individual clotting factors. Such tests are used, especially when factor VIII or factor IX deficiency diseases (haemophilia) or dicumarol poisoning are suspected.

■ Physiological anticoagulation and fibrinolysis

The processes of haemostasis are countered by equally complex **antithrombotic** and **anticoagulatory** as well as **fibrinolytic** mechanisms in intact vessels. Many of these functions are mediated by the **endothelium**.

Endothelial cells separate blood from the subendothelial matrix, preventing platelet adhesion and activation of

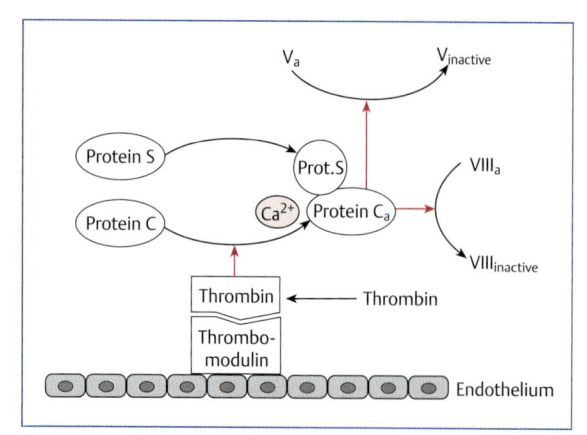

Fig. 9.9 Anticoagulant mechanisms. Under physiological conditions, numerous mechanisms prevent clotting. One of the most important pathways is binding of thrombin to thrombomodulin expressed on endothelial cells. Thrombin bound in this way changes its substrate specificity and now activates protein C to form activated protein C_a. Protein C_a, in complex with protein S, has an anticoagulant effect by inactivating factors Va and VIIIa. Red arrows = enzymatic effect (proteolysis), black arrows = conversion.

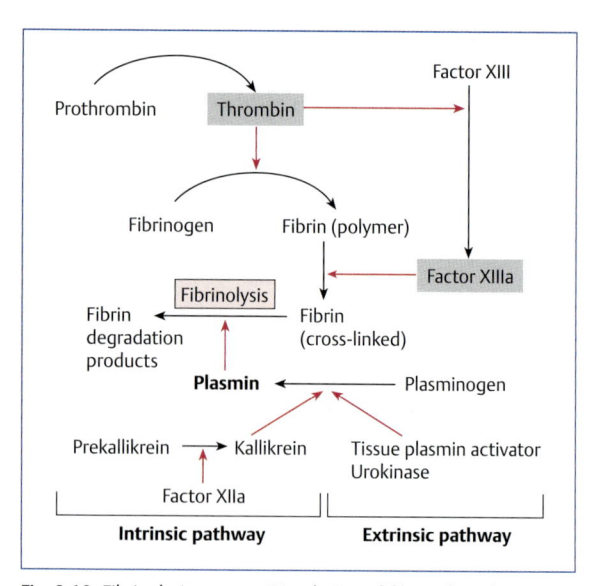

Fig. 9.10 Fibrinolysis system. Dissolution of fibrin clots also occurs through activation of plasmatic factors (intrinsic pathway) and tissue factors (extrinsic pathway). Both systems activate plasminogen to plasmin, which degrades fibrin into cleavage products. The latter are detectable in plasma and are diagnostically important. Red arrows = enzymatic effect, black arrows = conversion.

plasmatic coagulation by these structures. In addition, the cell surface of endothelial cells is strongly negatively charged. This repels thrombocytes, which are also negatively charged. The additional secretion of prostaglandin I_2 (PGI_2) and nitric oxide (NO) prevents intravascular **aggregation of thrombocytes**, a mechanism that is particularly important in the vicinity of already formed blood clots.

Thrombin is the key enzyme in the coagulation cascade. Formation of small amounts of thrombin leads to a strong positive feedback activation of the system. This is because thrombin, once formed, activates factor VII to VIIa, cofactors V and VIII to Va and VIIIa, and factor XI to XIa. In order to prevent fibrin formation under physiological conditions, correspondingly effective mechanisms for inhibiting thrombin activity must be present. On the luminal surface of endothelial cells, a protein, **thrombomodulin**, is expressed (**Fig. 9.9**), which binds thrombin and thus inhibits procoagulant activity. This **thrombomodulin-thrombin complex** is also a strong activator of the protease, "protein C". Activated protein C (C_a) inactivates factors Va and VIIIa and also has a fibrinolytic effect. The enzymatic activity of **protein C_a** can be further enhanced by the binding of protein S to protein C_a. Also found on the endothelial cell membrane is **heparan sulphate** (Table 9.9). This binds the plasma **antithrombin III** (ATIII). Free ATIII, to a small extent, is able to inactivate thrombin. Binding to heparan sulphate leads to a significant increase in the thrombin-inhibiting effect. In the same way, **heparin**, which is produced and released by endothelial cells and mast cells, can increase the ATIII effect by about 1000-fold when not bound to the membrane. Heparin is therefore also used therapeutically as a potent anticoagulant (**Table 9.9**).

> **IN A NUTSHELL**   !
>
> Antithrombotic and anticoagulant mechanisms are mediated by the vascular endothelium.

Clots, that have been already formed, are dissolved again by the **fibrinolysis system** (**Fig. 9.10**). Proteolytic degradation of fibrin is catalysed by a serine protease, **plasmin**. Plasmin is formed from its inactive precursor, plasminogen, under the influence of various activators. Plasminogen is already incorporated into the fibrin network during clot formation. With a precisely timed delay compared to fibrin formation, a plasminogen activator is released from damaged tissue and endothelial cells, resulting in the formation of plasmin in the fibrin network. In addition to this **tissue activator** (**extrinsic pathway**), there are also **blood activators** (**intrinsic** pathway of fibrinolysis). The most important blood activator is factor XIIa, which converts prekallikrein to **kallikrein**. Kallikrein then activates plasminogen to plasmin. However, plasmin does not only have a fibrinolytic effect. By degrading the coagulation factors Va and VIIIa, it also counteracts formation of new thrombin and thus of fibrin.

> **IN A NUTSHELL**   !
>
> The protease plasmin has a fibrinolytic and anticoagulant effect.

9.4.4   Pathophysiology

MORE DETAILS   Functional failures in the thrombocyte system or in plasmatic coagulation can lead to bleeding that is sometimes life-threatening. Both systems can be affected by congenital and acquired diseases. On the thrombocyte side, the most common causes are **thrombocytopenias** with platelet counts below 50000 μl^{-1} blood or genetic **disorders** in the formation of the von Willebrand factor (p. 235) (**Fig. 9.5**). The latter have been observed particularly in Doberman-Pinschers. Congenital defects in the plasmatic coagulation system can basically affect all factors. By far the most common are diseases with deficiency of factors VIII (**haemophilia A**) and IX (**haemophilia B**). Acquired factor deficiency is also seen clinically, in poisoning from ingestion of coumarin derivatives contained in rodenticides. As previously explained, these substances inhibit vitamin K-dependent γ-carboxylation of numerous coagulation factors (including II, VII, IX, X). This coumarin effect can be antagonised by high doses of vitamin K.

In contrast to this are the **hypercoagulopathies** in which an unphysiological activation of the coagulation system occurs throughout the entire organism. This is observed particularly frequently in systemic inflammatory reactions (e.g. sepsis), as a result of which so-called disseminated intravascular coagulation (DIC) can occur. The formation of **microthrombi** throughout the body leads to multiple organ failure and thus very often to the death of the affected individual.

Suggested reading

Gentry P, Burgess H, Wood D. Hemostasis. In: Kaneko JJ, Harvey JW, Bruss ML, eds. Clinical Biochemistry of Domestic Animals. San Diego: Academic Press; 2008: 287–330

Hoffman R, Bruce F, Edward J, Benz JR, McGlave PH, Silberstein LE, Shattil SJ, eds. Hematology – Basic Principals and Practice. 4th ed. Philadelphia: Churchill Livingston; 2005

Okhota S, Melnikov I, Avtaeva Y et al. Shear stress-induced activation of von Willebrand factor and cardiovascular pathology. Int J Mol Sci 2020; 21 (20): 7804

Smith SA, Travers RJ, Morrissey JH. How it all starts: initiation of the clotting cascade. Crit Rev Biochem Mol Biol 2015; 50 (4): 326–336

van der Meijden PEJ, Heemskerk JWM. Platelet biology and functions: new concepts and clinical perspectives. Nat Rev Cardiol 2019; 16 (3): 166–179

9.5 Blood groups

Thomas Göbel, Bernd Kaspers

> **ESSENTIALS**   ✖
>
> **Erythrocytes**, like any other cell, carry numerous molecules on their cell surface.
> - Most of these membrane-bound molecules are either **glycoproteins** or **glycolipids** with many different physiological functions.
> - Some of these molecules are **encoded** by **genes** that exhibit **polymorphism**, which means that there are different alleles that encode different variants of the molecules.
> - The immune system is tolerant of the body's own antigens, and therefore does not react to them.
>
> In a **blood transfusion** between two **genetically different animals**, all molecules on the erythrocytes that differ between donor and recipient act as antigens. The recipient can form **antibodies** against these foreign structures. These antibodies bind the molecules **on the erythrocytes**, and **activate** the **complement system** and **phagocytosis**. Thus, they cause a very **rapid destruction** of the foreign erythrocytes.

> **IN A NUTSHELL**   !
>
> Blood group antigens are polymorphic antigenic structures on the erythrocyte surface.

9.5.1 The human AB0 system

In the AB0 system, terminal sugars moieties of **glycolipids** define the blood group. Blood group **A** is defined by **N-acetylgalactosamine**, **blood group B** by **galactose**, blood group **AB** by a combination of these sugar residues, and blood group **0** by the absence of both sugar residues. The blood group characteristics A and B are inherited dominantly (AA or A0; BB or B0; AB), so that blood group 0 only occurs in homozygous form (00).

The special feature of the **AB0 system** is formation of antibodies against blood group antigens even **before contact** with foreign blood. Thus, individuals with blood group A form **antibodies** against blood group antigen B (Table 9.10). The reason for this antibody formation are substances that are ingested with food or produced by **intestinal bacteria** and have the same sugar structure as the blood group antigens. The immune system reacts to these foreign substances from the intestine by forming antibodies. Production of antibodies against blood group A is prevented in persons with blood group A by the fact that **autoreactive** lymphocytes (p.252) are removed by selection. Conversely, individuals with blood group B form antibodies against blood group A. People with blood group 0 form both anti-A and anti-B antibodies. In contrast, persons with blood group AB do not show antibodies against blood group A or B in their serum. In blood **transfusions** with blood of other blood groups, these antibodies bind to blood group antigens on the erythrocyte membrane and **agglutination and haemolysis** occur, due to complement activation (p.247). Since blood group antigens are glycolipids, the immune system almost exclusively forms **IgM antibodies**. The IgM antibodies (p.252) have a very strong agglutinating effect due to their ten binding sites, but they cannot pass the placental barrier. Therefore, they do not trigger any intolerance in the embryo.

Table 9.10 AB0 blood groups.

Blood group	Genotype	Serum antibodies
A	AA, A0	Anti-B
B	BB, B0	Anti-A
AB	AB	–
0	00	Anti-A, Anti-B

> **IN A NUTSHELL**   !
>
> The AB0 blood group antigens induce the formation of IgM antibodies.

9.5.2   Rhesus system of the human being

The **rhesus system** is characterised by different **rhesus antigens**, of which the **D antigen** is the most important. If the D antigen is missing from the erythrocyte membrane, the blood is called **rhesus negative**. In the rhesus system, in contrast to the AB0 system, there is no **cross-reactivity with antigens from the intestine**. Therefore, antibodies are only formed in rhesus negative persons after contact with rhesus positive blood. In repeated **pregnancies of rhesus negative mothers** with a **rhesus positive child**, production of antibodies against the D antigen is stimulated. This leads to rhesus incompatibility. In the first pregnancy, rhesus positive erythrocytes of the child enter maternal circulation during birth and stimulate the immune system there to form IgM antibodies against D antigen (= primary response). When the mother is re-immunised with D antigen during the next pregnancy, the Ig class switch leads to the massive production of IgG antibodies (p. 256) (= secondary response). These antibodies pass through the placenta, bind to D antigen on foetal erythrocytes and thus lead to haemolysis in the foetus. For **prophylaxis**, rhesus negative mothers are given an anti-D antiserum after each pregnancy, which binds to the rhesus positive erythrocytes of the child that have passed over, thus preventing the mother's immune response to the Rh antigen.

> **IN A NUTSHELL**   !
>
> Rhesus antigens induce IgG antibody formation in rhesus negative mothers.

9.5.3   Blood groups of animals

Domestic animals have **different blood group systems** of varying complexity. The naturally occurring antibodies are rarely of clinical significance in domestic mammals. However, in some animal blood group systems, naturally occur-

ring antibodies can form against blood group antigens. The actual structures that trigger antibody formation are carbohydrate residues. Many surface receptors on the erythrocyte membrane are modified by carbohydrate residues. Coincidentally, identical carbohydrate residues are also found on the surface of foreign intestinal bacteria. Those structures that are identical on both endogenous erythrocytes and gut bacteria do not trigger antibody formation, but allelic variants that do not occur on endogenous cells do. These natural antibodies can trigger incompatibilities in blood transfusions. In particular, natural antibodies against bovine J antigens and porcine A antigens have been described.

In domestic animals, there are very simple systems, such as the L system of cattle, which consists of only two alleles, up to very complex systems, such as the bovine B system with several hundred different alleles (**Table 9.11**). Together with other bovine blood group systems, this results in several million possible combinations in cattle. Some blood group antigens are not products of erythrocytes at all, but soluble serum components that bind passively to the erythrocyte membrane. Examples are DEA7 antigen (dog), J antigen (cattle), A antigen (pig) and R antigen (sheep). The presence of antibodies against some blood group antigens is possible even before contact with corresponding erythrocytes. These antibodies are also called **natural antibodies** or **isoantibodies**.

Similar to the rhesus system, there are also incompatibilities known as **neonatal isoerythrolysis** (**Fig. 9.11**). In this case, female animals have been immunised with foetal blood group antigens during pregnancy or at birth. After repeated contact, large quantities of IgG antibodies are formed, which, depending on species, are either transferred via the placenta, into the foetus or via the **colostrum** into the new-born. These antibodies cause **haemolytic anaemia**. Neonatal isoerythrolysis can occur, especially in horses.

Table 9.11 Blood group systems in domestic animals.

Animal species	Number	Names	Notes
Dog	8	DEA 1, 2, 3, 4, 5, 6, 7, 8	Five further blood group systems have been described (special feature: DEA7 not membrane-bound, but soluble serum component)
Cat	1	AB	Natural antibodies!
Horse	7	EAA, EAC, EAD, EAK, EAP, EAQ, EAU	EAC, EAK and EAU: only two alleles each, the Aa antigen of the EAA system is very important in neonatal isoerythrolysis
Cattle	11	A, B, C, F, J, L, M, R', S, T', Z	J soluble, B and C systems very complex with many alleles
Sheep	6	A, B, C, D, M, R	R soluble, B very complex
Pig	16	EAA to EAP	EAA soluble, natural antibodies against EAA

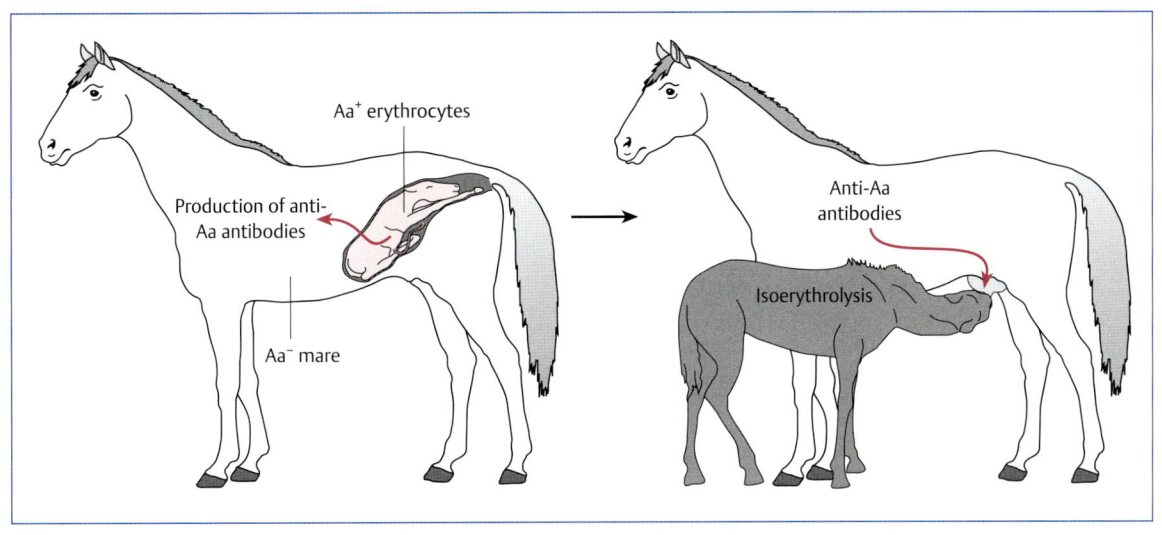

Fig. 9.11 Steps involved in neonatal isoerythrolysis. Immunisation of the mother usually occurs at birth, through contact with foetal erythrocytes carrying the A antigen. The mother then forms antibodies against the A antigen. In a subsequent pregnancy with a blood group antigen A positive foal, a new immunisation takes place. Antibodies against the A antigen are absorbed by the foal via the colostrum, then bind to erythrocytes and lyse them.

MORE DETAILS   In dogs, DEA1 antigen has a particularly important role. About 60% of all dogs are DEA1 positive. Antibodies against DEA1 are only formed after contact with DEA1 positive erythrocytes. When transfusing blood, care should be taken never to transfuse DEA1 positive blood to DEA1 negative recipients, as this antigen is very immunogenic and strongly induces antibody formation. Therefore, after a subsequent transfusion, intolerance reactions occur. In cats, there is only the AB blood group system with A, B or AB. About 75–95% of all cats are A positive and 5–25% B positive. However, there is a great variability depending on breed and country. Severe transfusion reactions can occur in the cat, as almost all B positive cats have natural anti-A antibodies. Even infusion of 1 ml of blood can cause severe shock.

Apart from these well-known blood group incompatibilities, there are usually few incidents with blood transfusions. With a first blood transfusion, it is very unlikely that antibodies against foreign blood group antigens are already present. This is only likely in the cases mentioned above. Therefore, the recipient of a blood transfusion will only form antibodies against foreign antigens on the surface of erythrocytes after the transfusion. Since not every blood group antigen is equally immunogenic, strong antibody formation only occurs with some antigens. Only after repeated infusions with blood from the same donor is there then a risk of a massive transfusion reaction. Therefore, firstly, it is advisable to change donors, and secondly, a crossmatching should always be carried out before a blood transfusion in order to exclude possible transfusion reactions.

IN A NUTSHELL   !

Blood group antigens can induce the formation of specific antibodies that trigger transfusion reactions.

Suggested reading

Schmid DO, Buschmann HG, Hammer C, eds. Blood Groups in Animals. Lengerich: Pabst Science Publishers; 2003

10   Immune defence – the immune system

Thomas Göbel, Bernd Kaspers

10.1   Functions of the immune system

ESSENTIALS   ✖

The immune system protects the body from infections, and it eliminates degenerate and dying cells. The **innate immune system** is responsible for immediate recognition and defence at the ports of entry of pathogens. In addition, it alerts the acquired immune system. Important elements of innate immunity are:
– Soluble factors such as the complement system, interferons and antibacterial proteins
– Phagocytes such as macrophages, granulocytes and dendritic cells

Acquired immune mechanisms are only activated several days after an infection. They form an immunological memory. Important elements of the acquired immune system are:
– B lymphocytes producing different antibodies (IgM, IgG, IgA and IgE)
– Cytotoxic T lymphocytes, which recognise and kill virally infected cells
– T helper cells, which regulate immune reactions by secreting soluble chemical messengers

10.2   Introduction – Cells and chemical messengers of the immune system

10.2.1   Pathogens activate the immune system

When looking at the immune system, two features stand out: **recognition** and a subsequent **reaction**. How does the immune system distinguish healthy from diseased cells and harmless microorganisms from dangerous pathogens? How are appropriate measures initiated after recognition, ranging from local reactions to systemic inflammation? Which immunoregulatory systems shape differentiated immune response to pathogens, the body's own cells, environmental antigens or foreign objects?

Humans and animals constantly come into contact with a multitude of microorganisms. An estimated 10^{14} bacteria live in human intestine, and the number is probably far greater in the cow's rumen. Most of these microorganisms are completely harmless inhabitants of the body. In contrast, invasion and multiplication of pathogens must be prevented as early as possible. One of the most important

features of the immune system is the ability to distinguish between **foreign**, potentially harmful structures that are recognised and destroyed by the immune system, and harmless or **endogenous** structures that the immune system ignores. The latter process is known as **tolerance**. For example, pathogenic infectious organisms activate immune defence, while the natural bacterial microbiome of the skin or intestine are tolerated by the immune system. In contrast, there are a number of pathogens that enter the body through external and internal body surfaces and cause disease. They have to be recognised and eliminated by the immune system.

Pathogens are divided into bacteria, viruses, fungi and parasites. For recognition by the immune system, it is particularly important where infectious agents multiply. While many bacteria, fungi or intestinal parasites multiply extracellularly, other pathogens such as viruses are found intracellularly. The **immune response** against **extracellular** and **intracellular pathogens** is different, since extracellular pathogens can be attacked directly, while intracellular infections require the body's own infected cells to be eliminated.

Any substance that causes a reaction of the acquired immune system is called an **antigen** (origin: antibody generating). Antigens, therefore, can comprise a very diverse range of chemical structures, for example synthetic substances, structures on the surface of pathogens or even soluble molecules, such as tetanus toxin.

> **IN A NUTSHELL**   !
>
> The immune system distinguishes between pathogens, harmless microbes and the body's own structures.

10.2.2   Innate and acquired immunity

The immune defence is based on two closely interconnected functional units, the **innate and the acquired immune system** (Fig. 10.1). These systems are jointly involved in immune responses. They differ primarily in the way how they recognize foreign structures, as well as in timing of the immune response, and the mechanisms of pathogen control. Thus, the **innate** defence mechanisms are responsible for immediately combating invading pathogens, within a few minutes. Cells of the innate immune system are therefore located directly at entry sites of pathogens, such as the lamina propria below an epithelium. The **acquired immune** system is activated only after a few days, in the regional lymph nodes. It forms an immunological memory in long-lived memory cells, which, with a repeated infection, provides immediate protection.

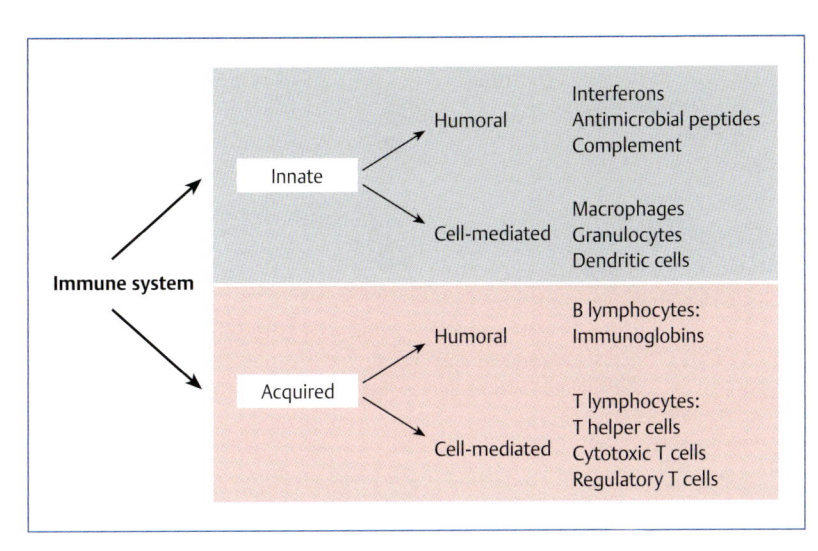

Circulation, respiration

Fig. 10.1 Components of the immune system.

In both systems, **soluble** (humoral) and **cell-mediated** immune mechanisms are involved (**Fig. 10.1**). In the innate immune system, these are the complement system and various phagocytes. In the acquired system, antibodies are formed by B lymphocytes, and various types of T lymphocytes perform cell-mediated immune reactions and release soluble chemical messengers. All cells of the immune system are equipped with a multitude of **receptors** for recognition of pathogens. These receptors recognise foreign structures on pathogens and they then activate cells.

> **IN A NUTSHELL**　　　　　　　　　　　　!
>
> The innate and acquired immune systems cooperate in the immune response. In both systems, there are cellular and soluble defence components. Immunological memory is formed by long-lived memory cells of the acquired immune system.

10.2.3　Blood cell differentiation

All blood cells are derived from pluripotent stem cells in the bone marrow (p. 224). Stem cells can form many different cell types. They are **undifferentiated** and have unlimited **ability to divide**. When stem cells divide, they give rise to daughter cells that either form new stem cells or, under the influence of numerous **colony-stimulating factors**, finally differentiate and lose the capabilities of stem cells (**Fig. 10.2**).

Leukocytes (p. 233) (Greek leukos = white) are divided on the basis of morphology and stainability into lymphocytes, monocytes, and neutrophil, eosinophil and basophil granulocytes. The **white blood cell count** differs between species with values of 3000–30000 cells per µl blood (**Table 9.8**). An increase in the total number of leukocytes is referred to as **leukocytosis** and a decrease is called **leuko(-cyto)penia**.

MORE DETAILS　The **leukocyte differential count** provides additional information about the percentage distribution of each cell type within the white blood cell count. Humans, horses, dogs and cats have more granulocytes than lymphocytes. In contrast, in ruminants, pigs, rodents and birds, lymphocytes are the dominant white blood cell, as they represent more than 50% of leukocytes in these species.

After their formation in bone marrow, various cells are released into blood. Some cells, such as erythrocytes, thrombocytes and granulocytes, are already fully functional at this stage. Other cell types only mature fully in tissues (monocytes) or in specialised organs (lymphocytes).

> **IN A NUTSHELL**　　　　　　　　　　　　!
>
> Depending on the species, granulocytes or lymphocytes dominate the leukocyte differential count.

10.2.4　Cytokines

After activation of the cells involved in immune defence, they release soluble chemical messengers. The nomenclature of these chemical messengers has varied over the years, and therefore is not standardised. The term **cytokines** is used as an umbrella name for these chemical messengers (**Fig. 10.3**). The **cytokines** can be further subdivided into **interferons** (named because of their "interference" with the multiplication of viruses), **tumour necrosis factor** (named after their effect on some tumour cell lines), **colony-stimulating factors** (named after their promoting effect on the development of certain blood cell lines), **chemokines** (named after their chemotactic effect), and **interleukins** (which serve, among other things, for communication between leukocytes or other cells of the immune system). Individual types of interleukins are numbered consecutively (example: interleukin-2, abbreviated IL-2). Cytokines often have multiple (pleiotropic) functions, and they are crucial in immune regulation. Some cytokines have a predominantly autocrine (p. 531) effect such as **IL-2**, which is produced by T lymphocytes and stimulates these cells to proliferate. Other cytokines have a **paracrine** effect (**IL-4** during interaction between B and T lymphocytes; **Fig. 10.15**) or **endocrine function** like **IL-1** during fever induction (**Fig. 10.6**).

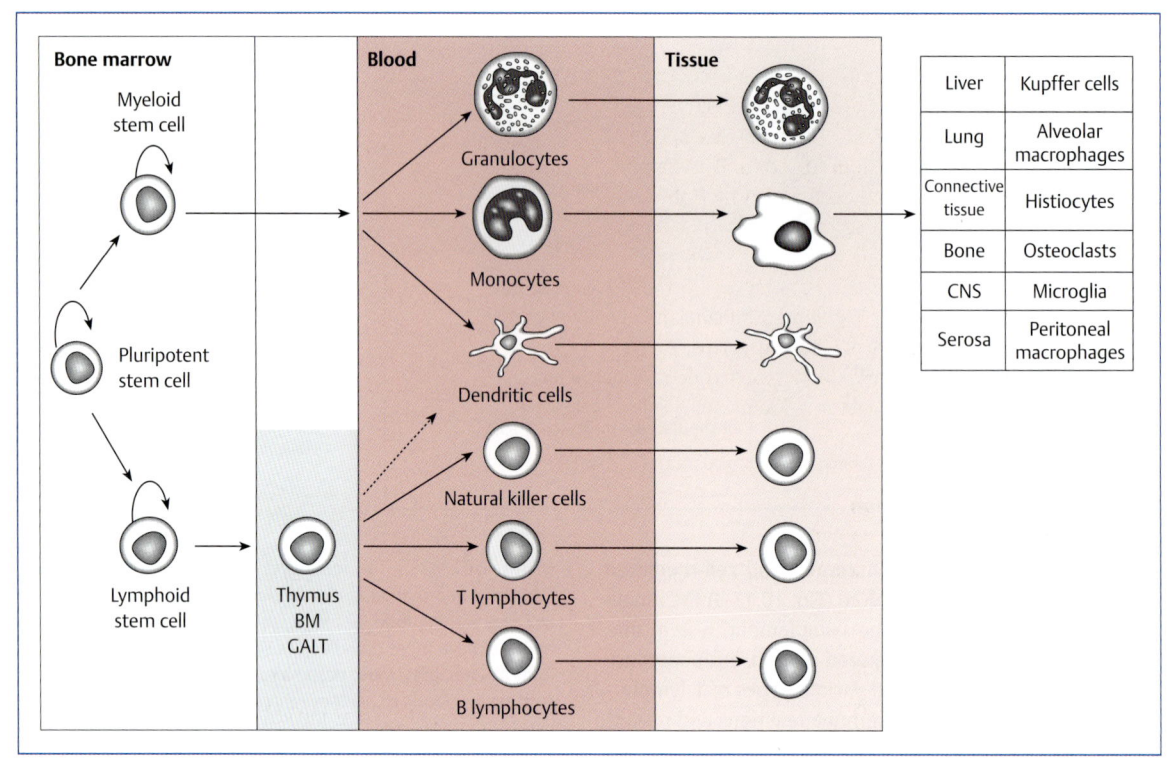

Fig. 10.2 Scheme of immune cell formation. BM = bone marrow; GALT = gut associated lymphoid tissue.

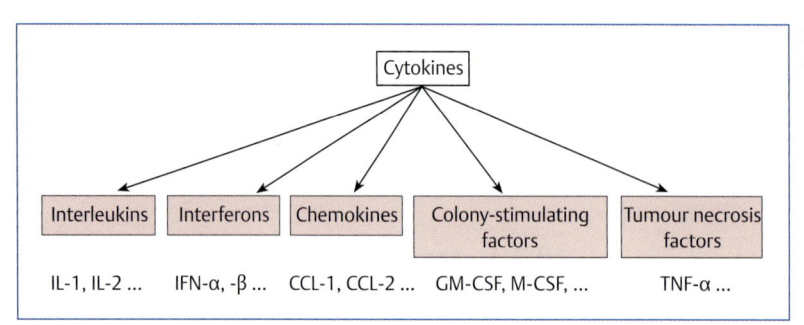

Fig. 10.3 Chemical messengers of the immune system.

<table>
<tr><td colspan="2">IN A NUTSHELL</td></tr>
</table>

> **IN A NUTSHELL** !
>
> Cytokines are soluble chemical messengers of the immune system. They have a variety of tasks (pleiotropic) and mostly have an auto- or paracrine effect.

10.3 Innate immune mechanisms

The term **innate immunity** covers a very wide range of mechanisms, all of which are already developed prenatally and are thus immediately available for immune defence after birth. Innate immunity includes a broad spectrum of different defence strategies, ranging from defence against infections by epithelial cells to the activity of specialised phagocytes.

Innate defence mechanisms react to widespread molecular structures that are only present on pathogens, and not on the body's own cells. After recognition of such **exoge-**nous structures, a constant (non-adaptive) immune reaction occurs. The advantage of this recognition strategy is the activation and destruction of pathogens within a few hours, as **no adaptation to** the particular **pathogen** is needed. These early defence mechanisms limit the spread of infectious agents and any associated tissue damage. In many cases, however, the innate immune mechanisms are not sufficient to completely eliminate an infection. Moreover, since the innate immune system does **not** induce an **immunological memory**, the immune response remains unchanged even after repeated infection with the same pathogen. Therefore, no improvement of the immune reaction against recurrent infections is achieved.

> **IN A NUTSHELL** !
>
> Innate defence mechanisms react immediately, but do not induce an immunological memory.

10.3.1 Natural barriers

The natural barriers of the body are very important **protective mechanisms** against infections, as they effectively prevent the entry of pathogens (**Table 10.1**). Any disruption of these barriers increases the risk of infection. For example, epithelial cells, which are tightly connected by **tight junctions**, protect the inner and outer surfaces of the body from the entry of pathogens. The continuous **exfoliation of epithelial cells**, or the flow of fluid and air prevent the adhesion of infectious agents. The **movement** of **cilia** also enables the retrograde transport of dirt and germs. All mucous membranes are protected by viscous **mucus** that prevents direct contact of pathogens with epithelial cells.

Table 10.1 Non-specific protection mechanisms.

Protective mechanism	Through ...
Mechanical	<ul><li>Epithelial cell tight junctions</li><li>Exfoliation</li><li>Liquid, air flow</li><li>Cilia movement</li></ul>
Chemical	<ul><li>Mucus</li><li>Fatty acids</li><li>Acidic pH value in the stomach</li><li>Enzymes</li></ul>
Microbiological	<ul><li>Physiological bacterial microbiome</li></ul>

The colonisation of body surfaces with the **natural bacterial microbiome** leads to displacement of pathogens through competition for nutrients. Infectious agents can also be inactivated and degraded by **fatty acids** of the skin, the **acidic pH** of the stomach, and by various **enzymes** of the digestive tract. Any impairment of these protective mechanisms, such as destruction of the epithelium in heat or chemical burns, cuts, animal or insect bite wounds, and also reduction of the natural bacterial microbiome through the use of antibiotics, all lead to increased susceptibility to infection.

> **IN A NUTSHELL** !
>
> Natural protective barriers prevent infections.

10.3.2 Soluble factors

Epithelial cells and granulocytes produce a variety of different small peptides with **antibacterial activity**. One group of these antibacterial substances is called **defensins**. These are small, strongly positively charged peptides that insert themselves into the negatively charged bacterial cell membranes and destroy the bacteria. Also, some **surfactants** (A and D) of the lungs have antibacterial properties.

Lysozyme, an antibacterial enzyme, is found in all body fluids except sweat and cerebrospinal fluid. Particularly high amounts are secreted into the egg white. Lysozyme is an enzyme of lysosomes and cleaves peptidoglycans, an essential component of the cell wall of many bacteria.

The protein **lactoferrin** binds iron and thus deprives bacteria of an important factor for their metabolism and colony formation on mucous membranes. Lactoferrin (p.610) is found intracellularly in granulocytes and macrophages. It is secreted into milk. Another protein that deprives bacteria of an essential nutrient is vitamin B_{12}-binding protein.

Interferons are another group of glycoproteins. They are produced by almost all animal cells within a few hours after a virus infection. They prevent virus replication in neighbouring cells. This **antiviral activity** is mainly attributed to group of type I interferons (α, β, ω and others), which inhibit viral replication in cells. **Interferon γ** is the only representative of type II interferons. It has a strong activating effect on macrophages.

> **IN A NUTSHELL** !
>
> Lysozyme, defensins and lactoferrin are soluble antibacterial factors. Interferons are soluble antiviral factors.

10.3.3 Complement system

The complement system includes about 20 different plasma proteins, the so-called complement factors. The complement system enhances or complements (hence the name!) the effect of antibodies in bacterial infections. Many complement factors are present as inactive **pro-enzymes** that are first activated by proteolytic cleavage. Subsequently, they cleave and thereby activate other complement factors. Comparable to plasmatic blood coagulation, recognition of infectious agents leads to a cascade-like activation of the complement system. The key results of complement activation are destruction of bacteria (**bacteriolysis**), attraction of inflammatory cells (**chemotaxis**) and an increase in phagocytosis (**opsonisation**).

MORE DETAILS There are three different pathways for activating the complement system: the **classical** pathway, the **alternative** pathway and the **lectin** pathway (**Fig. 10.4**). In the **alternative pathway**, the complement system is activated by attachment of complement factors B and D (stabilised by properdin (P)) to bacterial surfaces. Binding of antibodies to antigens triggers the "**classical pathway**" of complement activation with factors C1, C2 and C4. Certain sugar residues on bacterial surfaces can initiate the **lectin pathway** after binding to "mannose-binding protein". Activation of complement factors is by proteolytic cleavage into a small, soluble fragment and a large, membrane-bound fragment. The smaller fragment is labelled with the letter "a", the larger with the letter "b". All three pathways of complement activation eventually result in the formation of an enzyme complex known as **C3/C5 convertase**, which cleaves complement factors C3 and C5, leading to the **accumulation of large amounts of C3b and C5b** on the bacterial surface. C3b serves to mark antigens for the phagocytic cells, which are thereby stimulated to carry out phagocytosis. The attachment of C5b to the membrane leads to the formation of the **membrane attack complex**, in which additional complement factors (C6–C9) eventually form pores in the membrane. As a result, ion gradients at the membrane and the electrical energy stored therein are lost and cellular homeostasis can no longer be maintained. The soluble fragments **C3a** and **C5a** formed during cleavage act as **inflammatory mediators**. They attract further phagocytes to the

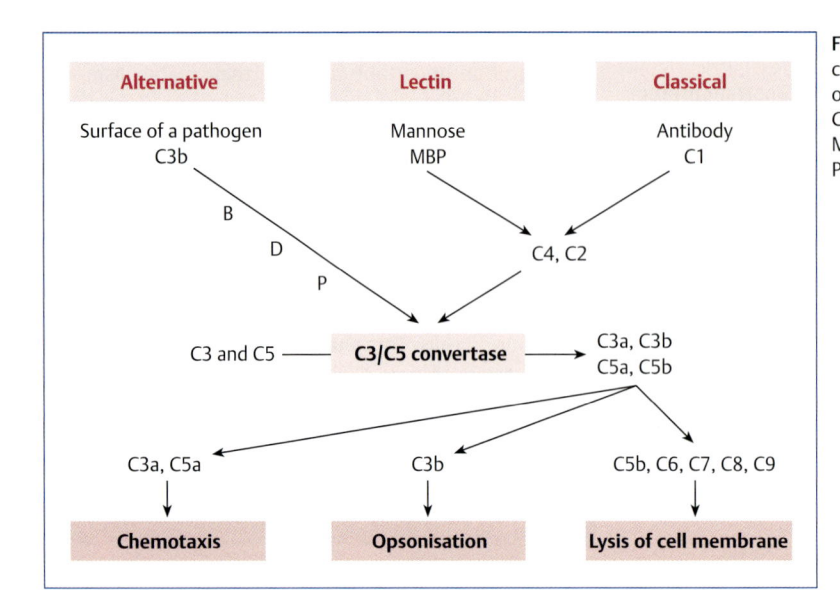

Fig. 10.4 Activation and functions of the complement system with the main effects of the individual complement factors B, C1–C9 and D.
MBP = Mannose-binding protein,
P = Properdin.

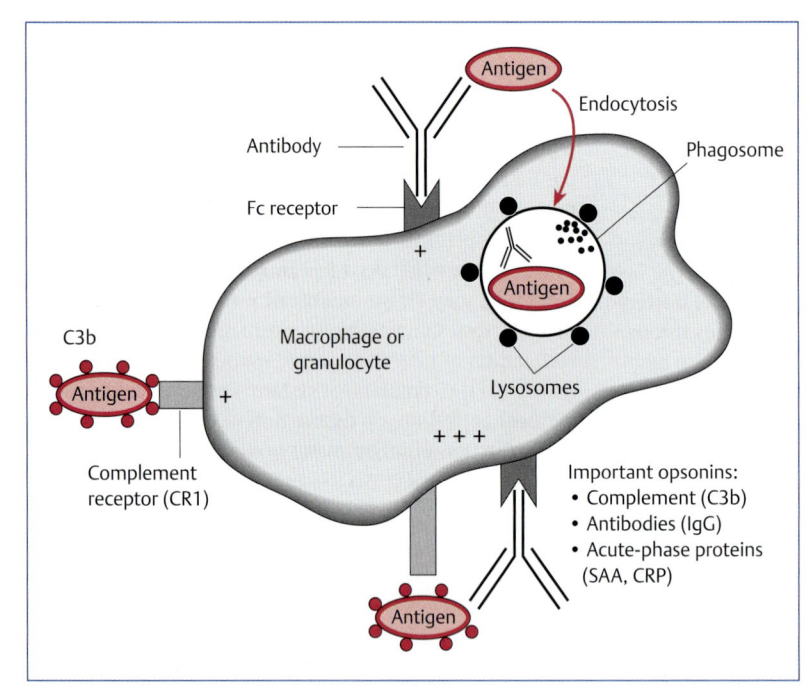

Fig. 10.5 Mechanism of opsonisation and phagocytosis.
" + " (weak) and " + + + " ("strong") indicate the strength of opsonisation by complement, antibody or combinations of both.
CRP = C-reactive protein, SAA = serum amyloid A.

region of inflammation (**chemotaxis**). C3a binds to mast cells, which then release histamine and thus increase vascular permeability.

IN A NUTSHELL   !

The main functions of the complement system are opsonisation, chemotaxis and cell lysis.

10.3.4 Opsonisation and phagocytosis

After bacteria or fungi have invaded the body, they can more effectively be attacked by **phagocytes** if they have been marked as "foreign" by attachment of various proteins to the microbial surface (**opsonisation**). Although there are different types of opsonisation, the basic princi-

ple is always the same. Proteins, known as **opsonins**, attach themselves to the surface of microbes. **Phagocytic cells** recognise these opsonised microbes via membrane receptors and are thereby stimulated to **phagocytose** (Fig. 10.5).

Antibodies and the complement fragment **C3b** are the most important factors for opsonisation. Phagocytes have receptors that are specific for C3b (**complement receptors**, e.g. **CR1**) or the Fc part of an antibody (Fc receptors (p.252)). After antibodies bind to the microbial surface, complement is then added through the classical pathway of complement activation. This combined opsonisation of antibody and C3b is the most powerful stimulus for phagocytosis by macrophages and granulocytes. Other serum proteins such as C-reactive protein (CRP) can also opsonise pathogens.

After opsonisation and recognition by phagocytic cells, phagocytosis then follows, so that bacteria, cell debris or foreign objects are taken up into a vacuole known as a **phagosome**. The fusion of the phagosome with the cell's **lysosomes**, forms the so-called **phagolysosome**, where phagocytised particles are degraded by constituents of the lysosomes (lysozyme, defensins, neutral proteases, acid hydrolases and others).

> **MORE DETAILS** Opsonisation is also responsible for removal of immune complexes from blood. When antibodies bind soluble antigen, this creates immune complexes that must be removed from blood. Binding of antibodies triggers the complement cascade and C3b binds to the immune complexes. Erythrocytes carry specific complement receptors that recognise and bind these immune complexes marked by complement and transport them to the spleen. There, macrophages phagocytose the immune complexes from the surface of erythrocytes without destroying the erythrocytes.

> **IN A NUTSHELL** !
>
> Opsonisation by antibodies and complement factors facilitates phagocytosis.

10.3.5 Recognition of pathogens by toll-like receptors

The most important defence cells of innate immunity are **granulocytes**, **macrophages** and **dendritic cells**. They are all activated by contact with pathogens. To recognise pathogens, these cells are equipped with various receptors on their cell surface or in cytoplasm. Some of these receptors recognise opsonins on the surface of pathogens, as described earlier. For example, complement receptor 1 (CR1) on granulocytes binds to complement fragment C3b on bacterial membranes and thus activates phagocytosis.

In addition to these receptors for opsonins, there is another large group of receptors, the so-called **toll-like receptors (TLR)**. These TLRs are highly conserved in animals and can even be detected in plants. They play a central role in the recognition of pathogens. So far, more than ten different TLR have been described (**Table 10.2**). Each of these TLRs binds a specific molecular pattern, the so-called **pathogen-associated molecular patterns**, that only occurs on pathogens, and not on the animal's own cells. These molecular patterns are structures that usually occur on entire groups of pathogens and also represent vital structural molecules that cannot be changed by mutation. For example, a lipopolysaccharide is an essential component of all Gram-negative bacteria. It is not found on eukaryotic cells. This lipopolysaccharide is recognised by TLR4. Other TLRs bind peptidoglycans, bacterial DNA or viral double-stranded RNA.

Table 10.2 Examples of Toll-like receptors and ligands.

TLR	Detected structure	Microorganism
TLR2	Peptidoglycan	Bacteria
TLR4	Lipopolysaccharide	
TLR5	Flagellin	
TLR9	Bacterial DNA	
TLR2/6	Zymosan	Fungi
TLR3	Double stranded RNA	Viruses
TLR7, TLR8	Single stranded RNA	

> **IN A NUTSHELL** !
>
> TLRs on phagocytes bind structures on pathogens and thus activate cells of the innate immune system.

10.3.6 Effector functions of cells of the innate immune system

The binding of TLRs to pathogens leads to the activation of effector functions in cells of the innate immune system. Depending on cell type, different defence responses are triggered. Particularly important mechanisms for elimination of pathogens are phagocytosis, **cytokine secretion**, release of toxic substances, and alerting of the acquired immune system.

The main function of **granulocytes** is **phagocytosis**. Granulocytes are also capable of producing toxic **reactive oxygen species**. Within seconds after microorganisms bind to the cell membrane of granulocytes, several enzymes are activated: NADPH oxidase, superoxide dismutase, myeloperoxidase, which form superoxide (O_2^-), H_2O_2 and OCl^- ("**respiratory burst**"). **Neutrophil granulocytes** are very short-lived. They usually die directly after phagocytosis at the site of infection. In contrast to neutrophil granulocytes, eosinophil and basophil granulocytes are only found in small numbers in the blood. **Eosinophil granulocytes** are mainly involved in defence against parasites, and they play a role in allergies. Eosinophilia therefore often indicates parasitoses or allergies. **Basophil granulocytes** and a related cell type, the **mast cells**, are found underneath epithelia and are involved in inflammatory reactions (p. 250) by releasing soluble mediators, especially histamine.

Monocytes leave blood after a short time and – depending on the tissue – differentiate into various cell types, especially into tissue macrophages. After recognising pathogens, phagocytosis is started and macrophages secrete a variety of cytokines that initiate an inflammatory response (p. 250). However, macrophages also engulf the body's own cells that are produced during normal cell renewal, or as a result of tissue damage. Since the body's own cells do not activate the TLR, cytokines are not released, and the immune system is not alerted. Thus, there is no inflammatory response.

Dendritic cells differentiate from either myeloid or lymphoid progenitor cells (**Fig. 10.2**). They have a characteristic morphology with numerous membrane protrusions. In skin, they are called Langerhans cells. Dendritic cells are located directly under epithelia of external and internal body surfaces. They are therefore the first cells to come into contact with pathogens during an infection. Thus, they represent a kind of **guard** and an **alarm part** of the immune system. After recognition and phagocytosis of pathogens, dendritic cells produce cytokines. Subsequently, they migrate to regional lymph nodes. There they meet lymphocytes and play an essential role in the activation and further maturation of lymphocytes.

> **IN A NUTSHELL** !
>
> Granulocytes, macrophages and dendritic cells eliminate pathogens and alert the immune system.

10.3.7 Inflammatory response

MORE DETAILS If microorganisms succeed in overcoming the mechanical and chemical barriers at the body's surfaces, they penetrate into tissues. There, they encounter resident **macrophages**, **mast cells**, and **dendritic cells**. These cells recognise microorganisms with the help of their TLR, or after opsonisation (p. 248) of the microorganisms. Their response consists in the secretion of numerous soluble **inflammatory mediators**. Among them are vasodilatory substances such as **histamine, prostaglandins, leukotrienes** and numerous chemical messengers that trigger pain (**bradykinin, serotonin, prostaglandins**). As a result of vasodilation, hyperaemia occurs and plasma components leak into the tissue. Complement components thus reach the site of infection, opsonise microorganisms and increase phagocytosis.

New inflammatory cells (granulocytes and macrophages) are attracted from blood into the tissue by cleavage products of complement factors (C3a, C4a, C5a) and by **chemokines** (chemotactic cytokines) such as **interleukin-8 (chemotaxis)**. The prerequisite for this is not only the presence of a chemotactic gradient but also an **activation** of the **endothelium**. One of the most potent activators is **tumour necrosis factor α (TNF-α)** which is released by activated macrophages. TNF-α causes formation of new **adhesion molecules** on the endothelium. This allows gran-

ulocytes and monocytes to adhere to the endothelium and to migrate between the endothelial cells into the tissue (**diapedesis**). As a result of this cell migration from blood into tissue, large numbers of granulocytes are lost from blood and are replaced by new, juvenile cells from bone marrow. These have a characteristic non-lobed nucleus. The increased number of such band cells is called a **leftward shift**. It is important diagnostically as an indicator of bacterial infection.

The processes described all aim to eliminate microorganisms, but they also cause the classic **signs** of **inflammation**: redness, warmth, pain, swelling and loss of function.

In severe bacteria-induced inflammation, there is massive activation of macrophages and subsequent formation of large quantities of **cytokines**, that also become systemically active (Fig. 10.6). **IL-1, IL-6** and **TNF-α** induce fever (p. 508) in thermoregulatory centres of the hypothalamus. The increase in body temperature slows down bacterial growth. These cytokines also trigger a reaction in brain known as "**sickness behaviour**". It is characterised by symptoms such as **loss of appetite** (inappetence), **tiredness** (somnolence), dizziness and other symptoms. IL-6 also initiates the **acute-phase response** with increased synthesis of many proteins in the liver, including complement factors, coagulation factors and two proteins with opsonising properties: **C-reactive protein** (CRP) and **serum amyloid A** (SAA). Increases in the concentrations of acute-phase proteins are very effective at limiting inflammation and eliminating microorganisms.

The various proinflammatory reactions can be suppressed by several anti-inflammatory mechanisms. For example, IL-1 in the hypothalamus stimulates the release of CRH, which in the anterior pituitary stimulates synthesis of αMSH and ACTH from proopiomelanocortin. Glucocorticoids released from the adrenal gland after ACTH stimulation as well as αMSH inhibit cytokine secretion from macrophages. Stimulation of efferent fibres of the autonomic nervous system by cytokines and inflammatory mediators leads to the release of acetylcholine and catecholamines in the site of inflammation. This has an inhibitory effect on cytokine secretion via nicotinic and β adrenergic receptors (p. 116).

> **IN A NUTSHELL** !
>
> Cytokines induce endothelial cell changes and an inflammatory response.

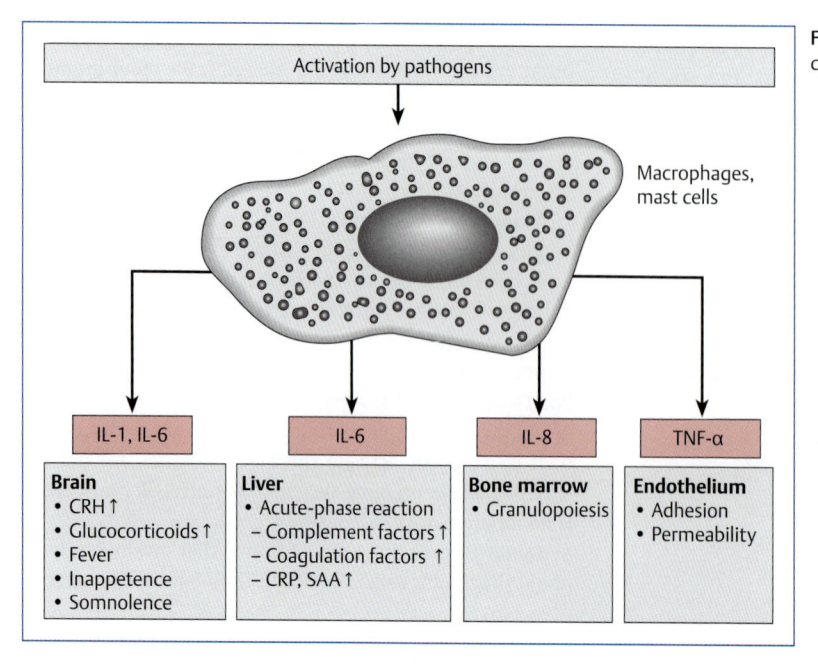

Fig. 10.6 Effect of proinflammatory cytokines.

Activation by pathogens

Macrophages, mast cells

IL-1, IL-6	IL-6	IL-8	TNF-α
Brain • CRH ↑ • Glucocorticoids ↑ • Fever • Inappetence • Somnolence	**Liver** • Acute-phase reaction – Complement factors ↑ – Coagulation factors ↑ – CRP, SAA ↑	**Bone marrow** • Granulopoiesis	**Endothelium** • Adhesion • Permeability

10.4 Acquired immune mechanisms

10.4.1 Features of acquired immune mechanisms

The cells responsible for the acquired immune response are **lymphocytes**. These cells have receptors which recognise antigens. These **antigen receptors** are highly variable, in contrast to TLRs on the cells of the innate immune system (**Fig. 10.7**). This means that each lymphocyte can recognise an **individual antigen** from its specific molecular structure. This antigen specificity is determined individually for each cell during maturation of lymphocytes. Since each lymphocyte has a different specificity, a very large number of structures can be recognised overall. However, this also means that the frequency of lymphocytes that are specific for any particular antigen is very low (about 1 lymphocyte in 10000–100000 lymphocytes). In order to increase the probability that the few lymphocytes with a particular antigen specificity will interact with that antigen, lymphocyte activation occurs exclusively in the lymphoid organs. Lymph nodes thus represent a kind of meeting point for lymphocytes and antigens, in which optimal conditions for lymphocyte activation prevail.

When a lymphocyte comes into contact with the antigen matching its receptor, activation, multiplication, and maturation of that line of lymphocytes takes place in the **lymphoid organs (lymph nodes, spleen, etc.)**. Thus, there is a considerable increase in the number of lymphocytes specific for that particular antigen. In this process, not only are highly specific **effector cells** formed, but also long-lived

memory cells. These are immediately available in the event of renewed contact with the same antigen and very quickly render the infectious agent harmless, ideally even before a disease is triggered. This part of the immune system is called the **acquired** or **adaptive immune system**, since a small number of specific lymphocytes are only stimulated to divide, differentiate and form an immunological memory by contact with antigens. The adaptive immune system "learns" throughout life and constantly adapts to the environment. All **vaccinations** (active immunisations) are based on the principle of formation of memory cells. Another characteristic of acquired immunity is **maternal immune protection** mediated by antibodies that are transferred either during pregnancy via the placenta, or shortly after birth via colostrum (p. 604).

B lymphocytes are the cells finally responsible for the **humoral** adaptive **immune response**. After antigen stimulation, they form highly specific proteins, the so-called **immunoglobulins or antibodies**. Each class of antibodies has different functions, such as local immune protection, complement activation and neutralisation. The **T lymphocytes** are responsible for the **cell-mediated** adaptive **immune response**. There are different subpopulations of T lymphocytes called cytotoxic T lymphocytes, T helper lymphocytes and regulatory T lymphocytes, all of which have different functions.

> **IN A NUTSHELL**   !
>
> The cells responsible for the acquired immune response are the lymphocytes.

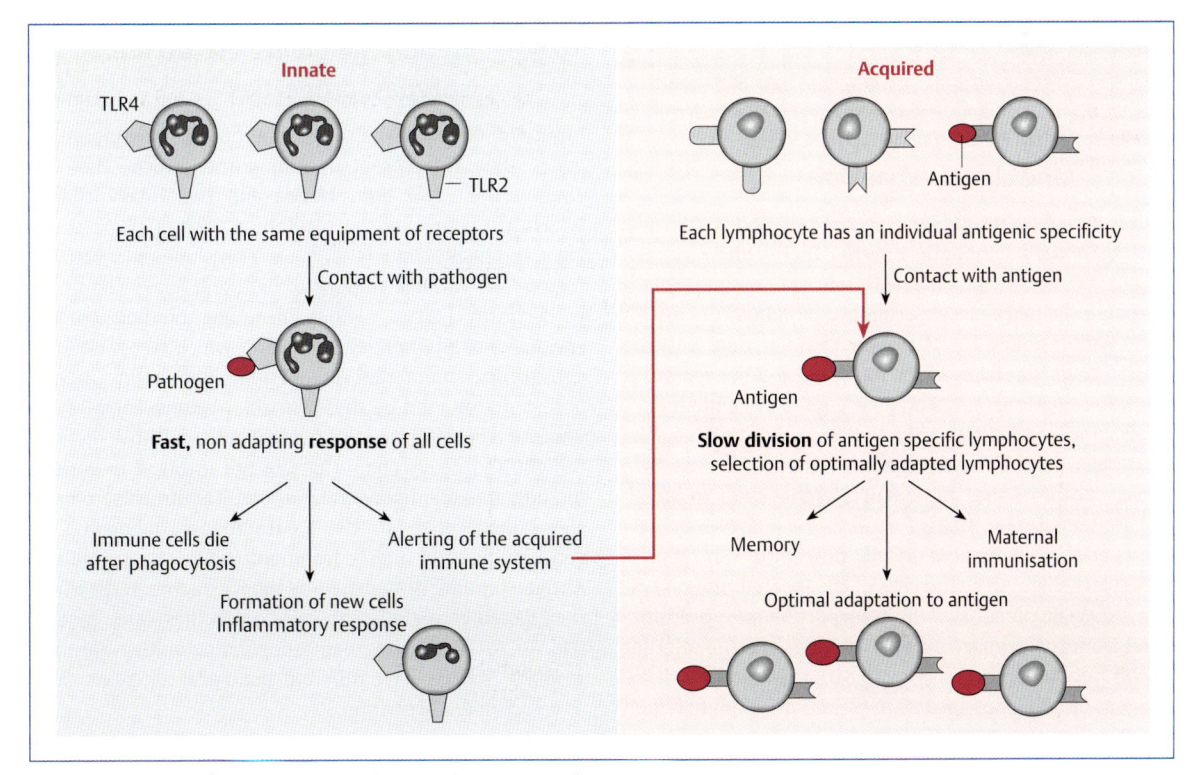

Fig. 10.7 Differences between innate and acquired immune mechanisms.

10.4.2 Formation and maturation of lymphocytes

Lymphoid stem cells mature into three different types of lymphocytes: **B lymphocytes** (B cells), **T lymphocytes** (T cells) and **natural killer cells** (NK cells) (**Fig. 10.2**). The precursors of the T cells (pre-T cells) reach the thymus in blood. B lymphocytes originate from pre-B cells. In humans and in mice, they mature in the bone marrow.

In sheep, cattle and rabbits, the lymphoid organs of the intestine are involved in lymphocyte maturation. These lymphoid organs are called **"gut-associated lymphoid tissue" (GALT)**. B cells of birds mature in the bursa of Fabricius, a protrusion of the proctadeal region of the cloaca. Early studies of **lymphocyte development** in birds gave the names of lymphocytes: **T** for **thymus-dependent** and **B** for **bursa of Fabricius-dependent** lymphocytes. Natural killer cells also develop from lymphoid stem cells.

Organs involved in the formation and development of lymphocytes are called **central** or **primary lymphoid organs**. These are **bone marrow**, **thymus** and, depending on the species, the **GALT**. In these organs, in addition to multiplication and maturation of lymphocytes, selection processes (p. 257) occur, so that ultimately only about 5–10 % of all cells are released into blood as mature lymphocytes. During **selection**, those lymphocytes that react with the body's own structures are eliminated by programmed cell death (**apoptosis**). This process is known as **central tolerance induction** or **negative selection**. In addition, non-functional lymphocytes (p. 250) are eliminated.

> **IN A NUTSHELL** !
>
> During maturation in thymus, bone marrow and GALT, autoreactive and non-functional lymphocytes are selectively eliminated.

10.4.3 Migration of lymphocytes and clonal expansion

Mature lymphocytes are transported in blood to (peripheral) **secondary lymphatic organs**. There, upon antigen contact, **activation** and **differentiation** of lymphocytes into **effector cells** takes place. Secondary lymphoid organs include **lymph nodes**, the **Waldeyer tonsillar ring** with the **tonsils**, **Peyer's patches** of the intestine, and the **spleen**. In addition to peripheral lymphoid organs, a large number of small lymphoid follicles are found in various tissues. The endothelial cells of these secondary lymphoid organs have special receptors that allow naive lymphocytes to attach and accumulate (**Fig. 10.8 a**).

In peripheral lymphoid organs, antigen concentration is particularly high, since the cells of the innate immune system, especially dendritic cells, transport phagocytised material from the primary inflamed regions, via the **afferent lymph** into lymph nodes (**Fig. 10.8 b**). In addition, soluble antigens or infectious agents are carried in lymph to lymph nodes, or are transported in blood to the spleen. Lymphocytes migrate through lymph nodes and are then trans-ported back into blood via the **efferent lymph**. From there, they can migrate again, at random, into any of the lymph nodes (**recirculation**; **Fig. 10.8 a**).

After a few days, lymphocytes die and are replaced by new ones. Thus, in peripheral lymphoid organs, antigens, inflammatory cells, and lymphocytes all congregate together. This creates an optimal milieu for **activation of lymphocytes**.

After successful binding with the specific antigen, **clonal expansion** of lymphocytes occurs in the lymph node. This means activation and proliferation of the antigen-specific cells. As a consequence, a large number of identical lymphocytes are formed (**Fig. 10.9**). These lymphocytes differentiate either into **effector cells** with different tasks, or into long-lived **memory cells** which are immediately available upon renewed contact with the same antigen. The effector cells of B lymphocytes are the **plasma cells** which secrete large quantities of soluble antibody molecules. T effector cells can generally be divided into **T helper cells**, **cytotoxic T cells** and **regulatory T cells**. These effector cells leave the lymph nodes after differentiation and migrate via blood directly to the site of infection, such as after a cut in the skin. The phenomenon that certain lymphocyte populations accumulate in certain organs is called **"homing"**. This behaviour is mediated by homing receptors on lymphocytes and cell adhesion molecules on the vascular endothelium.

> **IN A NUTSHELL** !
>
> Clonal expansion increases the population of antigen-specific lymphocytes, which subsequently develop into effector and memory cells.

10.4.4 Immunoglobulins – structure, isotypes, properties

Immunoglobulins are also called antibodies or **γ globulins**. When they are present in a monomeric form, they are composed of two **light chains** and two **heavy chains**, which are connected by disulphide bridges (**Fig. 10.10**). Light and heavy chains each have a constant and a variable region. The **variable regions** of light and heavy chains together form the two regions for antigen binding. Antigen specificity of B lymphocytes (p. 255), which recognise antigens through membrane-bound immunoglobulins (p. 249), is thus determined by these variable regions. Each B lymphocyte is specific for an individual antigen. Those sections in light and heavy chain that are not involved in antigen binding are called **constant regions**. The protease **papain** cleaves antibodies into two F_{ab} **fragments** (fragment antigen-binding) and one **Fc fragment** (fragment crystalline). Antigen binding is mediated by the F_{ab} fragments, in which the variable regions of the antibodies are located (**Fig. 10.10**). The Fc fragments, depending on the immunoglobulin isotype, have different biological functions, such as complement activation.

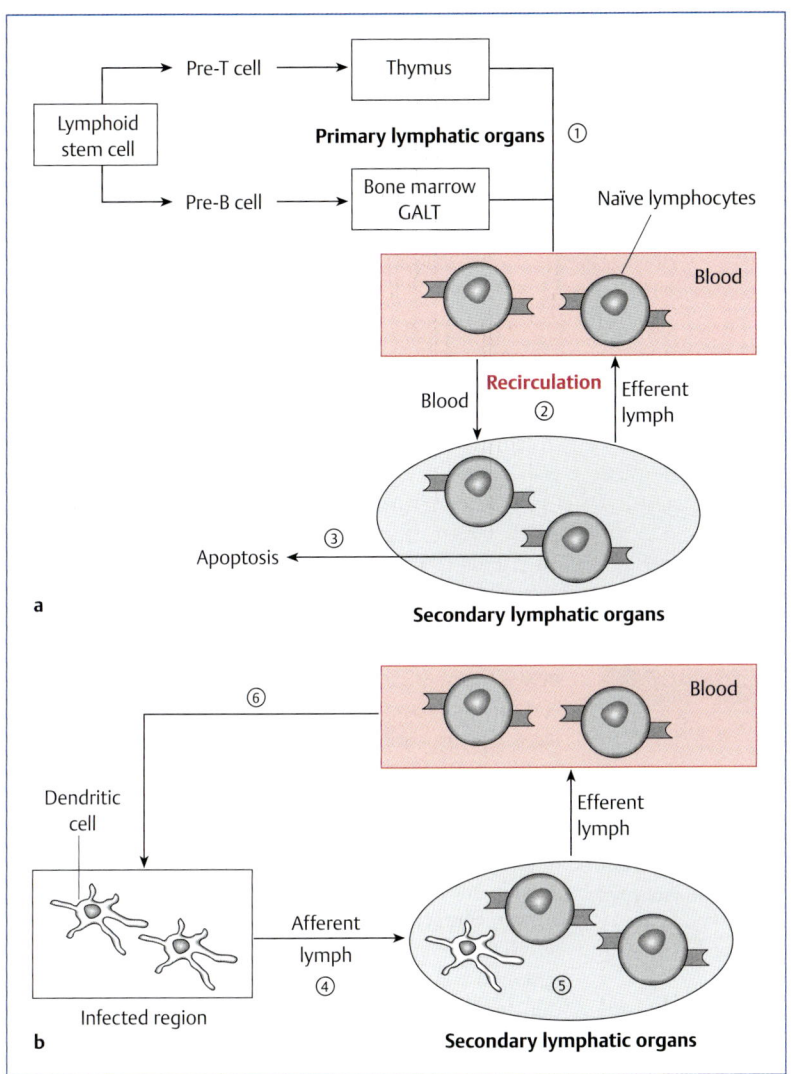

Fig. 10.8 Recirculation of lymphocytes.
a The different stages of lymphocyte maturation and migration are shown.
1: After differentiation in central lymphoid organs, mature but naïve lymphocytes are released into blood. **2:** Naive lymphocytes recirculate between blood and secondary lymphoid organs. **3:** If no activation occurs after 7–10 days of recirculation, lymphocytes die by apoptosis.
b Lymphocyte activation in secondary lymphoid tissues. **4:** Antigen from the site of infection is transported by dendritic cells via afferent lymph into the secondary lymphoid organs. **5:** Activation of specific lymphocytes occurs in these lymphoid organs. **6:** Activated lymphocytes then migrate via the blood directly to the site of infection.

Circulation, respiration

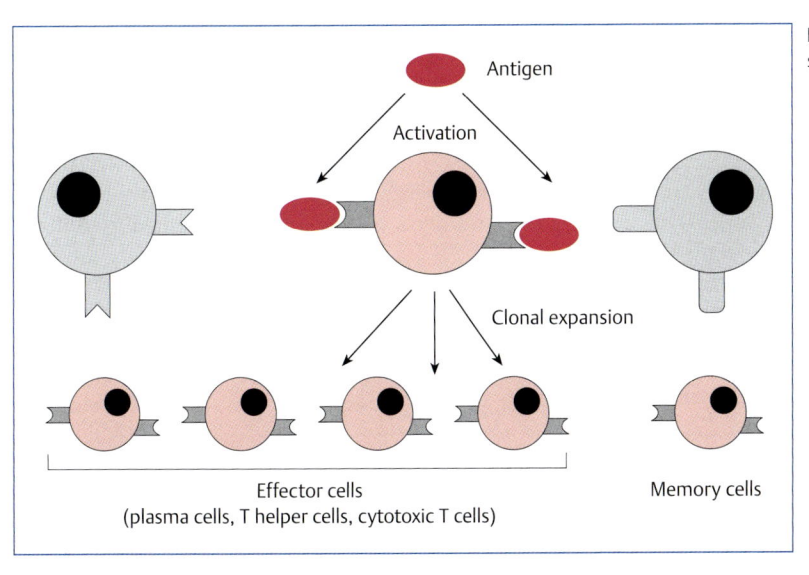

Fig. 10.9 Clonal expansion after antigen stimulation.

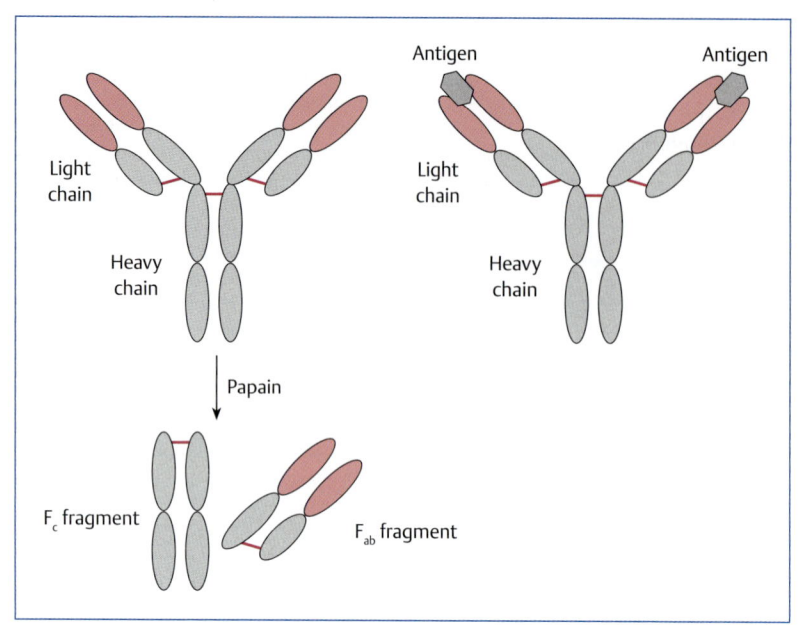

Fig. 10.10 Structure of an immunoglobulin molecule. The intermolecular disulphide bridges are marked by red lines. Individual domains of the Ig molecule are shown as ellipses. The variable domains are marked in red. The interaction of an antigen with the variable domains of light and heavy chains is shown on the right. After cleavage with the protease papain, Fc and F_{ab} fragments are formed.

IN A NUTSHELL   !

Antibodies have heavy and light chains with variable and constant domains.

A distinction is made between a total of five different forms of the constant regions. Depending on these five different constant regions, the five **immunoglobulin isotypes** IgM, IgG, IgA, IgE and IgD are distinguished (Table 10.3). **IgD** is only found in primates and rodents. Its function in domestic animals is largely unknown.

IgM is formed as the first antibody molecule after antigen contact. It is therefore also called the primary response antibody. IgM is present as a pentamer, i.e. five antibody molecules with a total of ten antigen binding sites are linked together. Antigen binding affinity of IgM is limited. IgM is mainly secreted into blood and onto mucosal surfaces. Certain antigens only induce formation of IgM antibodies, even after repeated contact. In most cases, these are sugar residues (e.g. blood group antigens of the ABO system (p.241). **IgG** represents a monomer that is localised in serum and tissue. It is the most important immunoglobulin in serum and is mainly formed after repeated antigen contact (**secondary response**). The binding affinity of IgG to the antigen is much higher compared to that of IgM. IgM and IgG are both important in **neutralisation**. In this process, they bind bacterial toxins or prevent viruses from attaching to receptors and thus prevent infection. IgM and IgG both activate the **classical pathway** of the **complement cascade**.

Table 10.3 Immunoglobulin isotypes.

Isotype	IgM	IgG	IgA	IgE
Structure				
Serum concentration $(mg \cdot ml^{-1})$	1	12	0.5	0.003
Complement activation	+++	++	+	–
Opsonisation	–	+++	+	–
Neutralisation	+	++	++	–
Mucosal protection	+	–	+++	–
Placenta transfer	–	+[1]	–	–
Colostrum	–	++[2]	+	–
Mast cell degranulation	–	–	–	+++

[1] Placental transfer only in primates, dogs, cats, rabbits, guinea pigs, depending on the form of placentation.
[2] Percentage of immunoglobulin isotypes in colostrum: 80% IgG and 10% each IgM and IgA.

IgA is the most important immunoglobulin on all **mucosal surfaces**. After its formation, two monomers are linked via a **J-chain** to form a **dimer**. IgA is actively transported through epithelial cells and is released at the luminal side of mucosal surfaces. In this process, IgA binds to **polymeric immunoglobulin receptors** on the basolateral side of epithelia. Part of the polymeric immunoglobulin receptor remains attached to the IgA molecule. This part is called the **secretory component**. It protects IgA from proteolytic degradation. IgA prevents pathogens from attaching to the epithelium in the intestine. Infectious agents that have already penetrated the epithelium are bound to IgA in the lamina propria of the intestine and transported back into the lumen.

IN A NUTSHELL !

IgM is formed in the primary immune response. IgG is the most important immunoglobulin of serum and tissue. IgA serves as immune protection on mucosal surfaces.

Many biological properties of antibodies are mediated by their binding to so-called **Fc receptors**. These receptors are specific for the Fc part of the antibody (e.g. FcγR for IgG). The Fc receptors are mainly located on cells of the innate immune system. There, they bind **antigen-antibody complexes** and thus induce cells to undergo phagocytosis (**Fig. 10.5**). Here, the interconnectedness of the innate immune system (macrophages, granulocytes and dendritic cells with Fc receptors) and the acquired immune system (formation of immunoglobulins that bind to Fc receptors) becomes very clear. The "non-specific" phagocytes thus receive individual antigen specificity from the acquired immune system via binding of highly specific antibodies to membrane-bound Fc receptors.

A special Fc receptor is the so-called **neonatal Fc receptor** (FcRn). It mediates **placental IgG transport** in primates and carnivores as well as transport of IgG from **colostrum** through the intestinal epithelium. The Fc receptor is formed on the epithelium for only a few hours to a few days postnatally. Therefore, the immediate intake of colostrum after birth is crucial for the immune protection of the new-born. The FcRn is also found on endothelial cells of blood vessels. There it binds serum IgG and leads to uptake of IgG into endothelial cells. In addition to binding to IgG, FcRn also binds to serum albumin. This constant uptake into endothelial cells and release back into blood or tissue greatly increases the half-life of IgG and albumin.

IN A NUTSHELL !

Fc receptors bind antigen-antibody complexes and activate cells of the innate immune system.

MORE DETAILS IgE is very important in the immune defence against multicellular pathogens (e.g. intestinal parasites). It is also significantly involved in the pathogenesis of type I allergy (immediate hypersensitivity). Sensitization occurs during the initial contact with allergens. In this phase, allergen-specific IgE antibodies are formed, which bind to Fcε receptors on eosinophil and basophil granulocytes and mast cells in tissue. After repeated allergen contact, IgE antibodies on the cell surface are cross-linked by the antigen. This results in cell activation and an explosive degranulation of intracellular granules. Chemical messengers released from granules (especially histamine) as well as prostaglandins and leukotrienes formed from arachidonic acid, cause, within seconds, the sometimes life-threatening symptoms such as conjunctivitis, oedema, hives, asthma or even shock.

While the pathogenesis is well studied, very little is known about the causes of allergy. Why do certain people and animals react to harmless environmental antigens with excessive IgE production? Certainly, allergy is a multifactorial disease in which both genetic predisposition and the environment play major roles. In recent decades, a steady increase in allergies in humans, and also in dogs and cats, has been observed in industrialised countries. In contrast, the incidence of allergies in developing countries is much lower. The so-called hygiene hypothesis is an attempt to explain this phenomenon: Because of excellent preventive medicine, young children in industrialised countries develop illnesses much less frequently than in developing countries. The immune system is clearly of great influence in early childhood. If viral or parasitic infectious diseases occur frequently at this stage of life, this strengthens **cell-mediated immunity**, while a low frequency of such diseases in this developmental phase promotes the tendency of the immune system to form **antibodies** and **IgE**.

IN A NUTSHELL !

IgE is involved in the defence against multicellular pathogens, and in the pathogenesis of allergic reactions.

10.4.5 Antigen-specific receptors of B and T lymphocytes

MORE DETAILS **B lymphocytes** use **membrane-bound** monomeric **immunoglobulin** of the IgM isotype, as antigen **receptors**, also known as the **B cell receptor (BCR)**. The antigen receptors on **T lymphocytes** are called **T cell receptors (TCR)** (**Fig. 10.11**). In contrast to the immunoglobulin molecule, TCR consists of only two proteins: the TCR α-chain and the TCR β-chain. These together form the αβ TCR on the surface of T lymphocytes. In addition, there is also so-called γδ TCR consisting of a γ- and a δ-chain. This γδ TCR is found on a subpopulation of T lymphocytes where the function is not known.

In addition to receptors for antigen recognition, lymphocytes need other molecules to transmit signals into the interior of a cell after antigen binding. In the case of TCR, these are various molecules known as the **CD3 complex**. The immunoglobulins on the membrane of B lymphocytes, on the other hand, are linked to the **Igα** and **Igβ** proteins. After antigen binding, there is a conformational change of the receptors and the associated proteins, which are then phosphorylated at cytoplasmic tyrosine residues. This phosphorylation triggers an intracellular cascade with subsequent activation of lymphocytes.

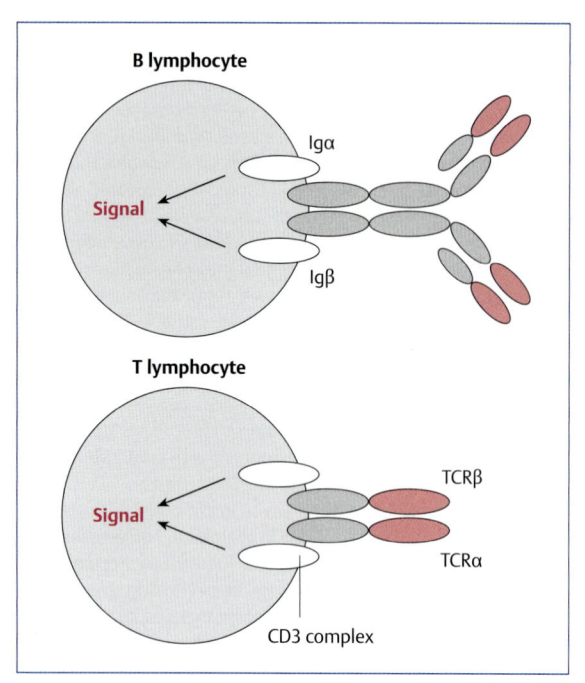

Fig. 10.11 Antigen receptors on B and T lymphocytes. The variable regions are marked in red, the constant regions in grey, the components for signal transmission in white.

10.4.6   Receptor diversity

Antigen recognition by the acquired immune system, in contrast to recognition of pathogenic patterns by the innate immune system, is much more flexible and covers an almost unlimited number of possible antigen specificities. In the innate immune system, there are only a limited number of different receptors. Each receptor in the innate immune system is encoded by a gene and is specific to a particular structure found only on pathogens. In the acquired immune system, there are only two basic structures of antigen receptors (T and B cell receptors), but these have a **variable part** that is newly formed during the development of lymphocytes and has its own **individual antigen specificity**. In total, several billion different Ig and TCR molecules are formed in each individual by a process known as **somatic recombination**.

> **MORE DETAILS** In somatic recombination, the Ig and TCR genes are assembled from small **gene segments** to form a complete gene (**Fig. 10.12**). The variable region of the **light chain** of an immunoglobulin molecule is encoded by **V segments** (V = variable) and **J segments** (J = joining), while the constant region is

transcribed by the **C segment** (C = constant). In the genome, 10 to more than 200 different V and J segments are located in sequence on a chromosome, depending on species. In each lymphocyte, one of each segment is randomly selected from many V and J segments during maturation. This results in an enormous **combinatorial diversity** of antigen receptors. At the junctions of the gene segments, additional deletions or nucleotide insertions occur, so that variability is further increased at junctions.

The composition of the genes for the **heavy chain** is similar, except that here the variable part is encoded not only by V and J segments, but by an additional gene segment called **D segment** (diversity). Since the **antigen binding site** is formed jointly by variable regions of the heavy and light chains, a further increase in variability occurs when the two randomly formed chains are combined. The **TCR repertoire** is formed by the same mechanisms, the TCR α-chain behaves analogous to the Ig light chain and the TCR β-chain corresponds to the Ig heavy chain. Somatic recombination only occurs during maturation of lymphocytes in primary lymphoid organs, after which each lymphocyte has its individual antigen specificity.

In contrast to the high number of different gene segments encoding the variable part of the antigen receptors, there are only a small number of **C segments**. In T lymphocytes, four TCR α, β, γ and δ C segments encode the corresponding TCR chains. In the immunoglobulin gene locus, there are five C segments designated as μ, δ, γ, ε, α, which represent the corresponding **immunoglobulin isotypes IgM, IgD, IgG, IgE and IgA**. The rearranged V(-D-)-J segment is joined to a C segment by RNA splicing during transcription (**Fig. 10.12**).

In addition to the five heavy chains of immunoglobulins, there are also two types of **light chains** called λ and κ, both of which can associate with all heavy chains. There are thus two possible combinations per heavy chain, for example IgG with κ or λ type light chains. However, there are considerable differences between animal species in the frequency of each light chain. Thus, cattle, horses, dogs and cats predominantly use λ chains, whereas humans, mice and rats mainly use κ chains. The relevance of these differences is unknown.

Because of this modular structure of the Ig molecule, biological properties can vary while the antigen specificity remains the same, by exchanging the constant region (**Fig. 10.12**). When B lymphocytes first come into contact with antigens, IgM antibodies are always formed (**primary immune response**). After repeated contact with antigens, there is a so-called **immunoglobulin class switch** from IgM to one of the other isotypes (**secondary immune response**). This occurs in specialised lymph follicles, called germinal centres, within lymph nodes. Direct cell contact is necessary between T helper cells, dendritic cells and B lymphocytes. Under the influence of various cytokines secreted by these cells, immunoglobulin class switch occurs. At the same time, in **germinal centres**, **somatic hypermutation** takes place, in which the variable region of the immunoglobulin molecule undergoes further mutation. Thus, antibodies with a higher affinity for the antigen are selected. These reactions in germinal centres thus lead to formation of **high affinity antibodies** of the IgG, IgA or IgE isotypes.

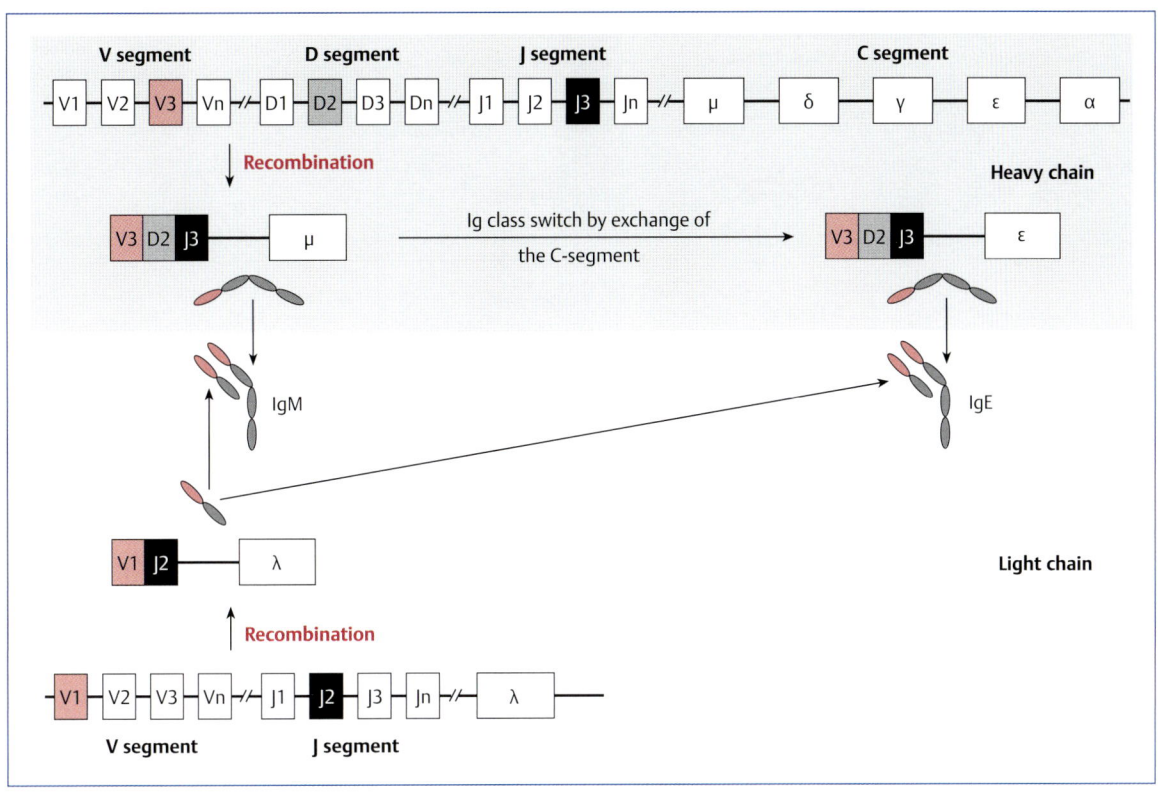

Fig. 10.12 Somatic recombination and Ig class switch. Different gene fragments are indicated by boxes. The gene locus for the heavy chain is highlighted in grey, and that for the light chain is shown below. The left half shows formation of an IgM isotype, the right half an IgE isotype after Ig class switch. In each B lymphocyte, an individual specificity is established by a new combination of fragments. Explanations are given in the text.

10.4.7 MHC proteins and selection in the thymus

In contrast to B lymphocytes, **T lymphocytes** do not recognise soluble antigens with their TCR, but instead recognise only small **peptide fragments** that are bound to so-called **MHC** (major histocompatibility complex) proteins. MHC proteins are membrane-bound proteins. They are composed of two polypeptide chains, with a groove on the surface where short peptides (i.e. potential antigens) are bound. Another special feature of MHC molecules is their great **polymorphic diversity**. This **polymorphism** is achieved by MHC molecules being encoded by different genes and each of these genes has many different **alleles** in the population.

> **MORE DETAILS**   In humans, there are three genes for MHC I, each with many alleles. Since the MHC proteins are transcribed equally from both chromosomes (codominant), six different versions are produced (two different alleles of the three genes). The MHC proteins are the main factors that lead to rejection of tissue or organ transplants. Therefore, for successful transplantation, it is necessary to find donors and recipients with similar or identical MHC alleles of the three genes.

In **thymus**, T lymphocytes with a TCR of only low binding affinity to the body's own MHC proteins, are weakly activated. This activation leads to final maturation of T lymphocytes (**positive selection**). T lymphocytes that do not bind at all to the body's own MHC proteins are eliminated

in the thymus. In the process of **negative selection**, T lymphocytes that are too strongly activated after binding to MHC proteins, and would therefore be **autoreactive**, are finally eliminated (**Fig. 10.13**).

> **MORE DETAILS**   In some autoimmune diseases, this selection of autoreactive cells in the thymus does not function correctly. Therefore, T lymphocytes directed against the body's own antigens are released into blood and are activated by self-antigens. Severe chronic inflammatory reaction and massive tissue damage often follow. Up to now, these diseases can only be treated by strong immunosuppression, for example with glucocorticoids.

There are two classes of MHC, known as **MHC I** and **MHC II**. Each of them activates different T lymphocyte subpopulations. These different T lymphocytes can be phenotypically differentiated by additional surface proteins. T lymphocytes that express **CD4 protein** on their surface are called **T helper cells**. They bind to MHC II proteins. In addition, there are T cells that are characterised by **CD8 antigen**. They bind to MHC I proteins and have a **cytotoxic function**. CD4 and CD8 proteins do not occur together on T cells, which means that most T cells can be classified as either CD4+ or CD8+ T cells.

> **IN A NUTSHELL**   !
>
> MHC molecules present peptides on the cell surface. Thereby they can stimulate T lymphocytes.

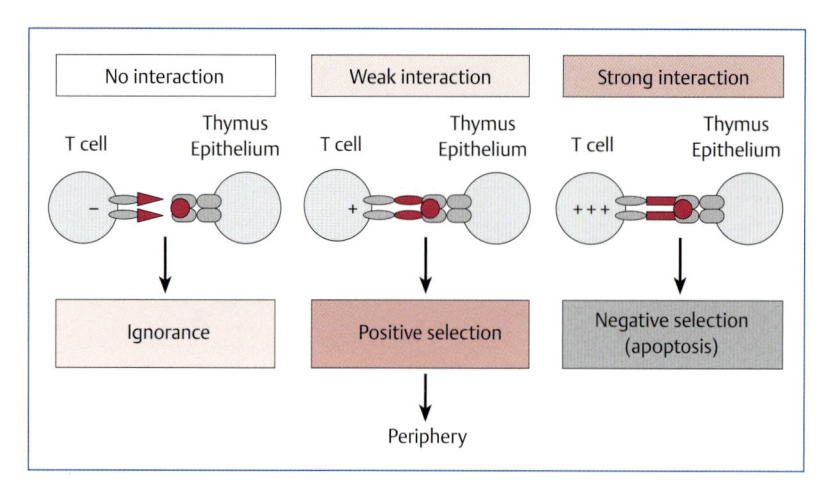

Fig. 10.13 Thymus selection. The strength of the TCR signal ("-" to "+++") influences whether cells are eliminated in the absence of function or due to selection.

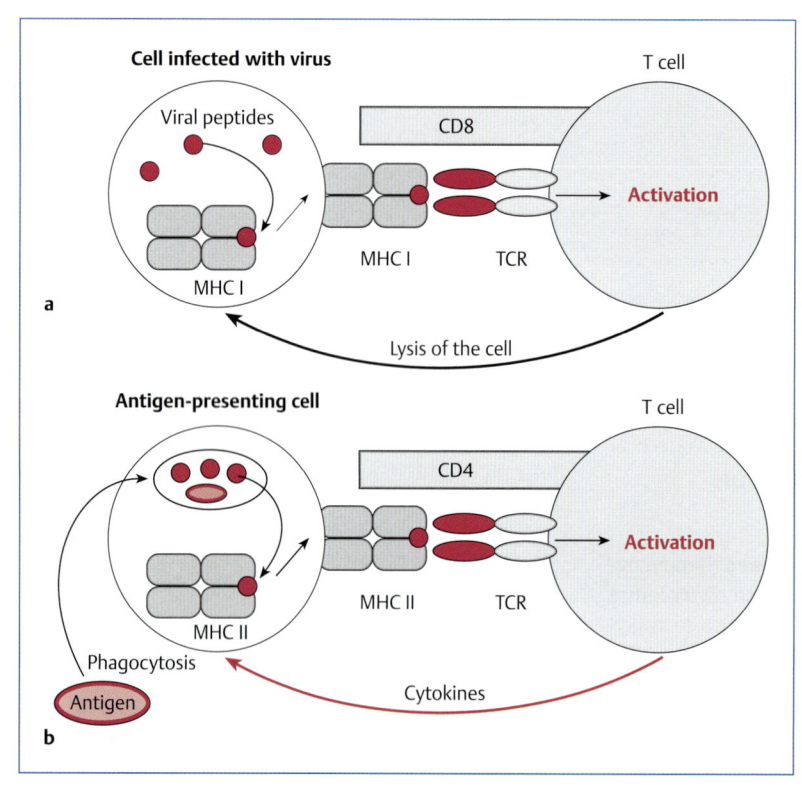

Fig. 10.14 Function of cytotoxic and T helper cells.
a Cytotoxic T cells destroy target cells after activation by the peptide-MHC I complex.
b Interaction between a T helper cell and an antigen-presenting cell, which, after activation, produces cytokines for further activation of the immune system.

10.4.8   MHC I proteins and cytotoxic T cell response

MHC I proteins are found on all **nucleated cells**. In normal cell metabolism, there is constant intracellular degradation of cellular proteins by an enzyme complex known as a **proteasome**. Proteolytic digestion of proteins produces short peptide fragments that are transported into the lumen of the endoplasmic reticulum where they bind into the **groove of MHC I molecules**. Normal body cells thus carry MHC I proteins with peptides from the body's own proteins. However, if a viral infection occurs so that viral proteins are being produced in cells, **viral peptide fragments** are also bound to MHC I proteins and presented on the cell surface. This identifies virus-infected cells for the immune system. **CD8⁺ T lymphocytes** permanently scan MHC mol-

ecules on the surfaces of cells with their TCR. They are activated by MHC molecules with foreign peptides and lyse those cells presenting foreign peptides (**Fig. 10.14 a**). Again, primary activation of cytotoxic lymphocytes occurs in lymphoid organs after virally infected cells have been transported there, or after **dendritic cells** have migrated into lymphoid tissue, for example, after a viral infection. After **activation** and **clonal expansion** in lymph nodes, lymphocytes migrate directly into the region of infection to destroy all virally infected cells, such as epithelial cells.

MORE DETAILS   Many viruses have developed mechanisms to escape this destruction by the host immune system. In particular, synthesis of MHC I molecules can be suppressed by various viral proteins. If MHC I molecules are no longer expressed in the cell surface, cytotoxic T lymphocytes are also no longer activated. Thus, viral infection can spread unhindered. This immunity gap is closed by other cells, the **natural killer** (NK) cells. The NK cells are specialised in recognising and destroying MHC I negative cells. In addition, NK cells are highly activated for cytolysis by proteins on the cell surface that are only produced by stress reactions such as infection or tumour degeneration. The mechanisms used by cytotoxic T lymphocytes and NK cells to destroy target cells are identical. They release the contents of **granules** with cytolytic substances such as **perforin**. They also can induce **apoptosis** in the target cells via direct cell-cell interaction.

> **IN A NUTSHELL**   **!**
>
> CD8$^+$ cytotoxic T lymphocytes lyse virus-infected cells.

10.4.9 MHC II proteins and CD4$^+$ T helper cells

CD4$^+$ T lymphocytes bind with their TCR to an **MHC II protein**. MHC II proteins are found on specialised cells such as **macrophages, dendritic cells** and **B lymphocytes**. These cell types are therefore referred to as **antigen-presenting cells** (Fig. 10.14b). In contrast to MHC I proteins, MHC II proteins bind only those peptides that are incorporated into cells from the extracellular space by phagocytosis or **endocytosis**. Shortly after MHC II synthesis, the peptide binding site is blocked in the endoplasmic reticulum and MHC II molecules with an empty peptide binding site are stored intracellularly in vesicles. After phagocytosis or endocytosis of antigens, these vesicles fuse with **phagolysosomes** and there bind peptide fragments that originate from the degradation of antigens. The peptide-loaded MHC II molecules are then transported to the surface of cells and there stimulate the **CD4$^+$ T lymphocytes**.

In order for CD4$^+$ T cells to be fully activated and to mature into specialised helper cells, they require further signals, especially those mediated by **cytokines**. Depending on their differentiation, T helper cells can be divided into different subpopulations, such as type 1 helper T cells and type 2 helper T cells. After stimulation e.g. by microorganisms, macrophages and dendritic cells produce **IL-12**, which stimulates CD4$^+$ T lymphocytes to differentiate into **type 1 helper T cells** (Th1). These type 1 T helper cells mainly produce **interferon-γ** (IFN-γ; Fig. 10.15). Interferon-γ is a cytokine that activates macrophages as well as CD8$^+$ T lymphocytes and NK cells and thus strongly stimulates **cell-mediated defence mechanisms** against **intracellular pathogens**.

In contrast, endocytosis of antigens after binding by antibodies on B lymphocytes leads to stimulation of so-called **type 2 T helper cells** (Th2). These type 2 T helper cells secrete the cytokines **IL-4** and **IL-13**, among others, and in turn stimulate B lymphocytes to differentiate into **plasma cells** and to secrete **antibodies**. The **humoral immune response** is thus important in the fight against extracellular pathogens. In recent years, additional T cell subpopulations have been identified based on their specific cytokine secretion. For example, Th17 cells produce IL-17, which is important in fungal infections, and regulatory T cells (Treg) secrete the immunosuppressive IL-10.

> **MORE DETAILS** In some autoimmune diseases the ratio between Th1 and Th2 cells seems to be disturbed. In autoimmune diseases, such as pemphigus vulgaris, which are triggered by autoreactive antibodies, an excessive Th2 reaction is observed. This favours the formation of antibodies. In allergy of the immediate hypersensitivity type, the Th2 reaction and thus the formation of IgE antibodies also predominate. Conversely, dominant Th1 reactions are found in cell-mediated autoimmune diseases, for example autoimmune mediated thyroiditis.

> **IN A NUTSHELL**   **!**
>
> CD4$^+$ T helper cells produce cytokines and modulate the immune response.

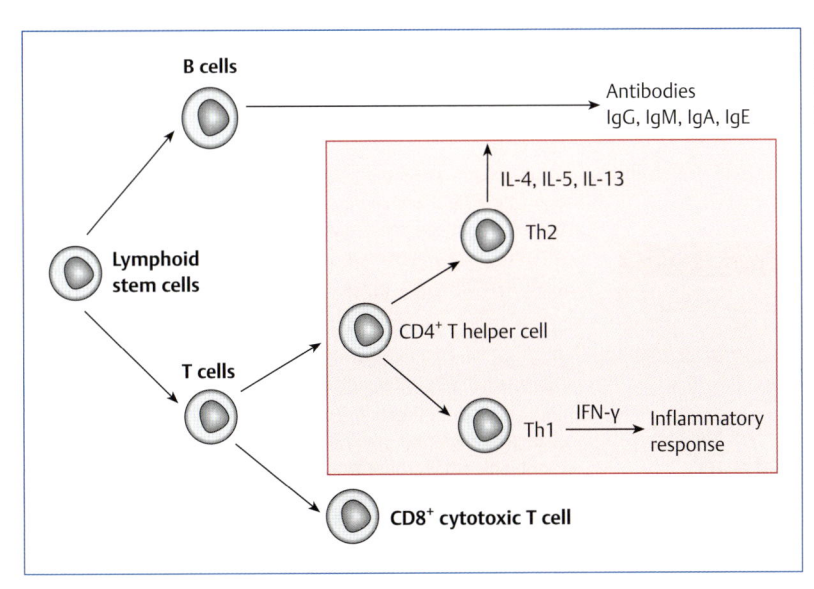

Fig. 10.15 Th1 and Th2 function. The central function of the CD4$^+$ T helper cells in the regulation of the immune response is highlighted in red.

Table 10.4 Important cytokines.

Cytokine	Production by:	Main effect
IL-1	Macrophages	Fever
IL-6	Macrophages	Acute-phase reaction
TNF-α	Macrophages	Endothelial changes
IL-8	Macrophages a. o.	Chemotaxis
IL-2	T cells	Proliferation
IL-12	Macrophages	Activation of macrophages and Th1 cells
IFN-γ	Th1 cells, NK cells	Macrophage activation
IL-4	Th2 cells	Humoral immunity
IL-13	Th2 cells	Humoral immunity
IL-10	Th2 cells, regulatory T cells	Immunosuppression
TGF-β	Regulatory T cells	Immunosuppression
Type I interferons (IFN-α/-β)	Every body cell	Antiviral

10.4.10   Immune regulation

The **activation** or **inhibition of immune responses** is mediated either by direct contact between different cells or by **cytokines**. In addition to the proteins described so far, involved in cellular contacts, such as the interaction between MHC peptide complexes with TCR, there are numerous other activating or inhibiting receptor-ligand systems that influence immune responses. During activation of T lymphocytes, the signal via the TCR is not sufficient for full activation. Clonal expansion and differentiation is only made possible by additional **co-stimulatory signals** such as the **CD28 protein** on T lymphocytes that binds to a protein known as **B-7** on dendritic cells. These additional requirements for lymphocyte activation prevent stimulation of **autoreactive cells**, which, despite **tolerance**, reach the periphery of the body in small amounts. In addition to these activating co-stimulatory proteins, there are a large number of inhibitory receptor-ligand systems that regulate maturation and function of lymphocytes. Also, so-called **regulatory T lymphocytes** are specialised in preventing **autoreactivity** via direct cell contacts and in particular via **immunosuppressive cytokines** such as **IL-10** and **transforming growth factor-β** (TGF-β).

Table 10.4 gives an overview of some cytokines and their main effects.

> **IN A NUTSHELL**   !
>
> The immune response is regulated by numerous soluble factors and receptor-ligand systems.

10.5   Innate and acquired immune mechanisms cooperate in immune defence

MORE DETAILS   After reviewing individual defence mechanisms, the close interconnection of the individual immune components in the **immune response** will be briefly illustrated using the example of **infections**.

The first stage of an infection is always overcoming of natural barriers by the pathogen. When pathogens enter a tissue, they encounter guardian cells of the innate immune system, especially macrophages, mast cells and dendritic cells. This first contact between the pathogen and the innate immune system is essential and initiates the subsequent immune response. There are numerous variables in this step, particularly the pathogen species, the multiplication strategy of the pathogen (intracellular, extracellular), the cell type of the immune system that has contact with the pathogen, and the type of molecular patterns on the pathogen that bind certain TLRs of animal cells. All these variables ultimately influence the expression of a wide variety of co-stimulatory proteins on cells, and the secretion of different cytokines. Thus, at the site of infection, very specific subpopulations of antigen-presenting cells are generated, which then activate individual lymphocyte subpopulations after migrating to regional lymph nodes. In other words, cells of the innate immune system are modified by their initial contact with the pathogen. They pass this information on to lymphocytes in lymph nodes by means of the changes in receptor and cytokine profile induced by pathogen contact.

In the entry ports of pathogens, cytokines trigger an inflammatory response, which leads to supply of blood with complement factors and various opsonins, via changes in the local vascular endothelia. These changes in the endothelium, together with the release of chemokines, lead to accumulation of more inflammatory cells.

This creates increased physical pressure in the region of infection (more fluid and more cells), which in turn promotes migration of stimulated cells via afferent lymph vessels to the regional lymph node. Pathogens are also carried away in lymph and then enter a lymph node, where activated antigen-presenting cells migrate to specialised regions that contain many lymphocytes. This concentration of antigen-presenting cells as well as native lymphocytes in a tiny region of the lymph node, allows very small numbers of antigen-specific lymphocytes to find their matching antigen. If this "meeting point lymph node" did not exist, the chance of a lymphocyte finding its "matching antigen" would be vanishingly small. Those lymphocytes that are specific for respective antigens divide and differentiate into effector and memory cells. In infections with extracellular pathogens, mainly type 2 T helper cells and B lymphocytes are activated in the lymph node. This leads to the production of highly specific antibodies, which reach the site of infection in blood. There, antibodies promote phagocytosis and neutralise the pathogens.

In infections with intracellular pathogens, such as viruses, cell lysis first occurs at the site of infection during virus replication. These dead cells are in turn taken up by phagocytes, which then migrate to regional lymph nodes. In addition, dendritic cells can be infected by a variety of different viruses and migrate to regional lymph nodes after infection. Intracellular infections and presentation in MHC I proteins is the main activation stimulus for type 1 T helper cells and cytotoxic T cells. Cytotoxic T cells migrate via efferent lymphatic vessels back into blood and from there directly to the site of infection, where they destroy infected cells.

When lymphocytes multiply in the lymph node, a small number of memory cells are always produced, in addition to effector cells. These memory cells have the same antigen specificity as the effector cells, i.e. they recognise an antigen that has previously entered the body. Memory cells of the B lymphocyte type are long-lived plasma cells that settle in bone marrow and continuously secrete small quantities of antibodies into blood. Memory cells of the T lymphocyte type remain in lymph nodes or at the site of entry of an infection. If there were to be a renewed contact with the same infectious agent, there is rapid recognition and elimination of the pathogen before it can multiply, because of specific antibodies in blood, secreted by plasma cells, and/or the increase in the number of specific T lymphocytes.

Vaccinations (active immunisations) are based on immunological memory. Many vaccinations use attenuated pathogens that can still multiply in the animal but no longer cause disease. The immune system reacts to these attenuated pathogens with an adequate immune response and the formation of **memory cells**. If there is contact again with the highly pathogenic "original" pathogen, memory cells can eliminate it immediately.

In addition to attenuated pathogens, **inactivated pathogens** are also used as vaccines. Since the pathogen can no longer reproduce, the amount of antigen is usually quite limited. The immune system usually reacts more slowly to such vaccinations. Therefore, several boosters must be given, until robust vaccine protection is achieved. Another group of **vaccines** consists only of individual **antigens** of the pathogens (subunit vaccines). They have the advantage of being very safe because there is no risk of infection. The immune system reacts very weakly to these vaccines, partly because of the small amount of vaccine antigen available, and partly because purified antigens do not activate TLR on the cells of the innate immune system. This means that the necessary cytokines are not released, and co-stimulatory proteins are not produced. To increase the immune response, so-called **adjuvants** are added to these vaccines. These adjuvants are mostly bacterial products with TLR ligands, which ensure sufficient stimulation of the antigen-presenting cells.

IN A NUTSHELL !

The initial contact between the pathogen and the innate immune system determines the immune response.

Suggested reading

Callahan GN, Yates RM. Basic Veterinary Immunology. Colorado: University Press; 2014

Day MJ, Schultz RD. Veterinary Immunology: Principles and Practice. Boca Raton: CRC Press; 2010

Tizard IR. Veterinary Immunology. 10th ed. Philadelphia: Saunders; 2018

11 Respiration

Gerolf Gros, Michael Pees, Helga Pfannkuche

11.1 Gas exchange

Gerolf Gros

ESSENTIALS ✗

Respiration refers to all the processes that are necessary to bring oxygen from the medium surrounding the animals (air or water) to the mitochondria of cells, and conversely to release the CO_2 produced in mitochondria into the environment. In mammals, respiration includes
- the upper airways, followed by the bronchial system, directing air from the environment to the alveoli of the lungs by convection,
- the transfer of O_2 from the alveoli into the pulmonary capillary blood by diffusion,
- convective transport of O_2 in the bloodstream to the tissues,
- diffusion of O_2 from the blood capillaries in the tissue to the mitochondria in cells.

The release of CO_2 occurs through the same processes in reverse order. The prerequisite for gas exchange is that the concentration and partial pressure of O_2 in air are higher than in the animal while those of CO_2 are lower (see **Table 11.1**). In fish, lungs are replaced by gills, and in amphibians, to a certain extent, by the skin.

Vertebrates have **four types of gas exchange**; their principles are outlined in **Fig. 11.1**:
1. **Gas exchange** in the **gills** of fish. The O_2 and CO_2 exchange takes place between the blood capillaries of the secondary lamellae of the fish gills and the water flowing over these lamellae. Blood and water flow in opposite directions in the gills ("countercurrent system").
2. **Gas exchange** in the lungs of **birds**. Gas exchange takes place between the blood capillaries and the parabronchi through which the gas flows, with the two directions of flow being perpendicular to each other ("cross flow").

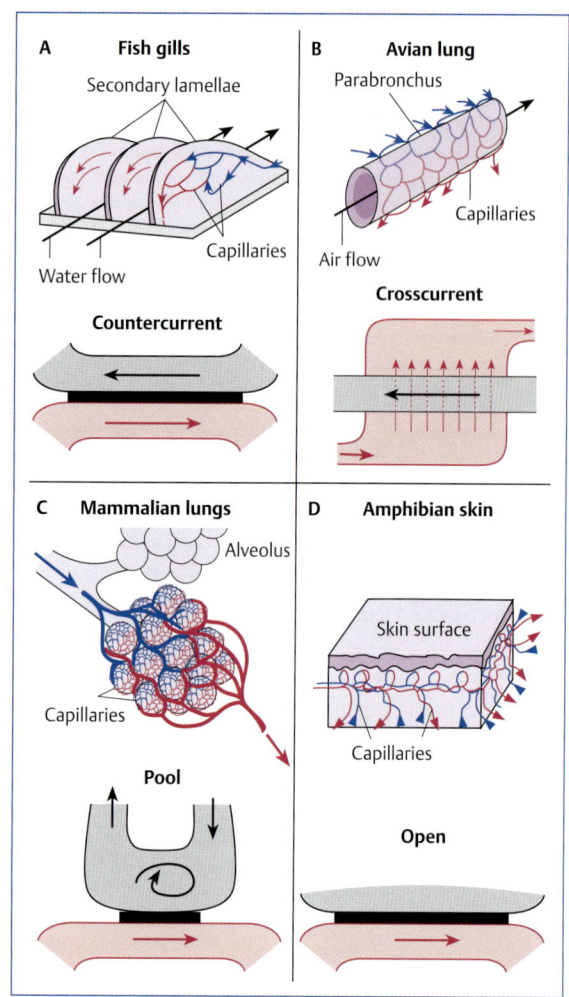

Fig. 11.1 Principles of gas exchange in the respiratory organs of various vertebrates, arranged in order of decreasing exchange efficiency: A Fish gills (countercurrent system), B Avian lungs (crosscurrent system), C Mammalian lungs (pool system), D Amphibian skin (open system Black arrows indicate the direction of flow of the O_2-carrying medium, water or air, red or blue arrows the direction of the O_2-receiving capillary blood flow. Blue coloured capillaries = venous capillary component, red coloured capillaries = arterial capillary component. Skin respiration in the "open system" is particularly inefficient because the diffusion resistance between capillaries and ambient air is very high due to the thickness of the skin.

3. **Gas exchange** in the **mammalian lung**. Here, the gas exchange takes place between the blood capillaries of the pulmonary alveoli and the alveolar space ("pool system", as there is a large, but still limited supply of oxygen available in the alveoli).
4. **Gas exchange** via the **skin**, which is important in amphibians. Here, oxygen and carbon dioxide are exchanged between the blood capillaries of the skin and the surrounding air ("open system" as the surrounding air space is practically unlimited).

First, the function of the mammalian lung is discussed in detail. In ch. 11.10, ch. 11.11 and ch. 11.12, the special features of gill respiration in fish, and respiration in reptiles and in birds are discussed.

11.2 Morphological basis of lung respiration in mammals

Gerolf Gros

Fig. 11.2 shows the processes required for mammalian respiration ("**external respiration**" and "**internal respiration**"):
1. O_2 is transported by the respiratory gas flow from the ambient air to the alveoli, CO_2 from the alveoli to the ambient air. This transport takes place by **convection**. This convective transport of gas is called **ventilation**.
2. O_2 passes, by **diffusion**, from the lumen of the alveolus into the blood of the alveolar capillary through the thin separating wall between the alveolus and the blood capillary: the alveolocapillary barrier. CO_2 moves in the opposite direction, also by diffusion.
3. Gas transport between alveolar capillaries and O_2-consuming tissues is via the bloodstream (pulmonary and systemic circulation), i.e., via **convection** by blood. The transport is very efficient because blood has a high binding capacity for both O_2 and CO_2.
4. The last step of gas exchange is diffusion of O_2 from blood into cells to reach the O_2-consuming and CO_2-producing mitochondria ("**internal respiration**").

11.2.1 Airways

The mammalian **airway system** consists of the "upper or extrathoracic" and "lower or intrathoracic" airways. The upper airway includes the nasal cavity, oral cavity, pharynx, larynx and the extrathoracic part of the trachea (**Fig. 11.17**). The lower airway includes the intrathoracic tracheobronchial system consisting of the intrathoracic trachea, bronchi, bronchioles and alveoli. The tracheobronchial system branches 23 times (23 "airway generations") or more. The "conduction zone" of this system extends to the 16th generation and includes trachea, bronchi, bronchioles and terminal bronchioles. In this region, as in the upper airways, **no gas exchange** takes place (**dead space**). The conduction zone is followed by the transition zone (three generations), in which the respiratory bronchioles allow limited gas exchange. The last four branches form the "**respiratory zone**" with the ductuli and sacculi alveolares, which is where **gas exchange** mainly takes place. The total cross-section of the respiratory tree is initially small and increases considerably from generation to generation.

An important task of the airways is to **clean** the inspired air. Smaller particles get stuck on the mucus layer of the bronchial epithelium. They are carried by the cilia of the epithelial cells towards the epiglottis. Larger particles trigger the cough reflex by irritating receptors in the mucous membranes of the airways. In this process, particles are exhaled by the strongly accelerated respiratory gas flow. In addition, the mucous membranes of the respiratory tract contribute to **warming** and **moistening** the inhaled air so that it arrives in the alveoli saturated with water vapour and at a temperature of approx. 37 °C (at physical rest).

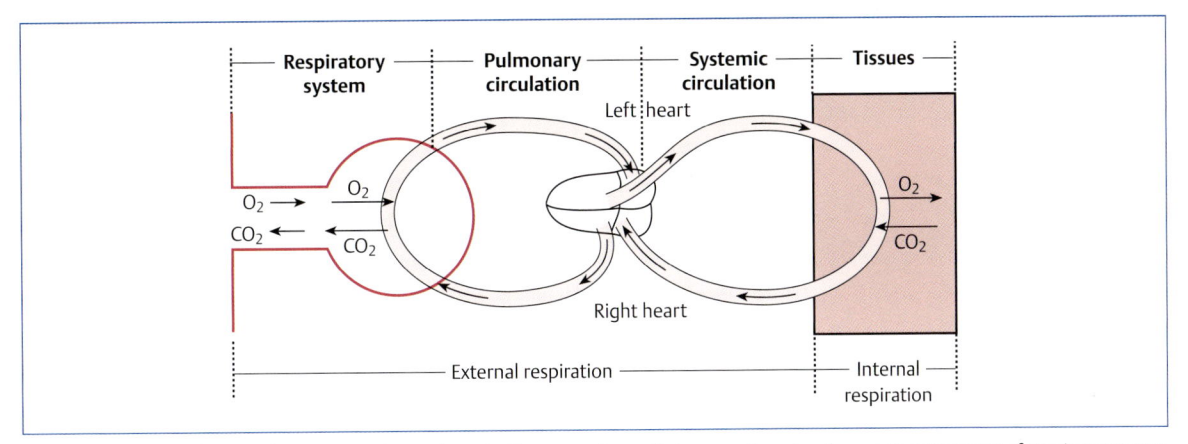

Fig. 11.2 External and internal respiration. External respiration comprises a first convection step (convective transport of respiratory gases through the respiratory tract), a diffusion step (diffusion of respiratory gases across the separating membrane between air and blood, or, in the case of fish and aquatic reptiles, between water and blood) and a second convection step (convective transport of O_2 and CO_2 through the blood of the pulmonary and systemic circulation from the respiratory organ to the O_2-consuming tissue and vice versa). Internal respiration (tissue respiration) includes a second diffusion step (diffusion of respiratory gases between tissue capillaries and mitochondria of the cells of the tissues) and the O_2-consuming processes taking place there. The two diffusion steps take place for O_2 and for CO_2 only as physically dissolved gases. Transport in blood takes place mainly in the form of chemically bound gases.

11.2.2 Morphological basis of inspiration and expiration

Air flow through the airways and into the alveolar space, i.e., ventilation, comes about through **changes in the volume** of the **intrathoracic space**. These are caused by rib movements ("**thoracic respiration**") and by diaphragmatic contractions ("**abdominal respiration**").

■ Thoracic respiration

Due to the position of the axis of rotation in the articulated connections between vertebrae and ribs, a cranial movement of the costal arches results in an enlargement of the thoracic cross-section laterally and, as can be seen in **Fig. 11.3**, especially ventrally. Enlargement leads to inspiration. The inspiratory movement of the ribs is caused by contraction of the "inspiratory muscles": Intercostales externi (**Fig. 11.4a**), intercostales interni intercartilaginei (**Fig. 11.4b**) and the scaleni. The expiratory caudal movement of the ribs is predominantly passive at rest, supported by contraction of the inner intercostal muscles (**Fig. 11.4 c**). The different action of the intercostal muscles is due to the different torques they exert on the posterior and anterior ribs respectively; it is greatest where the muscle insertion is furthest from the pivot point on the spine or sternum.

■ Abdominal respiration

Contraction of the diaphragm leads to expansion of the thoracic cavity towards the abdomen. It is the more effective of the two inspiratory mechanisms and is always involved in inspiration, both at rest and under physical exertion. In the expiratory phase, the diaphragm relaxes and curves more strongly into the thoracic cavity (**Fig. 11.3**). Most mammals use both thoracic and abdominal respiration. In the dog, thoracic respiration predominates, while in horses and ruminants abdominal respiration is more important. The type of respiration is of diagnostic significance. Stomach overfill and pregnancy hinder abdominal respiration and therefore make thoracic respiration more prominent. Rib fractures lead to an emphasis on abdominal respiration.

When there is increased ventilation, such as during physical activity, inspiration as well as expiration can both be supported by the auxiliary respiratory muscles. Auxiliary muscles are the pectoralis major and minor, scaleni, sternocleidomastoid and serrati muscles; they contribute to the cranial movement of the ribs. Auxiliary expirators are the abdominal muscles that pull the ribs backwards (caudally) and push the abdominal viscera cranially, thus allowing the diaphragm to press into the thoracic cavity.

> **IN A NUTSHELL**   !
>
> Inspiration occurs through "abdominal respiration" (diaphragmatic contraction) and through "thoracic respiration" (enlargement of the thoracic cross-section through cranial movement of the ribs). Expiration is passive at rest.

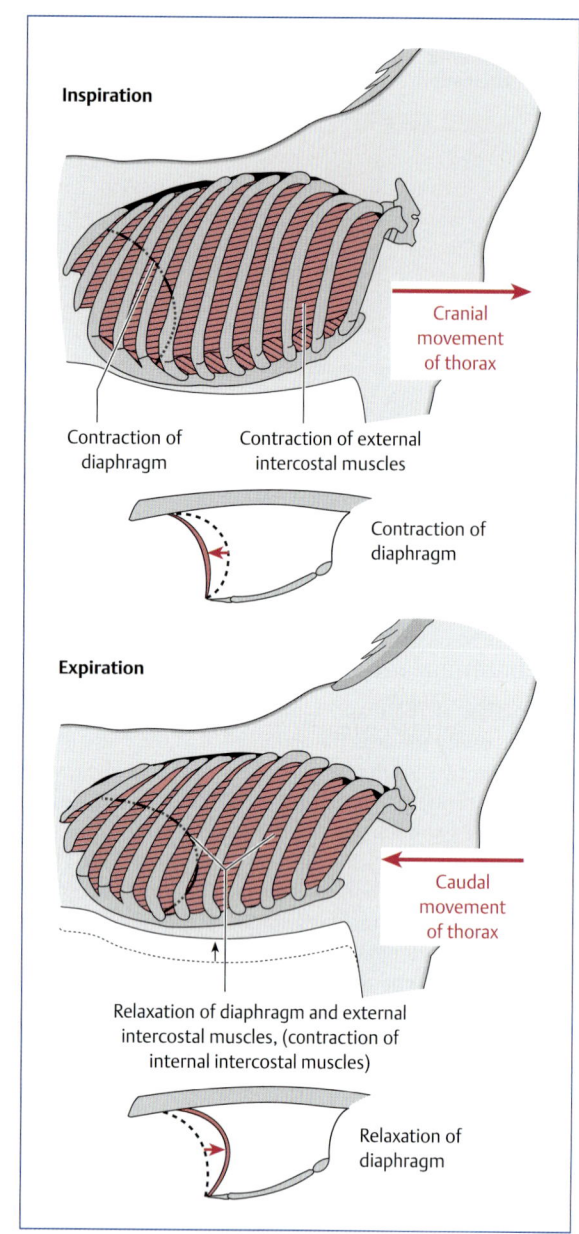

Fig. 11.3 Expansion of the intrathoracic space during thoracic respiration. Cranial movement of the rib arches by the inspiratory muscles causes the ribs to rotate about the rib-neck axes on the spine, expanding the thoracic cross-section laterally and ventrally (top). The lower part of each illustration shows the abdominal respiration that occurs simultaneously with the thoracic movement through diaphragmatic contraction (inspiration) and diaphragmatic relaxation (expiration).

11.2.3　Transmission thorax – lungs – pleurae

Why do the lungs follow the thoracic movements so completely that the gap between the parietal pleura and the visceral pleura is always narrow? The **pleural cavity** contains a thin film of fluid and is completely free of air. Since the fluid film is neither compressible nor expandable, the lung is forced to follow every change in size and shape of the thorax. Compared to an adhesion of the parietal to vis-

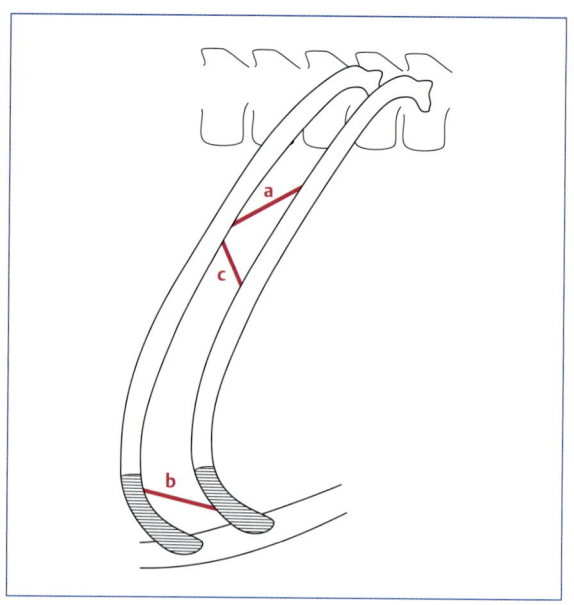

Fig. 11.4 Intercostal muscles. Cranial movement of the ribs and inspiration by mm. intercostales externi (**a**) and mm. intercostales interni intercartilaginei (**b**), caudal movement during active expiration by mm. intercostales interni (**c**).

ceral pleura, this construction has the advantage that the lung can move freely against the inner wall of the thorax. This is the only way to ensure uniformity of lung expansion during inspiration. In mammalian species in which the parietal and visceral pleura are partially fused together (elephant, tapir, etc.), ventilation is almost exclusively driven by diaphragmatic activity. Two mechanisms are responsible for maintaining the capillary fluid film in the pleural space:

- The epithelial cells that line the pleurae (mesothelium) balance **fluid reabsorption** from and **secretion** into the **pleural space** so that the amount of fluid in the space is usually kept constant.
- The total gas pressure (sum of all gas partial pressures) at the end of the pleural capillaries is lower than that in the atmosphere and in the alveolar space. Therefore, no gas bubbles can form in the pleural space and **gas** that has entered the pleural space during an injury (pneumothorax) is **reabsorbed**.

> **IN A NUTSHELL**　　　　　　　　　　　　　　　　　!
>
> The separation of visceral and parietal pleurae by the thin fluid-filled pleural space ensures that the lung follows all thoracic movements, and that the lung surface can slide against the inner thoracic wall.

11.2.4　Alveolocapillary barrier

After oxygen in the inspired air has reached the alveoli, it enters the blood of the alveolar capillaries by diffusion (Fig. 11.2).

The mammalian lung offers ideal conditions for high efficiency diffusion across the alveolocapillary barrier:

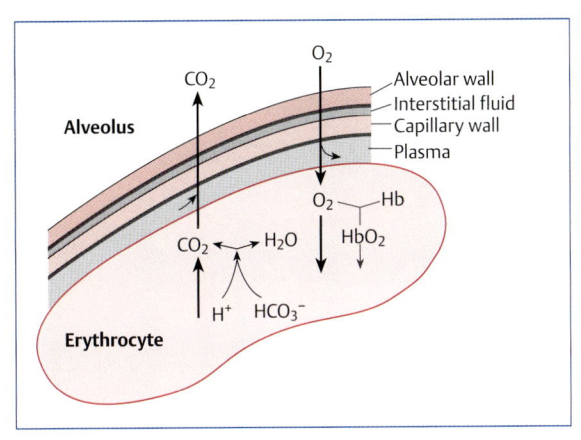

Fig. 11.5 The alveolocapillary barrier and the O_2 and CO_2 exchange between the alveolar space and the alveolar capillary. Thickness of the barrier: 0.5–1 μm.

- The **barrier** is very **thin**, < 1 μm, although it consists of alveolar epithelium, interstitial space or basal lamina and capillary endothelium (**Fig. 11.5**).
- The **contact area** between alveoli and alveolar capillaries is very **large**. As **Fig. 11.1** shows, the alveoli are surrounded by a dense capillary network. As a result of the small size of the individual alveoli (diameter approx. 0.2 mm) and their high number, the total alveolar surface area is large. The lung of a human, sheep or large dog has a total alveolar surface area of 120–140 m². The size of the exchange surface for O_2 and CO_2 and the thin alveolocapillary barrier ensure that diffusion between alveoli and capillary blood is completed by the time the blood leaves the lung.

> **IN A NUTSHELL**   !
>
> The alveolocapillary barrier is extremely thin at < 1 μm and, together with the large alveolar surface, ensures ideal diffusion conditions for O_2 and CO_2 between the alveolus and the blood.

11.3 Ventilation and lung volumes

Gerolf Gros

Ventilation describes the gas volume that flows into or out of the lungs per unit of time. **Lung volumes** are defined as partial volumes of the maximum total volume contained in the lungs. **Lung capacities** are composed of two or more of these lung volumes.

11.3.1 Volumes and capacities

Fig. 11.6 gives an overview of volumes and capacities (numerical values for horse, dog and cat):

- **Tidal volume, TV** or **V_{exp}:** Volume inspired or expired per single breath, approx. 6 l in horses at rest (approx. 0.5 l in humans (70 kg)).
- **Inspiratory reserve volume:** Volume that can still be inspired after a normal inspiration (at rest) at maximum effort. In the horse, this volume is approx. 24 l.
- **Expiratory reserve volume:** Volume that can still be expired after a normal expiration (at rest) at maximum effort. In the horse, this volume is approx. 15 l.
- **Residual volume, RV:** Volume that cannot be exhaled even during maximum exertion and always remains in the lungs. The physiological meaning of a residual volume is, among other things, that gas which is still present in the lungs even after the deepest expiration. Thus, O_2 can still be taken up by the lung capillary blood and CO_2 can still be released at the time of deep expiration. Residual volume is approx. 10 l in the horse.
- **Inspiratory capacity:** Sum of resting tidal volume and inspiratory reserve volume. Describes the maximum possible inspiratory volume after normal expiration, in horses about 30 l.
- **Functional residual capacity, FRC:** Sum of residual volume and expiratory reserve volume. FRC thus represents the volume of air present in the lungs at the end of passive expiration. FRC in the horse is about 25 l.

Circulation, respiration

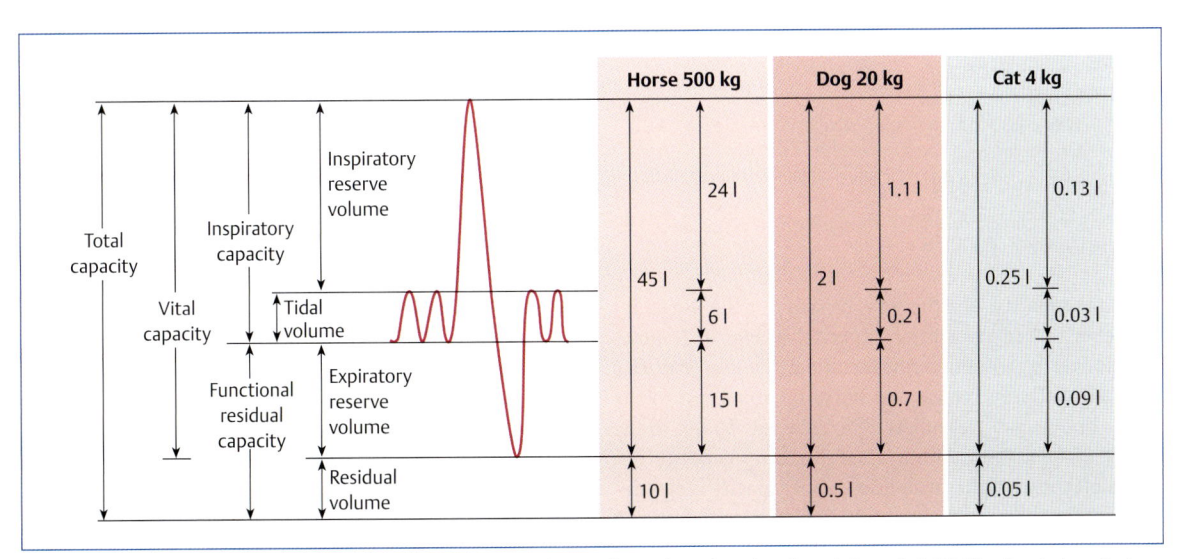

Fig. 11.6 Lung volumes and lung capacities in healthy horses, dogs and cats; based on data from Lekeux P, Art T. The Respiratory System: Anatomy, Physiology and Adaptation to Exercise and Training. In: Hodgson DR, Rose RJ (eds). The Athletic Horse. Philadelphia: Saunders Company, 1994; Hogg JC, Nepszy S. Regional lung volume and pleural pressure gradient estimated from lung density in dogs. J Appl Physiol 1969; 27: 198-203 and Stahl WR. Scaling of respiratory variables in mammals. J Appl Physiol 1967; 22: 453-460

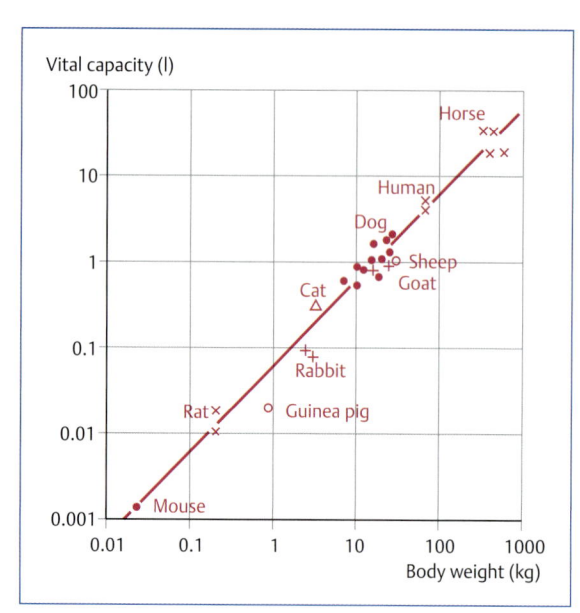

Fig. 11.7 The vital capacity (VC) of domestic and laboratory animals as a function of body weight. Double logarithmic plot. The following correlation results: VC (l) = 0.056 · body weight (kg)$^{1.02}$, i.e., an almost linear relationship (exponent: 1.02); based on data from Hörnicke H. Atmung und Gaswechsel. In: Lenkeit W, Breirem K, Crasemann E (eds). Handbuch der Tierernährung. Vol. I. Hamburg, Berlin: Paul Parey; 1969: 298–326

- **Vital capacity, VC:** Sum of resting tidal volume, inspiratory and expiratory reserve volume. VC indicates the maximum tidal volume and is therefore an important parameter of physical performance. In horses it is about 45 l.
- **Total capacity, TC:** Sum of all lung volumes: the maximum volume of gas that a lung can hold, approx. 55 l in horses. Similar to the vital capacity (**Fig. 11.7**), the total capacity increases across the different mammalian species approximately in proportion to their body weight.

The **tidal volume** at physical rest for various animal species is approximately as follows:
- rabbit (3 kg): 20 ml
- cat (4 kg): 30 ml
- dog (20 kg): 200 ml
- goat (40 kg): 350 ml
- human (70 kg): 500 ml
- cattle (500 kg): 3800 ml
- horse (500 kg): 6000 ml

The **vital capacity**, like the total capacity of the lungs, increases with body weight of a species. As **Fig. 11.7** shows in a double logarithmic representation, the vital capacity increases between mouse and horse by about ten to the power of four, just as body weight increases by ten to the power of four. Even within a species, vital capacity depends on body weight. In addition, vital capacity is age-dependent, initially increasing until growth is complete and then decreasing with age. The vital capacity is diagnostically important in detection of restrictive (p. 273) and also obstructive lung dysfunctions (p. 274) (**Table 11.2**). Func-

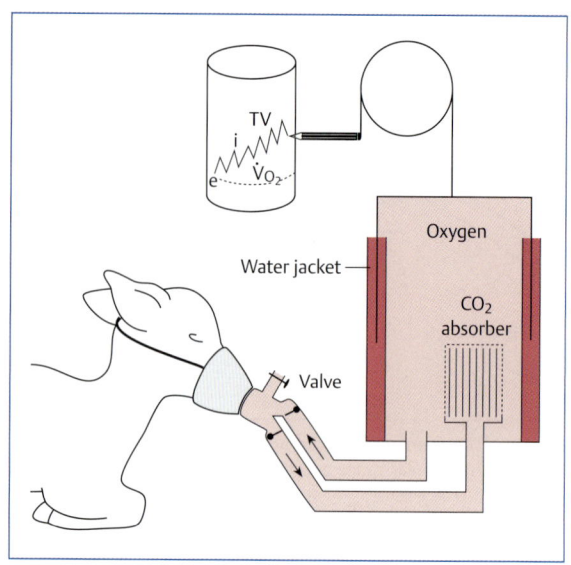

Fig. 11.8 Spirometer. A cylindrical bell is immersed in a water jacket of a likewise cylindrical container and thus makes an airtight seal of the variable interior of the spirometer. A recording lever attached to the bell records the respiratory movements. The animal is connected to the spirometer via a well-sealed mask (possibly via a tracheal tube in the case of anaesthetised animals). Inlet and outlet air are guided separately via flaps. If resting respiration is registered over a longer period of time, the spirometer volume decreases due to the animal's O_2 uptake (see tracing on the recording drum). The slope of the line reflects the oxygen consumption of the animal ($\dot{V}_{O_2}$). e = expiratory peak, i = inspiratory peak, the amplitude of each respiratory movement represents its tidal volume V_{exp}.

tionally, it is important because it represents the maximum tidal volume of an animal.

> **IN A NUTSHELL** !
>
> Vital capacity is the maximum possible tidal volume. It is reduced especially in restrictive, and also in obstructive lung dysfunction.

11.3.2 Measurement of lung volumes and capacities

The simplest procedure is **spirometry** (**Fig. 11.8**). This involves breathing from and into an enclosed space, with the bell of the spirometer moving downwards or upwards as a result of inhalation or exhalation. The exhaled gas is passed through a CO_2 absorber filled with soda lime, which removes CO_2 from the expired gas so that the spirometer remains CO_2-free. Before starting the measurement, the spirometer is filled with pure oxygen. While the animal breathes, only O_2 remains in the spirometer, hardly any N_2 is present and no CO_2 is added. As the animal's O_2 intake continues, the volume decreases. The mean volume decrease corresponds to the O_2 uptake. The volume changes in the spirometer are recorded by a recording lever connected to the bell. This creates the curve shown in **Fig. 11.6** and thus records the O_2 consumption of the animal as well as all lung volumes and capacities, except for the residual volume and the functional residual capacity. The proce-

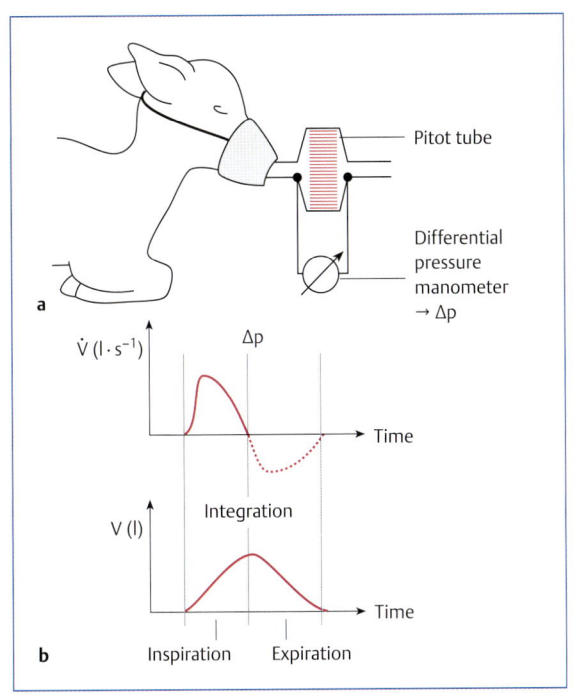

Fig. 11.9 a Principle of the pneumotachograph. The animal breathes through a "pitot tube" with a flow resistor through which it must breathe. The difference in pressures (Δp) upstream and downstream of the flow resistance is measured with a differential pressure manometer. **b** As a function of time, Δp provides the respiratory gas flow $\dot{V}$ (**b**, above), since the two variables are proportional to each other by analogy to Ohm's law for a given resistance. Electronic integration over time yields the tidal volume (V) as a function of time (**b**, bottom).

dure can be performed on anaesthetised or trained animals.

An alternative to spirometry is the **pneumotachograph**. **Fig. 11.9 a** shows the principle. Breathing in and out is done through a "pitot tube", which is connected either with a mask or a tracheal catheter (anaesthetised animals or animals used to a mask). The pitot tube creates a certain flow resistance due to the closely arranged lamellae. The pressure difference in front of and behind the lamellae resistance is measured. Analogous to Ohm's law (p. 193) ($\dot{V}=\Delta p/R$), the gas flow $\dot{V}$ can be measured. Δp is the pressure difference before and behind the lamellae and R is the existing flow resistance of the lamellae. The measured Δp is therefore proportional to the gas flow $\dot{V}$. By electronic integration of $\dot{V}$ over time, the volume is obtained. In addition to gas flow, all volumes that can be determined with a spirometer can also be recorded by a pneumotachograph (**Fig. 11.9 b**, lower part).

IN A NUTSHELL   !

Lung volumes and capacities can be measured with a spirometer (closed system) or with a pneumotachograph (open system). Respiratory gas flows are mostly recorded directly with the pneumotachograph.

MORE DETAILS   The **functional residual capacity** (FRC) and the residual volume can both be determined with the **Helium-wash-in method**. A spirometer is used as in **Fig. 11.8**, but this spirometer (volume V_{sp}) contains, in addition to O_2, a low concentration of helium ($C_{initial}$). A measuring device records the He concentration. At the end of a normal expiration of the animal, only the volume of the functional residual capacity [V_{FRC}, **Fig. 11.6**] is present. At that point, a valve is opened so that the animal now begins to get gas from the spirometer. Respiration of the animal distributes the helium evenly between the spirometer volume and the lung volume. The new helium concentration (C_{end}) is then measured and a mass balance for helium is formed, as the total amount of helium is largely unchanged. Since quantity equals concentration times volume, the volume of the FRC can be determined from the known V_{sp} and the measured He concentrations $C_{initial}$ and C_{end}.

Helium is a particularly suitable gas for this determination because its solubility in water is very low and therefore almost no helium is released from the alveolar space into blood and body tissues. Therefore, the assumption of an almost constant amount of He is justified:

$$V_{sp} \cdot C_{initial} = (V_{sp} + FRC) \cdot C_{end} \qquad (11.1)$$

The **residual** is obtained by subtracting the expiratory reserve volume from the FRC.

11.3.3   Dead space

The **anatomical dead space** is defined as the volume of the respiratory tract that is ventilated, but in which **no gas exchange** can take place. This is the space from the mouth or nose to the terminal bronchioles. This space must first be "purged" during both inspiration and expiration before an exchange of ambient air and alveolar gas can take place. The anatomical dead space varies somewhat with the respiratory cycle. During inspiration, lung and airway volume increases and sympathetic tone rises, both of which lead to bronchial dilation. Conversely, during expiration, along with the decrease in lung volume, there is some decrease in airway volume due to bronchoconstriction, which is exacerbated by an increase in parasympathetic tone (**Table 4.1**). The physiological task of the dead space is cleaning, humidification and warming of the respiratory air (p. 262).

The **functional dead space** is defined as the volume of the respiratory tract that is ventilated and in which **no gas exchange** takes place. It is equal to or greater than the anatomical dead space. In lung disease, there may be alveolar regions that are ventilated, but not perfused and thus do not contribute to gas exchange. Such pulmonary regions contribute to an increase in functional dead space. When an animal is intubated for artificial ventilation, the dead space increases by the volume of the catheter tube, which decreases the efficiency of ventilation.

MORE DETAILS

Measurement of the dead space

As in the case of residual volume determination, a volume balance is established for one indicator gas, in this case CO_2. Each expired breath volume (V_{exp}) consists of a primary portion V_{dead}, which originates from the dead space, followed by a secondary portion V_{alv}, which originates from the alveolar space:

$$V_{exp} = V_{dead} + V_{alv} \tag{11.2}$$

The quantity (m) of CO_2 exhaled with V_{exp} then applies accordingly:

$$m_{exp,CO_2} = m_{dead,CO_2} + m_{alv,CO_2} \tag{11.3}$$

Since at the end of an inspiration the dead space is filled with fresh air, which is practically devoid of CO_2 ($0.0004 \, ml \, CO_2 \cdot ml^{-1}$), the dead space portion V_{dead} of the subsequent expiration is also CO_2-free and therefore $m_{dead,CO_2} \approx 0$. All exhaled CO_2 thus comes from the alveolar fraction V_{alv}. If we now replace all CO_2 quantities m by CO_2 concentrations times gas volumes, it follows:

$$V_{exp} \cdot C_{exp,CO_2} = V_{dead} \cdot C_{dead,CO_2} + V_{alv} \cdot C_{alv,CO_2} \tag{11.4}$$
$$\text{(Bohr's formula)}$$

C_{exp,CO_2} is the CO_2 concentration in the total expired gas and C_{alv,CO_2} the CO_2 concentration in the alveolar space.

V_{exp} can be determined with a spirometer or pneumotachograph. If then C_{exp,CO_2} and C_{alv,CO_2} are measured, V_{alv} can be calculated from the above equation. This is possible because C_{dead,CO_2} is practically zero at the end of an inspiration (see above). Thus, the product $V_{dead} \cdot C_{dead,CO_2}$ is also practically zero, i.e., negligible.

The mean expiratory CO_2 concentration, C_{exp,CO_2}, is measured by collecting all expired gas from several respiratory cycles in a plastic bag, the "Douglas bag", and then measuring the CO_2 concentration of this gas, for example with an infrared analyser (absorption of infrared radiation by CO_2).

The alveolar CO_2 concentration, C_{alv,CO_2}, is determined by inhaling and exhaling through a CO_2 analyser. In accordance with what has already been said above, **Fig. 11.10** shows that at the end of an inspiration there is ambient air in the CO_2 analyser, i.e., $C_{CO_2} \approx 0$. After the onset of expiration, the CO_2 concentration increases continuously and reaches a plateau as soon as pure alveolar gas reaches the CO_2 analyser. The plateau occurs because the CO_2 concentration is the same everywhere in the very large volume of the alveolar space. The CO_2 concentration of this "alveolar plateau" is therefore approximately equal to C_{alv,CO_2}.

Typical values for these concentrations are $C_{exp,CO_2} = 0.04 \, ml$ $CO_2 \cdot (ml \, gas)^{-1}$ and $C_{alv,CO_2} = 0.056 \, ml \, CO_2 \cdot (ml \, gas)^{-1}$. V_{exp} can be obtained by spirometry. With these gas concentrations and $V_{exp} = 500 \, ml$, Bohr's formula gives a dead space volume V_{dead} of 140 ml, which is the normal anatomical dead space in humans. It accounts for approx. 30% of the resting tidal volume. The dead space is also about 25–40% of the tidal volume in domestic mammals at rest (but this does not apply to animals when panting (p. 293))!

> ### IN A NUTSHELL
>
> The **residual volume** is the volume of lung that cannot be decreased even with maximum exhaling effort. The **functional dead space** is the space that is ventilated, but does not contribute to the gas exchange of the lungs. It is equal to the anatomical dead space in healthy animals. Residual volume and anatomical dead space are determined by the volume distribution of an indicator gas: the residual volume with He, the dead space with CO_2.

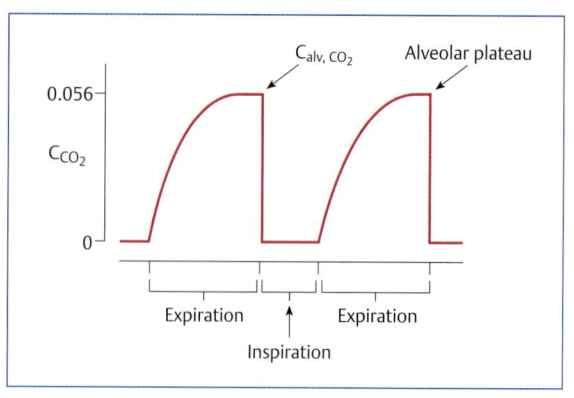

Fig. 11.10 Continuous recording of the CO_2 concentration (= C_{CO_2}) in front of the mouth with a CO_2 analyser, through which the exhaled gas passes. During expiration C_{CO_2} increases at first. In this phase, the dead space gas and the alveolar gas mix then reach an approximately constant value, the alveolar plateau (C_{alv,CO_2}). The CO_2 concentration corresponding to this plateau is also called the end-expiratory CO_2 concentration and approximates the CO_2 concentration in the alveolar space.

11.3.4 Ventilation

The volume of air inspired or expired over a defined period of time is also called **respiratory time volume** (or **respiratory minute ventilation**), $\dot{V}_E$. It is the product of the tidal volume (V_{exp}) times the respiratory rate (v):

$$\dot{V}_E = V_{exp} \cdot \nu \tag{11.5}$$

The **respiratory rate** depends on the body weight of an animal and decreases with increasing body weight (**Fig. 11.11**). The **resting respiratory minute volume** also depends mainly on body weight. It increases with increasing body weight (**Fig. 11.12**).

Ventilation of the alveolar space is called **alveolar ventilation** ($\dot{V}_{alv}$), while that of the dead space is **dead space ventilation** ($\dot{V}_{dead}$). Both together result in the respiratory time volume:

$$\dot{V}_E = \dot{V}_{dead} + \dot{V}_{alv} \tag{11.6}$$

Since the anatomical dead space is a less variable quantity, the "shallower" the breathing, i.e., the smaller the tidal volume in relation to the dead space volume, the smaller the alveolar ventilation. Panting (p. 293) is an example of extremely shallow breathing, where alveolar ventilation can drop to only a few percent of dead space ventilation. This allows a very high respiratory rate and high respiratory time volume with normal CO_2 exhalation (normal $\dot{V}_{alv}$), but large heat release from the airways. Conversely, "deep" breathing is the most efficient way to achieve high alveolar ventilation.

If the term $V_{dead} \cdot C_{dead,CO_2}$ is deleted from Bohr's formula and replaced by the volumes V_{exp} and V_{alv} with total ventilation and alveolar ventilation, respectively, we get:

$$C_{alv,CO_2} = C_{exp,CO_2} \cdot (\dot{V}_E / \dot{V}_{alv}) \tag{11.7}$$

Since the product $C_{exp,CO_2} \cdot \dot{V}_E$ is equal to the CO_2 output of an animal $\dot{V}_{CO_2}$ which is constant at constant O_2 consumption, the alveolar CO_2 concentration is inversely proportional to the alveolar ventilation under this condition:

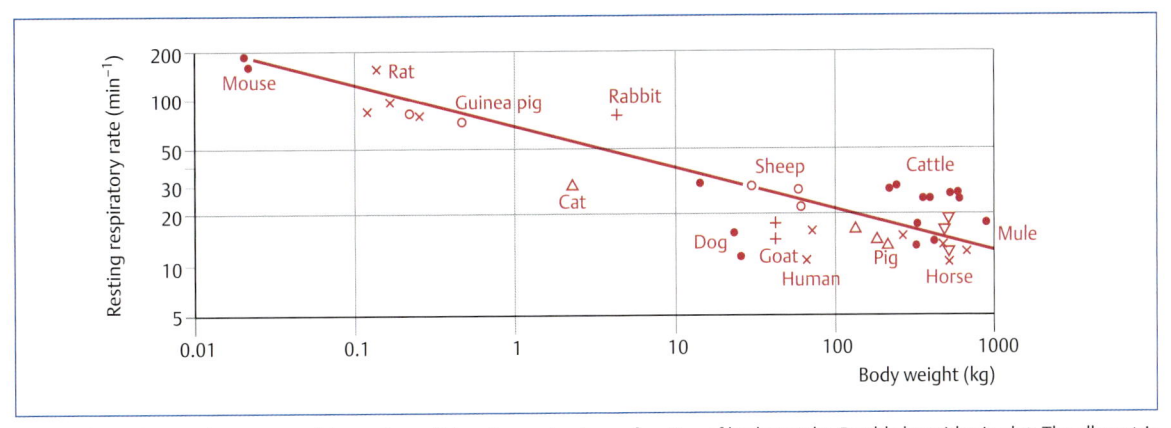

Fig. 11.11 Resting respiratory rate of domestic and laboratory animals as a function of body weight. Double logarithmic plot. The allometric relationship is described by the following regression line:
resting respiratory rate (min^{-1}) = 70 · body weight (kg)$^{-0.25}$; i.e., the smaller the animal, the higher the resting respiratory rate; based on data from Hörnicke H. Atmung und Gaswechsel. In: Lenkeit W, Breirem K, Crasemann E (eds). Handbuch der Tierernährung. Vol. I. Hamburg, Berlin: Paul Parey; 1969: 298–326

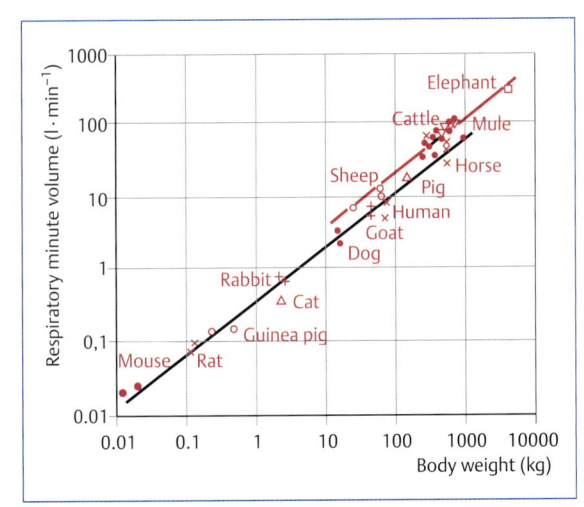

Fig. 11.12 Respiratory minute volume at rest of domestic and laboratory animals as a function of body weight. The larger the animal, the higher the resting respiratory minute volume ($\dot{V}_E$). The relationship for the lighter weight animals (black straight line) is: $\dot{V}_E$ (l·min^{-1}) = 0.38 · body weight (kg)$^{0.75}$, for the heavier animals (red straight line): $\dot{V}_E$ (l·min^{-1}) = 0.73 · body weight (kg)$^{0.75}$. The exponent of the two allometric relationships is therefore 0.75. From the exponent 0.75 value for the respiratory minute volume and the exponent of −0.25 for the resting respiratory rate (**Fig. 11.11**), it follows that the resting tidal volume depends on body weight with an exponent of 1.0., a tenfold increase in body weight is accompanied by a tenfold increase in resting tidal volume, while the resting respiratory minute volume increases somewhat less with body weight; based on data from Hörnicke H. Atmung und Gaswechsel. In: Lenkeit W, Breirem K, Crasemann E (eds). Handbuch der Tierernährung. Vol. I. Hamburg, Berlin: Paul Parey; 1969: 298–326

$$C_{alv,CO_2} \approx 1/\dot{V}_{alv} \qquad (11.8)$$

Gas concentration (C) and gas partial pressure (p) are proportional to each other. The relationship between the two is as follows:

$$p = C \cdot (p_{baro} - p_{H_2O}) \qquad (11.9)$$

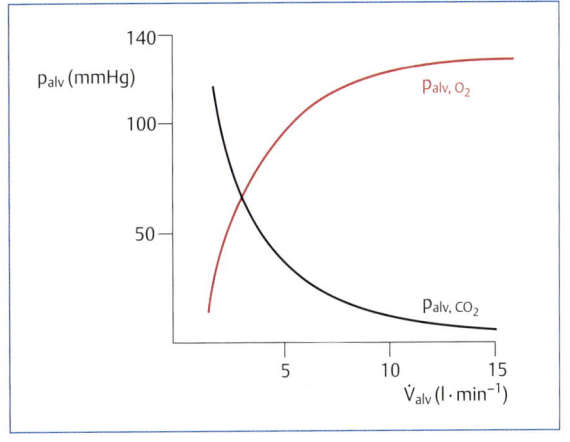

Fig. 11.13 Relationship between alveolar partial pressures p_{alv} and alveolar ventilation $\dot{V}_{alv}$ in humans. The points corresponding to normoventilation are at $\dot{V}_{alv}$ = 5 l·min^{-1}, p_{alv,CO_2} = 40 mmHg (= 5.3 kPa) and p_{alv,O_2} = 100 mmHg (= 13.3 kPa).

P_{baro} is the total pressure or barometer reading, p_{H_2O} the water vapour pressure. From these last two equations, the following applies:

$$p_{alv,CO_2} \approx 1/\dot{V}_{alv} \qquad (11.10)$$

Correspondingly, the relationship between the **alveolar CO$_2$ partial pressure** p_{alv,CO_2} and alveolar ventilation ($\dot{V}_{alv}$) is hyperbolic (**Fig. 11.13**): With increasing alveolar ventilation, the pressure p_{alv,CO_2} approaches zero. At very low $\dot{V}_{alv}$, p_{alv,CO_2} increases greatly. **Fig. 11.13** also illustrates that p_{alv,O_2} behaves as a mirror image of p_{alv,CO_2} when $\dot{V}_{alv}$ changes. After the passage of blood through the lungs, the blood partial pressures are equal to the alveolar partial pressures. Consequently, the following approximation also applies:

$$P_{art,CO_2} \approx 1/\dot{V}_{alv} \qquad (11.11)$$

P_{art,CO_2} stands for **arterial CO$_2$ partial pressure**. This equation helps to diagnose a pathological situation where there is a very large functional dead space, but only small alveolar ventilation. CO_2 release can then become so inefficient that p_{art,CO_2} (as well as p_{alv,CO_2}) becomes very high. The condition of increased CO_2 partial pressure in the arterial blood is called **hypercapnia**. Too low alveolar ventilation that leads to hypercapnia is called **hypoventilation**. Since the normal arterial p_{CO_2} is 40 ± 5 mmHg (40 mmHg = 5.3 kPa), the following definitions apply:

$$p_{art,CO_2} > 45 \text{ mmHg} = \text{hypercapnia} = \text{hypoventilation} \qquad (11.12)$$

$$p_{art,CO_2} < 35 \text{ mmHg} = \text{hypocapnia} = \text{hyperventilation} \qquad (11.13)$$

$$p_{art,CO_2} = 40 \pm 5 \text{ mmHg} = \text{normocapnia} = \text{normoventilation} \quad (11.14)$$

At **normoventilation**, ventilation is fully adapted to the existing metabolic rate. In **hypoventilation** or **hyperventilation** ventilation is too low or too high in relation to the CO_2 production rate. A distinction must be made between the terms **hyperpnoea** or **eupnoea**. Eupnoea is the normal resting ventilation of a species, while hyperpnoea is increased ventilation. For example, hyperpnoea is normal during physical exertion, but since p_{art,CO_2} remains normal in many cases, it is not considered to be hyperventilation, but normoventilation. The term **dyspnoea** does not refer to a specific tidal volume, but to the subjective sensation of **breathlessness**, which generally accompanies a reduced arterial pressure p_{O_2}.

> **IN A NUTSHELL**   !
>
> Alveolar ventilation is the decisive parameter of lung ventilation for gas exchange. If it is increased, this may be due to hyperventilation (with decreased p_{art,CO_2}) or hyperpnoea (with normal p_{art,CO_2}).

11.4 Mechanics

Gerolf Gros

When lung volume increases during inspiration, and also when it decreases during expiration, mechanical resistances must be overcome. Distinction has to be made between **elastic** and **viscous resistances**.

   Elastic resistances are effective both during respiratory activity and during respiratory rest; they include:

- **elastic structures** of the lung and thorax, i.e., mainly elastic fibres
- **surface tension** of the alveoli, which is effective at the interface of alveolar epithelium and alveolar gas and is reduced by surfactant (p. 272).

Both components of the elastic resistances lead to extensive lung collapse of an isolated lung.

   Viscous resistances are only effective during the ventilation process. They include:

- **flow resistance** of the airways ("resistance")
- **tissue resistance** (resistance that the lungs and thorax offer to non-elastic "plastic" deformation). Plastic deformation is comparable to the deformation of plasticine, which requires force, but is not spontaneously reversible.

Tissue resistance accounts for no more than 10% of viscous resistance, so it is mainly airway flow resistance that needs to be considered here.

> **IN A NUTSHELL**   !
>
> Elastic resistances are also effective when the lung-thorax system is at rest and are based on:
> - elastic structures (elastic fibres)
> - surface forces at the gas-water phase boundary of the alveoli
>
> Viscous resistances are only effective while there is a flow of respiratory gas. They are essentially due to airway resistance (flow resistance).

11.4.1 Elastic resistances

Elastic fibres of the lungs are always under tension. This and the surface tension of (p. 272) the alveoli both lead to a tendency of the lungs to shrink. One consequence of this is that normal resting expiration can occur passively through the "elastic retraction" of the lungs. After a deep inspiration, the thorax tends to decrease in volume, so that the lungs and thorax work together. In the resting position, however, i.e., after a normal expiration, the thorax offers considerable resistance to any further reduction in lung volume. Here, the retraction force of the lung is compensated for by an equal and opposite force of the thorax, so that the thorax-lung system is in balance. Therefore, a further reduction of lung volume requires the help of the expiratory muscles to overcome the resistance of the thorax. The strong retraction force of the lung itself is impressively demonstrated when a massive pneumothorax develops or when a lung is removed from the thorax during dissection, its gas volume drops to approx. 5% of its total capacity, i.e., to far less than the residual volume.

■ Intrapleural pressure

In vivo, the lungs always tend to reduce in volume and thus always exert a **retraction force** through elastic fibres and surface tension. Thus, during resting respiration, there is a **"negative" intrapleural pressure** in the very small gap between the visceral and parietal pleurae, a pressure that is lower than atmospheric pressure. If the pleural space is punctured (Fig. 11.14), this negative pressure can be measured. In the inspiratory position, the lung tissue is under greater elastic tension, so that the intrapleural pressure is "more negative" (−7 cm water column compared to atmospheric pressure) than in the expiratory position (−4 cm H_2O).

> **MORE DETAILS**   Opening of the pleural space, either from the alveolar space (e.g., due to bursting of an emphysema bubble) or from the outside (e.g., due to an accident), leads to an inflow of air into the pleural space and thus to lung collapse or **pneumothorax**. The affected lung no longer follows the thoracic and diaphragmatic movements and therefore no longer participates in ventilation and gas exchange. If only the lung on one side is affected, sufficient respiratory function can still be maintained by the contralateral lung.

Because of the risk of pneumothorax, measurements of intrapleural pressure by puncturing the pleural space should only be performed in exceptional cases. Instead, changes in pleural pressure can be well detected by measuring the respiratory changes in **oesophageal pressure**. This is possible because the oesophagus, like the pleural space, lies outside the lungs, but inside the thorax. The oesophageal wall is very soft and transmits the surrounding pressure well. For measurement, a catheter with a small balloon at the end is inserted into the oesophagus. The balloon is inflated until it lies snugly against the inner wall of the oesophagus (**Fig. 11.15 a**). A manometer is connected to the end of the catheter outside the mouth.

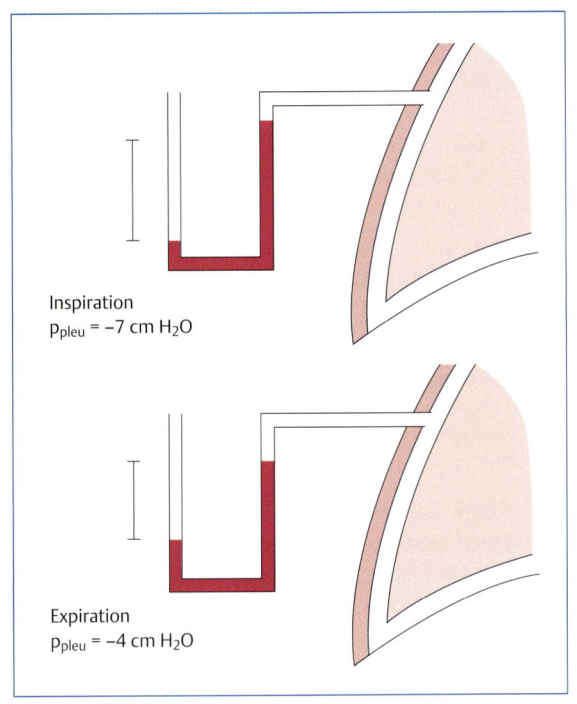

Fig. 11.14 Intrapleural pressures in normal inspiratory and expiratory positions. During inspiration, the pressure between the visceral and parietal pleurae becomes more negative as the elastic retraction force of the lung increases.

Inspiration
$p_{pleu} = -7$ cm H_2O

Expiration
$p_{pleu} = -4$ cm H_2O

> **IN A NUTSHELL** !
>
> Due to elasticity and surface tension, the lungs in the thoracic cavity develop a tensile stress on the inner wall of the thorax. This creates a negative pressure in the pleural space in the mid-respiratory position and during deep inspiration. A lung that is not stretched in the intact thorax collapses almost completely.

■ Lung compliance – pressure volume curve

The **pressure volume curve** of the lung describes the relationship between lung volume and transpulmonary pressure, which is the pressure difference between the gas space in the lung and the external environment. The slope of the pressure volume curve is a measure of the **volume expandability** of the lung which is called **compliance**. It is usually determined in the mid-respiratory position (at the FRC). In vivo, lung compliance is the ratio of the change in volume (ΔV_{pul}) to the change in transpulmonary pressure $\Delta(p_{pul} - p_{pleu})$ that determines expansion:

$$\Delta V_{pul}/\Delta\left(p_{pul} - p_{pleu}\right) = \text{Lung Compliance} = C_{lung} \qquad (11.15)$$

Note that p_{pul} is defined as the pressure difference between the space in the lungs and the atmosphere, and p_{pleu} as the pressure difference between the pleural space and the atmosphere. $p_{pul} - p_{pleu}$ thus represents the difference between two pressure differences.

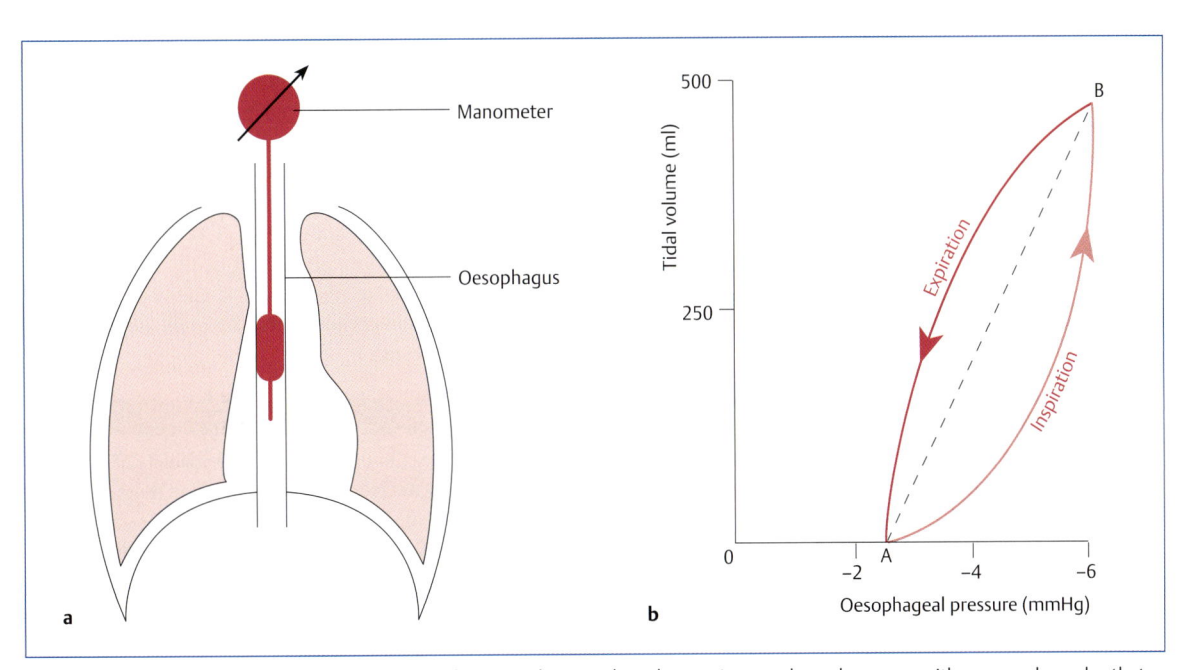

Fig. 11.15 a Measurement of changes in intrapleural pressure by recording changes in oesophageal pressure with an oesophageal catheter. **b** Determination of lung compliance from a respiratory loop. Tidal volume is measured with a spirometer or pneumotachograph, and pleural pressure changes are measured from oesophageal pressure (with an oesophageal catheter as in **a**). The slope of the line connecting the inspiratory endpoint (B) with the expiratory endpoint (A) gives the lung compliance (a measure of the elastic resistances of the lungs only), since in A and in B the respiratory gas flow is suspended and viscous resistances do not play a role at this moment.

If lung volume changes are related to the change in pressure difference between the pleural space and the atmosphere (Δp_{pleu}), the pressure volume curve and **compliance** of the **thorax** are determined. If lung volume changes are related to the change in pressure difference between lung and atmosphere (Δp_{pul}), the pressure volume curve and **compliance** of the entire **lung-thorax system** are obtained.

> **MORE DETAILS**   In vivo, the difficulty in determining compliance is to measure p_{pul} (the difference between intrapulmonary and atmospheric pressure) at different lung volumes. To do this, the lung volume is adjusted to a defined value by respiration from a spirometer, and then the connection to the spirometer is closed. Since there is now no more gas flow, the intrapulmonary pressure is indicated by the oesophageal pressure sensor. However, the pressure determined in this way can only be used if the glottis remains open and the respiratory muscles are completely relaxed. Both require the active cooperation of the test subject and are not possible on animals.
>
> A **simplified method** of determining **lung compliance** can also be performed without the active cooperation of the subject and thus is also possible in domestic animals. Lung volume changes can be recorded with the spirometer (or with a pneumotachograph) and intrapleural pressure changes with an oesophageal catheter during normal resting respiration. An example of such a recording shows **Fig. 11.15 b**. Each respiratory cycle results in a "respiratory loop". The two end points of the respiratory loop represent respectively the end of an inspiration (point B) and the end of an expiration (point A). When changing from one phase of the respiratory cycle to the other, there is a short pause in respiration each time, during which no gas flows. This means that at these two turning points the intrapulmonary pressure is equal to the atmospheric pressure, i.e., $p_{pul} = 0$, and the transpulmonary pressure difference is then $p_{pul} - p_{pleu} = -p_{pleu}$. Thus, the slope of the dashed line connecting A and B in **Fig. 11.15 b** represents:
>
> $$\Delta V_{pul}/\Delta p_{pleu} = C_{lung} \qquad (11.16)$$
>
> Values of C_{lung} change within mammalian species like vital capacities (**Fig. 11.7**) and are proportional to body weight.
>
> Lung compliance is reduced if, for example, after pneumonia, the lung tissue contains more connective tissue and poorly stretchable collagen fibres (pulmonary fibrosis). If a reduced compliance of the thorax is found with the above-mentioned more elaborate procedure, this may be due to a deformation of the thoracic rib cage.

■ Contribution of alveolar surface tension to elastic resistance – surfactant

The surface tension that prevails at the phase boundary between the alveolar gas space and the liquid film on the surface of the alveolar epithelium creates a force that acts to **reduce** the **size** of the **alveoli**. If the full surface tension were effective, as would be expected at a water-gas phase boundary, this would lead to the collapse of many alveoli and thus to a reduction in the gas exchange area of the lung. Lung areas in which the alveoli have collapsed are called **atelectases**. The development of atelectasis is prevented under physiological conditions by reducing the al-

veolar surface tension to approx. 1/10 of the value that would exist if the liquid film on the alveolar surface consisted of pure water. These surface-active substances are called surfactants and consist mainly of phosphatidylcholine, but also of other lipids and proteins. The surfactant is synthesised in the **type II alveolar cells** and coats the epithelial surface of the alveoli as a thin continuous film, where it acts as a detergent at the water-gas phase boundary. During ontogenesis, the production of surfactant increases continuously; the full production capacity is only reached in the mature new-born. Therefore, in an immature **preterm infant, surfactant deficiency** is a problem, leading to atelectasis and inadequate oxygenation of the blood (neonatal respiratory distress syndrome, NRDS).

> **MORE DETAILS**   A functional lack of surfactant can also occur in adult humans and other mammals through damage to the alveolocapillary barrier with plasma leakage from the alveolar capillaries into the alveoli. Formation of a fibrin layer on the alveolar surface and consequent inactivation of the surfactant also leads to massive atelectasis and consequent inadequate oxygenation of blood (acute respiratory distress syndrome, ARDS). ARDS can occur in lung shock in circulatory shock, polytrauma, massive pneumonia or sepsis.

The alveolar surface tension, which is still present even with adequate surfactant, must be overcome by applying force when the lungs are expanded, and the alveoli are enlarged in the process. Thus, surface tension contributes to the elastic resistances. The magnitude of this contribution becomes clear if one compares the pressure volume curve of the gas-filled lung with that of a liquid-filled lung (**Fig. 11.16**). The left dark red curve in **Fig. 11.16 a** shows the pressure volume relationship of a saline-filled lung, the right pink curves the same relationship for an air-filled lung. For the air-filled lung, lung filling and lung emptying occur at significantly different pressures. The pressure volume curve of the air-filled lung is over a range of higher pressures than the pressure volume curve of a fluid-filled lung. The curve of the fluid-filled lung is determined solely by the resistance of the elastic tissue components of the lung (mainly elastic fibres; **Fig. 11.16 b**, left curve). In the case of the air-filled lung, the resistance caused by the alveolar surface tension is added (**Fig. 11.16 b**, right curve).

As an approximation, about **half** of the **elastic retraction force** (and elastic resistance) of the normal lung is due to elastic **tissue components**, the other **half** is due to alveolar **surface tension**.

> **IN A NUTSHELL**   !
>
> Compliance describes the volume expandability of the lung alone, the thorax alone or the lung and thorax together. The compliance of the lung is a reciprocal measure of the total elastic resistance from the elastic components and the surface tension of the alveoli.

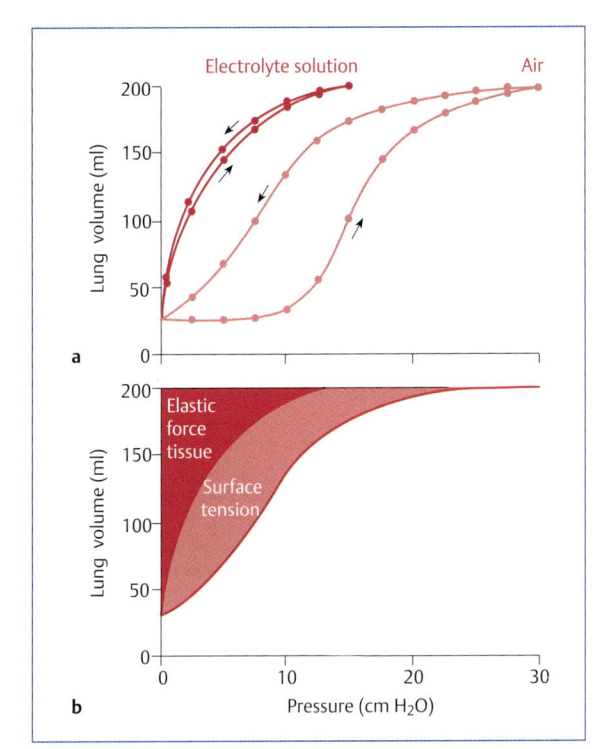

Fig. 11.16 a Pressure volume curves of an isolated fluid (electrolyte solution)-filled human lung (left, dark red curves) and an isolated air-filled lung (right, pink curves). The latter curve shows considerable hysteresis, i.e., shift of the curve between inspiratory filling and expiratory emptying. **b** On average, it is clear that the pressure volume curve of the air-filled lung (pink) runs further to the right than that of the fluid-filled lung (red). This is due to the contribution of the surface tension of the alveoli to the elastic resistances of the lungs, which is present in the air-filled lungs and absent in the fluid-filled lungs. The surface tension on average approximately doubles the pressure necessary to reach a certain volume. The lung volume changes are plotted against the intrapulmonary (= transpulmonary) pressure (measured at rest). [Source: Murray JF. Respiration. In: Smith LH, Thier SO (eds.). Pathophysiology - The Biological Principals of Disease. Section XI. Philadelphia: W. B. Saunders; 1985: 753-854]

■ Pathophysiological significance of compliance

MORE DETAILS Compliance is the key parameter for a whole group of pulmonary dysfunctions. Any pathological reduction in compliance – either of the lungs or of the thorax – is called **restrictive lung dysfunction**. In this group of disorders, increased force must be used to augment thoracic and lung volume during inspiration, so that the expansion capacity of the thorax or lungs is reduced. The maximum achievable lung volume is also typically reduced. This also diminishes the vital capacity. Reduced VC is thus another leading symptom of restrictive lung dysfunction in addition to reduced compliance. One example of restrictive lung dysfunction is lung fibrosis, in which increased collagen fibres have been deposited in the lung tissue.

> **IN A NUTSHELL** !
>
> In restrictive lung dysfunction, compliance is reduced, and vital capacity is decreased.

11.4.2 Viscous resistances

The elastic resistances determine the pressure volume curve of the lung, i.e., they define the relationship between lung volume and intrapulmonary pressure when there is no respiratory gas flow ("at rest"). While the lungs are being filled or emptied, i.e., gas is flowing through the airways, additional resistances have to be overcome: the viscous resistances. The most important part of this is the **airway resistance = flow resistance** of the **airways**, which is expressed analogous to Ohm's law (p. 193) $I = U/R$:

$$\dot{V} = p_{pul}/R \tag{11.17}$$

R is the **airway resistance**, $\dot{V}$ the respiratory gas flow and **p_{pul}** the difference between intrapulmonary and atmospheric pressure. The latter represents (by analogy with electrical voltage) the pressure difference driving the respiratory gas flow.

> **MORE DETAILS** The determination of resistance requires: a) measurement of the respiratory gas flow $\dot{V}$ and b) determination of intrapulmonary pressure. While the gas flow can be measured with a pneumotachograph, the pressure in the alveolar space of the lung is not accessible to direct measurement. This problem can be solved with the **body plethysmograph**, an airtight box in which the test subject sits and in which a highly sensitive manometer measures the pressure. A decrease in intrapulmonary pressure, such as that associated with an increase in lung volume (and thorax), is reflected in an increase in pressure in the plethysmograph box.
>
> For pets, and also for humans, the following alternatives for resistance determination can be used:
>
> **Resistance measurement from respiratory flow and pleural pressure**
>
> For a given lung volume, for two different breath flows $\dot{V}$ the corresponding pleural pressures p_{pleu} are measured. The resistance is then calculated from the change in pleural pressure per change in respiratory gas flow:
>
> $$R = \Delta p_{pleu}/\Delta \dot{V} \tag{11.18}$$
>
> This is based on the following consideration: If – at a given lung volume (for example at the FRC) – expiratory gas flow is increased by $\Delta\dot{V}$ then the observed increase in p_{pleu} is identical to the increase in intrapulmonary pressure required to achieve this. For a given lung volume, the elastic forces of the lung and thorax, and hence the transpulmonary pressure difference, are always the same. Under this condition the above equation is identical $R = \Delta p_{pul}/\Delta \dot{V}$.
>
> **Resistance measurement by means of pressure oscillation**
>
> Pressure waves are generated with a loudspeaker. The respiratory gas flow values and pressures measured at the mouth or nose allow an estimation of the airway resistance. Such devices are used in horses, ruminants and also in humans. Portable devices can also be used under field conditions.

In horses, about 75% of **airway resistance** comes from the **upper airways**, and 25% from the **lower airways** (**Fig. 11.17 a**). In humans, the upper airways are responsible for about 45% of the resistance, the lower for 55%. In the upper airways, the nasal cavity and the glottis are the places of greatest flow resistance.

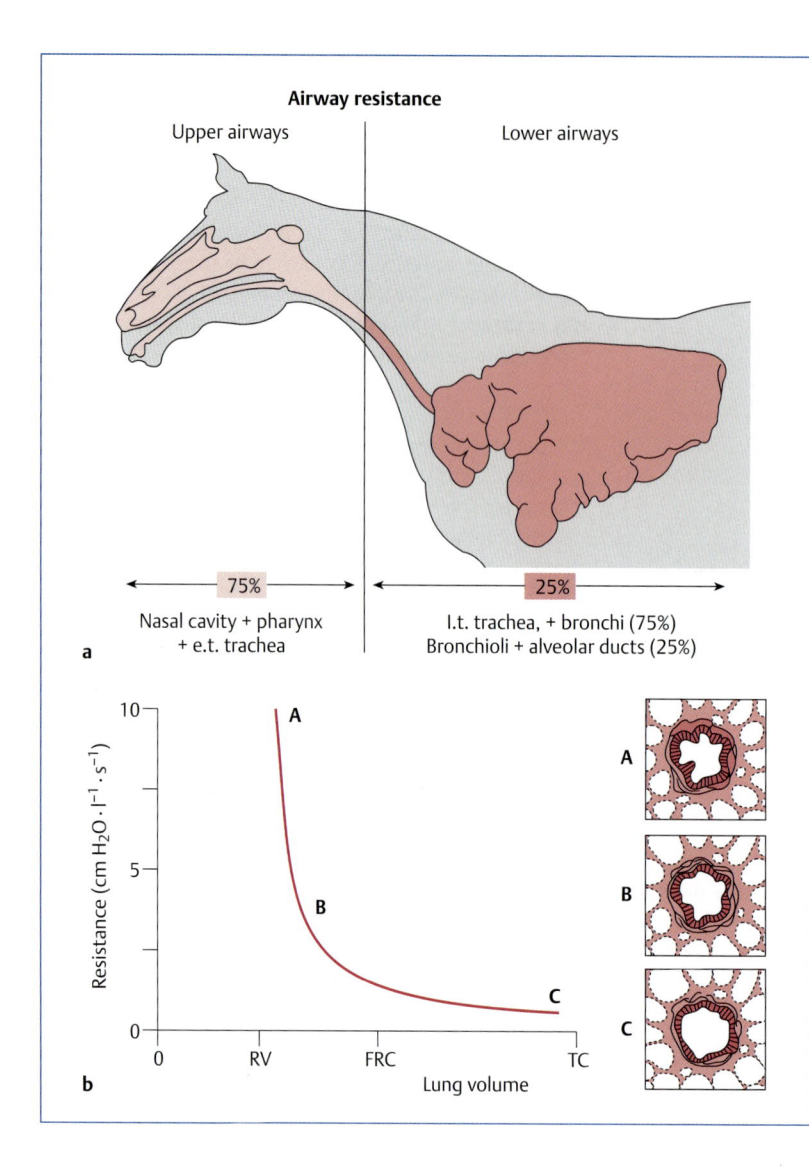

Airway resistance

Upper airways   Lower airways

75%   25%

Nasal cavity + pharynx   l.t. trachea, + bronchi (75%)
+ e.t. trachea   Bronchioli + alveolar ducts (25%)

a

b   Resistance (cm H₂O · l⁻¹ · s⁻¹) vs Lung volume (0, RV, FRC, TC), curve points A, B, C

Fig. 11.17 **a** Distribution of airway resistance in the horse. The upper airways with nasal cavity, pharynx, larynx and extrathoracic (e.t.) trachea account for about 75% of the total airway resistance. The lower airways with intrathoracic (i.t.) trachea, bronchi, bronchioles and alveolar ducts are responsible for 25%. The smallest airways, bronchioles and alveolar ducts, make the smallest contribution to resistance (25% of the flow resistance of the lower airways, i.e., only approx. 6% of the total airway resistance).
b Resistance of the lungs as a function of lung volume. Normally, the resistance of the lungs is measured and indicated at the functional residual capacity (FRC). In humans it is approx. 2 cm H₂O · l⁻¹ · s⁻¹. The figure illustrates that the resistance (R) depends considerably on the state of expansion of the lungs: At maximum inspiration R still decreases somewhat, at maximum expiration the resistance becomes "infinite", i.e., when the residual volume (RV) is reached the lower airways are closed, which ends the expiration process. The cause lies in the lung volume-dependent traction effect of the elastic fibres on the lower airways, as indicated by the airway cross-sections shown on the right edge. [Source: (a) Klein BG. Cunningham's Textbook of Veterinary Physiology. 5th ed., New York: Elsevier; 2012 and Lekeux P, Art T. The Respiratory System: Anatomy, Physiology and Adaptation to Exercise and Training. In: Hodgson DR, Rose RJ (eds). The Athletic Horse. Philadelphia: Saunders Company; 1994, (b) Murray JF. Respiration. In: Smith LH, Thier SO (eds.). Pathophysiology - The Biological Principals of Disease. Section XI. Philadelphia: W. B. Saunders; 1985: 753-854]

The **resistance depends** on **expansion of the lung** and thus on **lung volume**. Fig. 11.17 **b** shows that airway resistance rises considerably with decreasing lung volume. The upper airways are also involved in this, since a decrease in lung volume leads to a narrowing of the glottis and a bending of the larynx, which increases resistance. However, the main cause of the strong volume dependence of resistance lies in the region of the lower airways. As the volume of the lungs decreases, the stretch and tensile force of the elastic fibres of the lung tissue decrease. Since this tensile force also acts on the lower airways and is important for keeping them open, the lumen of the lower airways becomes increasingly narrowed as the tensile force falls until the lower airway system is closed when the residual volume is reached. In a normal respiration position (= normal expiratory position = FRC, functional residual capacity; Fig. 11.6), the volume dependence of the resistance is mainly determined by the larger of the lower airways down to the 10th generation. The smaller airways such as the bronchioles contribute little to total flow resistance (Fig. 11.17 a), since in this region the total cross-sectional space of the airways increases substantially.

■ Pathophysiological significance of resistance

MORE DETAILS   An increase in resistance characterises **obstructive lung dysfunctions**. In the lower airways, swelling of the airway epithelium, increased mucus secretion from the airway epithelia and/or spasm of the bronchial smooth muscle can all lead to a narrowing of the lumen of the bronchi and bronchioles. According to the Hagen-Poiseuille law (p. 193), this results in an increase in flow resistance proportional to the decrease in the fourth power of the radius. Examples of such diseases are COPD (chronic obstructive pulmonary disease) of horses, bronchial asthma and chronic bronchitis. Airway resistance is physiologically controlled by the autonomic nervous system. The sympathetic nervous system causes the bronchial smooth muscle to relax by activating the β₂ receptors, thus dilating the airways and reducing airway resistance. The parasympathetic nervous system constricts the airways by increasing smooth muscle tone, thus increasing airway resistance. As a result of the day-night rhythm of autonomic tone, bronchoconstriction and increased airway resistance occur during sleep. In the upper respiratory tract, pugs and bulldogs are particularly prone to obstruction (p. 294), but so are cats, other dogs, pigs, and horses.

Cystic fibrosis

The secretion of seromucous glands (gll. bronchiales) is important for the maintenance of a fluid film on the surface of the bronchi and thus for the transport of particles through the kinocilia towards the pharynx. The production of serous secretion is impaired in cystic fibrosis, the most common congenital autosomal recessive disease in humans in northern Europe (1:2500), with symptom-free heterozygous gene carriers occurring at a frequency of 1:25. A mutation alters the **CFTR** (cystic fibrosis transmembrane regulator) gene, which is responsible for the synthesis of a **chloride channel**. The channel is present in the apical membranes of epithelial cells in the pancreas, intestine, salivary and sweat glands and bronchi (especially bronchial glands). In the bronchi, the chloride channel, which is controlled by cAMP-dependent **protein kinase A**, mediates the **secretion** of Cl^- and thus also of **fluid**. A disturbance of the channel therefore leads to impaired fluid secretion. This causes a viscous mucus to form in the bronchial tubes, which hinders the "self-cleaning" of the respiratory epithelium and leads to chronic bacterial infection of the bronchial system. Serious obstructive symptoms develop, which are difficult to influence therapeutically and often lead to the death of the patients in early to middle adulthood. In milder cases survival can be for longer.

> **IN A NUTSHELL** !
>
> Flow resistance of the airways is primarily determined by the upper airways and, in the lower airways, mainly by the upper ten generations of the tracheobronchial tree. Increased flow resistance is the main symptom of obstructive pulmonary dysfunction.

11.5 Gas transport in blood

Gerolf Gros

The purpose of ventilation is to bring O_2 from the air by convection into the alveoli, from where it enters the blood through pulmonary gas exchange (p. 282). O_2 is then transported in blood to the O_2-consuming tissues.

Both oxygen and carbon dioxide are present in blood a) **chemically bound** and b) **physically dissolved**. The chemically bound proportion predominates by far for both gases. Nevertheless, the physically dissolved component is very important because it is mainly the dissolved gas that diffuses into fluids and across cell membranes. The concentration of the physically dissolved gas (C_{Gas}) is directly related to the prevailing partial pressure of the gas. (p_{Gas}; **Henry-Dalton law**):

$$C_{Gas} = \alpha_{Gas} \cdot p_{Gas} \tag{11.19}$$

α is the "solubility coefficient" of the gas in blood or in aqueous solution. The concentrations of the dissolved gases determine

- the diffusion of gases across the alveolocapillary barrier (**Fig. 11.5**),
- the diffusion of gases from capillary blood of tissues to the cell mitochondria (or vice versa) and
- the concentrations of the chemically bound gases in blood.

An important difference between O_2 and CO_2 is the value of the solubility coefficient α:

$$\alpha_{CO_2} \approx 20 \cdot \alpha_{O_2} \tag{11.20}$$

This means that CO_2 is 20 times more soluble in aqueous medium than O_2. This also means that the diffusion of CO_2 in aqueous medium is 20 times faster than that of O_2 at the same partial pressure difference.

> **IN A NUTSHELL** !
>
> The diffusion of gases takes place when physically dissolved. The concentration of the physically dissolved gases is proportional to the gas partial pressure. At the same partial pressures, 20 times more CO_2 than O_2 is dissolved in an aqueous medium.

11.5.1 Oxygen transport

O_2 is present in blood either **physically dissolved** or **chemically bound to haemoglobin**. For blood at 37 °C, α_{O_2} equals to 0.037 ml $O_2 \cdot$ (l blood)$^{-1} \cdot$ mmHg^{-1}. At an arterial O_2 partial pressure of 100 mmHg, the concentration of **dissolved oxygen in the blood** (C_{O_2}) amounts to

$$C_{O_2} = 3.7 \text{ ml } O_2 \cdot (\text{l blood})^{-1} \tag{11.21}$$

A much higher O_2 concentration is that **bound to haemoglobin** (HbO$_2$). With a haemoglobin concentration in the blood (C_{Hb}) of 150 g $\cdot$ l^{-1} and full O_2-loading of haemoglobin, then:

$$C_{HbO_2} = 200 \text{ ml } O_2 \cdot (\text{l blood})^{-1} \tag{11.22}$$

This is about **50 times** more than the concentration of **physically dissolved** oxygen.

Haemoglobin (p. 229) is a protein consisting of four polypeptide chains (globins) with a molecular weight of 64500 (**Fig. 11.18**). Hb in vertebrates is present exclusively within erythrocytes at a concentration of approx. 350 g $\cdot$ l^{-1} (MCHC in **Table 9.6**). Each of the two α- and two β-chains of the adult haemoglobin tetramer (left in **Fig. 11.18**) contains a haem (on the right in **Fig. 11.18**). In the centre of the haem structure a divalent iron is held by the N atoms of the four pyrrole rings, which in turn are connected by methine bridges and represent the porphyrin ring of the haem. In addition, the iron is connected to the so-called "proximal" histidine of the globin. Through this connection, conformational changes of the haem are transferred to the globin and those of the globin to the haem, so that there is a close interaction between haem and globin. The valence of iron allows a reversible accumulation of molecular oxygen, a process called **oxygenation**, with the valence of the iron remaining unchanged. In contrast, **oxidation** can alternatively take place, converting the divalent iron into trivalent iron; this produces **methaemoglobin**, which can no longer bind oxygen. Each haemoglobin molecule can reversibly bind four molecules of O_2, resulting in the transformation of **deoxyhaemoglobin** into **oxyhaemoglobin**. The maximum binding capacity of haemoglobin for

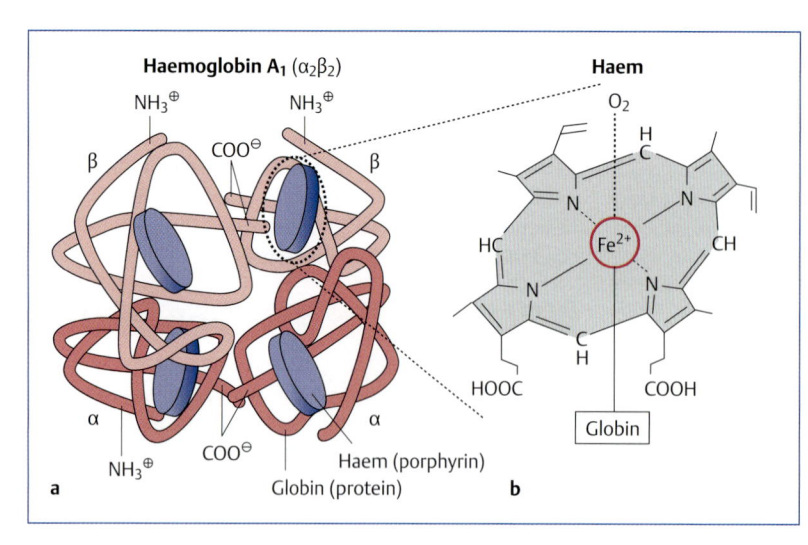

Fig. 11.18 Structure of haemoglobin.
a Three-dimensional arrangement of the 4 polypeptide chains (globins) of adult Hb with two α-chains and two β-chains. The four globins each have an N-terminal (NH_3^+) and a C-terminal (COO^-) end. At the centre of each chain is a haem (blue disc). **b** Haem consists of a porphyrin ring with an iron ion (usually Fe^{2+}) at its centre. The iron is held by two major and two minor valences from the porphyrin ring. There is also a firm bond of Fe to the "proximal histidine" of the associated globin chain, and O_2 can be reversibly attached by means of another minor valence of Fe. When iron is oxidised to Fe^{3+} (methaemoglobin formation), the ability to bind O_2 is lost.

O_2 is 4 mol·mol^{-1}, which corresponds to an **O_2 binding capacity** of **1.34 ml $O_2 \cdot$ (g Hb)$^{-1}$ (Hüfner's number)**.

The **O_2-carrying capacity** of **blood** is determined by the haemoglobin concentration of blood and Hüfner's number:

Hb concentration · Hüfner's number
= O_2-carrying capacity
$$(11.23)$$

The following therefore applies to the O_2-carrying capacity in human blood (Hb ≈ 150 g·l^{-1}):

150 g Hb · (l blood)$^{-1}$ · 1.34 ml O_2 · (g Hb)$^{-1}$
= 200 ml O_2 · (l blood)$^{-1}$
$$(11.24)$$

This concentration of bound oxygen is physiologically almost, but not quite, reached in arterial blood. The haemoglobin concentration in blood of most domestic animals and also in poultry is in the approximate range of 70–190 g·l^{-1} (**Table 9.5**), the O_2-carrying capacity is correspondingly between 100–255 ml·l^{-1}. As can be seen from **Table 11.1**, the O_2-carrying capacity of blood is in the same order of magnitude as the O_2 concentration of the air.

The **oxygen saturation of blood**, S_{O_2}, represents the relative proportion of total haemoglobin that is oxyhaemo-

globin. **Table 11.1** shows that blood is desaturated from near full saturation of 98% in arterial blood as it passes through the O_2-consuming tissues to a mean saturation of 73% in the mixed venous blood of the right atrium.

> **IN A NUTSHELL**   !
>
> 98% of the O_2 in blood is bound to haemoglobin, 2% is physically dissolved. One haemoglobin tetramer can bind four O_2 molecules, i.e., 1 g haemoglobin binds 1.34 ml O_2.

The **oxygen dissociation curve** describes the relationship between the oxygen saturation of haemoglobin (or concentration of HbO$_2$) and the existing O_2 partial pressure (**Fig. 11.19**). Its course has a characteristic **S-shape**. Fig. 11.19 also shows the O_2 dissociation curve of the red muscle pigment **myoglobin** (Mb) which has a **hyperbolic shape**, as is typical for a simple reaction of the type:

$$Mb + O_2 \leftrightarrow MbO_2 \qquad (11.25)$$

O_2 dissociation curve for myoglobin lies much further to the left than that for haemoglobin.

Table 11.1 Blood gases in arterial and mixed venous blood of dogs at physical rest. Corresponding partial pressures and concentrations in atmospheric air and in the alveolar space are also listed.

	P_{O_2}	S_{O_2}	$[O_2]$	P_{CO_2}	$[CO_2]$	pH
Arterial blood	90	98%	200	40	480	7.40
Venous blood	40	73%	150	46	520	7.37
Arteriovenous difference (avD)	–	25%	50	–	40	–
Atomspheric air	155	–	209.5	0.3	0.4	–
Alveolar space (at rest):	100	–	141	40	56	–

P_{O_2} and P_{CO_2} in mmHg, $[O_2]$ and $[CO_2]$ in blood: ml gas · (l blood)$^{-1}$; $[O_2]$ and $[CO_2]$ in gas mixture: ml gas · (l gas mixture)$^{-1}$ (1 mmHg = 0.133 kPa). In addition to O_2 and CO_2, air contains 781 ml · l^{-1} of N_2, and just under 10 ml · l^{-1} of other gases (especially the inert gases argon, neon and helium). In gases, part of the barometric pressure is accounted for by water vapour. The water vapour pressure in the alveoli at 37 °C is 47 mmHg, in air it is considerably lower at room temperature and varies with the humidity.

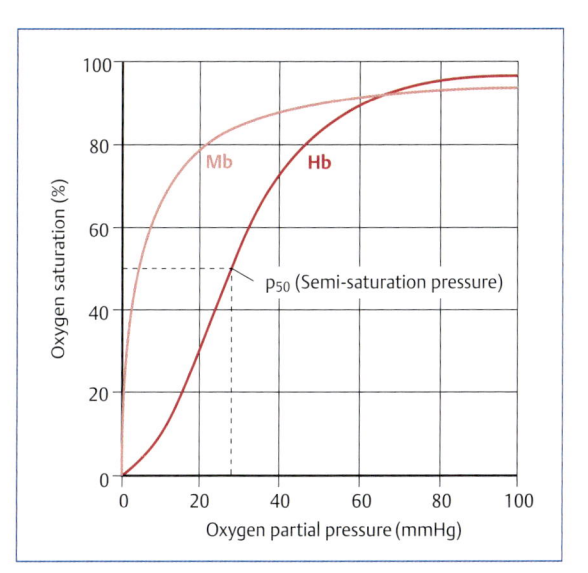

Fig. 11.19 Oxygen dissociation curves of haemoglobin (Hb) and myoglobin (Mb). Hb is a tetrameric protein and shows cooperativity in O_2 attachment, while Mb is a monomeric protein without cooperativity. In addition, the intrinsic O_2 affinity of the haem of Mb is greater than that of the haem of Hb, which places the Mb dissociation curve further to the left compared to the Hb dissociation curve. The O_2 affinities are characterised by the semi-saturation pressure p_{50} (about 27 mmHg for equine Hb, about 5 mmHg for myoglobin). [Source: Pape H-C, Kurtz A, Silbernagl S. Physiology. Stuttgart: Thieme; 2019]

The **S-shape** of the **O_2 dissociation curve** of **haemoglobin** is due to a **conformational change** of the **Hb molecule** induced by the attachment of the first O_2 to an iron in the centre of the haem (**Fig. 11.18b**). When Hb is fully deoxygenated, the four haem structures of the tetramer have a low affinity for O_2, so the initial part of the curve rises only slowly at first with increasing p_{O_2} ("foot" of the S). After the first O_2 molecule has attached to the tetramer, a **conformational change** occurs in the affected polypeptide chain as described above. This change is then transferred to the conformation of the other three chains and the en-

tire tetramer through interactions between the four globins. The changed conformation of the other three globins has now been reversed via the binding of the iron shown in **Fig. 11.18b**. As a result, the iron of the three still free globins increases their affinity for oxygen. As a result, the O_2 dissociation curve now "bends" into the **steep middle section**. The influence of the three not yet oxygenated haems by the O_2 loading of the first haem is called **cooperativity**. It can only occur in a protein molecule that consists of more than one subunit. Therefore, the O_2 dissociation curve of monomeric **myoglobin** (molecular weight 17000) does **not show an S-shape**.

The **biological meaning** of the **S-shaped course** is as follows: The steep middle part of the curve is **shifted** to the **right** by the flat initial part of the curve. This means that physiological desaturation in tissues takes place relatively far to the right, i.e., at relatively high O_2 partial pressures. Thus, there is a high pressure in the capillary p_{O_2} and thus a high driving force for the diffusion of dissolved oxygen from blood to the mitochondria. The delivery of O_2 to the tissue is favoured if the middle part of the dissociation curve is further to the right. On the other hand, the curve should not be so far to the right that at a p_{O_2} of 100 mmHg, as is present in the alveolus, the haemoglobin is no longer nearly completely saturated. The O_2 dissociation curve in **Fig. 11.19** represents a compromise between these requirements.

The **oxygen affinity** of **haemoglobin** is expressed in its position in the S_{O_2}-p_{O_2}-diagram. A shift to the right means low affinity, as high partial pressures are necessary to reach a certain O_2 saturation (S_{O_2}). Oxygen affinity is usually expressed by the partial pressure required to saturate haemoglobin to 50%. This **semi-saturation partial pressure** is called **p_{50}. High p_{50}** means **low** affinity, and **low p_{50}** value **high affinity**. Fig. 11.20 shows the different O_2 affinities of blood of some mammalian species. It can be seen that there is a clear allometric relationship between p_{50} and body weight: the greater the body weight, the lower the p_{50}, i.e. the higher the O_2 affinity. This means that the dis-

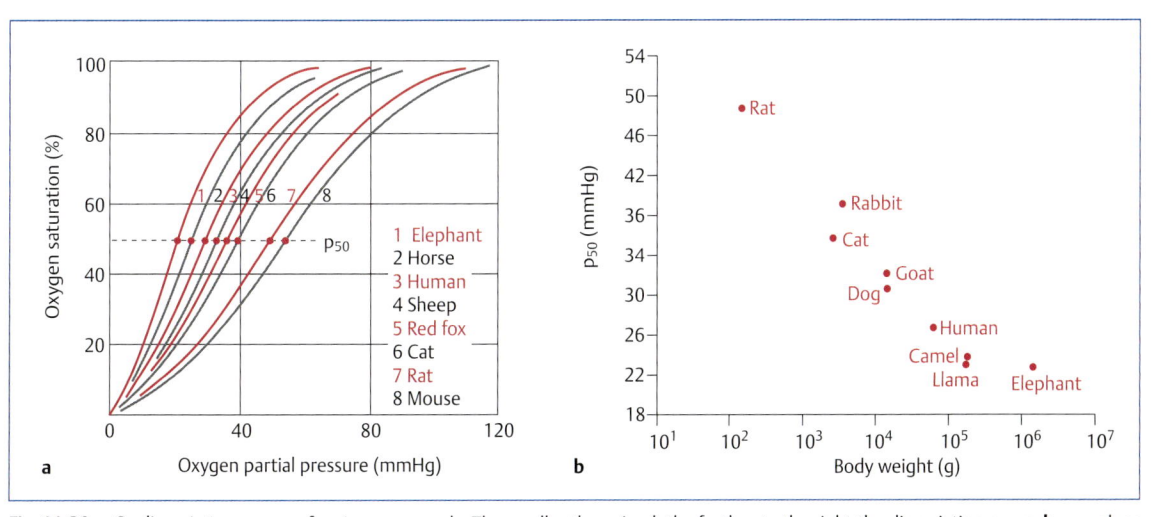

Fig. 11.20 a O_2 dissociation curves of various mammals. The smaller the animal, the further to the right the dissociation curve. **b** p_{50} values of the blood of various mammals. There is an allometric relationship showing an increase in p_{50} with decreasing body weight. [Source: Schmidt-Nielsen K. Scaling: Why is Animal Size so Important? Cambridge: University Press; 1984]

sociation curve lying further to the right in smaller animals is an adaptation to their higher specific O_2 consumption (p.490). A higher capillary pO_2 favours O_2 release into the tissue. The p_{50} values of birds are in a similar range to those of mammals. In contrast, the p_{50} values of fish (p.295), corresponding to the less favourable conditions of O_2 uptake from water, are considerably lower at about 5–18 mmHg, which favours the uptake of O_2 in the gills.

IN A NUTSHELL !

The O_2 dissociation curve of haemoglobin is S-shaped due to cooperativity of the O_2 dissociation of the four haemoglobin subunits. The resulting shift of the steep middle part of the O_2 dissociation curve to the right enables O_2 delivery to the tissue at relatively high O_2 partial pressures. A measure of the position of the O_2 dissociation curve, and thus of O_2 affinity, is the O_2 semi-saturation pressure p_{50}.

Regulation of O_2 affinity

O_2 affinity is not completely fixed, but can be modulated by various parameters. **Fig. 11.21** illustrates the variables influencing O_2 affinity in mammals: **Temperature**, blood **pH**, blood **CO_2 partial pressure** and the intraerythrocytic concentration of **2,3-bisphosphoglycerate (2,3-BPG)**. 2,3-BPG is a product of glycolysis metabolism, present in exceptionally high concentrations in erythrocytes.

The effects of the four variables can be summarised as follows:

- **increase** in **temperature** → **increase** in **p_{50}** = right shift of the dissociation curve
- **increase** in **H^+ concentration** (= **decrease** in **pH**) → **increase** in **p_{50}** = right shift of the dissociation curve
- **increase** of p_{CO_2} → **increase** of **p_{50}** = right shift of the dissociation curve
- **increase** in **2,3-BPG** → **increase** in **p_{50}** = right shift of the dissociation curve

Temperature effect

The temperature effect is because oxygenation of haemoglobin is inversely dependent on temperature (**Fig. 11.21 a**). Especially during physical work, blood temperature in the **lungs** is lower than the core temperature because of the increased ventilation rate, which favours **O_2 binding**. In the **working muscles**, the temperature can be several degrees above the core body temperature (**Fig. 26.17**), which lowers the affinity and promotes **O_2 release to the tissue**.

Effect of pH

The effect of pH is called the **Bohr effect**, and is based on oxygenation of haemoglobin being accompanied by dissociation of H^+ so that qualitatively:

$$Hb + O_2 \leftrightarrow HbO_2 + H^+ \tag{11.26}$$

This dissociation of protons from haemoglobin is due to a shift of pK_a of Hb. pK_a of amino acid residues of Hb changes downward with the conformational change of haemoglobin associated with oxygenation. Conversely, the release of H^+ and subsequent increase in H^+ concentration shifts the reaction equilibrium towards deoxyhaemoglobin, i.e., decreases O_2 affinity and shifts the O_2 dissociation curve to the right (**Fig. 11.21 b**). The physiological benefit of the Bohr effect is seen both in **O_2 uptake** of the **blood** in the **lungs** as well as in **O_2 release** in the **tissues**. In the lungs, CO_2 is released, which raises the pH and also O_2 affinity. In the tissues, CO_2 and (during anaerobic metabolism) lactate (p.627) are produced. The CO_2 is largely converted to HCO_3^- and H^+. Lactate production is accompanied by an equimolar release of H^+, i.e., formation of acid. Both the entry of CO_2 and lactic acid into blood causes pH to fall. This decreases the O_2 affinity and facilitates O_2 release into the tissues.

Effect of the carbon dioxide partial pressure

The effect of CO_2 is largely due to the **Bohr effect**, since a change in the p_{CO_2} is accompanied by a change in pH. A smaller influence is from carbaminohaemoglobin, i.e., CO_2 being bound by the N-terminal amino groups of haemoglobin, which promotes the deoxy conformation of the Hb tetramer. Thus, CO_2 also directly diminishes O_2 affinity (**Fig. 11.21 c**). Physiologically, this effect is in addition to, and in the same direction, as the Bohr effect.

Effect of 2,3-bisphosphoglycerate

2,3-BPG binds preferentially to deoxyhaemoglobin and stabilises the corresponding conformational state of the Hb tetramer, i.e., it shifts the Hb-O_2 equilibrium towards deoxyhaemoglobin and the O_2 dissociation curve to the right. At high altitudes (with low O_2 pressure) there is an increase in 2,3-BPG in erythrocytes and a rightward shift of the dissociation curve, which **facilitates O_2 release** to the tissues (**Fig. 11.21 d**).

MORE DETAILS Only in some non-mammals, such as crocodiles and hagfishes (*Myxinidae*), is O_2 affinity of blood regulated mainly by HCO_3^-.

IN A NUTSHELL !

The O_2 affinity of haemoglobin, i.e., the position of the dissociation curve, can be changed by a number of effectors. Such effectors are pH (Bohr effect), p_{CO_2}, 2,3-BPG and temperature.

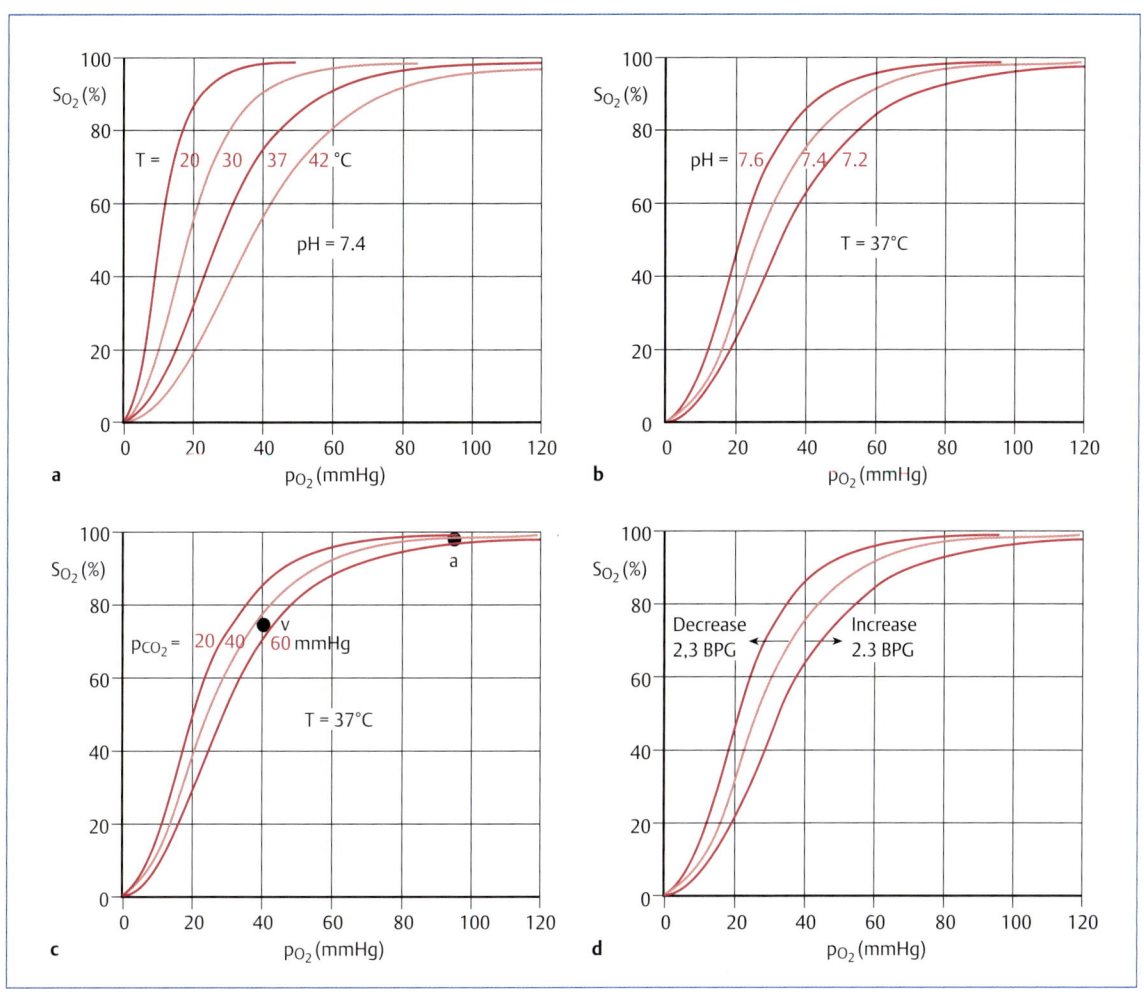

Fig. 11.21 Factors influencing O_2 affinity of blood.
a O_2 dissociation curve at different **temperatures**. An increase in temperature causes a rightward shift of the curve, i.e., a decrease in O_2 affinity.
b O_2 dissociation curve at different **pH values**. pH decrease (= increase in [H⁺]) causes a rightward shift (= **Bohr effect**).
c O_2 dissociation curve at different **CO_2 partial pressures**. Increase of the p_{CO_2} causes a rightward shift.
d O_2 dissociation curve at different concentrations of **2,3-BPG**. An increase in the intraerythrocytic BPG concentration also causes a rightward shift of the O_2 dissociation curve.
Points **a** and **v** in Figure **c** mark the situation in arterial blood (a) and in the mixed venous blood of the right atrium (v). Starting at an arterial O_2 saturation of 98%, the saturation drops to 73% on average during passage of blood through the tissues, i.e., the blood releases approx. ¼ of the bound O_2 under conditions of physical rest. O_2 release in the tissue is facilitated by the venous pH and venous p_{CO_2}. The venous pH is lower (especially in working muscle) than arterial pH (Bohr effect; b). Venous p_{CO_2} is higher than arterial p_{CO_2} (c). [Source: Schmidt RF, Lang F. Thews G. Physiologie des Menschen. 29th ed., Heidelberg: Springer; 2005]

■ O_2 transport in mother and foetus

Mother and foetus of mammals characteristically have **different** types of **haemoglobin**. Fig. 11.22 shows the change from the embryonic state (**embryonic haemoglobin, ε-chain**) to the foetal state (**foetal haemoglobin, γ-chain**) and then to the postnatal state (**adult haemoglobin, β-chain**) in the human new-born. At birth, foetal haemoglobin, a tetramer composed of two α-chains and two γ-chains, still dominates. Postnatally, the foetal Hb disappears within a few months and is replaced by adult haemoglobin, which consists of two α- and two β-chains. Such a change from foetal to adult haemoglobin is characteristic of some mammals, including primates, but not of horses, pigs, dogs and cats, nor of the laboratory animals, rabbits, guinea pigs, and rats, which have embryonic, but no foetal haemoglobin.

The **transfer of O_2** from maternal to foetal blood across the placenta is more difficult than oxygenation of blood in the lungs. In the alveolus, p_{O_2} remains practically constant because oxygen taken up by blood is continuously replaced by ventilation. In contrast, O_2 transfer from maternal to foetal blood, lowers the p_{O_2} of maternal blood which limits O_2 transfer. To compensate for this, various mechanisms exist:

• The **O_2 affinity** of **foetal blood** is **higher** than maternal blood:
  – by a higher O_2 affinity of the foetal compared to the adult haemoglobin (this being an intrinsic property of the foetal Hb (e.g., in sheep and goats where the foetal p_{50} is 10–20 mmHg lower than the maternal)) or
  – by foetal haemoglobin not binding 2,3-BPG (therefore, foetal Hb has a higher O_2 affinity than adult Hb,

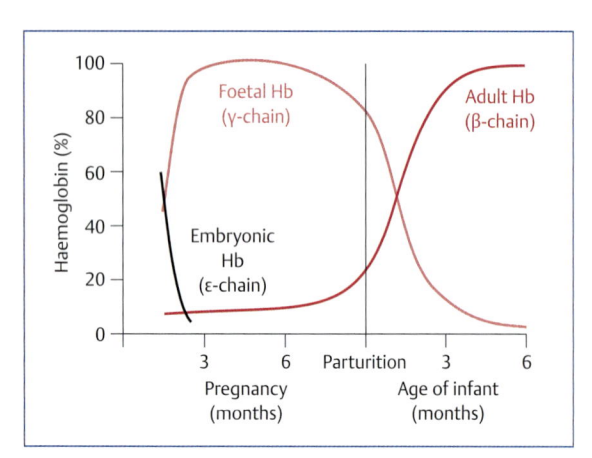

Fig. 11.22 Change of haemoglobin isoforms during human onto-genesis. During foetal life, the initially expressed embryonic Hb (ε-chain) is replaced by foetal Hb, HbF, which consists of two α- and two γ-chains. Postnatally, foetal Hb is replaced by adult Hb, HbA, which is composed of two α- and two β-chains. The proportions of the Hb isoforms are each expressed as a percentage, but the Hb concentration of foetal blood in absolute terms is considerably higher (180 g · l⁻¹) than the Hb concentration after the first year of life (150 g · l⁻¹). In some species (e.g., horse, pig), there is an immediate switch from embryonic Hb to adult Hb, so that new-borns only have adult Hb only. [Source: Young M. Changes in human haemoglobin with development. In: Altman PL, Dittmer DW (eds.). Respiration and Circulation. Bethesda: Fed Amer Soc Exp Biol; 1971]

although the intrinsic p_{50} values of the two haemoglobins are approximately the same (e.g., in some primates)) or
- by absence of 2,3-BPG even in foetal erythrocytes containing adult haemoglobin (because 2,3-BPG is absent from foetal erythrocytes, while present in adult erythrocytes, the O_2 affinity of foetal erythrocytes is therefore higher than that of adult (maternal) erythrocytes (e.g., horses and pigs)).

- The **O_2-carrying capacity** of **foetal blood** is **higher** than that of adult (maternal) blood, because foetal blood has a higher haemoglobin concentration than maternal blood. This is found in calves and lambs, and is particularly pronounced in humans, where the blood of new-borns has a Hb concentration of 180 g · l⁻¹ and maternal blood has a Hb concentration of only 120 g · l⁻¹ ("maternal pregnancy anaemia").

Both mechanisms of higher O_2 affinity and higher O_2-carrying capacity, favour O_2 uptake by the foetal blood by helping to "snatch" oxygen from the maternal blood. They occur together in some species and individually in others. In humans, for example, the affinities are practically the same, but the O_2-carrying capacities are particularly different.

IN A NUTSHELL   !

O_2 uptake by the foetus across the placenta is greatly enhanced by foetal blood having either a higher O_2-carrying capacity or a higher O_2 affinity or both, compared to maternal blood.

■ Blockage of O_2 transport

CO is extremely toxic because its affinity to haemoglobin is 350 times greater than that of O_2. Even at an ambient concentration of CO in air of only 0.004%, as can occur in dense car traffic (compared to 20.95% of O_2), 5% of the Hb is present as HbCO. In heavy smokers, up to 15% HbCO can be found, i.e., 15% of the available haemoglobin is lost for O_2 transport. **Methaemoglobin** (iron oxidised to Fe^{3+}) physiologically makes up about 1% of the total Hb, but in methaemoglobinaemia a considerable proportion of Hb becomes unavailable for O_2 transport.

11.5.2 CO_2 transport

CO_2 in blood is in three states: **physically dissolved** as CO_2, as HCO_3^- and, linked mainly to haemoglobin, as **carbaminohaemoglobin**. In blood, the solubility coefficient of CO_2 (α_{CO_2}) at 37 °C is 0.64 ml $CO_2 \cdot$ (l blood)⁻¹ · mmHg⁻¹. With an arterial CO_2 partial pressure of 40 mmHg (**Table 11.1**), the concentration of dissolved carbon dioxide in blood is

$$C_{CO_2} = 26 \text{ ml } CO_2 \cdot \text{(l blood)}^{-1} \qquad (11.27)$$

This is almost 10 times the concentration of dissolved oxygen in arterial blood, despite the 2.5 times lower partial pressure of CO_2 compared to O_2.

The other two states of CO_2 are also, like the bound state of O_2, found in much higher concentrations than the dissolved amount. **Table 11.1** shows that arterial blood contains a total of 480 ml $CO_2 \cdot$ (l blood)⁻¹, so that the physically dissolved gas accounts for only about 5% of total CO_2. Carbamino-CO_2 accounts for about 5% of total CO_2. This means that HCO_3^- is by far the greatest proportion and accounts for 90% of the CO_2 in blood.

The conversion of CO_2 to bicarbonate proceeds according to the following reactions:

$$CO_2 + H_2O \leftrightarrow H_2CO_3 \leftrightarrow HCO_3^- + H^+ \qquad (11.28)$$

The first step, CO_2 hydration (formula (11.28)), is quite slow without a catalyst, and takes about one minute to complete. In contrast, the second step, the dissociation of carbonic acid H_2CO_3, occurs extremely quickly. Since the transit time of an erythrocyte through the capillaries (contact time) is about 0.7 s, the speed of the hydration reaction of CO_2 would be far from sufficient to convert enough CO_2 into bicarbonate during the tissue passage of erythrocytes and, conversely, conversion of bicarbonate into CO_2 during passage through the capillaries of the lung. Therefore, it is essential for CO_2 uptake into and release from blood that the enzyme **carbonic anhydrase** (CA) is present in erythrocytes. It accelerates the first step of the above reaction by a factor of about 20000.

The reaction equilibrium can be described by the law of mass action:

$$\frac{[H^+][HCO_3^-]}{[CO_2]} = K_1' \qquad (11.29)$$

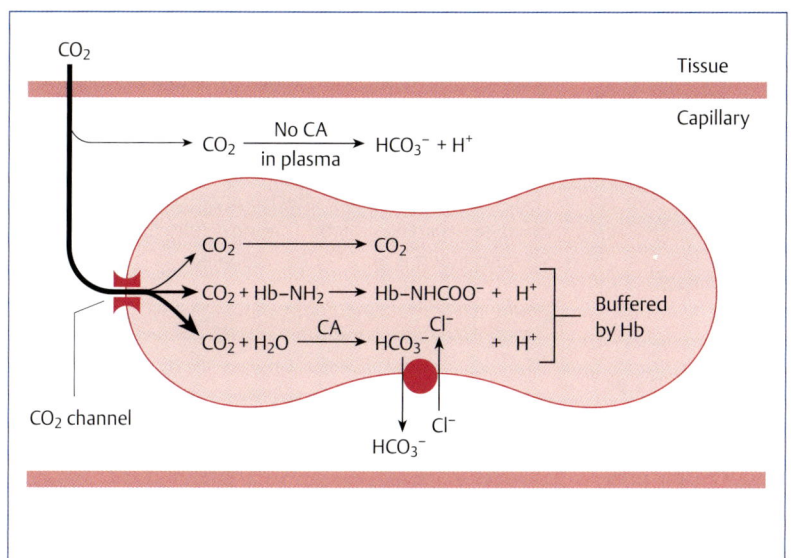

Fig. 11.23 CO_2 uptake by an erythrocyte in a tissue capillary. CO_2 diffuses into the blood capillary in a physically dissolved form. It does not react significantly with water in plasma, as there is no carbonic anhydrase (CA) present. Thus, little CO_2 hydration occurs while in the capillary. However, CO_2 enters erythrocytes via CO_2 membrane channels, where a small proportion remains physically dissolved, another small proportion reacts with the N-terminal NH_2 groups of haemoglobin to form carbaminohaemoglobin and the largest proportion forms bicarbonate by catalysis of carbonic anhydrase. The protons produced along with HCO_3^- are mainly buffered by haemoglobin. More than half of the HCO_3^- then exits erythrocytes into plasma in exchange for chloride via the HCO_3^-/Cl^- exchanger (Hamburger shift). In the lungs, all these processes take place in reverse order.

Circulation, respiration

The concentration of carbonic acid is proportional to the concentration of dissolved CO_2. It is, however, much lower than that of dissolved CO_2 and can therefore be neglected. K_1' is called the first apparent dissociation constant of carbonic acid. The logarithm of this gives the mass action relationship known as the Henderson-Hasselbalch equation (p. 347):

$$pH = pK_1' + \log_{10} \frac{[HCO_3^-]}{[CO_2]} \qquad (11.30)$$

The pK_1' value is 6.10 at 37 °C. From this it follows that the ratio of HCO_3^- to CO_2 at the normal blood pH of 7.40 is 20:1. This explains the large contribution of bicarbonate to the total blood CO_2 content. The Henderson-Hasselbalch relationship makes it possible to calculate the **bicarbonate concentration** from the easily accessible measurement of **pH** and **p_{CO2}** (and thus the dissolved [CO_2]).

The reaction of chemically bound CO_2 as carbamate (carbaminoHb) proceeds as follows:

$$HbNH_2 + CO_2 \leftrightarrow HbNHCOO^- + H^+ \qquad (11.31)$$

The amino groups participating in this reaction are only the four N-terminal amino groups of the haemoglobin tetramer. The CO_2 affinity of these amino groups decreases with oxygenation, so that the carbamino bond of haemoglobin is called **oxylabile**.

IN A NUTSHELL   !

5% of CO_2 in blood is physically dissolved, 5% is as carbaminohaemoglobin and 90% is bicarbonate.

The process of **CO_2 uptake** into **blood** is shown in **Fig. 11.23**. Dissolved **CO_2 diffuses** from the tissue through cell membranes, capillary walls, and blood plasma into the erythrocytes. CO_2 passes through the erythrocyte membrane with the help of membrane proteins that function as

gas channels. CO_2 channels are the erythrocytic aquaporin1, (which is permeable not only to water, but also to CO_2), and the rhesus protein. Inside erythrocytes, a small proportion remains physically dissolved, and a second, also small, proportion forms carbaminohaemoglobin. The greatest proportion forms **bicarbonate**, accelerated by the high **intraerythrocytic carbonic anhydrase activity**. The H^+ ions produced during carbamate and bicarbonate formation are buffered by haemoglobin (**Table 15.2**). In plasma, very little hydration of CO_2 occurs because there is no carbonic anhydrase in plasma. Bicarbonate formation and the presence of both haemoglobin and carbonic anhydrase inside erythrocytes facilitate the removal of CO_2, as haemoglobin is by far the most important non-bicarbonate buffer in blood. The protons are thus released into the erythrocyte cytosol where they can be buffered immediately. Since HCO_3^- is produced only in erythrocytes, an electrochemical gradient for bicarbonate from the inside to the outside is created. Following this, the greater part of the newly formed bicarbonate passes from the inside of the erythrocyte into blood plasma through the mediation of a **HCO_3^-/Cl^- exchanger** (antiport) in the **erythrocyte membrane**. As a result, the greater part of the bicarbonate produced is ultimately **transported** in **plasma**, and **not** in **erythrocytes**. The same process occurs in **reverse** during CO_2 release during erythrocyte passage through the **pulmonary capillaries**. The entire process takes about 0.5 s to complete, i.e., with a contact time of an erythrocyte in the capillary of 0.7 s, the entire process is sufficiently fast to enable CO_2 to pass into the alveolar air.

MORE DETAILS The process shown in **Fig. 11.23** is present in the blood of all mammals and birds and most fish. An exception are the erythrocytes of lampreys and hagfishes, which contain haemoglobin and carbonic anhydrase, but no HCO_3^-/Cl^- exchanger. Thus, their erythrocyte membrane is practically impermeable to bicarbonate.

IN A NUTSHELL   !

The following applies to CO_2 transport in the blood of most vertebrates:
- HCO_3^- and H^+ are formed rapidly from CO_2 almost exclusively within erythrocytes because of the presence of carbonic anhydrase.
- The resulting H^+ ions are almost completely buffered by haemoglobin.
- Subsequently, the greater part of the HCO_3^- is transferred into plasma in exchange for Cl^-.

The **CO_2 dissociation curve** of **blood** is shown in **Fig. 11.24**. The CO_2 content of arterial blood is about twice as high as its O_2 content (**Table 11.1**). The CO_2 dissociation curve is practically linear in the range of physiological partial pressure (40 – 46 mmHg). It is very different from the O_2 dissociation curve (**Fig. 11.19**; **Table 11.1**). O_2 dissociation curve deviates markedly from a linear course between 90 mmHg (p_{O_2} arterial) and 40 mmHg (p_{O_2} venous) with a flat end part.

The other important information in **Fig. 11.24** is the difference between the CO_2 dissociation curves of deoxygenated and oxygenated blood. Deoxygenation of the blood increases its capacity to absorb CO_2. This property of blood is known as the Christiansen-Douglas-Haldane effect or **Haldane effect** for short. The physiological **benefit** occurs in the tissues when **O_2 release facilitates CO_2 uptake**. Conversely, in the **lungs**, CO_2 release is facilitated by the simultaneous O_2 uptake.

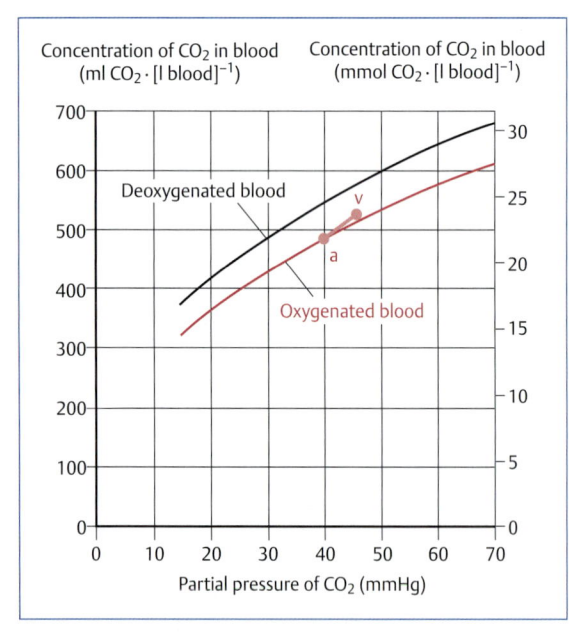

Fig. 11.24 CO_2 dissociation curves of blood (human, 37 °C). The curves are almost linear between the values of partial pressure of CO_2 detected in arterial (a) and mixed venous (v) blood. Fully deoxygenated blood can absorb approx. 10% more CO_2 than fully oxygenated blood (Haldane effect). In vivo, only part of the Haldane effect is apparent, as mixed venous blood is only about 25% deoxygenated, as shown by points a and v in Fig. 11.24. [Source: Schmidt RF, Lang F. Thews G. Physiologie des Menschen. 29th ed., Heidelberg: Springer; 2005]

The Haldane effect has two molecular mechanisms:
- During oxygenation, H^+ ions are released which, by reacting with HCO_3^-, lead to the formation of CO_2, and so enhance the release of CO_2.
- During oxygenation, CO_2 is cleaved from carbamate, which additionally increases CO_2 release. As shown in **Fig. 11.24**, the Haldane effect is only partially effective in vivo, since arterial blood is almost fully oxygenated, but venous blood is only ¼ deoxygenated.

IN A NUTSHELL   !

The Haldane effect facilitates the uptake of CO_2 from the tissues into blood by the simultaneous release of O_2 from blood to the tissues. The reverse process takes place in the lungs.

11.6   Gas exchange

Gerolf Gros

After ventilation of the alveoli, the next step in gas exchange is the diffusion of O_2 and CO_2 across the alveolo-capillary barrier, which is crucial for gas exchange with blood. The alveolocapillary barrier consists of alveolar epithelium, interstitium with basement membrane and capillary endothelium. Its thickness is only 0.5–1 μm (**Fig. 11.5**). The dissolved gases can only pass through this barrier by diffusion. This diffusion process follows **Fick's 1st law of diffusion** (**Fig. 1.6**):

$$\frac{dm}{dt} = -D \cdot A \cdot \frac{\Delta C}{d} \qquad (11.32)$$

Where dm/dt represents the amount of substance diffusing across the barrier per unit time. D is the diffusion coefficient characterising the diffusion rate of the substance. A is the available diffusion area. ΔC is the concentration difference driving the diffusion process and d is the thickness of the diffusion barrier.

Since the alveolar-blood barrier lies at a gas/liquid phase boundary, the above form of Fick's diffusion law cannot be directly applied because the **concentrations** of the **gas in the gas phase** and in the **blood never equalise**, as predicted by the diffusion law. Instead, gas partial pressures must be considered. Using the **Henry-Dalton law** (11.19) one can rewrite Fick's law as follows:

$$\frac{dm}{dt} = -\alpha \cdot D \cdot A \cdot \frac{\Delta p}{d} \qquad (11.33)$$

α is the solubility coefficient of the gas in the tissue of the alveolocapillary barrier and Δp is the partial pressure difference between the alveolus (p_{alv}) and the capillary (p_{cap}):

$$\Delta p = p_{cap} - p_{alv} \qquad (11.34)$$

The **diffusion capacity** of the **lung** characterises the diffusion properties of an individual lung without the need to determine the in vivo inaccessible parameters α, D, A and d. The diffusion capacity D_{lung} is defined by the following form of Fick's diffusion law:

$$\frac{dm}{dt} = D_{lung} \cdot (p_{cap}-p_{alv}) \qquad (11.35)$$

D_{lung} thus combines the "material constants" of the lung α, D, A and d into one quantity.

> **MORE DETAILS** To obtain the diffusion capacity of a lung, the following must be determined:
> 1. dm/dt, which in the case of D_{lung,O_2} is equal to the O_2 consumption of an animal $\dot{V}_{O_2}$, taking place entirely in the lungs.
> 2. p_{alv} can be determined as end-expiratory partial pressure as described above (**Fig. 11.10**).
> 3. p_{cap} can only be estimated from the mixed venous and arterial partial pressure using complex calculation procedures.
>
> The O_2 consumption ($\dot{V}_{O_2}$) can be calculated from the slope of a spirometer recording $\Delta V/\Delta t = \dot{V}_{O_2}$ (**Fig. 11.8**), see ch. Indirect calorimetry (p. 486).

The difficulty of obtaining p_{cap} is generally **circumvented by not determining** the **diffusion capacity** for O_2, **but instead** for that of **CO** at low concentrations. Since the affinity of Hb for CO is extremely high, $p_{cap,CO}$ remains practically $= 0$ in this measurement, so that the above equation is simplified and the determination of p_{cap} is omitted. $D_{lung,CO}$ is then used to estimate D_{lung,O_2}:

$$D_{lung,O_2} = 1.23 \cdot D_{lung,CO} \qquad (11.36)$$

This takes into account the slightly lower value of D_{lung} for CO compared to O_2. $D_{lung,CO}$ in the dog is 7 ml $\cdot$ (mmHg $\cdot$ min)$^{-1}$. D_{lung,O_2} thus results in 8.6 ml $\cdot$ (mmHg $\cdot$ min)$^{-1}$. In mammals, there is approximate proportionality between the size of the diffusion capacity of the lungs and body weight.

Under pathological conditions, D_{lung} may be decreased firstly because the total exchange area (A) of the pulmonary alveolar space is reduced or secondly because the thickness (d) of the alveolocapillary barrier is increased. An example of an increase in d is **pulmonary fibrosis**, where more connective tissue accumulates in the interstitium of the alveoli. Therefore, the clinical signs of restrictive lung dysfunction often include reduced diffusion capacity of the lung. One example of a reduction in A is **emphysema**, in which lung tissue is fused, creating large holes in the lung parenchyma, the so-called bullae (emphysema bubbles), in which both alveoli and blood capillaries have been lost. Therefore, the total alveolar surface area, and thus also D_{lung} are reduced.

> ### IN A NUTSHELL   !
>
> The diffusion capacity D_{lung} encapsulates the diffusion properties of a lung, for example for O_2, D_{lung} is the diffusion coefficient D, times the solubility α, times the diffusion area A, all divided by the diffusion distance d.

Contact time in pulmonary capillaries. In addition to α, D, A, Δp and d, the contact time (dt in Fick's equation) available to an individual erythrocyte for gas exchange with the alveolus also determines the total amount of gas passing over the alveolocapillary barrier. **Fig. 11.25** shows the intracapillary course of the O_2 partial pressure during the mean contact time in the lung of 0.75 s.

Diffusion capacity of the lungs for O_2. The solid curve in **Fig. 11.25** applies to lungs with a normal **diffusion capacity** for **oxygen**. The dotted curve is that for a lung with reduced diffusion capacity (e.g., due to pulmonary fibrosis) where O_2 uptake by blood is much slower. **Fig. 11.25** shows

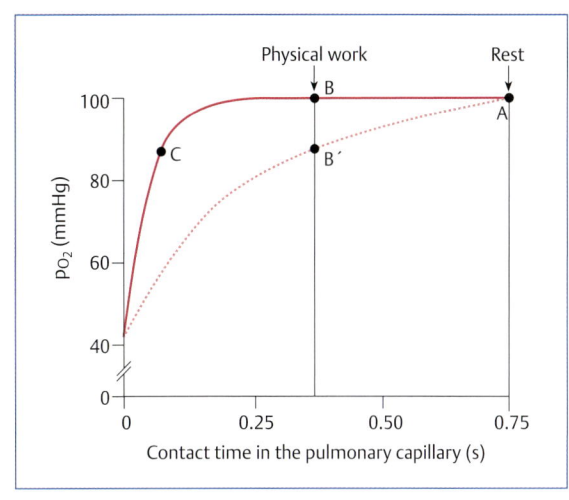

Fig. 11.25 O_2 partial pressure equalisation in the lung as a function of contact time in the pulmonary capillary. Solid curve: normal lung (up to point A) or emphysema lung (up to point B), dotted curve: lung with fibrosis and thickened alveolocapillary barrier. The contact time of the healthy lung at rest (A) is 0.75 s. Physical work with increase in cardiac output can halve the contact time (B and B'), leading to deficient O_2 loading of blood when the alveolocapillary barrier is thickened (B'). Loss of pulmonary capillaries in emphysema can also reduce contact time significantly (B), with further shortening of contact time through work (C) then limiting oxygenation of blood. [Source: Murray JF. Respiration. In: Smith LH, Thier SO (eds.). Pathophysiology - The Biological Principals of Disease. Section XI. Philadelphia: W. B. Saunders; 1985: 753–854]

the effect of some physiological and pathological situations on O_2 uptake:

- In healthy lungs, O_2 uptake is completed after approx. 0.2 s, so that the contact time at physical rest (point A) is adequate.
- During physical work, the cardiac output increases and the contact time is reduced by about 50% due to the increased flow velocity of blood in the lungs. Nevertheless, in the healthy lung with full diffusion capacity between alveolar air and capillary blood, normal p_{O_2} can still be maintained during physical work (B).
- Where there is reduced diffusion capacity due to thickened alveolocapillary membranes (e.g., pulmonary fibrosis), the contact time at rest is just sufficient (dotted curve, A), but when the contact time is shortened by physical work, it is no longer sufficient (B'). Under physical stress, arterial hypoxaemia occurs, which is accompanied by dyspnoea.
- If the pulmonary capillary bed is partially obstructed (e.g., embolism) or partially destroyed (e.g., emphysema), the flow velocity in the remaining capillaries is increased and the contact time is shortened, so that a partial pressure equalisation can still be achieved at rest (B). However, if the contact time is then further shortened during physical work (C), a partial pressure equalisation between alveolar air and capillary blood is no longer possible, resulting in arterial hypoxaemia, again accompanied by dyspnoea.

Thus, both with a thickened alveolocapillary barrier (generally in conjunction with reduced exchange surface A and reduced contact time in the pulmonary capillaries), gas exchange and exercise capacity can be drastically reduced. In healthy lungs, however, the contact time and diffusion capacity are sufficient for O_2 uptake in the lungs, and this is still true even if the contact time is approximately halved during physical work.

> **IN A NUTSHELL**   !
>
> In addition to the diffusion capacity of the lung, the contact time of an erythrocyte in the pulmonary capillary is critical for adequate gas exchange. In healthy lungs the contact time is normally sufficient, but it can become inadequate when the size of the pulmonary capillary bed is pathologically diminished and cardiac output is increased.

Diffusion capacity of the lungs for CO_2. While the diffusion coefficients D for O_2 and CO_2 are very similar, the solubility coefficients α, differ by a factor of 20. Therefore:

$$D_{lung,CO_2} = 20 \cdot D_{lung,O_2} \tag{11.37}$$

Diffusion disorders of the lung with reduced diffusion capacity therefore primarily affect O_2 uptake. Only when diffusion capacity is highly restricted is CO_2 release in the lung also affected. Therefore, the following arterial blood gas findings are characteristic for a diffusion disorder at first:

$$P_{art,O_2} \Downarrow; \; P_{art,CO_2} =; \; \text{named } \textbf{partial insufficiency} \tag{11.38}$$

Only when there are very severe diffusion disturbances will the following situations develop:

$$P_{art,O_2} \Downarrow; \; P_{art,CO_2} \Uparrow; \; \text{named } \textbf{global insufficiency} \tag{11.39}$$

> **IN A NUTSHELL**   !
>
> Diffusion disturbances initially produce a partial insufficiency with reduced p_{art,O_2} and normal p_{art,CO_2}. Only when there are massive disturbances will a global insufficiency of both O_2 and CO_2 result.

Lung circulation. Since the entire cardiac output must flow through the pulmonary vessels, the pulmonary perfusion ($\dot{Q}$) is equal to the cardiac output at rest: approx. 38 in horses, approx. 6 in humans, approx. $4.4 \, l \cdot min^{-1}$ in greyhounds.

Physiological right-left shunt. A small part of the bronchial vessels sends venous blood into the pulmonary vein (carrying arterial blood), and a small part of the coronary venous blood enters the bronchial vessels already oxygenated – i.e., the blood that has already passed through the alveolar capillaries receives an **admixture** of some **venous blood**. This admixture physiologically accounts for about 2% of the cardiac output (physiological shunt). It is responsible for a drop in arterial p_{O_2} by 5 mmHg, even though the end-capillary p_{O_2} of the lung is completely equal to the alveolar p_{O_2} of 100 mmHg. The normal alveolo-arterial p_{O_2} difference ($AaDp_{O_2}$) of 10 mmHg is therefore half due to the physiological shunt. A pathological shunt, such as in a ventricular septal defect, results in greatly reduced p_{art,O_2} and a considerably increased $AaDp_{O_2}$.

Blood perfusion of the lung during physical work. As shown in **Fig. 26.16**, an increase in cardiac output of more than 9 times that at rest, can be observed in horses during heavy exercise. In untrained humans the cardiac output can increase to a maximum of about 4-fold, and in highly trained humans up to 8-fold. How is this increase in pulmonary perfusion achieved? Firstly, the pulmonary blood pressure increases (pulmonary hypertension), which increases the driving pressure difference for lung perfusion. Secondly the vascular resistance decreases as the pressure-passive pulmonary vessels dilate (ch. 8.7 (p.213), **Fig. 8.21**) and the pulmonary capillary blood volume also increases. This means that the contact time in the pulmonary capillaries does not decrease in inverse proportion to the increasing cardiac output. Therefore, the halving of contact time as shown in **Fig. 11.25** is realistic, even during heavy physical work.

Ventilation and blood perfusion. The blood supply to the lungs is not homogeneously distributed. In standing animals at rest, the ventral parts of the lungs are more perfused than the dorsal parts. In horses this ventral-dorsal perfusion difference is in a ratio of about 3:1. The main reason for this is the markedly pressure-passive behaviour of the pulmonary vessels, which causes the vessels to dilate at the higher hydrostatic pressure in the lower parts (ch. 8.7 (p.213), **Fig. 8.21**), while the opposite occurs in the upper parts of the lungs.

In a similar way to lung perfusion, lung ventilation is unevenly distributed in the standing horse. Ventilation is higher in the ventral lung areas than in the dorsal; the ratio of alveolar ventilation to perfusion ($\dot{V}_{alv}/\dot{Q}$) is approximately the same in all regions of the lung. In the standing human, as in the horse, the basal part of the lung is better perfused and ventilated than the apical part.

The good coordination between ventilation and perfusion in all parts of the lung is due to the **Euler-Liljestrand mechanism** (hypoxic vasoconstriction of the pulmonary vessels). In contrast to muscle, where decreased p_{O_2} or increased p_{CO_2} cause a vasodilation leading to an increase in blood flow (p.209), the pulmonary vessels behave the other way round. If an alveolar region is poorly ventilated and p_{O_2} falls and p_{CO_2} rises, the vessels of this area react with vasoconstriction. Hypoxic vasoconstriction of the lung is thus an important mechanism that ensures that ventilation and perfusion are matched. This prevents an alveolus from being heavily perfused even though it is not being ventilated, or vice versa.

MORE DETAILS   Despite the Euler-Liljestrand mechanism, the coordination between alveolar ventilation ($\dot{V}_{alv}$) and perfusion ($\dot{Q}$) is physiologically not as perfect in all species as it is in the horse. In humans, the ventilation-perfusion ratio of the lung is about 0.8 that of the horse, but this ratio is not completely homogeneously distributed within the lung. There are regions of the lungs with either a higher or a lower ventilation-perfusion ratio. $\dot{V}_{alv}/\dot{Q}$ reaches a value of 0.8 only on average. In healthy animals, such a moderate uneven distribution of $\dot{V}_{alv}/\dot{Q}$ is called a "physiological distribution disorder". This can be responsible for 50% of a normal alveolo-arterial p_{O_2} difference of 10 mmHg at rest, thus reducing the p_{art,O_2} by 5 mmHg. In the horse, on the other hand, the alveolo-arterial p_{O_2} difference is only 5 mmHg, which is solely due to the "physiological shunt".

IN A NUTSHELL !

The good, although not perfect, balance between ventilation and blood perfusion in the lungs of all species, is mediated by the Euler-Liljestrand mechanism (hypoxic vasoconstriction).

MORE DETAILS

Distribution disorders

A distribution disorder is an inhomogeneity, beyond physiological levels, of the distribution of $\dot{V}_{alv}/\dot{Q}$ in the lung tissue. In such a condition, the mean $\dot{V}_{alv}/\dot{Q}$ can be completely normal. Nevertheless, such a distribution disorder leads to severe disturbances of gas exchange in the lungs with the main symptom being arterial hypoxaemia (= reduced p_{O_2} in the arterial blood). It can occur in a wide range of lung diseases, such as pneumonia, bronchitis, pulmonary vascular thrombosis, and embolism. It can also be very pronounced under anaesthesia.

Why does an inhomogeneous distribution of $\dot{V}_{alv}/\dot{Q}$ lead to a reduced oxygen exchange? The situation is illustrated in **Fig. 11.26** for a horse with a mean cardiac output (CO) of 38 l·min^{-1} at rest. We can think of the whole lung as divided into two compartments, **A** and **B**. Both compartments are of equal size and equally well perfused; i.e., each compartment receives half of the total lung perfusion (=1/2 CO) of 19 l·min^{-1}. However, their ventilations are extremely different. Compartment **A** with $\dot{V}_{alv}$ = 25 l·min^{-1} receives 5/6 of the total alveolar ventilation of 30 l·min^{-1}. Compartment **B**, on the other hand, with $\dot{V}_{alv}$ = 5 l·min^{-1}, receives only 1/6 of the total alveolar ventilation. The mean ventilation-perfusion ratio of this lung is 30/38 = 0.8, i.e., completely normal. Nevertheless, there is a major problem of gas exchange due to the fact that compartment **A** has a $\dot{V}_{alv}/\dot{Q}$ ratio of 25/19 = 1.3, but compartment **B** has a ratio of only 5/19 = 0.26. The very good ventilation in compartment **A** brings about a slight increase in alveolar p_{O_2} from 100 to 110 mmHg. As can be seen from the oxygen dissociation curve of **Fig. 11.19** this does not lead to a further increase in the O_2 saturation of the blood leaving the alveolar capillary. S_{O_2} is still 98% as in the normal lung (**Table 11.1**). In compartment **B**, on the other hand, the p_{art,O_2} is drastically reduced from 100 to 50 mmHg. Again, it can be seen from **Fig. 11.19** that S_{O_2} is now only 85% instead of 98%. If these two regional bloods mix 1:1 in the pulmonary vein, the average saturation in this blood and then also in the arterial blood is 91.5%, which is significantly below normal arterial saturation. Which p_{O_2} is the result in this mixed blood? This is not determined by the O_2 partial pressures of the blood from the two compartments, nor by their concentrations of dissolved oxygen. Rather, it is determined by the loadings of their haemoglobin with O_2. The reason is that 50 times more O_2 is bound to Hb (p. 275) than is physically dissolved, so the bound O_2 is far more dominant. Therefore, the p_{O_2} of the arterial blood simply results from the saturation of the mixed blood. For S_{O_2} = 91.5%, one reads from the O_2 dissociation curve an arterial p_{O_2} of only 66 mmHg. This means very considerable arterial hypoxaemia – and this despite normal total lung ventilation, despite normal lung perfusion and despite a normal mean $\dot{V}_{alv}/\dot{Q}$ ratio. It is only the inhomogeneous distribution of these parameters across the lung tissue that is responsible for the severe disturbance of gas exchange. The slight, so-called "physiological distribution disor-

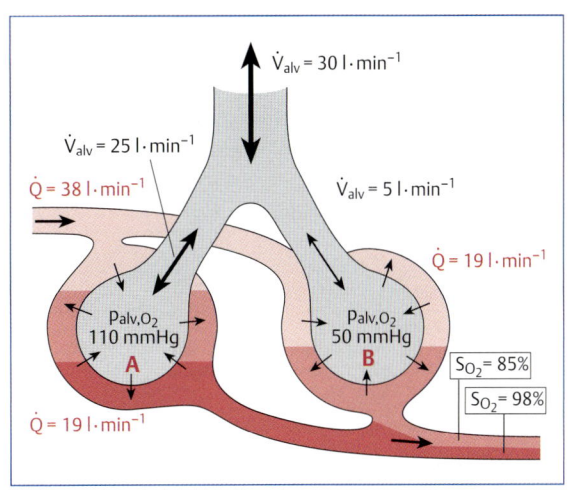

Fig. 11.26 Schematic representation of a distribution disorder of the lung in a horse. The lung consists of two compartments of equal size, which are equally well supplied with blood (each half of $\dot{Q}$ = 38 l·min^{-1}), but are ventilated very differently. $\dot{V}_{alv}$ in compartment **A** amounts to 25 l·min^{-1}, $\dot{V}_{alv}$ in compartment **B** is only 5 l·min^{-1}. As a result, there is a moderately increased p_{alv,O_2} in compartment A (which, because of the dead space, does not correspond to the p_{O_2} of 140 mmHg due to the dead space) and a drastically lower p_{alv,O_2} in compartment in B. As a result, blood leaves the alveolar capillaries of compartment A with an O_2 saturation of 98%, while that of compartment B has S_{O_2} = 85%. The mixed blood that then enters the arterial system has an O_2 saturation of 91.5% and a p_{O_2} of 66 mm Hg (**Fig. 11.19**). This is a situation of severe arterial hypoxaemia (**Table 11.1**). The small arrows symbolise the exchange of O_2 and CO_2 across the alveolocapillary barrier.

der", which is present in humans and several other species, leads to a moderate reduction in the p_{art,O_2} compared to the p_{alv,O_2} by 5 mmHg.

The fact that the mixture of blood from compartments **A** and **B** does not result in a normal mean p_{art,O_2} is due to the non-linear course of the O_2 dissociation curve in the range between 110 and 50 mmHg (**Fig. 11.19**). Since, as mentioned (**Fig. 11.24**), the CO_2 dissociation curve is practically linear in the range of CO_2 partial pressures occurring in vivo, a distribution disturbance remains without consequences for the p_{art,CO_2}. It is therefore a characteristic feature of a distribution disturbance that the p_{art,O_2} is greatly reduced, but the p_{art,CO_2} is normal, i.e., there is **partial insufficiency**. This is accompanied by an **increased alveolo-arterial O_2 partial pressure difference (AaDp$_{O_2}$)**. In our case the mean p_{art,O_2} of 100–66 = 34 mmHg: a value that is normally only 5–10 mmHg.

Extreme cases of distribution disorders are lung compartments that are well supplied with blood, but are not ventilated (**functional shunt**), or those that are well ventilated, but are not perfused (**functional dead space**).

IN A NUTSHELL !

Even if the global ventilation and perfusion of a lung are normal, inhomogeneities in the distribution of the ventilation-perfusion ratio (distribution disorder) can lead to severe disturbances in gas exchange, mainly affecting the p_{art,O_2}.

Circulation, respiration

Table 11.2 Characteristics of gas exchange in different lung dysfunctions.

Pulmonary dysfunction	P_{art,O_2}	$AaDp_{O_2}$	P_{art,CO_2}	Increase of p_{art,O_2} when inspirating 100% O_2	Blood gases
Restrictive ventilation disorder (without diffusion disorder!)	↓	=	↑	clearly	Global insufficiency
Obstructive ventilation disorder	↓	=	↑	clearly	Global insufficiency
Diffusion disorder	↓	↑	=	clearly	Partial insufficiency
Pathological shunt	↓	↑	=	hardly	Partial insufficiency
Distribution fault	↓	↑	=	clearly	Partial insufficiency

↓ decreased, ↑ increased, = remains the same

MORE DETAILS

Gas exchange in various lung dysfunctions

Common to all disorders is the leading symptom of arterial hypoxaemia, i.e., reduced p_{art,O_2}. Differences exist between P_{art,CO_2} and the alveolo-arterial p_{O_2} difference. In addition, an increase in inspiratory oxygen concentration exerts different effects on the O_2 pressure in the arterial blood when comparing diseases (**Table 11.2**).

Global insufficiency is characteristic of all ventilatory disorders. Shunt, diffusion and distribution disorders are characterised by partial insufficiency. For the differential diagnosis of shunt distribution disorder, the effect of an increased inspiratory O_2 concentration on the AaD for p_{O_2} can be used. Under 100% oxygen breathing, the AaD largely disappears in distribution disorders, whereas it remains or even increases in the case of pathological shunt (= 100% oxygen test).

11.7 Tissue respiration (internal respiration)

Gerolf Gros

11.7.1 O_2 supply and O_2 consumption in the tissues

■ Diffusion of respiratory gases in the tissues

After oxygen in blood arrives in the tissue capillaries (**Fig. 11.2**), "**tissue respiration**" follows. This is the transport of O_2 from the capillary to the cell mitochondria and its utilisation, with conversely the formation of CO_2 in the cell and its removal to the capillary. As in the alveolocapillary barrier of the lung, O_2 transport into the **tissue** must travel the distance by diffusion of the physically dissolved gas. In contrast to the **lung**, however, where the diffusion distance is only 0.5 μm, much greater distances have to be overcome. These are the distances between capillaries in the tissue. The **distance** between two capillaries must then be overcome by diffusion from each so that all cells in the region are supplied with O_2. Capillary distances are approx. 25 μm apart in cardiac muscle, approx. 40 μm in cerebral cortex and approx. 80 μm in skeletal muscle. These large diffusion distances can be overcome by **diffusion** of **O_2**, because **large partial pressure gradients** exist even between the capillary and the margins of its supply region. Since mitochondrial cytochrome oxidase is still oxidised at O_2 partial pressures as low as 0.1 mmHg, the minimum

p_{O_2} in the tissue is near zero. This situation is described in **Fig. 11.27**, illustrating the classical concept of the Danish physiologist August Krogh (1874–1949). The tissue to be supplied is assumed to be composed of many "supply cylinders", with a capillary running in the centre of each cylinder. The radius of the cylinder corresponds to the largest diffusion distance to be overcome, 30 μm in the example of the **Fig. 11.27** (the distance between the capillaries is set to 60 μm). At the arterial end, the p_{O_2} of blood in the capillary is 90 mmHg, while at the venous end only 30 mmHg. This difference reflects the amount of O_2 delivered to the tissue by diffusion along the course of the capillary. From the capillary towards the periphery of the cylinder, the p_{O_2} drops by approx. 30 mmHg, which means that the tissue reaches a lower p_{O_2} the greater the distance from the capillary. This shows that diffusion has a limit. At the venous

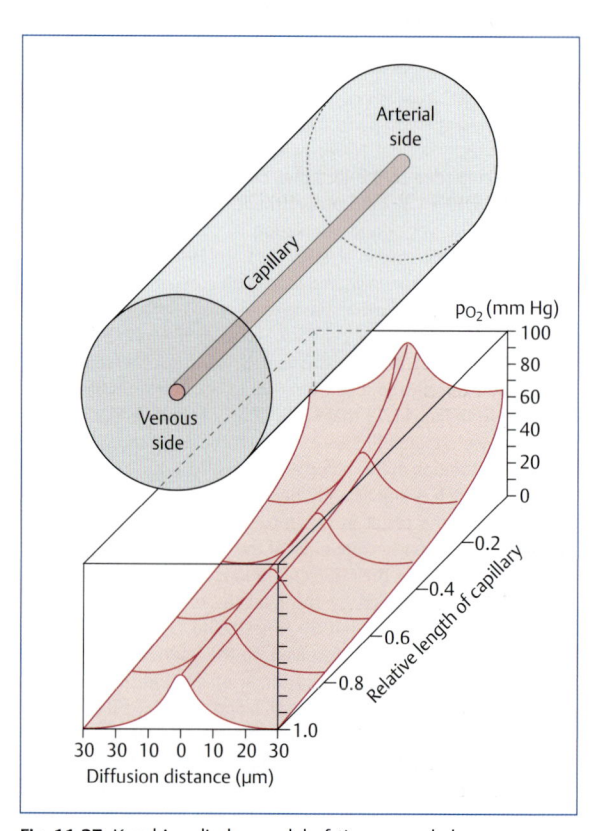

Fig. 11.27 Krogh's cylinder model of tissue supply by oxygen diffusion from the blood capillary. Y-axis: p_{O_2} in capillary or tissue. The diffusion process causes a drop in the p_{O_2} from the capillary towards the periphery of the cylinder by approx. 30 mmHg.

end of the cylinder, the p_{O_2} can drop to 0 mmHg in the periphery of the cylinder. The partial pressures in the tissue therefore vary between an arterial value of about 90 mmHg (immediately at the entry of a capillary) to very low values (at the edge of the supply region). The p_{O_2} is therefore very unevenly distributed throughout the tissue. If the O_2 supply deteriorates, the regions at greatest distance from a capillary, especially at its venous end, will therefore be the first to become anoxic, while those close to the capillary are still sufficiently supplied.

The **diffusion** of **CO_2** is about 20 times faster than that of O_2 due to its higher solubility. Since CO_2 has to diffuse the same distances as O_2, but in the opposite direction, the **CO_2 partial pressure gradients** in the tissue are much smaller than those for O_2.

■ O_2 supply

The O_2 supply is the amount of O_2 transported by blood per unit of time. It depends on the arterial O_2 concentration (C_{art,O_2}) and the blood flow to the tissue:

$$O_2 \text{ supply} = C_{art,O_2} \cdot \text{blood flow} \tag{11.40}$$

Or, since almost the entire O_2 content of blood is bound to haemoglobin,

$$O_2 \text{ supply} = S_{art,O_2} \cdot C_{Hb} \cdot 4 \cdot \text{blood flow} \tag{11.41}$$

S_{art,O_2} is the arterial oxygen saturation of haemoglobin and C_{Hb} is the haemoglobin concentration of blood in $mol \cdot l^{-1}$ (tetramer! =4). This shows that O_2 supply to the organs can be endangered if the arterial saturation of haemoglobin (in lung dysfunction) or the haemoglobin concentration of blood (in anaemia) are severely reduced, or if the blood supply to the organ is insufficient (in lowered arteri-

al blood pressure or strong vasoconstriction). On the other hand, there is a **reserve O_2 supply** because O_2 consumption in the tissues is normally less than the supply. Under resting conditions, venous blood still contains a considerable O_2 concentration: **mixed venous blood** from the right atrium still has an **O_2 saturation** of **73%** (Table 11.1).

The O_2 supply to the heart varies greatly during systole when, as a result of contraction of the ventricles, the heart vessels are compressed and the coronary blood flow drops very sharply; see ch. on cardiac energetics (p. 180) and blood pressure. During systolic contraction, the heart must take its oxygen from the available supplies. These are physically dissolved O_2, the oxyhaemoglobin of the blood present in the capillaries and the oxygen bound by the **myoglobin** of the heart muscle cells. Myoglobin is particularly important for this function because of its low p_{50} (5 mmHg; **Fig. 11.19**, light pink curve). It is almost fully loaded with O_2 under normal conditions and can thus release a lot of O_2 in case of O_2 deficiency.

■ O_2 consumption

The O_2 consumption of an organ is determined from the arteriovenous concentration difference for O_2 (avD_{O_2}) and the rate of blood flow:

$$O_2 \text{ consumption} = avD_{O_2} \cdot \text{blood flow} \tag{11.42}$$

avD_{O_2} is defined as ($C_{art,O_2} - C_{ven,O_2}$). C_{ven,O_2} applies to the venous blood of an organ. This is an application of **Fick's principle** (mass balance for O_2), which enables the O_2 consumption of an organ to be determined from measurements of blood flow and arterial and organ venous O_2 concentration or saturation. **Table 11.3** shows O_2 consumption and blood flow for some organs.

Table 11.3 Specific O_2 consumption and specific blood flow of various organs in humans. Mean values under resting conditions (except cardiac and skeletal muscle). O_2 consumption and blood flow are given per kg tissue wet weight.

Organ	Organ weight (kg)	O_2 consumption $(ml \cdot min^{-1} \cdot kg^{-1})$	Blood flow $(ml \cdot min^{-1} \cdot kg^{-1})$	avD_{O_2} $(ml \cdot (100\,ml)^{-1})$	O_2 utilisation
Skeletal muscle	30	–			
▪ At rest	–	2	40	5	25%
▪ Heavy exercise	–	200	1200	17	85%
Heart	0.3	–			
▪ At rest	–	100	700	15	75%
▪ Heavy exercise	–	up to approx. 500	up to approx. 3000	17	85%
Liver	1.5	56	1000	5.6	28%
Brain (total)	1.5	35	500	7	35%
▪ Cortex	–	80	800	–	–
▪ Medulla	–	15	250	–	–
Kidney (total)	0.3	60	4000	1.5	7.5%
▪ Cortex	–	90	5000	–	–
▪ Outer medulla	–	60	1200	–	–
▪ Inner medulla	–	4	250	–	–
Skin	0.5	0.9	100	0.9	4.5%

Specific O_2 consumption in $ml\ O_2 \cdot min^{-1} \cdot (kg\ wet\ weight)^{-1}$; specific blood flow in $ml\ blood \cdot min^{-1} \cdot (kg\ wet\ weight)^{-1}$; avD_{O_2} = arteriovenous concentration difference for O_2 in $ml\ O_2 \cdot (100\ ml\ blood)^{-1}$. Utilisation is calculated using C_{art,O_2} = 200 ml $O_2 \cdot (l\ blood)^{-1}$ (**Table 11.1**) (data based on Schmidt RF, Lang F. Thews G. Physiologie des Menschen. 29th ed. Heidelberg: Springer; 2005).

Both O_2 consumption and blood flow depend very strongly on the metabolic activity of the organs. A reduction in C_{ven,O_2} increases the avD_{O_2} and thus, apart from an increase in blood flow, the O_2 consumption of an organ can also increase. The O_2 consumption rates of skeletal and cardiac muscles increase particularly strongly during physical work.

Table 11.3 also shows that there are **regional differences** in O_2 consumption within organs. Examples are the brain where the cortex has a higher consumption than the medulla. In the kidney the blood flow into the inner medulla is 20 times less than into the renal cortex.

The **O_2 utilisation** describes the relationship between O_2 consumption and O_2 supply by their quotients:

$$O_2 \text{ utilisation} = \frac{O_2 \text{ consumption}}{O_2 \text{ supply}}$$
$$= \frac{avD_{O_2} \cdot \text{blood flow}}{C_{art,O_2} \cdot \text{blood flow}} = \frac{avD_{O_2}}{C_{art,O_2}} \qquad (11.43)$$

Since O_2 utilisation is the ratio of avD_{O_2} to arterial O_2 concentration, it indicates the extent to which the O_2 content of arterial blood has been "exhausted". If the O_2 utilisation has a value of 25%, as in resting muscle, this means that 25% of the O_2 content of arterial blood has been depleted. O_2 utilisation is very different in different organs under resting conditions (Table 11.3). The kidney has a particularly low utilisation of only 7.5%, so the renal venous blood has a particularly high O_2 saturation of 90.7%. Low oxygen utilisation is mainly due to extraordinarily high blood flow rate through the kidney. The heart, on the other hand, has a particularly high utilisation of 75% even at physical rest. Consequently, the coronary venous blood has a particularly low O_2 saturation of only 25%, which is only slightly lowered further during exercise.

■ Increased O_2 consumption of organs with increased metabolic activity

Increased O_2 consumption occurs with an **increase in blood flow**, which increases O_2 supply, and an **increase in O_2 utilisation by the perfused tissue**. Table 11.3 shows the values of resting and working skeletal muscle. During work, blood flow can be increased by a factor of 30 in men (Table 11.3), and in a sport horse even by a factor of 70 (Fig. 26.16). The avD_{O_2} is elevated at the same time by a factor of 3.4. This means that the O_2 consumption of working muscle can be increased by a factor of more than 100–200. In the heart, on the other hand, an increase in O_2 consumption is only possible to a maximum of 5 times. This is essentially achieved by increasing coronary blood flow.

IN A NUTSHELL !

The oxygen supply to tissues exceeds their O_2 consumption: about 0.2 times in the heart during exercise, about 4 times in muscle at rest, and up to 20 times in skin. Through a combination of increased organ perfusion and an increase in the arteriovenous O_2 concentration difference, a massive increase in O_2 supply can be achieved.

11.7.2   Disorders of O_2 supply

Tissue hypoxia (p_{O_2} < normal) or even **tissue anoxia** (p_{O_2} = 0) is caused by inadequate O_2 supply to organs. It can be caused by arterial hypoxaemia (reduced p_{art,O_2}), ischaemia (insufficient blood supply) or anaemia (reduced O_2-carrying capacity of blood). All three disorders lead to a reduction in O_2 supply. However, disorders of O_2 supply can also be caused by disorders of O_2 utilisation in cells, such as by poisoning of enzymes of the respiratory chain.

MORE DETAILS

Hypoxaemic tissue hypoxia

This disorder is due to **reduced oxygen saturation** of **arterial blood**. The typical cause is impaired lung function due to hypoventilation resulting from restrictive or obstructive ventilation disorders, distribution disorders, or diffusion disorders. The same problem can occur at high altitudes because of reduced p_{O_2} in the inspired air. This is illustrated in **Fig. 11.28a**, which shows the effect of arterial hypoxia on O_2 supply to a tissue (p_{art,O_2} 40 instead of 90 mmHg). The O_2 content of arterial blood is markedly reduced, which is partly compensated for by the blood in the tissues releasing more oxygen than normal. Nevertheless, capillary p_{O_2} as well as venous p_{O_2} both decline. This results in a reduction in the O_2 partial pressure gradient between a capillary and the cells of a tissue. At the arterial end, the capillary blood has a p_{O_2} of only 40 mmHg, and at the venous end only about 20 mmHg. This reduces the capillary blood flow according to Fick's diffusion law (ch. 11.6 (p. 282), formula (11.32)), and the diffusion rate of O_2 into the tissue (**Fig. 11.27**). A decrease in the arterial O_2 content thus necessarily causes deterioration in O_2 supply, which can lead to tissue hypoxia and finally to anoxic regions in the tissue. With prolonged arterial hypoxaemia, erythropoiesis is stimulated. The resulting increase in the haemoglobin concentration of blood, with a consequent increase in blood O_2-carrying capacity, can partially compensate for this disturbance.

Anaemic tissue hypoxia

In this disorder, O_2 supply to the tissues is reduced due to the **lowered O_2-carrying capacity** of blood. Anaemia can be caused by blood loss or a disorder of erythrocyte production or a shortened life span of erythrocytes. Increased concentration of methaemoglobin or an increased amount of carbon monoxide-loaded haemoglobin (functional anaemia) also lead to a decrease in the O_2-carrying capacity. The consequences are illustrated by the O_2 dissociation curve in **Fig. 11.28b** for the heart. If the haemoglobin concentration of blood is reduced from 150 g/l to 100 g/l the arterial O_2 content and thus the O_2 supply is reduced even with normal lung function. This is partially compensated for by a reduction in venous O_2 content. In the example of **Fig. 11.28b**, this leads to a reduction of the organ venous p_{O_2} from 25 to approx. 19 mmHg. This in turn diminishes the oxygen supply to a tissue by diffusion.

Ischaemic tissue hypoxia

Ischaemia is **restricted organ perfusion**, which also leads to a reduction in the O_2 supply. The resulting hypoxia, like the other two disorders, is accompanied by a marked decrease in venous p_{O_2} and venous O_2 saturation, which only partially compensates for the decrease in O_2 supply. **Fig. 11.28c** illustrates the situation. Hb concentration of blood and lung function are both normal, but because of deficient perfusion, the blood becomes more desaturated during tissue passage, the avD_{O_2} is thus increased. The illustration shows that this in turn leads to a reduced end-capillary venous blood supply and thus reduced tissue supply through O_2 diffusion, which results in tissue hypoxia. Ischaemia can occur in many organs simultaneously through a drop in arterial pressure (circulatory shock) or in only one organ, e.g., due to vascular occlusion (infarct, thrombosis, embolism).

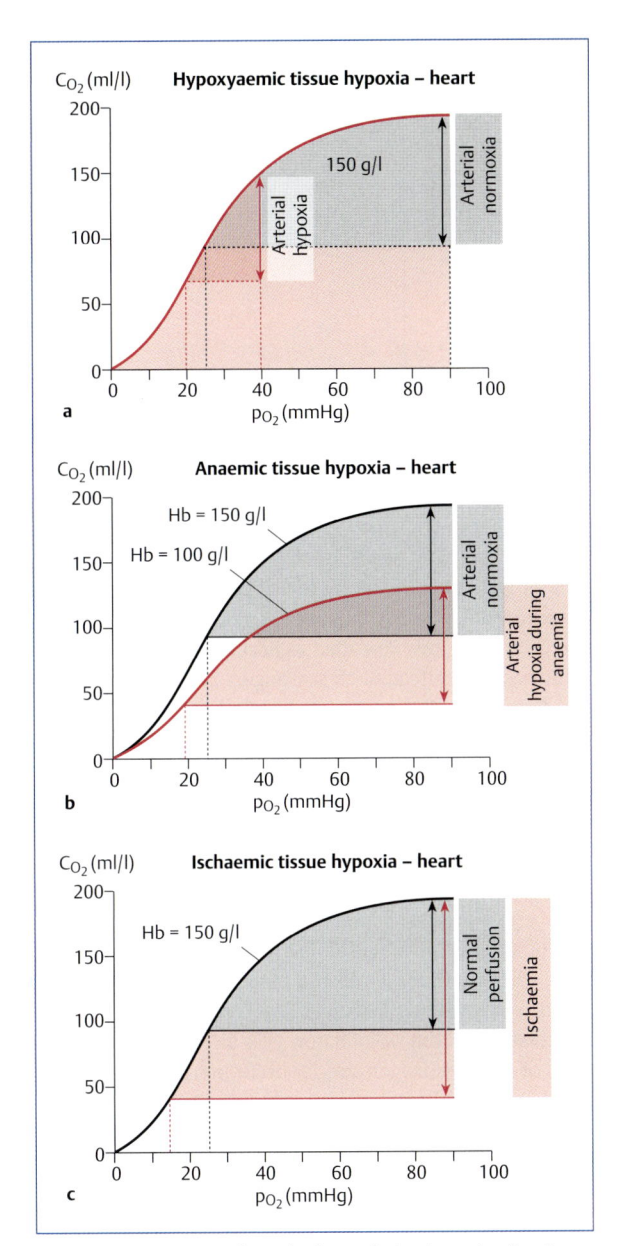

Fig. 11.28 Oxygen supply to the heart during hypoxia of various causes.

a Effect of arterial hypoxia on tissue O_2 supply illustrated by the haemoglobin oxygen dissociation curve for the heart. Regarding blood supply to the heart, at physical rest and at normal p_{art,O_2} of 90 mmHg, the p_{O_2} at the venous end of the capillary drops to 25 mmHg, which can be interpreted as an expression of the particularly large avD_{O_2} in the heart (**Table 11.3**). When arterial p_{O_2} drops to 40 mmHg, the venous p_{O_2} then drops to as low as 20 mmHg. The result is a reduced p_{O_2} slope towards the tissue and thus a reduced O_2 supply of the tissue by diffusion (**Fig. 11.27**, see formula (11.32)). [Source: Schmidt RF, Thews G. Physiologie des Menschen. 23rd ed., Heidelberg: Springer; 1987]

b Effect of anaemia on tissue O_2 supply. As the arterial O_2 content of blood is reduced in anaemia, even with normal lung function, the blood in the tissues is desaturated further than normal, resulting in a reduced end-capillary p_{O_2}. The latter results in a deteriorated supply of O_2 to the tissues. [Source: Schmidt RF, Thews G. Physiologie des Menschen. 23rd ed., Heidelberg: Springer; 1987]

c Effect of ischaemia on the O_2 supply to the heart. The reduced organ perfusion leads to an increased D_{O_2} and thus to decreased end capillary p_{O_2}. This results in tissue hypoxia as shown in **Fig. 11.28a** and **Fig. 11.28b**.

11.7.3 Tissue hypoxia in diving mammals

MORE DETAILS During **diving**, air-breathing vertebrates are cut off from their O_2 supply. They depend on their body's O_2 stores, which are mainly the haemoglobin in blood, the myoglobin of muscles and the gaseous O_2 in the lungs. Many diving species (e.g., dolphins, whales, seals) have much higher amounts of myoglobin and haemoglobin than humans and thus have a much larger storage capacity for O_2 in their bodies. The O_2 content of the lungs is usually not very important, since the lungs of many diving species are small (e.g., 1% of body volume in the duck whale) and since some species, such as the Weddell seal, exhale before they submerge. The purpose of the last two adaptations is to keep the volume of gas in the alveolar space as low as possible.

The latter adaptation minimises the effect of increased alveolar gas pressure during diving. The high-pressure gas of the alveoli diffuses into blood and tissues in correspondingly large quantities, which can lead to the formation of gas bubbles during a rapid ascent to the surface and an accompanying rapid reduction of the gas partial pressures in the body. In the blood capillaries, the formation of gas bubbles has the effect of embolism, i.e., blockage of organ perfusion (Caisson's disease or decompression sickness). The less gas in the alveoli, the less likely it is that Caisson disease will occur. In humans, the problem of Caisson disease can be reduced if, when diving with a gas cylinder to supply oxygen, the inspiratory and alveolar gas contains helium instead of N_2, the major component of air. Since helium is much less soluble in water than N_2, the risk of gas bubbles forming during surfacing is significantly reduced. This allows professional divers to reach diving depths down to 600 m.

An increase only in the O_2 stores of haemoglobin and myoglobin in diving animals, however, would not be sufficient to sustain diving times of 2 h (duck whale), 1.5 h (sperm whale) or even only 15 min (Weddell seal) compared to the maximum 2 min possible for (untrained) humans (however: record in apnoea time diving: 11 min 35 s; 2009). Therefore, all diving species reduce blood flow to the peripheral organs, except the heart and brain, and thus reduce O_2 utilisation to the bare minimum, thus allowing a kind of ischaemic hypoxia. The resulting decrease in cardiac output is reflected by bradycardia during diving. Only a few animal species switch to anaerobic metabolism in the peripheral organs. This would lead to a lactate acidosis which is unfavourable for the rapid O_2 uptake of blood in the lungs, necessary after ascent to the atmosphere (**Fig. 11.21 b**).

11.7.4 Time course of cell damage in acute anoxia

Acute anoxia in one or more organs may lead to death of the organ(s) or of the animal. After an **initial interval** during anoxia in which no functional changes occur, a phase of **restricted cell function** follows. This is followed by a phase of **complete failure** of **cell function**, although the cell structure is still maintained. Until the end of this phase, the damage is still reversible and resuscitation is still possible. Thereafter, **irreversible damage** and **cell death** occur. The irreversible phase is characterised by increasing damage to cell structures. The chronological sequence of these consequences of anoxia is shown schematically in **Fig. 11.29**. The different phases are explained in more detail below.

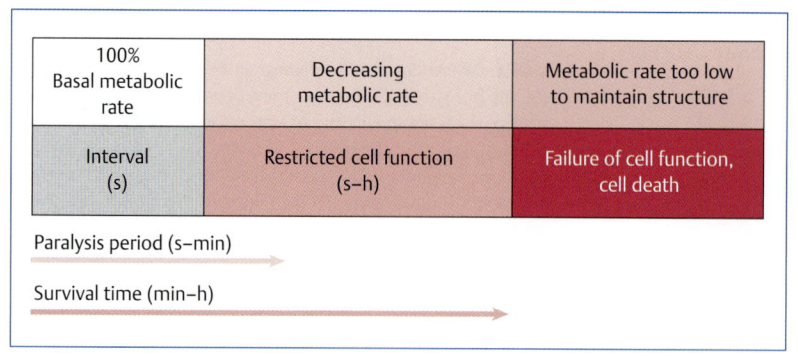

Fig. 11.29 Cell metabolism and cell function after acute onset of (usually ischaemic) tissue hypoxia. See text for definitions of terms.

MORE DETAILS The time interval of anoxia until the onset of cell death varies because cells have several **energy reservoirs**. There are limited reserves of energy-rich phosphates such as ATP and creatine phosphate (**Fig. 6.13**, **Fig. 26.1**). O_2 reserves are initially still present as physically dissolved O_2, but are also bound to haemoglobin in the tissue capillaries. Myoglobin in the heart and muscle fibres may also act as oxygen stores. When these small O_2 reservoirs are depleted, many tissues can gain energy through anaerobic glycolysis. This energy source is limited by the supply of glucose in the cell and by the fact that the end-product is lactic acid, which causes intracellular acidosis. After all these energy sources have been used up, structural damage and cell death occur.

Organ failure and survival times

The anoxic failure time is from the onset of anoxia to the onset of complete failure of all cellular functions. The survival time is the time interval from the onset of anoxia to the onset of irreversible damage. Within this latter period, recovery of full organ function is possible.

The **survival time** of resting skeletal muscle, and also the resting heart, is many hours. This makes heart transplants possible. Kidney and liver have survival times at body temperature of about four hours. The brain, on the other hand, has a survival time of only about ten minutes. This makes it the organ most susceptible to O_2 deficiency. The **anoxic tolerance time** of the brain is about ten seconds. Thereafter the electrical activity of the brain ceases (zero-line EEG). The paralysis time of the beating heart is four minutes. Consequently, the **survival time** of the **whole animal** is also about **four minutes**. If the heart beats again in anoxia after four minutes, the ejection rate during the following (six or more) minutes is low. The resulting very low arterial pressure does not ensure sufficient perfusion of the brain; the survival time of the brain (ten minutes) is exceeded.

11.7.5   Cell damage due to reactive oxygen species

Reactive oxygen species are highly **reactive oxygen compounds**. Reactive oxygen species include the superoxide anion O_2^- which is formed by O_2 taking up an electron, as well as hydrogen peroxide H_2O_2, and the hydroxyl radical OH^-. Superoxide anions are also formed under normal conditions in low concentrations in the respiratory chain of cells as well as in leukocytes and endothelia by NAD(P)H

oxidase when it oxidises NAD(P)H to NAD(P)$^+$. From two O_2^- molecules and two H^+ ions, **superoxide dismutase** can produce H_2O_2. **Catalase** in the peroxisomes of cells degrades H_2O_2 to H_2O and O_2. The cooperation of these two enzymes therefore leads to the elimination of both O_2^- ions as well as H_2O_2, so these are **protective antioxidant enzymes** which normally keep the concentration of reactive O_2 species low. So-called **radical scavengers** also have an antioxidant effect. Such scavengers are **vitamin E, vitamin C** and **glutathione**, see ch. Metabolism of erythrocytes (p.232) and biotransformation by chemical modification (p.474). **Metal ions**, such as iron and copper, promote oxidation and the formation of reactive oxygen species, therefore metal chelators also have an antioxidant effect.

Reactive oxygen species (in normal low concentrations) are important for some signal transduction processes in cells (e.g., phosphorylation of the insulin receptor, activation of several transcription factors). In higher concentrations, they can damage cell and mitochondrial membranes, impair enzymes and DNA and DNA synthesis, and lead to inactivation of the vasodilator, NO. Increased concentrations of reactive oxygen species occur in hyperoxia as a result of increased oxygen concentration in the inhaled air, which leads to cell damage in the longer term, especially in the lungs.

MORE DETAILS Another pathophysiological example of the harmful effect of reactive O_2 species is the so-called **reperfusion damage**, which can occur after a prolonged **circulatory standstill** with tissue anoxia. When blood flow is restored, this leads to a rapid increase in p_{O_2} in the tissue. As a consequence, there is an increased production of O_2^- and H_2O_2 resulting in severe tissue damage that is more serious than the anoxic damage alone. This can occur when vessels are reopened after an infarction, but also when a transplanted organ is connected to the recipient's circulation.

Apart from the variable formation of reactive oxygen species, varying O_2 partial pressures in tissues have important direct signalling functions. The p_{O_2} regulates the width of the resistance vessels of many vascular beds and, via the transcription factor HIF1α, regulates vessel proliferation or angiogenesis, erythropoiesis and the proportion of anaerobic glycolysis relative to oxidative metabolism.

11.8 Regulation of respiration

Gerolf Gros

11.8.1 Rhythmogenesis

Two regions in the medulla oblongata are involved in the control of respiration (**Fig. 5.11**): the neurons of the ventral respiratory group and the neurons of the dorsal respiratory group in the nucleus tractus solitarius. The ventral respiratory group represents the actual respiratory centre where rhythmogenesis takes place. In the nucleus tractus solitarius, the afferent inputs for cough, Hering-Breuer and chemosensory reflexes are managed. The neurons of the pontine respiratory group have (inhibitory) influences on the ventral respiratory group.

A large number of respiratory neurons with different properties form a network in the ventral respiratory group generating the respiratory rhythm. The neurons of the network are responsible for three phases of the respiratory cycle:

- **inspiratory neurons**:
  - activation of the phrenic nerve and the nn. intercostales externi
  - diaphragmatic contraction and contraction of the mm. intercostales externi
  - → inspiration
- **postinspiratory neurons**:
  - termination of the contraction of the diaphragm and mm. intercostales externi
  - → post-inspiration = passive expiration
- **expiratory neurons**:
  - activation of the expiration mm. intercostales interni and the abdominal muscles
  - → "active" expiration phase. At rest, expiration is predominantly passive.

> **IN A NUTSHELL** !
>
> The respiratory rhythm with constant alternation between inspiration and expiration is generated by a network of respiratory neurons (= respiratory centre) in the medulla oblongata.

11.8.2 Respiratory reflexes

■ Inflation reflex, Hering-Breuer reflex

Pulmonary stretch sensors are located in the bronchial tree. Their signals are transferred via the vagal nerve. The receptors influence respiratory activity via neurons of the dorsal respiratory group in the nucleus tractus solitarius. **Expansion** of the lungs during inspiration leads, via these afferents, to an **inhibition** of **inspiration** and an activation of post inspiration. The purpose is to **protect** the lungs from **over-expansion**. When the afferents of these stretch receptors are switched off, the depth of breathing increases combined with a decrease in respiratory frequency.

■ Protective reflexes

Mechanical or chemical irritation of receptors in the submucosa of the nasal mucosa triggers the **sneezing reflex**. Similarly, mechanical or chemical stimulation of subepithelial receptors in the larynx and trachea trigger the **cough reflex**. During coughing, very high velocities of expiratory airflow are generated, which are associated with turbulence that expels particles from the trachea and larynx.

■ Deflation reflex, Head reflex

Deflation reflex is the mirror image of the lung inflation reflex. A marked decrease in lung volume ("deflation") triggers an increase in the rate of respiration, i.e., hyperpnoea, as a result of reduced activity of the lung stretch sensors and probably other lung sensors. This reflex could play a role in the occasional spontaneous single very deep breaths ("**sighs**"), which occur at irregular intervals during normal quiet respiration and contribute to the **prevention** of **atelectasis**.

> **MORE DETAILS**
>
> **J-Reflex**
>
> In close relation to the alveolar capillaries (juxtacapillary), free nerve endings of C fibres are located in the lung interstitium, which are activated when the extracellular space of the lung increases (e.g., in pulmonary oedema, congestive pulmonary oedema, pulmonary hypertension). The result is a depression of respiratory activity ending in apnoea, as well as bradycardia and arterial hypotension. It is assumed that this reflex is responsible for respiratory disorders in pulmonary oedema, pulmonary congestion, etc. It also possibly limits exertion during exercise, when the pressures in the pulmonary vascular system increase giving rise to dyspnoea during physical exertion.

> **IN A NUTSHELL** !
>
> The activity of the respiratory centre is modulated by the afferents of respiratory reflexes such as the lung expansion reflex (Hering-Breuer) and protective reflexes (cough reflex, sneeze reflex).

11.8.3 Chemical respiratory regulation

Chemical regulation is the essential mechanism that adjusts the respiratory minute volume under conditions of physical rest so that it adapts to the metabolic state. Chemosensors measure the arterial blood gas parameters p_{art,CO_2}, pH_{art} and p_{art,O_2}. These sensors are the **peripheral (arterial) chemosensors** in the **glomera carotica** (at the carotid bifurcations) and in the **glomera aortica** (in the aortic arch). They register p_{art,CO_2}, p_{art,O_2} and pH_{art}. **Central chemosensors** in the **medulla oblongata** register p_{art,CO_2} and pH_{art}. The information is used in the respiratory centre in the medulla (p.291) to control respiratory rate and volume.

Peripheral (arterial) chemosensors are the type I glomus cells, which are secondary sensory cells in the glomera of the carotid bifurcations and aortic arch. A cellular O_2 sensor regulates K^+ channels in these cells. At low arterial O_2 partial pressure, the K^+ channels are closed leading to depolarisation of the cell. This leads to a Ca^{2+} influx via potential-controlled Ca^{2+} channels, whereupon the type I glomus cell releases more transmitters and thereby excites the afferent fibres that run in the glossopharyngeal nerve (glomus caroticum) and in the vagus nerve (glomus aorticum). The information is sent to neurons of the nervus tractus solitarii in the medulla oblongata; see Rhythmogenesis (p. 291). An increase in p_{art,CO_2} and a decrease in pH_{art} resulting in intracellular acidification of the type I glomus cells. This leads to an influx of Na^+ by increasing the transport rate of a Na^+/H^+ exchanger, which activates a Na^+/Ca^{2+} exchanger and thus increases the intracellular Ca^{2+} concentration and transmitter release. Therefore, p_{O_2} decrease as well as rise in p_{CO_2} and fall in pH, all cause an increase in the pulse frequency of the afferent nerves and consequently an increase in ventilation.

MORE DETAILS   The central chemosensors trigger an increase in ventilation when there is a rise in p_{art,CO_2} and decrease of pH_{art}. A change from p_{art,CO_2} due to the good diffusion properties of CO_2 also leads rapidly to corresponding changes of p_{CO_2} and pH in the extracellular space of the brain and in the cerebrospinal fluid detected in an unknown way by the central chemosensors.

Fig. 11.30 shows the respiratory responses to changes in p_{art,CO_2}, pH_{art} and p_{art,O_2}. It shows that p_{art,CO_2} has a particularly **pronounced effect** on ventilation. In humans, when p_{art,CO_2} rises from 40 to 60 mmHg, the respiratory minute volume is increased almost 10-fold from $7 \, l \cdot min^{-1}$ to $60 \, l \cdot min$. At 70 mmHg, maximum respiratory minute volume of $75 \, l \cdot min^{-1}$ is reached. At partial pressures > 70 mmHg, CO_2 has a respiratory depressing effect (until finally "CO_2 narcosis"). **Lowering** the **pH_{art}** leads to a

weaker effect on ventilation. Ventilation is increased by about 50% at $pH_{art} = 7.2$ (red curve). The effect of **hypoxaemia** is much less pronounced. Up to a p_{art,O_2} of 50 mmHg, there is **hardly** any **increase in ventilation**. Only in the case of very severe hypoxaemia with a considerable reduction in O_2 saturation does ventilation increase markedly. At an extremely low p_{art,O_2} of 20 mmHg, it reaches about twice the normal resting ventilation (red curve). The respiratory drive by O_2 is therefore only important in the case of pronounced hypoxaemia (e.g. at high altitudes). It is also decisive in chronic hypercapnia (e.g. chronic ventilation disorder), when the respiratory centre adapts to high p_{art,CO_2} values and thus O_2 supply becomes the main stimulus.

Chemical respiratory drives can cause about a tenfold increase in respiratory minute volume, while the maximum possible ventilation (voluntary in humans) is 25 times the normal resting ventilation. Maximum physical work in humans leads to a respiratory minute volume of about 15 times the value of resting ventilation. In horses this increase is about 23 times that of resting ventilation (**Table 26.4**).

> **IN A NUTSHELL** !
>
> Chemical respiratory regulation adjusts the activity of the respiratory centre (and ventilation) to metabolic needs. Mainly it is p_{art,CO_2} and to a lesser extent pH_{art} and p_{art,O_2} that provide afferents to the respiratory centre via peripheral and central chemosensors.

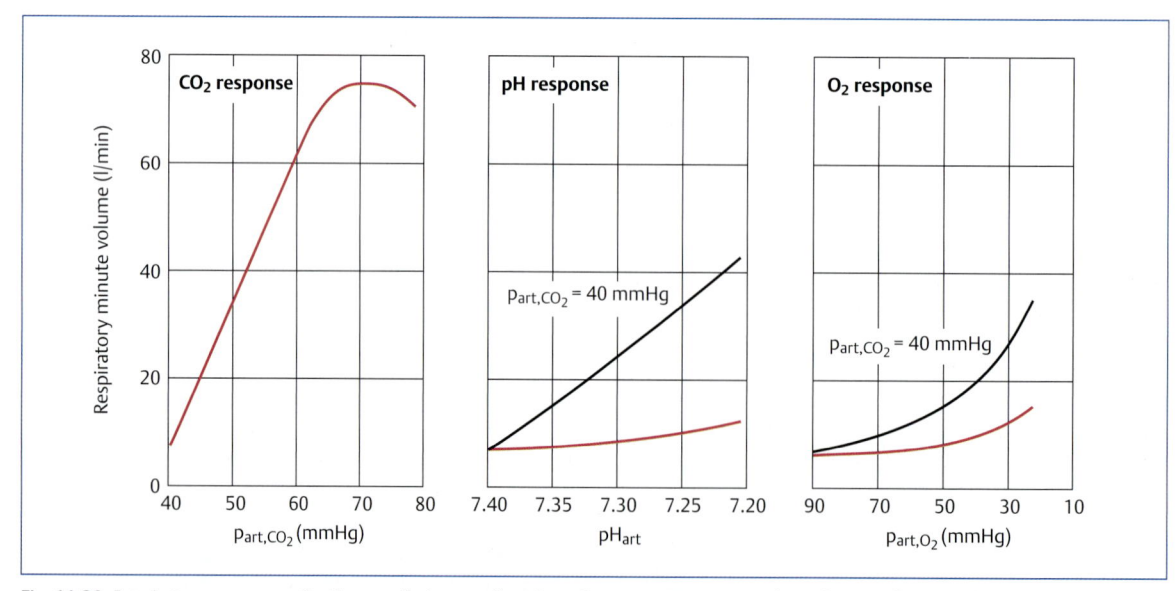

Fig. 11.30 Respiratory responses: Resting ventilation as a function of p_{art,CO_2}, pH_{art}, p_{art,O_2}. The red curves for pH_{art} and p_{art,O_2} represent the ventilation when arterial pH falls and when the inspiratory O_2 partial pressure is reduced (at high altitude). When pH or p_{O_2} are lowered, the subsequent increase in ventilation is accompanied by increased expiration of CO_2, with a consequent reduction in the CO_2-related respiratory drive. Only if p_{CO_2} is kept constant at 40 mmHg, will the respiratory responses to a decrease in pH or p_{O_2} become stronger (black curves). The difference between the red and black curves illustrates the major importance of p_{CO_2} in ventilation control. p_{CO_2} represents the strongest "chemical" signal in regulating respiratory action. [Source: Schmidt RF, Lang F. Thews G. Physiology des Menschen. 29th ed., Heidelberg: Springer; 2005]

11.8.4 Respiratory regulation at work

In humans, and in domestic animals as far as they have been investigated, the arterial blood gas parameters P_{art,CO_2}, P_{art,O_2} and pH_{art} remain largely unchanged during submaximal physical exertion, i.e., work that is significantly below the endurance limit. Therefore, changes in blood gas pressures or pH cannot be the cause of the increased ventilation observed during exercise. Only at workloads close to the endurance limit is there a drop in the P_{art,CO_2} due to hyperventilation at high workload and also a definite drop in p_{art,O_2} (deficient oxygenation of the blood in the lungs with reduced contact time). These changes have been observed in horses as well as in humans. Neither though, can be responsible for an increase in ventilation during submaximal physical exertion. Instead, two neural mechanisms seem to be involved during submaximal physical exertion:

- **Central coinnervation:** At the onset of work, the respiratory centre (as well as the circulatory centre) is "coinnervated" by activation of the sensorimotor system. This also explains why ventilation and cardiac output are both immediately increased at the start of work.
- **Re-afference principle:** Fine-tuning of ventilation and circulation for the actual work performed is via feedback from the working muscles. Chemosensors and/or mechanosensors are thought to be the sensors in the muscle tissue.

■ Synchronisation of respiration and locomotion in horses and dogs

This is a special form of breath control for galloping horses and dogs. Leg movement and respiratory rate are approximately in synchrony during galloping (**Fig. 26.9a**), thus facilitating ventilation. Furthermore, there is a linear relationship between tidal volume and jump length (**Fig. 26.9b**). This leads to linear coupling of ventilation with speed and represents an efficient way of adapting ventilation to workload. There is also a linear relationship between speed and O_2 consumption (**Fig. 26.6**). The resting horse has a respiratory minute volume of about $60 \, l \cdot min^{-1}$ and a respiratory frequency of about $12 \, min^{-1}$. At a gallop, the respiratory minute volume can increase to $1400 \, l \cdot min^{-1}$, i.e., 23 times the resting value, and the respiratory rate can increase 10-fold to $120 \, min^{-1}$ (**Table 26.4**).

In addition to the adaptation of ventilation during galloping to O_2 consumption, the 1:1 coupling of the pattern of leg movement and respiration frequency also provides a mechanical advantage during inhalation and exhalation. **Fig. 11.31** illustrates this for the dog. During galloping, inspiration causes the body to stretch and the lumbosacral joint to extend, which is associated with a caudal tilting of the pelvis. Both changes lower the pressure in the abdominal cavity and thus favour expansion of the lungs. During expiration, these mechanisms work in the opposite directions. They cause compression of the abdominal space and thus a reduction in the volume of the lungs. This means that changes in body shape while galloping are of considerable benefit in assisting ventilation of the lungs.

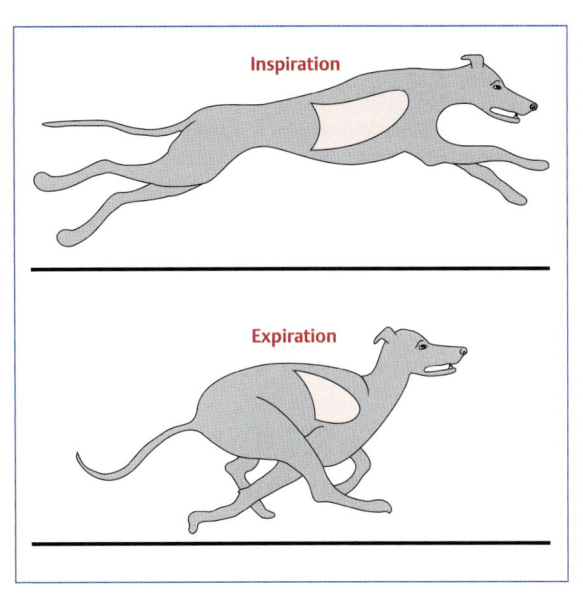

Fig. 11.31 Changes in the body shape of a galloping dog alternately support compression and expansion of the lungs. Since phases of movement and respiration are strictly coupled, extreme flexion of the extremities and lumbosacral joint with shortening of body length contributes to an increase in intrapulmonary pressure that supports expiration. Extreme extension of the body and all the extremities contribute to a decrease in intrapulmonary pressure that supports inspiration.

In the galloping horse there is also a 1:1 coupling between respiratory rate and the pattern of leg movement. Here too, ventilation is thought to be supported by the changes in body shape, but the details have yet to be defined. More information on this is given in ch. 26.3.2.

MORE DETAILS A prerequisite for the coupling of leg movement pattern and respiratory rate is that horses and dogs can finish the expiratory phase in the time interval of a canter jump. In a healthy horse, half of this period is sufficient for complete expiration. In horses suffering from chronic obstructive bronchitis (COPD, chronic obstructive pulmonary disease) the expiratory phase is prolonged due to increased airway resistance. This reduces the maximum respiratory rate and thus the maximum walking speed in COPD affected horses.

11.8.5 Panting

The regulation of respiration is closely related to the regulation of temperature and water balance. In dogs, pigs, sheep, and also in poultry and rabbits, the mechanisms of respiratory regulation can have thermoregulatory commands superimposed upon them. The trigger here is the rise in body core temperature above a certain "panting threshold". High frequency respiration becomes established. Thus, the respiratory rate can increase to about 240 breaths per minute in sheep, to 400 in pigs and up to 700 in rabbits. In dogs, 300–400 breaths per minute can be achieved compared to about 20 per minute at rest (**Fig. 11.11**). The high respiratory frequencies are accompanied by a marked reduction in the depth of breathing, i.e., "shallow breathing" develops. Alveolar ventilation is not greater than during resting respiration. Therefore, there is no increased CO_2 exhalation and no respiratory alkalosis. The increase in ventilation is actually an increase in "dead space ventilation" (ch. 11.3.3 (p.267)). Thus, the process of panting is not hyperventilation, but hyperpnoea. However, if the core temperature exceeds critical ranges (2nd phase of panting), the respiratory rate decreases and the tidal volume increases, which then leads to critical respiratory alkalosis (a condition that can be found in dogs that have been left in a sun-exposed closed car for a long time).

Panting can also be observed in cats, but is then a sign of extreme stress. The importance of panting for thermoregulation is described in more detail in ch. 20.7.2.

11.9 Comparative pathophysiology of lung function in domestic animals

Gerolf Gros

11.9.1 Obstructive lung diseases

MORE DETAILS   Airway obstructions can be divided into three classes according to their cause:

Intraluminal causes

Mainly excessive secretion of mucus into the bronchial lumen, for example in COPD.

Intramural causes

Here the cause is in the wall of the airways. It may be due to severe constriction of the bronchial smooth muscle, hypertrophy of the mucous glands as in COPD, or thickening of the laryngeal or bronchial walls due to inflammation and oedema in laryngitis or bronchitis.

Extraluminal causes

An important disease is emphysema, in which lung tissue weakens and ruptures. Because of the associated loss of elastic fibres, less radial tension is exerted on the airways so that the airway lumina are reduced. In this respect, emphysema is also an obstructive disorder. A second disease that (also) has an extraluminal effect is **COPD** (chronic obstructive pulmonary disease). Because of impeded expiration, an increased pressure is generated in the lungs, which transmits to the interstitium and thus leads to a compression of intrathoracic airways, which further impedes expiration.

The main functional consequence of obstructive lung disease is increased resistance, increased residual volume (due to premature airway closure during expiration) in conjunction with reduced vital capacity at normal total capacity.

Obstructive diseases are further subdivided according to the location of the obstruction in the respiratory system. **Obstruction** of the **upper respiratory** tract can occur in the nose, pharynx, larynx or the extrathoracic trachea. Paralysis of the larynx is particularly common in horses and dogs, brachycephaly is common in pugs and bulldogs, acute laryngitis can be observed in cattle, atrophic rhinitis is found in pigs and chronic nasal infections in

cats. Since the upper respiratory tract contributes particularly to the total resistance (**Fig. 11.17 a**), the main consequence is an increase in airway resistance with a considerable increase in the mechanical work of respiration. **Obstructions** of the **lower airways** refer to the intrathoracic trachea, the bronchi and bronchioles. The main symptoms here, in addition to increased airway resistance, can be an irregular pattern of ventilation and considerable impairment of ventilation-perfusion, with resultant arterial hypoxaemia. Because of hypoxic vasoconstriction in the poorly ventilated regions of the lung, pulmonary hypertension can also occur. Examples are chronic bronchitis, which is particularly common in horses, dogs and cats, and allergic bronchospasm in cattle.

The most common lung disease in horses is COPD (chronic obstructive pulmonary disease). It is considered to be hyperresponsiveness of the airways to inhaled particles or inhaled allergens such as fungal spores, and chemicals such as ammonia and H_2S. It affects the lower airways, which generally also become infected with bacteria. The obstruction is from increased mucus secretion, pus, bronchoconstriction and chronic inflammation of the bronchioles with hyperplasia of the epithelium, causing affected horses to cough. The increased airway resistance can lead to distributional disturbances with arterial hypoxaemia and consequential pulmonary vasoconstriction, with pulmonary hypertension and right heart hypertrophy. In the long term, chronically elevated airway resistance leads to the development of pulmonary emphysema with loss of lung tissue (**rupture and collapse**). Dogs and cats can also develop allergic bronchitis (**feline asthma**).

11.9.2 Restrictive lung diseases

MORE DETAILS   The main symptoms are reduced lung compliance, severely reduced vital capacity, and reduced total capacity. Resistance is normal.
- **Interstitial lung diseases:** They are characterised by progressive fibrosis of the lung from unknown causes or as a result of inflammation of lung tissue. Deposits of collagenous fibres in the lung interstitium limit the volume expandability of the lung. While these diseases are common in humans, they are rarely observed in domestic animals.
- **Intraparenchymal restrictive diseases:** Microbial pneumonias (lung infections) reduce volume expandability because of fluid accumulation and cell infiltration. Malignant lung tumours or lung metastases also belong to this group of diseases.
- **Extraparenchymal restrictive diseases:** Restrictions of the expansion capacity of the lungs or thorax can be caused by pleural effusion (fluid accumulation in the pleural space), pneumothorax (collapse of the lung due to air entering the pleural space, after injuries to the thoracic wall or rupture of emphysema bubbles), deformities of the bony thorax or weakness of the respiratory muscles.
- **NRDS (neonatal respiratory distress syndrome):** NRDS is observed in premature lambs, pigs, calves, foals, and dogs. Due to surfactant deficiency, volume expandability of the lungs is reduced. Atelectasis and poor oxygenation of blood in the lungs may also occur.

11.10   Respiration in fish

Helga Pfannkuche, Michael Pees

ESSENTIALS ✗

Fish must obtain the oxygen they need from water. Since simple diffusion through the body surface into the animal would be too inefficient, specialised gas exchange organs, the gills, have developed for this purpose. The fact that blood and water flow past each other in countercurrents in the gills makes an efficient exchange of gases possible. Regulation of respiration in fish is less modulated by CO_2 concentration in blood than it is in mammals, but instead it is mainly influenced by the oxygen saturation of blood.

11.10.1   Gas exchange in water

Microorganisms that live in water can meet their oxygen demand by the diffusion of dissolved oxygen directly through their external surface. This also applies to some extent in amphibians and reptiles (p. 297) during hibernation when there is less **oxygen demand**. Fish, which must obtain oxygen dissolved in water, are too large to extract oxygen by this means, as their body surface area is too small and the diffusion distances are too long. Therefore, fish have developed special organs, the **gills**, which enable

enough dissolved oxygen to pass into the bloodstream and thus be available to supply the internal organs. Nevertheless, a particular challenge is the **lower availability** of **oxygen** in water compared to that in air. Water has a 30-fold lower concentration of oxygen compared to air. Consequently, the gills must be perfused 30 times more than an alveolar surface of comparable area must be ventilated. Another challenge is the reduced solubility of oxygen as water temperature increases. Water at 40 °C has only half the oxygen content of water at 0 °C. The salt concentration in the water also affects the oxygen content. Thus, seawater is significantly less oxygenated than freshwater at the same temperature.

11.10.2   Ventilation

In contrast to the mammalian lung (p. 261), in which oxygen uptake takes place via a "pool system", oxygen from water is exchanged during a continuous fluid flow in a **countercurrent system** (Fig. 11.33) along the gills. This type of ventilation is energetically more favourable for the animal than a pool system exchange, as water has a higher viscosity than a gaseous medium.

During ventilation, the water flows in through the **mouth** and out through the **gill slits**. Entry of water is initiated by lowering the floor of the oral cavity, and thus increasing its volume, with a resultant decrease in pressure.

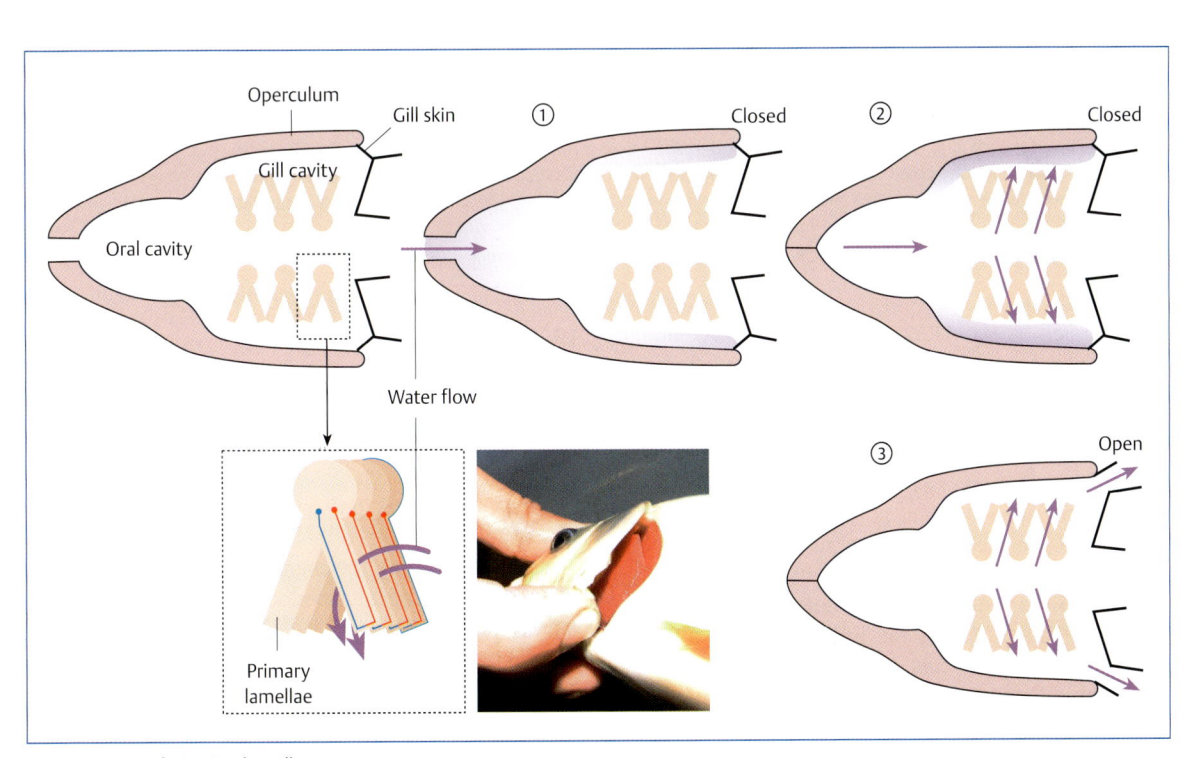

Fig. 11.32 Ventilation in the gills.
(**1**) The mouth is open, and the mouth cavity is dilated. Thus, the pressure in the mouth cavity drops and water flows in. The gill cavity starts to expand.
(**2**) The mouth closes and the gill cavity expands by lifting the gill operculum. The mouth cavity narrows again. This forces the water between the gill lamellae. The gills are made up of stacks of primary lamellae anchored to the gill arch.
(**3**) The operculum opens by lifting the gill skin and the gill cavity narrows. This causes the water to flow outwards between the lamellae. Then the mouth cavity opens again and widens. The cycle begins again.
  The photograph shows a "stack" of primary lamellae under the gill operculum of a koi carp. [Source: Prof. Dr. Michael Pees, Klinik für Heimtiere, Reptilien und Vögel, Stiftung TiHo Hannover]

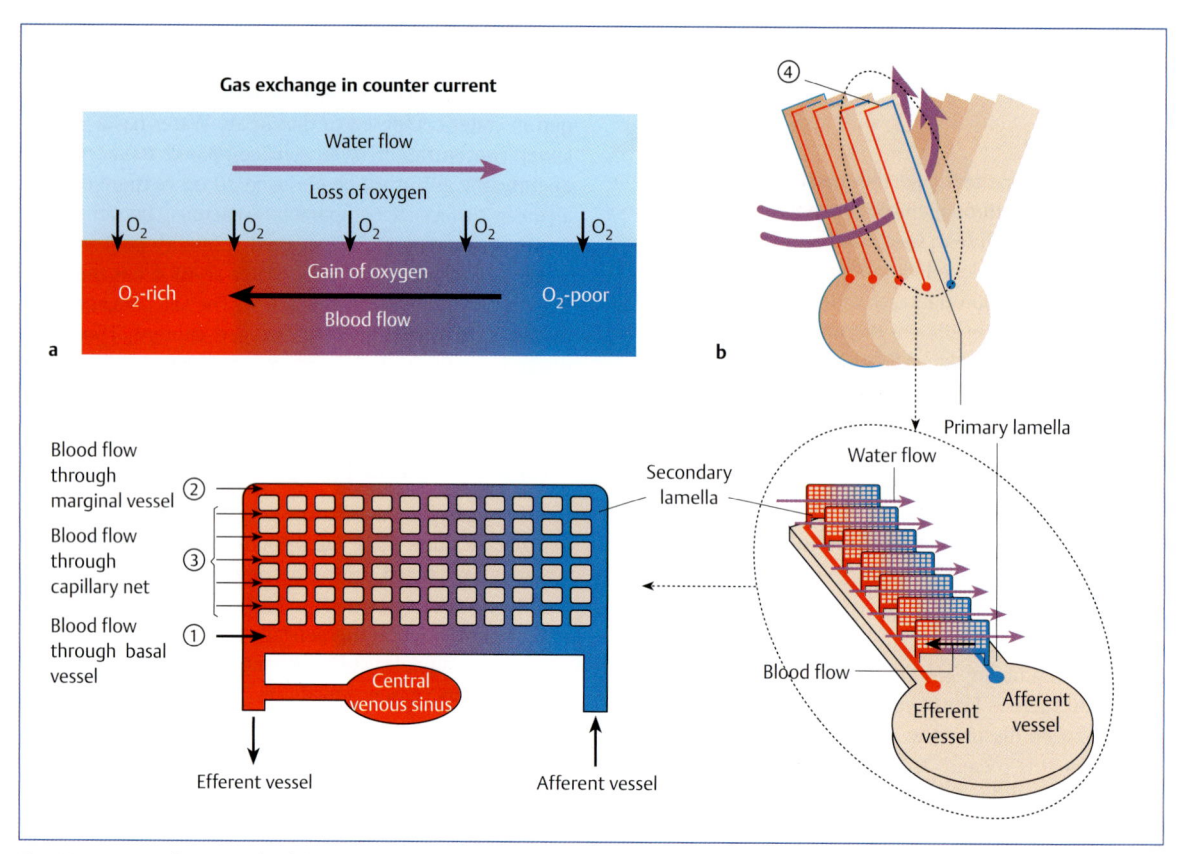

Fig. 11.33 Gas exchange in the fish gill.
(**a**) The exchange of respiratory gases between blood and water takes place by countercurrent diffusion with opposite direction of flow of the two media. It should be noted that over the entire exchange distance, the oxygen concentration of the water is always higher than in the neighbouring blood. This allows oxygen uptake over the entire contact distance (further explanation in the text).
(**b**) In the secondary lamellae, particular vessels increase the efficiency of gas exchange. ① During blood flow through the basal vessel, the contact surface for exchange is only small. ② Preferential blood flow through the marginal vessels of the secondary lamellae increases the contact surface and prolongs the contact time, which increases the diffusion possibilities for the respiratory gases. ③ The greatest possible exchange of respiratory gases between blood and the passing water is achieved by increasing blood flow in the capillary networks within the secondary lamellae. ④ Further reduction of blood flow in the secondary lamellae can be achieved by direct flow from the afferent to the efferent vessel at the edge of the primary lamellae.

As illustrated in **Fig. 11.32** the water flows out of the mouth cavity between the lamellae of the gills because of the lower **pressure** in the gill cavity. The water then flows outwards under the open opercula.

Some fish species (e.g., some sharks and tunas) use the water inflow that occurs when they swim forward with their mouths open (dynamic pressure ventilation). Such a **"pitot ventilation"** is beneficial because no additional energy is needed to actively move water through the gills.

In **bony fish** the opening and closing of the **gill opercula** forces ventilation. During the influx of water into the mouth cavity, the opercula are initially closed by the gill skin. They only open after the water is forced between the gill **lamellae** by the increase in pressure in the oral cavity (function of a pressure-suction pump). **Cartilaginous fish** that do not have opercula also direct water between the gill lamellae by contraction of muscles around the oral cavity. Because of the absence of opercula, there is no decrease in pressure in the gill cavity to enhance the flow of water.

11.10.3 Gas exchange

The actual gas exchange takes place at the so-called **secondary lamellae**. These are folds in the **primary lamellae** which are covered with a thin epithelium, with capillaries directly below. (**Fig. 11.33**). Since the **diffusion barrier** for the respiratory gases thus consists only of the capillary wall and a single-layer epithelium, the diffusion distance is very short (1–10 μm). The course of the capillaries and the direction of flow of the blood are opposite to that of the water along the secondary lamellae. This opposite flow of the two media leads to an extremely efficient **countercurrent** gas exchange (**Fig. 11.33**). Oxygen-poor blood takes up oxygen diffusing from the water down a concentration gradient to the blood. As the partially oxygenated blood continues through the gill capillaries, it meets the continuous inflowing water with a higher oxygen concentration, so that the oxygen content continues to increase as blood flows along the entire contact surface.

11.10.4   Regulation of respiration

The oxygen concentration in water is more variable than that in air. Warming of water and the cessation of photosynthesis by aquatic plants at night can lead to significant decreases in available oxygen. As a result, fish must be sensitive to changes in **oxygen concentration** in blood. When there is a decrease in the O_2 partial pressure of blood there is an increase in water flow through the gills and also a body movement to be closer to the water surface. It is more oxygen-rich water at the interface between air and water. Fish also actively seek out a water inlet or the aerator in artificial aquaria to supply themselves with oxygen-rich water.

Reducing oxygen consumption through inactivity and moving to colder water, thus reducing metabolic activity, are also strategies to counteract hypoxia.

Modulation of **blood flow in the gills** also plays an important role in adapting oxygen uptake to demand and availability. (**Fig. 11.33**). This must be controlled so that there is sufficient exchange of respiratory gases. Perfusion, however, is limited for osmoregulatory reasons, as the thin diffusion barrier in the gill epithelium (p. 463) also leads to the loss of electrolytes through diffusion.

The gill lamellae are innervated both afferently and efferently. O_2 concentration in blood can be determined so that blood flow to the filaments can be adjusted. In **Fig. 11.33** different possibilities of blood flow in the primary and secondary lamellae are shown. If the O_2 supply is reduced, or the O_2 concentration in blood decreases, oxygen uptake can be increased by constricting the **efferent vessels** and directing more of the incoming blood through the **capillary networks** of the secondary lamellae (**3** in **Fig. 11.33**). The blood flows mainly into a **central venous sinus** after perfusion of the secondary lamellae. This is important for osmoregulation of fish (p. 341), such as for the uptake of sodium from water in freshwater fish. Such efferent vasoconstriction occurs in hypoxia. Vasoconstriction is mediated by acetylcholine. As well as **acetylcholine**, **adrenaline** and **noradrenaline** are also involved in the regulation of blood flow to the gills. The catecholamines have a vasodilatory effect on the efferent vessels (involvement of β receptors) and, by stimulating α receptors, a vasoconstrictor effect on the anastomoses leading to the central venous sinus. Acetylcholine and norepinephrine thus have opposite effects, particularly on osmoregulation (p. 341).

Another form of modulation of the gas exchange surface is found especially in hypoxia-tolerant fish species. When O_2 consumption is low in oxygen-rich water, these species even reduce the contact surfaces between the secondary lamellae and water, by filling the spaces between the secondary lamellae with undifferentiated cells. This not only saves energetic effort for osmoregulation, but also protects the gills from pollutants, parasites, and oxygen radicals. However, this adaptation also means that sudden changes in water quality can lead to acute anoxic health problems, as the system cannot react rapidly.

In the long term, hypoxia increases the **haemoglobin concentration** in the blood of fish, similar to air-breathing species. This can also occur when the gills become "slimy"

due to disease. When this happens, the oxygen diffusion path between the capillary lumen and the gill water flow, which consists only of the capillary wall and a single-layer epithelium, is massively enlarged by the deposition of a slime layer so that oxygen uptake becomes more difficult. Therefore, the gills must also be assessed during a clinical examination. Unlike in mammals, the $\mathbf{p_{CO2}}$ hardly plays a role in the regulation of respiration because CO_2 is much more water-soluble than oxygen (see formula (11.20), ch. 11.5.1 and 11.5.2), so that CO_2 release is much easier than O_2 uptake.

> **IN A NUTSHELL**   !
>
> In fish, gas exchange takes place at the secondary lamellae of the gills.

MORE DETAILS   Over the course of evolution, air breathing has developed in some fish. These **lungfish** have both gills and simple lungs. When breathing air, the circulatory system of the lungfish directs the oxygen-rich blood from the lungs to the body tissues via modified gill arches, which are no longer capable of gas exchange. When the fish is underwater, the blood is conducted through functional gill arches, and from there to the body tissues and back to the heart.

11.11   Respiration in reptiles

Michael Pees, Helga Pfannkuche

> **ESSENTIALS**   ✖
>
> Reptiles, as exothermic animals, have a lower demand for oxygen than endothermic species. Their respiratory system has a smaller gas exchange area than that of mammals and birds. Depending on the physical activity of a reptile species, the lungs can have a very simple or a more complex structure. Of special practical importance is the irregular breathing rhythm in reptiles, which comprises episodes of increased ventilation and also of apnoea.

11.11.1   Structure of the respiratory tract

The respiratory system of reptiles is generally less efficient than that of mammals and birds. However, because of their lower metabolic activity and the high proportion of (facultative) anaerobic metabolic processes, the oxygen demand of reptiles is also significantly lower compared to endothermic animals (**Fig. 20.1**).

Within the class of reptiles, there are big differences between individual families and even between species of the same family. While the lungs of monitor lizards and turtles are rather highly specialised, some lizard species have very primitive lungs with a narrow range of functionality.

In all reptiles, the lungs have a wide lumen and consequently a smaller surface area (gas exchange area) than in endothermic species. There are neither alveoli nor air capillaries for gas exchange. The reptile lung functions rather like a more or less subdivided sac lined with respi-

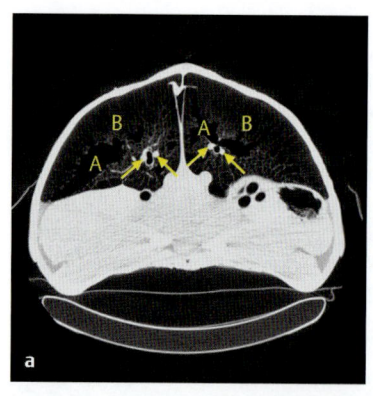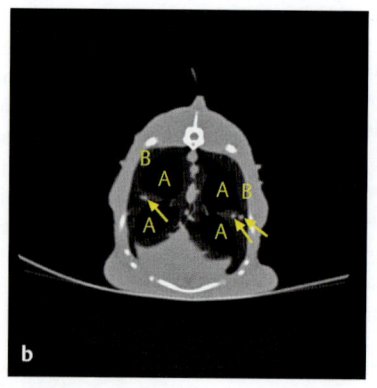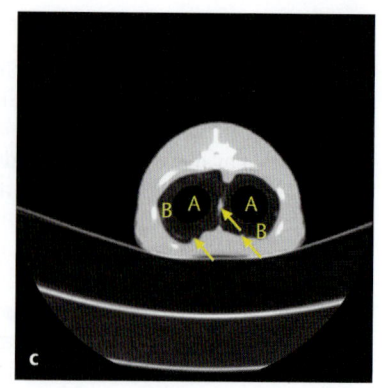

Fig. 11.34 Illustration of the lungs in a spurred tortoise, a green iguana, and a tiger python (from left to right). Computed tomography, axial section transverse to the longitudinal axis of the body.
The large central air spaces are shown, which branch finely into faveoli. In turtles there is an uneven central air space. In many lizards there is an upper and lower air space. In snakes there is a large central lumen running through the lung which becomes an air sac as the epithelium decreases caudally. A = air lumen, B = lung epithelium (faveoli), arrows = lung vessels. [Source: Dr. I. Kiefer, Klinik für Kleintiere, Universitat Leipzig]

ratory epithelium. This subdivision varies greatly, up to tightly packed tubules that increase the gas exchange surface (**Faveoli, Fig. 11.34**). Snakes in particular (but also other reptile species) have centrally arranged smooth muscle bars that mediate ventilation of these tubules from the large central lumen. Caudally, the lung usually merges into an **air sac** which only fulfils the function of an air reservoir (bellows) ventilating the faveoli, even during apnoea. This air sac is most pronounced in snakes. Of clinical importance is that the **mucociliary apparatus** (for cleaning the respiratory tract (p. 262)) is hardly developed in the reptile lung, which favours the development of infections and makes the removal of inflammatory material more difficult. The 11.11.2 in most species also makes removal of mucus more difficult, since coughing is not possible.

11.11.2   Ventilation

Reptiles do not have a diaphragm. Only crocodiles have a comparable structure, as in these species the liver is separated from the rest of the abdominal cavity by a septum. This septum is pulled caudally by a diaphragmatic muscle during inspiration, thus expanding the thoracic cavity. Inspiration in lizards and snakes occurs primarily through expansion of the thorax by means of the intercostal muscles. During undulating locomotion, the movement of the thorax may oppose the respiratory movement. In this case, inspiration can be supported by swallowing respiration (see below), like that in amphibians.

> **MORE DETAILS**
>
> **Swallowing respiration**
>
> Amphibians and some reptiles ventilate their lungs with the help of an **oral cavity pressure pump (swallowing respiration)**. For this purpose, outside air is sucked into the oral cavity through the mouth and nostrils. The epiglottis is closed and access to the lungs is thus blocked. The outside air flows into a depression in the floor of the oral cavity, where it is "temporarily stored". In the next step, the glottis opens and the used air from the lungs flows out through the oral cavity. The fresh "temporarily stored" air then enters the lungs. To do this, the oral cavity is closed, the epi-

glottis remains open, and the air is forced into the lungs by lifting the floor of the oral cavity. The epiglottis then closes again.

Ventilation is a particular challenge for snakes while devouring large prey. Breathing is made possible here by moving the cranial end of the trachea into the mouth cavity next to the prey. For turtles, expansion of the thoracic cavity by means of rib movements is not possible due to their rigid shell. In these species, expansion of the lungs during inspiration is achieved by contraction of special abdominal muscles. In addition, ventilation can also be supported by limb movements. This is particularly seen when breathing is difficult, such as when the abdominal cavity becomes distended.

In aquatic species, gas exchange via the **cloacal mucosa** also plays a role, especially in times of inactivity. This can be sufficient to meet the oxygen demand during periods of rest (winter torpor).

11.11.3   Gas exchange

Reptile lungs have only about 1% of the gas exchange surface of the lungs of mammals of the same body size. However, the efficiency of gas exchange across the lung wall depends not only on the available surface area, but also on the extent of the capillary bed. In many reptile lungs, the caudal lung regions are ventilated, but hardly have any capillaries (air sac, see above). This means that they are not available for gas exchange. This lower blood flow in combination with lower ventilation compared to mammals is a disadvantage when infections occur. Although the lung reacts by a rapid remodelling of the respiratory epithelium and the migration of inflammatory cells, this process takes longer due to the sparse capillary bed. The reduced ability to clear secretions (due to lack of coughing) can then lead to accumulation of pus and secretions. This can be observed especially in snakes with their deep-reaching faveoli system. They are therefore also more susceptible to lung diseases than turtles and lizards.

11.11.4   Regulation of respiration

The central neurons that regulate ventilation in reptiles are presumably located in the medulla oblongata, like those in mammals. Nevertheless, the respiratory rhythm of reptiles can by no means be equated with that of mammals. Ventilation and the cardiac-controlled blood flow, which serves either the pulmonary or the systemic circulation, must be (p. 216) closely coordinated.

As a result, reptiles often do not show a regular ventilation rhythm, but have alternate phases of increased inspiration and expiration, where the lungs are also supplied with more blood, along with phases with no ventilation.

These **apnoea phases** can be very long, up to more than 24 hours in aquatic species. These apnoea phases are of relevance in **inhalation anaesthesia** as this makes induction of anaesthesia and its control very difficult. Oxygen as a carrier gas lowers the respiratory rate even further, as the oxygen content in the lungs is an important regulator of the respiratory rate. Accordingly, assisted ventilation is usually necessary after intubation to ensure sufficient air exchange.

Since reptiles are exothermic animals, their activity level and thus their oxygen demand are in general greatly dependent on the ambient temperature. A high ambient temperature has a greater stimulatory effect on respiratory activity than the gas partial pressures in blood.

A special feature of reptiles is that they can switch to anaerobic metabolic processes in the event of oxygen deficiency. This makes acute suffocation unlikely, but the clinical manifestations of disease processes, and presentation for veterinary treatment, may be greatly delayed.

> **IN A NUTSHELL**   !
>
> The lungs of reptiles have a simple structure. The breathing rhythm is irregular.

11.12   Respiration in birds

Helga Pfannkuche, Michael Pees

> **ESSENTIALS**   ✕
>
> The respiratory system of birds is extremely efficient. Unlike in mammals, it is divided into an air-conducting/air-storing part (trachea, bronchi, air sacs) and a gas-exchanging part (lungs). In birds, both inspiration and expiration are active even under resting conditions. Gas exchange takes place in the lungs between the "air capillaries" and the adjacent blood capillaries. The diffusion barrier is very thin. High oxygen saturation of the blood can be achieved even during flights at high altitudes. The control of respiration has many parallels to that of mammals. However, birds additionally have intrapulmonary CO_2 sensors.

11.12.1   Subdivision of the respiratory system

The respiratory system of birds, like their cardiovascular system, is extremely efficient and is thus capable of meeting the high oxygen demand of flight. More clearly than in mammals, the avian respiratory system is divided into a **large-volume air-storing part** and a **smaller gas-exchanging part**. The **air sacs** make up the largest part of the entire respiratory system. They account for about 15% of the bird's total body volume. In contrast, the volume of the respiratory organs of mammals is only about 7% of body volume. However, in birds, the **lung** itself is small and, in comparison to the mammalian lung, it has a unidirectional flow. During inspiration and expiration, air flows in the same direction. The mammalian lung thus corresponds to a terminal station, whereas the avian lung corresponds to a more efficient and thus smaller transmission station (**Fig. 11.1**).

11.12.2   Ventilation

In principle, birds can breathe both through the nose and through the mouth. The latter also plays a role in thermoregulation for heat dissipation. As birds do not have sweat glands, heat dissipation by evaporation is implemented by panting: short, rapid breathing movements, usually together with the spreading or even rhythmic trembling of the wings (heat dissipation through the then barely insulated trunk wall).

Inspiration and **expiration** are active in the bird even under resting conditions. During inspiration, the thorax expands and air flows into the caudal air sacs (posterior thoracic and abdominal air sacs). At the same time, air flows through the lungs from caudal to cranial (**Fig. 11.35**). Birds do not have a diaphragm and the lungs do not follow the movements of the thorax (mammals: fluid film between the pleurae, see ch. Transmission thorax – lungs – pleurae (p. 264)). Instead, the lungs are fused to the thoracic wall and hardly change their volume during a respiratory cycle. The air sacs act as bellows that drive the air flow through the lungs. These are thin-walled and follow the expansion of the rib cage. As there are hardly any retraction forces, the **overall compliance** (compliance of the air sacs and compliance of the body wall) is high. Overall compliance plays a role in inspiration, i.e., a lot of air can flow into the air sacs without a significant increase in pressure (explanation of compliance see ch. lung compliance (p. 271)).

During inspiration, contraction of the intercostal external and costosternal muscles expands the thorax and moves the sternum ventrally (**Fig. 11.35**). In particular, this displacement of the **sternum**, which is attached cranially to the **coracoid** like a hinge, is essential for ventilation in birds. It is therefore important that the sternum remains ventrally movable when the bird is manually restrained.

Since the air sacs have practically no retraction forces, passive **expiration** as in mammals is not possible. Expiration therefore takes place actively, essentially by contrac-

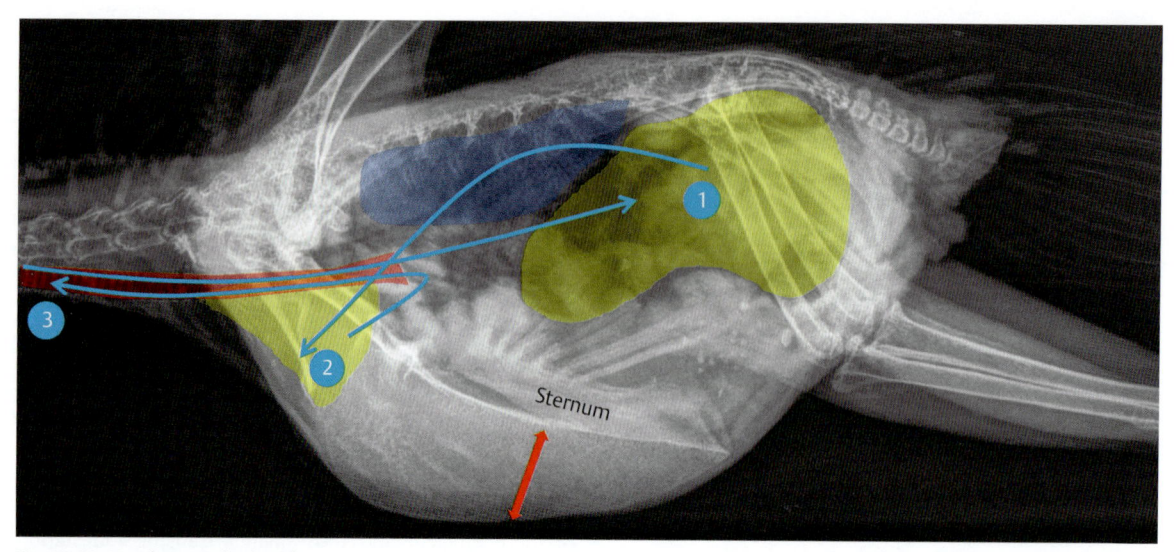

Fig. 11.35 Ventilation in birds. When inspirating, the air first flows into the abdominal air sac (**1**, highlighted in yellow), then via the lungs (highlighted in blue) into the cranial air sacs (**2**, highlighted in yellow) and is then exhaled via the trachea (**3**, highlighted in red). The lungs are thus perfused unidirectionally during inhalation and exhalation, which is an ideal arrangement to facilitate gas exchange. The red double arrow marks the direction of movement of the sternum during inhalation and exhalation. [Source: Prof. Dr. Michael Pees, Klinik für Heimtiere, Reptilien und Vögel, Stiftung TiHo Hannover]

tion of the mm. intercostales interni and the abdominal muscles. During expiration, the sternum shifts back in a dorsal direction, thus reducing the size of the thoracic cavity. During expiration, the air from the posterior air sacs is pushed cranially through the lungs. The air from the anterior air sacs (cervical, subclavian, and anterior thoracic air sacs) flows out through the trachea. Ultimately, during both inspiration and expiration, air flows through the lungs from caudal to cranial, ensuring continuous gas exchange.

During inspiration, the sternum must move ventrally, and during expiration it moves dorsally again. If that does not happen, for example when a bird lies on its back for a long period of time during anaesthesia (a supine position is physiologically not possible in birds), there is considerable strain on respiration, which can only be compensated with difficulty by the more strongly developed inspiratory musculature.

> **MORE DETAILS**   The unidirectional airflow from caudal to cranial is used therapeutically both in treatment of tracheal stenosis (narrowing of the trachea due to foreign bodies or infections) and for the introduction of anaesthetic gas. The abdominal air sac can be punctured, and oxygen/anaesthetic gas introduced. This then flows continuously through the lungs and then out through the trachea.

11.12.3   Gas exchange

Gas exchange takes place exclusively in the lungs. Despite their small size, the lungs have an enormous gas exchange surface, which is about ten times larger than that of a mammal of comparable body size. The structure of the lungs supports the efficient exchange of O_2 and CO_2. In birds, the two main bronchi, which conduct air into the lungs, originate in the region of the **syrinx**. The main bron-

chi open into the abdominal air sacs, while connections to the other air sacs branch off from the main bronchi beforehand. Air from the main bronchi enters the lungs via the **secondary bronchi**. Unlike in mammals, the secondary bronchi do not branch further, but merely serve as conduits to the **parabronchi**. These originate from the secondary bronchi and connect the dorsal and ventral secondary bronchi in an arc. Because of their parallel arrangement, the parabronchi are also called **lung pipes**. Their number differs significantly between species. While the domestic chicken has only about 300–500 lung pipes, the duck, as an efficient flyer, has about 1800 parabronchi.

The actual gas exchange takes place in the **air capillaries**. These are fine, blind-ended tubes that lead from the parabronchi through small funnels. In terms of their function, the air capillaries correspond in principle to the alveoli of mammals. However, their wall is even thinner and their lumen smaller than that of alveoli. Thus, air capillaries have a diameter of only about 3 µm, which corresponds to about one hundredth of the diameter of an alveolus. The use of such extremely thin-walled and fine-lumened structures in the avian lung is possible because the lung is subject to practically no volume changes during a respiratory cycle and is firmly fixed to the dorsal thoracic wall. Like mammalian alveoli, air capillaries are at risk of collapsing, which can be prevented by the production of a special surfactant (with a different composition to that of mammals).

The exchange of gas between the air capillaries and the surrounding blood vessels is made possible and perfected by a special arrangement of the vessels. Air capillaries and blood capillaries are positioned perpendicular to each other so that each air capillary is **"crossed"** by numerous blood capillaries (**Fig. 11.1**). These blood capillaries arise from vessels with a flow direction opposite to the air flow

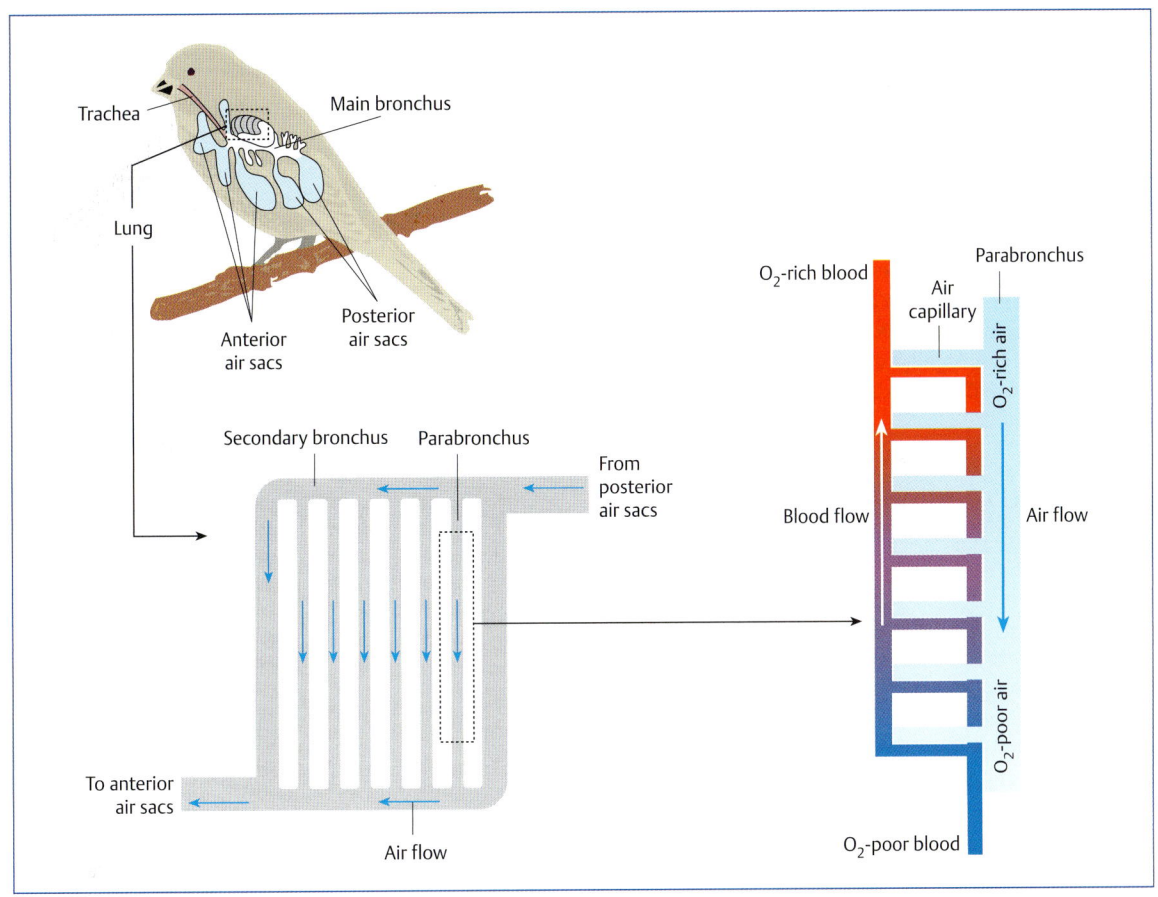

Fig. 11.36 Gas exchange in the avian lung: Air flows through the parabronchi from caudal to cranial. Gas exchange takes place between the blind-ending air capillaries and the adjacent blood capillaries. More details in the text.

in the air capillaries (**Fig. 11.36**). As a result, the air capillaries, which are the first to emerge from the parabronchi, i.e., carry air that is rich in oxygen and low in CO_2, meet blood that has already "completed" most of the gas exchange. This blood is therefore already largely saturated with oxygen. Nevertheless, there is still a concentration gradient between this blood and the fresh air in the air capillaries. This is because the O_2 partial pressure in the posterior air sacs is approx. 115 mmHg (when partial pressure of 145 mmHg in the inspiratory air), which is significantly higher than the O_2 partial pressure in the alveoli of mammals. Oxygen exchange in the direction of blood flow can therefore still take place. The air capillaries that emerge later from the parabronchi contain air that has already released considerable amounts of oxygen. Although the air is already mainly "used up", it still carries more oxygen (approx. 100 mmHg) than the oxygen-poor blood flowing into the lungs. Oxygen transfer into blood can therefore also take place here. This staggered diffusion of oxygen from the air capillaries into the blood capillaries makes the transfer particularly efficient and superior to the alveolar system of mammals. Nevertheless, this more efficient gas exchange does not result in higher partial pressure values for O_2 in the avian arterial blood compared to that in mammals (**Table 11.1**).

11.12.4 Regulation of respiration

The mechanisms of respiratory adaptation to physical load are similar in both birds and mammals (re-afference and central coinnervation, see ch. 11.8.4). Also similar to mammals (ch. 11.8.3 (p.291)), birds have arterial and central **chemosensors** which detect p_{O_2}, p_{CO_2} and the pH of blood. The most important information (as in mammals) is provided by the sensors for CO_2. In addition to the arterial and central CO_2 sensors, birds also have intrapulmonary CO_2 sensors, located along the parabronchi. These additional intrapulmonary sensors probably help to fine-tune ventilation.

However, ventilation is not exclusively controlled by p_{CO_2}. **Hypoxia** also leads to increased ventilation with an increase in the depth of breathing. However, for birds that fly at high altitudes, the problem of low oxygen supply leads to an increase in respiration rate, which then results in hypocapnia. Birds, like mammals, react to **hypocapnia** by reduced ventilation. Birds that frequently fly at high altitudes escape this dilemma by acclimatisation, which leads to a disproportionate increase in ventilation in hypoxia.

> **IN A NUTSHELL**
>
> In birds, unidirectional flow passes through the lungs during respiration. Gas exchange takes place at the air capillaries. The air sacs are used for ventilation.

11.13   Acknowledgement

Gerolf Gros thanks Dr Samer Al-Samir (Hanover) for his technical support with some of the illustrations newly designed or revised for this edition. He also owes special thanks to Prof. von Engelhardt for his intensive support in the consideration of pet-specific features in the respiratory chapter.

Suggested reading

Beadle RE. The Respiratory System. In: Jones WE, ed. Equine Sports Medicine. Chapter 6. Philadelphia: Lea & Febiger; 1989: 59–86.

Comroe JH, Forster RE, DuBois AB et al. The Lung. 2nd ed. Chicago/Il: Yearbook; 1962

Endeward V, Al-Samir S, Itel F, Gros G. How does carbon dioxide permeate membranes? A discussion of concepts, results, and methods. Frontiers in Physiology 2014; 4: 382

Fishman AP, ed. The Respiratory System. Vol. I–IV. In: Handbook of Physiology (Section 3). American Physiological Society; 1987

Geers C, Gros G. Carbon dioxide transport and carbonic anhydrase in blood and muscle. Physiol Rev 2002; 80: 681–715

Kitchen H, Brett I. Embryonic and foetal hemoglobin in animals. Ann N Y Acad Sci 1974; 29: 653–671

Klein, BG. Cunningham's Textbook of Veterinary Physiology. 5th ed. New York: Elsevier; 2012

Lekeux P, Art T. The Respiratory System: Anatomy, Physiology and Adaptations to Exercise and Training. In: Hodgson DR, Rose RJ: The Athletic Horse. Philadelphia: Saunders Company; 1994

Moyes CD, Schulte PM. Principles of Animal physiology. Pearson; 2008

Murray JF. Respiration. In: Smith LH, Thier SO, eds. Pathophysiology – The Biological Principles of Disease. Section XI. Philadelphia: W. B. Saunders; 1985: 753–854.

Randall D, Burggren W, French K. Eckert Animal Physiology. 4th ed. New York: EdWH Freeman and Comp.; 2001

Randall DJ, Burggren W, Fench K. Gas exchange and acid-base balance. In: Eckert's Animal Physiology. 5th ed. Chapter 13. New York: W. H. Freeman; 2002

Scanes CG, Dridi S. Sturkie's Avian Physiology. Philadelphia: Elsevier; 2021

Scheid P, Piiper J. Vertebrate respiratory gas exchange. In: Handbook of Physiology: Comparative Physiology. Am Physiol Soc Bethesda 1997; 309–356

Scheid P, Slama H, Piiper J. Mechanisms of unidirectional flow in parabronchi of avian lungs: measurements in duck lung preparations. Resp Physiol 1972; 14:83–95

Schmidt-Nielsen K. Animal Physiology: Adaptation and environment. Cambridge: University Press; 1979

Sjaastad ØV, Sand O, Hove K. Physiology of Domestic Animals. Oslo: Scandinavian Veterinary Press; 2012

Steel WR. Scaling of respiratory variables in mammals. J Appl Physiol 1967; 22:453–460

Wildgoose WH. BSAVA Manual of Ornamental Fish. New Jersey: Wiley & Sons; 2001

Young M. Changes in human hemoglobins with development. In: Altman PL, Dittmer DW, eds. Respiration and Circulation. Bethesda: Fed Amer Soc Exp Biol; 1971

Regulation of the internal milieu

12 Kidney

Gotthold Gäbel, Salah Amasheh; former collaboration: M. Fromm

12.1 Role of the kidney

> **ESSENTIALS** ✖
>
> The kidney has five main functions:
> 1. **Excretion** of **metabolic waste products** and foreign chemicals. These are either filtered exclusively (e.g., creatinine), filtered and only partially reabsorbed (e.g., urea), or filtered and additionally secreted (e.g., potassium, uric acid, NH_4^+, protons, toxins, drugs, food additives, pesticides).
> 2. **Conservation** of **substances** that are to be **retained in the body**. These are either not filtered at all (e.g., large-molecule proteins) or filtered and reabsorbed (e.g., electrolytes such as sodium and chloride, glucose, amino acids, water).
> 3. **Regulation** of **water** and **electrolyte balance** by excretion of a concentrated or diluted urine or adjustment of the excretion/absorption rate of the individual electrolytes.
> 4. **Regulation** of **acid-base balance** by excretion of an acidic or alkaline urine.
> 5. **Endocrine functions** through metabolism and production of hormones.

ular solutes and water pass into the tubules by **filtration** from the glomerulus capillaries. Then, through **tubular reabsorption**, all the particular solutes required for functions throughout the body are recovered by specific transport mechanisms. In addition, some solutes are released into the lumen by tubular secretion. The solutes that are not reabsorbed as well as those secreted solutes remain in the tubular system and are finally excreted in urine.

However, the kidneys do not only distinguish qualitatively between waste products and physiologically relevant substances. They also regulate the retention or excretion of essential solutes and water in order to maintain their physiological concentration in body fluids. This continuous maintenance of the internal milieu is mainly by regulation of tubular reabsorption of these solutes and water.

For their size of less than 1% of body weight, mammalian kidneys have an extremely high blood flow of 15–25% of cardiac output. Depending on the species, ⅕–⅓ of the plasma flow is filtered in the glomeruli. However, only less than **1%** of that filtrate volume is actually **excreted** as urine under conditions of whole-body water balance. More than **99%** of the filtrate is therefore **reabsorbed** in the tubules and thus remains in the body.

12.2 Basics

The kidney is essential for homeostasis of the internal milieu, and thus has an important function in development and in adaptation to different habitats. The kidney enables the excretion of a wide range of noxious and dispensable substances while at the same time conserving and maintaining water and electrolyte balance, blood pressure, and acid-base balance. A lot of **metabolic waste products** can only be excreted in significant quantities by the kidneys. The problem for this is that metabolic waste products do not differ in molecular weight, chemical properties, or electrical charge from substances that are not to be excreted.

The kidneys therefore use the following strategies to excrete a large number of substances: First, all low-molec-

12.3 Morphology

The kidney is made up of a large number of lobes, on which an outer cortex (cortex renis) and an inner medulla (medulla renis) can be seen in cross-section. The functional units of the kidney, the **nephrons**, are embedded in the lobes, and can only be distinguished microscopically. Each nephron is infolded at its beginning so that a double-walled capsule (**capsula glomeruli, Bowman's capsule**) is formed (**Fig. 12.5**). Embedded in Bowman's capsule is a compact tuft of interconnected capillaries, the **glomerulus**. The Bowman capsule tapers towards the **proximal tubule**. This consists of a longer initial segment which first becomes **convoluted** in the cortex and then merges into a shorter **straight** segment in the medulla. This straight segment of the proximal tubule is the first segment of a

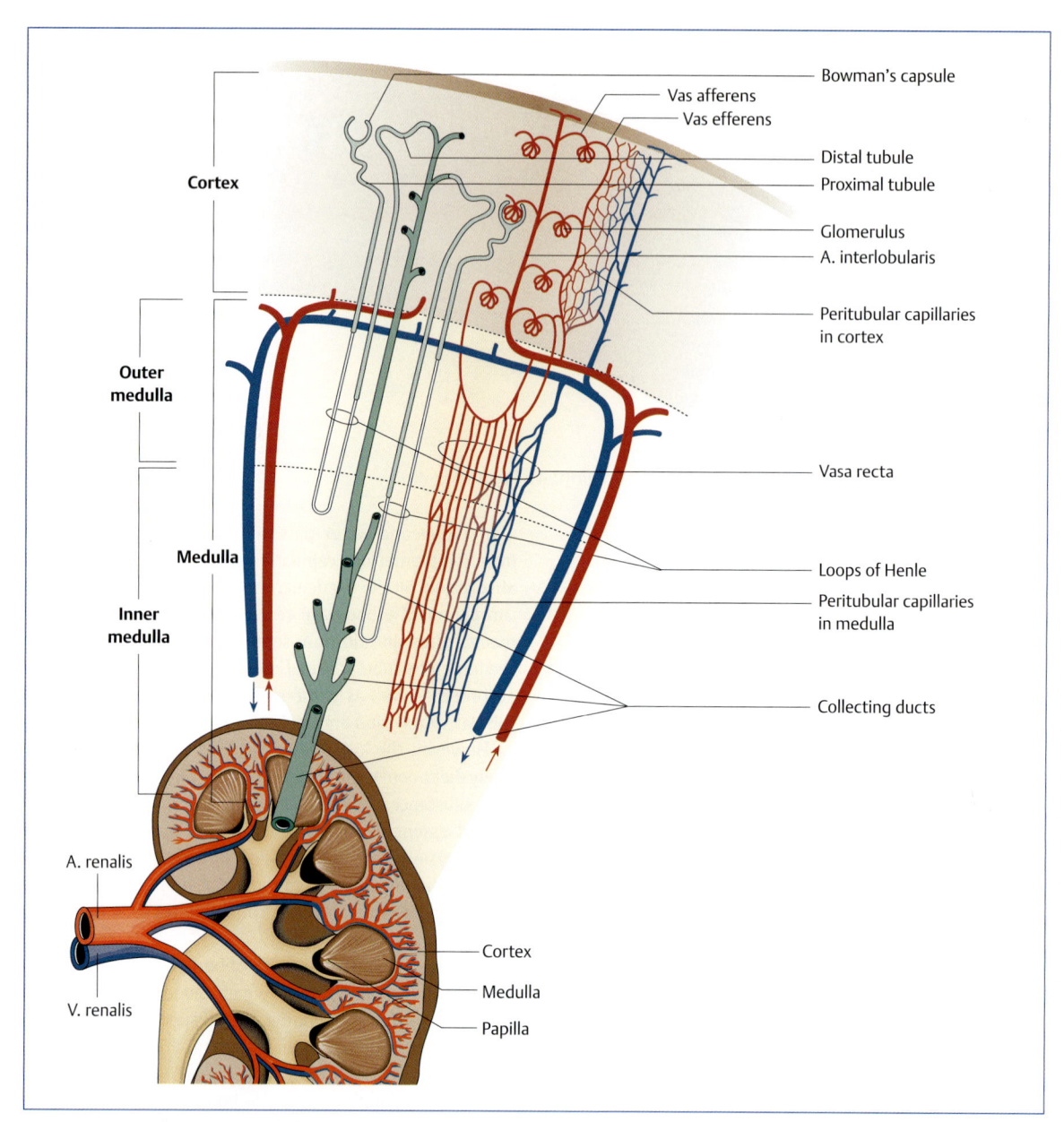

Fig. 12.1 Structural organisation of the kidney.
Left: Two nephrons with collecting tubule system. Superficial nephrons have short loops of Henle, whereas deep (juxtamedullary) nephrons have long loops that extend into the inner medulla. The glomeruli are followed by the proximal tubules, the loops of Henle and the distal tubules, which open into the collecting tubule system (for more detailed histology: see text).
Right: Arrangement of the vessels: Afferent arterioles (vasa afferentia) emerge from the interlobular arteries and pass into the glomerulus. From here, the blood is conducted by efferent arterioles (vasa efferentia) into peritubular capillary networks that surround the tubules of the cortex and medulla. The medullary capillary network along with the incoming arterioles and the outgoing venules are known as the vasa recta.

U-shaped loop, the **loop of Henle**. Here the proximal tubule tapers to a thin section, the **descending limb of the loop of Henle**. This either turns (in short loops) directly into the **thick segment of the ascending limb of the loop of Henle** or (in longer loops) it extends deeper into the medulla and passes first into the **thin segment of the ascending limb** and then into the **thick segment of the ascending limb**. The thick ascending segment runs back in a straight line to its own glomerulus and forms the **macula densa** at the point of contact. The thick ascending segment of the loop of Henle is part of the **distal tubule**. When a distinc-

tion is made in the following sections of this chapter between the loop of Henle and the proximal tubule or distal tubule, this is essentially a demarcation between the loop of Henle and the other parts of the proximal or distal tubule. The straight segment of the distal tubule is followed by the **convoluted distal tubule** which opens into the **collecting tubular system**. Although the arrangement of the **tubular structures** of the renal parenchyma always follows this same basic principle (**Fig. 12.1**), the length of the loops of Henle differs depending on their topographical position in the kidney: the superficial tubules form short loops,

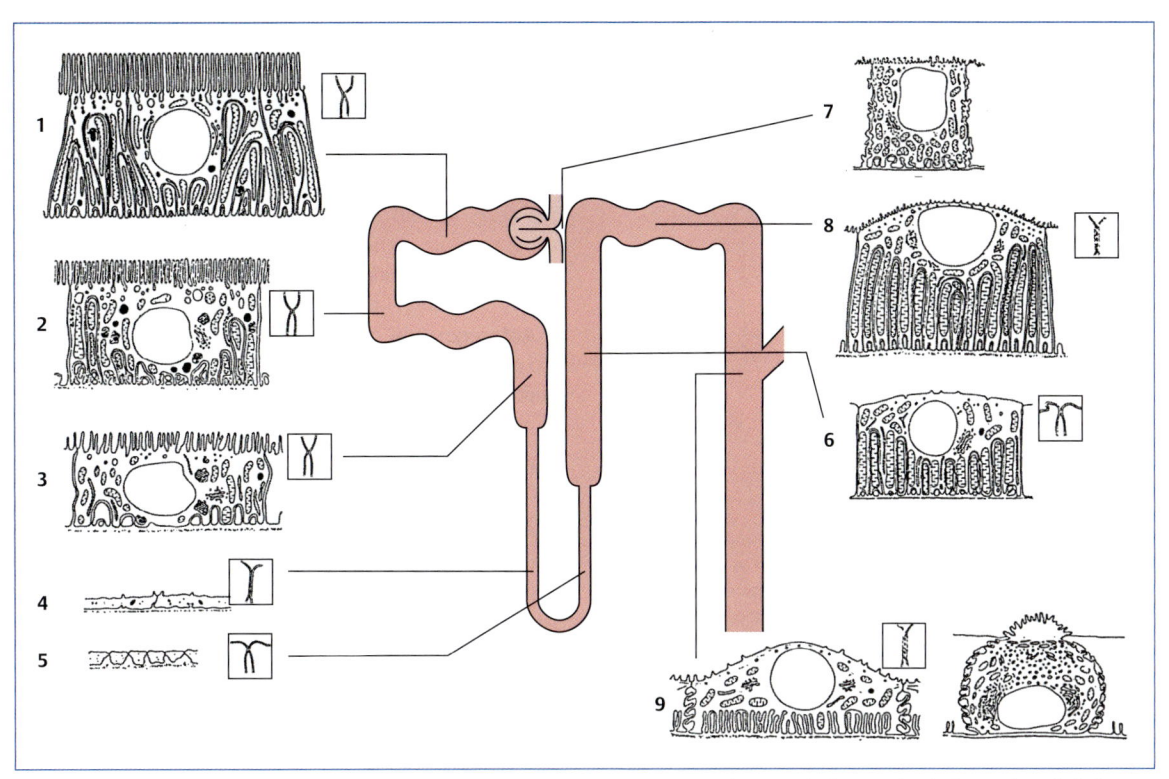

Fig. 12.2 Longitudinal heterogeneity of the tubular epithelia. The epithelial cells are shown with the apical side facing the tubule lumen upwards. The rectangular detail drawings are enlarged representations of the zonulae occludentes (tight junctions). **1** proximal convoluted tubule (segment S 1); **2** proximal convoluted tubule (segment S 2); **3** proximal straight tubule (pars recta, segment S 3); **4** thin descending part; **5** thin ascending part; **6** thick ascending segment of loop of Henle; **7** macula densa; **8** distal convoluted tubule; **9** cortical segment of collecting duct, right: "dark" principal cell, left: "light" intercalated cell.
Mitochondrial abundance indicates highly active transport processes (**1–2** and **6–8**). Small flat cells show no measurable active transport (**4–5**). Prominent infolding of the apical membrane (surface enlargement) and punctate zonulae occludentes are typical of "leaky" epithelia with high permeability, high transport rates and an inability to transport against appreciable concentration gradients (**1–2**). Pronounced zipper-like zonulae occludentes are typical of tight epithelia with lower permeability, lower transport rates and the ability to transport against steep gradients (**8–9**).

while the deep (= juxtamedullary) tubules have long loops that reach close to the tip of the papilla. The longer the loops, the greater their capability of concentrating urine.

The epithelium of each tubule segment differs in its ultrastructure (**Fig. 12.2**). The epithelial cells of the proximal tubule are linked by tight junctions which are more permeable than the apical cell membrane. In contrast, in the tightly linked epithelial cells of the distal tubules and the collecting ducts, the tight junctions are less permeable than the apical cell membrane. Tubule cells, with their highly active membrane transport systems, have numerous mitochondria in close proximity to the Na^+/K^+-ATPase in the basolateral membrane.

The arrangement of the **blood vessels** is schematically shown in **Fig. 12.1**. Blood supply to the kidneys is characterised by two capillary systems connected in series. Due to the **in-series connection** of vessels (afferent arterioles → glomerular capillaries → efferent arterioles → peritubular capillaries) blood is first filtered in the glomerular capillaries and then passes to the region of reabsorption and secretion in the peritubular capillaries.

Lymphatic vessels are mainly found in the renal cortex while in the renal medulla they are sparsely distributed and weakly developed. The kidney is supplied with **sympa-**thetic nerve fibres** from the coeliac plexus to the smooth muscle cells of the arteries and arterioles and to the juxtaglomerular apparatus.

> **IN A NUTSHELL** !
>
> Nephrons are the functional units of the kidney. They consist of a glomerulus and a tubular system. With the glomerulus capillaries and the peritubular capillaries, the kidney has two capillary systems connected in series.

12.4 Haemodynamics

12.4.1 Blood flow to the kidney

Although the kidneys represent less than 1% of body weight, renal blood flow is 15–25% of **cardiac output**. Thus, a 30 kg dog has a cardiac output of approximately $2.4 \cdot min^{-1}$ at rest (**Table 7.1**), of which $0.55 \cdot l \cdot min^{-1}$ supplies the kidneys. This high blood flow is necessary:
- to supply the kidney itself with nutrients and oxygen,
- to provide sufficient blood for filtration and
- to transport the substrates reabsorbed or secreted in the tubular system.

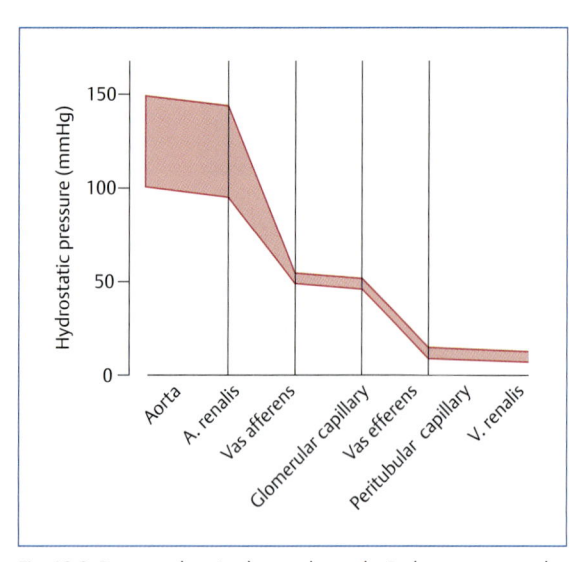

Fig. 12.3 Pressure drop in the renal vessels. Red area: autoregulatory levelling of different arterial pressures by the afferent arterioles. When the blood pressure in the aorta or renal artery fluctuates between 100 and 150 mmHg, autoregulation of the vas afferens keeps blood pressure in the glomerulus capillaries largely constant at 50 mmHg.

The blood supply to the kidney varies considerably from region to region. About 90% of the total flows through the renal cortex (in dogs, only about 80%), while only about 7% passes through the outer medulla and about 1% through the inner medulla.

The pressure curve along the renal vessels and its regulation is shown in **Fig. 12.3**. There is little drop in pressure in the glomerulus capillaries and in the peritubular capillaries. The main resistance vessels are the afferent and efferent arterioles, so that the pressure drop here is particularly high and regulated changes in resistance lead to marked changes in blood flow. The glomerular capillary network, where blood is filtered, is located between the afferent and efferent arterioles. The peritubular capillary network follows downstream from there. Consequently:

- an increase in resistance in the vas afferens leads to both reduced filtration and reduced blood flow overall. A reduction in resistance has the opposite effect (corresponding to the red area in **Fig. 12.3**),
- an increase in resistance in the vas efferens leads to increased filtration, but to reduced overall blood flow (not shown in **Fig. 12.3**).

> **IN A NUTSHELL**   **!**
>
> Renal blood flow is high, especially in the renal cortex. The high blood flow (15–25% of cardiac output) ensures efficient filtration in the glomerulus and also efficiency of the reabsorption processes in the tubular system. If resistance in the vas afferens increases, glomerular filtration becomes less efficient.

12.4.2 Regulation of renal blood flow

■ Autoregulation

The term **autoregulation** of renal blood flow refers to the fact that blood flow is kept relatively stable within a range of mean arterial pressure of 80–180 mmHg (**Fig. 12.3**, **Fig. 12.4**). Within the physiological fluctuation range of blood pressure, renal blood flow (RBF) or renal plasma flow (RPF) and glomerular filtration rate (GFR) remain mainly constant (**Fig. 12.3**, **Fig. 12.4**).

Autoregulation of **RBF** and **GFR is** mainly mediated by two mechanisms: the **Bayliss effect** and **tubuloglomerular feedback**.

Bayliss effect (myogenic mechanism)

The Bayliss effect (William M. Bayliss, 1860–1924; British physiologist) is particularly effective in the vas afferens. It is based on the reaction of vascular smooth muscle fibres to stretching which causes an increase in their tone. The particular significance of this mechanism is the rapidity of response (1–2 s) to an increase in blood pressure. The principle of this mechanism is described in more detail in ch. Autoregulation, myogenic tone (p. 208).

It is assumed that with increased vascular wall tension from the increased blood pressure a **Ca^{2+} influx** is triggered by stretch-activated cation channels (for the effect of Ca^{2+} in smooth muscle cells see ch. 6.3.3 (p. 162) Electromechanical coupling in smooth muscle).

Tubuloglomerular feedback

If blood pressure rises and the Bayliss effect only partially adjusts to this, then GFR increases. If, as a consequence, the reabsorption capacity of the tubular system for NaCl is also exceeded, the NaCl concentration in the thick segment of the loop of Henle increases. As a result of the increased NaCl flow, the uptake of NaCl in macula densa cells of the juxtaglomerular apparatus also increases (**Fig. 12.5**, **Fig. 12.6**). Various mediators such as adenosine cause constriction of the vas afferens which results in a reduction in GFR. However, the tubuloglomerular feedback will also respond to a drop in blood pressure or GFR and promote enhanced GFR. The reaction time of the tubuloglomerular feedback is 15–20 seconds.

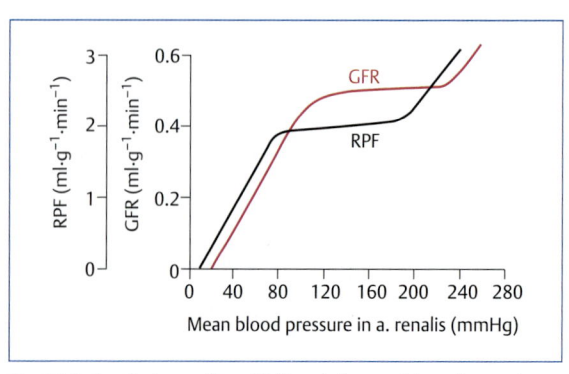

Fig. 12.4 Renal plasma flow (RPF) and the resulting glomerular filtration rate (GFR) are autoregulated. The figure shows the range of both variables in dogs.

Inner milieu

> **IN A NUTSHELL** !
>
> Cortical blood flow is autoregulated, i.e., largely independent of fluctuations in arterial blood pressure. Autoregulation is mediated by two mechanisms: the Bayliss effect and tubuloglomerular feedback. The Bayliss effect adjusts the diameter of the vas afferens.

MORE DETAILS

Shock kidney

"Autoregulation" does not mean that renal blood flow is completely independent of blood pressure. Thus, if there is a severe drop in blood pressure from blood loss, this could fall below the regulatory range of autoregulation (**Fig. 12.4**: at a blood pressure < 60 mmHg). This is a complication that could result in kidney damage from circulatory shock. In shock, the initial response to the pronounced fall in systemic blood pressure is activation of the sympathetic nervous system in the so-called pre-shock stage (compensated shock). However, this activation of the sympathetic nervous system further reduces blood flow to the kidneys. Thus, with strong activation of the sympathetic nervous system in the afferent renal vessels, norepinephrine acts on α_1 receptors (p. 117) causing a great increase in blood flow resistance. In advanced shock, in the so-called irreversible stage (decompensated shock), systemic activation of the sympathetic nervous system is largely ineffective, i.e., the drastic drop in blood pressure persists due to general vasodilation despite activation of the sympathetic nervous system. For the kidney, this means that blood flows in at a lower pressure, which is further reduced as a result of sympathetic activation in the afferent renal vessels, so that autoregulation is "overtaxed". This ultimately results in a drastic reduction in blood flow to the entire kidney. As a result of the reduced blood supply, the kidney suffers from functional deficiencies (oliguria to anuria) and ultimately to irreversible morphological changes (shock kidney).

■ Renin-angiotensin-aldosterone system

Renin is not involved in the mechanisms of tubuloglomerular feedback, but nevertheless has a strong effect on renal blood flow. Renin is produced from the granules of specialised smooth muscle cells of the juxtaglomerular apparatus (**Fig. 12.5**, **Fig. 12.6**). The release of renin can be triggered by pressure sensors in the kidney that respond to a drop in

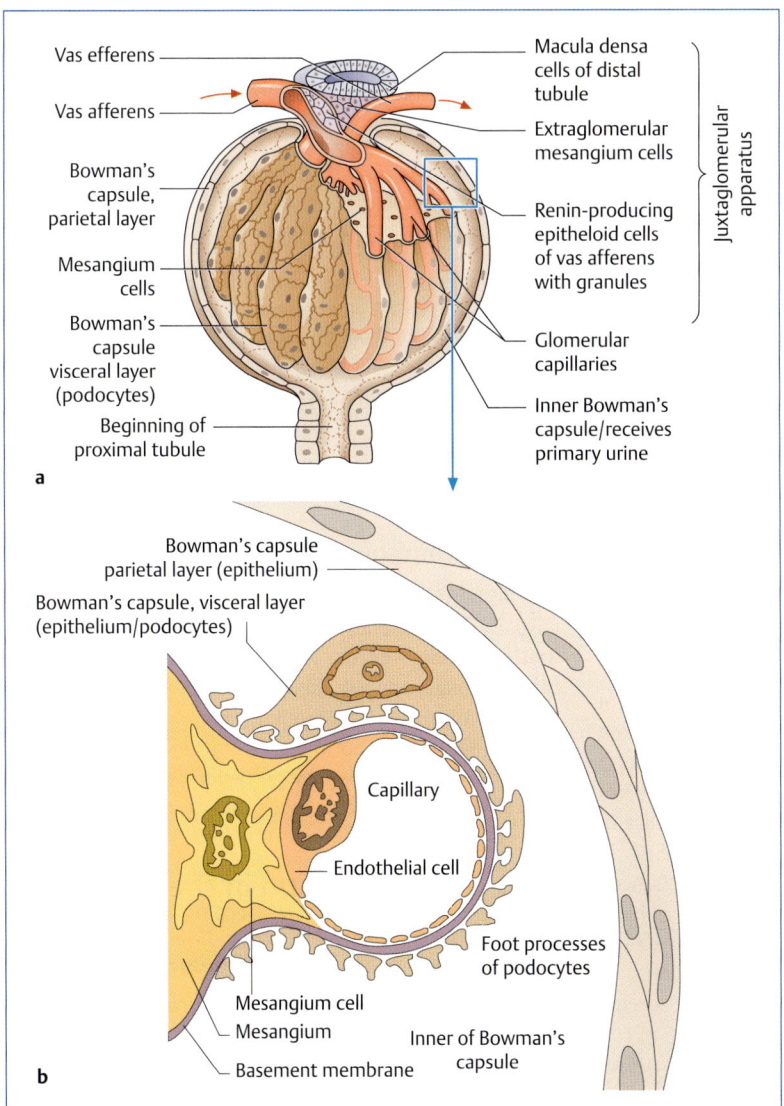

a

Vas efferens

Vas afferens

Bowman's capsule, parietal layer

Mesangium cells

Bowman's capsule visceral layer (podocytes)

Beginning of proximal tubule

Macula densa cells of distal tubule

Extraglomerular mesangium cells

Renin-producing epitheloid cells of vas afferens with granules

Glomerular capillaries

Inner Bowman's capsule/receives primary urine

Juxtaglomerular apparatus

b

Bowman's capsule parietal layer (epithelium)

Bowman's capsule, visceral layer (epithelium/podocytes)

Capillary

Endothelial cell

Foot processes of podocytes

Mesangium cell
Mesangium
Basement membrane

Inner of Bowman's capsule

Fig. 12.5 a Structure of a glomerulus with juxtaglomerular apparatus. The smooth muscle cells of the vas afferens have distinct granules in renin-producing epithelioid cells. The glomerular capillaries connect into an efferent arteriole (vas efferens).

b The vascular wall of the glomerular capillary loops consists of three layers: endothelial cells, a basement membrane and epithelial cells with foot processes of podocytes attached on the outer side. The podocyte arrangement stabilises the capillary loop and counteracts pressure-passive stretching.
Mesangium cells are located between the capillary loops and in between the arterioles and the macula densa segment of the distal tubule. [Source: (a) Schünke M, Schünke G. Nephron (funktioneller Aufbau). In: Schünke M, Faller A (eds.). Der Körper des Menschen. 18th, unamended ed. Aufl., Stuttgart: Thieme; 2020.
(b) Kellner U. Glomerulonephritiden. In: Krams M, Frahm S, Kellner U et al. (eds.). Kurzlehrbuch Pathologie. 2nd ed., Stuttgart: Thieme; 2018]

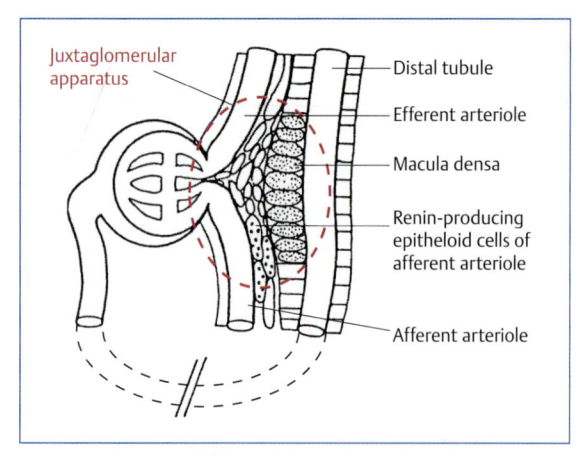

Fig. 12.6 Structure of the juxtaglomerular apparatus.

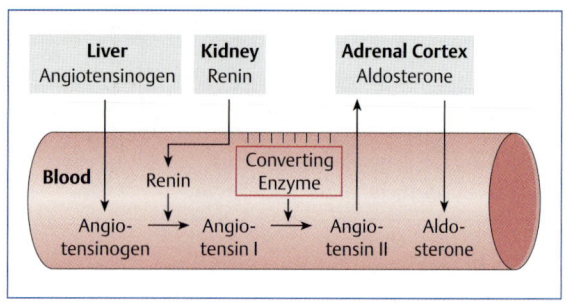

Fig. 12.7 The renin-angiotensin-aldosterone system. Renin is released from the kidney into blood and catalyses the conversion of angiotensinogen produced by the liver into angiotensin I. Angiotensin I undergoes a further conversion to angiotensin II by the angiotensin-converting enzyme (ACE). Angiotensin II stimulates the release of aldosterone from the adrenal cortex. ACE is located on the surface of endothelial cells of the capillaries. The plasma concentration of renin is the limiting factor in the reninangiotensin-aldosterone system and thus the main determinant of the plasma concentration of angiotensin II. The numerous effects of angiotensin II are described in the text.

blood pressure. However, renin release is also increased when there is a decrease in NaCl concentration at the macula densa, and also with sympathetic stimulation. As shown in **Fig. 12.7**, the only known substrate for renin action is angiotensinogen secreted by the liver into blood. Thus, renin release first leads to the formation of angiotensin I by cleaving a decapeptide from angiotensinogen. From angiotensin I, the octapeptide angiotensin II is formed by the endothelial angiotensin-converting enzyme (ACE) through the cleavage of two amino acids. ACE is expressed by almost all vascular endothelia throughout the body. Angiotensin II has numerous effects, and its effect on blood supply of the kidney is usually not due to its local, but its systemic action (see nos. 2–5 of the following list):

1. In the kidney, angiotensin II has a vasoconstrictor effect on both the vas afferens and the vas efferens. However, this local counter-regulatory effect does not play a significant role in the physiological regulatory range.
2. Angiotensin II has a systemic vasoconstrictor effect which is strong because it potentiates the action of norepinephrine and it activates angiotensin receptors in vascular smooth muscle leading also to constriction of the vessels. In this way, a general vasoconstriction is induced in the arteries, which in turn counteracts the drop in blood pressure and thus also the drop in GFR.
3. Angiotensin also leads to an increase in sympathetic nerve activity via an effect on the central nervous system.
4. In addition, angiotensin II can induce a sensation of thirst and a desire for salt and also a release of ADH from the pituitary gland. With these stimuli, the extracellular volume increases. Regulation of water and salt balance is described in more detail in ch. 13.8. This increase in extracellular volume in turn leads to an increase in blood pressure via the Frank-Starling mechanism (p. 170).
5. In addition to its direct effect on receptors of the vascular musculature, the increased release of angiotensin II also provokes secretion of aldosterone from the adrenal cortex (**Fig. 12.7**). Aldosterone causes a retention of Na^+ (p. 314) by the kidney (and in the colon) and thus subsequently also of water.

All these described effects, including that of aldosterone, result in an increase in intravascular volume and in blood pressure, and thus also prevent a drop in GFR. Angiotensin II can be considered one of the most potent agents for increasing systemic blood pressure.

MORE DETAILS

ACE inhibitors

The strong vasoconstrictor properties of angiotensin have pathophysiological significance in various diseases. In affected patients, it is necessary to minimise the effect of angiotensin II. This is done by pharmacological inhibition of the angiotensin-converting enzyme (ACE inhibitor) or via receptor antagonists. In small animal medicine, ACE inhibitors are used in chronic heart disease to minimise cardiac work. The focus here is on the general vasoconstrictor effect of angiotensin II or its suppression and thus minimisation of the load on the heart. Another indication is the symptomatic treatment of chronic renal insufficiency, for example in cats.

■ Other hormones modulating blood flow

Several hormones and transmitter substances also have a partially indirect effect on renal blood flow. **Atrial natriuretic peptide** (see ch. Regulation of sodium transport (p. 314)) dilates the vas afferens, increasing filtration pressure and thus GFR. This promotes the natriuretic and also diuretic effect of the hormone. Prostaglandins (p. 535) have a vasodilating effect, which can enhance blood supply to the kidneys, especially in the medullary region.

12.5　Ultrafiltration in the glomeruli

Filtration is the transport of solvent (water) and filterable solutes through a filter down a hydrostatic pressure gradient. A simple filter distinguishes between dissolved solutes and the solvent and undissolved particles. The pore size of the filter in the glomeruli is smaller than in simple filters, according to filter technology classifications, and the processes in the glomerulus are also referred to as **ul-**

trafiltration, particularly because proteins are retained in the capillary blood flow. The filtrate discharged into the Bowman capsule is called **primary urine**. The filtration capacity of the kidneys is enormous. For example, a dog with a cardiac output of approx. $2.4 l \cdot min^{-1}$ (Table 7.1) has a renal blood flow of about $0.55 l \cdot min^{-1}$ or about $800 l \cdot d^{-1}$ (Table 12.3). This corresponds to a renal plasma flow of approx. $440 l \cdot d^{-1}$ (haematocrit $0.45 l \cdot l^{-1}$). Through ultrafiltration in the glomeruli, a volume of approx. $140 l$ filtrate/day is produced, i.e., a multiple of the amount of plasma of the dog. However, this high filtration rate is necessary so that the end products of metabolism such as urea can be eliminated. The water of the primary urine is almost completely reabsorbed in the tubules, so that only about one hundredth of the filtered volume reaches the renal pelvis.

12.5.1 Filtration barrier

The **filtration barrier** (Fig. 12.5) consists of three layers (from the inside to the outside): fenestrated endothelial cells, basement membrane and epithelial podocytes. The three layers impede the passage of molecules depending on their **size** and **charge**. Small molecular weight solutes can pass through just as easily as water and thus are "freely filtered". Substances with a higher molecular weight, especially plasma proteins, are almost completely prevented from passing through. Blood cells are retained by the fenestrated endothelial cells of the capillaries (Fig. 8.16). Substances with a molecular weight of ≈ 200 kDa or more are retained in the three-layer basement membrane. The narrowest limiting point for the passage of solutes are the slit pores of the podocytes. Substances of > 65 kDa cannot normally pass through here.

In Table 12.1 the molecular weights and molecular sizes of some typical solutes are compared with their filterability. In addition to molecular size and shape, the plasma binding and charge of the solutes also play a role. When bound to plasma proteins, small molecular weight solutes avoid filtration. These include Ca^{2+}, Mg^{2+}, iron, various hormones (e.g., corticosteroids, thyroid hormones) and many drugs.

> **IN A NUTSHELL** !
>
> Only low-molecular weight substances normally pass through the glomerular filter. Larger molecules such as plasma proteins are retained. The same applies to molecules and ions that are bound to plasma proteins. They are not "freely filterable".

12.5.2 Net filtration pressure

The same forces that cause fluid to be squeezed out of capillaries by filtration into the surrounding tissue (Fig. 8.17) are responsible for fluid being squeezed out of the glomerulus loops into Bowman's capsule. Accordingly, the following forces act:

1. **Hydrostatic pressure:** acts in the direction of the Bowman's capsule
2. **Colloid-osmotic pressure:** Due to the filter, proteins are largely retained in the blood of the glomeruli and do not appear in the filtrate. This uneven distribution of proteins causes a colloid-osmotic pressure that is opposite to the hydrostatic pressure.

The **net filtration pressure** is the sum of the individual pressures and thus the net pressure that forces fluid through the glomerular membrane. According to the preconditions presented, the following relationship applies at the entry of blood into the capillaries of the glomeruli:

$$\text{net filtration pressure} = \Delta p - \Delta \pi \qquad (12.1)$$

$$15 = 40 - 25 \text{ (mmHg)}$$

Here Δp is the effective hydrostatic pressure and $\Delta \pi$ the effective colloid- osmotic pressure.

The glomerular filtration rate is most strongly influenced by changes in hydrostatic pressure. Therefore, in order to keep the GFR approximately constant when blood pressure drops or rises, renal blood flow is autoregulated, see ch. Autoregulation (p. 306).

Inner milieu

Table 12.1 Relationships between molecular weight, molecular size and glomerular filterability. Sucrose, inulin and egg albumin are substances that do not occur in blood under physiological conditions. They are listed here only to illustrate the differences in filterability. The molecular radius of each assumes an idealised "spherical shape".

Substance	Molecular weight (Da)	Molecular radius (nm)	Sieve coefficient ([X] filtrate / [X] plasma)
Water	18	0.10	1.0
Urea	60	0.16	1.0
Glucose	180	0.36	1.0
Sucrose	342	0.44	1.0
Inulin	5500	1.48	0.98
Myoglobin	17000	1.95	0.75
Ovalbumin	43500	2.85	0.22
Haemoglobin	68000	3.25	0.03
Serum albumin	69000	3.55	<0.01

based on data from Pitt's RF. Physiologie der Niere und der Körperflüssigkeiten. Stuttgart: Schattauer; 1972

Mesangium

The space between the capillary loops is filled by a mesangium (**Fig. 12.5**) consisting of mesangium cells and a mesangial matrix of collagen and fibronectin. The mesangium cells are contractile cells connected by gap junctions, thus forming a uniformly functioning syncytium. The mesangium is not bounded on the capillary side by a basement membrane, but only by fenestrated endothelium. This means that there is not a highly selective filter membrane towards the mesangium.

The mesangium is anchored to the juxtaglomerular apparatus by the contractile cells and attaches to the basement membranes of the capillaries via micro-tendons. Mesangial cells have autocrine, paracrine, and endocrine functions, i.e., they produce growth factors and hormones that influence the environment. Many vasoconstrictors lead to contraction of the mesangium cells and thus to a reduction in GFR. The hormones mainly causing vasoconstriction are antidiuretic hormone (=ADH), angiotensin II, endothelin, thromboxane and parathyroid hormone.

> **IN A NUTSHELL**   !
>
> The parameters that affect ultrafiltration are the size and permeability of the filtering surface as well as the transmural hydrostatic and colloid- osmotic pressure difference. The controlled parameter is the hydrostatic pressure.

12.5.3   Methods for assessing filtration

■ Determination of metabolic waste products in plasma

A decrease in excretion of a substance leads to its increased plasma concentration. Therefore, plasma analyses can to some extent be used to check renal function. However, an increase in plasma concentration of a substance may also indicate either increased dietary intake or increased endogenous production. Substances in plasma that can be used to indicate renal function are the concentrations of urea, creatinine, creatine, or uric acid, all derived from intermediary metabolism. They are all nitrogenous substances and are mainly excreted via the kidneys. Because they are easier to measure, urea and creatinine and symmetrical dimethylarginine (SDMA) are usually assayed in addition to electrolytes.

Urea is synthesised in the urea cycle (p. 472) in the liver from ammonia. It is the detoxification product of proteolysis and is normally excreted by the kidneys. However, the urea concentration in plasma is also subject to fluctuations independently of kidney function. For example, it can increase a few hours after protein-rich food intake or also in increased proteolytic degradation (fever, tissue breakdown, etc.). There is also the problem that urea in the glomerular filtrate is reabsorbed in the tubular system (p. 324), thus making it difficult to draw definite conclusions about glomerular filtration capacity from the plasma concentration of urea.

Creatinine is a product of muscle catabolism of creatine and is released into plasma at a mainly constant rate. Creatinine therefore has the analytical advantage over urea in that its plasma concentration is relatively constant and does not change with increased dietary protein intake or an increased rate of endogenous proteolysis. Another advantage of creatinine is that it enters the tubular system almost exclusively via filtration. Disturbances of renal filtration function therefore quickly lead to an increased concentration of creatinine in plasma.

Symmetrical dimethylarginine (**SDMA**) is formed by proteolysis in the cell nucleus. Like creatinine, it also enters the bloodstream at a constant rate, is filtered by the kidneys and excreted in urine. The plasma concentration correlates very closely with the glomerular filtration rate and, in contrast to creatinine, is not dependent on muscle mass. In dogs and cats, SDMA is increasingly used as an early marker for declining kidney function. An increased concentration of SDMA in plasma indicates reduced glomerular filtration capacity.

■ Renal clearance

The **renal clearance** value of a substance is the result of filtration and secretion minus its reabsorption. For example, a renal clearance value of $125\,ml \cdot min^{-1}$ means that 125 ml plasma volume is completely freed ("cleared") of the substrate in question in one minute during passage through the kidneys. From measurement of the renal clearance of various substances, it is thus possible to draw conclusions about the functional properties of the kidneys. In **Table 12.2**, renal clearance values for humans under normal conditions are presented. It can be seen that substances that are filtered and then completely reabsorbed, such as **glucose**, have a clearance value of **zero**, i.e., the plasma maintains the same concentration of glucose during passage through the kidneys. If there is a change in the excretion characteristics of such filtered substances, conclusions can be drawn about the reabsorption capacity. When reabsorption is no longer complete, the concentration of the filtered substance decreases in plasma, but increases in urine. However, if substances that are usually reabsorbed, are detected in urine, this does not necessarily indicate renal malfunction. Detection of glucose in urine usually indicates an increased plasma glucose concentration, so that the increased filtration exceeds the normal reabsorption capacity of the kidney for glucose.

Table 12.2 Typical renal clearance values in humans under normal conditions. Paraaminohippuric acid (PAH) and inulin are substances that are not present in blood under physiological conditions. To determine their renal clearance (and thus renal function), they must be infused intravascularly. For sodium and potassium, the clearance values vary over a wide range, as their excretion can be regulated, see ch. 12.7.3 and ch. 12.8.3.

Substance	Clearance ($ml \cdot min^{-1}$)
Glucose	0
Amino acids	0
Na^+	0.5–6.25
K^+	2–180
Urea	approx. 75
Inulin (creatinine)	125
PAH	650

based on data from Silbernagl S, Despopoulos A. Taschenatlas Physiologie, 7th ed. Stuttgart: Thieme 2007

■ Renal clearance of creatinine

Determination of the renal clearance of certain marker substances provides information about the functional capacity of the kidney. If a substance is entirely filtered, renal filtration capacity can be measured from the excretion characteristics of the substance. Determination of the renal clearance of creatinine therefore allows conclusions to be drawn about the GFR.

Thus, for the amount of creatinine filtered in the glomeruli per minute:

$$\text{filtered quantity} = \text{GFR} \cdot [\text{Cr}]_P \tag{12.2}$$

$[\text{Cr}]_P$ is the creatinine concentration in plasma.

The amount excreted in urine per unit time applies as follows:

$$\text{amount in urine} = V_U \cdot [\text{Cr}]_U \tag{12.3}$$

Where V_U = urine volume per time, $[\text{Cr}]_U$ = concentration of creatinine in the urine.

If creatinine is neither absorbed nor secreted in the tubular system, the amount eliminated from plasma per unit of time must be equal to the amount excreted in urine. Accordingly, the following applies:

$$\text{filtered quantity} = \text{excreted quantity}$$

or

$$\text{GFR} \cdot [\text{Cr}]_P = V_U \cdot [\text{Cr}]_U \tag{12.4}$$

The upper equation can be transformed according to the GFR:

$$\text{GFR} = V_U \cdot \frac{[\text{Cr}]_U}{[\text{Cr}]_P} \tag{12.5}$$

From this transformation, the value for the GFR can be read directly. By definition, the right-hand part of the equation denotes the creatinine clearance, i.e., the plasma volume per time that is completely freed ("cleared") of creatinine during passage through the kidneys. To determine GFR by measuring creatinine, the urine volume per time as well as the concentrations of creatinine in urine and in plasma must be measured.

Creatinine clearance has a small error, however, because creatinine is also – albeit to a small extent – secreted tubularly in many animals and therefore measurement of plasma and urine concentrations would indicate a somewhat too high GFR value. However, determination of creatinine has the advantage that the procedure can be simplified even further. Thus, GFR can also be estimated from the plasma concentration of creatinine alone without measuring excretion in urine.

This determination is methodologically based on an elegant simplification of the renal clearance of creatinine. Thus, the largely constant clearance of creatinine also means that $V_U \cdot [\text{Cr}]_U$, i.e., the numerator of the last equation, is almost constant. As a result, this equation can be simplified to leave an inverse relationship between GFR and $[\text{Cr}]_P$ (creatinine plasma concentration) (**Fig. 12.8**). The following can be read from the course of the curve shown in **Fig. 12.8**. If the GFR falls to half its normal value, the creatinine concentration in plasma would increase to twice

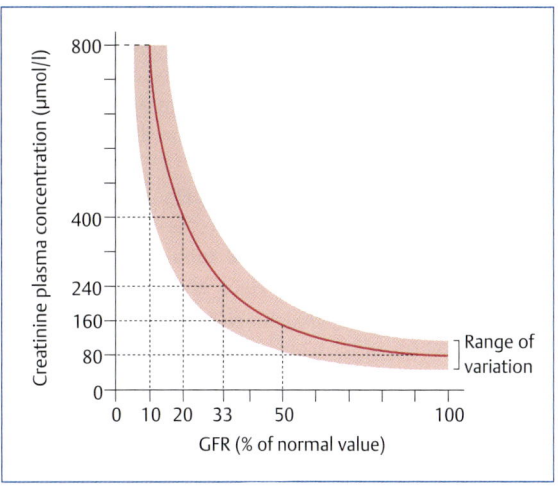

Fig. 12.8 Relationship between creatinine plasma concentration and glomerular filtration rate (GFR).

its normal value. Correspondingly, a decrease in GFR to $\frac{1}{3}$, $\frac{1}{5}$ or $\frac{1}{10}$ of the norm leads to an increase in $[\text{Cr}]_P$ by 3, 5 or 10 times the norm, respectively. This means that creatinine clearance does not necessarily have to be determined if renal failure is suspected.

Thus, just from the **plasma concentration** of **creatinine** alone the filtration capacities of the kidneys can be approximately determined. However, this can only be done, if **GFR** is severely restricted, because in the flat area of the curve (**Fig. 12.8**) the normal physiological variation prevents a reliable estimate.

If a substance is filtered unhindered and is additionally secreted completely into the tubules (example: paraaminohippurate, PAH), the **clearance** of this substance corresponds approximately to the **renal plasma flow** (**RPF**): C_{PAH} = RPF. The renal blood flow (RBF) is calculated from RBF = RPF/(1 – haematocrit).

> ### IN A NUTSHELL !
> Renal clearance is a substrate-related parameter and refers to the plasma volume that is completely cleared of a particular substance in a certain unit of time. The renal clearance of creatinine gives an assessment of the filtration capacity of the kidneys.

12.6 Tubular transport mechanisms: Overview

The **filtered primary urine** is – except for proteins – similar in composition to blood plasma. The tubules have the function of preparing the final urine from the primary urine. This is done by a series of complex mechanisms. After large quantities of solutes and water have been collected in the renal tubules by **glomerular ultrafiltration** additional solutes are added by **tubular secretion**. However, the main task of the tubule system is to retrieve essential substances from the filtrate by **reabsorption** to prevent their loss. These include many ions such as sodium, chloride, calcium, magnesium and organic molecules such as glucose and amino acids, and also water. There are a number of specific reabsorption transport mechanisms to recover these essential substances from the filtered primary urine, while "waste and foreign substances" continue for excretion in urine.

The differences in ultrastructure in **Fig. 12.2** are also reflected in the different functional properties of the different tubule sections. The **proximal tubules** are **leaky** and transport large amounts of NaCl and water, but only against small concentration gradients. The **distal tubule segments**, on the other hand, are **dense** (**tight**) and transport only small amounts, but possibly against steep concentration gradients. Hormonally controlled **fine-tuning** of the composition of urine takes place in the distal segments.

The relative reabsorption of Na^+, Cl^- and water compared to the filtered amount in the segments of the renal tubule in the **antidiuretic state**, i.e., with low water intake and excretion, is summarised in **Fig. 12.9**.

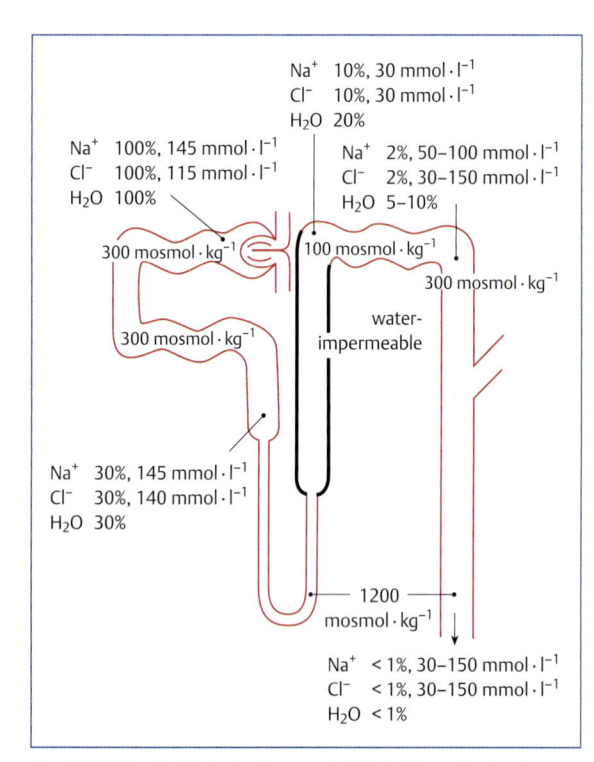

Fig. 12.9 Extent of tubular transport of Na^+, Cl^- and water in antidiuresis. The percentages refer to the amounts still present in the respective nephron segments in relation to the filtered amount ("filtered load" = 100%). In addition, local tubular concentrations and osmolalities are given. The tubular concentrations reflect reabsorption processes, especially of sodium, with chloride following passively as a counter anion. The reabsorption of chloride in the proximal tubule is slightly lower than that of sodium (due to the lumen-positive potential in the second half of the proximal tubule). This slightly shifts the concentration ratios of chloride to sodium at the end of the proximal tubule compared to the beginning.

12.7   Sodium and chloride movement in the nephron

12.7.1   Importance of the kidney for NaCl balance

The total body content of exchangeable Na^+ is **filtered** by the **glomeruli** about **10 times per day**. This means that in a horse of 500 kg ≈ 200 mol = 11 kg NaCl (!) per day passes into the renal tubules by filtration. Therefore, effective tubular reabsorption is necessary to prevent salt loss. Thus, of the filtered load in antidiuresis, > **99 % is reabsorbed** and only < 1 % is excreted. About 70% of the filtered Na^+ is reabsorbed in the proximal tubule.

Because the proximal tubule is very permeable, water follows the reabsorbed sodium and chloride by osmosis. As a result, the concentration of osmotically active components in the tubule fluid remains unchanged at approx. 280–300 $mosmol \cdot kg^{-1}$. This type of reabsorption is called **isoosmolar reabsorption**. In the loop of Henle, about 20% of the filtered sodium and chloride are further reabsorbed. However, since the ascending thick segment of the loop of Henle is almost water-impermeable, water remains in the tubule lumen. Thus, the fluid exiting the thick segment of the loop of Henle is hypoosmolar. In the subsequent parts of the distal tubule and in the collecting duct, the residual sodium and chloride of the 99% that entered the filtrate are finally reabsorbed. The kidney thus has minimum ability to reduce sodium and chloride excretion. Sodium reabsorption, especially in the distal nephron segments, is controlled by the adrenocortical hormone **aldosterone**.

12.7.2   Mechanisms of tubular NaCl transport

■ Principle

In principle, the reabsorption of NaCl, and indirectly also that of water, is mediated in all sections of the tubule system by a Na^+/K^+-ATPase on the basolateral membrane of the cells. This transporter keeps the sodium concentration inside the cell low. As a result, there is a chemical gradient from the tubule lumen to the cell interior, which drives sodium into the cell interior. In many electrogenic transporters, the transepithelial potential difference (negative on the inside of the cell) also acts as an additional driving force, drawing the positively charged sodium into the cell interior. While the **basolateral** outflow of sodium is generally mediated via the **Na^+/K^+-ATPase**, the type of **apical sodium transporter differs** in different segments of the tubule.

■ Proximal tubule

On the apical side of the **proximal tubule, Na^+** is taken up into the tubule cell predominantly by **cotransport** with other substances, mainly glucose (sodium glucose linked transport = SGLT), but also with neutral and acidic amino acids (**Fig. 12.10**). This means that the reabsorption of sodium is linked to the retrieval of other essential solutes.

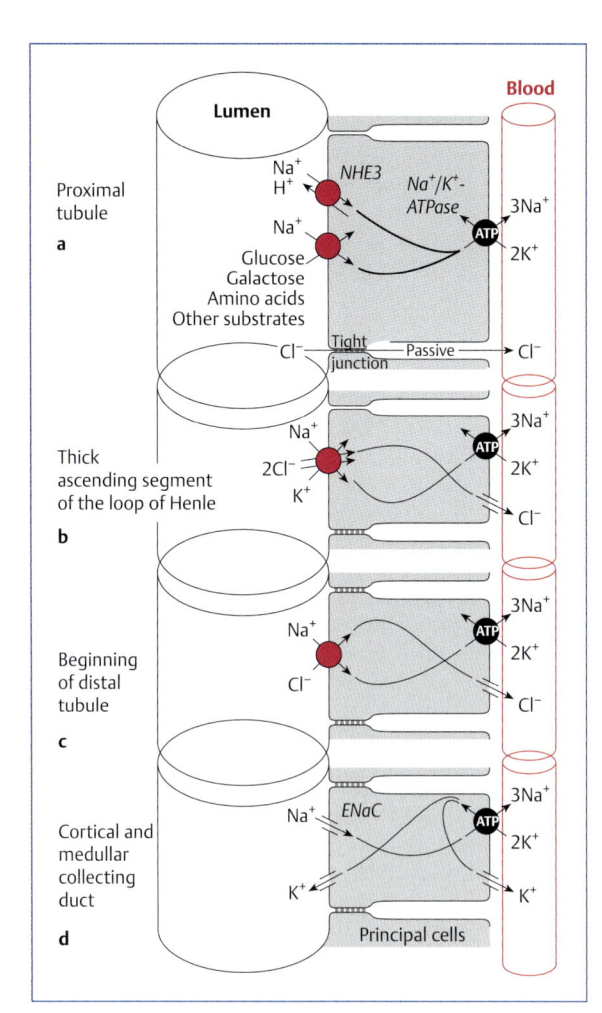

Fig. 12.10 Cell models of tubular transport of Na⁺ and Cl⁻. NHE3 = Na⁺/H⁺ exchanger 3; ENaC = epithelial Na⁺ channel.

Phosphate, sulphate, mono- and dicarboxylic acids are also reabsorbed under the influence of the sodium gradient.

The **symport** of **sodium** with **glucose** and **amino acids** is **electrogenic**. The transport of sodium ions transfers positive charges from the lumen to the blood. In this way, the lumen in the first section of the proximal tubule becomes negatively charged and the blood side of the epithelium becomes positively charged (about 2 mV potential difference), which is a driving force for chloride diffusion. However, this chloride diffusion causes a lumen positive potential in the later sections of the proximal tubule, which slightly limits the reabsorption of anions, including chloride, and promotes the reabsorption of cations. In addition to the symporters, sodium ions are also reabsorbed by means of a **Na⁺/H⁺ antiporter** (NHE3 = Na⁺/H⁺ exchanger 3) from the tubule lumen into the tubule cells. The uptake of sodium by this mechanism promotes the release of protons from the cells into the tubule lumen. The Na⁺/H⁺ antiporter represents an essential mechanism in the maintenance of a stable acid-base status (p. 326).

Cl⁻ is reabsorbed in the first section of the proximal tubule entirely **passively** and also by a paracellular pathway. There are three mechanisms for this:

1. by diffusion because of a lumen-negative transepithelial voltage of −2 mV,
2. by diffusion because of the increased luminal Cl⁻ concentration as water is being reabsorbed,
3. through solvent drag (**Fig. 12.10**).

The reabsorption of sodium and chloride and also of the other solutes drives **water reabsorption**. Other solutes are also absorbed by the solvent drag effect from the reabsorption of water. Due to the high paracellular permeability, most of the sodium and chloride is reabsorbed in this way.

> **IN A NUTSHELL** !
>
> In the **proximal tubule**, about ⅔ of the filtered Na⁺, Cl⁻ and water are reabsorbed. Na⁺ is mainly reabsorbed by an active process and, with its apical uptake into the cell, promotes the reabsorption of other solutes through numerous symports.

■ Loop of Henle

The **thin** descending segment of the **loop of Henle** consists of mitochondria-poor, small epithelial cells (**Fig. 12.2**); hence the tubule is "thin" here. The epithelial lining is very **permeable to water**, but there is no significant active transport. About 25% of filtered water is reabsorbed in this segment. Water reabsorption is driven by the increasing osmolality of the interstitium towards the medulla in the countercurrent multiplier system (p. 317) (**Fig. 12.14**).

In the **thick ascending segment** of the **loop of Henle**, 25–30% of the filtered Na⁺ and Cl⁻ are reabsorbed. Uptake of these ions is mediated by a symporter in the apical membrane that transports Na⁺, K⁺ and Cl⁻ in a 1:1:2 ratio. On the basolateral side, Na⁺ is released through the Na⁺/K⁺-ATPase and Cl⁻ is released through a channel into the interstitium. The thick ascending segment of the loop of Henle contains **no water channels** and is thus practically **water impermeable**. As a result, the **osmolality** of the tubular fluid decreases to about **100 mosmol · kg⁻¹** in the thick ascending loop of Henle towards the distal tubule. Therefore, the thick ascending segment is also called the **dilution segment** with the consequent increase in osmolality in the interstitial space. (**Fig. 12.9**).

■ Distal nephron and collecting duct

In the **distal convoluted tubule** about 10% of the filtered Na⁺ and Cl⁻ are reabsorbed. The apical membrane contains a Na⁺/Cl⁻ symporter. The considerable **water permeability** of the distal tubule causes the tubular fluid to soon become isoosmolar with blood plasma.

The cortical and the outer medullary collecting duct consist of two cell types:
- mitochondria-rich ("dark") principal cells
- intercalated cells with fewer mitochondria ("light").

The type A intercalated cells serve, depending on the metabolic state, either to acidify urine or to make it more basic (type B intercalated cells). They are described in more detail in ch. "Transport processes in the proximal tubule and the collecting duct" (p. 326).

In the principal cells, Na⁺ is taken up apically through a sodium channel (ENaC = epithelial Na⁺ channel). Synthesis of the channel and incorporation into the membrane is induced by **aldosterone**. The principal cells thus serve to finely regulate sodium balance. The mechanism of chloride reabsorption is not yet fully understood.

Although only a maximum of 5% of the filtered Na⁺ and Cl⁻ are reabsorbed in the collecting duct, this occurs against considerable concentration gradients.

In addition to NaCl balance, the principal cells also control water balance. Under the influence of antidiuretic hormone increasing the intracellular concentration of cAMP water channels (aquaporins) are introduced into the apical membrane. The basolateral membrane is inherently very permeable to water. Regulation of renal water reabsorption by antidiuretic hormone is described in more detail in ch. 12.9.1 and ch. 13.8.

12.7.3   Regulation of sodium transport

Regulation of renal Na⁺ reabsorption is predominantly by aldosterone and to a lesser extent by atrial natriuretic peptide (ANP = atriopeptin). **Aldosterone** promotes Na⁺ reabsorption towards the end of the distal tubule and in the cortical collecting ducts. Sodium excretion can vary over very wide ranges. At high plasma aldosterone levels, almost all sodium entering the distal tubules is reabsorbed, so that the urinary sodium concentration is very low. When plasma aldosterone levels are low, almost all the sodium that enters the far end of the distal tubule segments is not reabsorbed and is excreted in urine.

Aldosterone is produced in the zona glomerulosa of the **adrenal cortex**. Secretion is stimulated by the following factors – in order of importance:
1. **angiotensin II** (the regulation by the renin-angiotensin-[aldosterone] system is shown in **Fig. 12.7**)
2. **hyperkalaemi**a
3. **hyponatremi**a
4. **ACTH** or **glucocorticoids**
Steroid hormones are lipophilic. Therefore, aldosterone diffuses through the lipid phase of the cell membrane (① in **Fig. 12.11**) and binds intracellularly to a receptor protein ②. The receptor-hormone complex diffuses into the cell nucleus ③, where it activates DNA as a transcription factor to form proteins ⑤ coding mRNA ④. In particular, it induces the increased synthesis of two transporters: the apical **Na⁺ channel** (ENaC: Epithelial Na⁺ channel) ⑥ and the basolateral Na⁺/K⁺-ATPase ⑦. At the same time, aldosterone directly and indirectly stimulates K⁺ secretion ⑧⑨, described in more detail in ch. 12.8.3. The genomic effect of aldosterone from receptor binding to the incorporation of the transport proteins into the apical cell membrane has a latency period of several hours. Thus, a longer time elapses before a change in sodium and/or potassium

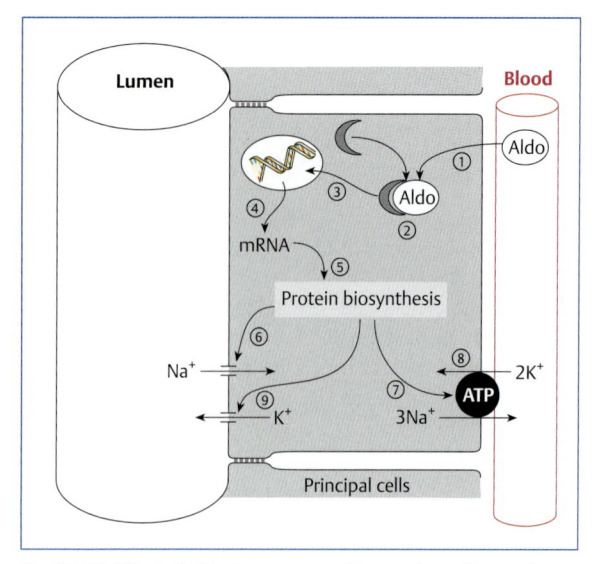

Fig. 12.11 Effect of aldosterone on sodium reabsorption and potassium secretion in the principal cells of the collecting ducts. Explanation of these processes in the text.

balance can be counter-regulated by aldosterone. The effect of aldosterone on sodium and potassium balance is not limited to the kidney. It also acts in the colon (p. 442) and the salivary glands, i.e., everywhere where ENaC channels are present.

Glucocorticoids (**Table 23.1**) can also bind to the aldosterone receptor and thus non-specifically influence sodium balance. However, the principal cells of the distal nephron protect against this by the action of hydroxysteroid dehydrogenase that degrades glucocorticoids.

Antagonists of aldosterone are the natriuretic peptides: **atrial natriuretic peptide** (ANP) and **brain natriuretic peptide** (BNP). ANP is produced in the atria of the heart, BNP in the ventricles of the heart. These peptides are released into blood when the heart muscle cells are stretched in response to increased venous return. The peptides inhibit the secretion or action of renin, aldosterone, and antidiuretic hormone, and have a dilating effect on the renal vessels, thus increasing GFR. All these effects of ANP and BNP, in addition to reducing the sodium concentration in the blood, also reduce blood volume and pressure. However, their half-life is only a few minutes, so that because of the long-term genomic mechanism of aldosterone, its effect is only briefly suppressed.

> ### IN A NUTSHELL   !
>
> The thick ascending portion of the loop of Henle is water-impermeable so that the tubular fluid is diluted by ion reabsorption. The distal sections of the nephron together with the collecting duct serve to fine-tune Na⁺ balance. Sodium reabsorption is regulated by aldosterone and atrial natriuretic peptide.

12.8 Potassium movement in the nephron

12.8.1 Importance of the kidney for potassium balance

There is little potassium in the extracellular fluid (**Table 1.4**). This means that even with moderate dietary potassium intake, the concentration of potassium in the extracellular fluid fluctuates considerably. This is particularly relevant for farm animals or herbivores, where the diet often contains several times the potassium requirement, mostly as a result of the use of potassium-rich fertilisers. The excitable cells of the body are extremely sensitive to changes in K^+ concentration in plasma (see ch. Diffusion potentials and K^+ balance (p.34)), as K^+ is an essential component of the membrane potential. If potassium concentration in extracellular fluid more than doubles (severe hyperkalaemia), cardiac arrest may occur (see ch. Electrolytes (p.190)). In certain regulatory disorders such as hyperaldosteronism, however, the potassium concentration in the extracellular fluid may fall. If, in extreme cases, its concentration falls to less than half the normal value (severe hypokalaemia), skeletal muscles can no longer contract and cardiac arrhythmias may develop.

Adjustment of K^+ **balance** is mainly by means of variation in renal K^+ excretion, as only about 10% of potassium ions in the body are physiologically excreted through the intestine. A high dietary intake of potassium therefore means that the kidney has to excrete more potassium to maintain a constant amount of potassium in the body. However, with very high potassium intakes, and thus high aldosterone levels, the intestine is also able to increase potassium excretion by up to 30% of the intake (see ch. Secretion of inorganic ions (p.443)).

12.8.2 Potassium: filtration, absorption and secretion

Potassium is filtered unhindered in the glomerulus. Reabsorption in the proximal tubule recovers about 60–70% of filtered K^+, and about 20–30% is reabsorbed in the loop of Henle, so that only about 5–15% reaches the distal tubule. In the distal tubule and collecting duct, net transport of K^+ is highly variable and can fluctuate between reabsorption and prolific secretion. Whether K^+ is secreted or reabsorbed in the distal tubule depends mainly on dietary K^+ intake or the amount of K^+ filtered in the nephron.

In the **proximal tubule**, potassium is almost exclusively reabsorbed passively by diffusion through tight junctions and by solvent drag (**Fig. 12.12**). Diffusion is promoted by the activity of the Na^+/K^+-ATPase. The ATPase receives potassium, which has diffused into the intercellular space via the tight junctions, and transports it into the cell interior. From the cell interior, potassium is then transported across the basolateral membrane through a potassium channel and via a K^+-Cl^- cotransporter. A small proportion of the reabsorbed potassium is transported back into the lumen via an apical potassium channel. Even though this return flow is quantitatively insignificant, it is important for the transfer of other substances. Thus, potassium transport into the lumen generates a membrane potential (negative inside the cell) that drives other electrogenic transport, such as the Na^+ glucose cotransporter (SGLT).

MORE DETAILS

Paracellular ion channels

The tight junctions are ion-selective as they contain specific paracellular channels. For example, potassium reabsorption occurs via claudin 2 proteins. The paracellular reabsorption of chloride (see ch. proximal tubule (p.312)) is also mediated by the protein claudin 17, which forms an anion channel within the tight junctions.

In the **thick ascending segment** of the **loop of Henle**, K^+ is transported into the cell by the apical Na^+-K^+-$2Cl^-$ symporter (**Fig. 12.12**).

In the **distal tubule** and the **collecting duct**, potassium can be both reabsorbed and secreted (**Fig. 12.12**). Reabsorption takes place via type A intercalated cells (explanation of intercalated cell types in ch. "Transport processes in the proximal tubule and the collecting duct" (p.326)). Potassium is transported from the lumen into the cytosol of the intercalated cells by an active K^+/H^+-ATPase. Basolaterally, it is discharged again via a potassium channel. Potassium secretion into the lumen occurs through the principal cells. Here, potassium crosses the basolateral membrane by the action of the Na^+/K^+-ATPase and is discharged into the lumen via apical channels.

If there is a need to secrete potassium, in the case of potassium excess, secretion into the tubule lumen predominates. Here, **aldosterone** is the controlling factor that stimulates potassium secretion.

12.8.3 Regulation of potassium excretion by aldosterone

In ch. 12.7.3 the active reabsorption of sodium in the cortical cells and distal tubule is described effectively being regulated by aldosterone. **Aldosterone** has the same efficiency in regulating potassium secretion as in regulating sodium transport, but its effect on potassium balance is opposite to its effect on sodium balance. It activates Na^+/K^+-ATPase in the principal cells, which provides the driving force to reabsorb sodium from the tubular fluid into the interstitium. In turn, potassium is transported in the opposite direction (⑧ in **Fig. 12.11**). Potassium that is increasingly taken into cells by the action of ATPase is then increasingly secreted via apical potassium channels. Aldosterone also stimulates the expression of potassium channels (⑨ in **Fig. 12.11**). As a result of these processes, potassium secretion into the tubular fluid increases greatly under the influence of aldosterone. The regulatory circuit that stimulates aldosterone production when there is an excess of potassium differs from that of the renin-angiotensin-aldosterone system. Thus, the cells of the adrenal cortex, which secrete aldosterone, are also able to monitor potassium concentration in the extracellular fluid. With an increased dietary intake of potassium, there is an initial increase in extracellular potassium concentration. This in

Inner milieu

turn stimulates aldosterone release from the adrenal cortex. The increased concentration of aldosterone in blood increases potassium secretion via the mechanisms described above and thus leads to an increased elimination of potassium from the body.

12.8.4 Interactions between potassium and acid-base balance

Independent of the aldosterone effect, changes in the extracellular and intracellular H^+ concentration have a strong influence on potassium excretion. Potassium excretion is increased in acute **alkalosis** and decreased in acute **acidosis**. In alkalosis, the H^+/K^+-ATPase in the collecting duct (**Fig. 12.12**) absorbs less potassium because fewer protons are available for exchange. In acidosis, on the other hand, more potassium is absorbed because more protons are then available for exchange. As a result, acidosis leads to hyperkalaemia and alkalosis to hypokalaemia.

The causes of acidoses/alkaloses are described in ch. 15.5, Disorders of acid-base balance (p. 352). For example, severe diarrhoea is often accompanied by acidosis, which in turn has an effect on excitable structures (heart) via the described changes in potassium balance. Apart from dehydration, this is the main reason why diarrhoea in young animals (especially calves and piglets) is associated with high mortality.

Conversely, potassium balance also has an effect on acid-base status. Hyperkalaemia leads to a depolarisation and consequently to a reduced outflow of HCO_3^- from cells (the outside of the cell becomes less positive and therefore less attractive for anions). Consequently, hyperkalaemia is followed by alkalinisation of the glomerular filtrate as a result of reduced activity of the Na^+/H^+exchanger and the H^+/K^+-ATPase and thus a general inhibition of proton excretion by the kidney. The result is thus general acidosis.

Hyperkalaemia is therefore often associated with acidosis and, conversely, acidosis with hyperkalaemia.

MORE DETAILS

Interactions between sodium and potassium

Both sodium and potassium are regulated by aldosterone, albeit in opposite directions. Increased potassium secretion is thus coupled with increased sodium reabsorption. The question inevitably arises as to whether this causes conflicts in homeostasis between the two ions when there is a sodium deficiency. The first response in sodium deficiency is increased secretion of aldosterone. Aldosterone then induces increased renal sodium reabsorption, but at the same time also an increased excretion of potassium, which can then lead to secondary hypokalaemia.

Conversely, excessive potassium intake, especially in herbivores (potassium fertilisation of pastures), can induce hypernatremia due to the resulting increase in aldosterone levels which stimulate sodium reabsorption. Care should therefore be taken to limit the potassium intake of farm animals.

Hypo- and hyperaldosteronism

Disturbances in aldosterone production or secretion lead to clinical signs, mainly related to the induced hypo- or hyperkalaemia. Thus, when aldosterone secretion is depressed (Addison's disease), the resulting retention of K^+ and hyperkalaemia are reflected by evidence of cardiac arrhythmia (p. 190). The parallel hyponatremia affects water balance (dehydration) among other things. Conversely, hyperaldosteronism, for example as a result of an adrenocortical tumour, leads to hypokalaemia, which is also noticeable as cardiac arrhythmia.

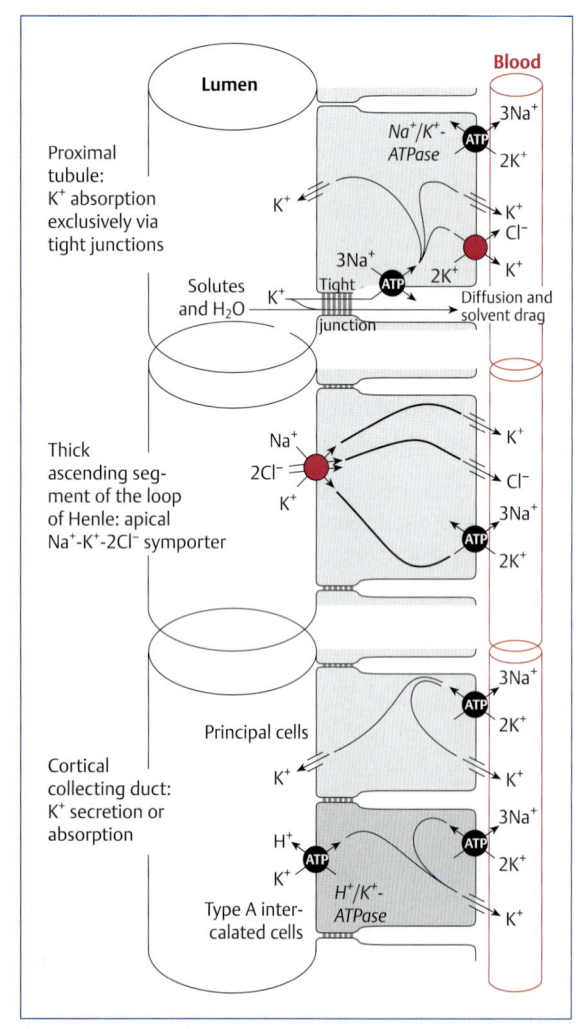

Fig. 12.12 Tubular transport mechanisms of potassium.

IN A NUTSHELL !

In the proximal tubule, 60–70% of filtered potassium is reabsorbed paracellularly; in the thick ascending segment of the loop of Henle, a further 25–35% is reabsorbed via the apical Na^+-K^+-$2Cl^-$ symporter. In the distal tubule and the collecting duct, K^+ transport is under the hormonal control of aldosterone. Aldosterone induces potassium secretion.

12.9 Water movement in the nephron and urine concentration

12.9.1 Quantity and mechanisms

The high glomerular filtration rates described in ch. 12.5 are necessary to eliminate unwanted substances and metabolic waste products. On the other hand, the water "lost" in the filtrate must be effectively reabsorbed again to keep the body's water balance in equilibrium. Thus, as explained in ch. 12.5, $\approx 140 l \cdot d^{-1}$ are filtered by the glomeruli in a 30 kg dog. If we assume a blood volume (p. 218) of approx. 2.4 l with a plasma content of 1.3 l (blood: 7.5% of body weight; haematocrit $0.45 l \cdot l^{-1}$; Table 7.1, ch. 9.1 (p. 218)), a GFR of $140 l \cdot d^{-1}$ (or $\approx 0.11 \cdot min^{-1}$) means that the entire plasma volume of the dog completely passes through the glomerular filter every 13 minutes. While this is an essential requirement for the kidney's cleansing function, it also means that the entire liquid portion of blood is temporarily "lost" to the animal in 13 minutes. Effective ultrafiltration must therefore be accompanied by equally effective reabsorption of water. Under physiological (markedly antidiuretic) conditions $139.5 l \cdot d^{-1}$, more than 99% of the filtered volume is reabsorbed in a dog with a GFR of $140 l \cdot d^{-1}$, so that only about $0.5 l \cdot d^{-1}$ is excreted in urine (Table 12.3).

Table 12.3 Changes in volume flow and osmolality over the course of the nephrons in a 30 kg dog. The data refer to both kidneys. The values for the final urine apply to the situation of pronounced antidiuresis.

Localisation	Volume flow $(l \cdot d^{-1})$	Osmolality $(mosm \cdot kg^{-1})$
Renal artery: RBF	800	–
Renal artery: RPF	440	300
Bowman's capsule: GFR	140	300
End proximal tubule	40	300
End Henle loop	25	< 100
Final Urine	< 0.5	> 1000

RBF = renal blood flow; RPF = renal plasma flow (of which approx. 80% is supplied to the filtration in dogs); GFR = glomerular filtration rate.

Water is mainly passively transported in the tubule system. For osmotic reasons, it follows the sum of all transported solutes in the ratio of 1 l of water per 300 mosm of solute (corresponding to the osmolality of blood plasma of $\approx 300 \, mosmol \cdot kg^{-1}$). Therefore, the transport rate of water is determined by the **sum** of all **solutes absorbed** and the **permeability for water** reabsorption ("hydraulic conductivity"). Because of the quantities of sodium and chloride, their reabsorption in particular has a modulating influence on water reabsorption. Water can be transported paracellularly and/or transcellularly depending on the permeability of the tubule segment. Due to the high water permeability of its epithelium, **isoosmolar** reabsorption occurs in the **proximal tubule**, i.e., so much water follows the reabsorbed solutes that the osmolality in the tubule lumen remains constant. Although the concentration of glucose and amino acids decreases to trace levels by the end of the proximal tubule, the concentrations of Na^+ and Cl^- remain almost constant. In this way, at the end of the proximal tubule, about 70% of the glomerular filtered water has already been reabsorbed (Fig. 12.9). In the **distal tubule segments**, the paracellular pathway becomes more and more impermeable, so that the transport is increasingly transcellular and can thus also take place **against** increasingly greater **concentration gradients**.

For the transcellular pathway, especially through the apical cell membrane, the lipid phase of the cell membranes of these cells has a very low water permeability, so that transcellular transport depends on water channels. Such channels called aquaporins are found in many cell types in various forms. However, there are two sections of the tubular system of the kidney that do not have aquaporins, or do not have them continuously. Thus, in the thick ascending segment of the loop of Henle, there are no water channels at all. In the apical membrane of the distal tubules and the collecting ducts, water channels are only incorporated and activated in the presence of antidiuretic hormone.

> **IN A NUTSHELL** !
>
> About 70% of the glomerular filtered water is reabsorbed in the proximal tubule. The driving force for this is the reabsorption of NaCl. The reabsorption of water is isoosmolar, i.e., the osmolality of the tubular fluid is not changed as it flows through the proximal tubule.

12.9.2 Countercurrent multiplier system and antidiuresis

■ Importance of urine concentration

The amount of urine excreted per unit time depends firstly on the amount of water ingested. Additional factors are high ambient temperatures and intense physical work, which increase water loss by other mechanisms. Young animals in the suckling phase take up considerably more liquid than adult animals, relative to body mass or body surface. Accordingly, the daily amount of urine is higher in young animals and they excrete urine with a lower osmolality. In addition, there are great variations in both urine volume and osmolality in different animal species. In general, the kidneys of all species are capable of concentrating urine, i.e., excreting urine with a higher osmolality than plasma. The high concentration capacity in felids and desert mammals is striking and enables them to survive with minimal water intake. However, this high concentration capacity of urine is problematic because felids have a high tendency to form urinary calculi (urinary bladder stones). In Table 12.4 the average amount of urine per day is compared to the maximum achievable osmolality of urine.

Table 12.4 Mean urine volume per day and maximum urine osmolality (during antidiuresis) in different species.

Species	Mean amount of urine per day ($ml \cdot d^{-1} \cdot kg^{-1}$)	Maximum urine osmolality ($osmol \cdot kg^{-1}$)
Cattle	17–45	1.0
Human	9–30	1.4
Pig	5–30	1.1
Horse	3–18	1.2
Dog*	20–40	2.8
Cat	10–20	>3

based on data from Altman PL, Dittmer D. Blood and other body fluids/analysis and compilation by Philip L. Altman; edited by Dorothy S. Dittmer; prepared under the auspices of the Committee on Biological Handbooks. Washington: Fed Amer Soc Exp Biol; 1961; Ketz, HA. Die Physiologie der Niere. In: Kolb E (ed.). Lehrbuch der Physiologie der Haustiere. 5th ed., Jena: Fischer; 1989; Kohn B, Schwarz G (eds). Praktikum der Hundeklinik: gegründet von Hans G. Niemand. 12th ed., Stuttgart: Enke; 2018; van Vonderen JK, Kooistra HS, Rijnberk A. Intra- and interindividual variation in urine osmolality and urine specific gravity in healthy pet dogs of various ages. J Vet Intern Med 1997; 11: 30–35
* The osmolality values of dogs were obtained from severely dehydrated animals.

As can be seen from **Table 12.4** urine can be concentrated up to 4–10 times plasma osmolality (**antidiuresis**), depending on the species.

■ Mechanisms of urine concentration

The ability to concentrate urine and thus minimise urine volume is related to the length of the loop of Henle and the effectiveness of the **countercurrent multiplier system**.
    The **anatomical structures** involved are (**Fig. 12.13**): 1. descending limb of the loop of Henle, 2. ascending limb of the loop of Henle, 3. collecting duct, 4. descending, and 5. ascending vessels of the vasa recta. Due to the structure

of the tubular systems, the following **two countercurrent multiplier systems** are created:
1. between descending and ascending limb of the Henle loop,
2. between the ascending limb of the Henle loop and the collecting duct.

For the countercurrent multiplier systems to work, different tubule sections have different **transport characteristics:**
- descending limb of the Henle loop: high water permeability
- thick ascending segment of the Henle loop: active Na^+ and Cl^- reabsorption
- entire ascending limb of the Henle loop: water impermeability
- collecting duct: high water permeability when ADH is active
- medullary collecting duct: urea reabsorption

IN A NUTSHELL   !

The urine is concentrated by two countercurrent multiplier systems:
1. Between descending and ascending limb of the Henle loop
2. Between the ascending limb of the Henle loop and the collecting duct

---

The concentration of urine is a dynamic process that develops during the flow of tubular fluid. The **basic principle** of **countercurrent concentration** is explained for the first countercurrent system: the **descending** and **ascending limbs** of the **loop of Henle**. The ascending limb of the loop of Henle acts as the driving force. This part of the nephron is characterised by NaCl (and K^+) being actively reabsorbed while the tubule cells are mainly impermeable to water. For a theoretical filtrate osmolality of $\approx 300 \ mosmol \cdot kg^{-1}$ this osmolality therefore declines (**Fig. 12.14**).

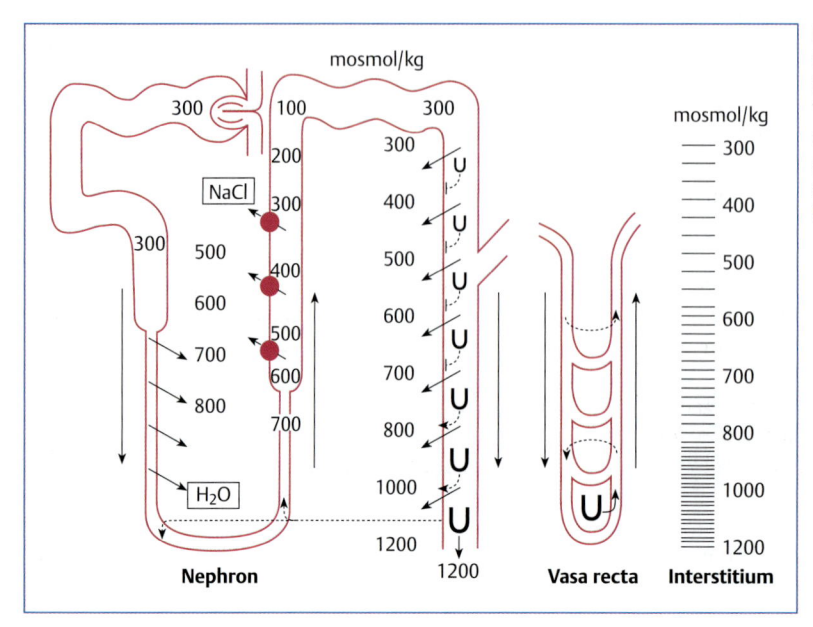

Fig. 12.13 Schematic representation of the concentration and dilution of urine by the countercurrent multiplier system. Tubular and vascular processes and the resulting corticomedullary osmotic gradient in the interstitium are shown separately. Explanations in the text. U = urea.

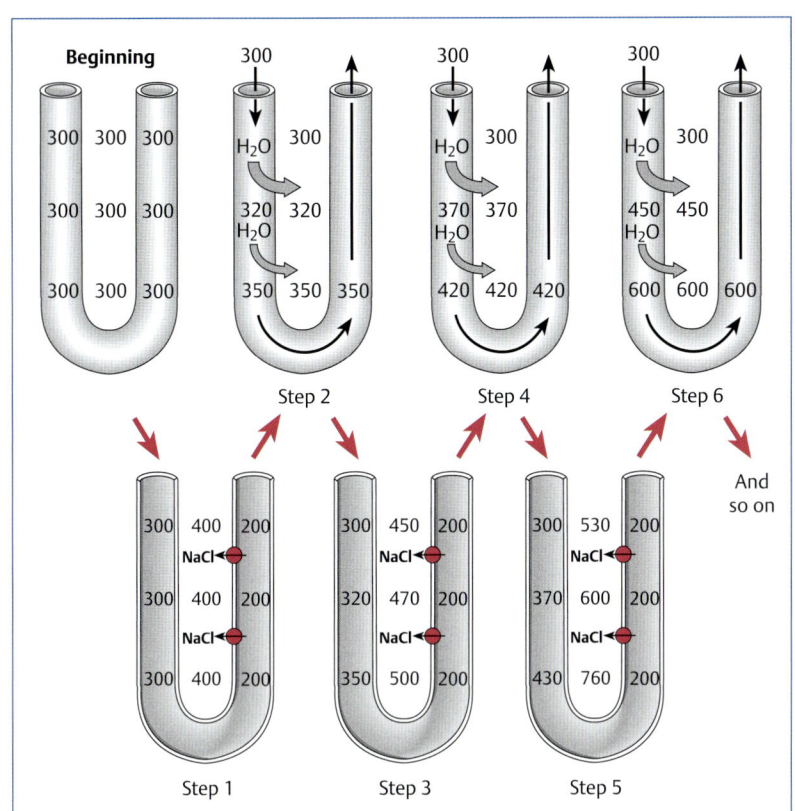

Fig. 12.14 Basic mechanism of counter-current concentration (explanation in the text). Only the loop of Henle is shown here. The descending limb is very permeable to NaCl and water. The ascending limb is water-impermeable and has reabsorption mechanisms for NaCl in the thick segment shown here. [Source: Klinke R, Pape HC, Kurtz A et al. Physiologie. Stuttgart: Thieme; 2009]

In the 1st step (**Fig. 12.14**), NaCl is reabsorbed from the ascending limb, but water cannot follow due to the water impermeability of the ascending limb. Therefore, in the example, the osmolality in the ascending limb decreases by $100 \, mosmol \cdot kg^{-1}$ from 300 to $200 \, mosmol \cdot kg^{-1}$. As a consequence, the osmolality of the interstitium increases to $400 \, mosmol \cdot kg^{-1}$.

At the end of the 1st step, there is initially a difference in osmolality of $100 \, mosmol \cdot kg^{-1}$ between the liquid in the lumen of the descending limb of the loop of Henle and the interstitium. This results in water flowing from the descending limb of the loop into the interstitium in the 2nd step. As a result, when the liquid flows through the descending limb of the loop of Henle, the osmolality increases accordingly from 300 to $350 \, mosmol \cdot kg^{-1}$.

In the 3rd step, NaCl is reabsorbed from the ascending limb (as in the first step), so that the osmolality in the ascending limb decreases (to $200 \, mosmol \cdot kg^{-1}$). In the interstitium, the absorbed electrolytes increase the osmolality from 400 to $500 \, mosmol \cdot kg^{-1}$.

In the 4th step, the liquid now continues to flow (as in the 2nd step). Water diffuses from the descending limb of the Henle loop, so that there are now $420 \, mosmol \cdot kg^{-1}$ in the lower segment of the ascending loop.

In the 5th step, NaCl reabsorption occurs again (as in the 1st and 3rd steps), so that the osmolality in the ascending limb decreases. In the interstitium, however, the osmolality increases to $760 \, mosmol \cdot kg^{-1}$.

In the 6th step (as in the 2nd and 4th steps) the liquid continues to flow, water is reabsorbed from the descending limb towards the interstitium due to the osmotic gradient, so that there are now $600 \, mosmol \cdot kg^{-1}$ in the lower segment of the ascending loop.

All the following steps are just repetitions of the steps explained above with higher and higher osmolarities until the upper end of the Henle loop is reached. It follows that the longer the Henle loop, the more pronounced the ability to concentrate.

The fluid leaving the ascending limb of the loop of Henle is thus always hypoosmolar to plasma (less than $100 \, mosmol \cdot kg^{-1}$). But how does the urine finally concentrate to the values listed in **Table 12.4**? To achieve this, the second countercurrent multiplier principle between the **collecting duct** and the **loop of Henle** come into effect. Because the collecting duct runs in the immediate vicinity of the loops of Henle, the second countercurrent multiplier principle concentrates the collecting duct fluid on its way to the renal medulla to the same extent as the first countercurrent multiplier principle described in **Fig. 12.14** for concentration of fluid in the descending loop of Henle. However, a prerequisite for the second countercurrent principle to work effectively is that the collecting duct becomes **water-permeable** through the action of **ADH**. Depending on the species, the excreted urine can be concentrated 3–10-fold in maximum antidiuresis compared to blood plasma (**Table 12.4**).

In the **inner medulla**, the concentration increases further, although no active NaCl reabsorption of the loop of Henle takes place here. In fact, in the inner medulla, it is not these two ions, but mainly **urea**, which increases the concentration (**Fig. 12.13**). The **cortical collecting duct** is **impermeable** to **urea, but** is **permeable** to **water under**

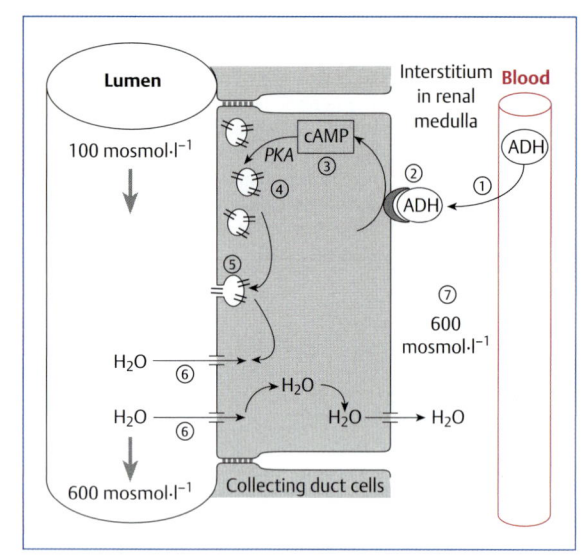

Fig. 12.15 Effect of ADH on water reabsorption in the collecting ducts. Explanation of the processes in the text. = Aquaporins.

the influence of ADH, so that water, but not urea is reabsorbed, thus increasing the concentration of urea in the cortical collecting duct. Only the medullary collecting duct has a specific transport protein for urea in the apical membrane, where urea can diffuse down a concentration gradient into the vasa recta and then into the thin segments of the loop of Henle. A proportion of the urea passing into the collecting ducts is thus subject to **recirculation**.

In total, more than 99% of the filtered water can be reabsorbed in the tubular system under the influence of ADH, so that the urine becomes so concentrated via the countercurrent system that its osmolality can increase to several times plasma osmolality. The corresponding control circuit is described in ch. 13.8.1. **ADH release** from the **posterior pituitary lobe** is triggered by an increase in plasma osmolality and/or a decrease in plasma volume. Under these circumstances, ADH secretion increases and reaches the collecting duct epithelial cells in blood (① in **Fig. 12.15**. There it binds to membrane receptors ② and stimulates the intracellular formation of cAMP and thus activation of protein kinase A (PKA) ③. Subsequently, more **aquaporin-2 water channels** are incorporated into the cell membrane ⑤. The protein structures of these channels were previously stored in vesicles ④. The consequence of the incorporation of the channels is an increase in water permeability in the cell membrane ⑥. The water movement is driven by the osmotic gradient that is built up in the interstitium by the activity of the ascending limb of the loop of Henle ⑦.

IN A NUTSHELL   !

The driving force for the outflow of water from the descending limb of the loop of Henle and from the collecting duct is increased osmolality in the interstitium due to NaCl reabsorption in the ascending limb of the loop of Henle. Near the renal pelvis, interstitial osmolality is also increased by urea transfer from the collecting duct.
The degree of urine concentration is controlled by ADH.

■ Diuresis

Diuresis refers to all conditions where there is increased urine excretion per time. Three forms are distinguished: water diuresis, osmotic diuresis, and pressure diuresis (**Fig. 12.16**).

Water diuresis and antidiuresis

As described above, under the influence of ADH, more than 99% of filtered water can be reabsorbed in the tubular system and the urine can become highly concentrated, so that its osmolality can increase to several times that of plasma.

Conversely, with decreasing ADH secretion, the incorporation of aquaporins into the apical membrane ceases, so that the collecting duct becomes increasingly water impermeable. If water cannot now follow the solutes reabsorbed in the collecting duct, the tubular fluid becomes **hypoosmolar**. An almost water-clear urine of low osmolality is excreted in large quantities per time (**Fig. 12.16b**). The transport rates of the solutes are not affected during water diuresis, as only water reabsorption in the collecting duct is reduced.

MORE DETAILS In **diabetes insipidus** either no ADH is formed and released (**diabetes insipidus centralis**) or ADH is released, but has no effect in the kidney (**diabetes insipidus renalis**).

IN A NUTSHELL   !

Water diuresis is caused by inhibition of ADH secretion. In the presence of ADH, aquaporins are incorporated into the apical membrane of the collecting ducts and antidiuresis occurs with a low urinary excretion rate.

Osmotic diuresis

Osmotic diuresis occurs when solute reabsorption is reduced or entirely absent and therefore these solutes remain in the tubular lumen along with an osmotically equivalent amount of water, and then drain into the renal pelvis as urine. Osmotic diuresis can be considerably stronger than water diuresis. However, the urine osmolality does not fall below the value of plasma osmolality ($\approx 300\ mosmol \cdot kg^{-1}$).

In principle, osmotic diuresis can have three causes:
1. Filtration of non-absorbable solutes (osmotic diuresis in the narrower sense; **Fig. 12.16c**). An example of a solute that is filtered, but for which no reabsorption transport mechanism is available is the sugar alcohol mannitol.
2. Exceeding the tubular transport maximum due to increased concentration in the filtrate (**Fig. 12.16d**). A typical example is the condition in diabetes mellitus (p. 547). When the concentration of glucose in plasma and in the ultrafiltrate increases to $> \approx 10\ mmol \cdot l^{-1}$ (cats: $\approx 15\ mmol \cdot l^{-1}$), glucose in the proximal tubule fluid can no longer be 100% absorbed.

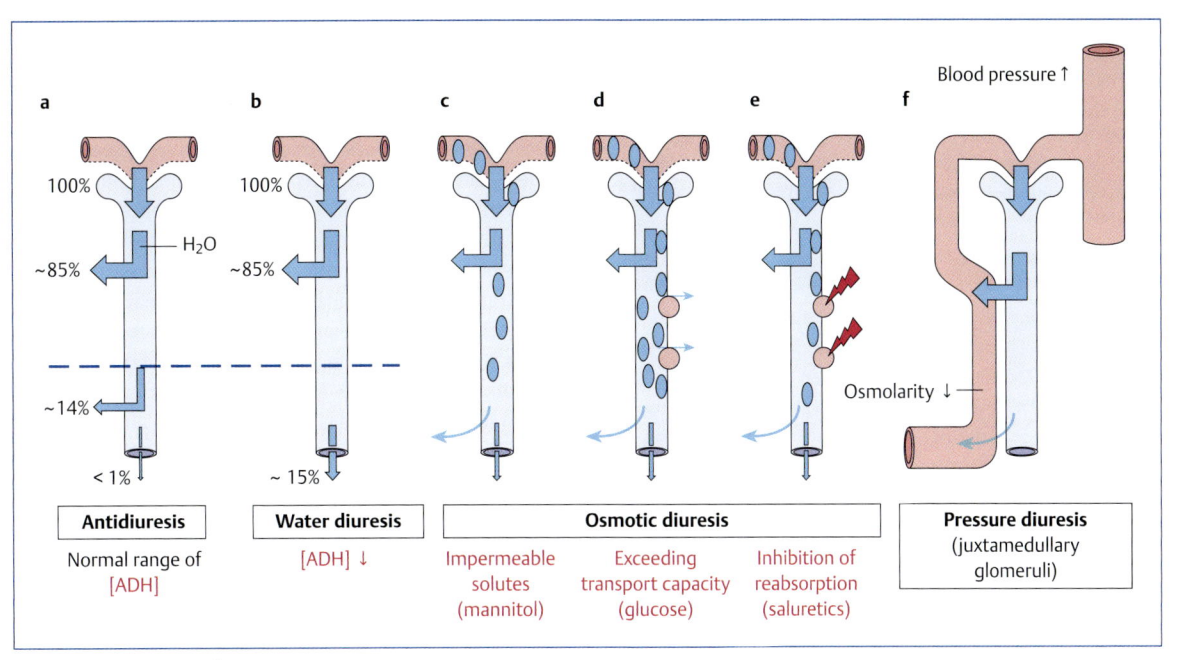

Fig. 12.16 Diuresis mechanisms.
a Normal state = antidiuresis: In the presence of antidiuretic hormone (ADH), about 14% of the ultrafiltrate (= 100%) is reabsorbed in the distal nephron. Less than 1% is excreted. Below dashed line: distal nephron.
b Water diuresis: In the complete absence of ADH, virtually no water is reabsorbed in the distal nephron.
c-e Forms of **osmotic diuresis:** Solutes that are not completely reabsorbed aid the retention of water in the tubular lumen by maintaining osmotic pressure and are thus excreted in urine together with water retained in the lumen. This can have three causes: **c** Filtration of impermeable substances (example: mannitol),
d Increase in filtered solutes in quantities exceeding the reabsorption transport capacity (example: hyperglycaemia), **e** Inhibition of the reabsorption mechanisms, e.g., by pharmaceuticals (saluretics).
f Pressure diuresis: Through pressure-passive increase in medullary blood flow, which flushes osmolytes out of the hyperosmolar medulla.

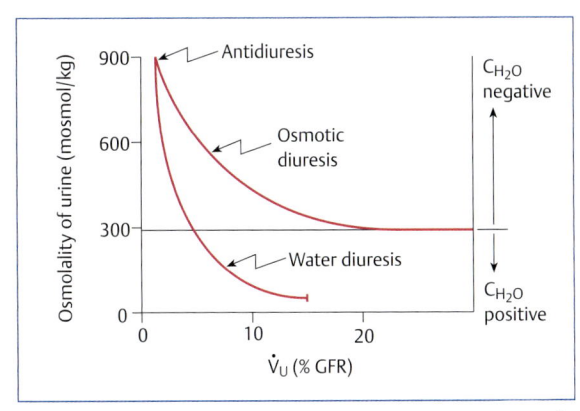

Fig. 12.17 Ratio of urine osmolality and urine excretion rate (= $\dot{V}_U$ in% of glomerular filtration rate) with increasing osmotic diuresis or water diuresis. C_{H_2O}: Free water clearance, i.e., difference between water excretion and the excretion of osmotically active substrates.

3. Inhibition of tubular ion reabsorption (**Fig. 12.16e**, **Fig. 12.17**). Diuretics that act by this mechanism are also called **saluretics**, because they cause an increase in the excretion of salts in plasma. Therapeutically, they are suitable for flushing out toxins (if filtered in the glomeruli) and oedema fluid (**Fig. 12.18**).

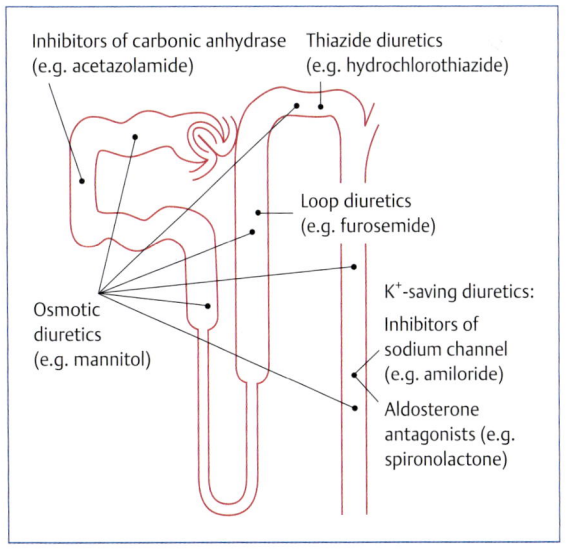

Fig. 12.18 Sites of action of diuretics.

MORE DETAILS

Saluretics

Saluretics are filtered, some are additionally secreted in the proximal tubule. Tubular water reabsorption then increases the concentration of saluretics to the point where they become diuretically effective. **Loop diuretics** are the most potent saluretics. They inhibit only one transport mechanism: the **Na⁺-K⁺-2Cl⁻ symporter** in the thick ascending segment of the loop of Henle (**Fig. 12.10**). Loop diuretics can therefore cause hypokalaemia.

Thiazide diuretics inhibit the **Na⁺-Cl⁻ symporter** localised in the distal convoluted tubule.

K⁺-saving diuretics have only a weak effect. They inhibit the **Na⁺ channel ENaC** localised in the principal cells of the collecting duct. Their importance lies in the fact that they also indirectly inhibit K⁺ secretion and are therefore often given in combination with loop and thiazide diuretics to compensate for the loss of K⁺ caused by these agents.

> **IN A NUTSHELL** !
>
> In osmotic diuresis, solutes are not reabsorbed, so that water is also not reabsorbed and is excreted in urine together with the solutes. Causes are: an increased amount of salt in the tubular system with diuretic administration, or an increased amount of glucose in the tubular system with diabetes mellitus.

12.9.3 Pressure diuresis

The Bayliss effect is less pronounced in the juxtamedullary glomeruli or their vasa afferentia than in the superficial glomeruli. The juxtamedullary glomeruli also feed the vasa recta (**Fig. 12.1**). As a result, **medullary blood flow** also tends to increase with elevated arterial blood pressure. An increase in blood flow in the vasa recta leads to an increased removal of solutes from the renal medulla. This reduces the osmolality of the renal medulla, which is the driving osmotic force for passive water efflux from the collecting ducts. Consequently, water reabsorption from the collecting ducts is reduced. This form of diuresis resulting from increased blood pressure is called **pressure diuresis**.

12.10 Movement of calcium and phosphate in the nephron

The functions of calcium are manifold. Accordingly, the body must be supplied with adequate amounts of this ion. The calcium requirement is greatly increased in production animals (laying hens, dairy cows), where large amounts are lost in the products (egg or milk). Increased amounts of calcium are also needed during growth to produce the hydroxyapatite mineral in the organic matrix of the skeleton. Depending on species, age, production status and the regulatory factors of calcium homeostasis, the absorption rate of calcium (p. 435) in the intestine can vary between 20 and 90%.

About 40% of calcium in blood plasma is bound to proteins. Therefore protein-bound calcium is not filtered by the glomeruli. Only about 60% of blood calcium is able to pass into the glomerular filtrate.

The proportions of filtered calcium that are reabsorbed are: 60% in the proximal tubule, 30% in the thick segment of the ascending limb of the loop of Henle and 9% in the distal segments. The residual 1% is excreted in urine.

Calcium is reabsorbed in the proximal tubule, mainly through the tight junctions by diffusion and solvent drag. Because of this, the Ca^{2+} concentration remains almost unchanged along the proximal tubule.

Active, transcellular transport takes place mainly in the distal nephron segments. The mechanisms here are similar to those in the small intestine (**Fig. 16.65**).

In addition to its involvement in bone formation, phosphate is also a component of energy-rich compounds (ATP, nucleic acids, phosphorylated proteins, phospholipids) and is essential as a buffering agent in extracellular fluid (ch. 15.3.1). In food, phosphorus is present either as inorganic phosphate or organically in phosphorus-containing compounds. Phosphorus absorption takes place mainly in the small intestine. The amount absorbed varies between 20 and 80% depending on its availability as phosphate.

In blood, phosphate is mainly present as hydrogen phosphate (HPO_4^{2-}), and is therefore filtered almost unhindered. Hydrogen phosphate is reabsorbed in the proximal tubule together with three Na^+ by a symporter against an electrochemical gradient. Coupling with sodium facilitates phosphate uptake into the cell, but has little effect on sodium recovery because of the comparatively small amounts in this process. On the basolateral side, inorganic phosphate (P_i) leaves the cell via an anion exchange mechanism and possibly a phosphate channel. There is no significant paracellular permeability in the proximal tubule.

The filtered hydrogen phosphate fulfils a special role in buffering (p. 346) the protons secreted in the proximal tubule.

Calcium and phosphate transport is influenced not only by their respective concentrations in plasma, but also by the hormones: **parathyroid hormone (PTH), calcitonin and 1,25-(OH)₂ D₃** (calcitriol). PTH leads to an increased reabsorption of calcium and an increased excretion of phosphate by inducing phosphate transporters. Calcitriol has a similar effect to PTH. Calcitonin, in contrast, has an inhibitory effect on the reabsorption of both phosphate and calcium, thus acting as an antagonist of PTH in calcium homeostasis and as a synergist of PTH in phosphate homeostasis. However, the effect of calcitonin is probably secondary to that of PTH and only noticeable at unphysiologically high doses. These hormones exert their actions not only in the kidney, but also in bone and intestine. The corresponding control circuit is described in ch. 23.2.4.

> **IN A NUTSHELL** !
>
> Calcium is not completely filtered due to its binding to plasma proteins. In the proximal tubule and in the thick ascending limb of the loop of Henle, it is mainly reabsorbed paracellularly. Phosphate is reabsorbed in the proximal tubule in symport with Na^+.
>
> Phosphate and calcium transport is regulated by **parathyroid hormone (PTH), calcitonin** and **1,25-(OH)₂ D₃** (calcitriol).

MORE DETAILS

Magnesium

In addition to being a component of bone mineral, magnesium is an activator and cofactor in numerous enzyme reactions, in nerve excitability, in muscle contraction, and in DNA and mRNA synthesis. The sites of absorption in monogastric animals are the small intestine and the large intestine. Ruminants absorb most magnesium in the forestomachs and some also in the large intestine (**Fig. 16.39**). Inadequate magnesium absorption leading to hypomagnesaemia causes tetany (p. 409).

In blood, some magnesium, like calcium, is bound to proteins. Because of this, about 50–80% of total plasma magnesium passes into the glomerular filtrate. The proximal tubule is less permeable to Mg^{2+} than all other small ions. Therefore, only 30–40% of Mg^{2+} is reabsorbed there. In the thick ascending limb of the loop of Henle, most (50–60%) of the ultrafiltered magnesium is reabsorbed mainly by a paracellular route. Like Ca^{2+} reabsorption, Mg^{2+} reabsorption is driven by the lumen-positive voltage generated by Cl^- reabsorption.

In the distal tubule, only 2–5% of filtered Mg^{2+} is reabsorbed, so that the remaining 5–10% is excreted in urine.

Sulphate

The characteristics of sulphate transport are similar to those of phosphate. It is taken up into the cell of the proximal tubule by a symporter together with three Na^+. On the basolateral side, sulphate leaves the cell down an electrochemical gradient through an antiporter that exchanges sulphate for other anions (but not phosphate).

Klotho

Klotho is a proteohormone of the kidneys anchored in the cell membrane. It is a cofactor of the FGF23 receptor, and when stimulated leads to an increase in phosphate excretion and reduced formation of calcitriol. Fibroblast growth factor FGF23 has hormonal effects and is produced in bone. This function in bone is another way that renal insufficiency has a negative effect on bone structure and function.

12.11 Glucose reabsorption

12.11.1 Importance of glucose transport

The physiological plasma concentration of D-glucose in monogastrics is $\approx 5\,mmol \cdot l^{-1}$ (values in the cat up to $\approx 10\,mmol \cdot l^{-1}$). Glucose is freely filterable, so the same concentration is initially present in the primary urine. At this concentration, D-glucose is completely absorbed in the first half of the proximal tubule (**Fig. 12.19**, black line). When the concentration in the filtrate increases due to rising plasma concentration, further sections of the proximal tubule are gradually included in this reabsorption process. The maximum reabsorption capacity is reached when the entire proximal tubule is functioning in glucose reabsorption (**Fig. 12.19**, red line).

12.11.2 Mechanism of glucose transport

All the transporters mentioned below are specific only for D-sugars and no L-sugars are able to be transported. Glucose and galactose, together with sodium, are taken up into the cell via a **secondary active transport mechanism**, the SGLT (sodium glucose linked transporter) **against** their **concentration gradients** (**Fig. 12.20**). The driving force is

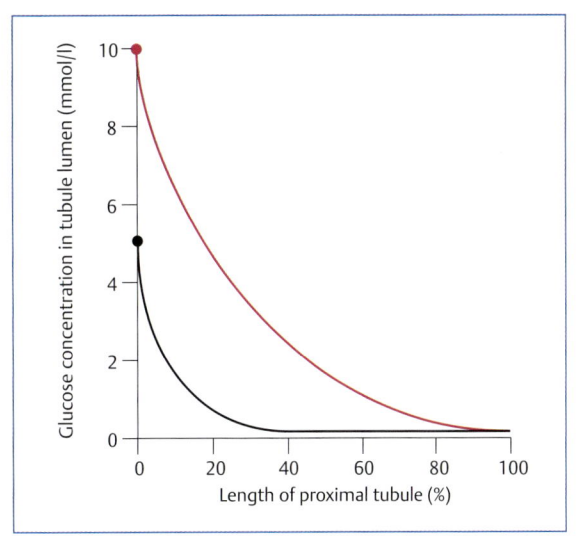

Fig. 12.19 Decrease in glucose concentration in the proximal tubule with normal (black line) and with increased glucose concentration in plasma (red line). [Source: Rhode R, Deetjen P. Die Glucoseresorption in der Rattenniere. Mikropunktionsanalysen der tubulären Glukosekonzentration bei freiem Fluss. Pfl Arch Physiol 1968; 302: 219–232]

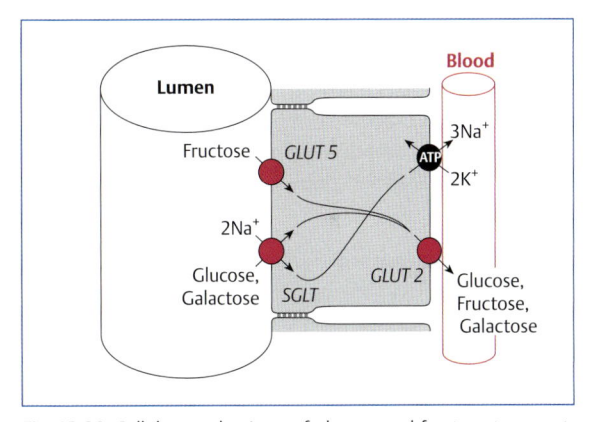

Fig. 12.20 Cellular mechanisms of glucose and fructose transport in the proximal tubule. SGLT = sodium glucose linked transporter; GLUT = glucose transporter.

the electrochemical gradient for Na^+, which is directed at sodium reabsorption and is exploited by coupling sugar uptake with that of Na^+. The **Na^+ gradient** is maintained by the basolateral Na^+/K^+-ATPase. The outflow of glucose from the cell takes place by facilitated diffusion through a GLUT2 (glucose transporter 2) present on the basolateral side.

It is important to emphasise that **glucose reabsorption** is **only** possible in the **proximal** parts of the nephron, so the glucose that cannot be reabsorbed in the proximal tubule remains in the tubule lumen, resulting in the excretion of glucose in urine = **diabetes mellitus**.

The filtered glucose can be almost completely reabsorbed up to a **threshold concentration**. In dogs, the threshold concentration is about $10\,mmol \cdot l^{-1}$, and in cats is significantly higher, about $15\,mmol \cdot l^{-1}$. When there is insulin deficiency or insulin resistance, glucose concentration in plasma does increase. This initially does not lead to glucose excretion in urine. However, as plasma glucose

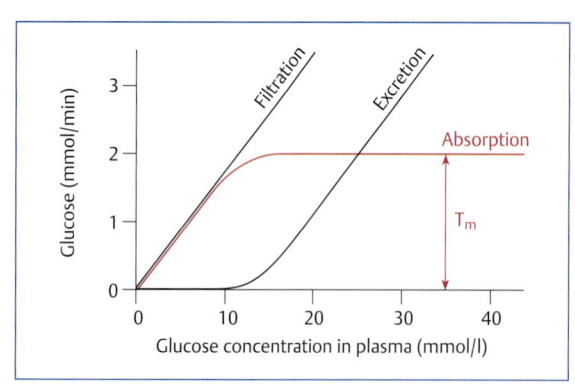

Fig. 12.21 Filtration, absorption, and excretion of glucose as a function of glucose concentration in plasma. T_m = Transport maximum.

concentration rises further, and thus its concentration in primary urine, the threshold concentration for reabsorption is then exceeded and glucose is detectable in urine. In the diabetic dog or cat, glucose is excreted in urine in increasingly larger quantities at plasma concentrations above the threshold concentration (glucosuria). This is shown in **Fig. 12.21**. It can be seen that the excretion rate is the difference between the filtration rate and the reabsorption transport rate. Since glucose remains in the tubule lumen when this transport rate is exceeded, it also has an osmotic effect. Therefore, with glucose, more water is excreted, which causes osmotic diuresis (polyuria) and at the same time thirst (polydipsia), a symptom that usually occurs in diabetes mellitus.

MORE DETAILS

Basis of the efficiency of glucose absorption

SGLT is found in two isoforms in the proximal tubule. In the first part of the proximal tubule, SGLT2 with a lower affinity for glucose is present and takes up Na^+ and glucose into the cell in a 1:1 ratio. Towards the end of the proximal tubule (straight segment), SGLT1 is found, which takes up Na^+ and glucose in a 2:1 ratio and can therefore still transport glucose at very low luminal concentrations. In addition to glucose, SGLT 1 also accepts galactose. An SGLT1 is also found in the small intestine (p. 424).

Reabsorption of other sugar monomers

For fructose there is only one simple transport protein in the apical membrane, the so-called GLUT5 (glucose transporter 5). This is a uniporter that only transports fructose, so that this sugar is passively transported by facilitated diffusion, driven by its concentration gradient (**Fig. 12.20**). The outflow of fructose and galactose from the cell, like that of glucose, is by facilitated diffusion through the basolateral GLUT2 transporter.

IN A NUTSHELL   !

Glucose filtration is unrestricted, but it is completely reabsorbed in the proximal tubule in secondary active cotransport with sodium, so that no glucose is detectable in the final urine under physiological conditions. When glucose concentrations in plasma or primary urine double, the transport maximum is exceeded, and glucose is excreted in the final urine and can be detected there (diabetes mellitus).

12.12 Movement of amino acids, oligopeptides and proteins in the nephron

Amino acids (as well as oligopeptides and polypeptides) are filtered unhindered, so that the normal plasma concentration of all amino acids of about $2–3\,mmol \cdot l^{-1}$ is also their concentration in the primary filtrate. Excretion of various amino acids in the final urine is 0.1–6% of the filtered amount.

Amino acids are mainly absorbed in the first segment of the **proximal tubule**. There are different transport systems depending on the properties of the amino acid (acidic, basic, neutral). Transport systems also exist for oligopeptides in the apical membrane.

Proteins are only filtered to a small extent and then are almost completely reabsorbed in the following tubule segments by endocytosis, so that only vanishingly small amounts appear in the final urine. Proteinuria, i.e., the detection of proteins in the final urine, can therefore possibly indicate damage to the glomerulus.

IN A NUTSHELL   !

Amino acids and oligopeptides are filtered unhindered and then (almost) completely reabsorbed, so that only traces are excreted.

12.13 Movement of end products of N metabolism and organic ions in the nephron

12.13.1 Urea

The nitrogen produced during the breakdown of proteins and amino acids must be excreted if it cannot be used for the resynthesis of amino acids. Nitrogen is excreted as three different end products according to animal species. While fish mainly excrete ammonia, reptiles, birds and mammals excrete urea and/or uric acid. Urea can be produced in two ways: in the urea cycle (p. 472) (e.g., mammals) or by the uricolytic pathway (e.g., bony fish). Urea production is related to the protein intake with food.

The kidney excretes urea very effectively, but its clearance is less than that of creatinine (**Table 12.2**). Initially, urea is filtered unhindered in the glomerulus. About half of the filtered amount is reabsorbed proximally by diffusion and solvent drag. The **distal tubules** and the **cortical collecting ducts** are almost **impermeable** to urea. Only the **medullary segment** of the **collecting duct** has specific transport proteins for urea in the apical membrane, so that urea can diffuse along a concentration gradient into the thin segments of the **loop of Henle**. A special transport protein for urea is again involved in the back diffusion into the loop of Henle. The back-diffused urea flows down the collecting duct with the tubule fluid and thus enters a **cycle** (**Fig. 12.22**). With this circulation, urea contributes significantly to the high osmolality in the renal medulla

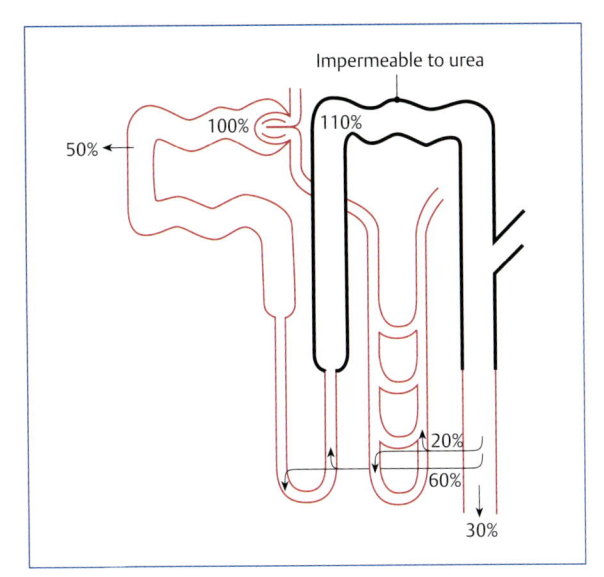

Fig. 12.22 Tubular transport of urea in antidiuresis. The percentages refer to the amounts still present in the respective nephron segments in relation to the filtered "load" (100%).

(Fig. 12.13) and thus reinforces the countercurrent multiplier principle.

Since urea transport in the medullary collecting ducts **depends** on the amount of water reabsorbed in the distal tubule segments, a reduction in **water excretion** causes reduced urea excretion. A pathological reduction in GFR therefore leads to an increase in plasma urea concentration (**uraemia**).

IN A NUTSHELL !

Urea is about 50% passively reabsorbed proximally. It is reabsorbed in the medullary segment of the collecting duct and then secreted back into the loop of Henle. This circuit contributes significantly to countercurrent concentrating mechanisms.

12.13.2 Uric acid, oxalate, allantoin and hippuric acid

Uric acid is mainly present in plasma as Na^+ urate. The solubility of urate is low, so that when there is an increased plasma concentration (**hyperuricaemia), calcium urate crystals** can form. The formation of such crystals in joint capsules leads to phagocytosis and inflammatory reactions known as **gout**.

Most mammals convert N-containing substances mainly into urea and therefore do not excrete significant amounts of uric acid (**ureotelic animals**). If uric acid accumulates in these animals during nucleic acid degradation, it is converted to **allantoin** catalysed by the enzyme uricase (uricolytic pathway). **Humans** or **apes** and the **Dalmatian dog** do not possess **uricase** and therefore also excrete larger proportions of nitrogen metabolism as uric acid. Terrestrial birds (p.338) and reptiles (p.340) excrete nitrogen predominantly as uric acid (**uricotelic animals**).

IN A NUTSHELL !

While mammals excrete only some nitrogen as uric acid, it is the most important nitrogen excretory product in reptiles and birds. The secretion mechanism is that for organic weak anions.

MORE DETAILS

Uric acid excretion: Mechanism

Most uric acid (70% in humans) is excreted in urine, with a smaller proportion being excreted into the intestine. Uric acid is filtered unhindered, but the transport properties in the proximal tubule differ in different animal species: In humans, chimpanzees and most dogs, about 90% of the filtered uric acid is reabsorbed in the renal tubules. With increased urate concentration in plasma or primary urine, uric acid is both increasingly reabsorbed and increasingly excreted. The reabsorption mechanism reaches a transport maximum at a urate concentration in the primary urine above $1\,mmol \cdot l^{-1}$. In **Dalmatian dogs**, unlike other dogs, uric acid is not reabsorbed proximally, but is secreted.

Allantoin and oxalate excretion: Mechanism

Allantoin appears to be excreted virtually exclusively by glomerular filtration in rats and dogs (exception: Dalmatians). In most mammals (not humans and apes), the uric acid formed during purine degradation is further degraded in the hepatocytes to allantoin or allantoic acid which are excreted via the kidney. Dalmatian dogs are an exception to this. They are not able to completely incorporate the uric acid produced into the peroxisomes of hepatocytes. They therefore excrete uric acid in urine.

Oxalate is formed in amino acid metabolism and is also absorbed from food, for example as a calcium salt. It is mainly secreted in the proximal tubule and only reabsorbed to a small extent. As a result, its concentration in urine may be sufficient to induce urinary stone formation.

Urinary stones

In dogs and cats, ammonium magnesium phosphate (**struvite**) and **calcium oxalate** are the most common types of kidney and urinary stones. Dietary factors and also a low urine volume and/or low micturition frequency are causative factors in the formation of urinary stones. They can also be the result of urinary tract infections with changes to the internal milieu.

Urate stones are formed when the metabolic conversion of uric acid into allantoin is limited, as in the Dalmatian.

12.13.3 Organic anions and cations

Many weak organic anions and cations are not only filtered, but are additionally secreted by tertiary active secretion mechanisms, predominantly in the proximal straight tubule (**Fig. 12.23**). These substances can be either endogenous or exogenous, and many drugs especially fall into the category of exogenous substances.

MORE DETAILS

Mechanism of anion and cation excretion

Organic anions such as **furosemide** (a diuretic; **Fig. 12.18**) and penicillin, an antibiotic, are taken up into the cell on the basolateral side by an α-ketoglutarate/organic anion antiporter against an electrochemical gradient (**Fig. 12.23**). The α-ketoglutarate gradient driving this transport is generated by a symporter that transports Na^+ against α-ketoglutarate or dicarboxylate. The apical efflux occurs through anion antiporters and uniporters that have not yet been structurally characterised.

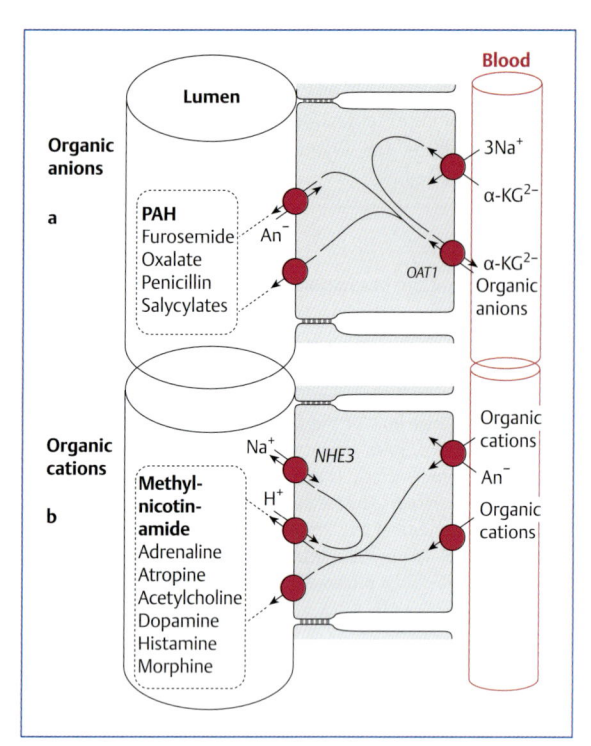

Fig. 12.23 Secretion of organic ions in the proximal straight tubule. **a** Organic anions. **b** Organic cations. The lists show some of the organic ions transported.
α-KG^{2-} = α-ketoglutarate (= 2-oxo-glutarate); An$^-$ = anion of unknown variety; NHE3 = Na$^+$/H$^+$ exchanger 3; OAT = organic anion transporter; PAH = paraaminohippuric acid.

Organic cations are taken up into the cell basolaterally down concentration gradients by symporters as well as by uniporters (**Fig. 12.23**). Apical efflux occurs through uniporters and H$^+$/org. cation antiporters. The H$^+$ gradient driving this tertiary active transport is generated by the apical Na$^+$/H$^+$ antiporter. Typical organic cations secreted in this way are atropine and morphine.

It must be emphasised here that this pathway of active secretion represents only part of the process of elimination. An essential requirement for elimination is that these substances are filtered by the glomeruli.

> **IN A NUTSHELL** !
>
> Several secretory transport systems exist in the proximal straight tubule for a large number of organic anions and cations, including many drugs.

12.14 Maintenance of the acid-base balance by the kidney

12.14.1 Kidney as part of the regulation of the acid-base balance

In addition to the respiratory tract and the liver, the kidney plays a decisive role in maintaining the pH of body fluids within a narrow range. How the different systems interact is described in ch. Regulatory Systems (p. 346). In contrast to the respiratory tract, the kidney is also able to excrete non-volatile acids and to vary the buffering capacity in the

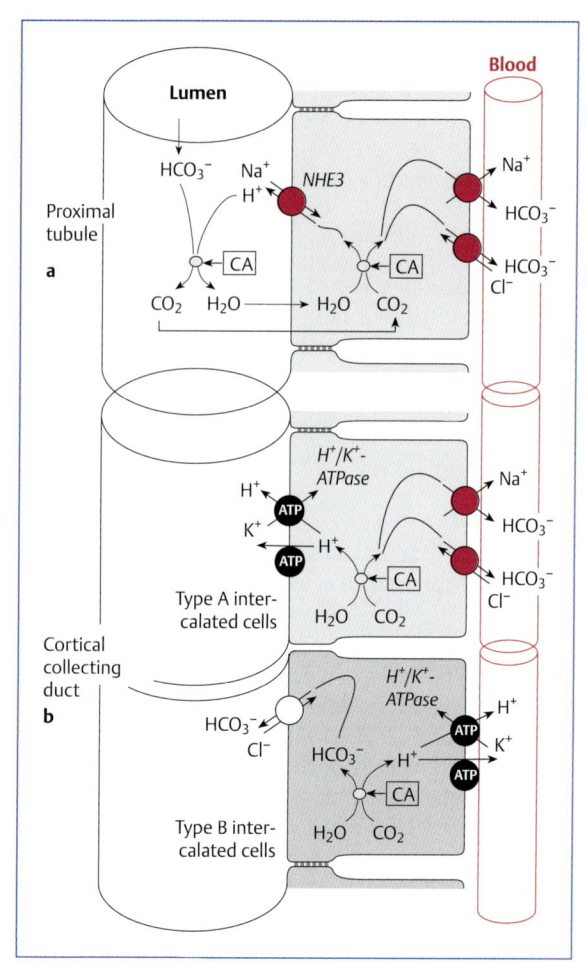

Fig. 12.24 Cellular mechanisms of renal H$^+$ transport. **a** Proximal tubule: apical Na$^+$/H$^+$ antiporter = NHE3 (Na$^+$/H$^+$ exchanger 3). **b** Cortical collecting duct: apical H$^+$/K$^+$-ATPase and H$^+$-ATPase in type A intercalated cells; basolateral H$^+$/K$^+$-ATPase and H$^+$-ATPase in type B intercalated cells.
CA = carbonic anhydrase.

body, especially the amount of bicarbonate (HCO$_3^-$), depending on the metabolic state.

Thus, depending on diet and metabolic state, either an acidic or alkaline urine is excreted. With a high-protein diet (dog, cat), there is a need for proton excretion, i.e., **carnivores** usually excrete an **acidic urine**. With **plant-based diets**, alkalising salts (fumarate, citrate) are ingested. Therefore, the acid-base balance of the body must be adjusted by excreting **alkaline urine**.

12.14.2 Transport processes in the proximal tubule and collecting duct

Various transport proteins are available in renal cells for the elimination of protons (**Fig. 12.24**). In the proximal tubule, protons are mainly eliminated via the secondary active **sodium/proton antiporter NHE3**. The proximal tubule is quantitatively the most important section of the nephron for proton elimination. In the far end of the distal tubule and the collecting duct, H$^+$ secretion is controlled by a (primarily active) **H$^+$-ATPase** and also an **H$^+$/K$^+$-ATPase** which is localised in the **apical membrane** of **type A inter-calated cells**. In alkalotic metabolic states, on the other hand, H$^+$-ATPase and H$^+$/K$^+$-ATPase are incorporated into the **basolateral membrane**, so that H$^+$ is reabsorbed (**type B intercalated cells**). On the opposite side of the cell there are HCO$_3^-$-transporting carriers (**Fig. 12.24**).

> **IN A NUTSHELL** !
>
> Protons are secreted in the proximal tubule via a Na$^+$/H$^+$ antiporter. In the distal nephron, protons can be secreted by the intercalated cells. In the distal tubule, however, protons can also be reabsorbed or bicarbonate is secreted if the metabolic state is alkaline. The proximal tubule is quantitatively the most important section of the nephron for proton elimination.

12.14.3 Proton excretion, bicarbonate reabsorption and production

Since the transport processes in the proximal tubule are critical for maintaining acid-base balance, they and their adaptation to the metabolic situation need to be understood. In the collecting duct, only small quantities of protons or buffer bases are transported. In the collecting duct, however, the fine adjustment of proton excretion takes place via the mechanisms described above.

■ Bicarbonate reabsorption in the proximal tubule

Before systemic regulation of acid-base balance takes place via the kidney, it is the principal task of the proximal nephron sections to reabsorb the filtered bicarbonate so that initially no buffer loss occurs. At normal HCO$_3^-$ plasma concentration (about 24 mmol · l^{-1}), practically no bicarbonate is excreted, since all that has been filtered is reabsorbed.

The mechanism of **HCO$_3^-$ recovery** in the proximal tubule is shown in **Fig. 12.25 a**. HCO$_3^-$ in the lumen is not taken up into the cell as such, but combines with secreted H$^+$ to form H$_2$CO$_3$ which then dissociates into CO$_2$ and H$_2$O. The luminal reaction H$^+$ + HCO$_3^-$ → H$_2$CO$_3$ → CO$_2$ + H$_2$O is catalysed by a **membrane-bound carbonic anhydrase**. CO$_2$ then diffuses through the lipid phase of the cell membrane into the cell. The CO$_2$ that reaches the intracellular space is converted by another intracellular carbonic anhydrase back into H$_2$CO$_3$. H$_2$CO$_3$ dissociates and releases H$^+$ to the Na$^+$/H$^+$ antiporter, which allows the proton to recirculate back into the lumen. The remaining HCO$_3^-$ diffuses via different transport mechanisms (**Fig. 12.25 a**) through the basolateral membrane into blood and is thus reabsorbed. This reabsorption of bicarbonate in the proximal tubule is found both in species that excrete an acidic urine due to their protein-rich diet (carnivores) and in species that excrete an alkaline urine due to their vegetation-rich diet (herbivores).

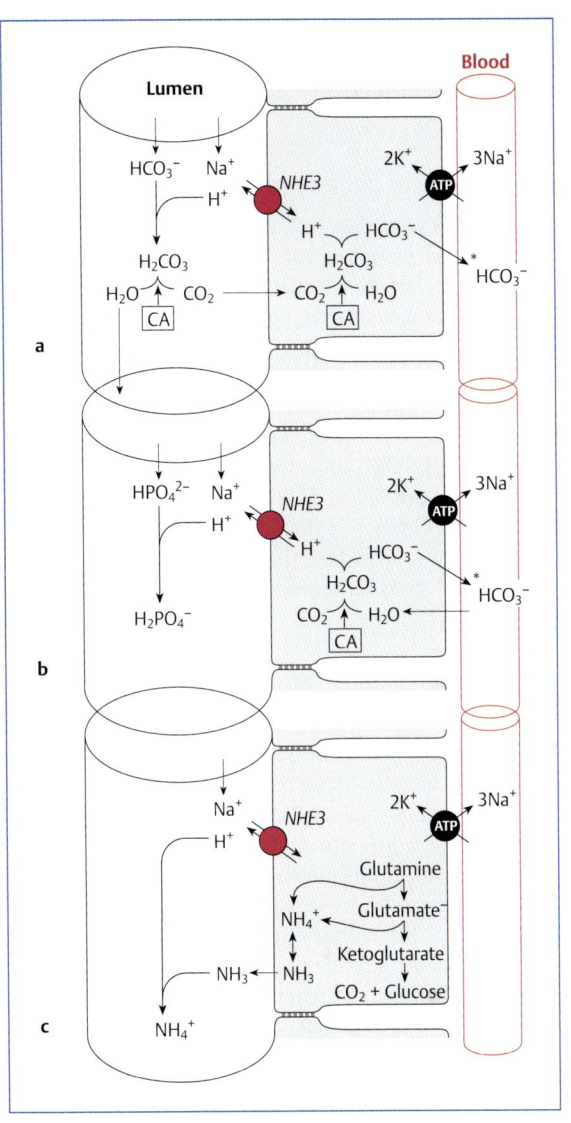

Fig. 12.25 Cellular mechanisms of HCO$_3^-$ recovery and H$^+$ secretion in the proximal tubule. **a** HCO$_3^-$ recovery. **b** Secretion of protons as H$_2$PO$_4^-$. **c** Secretion of protons as NH$_4^+$. The general mechanisms of HCO$_3^-$ excretion (*) from the cell into blood are shown in **Fig. 12.24**.

■ New bicarbonate formation and H$^+$ excretion

In addition to the basal recovery of HCO$_3^-$, the kidney in acidosis is capable of excreting increasing amounts of protons and to form new HCO$_3^-$. Thus, in respiratory acidosis, the p$_{CO_2}$ in blood increases. With increased p$_{CO_2}$ the influx of CO$_2$ into cells of the proximal tubule is also augmented. The increased influx of CO$_2$ also produces increased amounts of H$^+$ and bicarbonate due to the activity of intracellular carbonic anhydrase (formation of H$_2$CO$_3$ with subsequent dissociation). The increased formation of bicarbonate also leads to its increased reabsorption via the basolateral transporters (**Fig. 12.24**). The dissociation of H$_2$CO$_3$ not only produces bicarbonate, but also protons. The increased accumulation of protons is compensated by the apically localised Na$^+$/H$^+$ antiporter and leads via this transporter to an increased excretion of protons into the tubule lumen. The increased accumulation of protons in the tubule is in turn buffered by various systems as described below.

Acidification of urine by phosphate excretion

About 80% of phosphate (pK_a 6.8) in blood is in the form of the hydrogen phosphate ion (HPO_4^{2-}). In acidosis, phosphate is released from bones into the extracellular fluid and is increasingly filtered. It combines in the tubule with secreted H^+ to form dihydrogen phosphate ($H_2PO_4^-$). The transport system for phosphate (p.322) mainly accepts HPO_4^{2-} and very little $H_2PO_4^-$. Thus $H_2PO_4^-$ being largely unabsorbable, is excreted (**Fig. 12.25b**). At the same time HCO_3^- is reabsorbed and thus counteracts acidosis. The protons that are linked to buffer bases in urine can be measured by titration of the urine to the plasma pH value. The resulting value of the "titration acidity" or the "titratable acidity" gives an indication of acid-base imbalances (p.349).

Acidification of urine through ammonium excretion

The ammonia/ammonium buffer (NH_3/NH_4^+), with a pK_a of 9.2, has an even higher buffer capacity in the acidic range than the phosphate buffer. In the tubule epithelial cells NH_4^+ and NH_3 are formed from amide-containing amino acids, especially glutamine. Glutamine is converted into ketoglutarate with the release of $2 NH_4^+$. After dissociation of NH_4^+, NH_3 diffuses through the lipid phase of the apical membrane into the tubule lumen. NH_3 combines in the tubule fluid with H^+ to form NH_4^+ and, since it cannot be absorbed, is excreted as acid urine (**Fig. 12.25c**). The glutamine required for NH_3 production comes from the liver. In acidotic metabolic conditions, the liver can release more glutamine. The increased glutamine supply can then be used by the kidneys to increase the production of ammonium ions. The excretion of ammonium ions can increase up to 10-fold in acidosis. In this way, the liver indirectly participates in the adjustment of acid-base balance.

> **IN A NUTSHELL** !
>
> When acidosis develops, the kidneys compensate by excreting more acid and producing more bicarbonate.

12.15   Endocrine functions of the kidney

The kidney is not only the target organ of various hormones such as aldosterone (p.314), ANP (p.314), ADH (p.318) and PTH (p.322), but is also capable of producing various hormones and mediators itself or converting them from precursors into their active form.

12.15.1   Renin-angiotensin system

Renin is released from specialised smooth muscle cells of the afferent arteriole and acts as a peptidase that converts angiotensinogen to angiotensin I. The renin-angiotensin-aldosterone system is described in more detail in ch. Renin-angiotensin system (p.307).

12.15.2   Erythropoietin

Erythropoietin (EPO) is synthesised in the liver during foetal development, but almost exclusively in the kidney in adult animals. EPO is formed in the renal cortex, in a fibroblast population located between proximal tubule cells and peritubular capillaries. The release of EPO is mainly stimulated by a **decrease** in the **partial pressure of O_2** in the **kidney** itself. The stabilisation of a transcription factor, the **hypoxia-inducible factor** (HIF) (p.231), plays an important role here. EPO in blood, reaches its site of action, the bone marrow, where it stimulates erythropoiesis (p.230). Chronic renal insufficiency therefore leads to "renal" anaemia. Nowadays, this can be treated with genetically engineered EPO.

Why the kidney serves as an O_2 sensor triggering EPO release is not fully understood. It is conceivable that because of the high oxygen consumption of the kidney any decrease in oxygen supply is particularly noticeable here, i.e., a rapid change of p_{O_2} occurs.

> **MORE DETAILS**   Other hormones produced in the kidney that promote the formation of particular blood cells are thrombopoietin (TSF, thrombocytopoiesis-stimulating factor) and megakaryopoietin (MSF, megakaryocyte-stimulating factor). Both ultimately act on the formation of thrombocytes.

> **IN A NUTSHELL** !
>
> Renin, which is mainly produced in the epithelioid cells of the afferent arterioles, promotes the formation of angiotensin II. Erythropoietin (EPO) promotes haematopoiesis.

12.15.3   Vitamin D hormone, endothelins and eicosanoids

Vitamin D hormone (cholecalciferol, calcitriol, 1,25-dihydroxycholecalciferol)

The formation of active vitamin D takes place in three phases:

1. Vitamin D_3 is formed from 7-dehydrocholesterol in skin by the action of UV radiation, or is ingested with food.
2. It is hydroxylated in the liver to 25-OHD (calcidiol).
3. In the kidney, 25-OHD is hydroxylated to the active vitamin D hormone $1,25-(OH)_2 D_3$ (calcitriol). Intrarenal activation occurs in the mitochondria of the proximal tubule epithelium by a cytochrome P450 monooxygenase. This enzyme is stimulated differently in the two segments of the proximal tubule, in the convoluted segment by PTH and in the straight segment by calcitonin.

Vitamin D hormone promotes Ca^{2+} absorption in the intestine (p.435), reabsorption in the kidney (p.322) and mobilisation from bone mineral. The endocrine functions of vitamin D hormone are discussed in more detail in the chapter Calcitriol (p.549).

> **IN A NUTSHELL** !
>
> The kidneys are the site of formation of the active vitamin D hormone.

MORE DETAILS

Endothelins and eicosanoids

Endothelins (ET) are a group of tissue hormones that act as functional antagonists of EDRF (endothelium-derived relaxing factor (p.210) identical to NO). They are produced in the kidney in the endothelial cells of most arterial and venous vessels as well as in the glomerulus and the tubule cells of the renal medulla. ET mainly have a contractile effect on the mesangial system and the smooth muscle cells of blood vessels. This causes a decrease in GFR by decreasing the surface area for filtering.

The most important eicosanoids formed in the kidney under physiological conditions are the prostaglandins E_2, I_2 and $F_{2\alpha}$ and, to a lesser extent, thromboxane A_2. Eicosanoids are formed in almost all structures of the kidney, most notably in the arterial vessels. Eicosanoid receptors have also been detected in all of these structures. Hormonal stimuli for renal eicosanoid synthesis include angiotensin II, catecholamines (as well as sympathetic stimulation), kinins and ADH. The renally formed eicosanoids are inactivated in the renal cortex within seconds to minutes. The effects of eicosanoids are predominantly autocrine and paracrine. The main effects are: 1. vasodilation by PGI_2 and PGE_2 and vasoconstriction by TxA_2 and $PGF_{2\alpha}$; 2. inhibition of tubular Na^+ reabsorption by PGE_2 and PGI_2; 3. attenuation of the effect of ADH by PGE_2.

Suggested reading

Randall D., Burggren W, French K. Eckert Animal Physiology. 5th ed. Freeman; 2001

Schrier RW. Atlas of diseases of the kidney. 1999. Internet edition: www.kidneyatlas.org

Inner milieu

13   Water and sodium balance

Gotthold Gäbel

13.1   Functions of water and sodium

> **ESSENTIALS** ✗
>
> The body of mammals consists of 45–75% water. Only in an aqueous milieu can electrolytes dissociate, enzymes catalyse their reactions, and solutes diffuse. The water content of the body and the composition of extra- and intracellular fluid are kept constant within narrow limits. Water and electrolytes are ingested with food and then absorbed in an unregulated manner in the gastrointestinal tract (GIT). However, the excretory capacity of the kidneys is mainly regulated. Thus, the ADH regulatory system is triggered by changes in extracellular fluid volume, and particularly by changes in extracellular fluid osmolality. ADH increases the reabsorption of water in the distal sections of the nephron. Increased osmolality of extracellular fluid also promotes a sensation of thirst in the central nervous system.
>
> Sodium is quantitatively the most important ion of extracellular fluid. Hence, any changes in sodium concentration lead directly to changes in osmolality and thus to the volume of extracellular fluid, i.e., to hypo- or hypervolaemia. The renin-angiotensin-aldosterone system as well as atrial natriuretic peptide are the main regulators of sodium concentration in body water. Aldosterone induces increased sodium reabsorption in the kidney and thus has a sodium-conserving effect. Atrial natriuretic peptide is an antagonist and so reduces sodium reabsorption in the kidney. Disturbances in water and electrolyte balance are observed as dehydration or hyperhydration, depending on the direction of change in extracellular fluid volume. Increase or decrease in osmolality of extracellular fluid from the normal value are referred to as hypo- or hypertonic disturbances in water and electrolyte balance. Such imbalances can have acute life-threatening consequences.

13.2   The importance of water

Tissues and organs are only able to maintain their physiological functions in an aqueous medium. Organic substrates and ions dissolved in water surrounding the cells of organs are then available for metabolic conversions. Therefore, the quantity of water and the concentration of substances dissolved in it are kept constant.

13.3   Water balance

13.3.1   Water intake

Every animal species releases water in different ways from the body. Therefore, to keep a constant quantity of total body water, **water intake** must balance water output (p.330).

Mammals obtain their water requirements from three sources:

- water ingested with the **feed**
- **drinking water**
- **water** from oxidative metabolism

In **Table 13.1** the water balance of a lactating and a non-lactating cow is compared.

Table 13.1 Water balance of a cow in lactating and non-lactating condition (data in $l \cdot d^{-1}$) – with a low milk yield of $12 l \cdot d^{-1}$.

	Non-lactating	Lactating
Water intake		
Drinking water	26	51
Water in the feed	1	2
Oxidation water	2	3
Total	29	56
Water output		
Urine	7	11
Evaporation (skin/breathing)	10	14
Faeces	12	19
Milk	0	12
Total	29	56

Source: Reece WO, Erickson HH, Goff IP, Uemura EE (eds.). Duke's Physiology of Domestic Animals. 13th ed., Ames: Wiley-Blackwell; 2015

It is clear that when there is an increased need for more water input, such as when there is increased water output in milk, this is mainly supplied by an increase in drinking water intake.

The milk yield of the lactating cow in **Table 13.1** is at the lower end of normal for modern dairy production. In general, it can be assumed for most species that 2–5 litres of water must be consumed per kg of dry matter intake. This means that a high-yielding dairy cow with 20 kg dry matter intake per day must have 80–100 litres of water available to drink per day. In addition, water intake should be timed close to feed intake.

Water intake from the feed itself or from oxidative metabolism is quantitatively a minor source under most circumstances. Water of oxidation is always produced during organic substrate oxidation. For the complete oxidation of glucose, the following reaction equation applies:

$$C_6H_{12}O_6 + 6O_2 \rightarrow 6CO_2 + \mathbf{6H_2O} \tag{13.1}$$

$$180\,g + 192\,g \rightarrow 264\,g + \mathbf{108\,g}$$

It can be seen that approx. 0.6 g of water are produced per gram of oxidised glucose. Corresponding reaction equations result in approx. 1 g of water per gram of oxidised fat and approx. 0.4 g of water per gram of oxidised protein. O_2 is required for oxidation, which must be absorbed through respiration. In arid regions, water loss via the respiratory tract during the required O_2 uptake is often greater than the water gain from oxidation, i.e., oxidation water can then only partially contribute to water requirements in combination with other mechanisms.

13.3.2 Water loss

Terrestrial mammals lose water in the following ways:

- through the **skin**
- via the **respiratory tract**
- in **urine excretion**
- in **faecal excretion**
- in animal **products** such as milk etc.

Water is continuously released through evaporation from skin and from the epithelia of the respiratory tract (**perspiratio insensibilis**). The extent of this water loss depends on the ambient temperature and humidity, and it increases with sweating or with panting (**perspiratio sensibilis**). Water loss in faeces is low in carnivorous and omnivorous animals, but in herbivores there is usually a larger proportion of total water loss in faeces because of higher faecal water content. Water loss from animal products can be quite significant, especially for milk-producing animals.

Table 13.1 makes it clear that large amounts of water are "lost" with the milk of the lactating cow. Most mammals lose only small amounts of water from sweating, as only a few mammals have pronounced sweat production, the exceptions being humans and equids and Bovidae and Camelidae to a lesser degree. In working horses, the loss of water through sweat can be considerable. Sport horses (e.g., during endurance riding) lose up to 8% of their body weight in sweat over five hours of activity. A supply of water must therefore be provided to replenish such a loss. This considerable loss of water is also a problem because horse sweat contains a high concentration of electrolytes (especially NaCl), which must also be replenished (**Table 26.6**).

These processes of water loss are obligatory and thus can only be modified to a limited extent in the regulation of water balance. In contrast, the output of water in urine can be regulated, but only slightly, in faeces. However, there are limits to this regulation:

- related to the feed supply or the metabolic profile, because metabolic waste products are produced that have to be excreted in urine such as urea, uric acid, creatine, and creatinine.
- these metabolic waste substrates can only be concentrated in the kidneys up to a certain maximum value, so a minimum amount of water must always be excreted to eliminate these waste products in urine.

Table 12.4 shows the maximum concentrating capacity of the kidney and, in parallel, the range of variation in urine excretion in different domestic animals. It becomes clear that in most animal species the kidneys can concentrate urine to more than 4 times the plasma osmolality, i.e., up to 1400 mosmol $\cdot$ kg^{-1}. The comparatively high renal concentration capacity of the felid kidneys is striking, up to values > 3000 mosmol $\cdot$ kg^{-1}.

Regulation of water output is primarily through a change in the volume of urine. If there is a lack of drinking water supply, the volume of urine produced can be restricted. However, a minimum amount of water must always be excreted to enable the excretion of metabolic waste products.

13.4 Compartmentalisation of body water

On average, 45–75% of body mass consists of water. The higher values are found in young animals, and the lower end of this range are in older animals. As well as age, the proportion of water in the body also depends on its fat content. Fat tissue has a much lower water content (10–30%) than other tissues (striated muscle: 70–80%), so animals with a higher fat content have a lower water content than lean animals. In **Fig. 13.1** the distribution of body water is shown schematically.

Total water volume is divided into two compartments: **extracellular** and **intracellular** water. Water in cells accounts for about 60% of total body water. The extracellular water (approx. 40% of total) is divided into three further compartments. **Blood plasma** is the extracellular liquid portion of blood. **Interstitial water** is the water that surrounds cells in tissues. However, the interstitial space also contains collagens and proteoglycans, so that interstitial water is closely associated with these structures. This mixture of scaffolding substances and water is not liquid, but has a rather gel-like to even solid consistency. Plasma water and interstitial water are closely related, as water is effectively exchanged through the wall of capillaries. A sub-compartment of extracellular water is **transcellular water**. This is mainly the water in epithelium lined hollow organs (bladder, ureter, gastrointestinal tract, joints). Since this water is separated by a denser barrier compared to that of capillary endothelium, there is less water exchange between transcellular and other pools of extracellular water. Transcellular water can even serve as a reserve. For example, the forestomachs of ruminants, which contain a large amount of water, can also be considered a water reservoir, as the reticulorumen of a high-yielding dairy cow (600 kg bw) contains more than 150 litres of water, i.e., more than 25% of total body weight, see ch. 16.4.1).

45–75% of the body consists of water. Of this, approx. 60% is located intracellularly and approx. 40% extracellularly. In herbivores, the extracellular or transcellular water can make up a larger proportion, mainly because of the size of the gastrointestinal tract.

13.5 Composition of extracellular and intracellular fluid

In **Table 1.4** the ionic composition of extracellular and intracellular fluid is listed. The composition of the transcellular fluid usually varies greatly and therefore cannot be defined by typical numerical values.

The **extracellular fluid** contains mainly **sodium** as a cation, while **intracellularly potassium** is the most prominent cation. This uneven distribution is a consequence of the activity of Na^+/K^+-ATPase in cell membranes, which transports sodium to the extracellular and potassium to the intracellular compartment (**Table 1.4**). Extracellularly, the positive charge of sodium is mainly balanced by chloride, but intracellularly, the charge balance of potassium is mainly by largely impermeable anions (phosphate and negatively charged proteins). In addition to charge balancing, these organic ions fulfil diverse functions in cell metabolism. In addition to inorganic electrolytes (mainly sodium and chloride), extracellular fluid also contains bicarbonate as a buffering agent (p. 346) (**Table 15.2**), various proteins and other organic solutes.

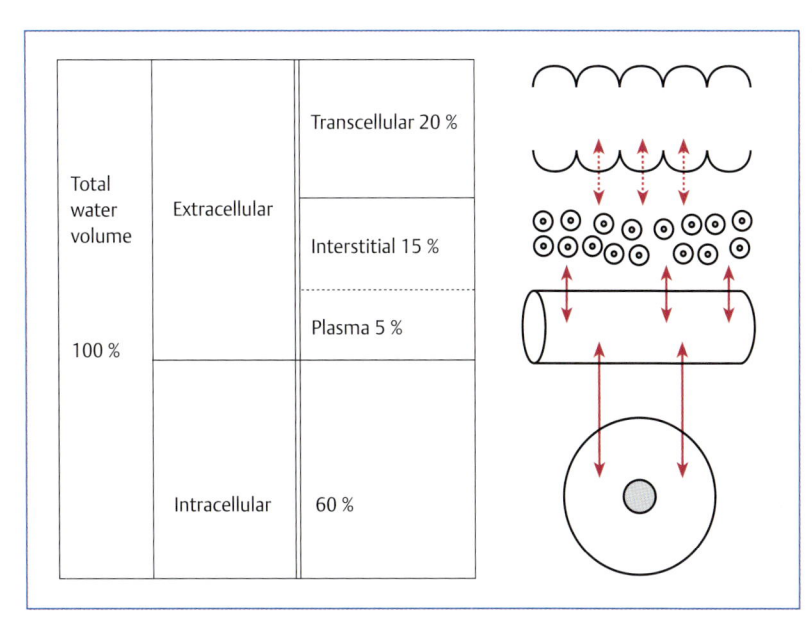

Fig. 13.1 Fluid spaces of the body and exchange of fluid between those spaces.

Inner milieu

The extracellular fluid is often referred to as the "**inner milieu**" which ensures the survival of cells. To fulfil this function, the composition of extracellular fluid must be precisely regulated, mainly by the kidneys, so that cells are immersed in a fluid that contains electrolytes and substrates in adequate, constant concentrations. Since water and low-molecular substances can easily pass through capillary endothelium, blood plasma (**Table 9.2**) and interstitial fluid have similar contents of low-molecular weight substances, but differ in their protein content. The latter is because proteins (albumin, globulins) are in higher concentrations in plasma than in the interstitium, and they cannot cross the endothelial barrier. In addition to their specific individual functions, plasma proteins (p. 220) also collectively maintain the colloid-osmotic (oncotic) pressure.

> **IN A NUTSHELL** !
>
> Extracellular fluid consists of transcellular water (especially in the gastrointestinal tract), blood plasma and the fluid between the cells, the interstitial fluid. Interstitial fluid is similar in composition to blood plasma, except for that of proteins.

13.6 Osmotic equilibrium and water movement

The components listed in **Table 1.4** are osmotically active, so that when there are osmotic imbalances between compartments, major water shifts can occur. In the following sections, the principles of osmotically induced water movement are discussed, and later how this is regulated.

In principle, osmotically induced water movement has two prerequisites:

- a selectively permeable membrane,
- a transmembrane osmotic gradient.

Osmotic water movement occurs when a membrane (e.g. the cell membrane) separates two fluid compartments (e.g. extracellular and intracellular fluid) and is selectively permeable to water, but not to dissolved substances. Furthermore, if the total concentration of dissolved, osmotically active substances on each side of the selectively permeable membrane is different, there will be a net diffusion of water to the side with the higher concentration of dissolved substances – a process called **osmosis**.

13.6.1 Osmolality, osmolarity and osmotic pressure

The concentration of all dissolved and thus osmotically effective substances is called **osmolality** (if related to **1 kilogram of solvent**) or **osmolarity** (if related to **1 litre of solvent**). It should be noted that the osmolality of a solution is determined by the molar concentration of the dissolved substances. For example, 180 g glucose (= 1 mol) dissolved in 820 g water (i.e., glucose + H_2O = 1 kg) produces 1 os-

mol · kg^{-1}. However, if substances dissociate (as is the case with salts), each of the dissociated molecules is osmotically effective. Thus, if 58 g NaCl (= 1 mol NaCl) is dissolved in 942 g water (i.e., water + NaCl = 1 kg), this dissociates (ideally) into 1 mol Na$^+$ and 1 mol Cl$^-$, i.e., the osmolality is 2 osmol · kg^{-1}.

In reality, osmolality calculated in this way does not correspond exactly to the actual osmolality. The reasons for this are an incomplete dissociation of the salt and/or mutual interactions of the molecules and ions (attraction or repulsion), which in turn influence their osmotic activities. Thus, the addition of the osmotically active substances listed in **Table 9.2** gives a value of 300 mosmol · kg^{-1}, but the actual measured value is about 290 mosmol · kg^{-1} for the reasons mentioned.

If water diffuses through a membrane that is selectively permeable to water to the side of higher osmolality, this osmotic movement of water can be balanced or even reversed by pressure exerted on the solution with higher osmolality. The pressure needed to just stop osmosis is called the **osmotic pressure**. The osmotic pressure of a solution at 37 °C can be approximately calculated by the following formula:

$$\text{osmotic pressure (kPa)} = 2.6 \cdot \text{osmolality} \left(\text{mosmol} \cdot \text{kg}^{-1}\right) \quad (13.2)$$

For physiological body fluids, this means that they can generate an osmotic pressure of 2.6 · 290 = 754 kPa. This corresponds to a water column of approx. 77 metres (1 kPa corresponds to 10.2 cm H_2O)!

Consequently, even small osmotic differences in the water compartments can lead to large shifts of water. To avoid such water transfer, osmotic differences must be prevented from occurring, i.e., osmolality must be regulated effectively and within narrow limits.

> **IN A NUTSHELL** !
>
> The osmolality of extra and intracellular fluid is about 290 mosmol · kg^{-1}. Osmotic gradients are the driving forces for water shifts.

13.6.2 Colloid-osmotic pressure

As shown in **Table 9.2** plasma proteins, especially albumin, are the main organic components of plasma. They exert a colloid-osmotic (= oncotic) pressure. Since vascular endothelium is generally poorly permeable to proteins, these proteins are only in plasma and not in the interstitium. Because of this, the colloid-osmotic pressure almost always acts in the direction of the plasma/blood and is the counterpart of hydrostatic pressure. However, these conditions are massively disturbed in proteinuria or where synthesis of plasma proteins is depressed, as in liver disease, and this results in osmotic imbalances between the compartments.

13.6.3 Water movement in an anisotonic environment

If cells or tissues are placed in a solution where the concentration of osmotically active, non-permeable substances matches that of the cytoplasm, then no osmotically induced net water movement takes place. Such a solution is defined as **isotonic**. A solution where the concentration of osmotically active, non-permeable substances is lower than that of cells is called **hypotonic**. Water is driven into cells from such a solution, inducing them to swell. In **hypertonic** solutions, because of higher osmolality in the extracellular space, a movement of water out of cells can be observed, so that cell volume shrinks.

A distinction must be made between isoosmolality and isotonicity. An isoosmolar solution, when added to blood for example, does not necessarily have to be isotonic. Thus, a urea solution of $300\,mmol \cdot l^{-1}$ ($\approx 280\,mosmol \cdot kg^{-1}$) is isoosmolar, but hypotonic for erythrocytes, because urea can quickly diffuse across the cell membrane into erythrocytes and thus osmotically draws water in. An isoosmolar 0.9% NaCl solution ($154\,mmol \cdot l^{-1}$ NaCl) is mainly isotonic to plasma or extracellular fluid, since NaCl cannot easily pass through the cell membrane. It is therefore often referred to as "**physiological saline solution**". The term "physiological" refers only to the osmolality of this solution and is therefore misleading.

13.7 Volume regulation of cells

Osmotic differences between intracellular and extracellular spaces can be minimised by two strategies:

- Extracellular osmolality must be regulated within relatively narrow limits and/or
- the cells must be able to adjust the osmolality of the intracellular space to that of the extracellular space.

To understand the intracellular setting of osmolality, one must first realise that intracellularly osmolality is determined primarily by potassium and large (protein) anions, and extracellularly primarily by NaCl. This ion distribution must be maintained. The intracellular anions are "fixed" in the cell due to their size. To maintain the concentration gradients of the smaller sodium, potassium and chloride ions, other mechanisms are required. For the general maintenance of ion distribution, the activity of **Na⁺/K⁺-ATPase** is essential. Through the pumping activity of this ATPase, sodium entering the cell is returned to the extracellular concentration, while potassium, in turn, is concentrated intracellularly. The high intracellular potassium concentration (and thus the activity of the Na⁺/K⁺-ATPase) has an indirect effect on the distribution of chloride. Thus, potassium diffuses from the intracellular to the extracellular fluid down a concentration gradient, and this generates a membrane potential. As the membrane potential approaches the chloride equilibrium potential, a net influx of chloride into the cell is prevented and an **osmotic equilibrium** is created. As a result, the osmotic effectiveness of the intracellular protein anions is not further enhanced by any chloride influx. A deficiency of energy or O_2, such as in

ischaemia, leads to reduced activity of the Na⁺/K⁺-ATPase. This increases intracellular sodium concentration and simultaneously decreases intracellular potassium concentration. As a result, the membrane potential can no longer be maintained and chloride flows in, increasing the osmolality of the cell. Water flows into the cell, resulting in "cell oedema".

Beyond these basic mechanisms, however, cells can also adapt to osmolality deviations of the extracellular fluid within certain limits. If **cells** are transferred into **hypertonic solutions**, the **shrinkage** described above can initially be observed. After some time, the cells return to their physiological volume, as the intracellular osmolality increases and thus adapts to the extracellular one. This increase in intracellular osmolality is based on two mechanisms:

1. An increase in sodium transport (mainly through activation of sodium cotransport systems). This results in an influx of sodium into the intracellular space.
2. Degradation of macromolecular substances into several low-molecular weight ones (e.g., degradation of proteins into amino acids).

The **cell swelling** that occurs in a **hypotonic solution** is counteracted in a corresponding manner by lowering the intracellular osmolality:

1. Activation of transport systems for potassium with the resulting discharge of potassium out of the cell.
2. Conversion of numerous low-molecular weight substances into fewer higher-molecular weight ones (e.g., protein synthesis from amino acids).

The mechanisms of these **regulatory volume changes** are summarised schematically in **Fig. 13.2**.

It must be emphasised, however, that cells (with the exception of cells in the kidney) are rarely exposed to large fluctuations in extracellular osmolality under physiological conditions, since the ADH system reacts very sensitively and rapidly and can keep extracellular osmolality constant within narrow limits, see ch. 13.8.1.

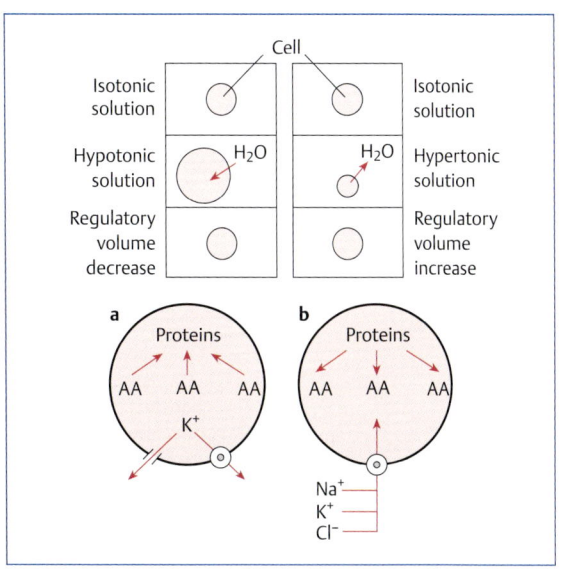

Fig. 13.2 Changes in cell volume in anisotonic medium and mechanisms of counter-regulation (AA = amino acids). **a** Intracellular osmolality decreases. **b** Intracellular osmolality increases.

Inner milieu

13.8 Regulation of fluid balance and osmolality in extracellular fluid

The most important regulatory organ for the regulation of fluid balance is the kidney, and the most important regu-lating hormone is **antidiuretic hormone (ADH)**. In addi-tion, **aldosterone** and a peptide hormone, the **atrial natri-uretic peptide**, are also involved in this regulation. The **renin-angiotensin system** also has an influence. Osmore-gulation takes precedence over volume regulation. The os-mosensors are much more sensitive than the volume sen-sors. Changes in plasma osmolality induce not only hormonal regulation, but also behavioural changes. Thus, the volume and osmolality of the extracellular fluid can also be kept constant by triggering thirst and an increased salt appetite.

ADH is also known as vasopressin. Under physiological conditions, however, **vasoconstrictor** effects of ADH do **not** occur.

13.8.1 Osmoregulation

The osmolality of plasma or extracellular fluid rarely varies by more than 1–2%. The monitoring and control systems are therefore extremely sensitive. **Fig. 13.3** shows the **con-trol circuit** for osmoregulation. As can be seen, the control loop is based on simple negative feedback. The regulating elements are the intake of water and water excretion via the kidneys. The regulation process corresponds to the fol-lowing cascade:

1. **Loss of hypoosmolar fluid** (e.g., panting) increases the osmolality of extracellular fluid.
2. Increased osmolality excites **osmosensors** in the hypo-thalamus and in the region of the portal vein.
3. Excitation of osmosensors in turn has two effects:
   a) Stimulation of **ADH production** in the supraoptic and paraventricular nuclei of the hypothalamus and in-creased ADH secretion from the posterior pituitary (**Fig. 5.21**).
   b) Stimulation of the **thirst centre**.
   c) An increased ADH level in plasma increases **water permeability** in the distal tubules and in the collecting ducts of the renal nephrons. This in turn results in in-creased water reabsorption and thus less water excre-tion.
   d) The **sensation of thirst** causes the animal to take in water.

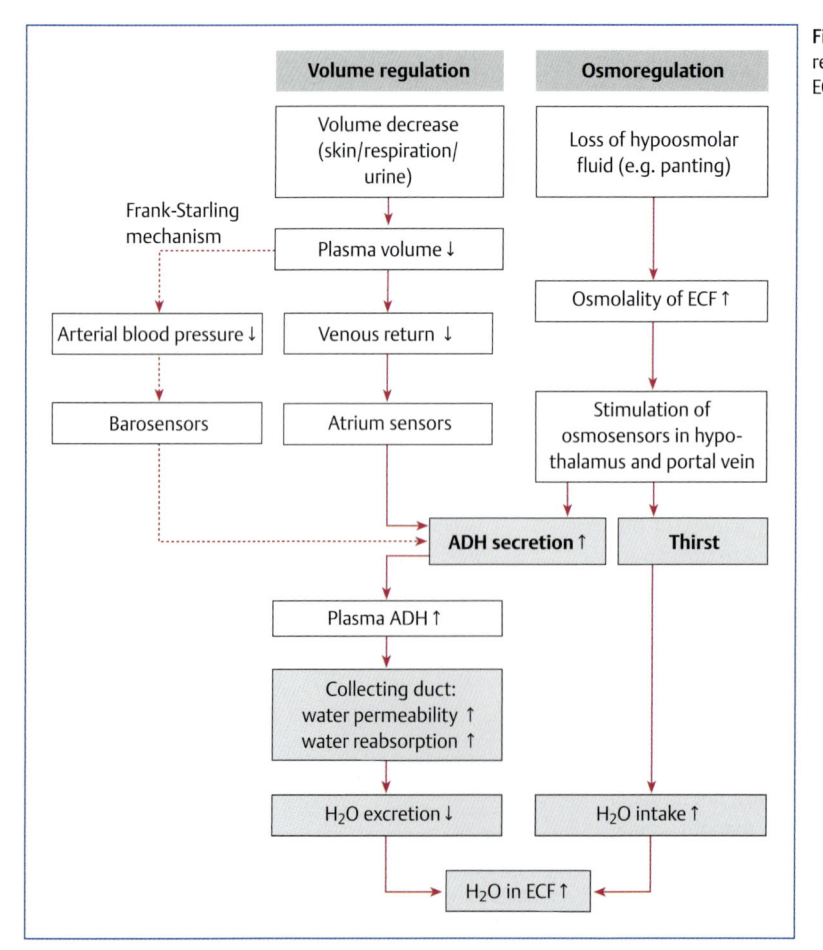

Fig. 13.3 Scheme of ADH-mediated regulation of osmolality and volume. ECF = Extracellular fluid.

A reduction in **H₂O excretion** or an increase in **H₂O intake** decreases the concentration of osmotically active solutes, so osmolality decreases.

13.8.2 Volume regulation

In **Fig. 13.3**, volume regulation is compared to osmoregulation.

If isoosmolar volume changes occur (i.e., the osmolality of extracellular fluid does not change), osmosensors cannot react.

The volume can be perceived indirectly via stretch sensors in the great venae cavae or in the atrium of the heart. If blood volume decreases drastically, as in haemorrhaging, there is a reduction in venous return. The reduced preload indirectly induces (p. 212) increased ADH secretion via the sensors in the right atrium (Frank-Starling mechanism (p. 170)).

The ADH control circuit reacts much more sensitively to changes in osmolality than to changes in volume. If a dog pants, the almost pure water loss associated with this leads to a great increase in osmolality and thus to a strong signal in the ADH control circuit. If a horse sweats, large amounts of electrolytes (ch. 26.5 (p. 627)) are secreted in sweat, so that the osmolality of plasma hardly changes or may even drop. Due to the absence of an osmotic signal, ADH secretion is not increased and the feeling of thirst is not induced sufficiently to promote a search for water. This should be taken into account when replenishing water and electrolyte losses, especially in (endurance) horses trained intensively.

With reduced circulating blood volume, the minimized preload of the heart affects cardiac output and thus arterial blood pressure (Frank-Starling mechanism), which in turn is detected by the barosensors (p. 211). In this way a decrease in arterial blood pressure can also increase ADH release and thus minimize water excretion. However, the influence of the barosensors on ADH release and water excretion is, like the effect of the volume sensors, much smaller than the response to the osmosensors.

> **IN A NUTSHELL**   !
>
> Antidiuretic hormone (ADH) is the most important hormone for osmo- and volume regulation. ADH stimulates water reabsorption in the collecting duct of the nephron, which results in urine becoming more concentrated.

■ Volume regulation by NaCl concentration

The regulation of water content and NaCl balance are interdependent. The consequence of any change in NaCl concentration is always a disturbance in water balance because of a shift in osmotic pressure. The **renin-angiotensin-aldosterone cascade** is central to the direct control of NaCl balance, and thus to the indirect control of water balance. The mechanism of action is described in detail in the chapters Renin-angiotensin system (p. 307) and Regulation of sodium transport (p. 314). Although aldosterone has a central role in the regulation of sodium balance, other factors are also involved. **Atrial natriuretic peptide** is particularly important here. It is synthesised by special cells in the right atrium of the heart (see ch. Distribution and regulation of blood volume (p. 212)).

If plasma volume increases, there is an increase in venous return and thus a stretching of the atria of the heart. This stretch is detected and causes those special cells in the right atrium to secrete atrial natriuretic peptide. This in turn acts in the kidneys to depress sodium reabsorption, so more sodium is excreted and plasma sodium level decreases. This results in a reduction of plasma volume by the osmotically induced shift in water distribution.

■ Thirst and salt appetite

The subjective **feeling of thirst** is mainly triggered by an increase in plasma osmolality, termed osmotic thirst. The osmosensors that trigger the thirst sensation in the hypothalamus are in the same region as the osmosensors that induce the release of ADH. A feeling of thirst can also be induced by a decrease in blood volume, which is then referred to as hypovolaemic thirst. A decrease in blood volume is detected by sensors in the right atrium, as described in the previous subchapter, and is transmitted to the hypothalamus via the vagus nerve. Furthermore, thirst can also be caused by angiotensin II which acts directly on the thirst centre in the brain. For further effects of the renin-angiotensin system see ch. Renin-angiotensin system (p. 307).

The centrally triggered feeling of thirst can be inhibited by peripheral sensors. It is known that sensors in the gastrointestinal tract can detect how much water is absorbed after drinking and this limits the feeling of thirst. A dehydrated animal given the opportunity to take in water will therefore only drink enough to compensate for the water deficit. This limiting of water intake occurs even before the water has been absorbed from the alimentary tract so that hyperhydration (p. 336) is prevented.

Thirst-inducing mechanisms are coupled with those of thermoregulation. It is known that dehydrated dogs and goats show less panting, but if they are given water to drink, the intensity of panting then increases. It is also known that the regulation of core body temperature depends on the hydration status of the animal.

Salt appetite, in addition to the hormonal regulatory mechanisms of aldosterone, is also involved in adjusting sodium balance. Aldosterone not only increases sodium reabsorption (p. 314) in the kidney, but also induces a salt appetite. Thus, animals in NaCl deficit seek to consume more NaCl under the influence of aldosterone, which can be exploited by offering salt licks. Angiotensin II, in addition to its indirect effect of inducing aldosterone secretion, and its subsequent stimulation of a salt appetite, can also directly induce a salt appetite by acting on special receptor regions in the brain.

13.9   Disturbances in water and NaCl balance

The regulatory mechanisms discussed in ch. 13.8 (p. 334) are quite efficient in counteracting an oversupply or undersupply of water or NaCl. However, disturbances in water and NaCl balance can occur if

- the regulatory mechanisms are stressed beyond a certain level and/or
- the regulatory systems fail partially or completely.

Disturbances in water and NaCl balance can greatly impair bodily functions and possibly even lead to death. For example, the excretion of metabolic waste products may be reduced, thermoregulation may be impaired, and blood perfusion of tissues may also be disturbed.

A negative water balance leads to **dehydration** (water deficit, volume loss). A positive water balance leads to **hyperhydration** (water surplus, volume increase). Depending on how the NaCl supply changes at the same time, the osmolality of body fluids also changes to become either hypertonic or hypotonic.

MORE DETAILS   A **lack of water intake** alone leads initially to a decrease in extracellular volume. The extracellular osmolality increases because there is a relatively greater deficiency of water than of electrolytes (**hypertonic dehydration**). Because of hyperosmolality of the extracellular fluid, intracellular water is osmotically drawn from cells so that both extracellular and intracellular volumes are reduced. However, hypertonic dehydration can occur not only as a result of reduced water intake, but also as a result of increased water excretion. When hypotonic sweat is secreted (humans), when panting develops (dogs), in diabetes insipidus (ADH deficiency) or in osmotic diuresis (e.g., glucosuria due to diabetes mellitus), more water is lost from the body via the skin, the respiratory tract or the kidney. If the water deficit is not corrected by fluid intake, hypertonic dehydration is the result.

When there is **excessive water intake** water intoxication occurs. In calves, as a result of excessive and too rapid drinking when switching to self-drinking, the increase in extracellular volume is initially accompanied by a decrease in osmolality (**hypotonic hyperhydration**). From the osmotic gradient that develops water flows into the cells. Hypotonic hyperhydration is therefore characterised by an increase in both fluid volumes. Hypotonic hyperhydration can also occur when there are excretory disorders of the kidney (e.g., excessive ADH secretion). When there is a **NaCl deficiency**, extracellular osmolality is first reduced. This is followed by an osmotic shift of water from the extracellular space into the cells, which is eventually reversed by the volume-regulatory mechanisms of cells (p. 333) described above. However, the extracellular volume remains reduced (**hypotonic dehydration**). Such a disturbance can be caused by insufficient **NaCl intake** or by severe **NaCl losses** (aldosterone deficiency, vomiting, loss of hypertonic sweat in horses). Severe, life-threatening losses of both NaCl and water are the leading symptomatology in secretory diarrhoea (p. 445) caused by infectious agents (*Clostridia*, *Escherichia coli*, *Salmonella* etc.). These pathogens form toxins that stimulate chloride secretion in the intestine and inhibit sodium reabsorption, causing more water to flow osmotically into the intestinal lumen. Depending on the ratio of water to electrolyte losses, dehydration from diarrhoea can be either hypotonic or hypertonic. Dehydration becomes life-threatening from a resulting cardiovascular disorder. With **excessive NaCl intake** (so-called salt poisoning, e.g., in calves and piglets consuming a large amount of NaCl in feed, while at the same time not having enough water intake), the increased extracellular osmolality initially shifts water out of cells into the extracellular fluid. The cellular mechanisms described above can only slightly counteract this shift, so that the increase in extracellular volume persists (**hypertonic hyperhydration**). In addition to a diet-induced increase in **NaCl intake**, pathological excess production of aldosterone can also cause an increase in NaCl retention and thus to the described shifts in the water compartments (hyperaldosteronism).

Suggested reading

Randall D., Burggren W, French K. Eckert Animal Physiology. 5th ed. Freeman; 2001

14 Excretion in birds and reptiles and osmoregulation in fishes

Helga Pfannkuche, Michael Pees

14.1 Excretion in birds

ESSENTIALS ✖

The most important excretory organ of birds is the kidney. Two functionally different types of nephrons are found in birds. One of these resembles and has similar functions to those of mammals. The other corresponds to the nephrons of reptiles and excretes uric acid or its salts. In addition to the kidneys, the cloaca and the posterior intestinal segments also contribute to the regulation of salt and water balance, so the urine passing into the cloaca is further concentrated there. Birds that depend on the intake of salt water for their water supply also have salt glands which can assist in excreting excess NaCl.

14.1.1 Principles of water absorption

As with mammals, the mechanisms for intake and conservation of water differ among bird species. In general, water can be obtained (p. 329) either by **drinking** or from **food** or as **oxidation water** from metabolism. The quantities ingested by drinking vary considerably. Very small species with body weights of 10–20 g consume approx. 50% of their body weight per day as drinking water, while species with body weights of 100 g or more consume only about 5% of their body mass as daily drinking water. However, it is not only the size of birds that determines their water requirement, but also the climatic conditions of their habitat. Birds living in arid regions have a significantly lower water intake than those in habitats where salt water is the main available source of water and which have salt glands for NaCl excretion.

Physiological stimuli for water intake are both an increase in Na^+ concentration in the cerebrospinal fluid (detected in the hypothalamus) and an extracellular volume deficit. Volume deficit is presumably detected by stretch receptors in the interstitium around blood vessels. As in mammals (p. 335), an increase in **angiotensin II concentration in plasma** also induces the drinking of water.

14.1.2 Kidneys

■ Structure

The kidney is the **most important excretory organ** in birds. Its function is supported by excretory and absorptive mechanisms of the intestine, the cloaca and possibly also the salt glands.

The avian kidney is paired, but a urinary bladder and a renal pelvis are absent. The kidneys are retroperitoneal, and are not strictly divided into lobules like mammalian kidneys, but are divided into **three larger lobes**: a cranial, a middle and a caudal lobe. The lobes are separated from each other by the renal vessels. A clinically relevant feature are nerve bundles that run through the renal parenchyma. If the **kidneys** are **damaged**, with resulting changes to these nerve structures, **restricted movement** of the **hind limbs** may follow.

As in mammals and reptiles, the functional units of bird kidneys are nephrons. Two types of nephron are found in bird kidneys, which are either similar to nephrons in the reptile kidney (p. 340) (ch. 14.2.1) or to those in the mammalian (p. 303) kidney. Accordingly, avian nephrons are classified as either a "reptile-type" or a "mammalian-type". There are also transitional forms between these two distinct types.

■ Blood supply to the kidney

The avian kidney is supplied with blood by three arteries: a. renalis cranialis, a. iliaca externa, a. ischiadica. These renal arteries divide into **afferent arterioles** and then into **glomerular capillaries**. After leaving the glomeruli, the blood vessels form peritubular capillaries and finally the venous system. In addition to this renal vascular system, which corresponds to that of mammals, there is also a **renal portal vein system**. This consists of a venous vascular ring into which veins from the posterior sections flow and from which smaller vessels lead to the peritubular capillaries. Flow through this system is controlled by valves located between the common iliac vein and the caudal vena cava. When the valves are open, blood coming from the common iliac vein flows directly into the vena cava. Valve closure is prevented by **noradrenalin** and **adrenalin**, which supports the flow of blood to the heart in stress situations. **Acetylcholine** causes the valves to close so that blood flows from the iliac vein into the portal vein system and thus into the small vessels. Often, however, the blood is only partially diverted.

Blood from the renal portal system mixes with that from the efferent glomerular vessels. The resulting mixture of venous (coming from the portal system) and arterial (coming from the glomeruli) blood supplies the peritubular capillaries. The inflow from the renal portal system can reduce fluctuations in the peritubular blood supply when the renal arterial blood supply is reduced. Also, the renal portal system participates in nitrogen recycling (p. 339) by transporting nitrogen-containing compounds from the posterior digestive tract to the kidney. The blood supply from the renal portal system is probably of greater importance, especially for capillaries of the peripheral tubules, which are associated with reptile-type nephrons.

Inner milieu

Glomerular filtration

Irrespective of the type of nephron, the formation of an **ultrafiltrate** in the glomeruli and the surrounding Bowman's capsule also occurs in the bird's kidney. Since the capillaries in birds have a larger diameter than those of mammals (because of the larger nucleated and thus less deformable erythrocytes), the capillary clusters in the glomeruli are also larger. In addition, the slit pores of the filter are larger in chicken glomeruli and the negative charge of the filter is lower than in the mammalian glomeruli. As a result, the urethral urine of birds contains more **protein** than that of mammals.

In general, due to a smaller filtration surface in the glomeruli, less plasma is filtered in a glomerulus in birds than in that of a mammal. However, the number of glomeruli is higher in birds, so that the total filtration capacity related to body mass does not differ between bird and mammalian kidneys.

The glomerular filtration rate (GFR) is more variable in birds than in mammals. It is mainly dependent on hydration status, with osmolality, rather than plasma volume, being the essential parameter for the regulation of filtration rate and reabsorption in the tubular system. The most important hormone regulating GFR is **arginine vasotocin** (**AVT**) from the neurohypophysis. The stimulus for its release is an increase in extracellular osmolality. A loss of volume also increases AVT release.

AVT leads to a reduction in GFR which seems to be caused by constriction of afferent arterioles at reptile-type nephrons with a subsequent reduction in the filtration rate. However, since urine volume decreases more under the influence of AVT than GFR, it is now assumed that AVT also affects the reabsorption processes by stimulating the incorporation of **aquaporins** into the cell membrane of tubular epithelial cells.

Tubular system

The processes that take place in the tubules after filtration depend on the type of nephron:

Reptile-type nephrons lie cortically in the outer layers of the renal parenchyma. They are more numerous than the mammalian-type nephrons. Their main function is to excrete **uric acid**, the primary end product of protein breakdown in birds. Reptile-type nephrons, unlike mammalian-type nephrons, have a proximal and a distal tubule, but no loop of Henle. They are therefore also called **"loopless nephrons"**.

Uric acid is the main product of nitrogen catabolism in birds. It is excreted with the help of the reptile-type nephrons. **70–80 % of waste nitrogen** is excreted in the form of uric acid. The rest is in the form of ammonia, creatinine, amino acids and urea. Nitrogen excretion in the form of uric acid is very efficient. Four nitrogen atoms are excreted per uric acid molecule (urea: two). However, the synthesis of uric acid is more energy-consuming than that of urea.

Uric acid is mostly formed in the liver and reaches the kidneys in blood. Uric acid has a pK$_a$ value of 5.6 and therefore 98 % of that in blood is **urate** anion.

Urate can easily pass through the fenestrated capillaries of the glomerulus, so it is **freely filtered**. While the mammalian nephrons do not allow efficient secretion of urate (p. 325), the reptile-type nephrons have effective secretion mechanisms. Thus, in addition to filtration, urate enters urine **via tubular secretion**, predominantly in the proximal tubule of the reptile-type nephrons. Approximately five times more urate is secreted than filtered. The blood, which feeds the peritubular capillaries from the renal portal system, plays a particularly important role in filtration.

In the lumen of the tubule system, the urate concentration is significantly higher than in blood plasma due to its active secretion and water reabsorption from urine. As a result, there is in principle a danger that with generally low solubility of urates and also uric acid, the solubility threshold is exceeded, and **urate crystals** could precipitate. This is largely counteracted by binding urate **anions** to **albumin**. As there is much more protein in bird urine (approx. 5 mg/ml) than in mammalian urine, there is sufficient albumin available to bind urate anions. The urates bound to albumin are not osmotically active, so unlike urea they do not contribute to urine osmolality. Under physiological conditions, **urate crystals** do not form and precipitate in the tubule lumen, but they are a part of a colloidal suspension which also contains mucoid components. The formation of this suspension also has the advantage that the amount of water needed for excretion is less than if the urates were in a true solution. This allows the bird to excrete nitrogen effectively even with a low intake of drinking water. The excreted uric acid can be observed as a white admixture on the bird's faeces.

Mammalian-type nephrons are localised in the kidney medulla and have a **loop of Henle**. These nephrons are capable of both urine production and concentration. They thus show more of the typical characteristics of the mammalian kidney. Due to their ability to **concentrate urine** and thus to conserve water, the medullary nephrons are particularly important for avian species in arid regions and are also particularly numerous in these birds.

Water and electrolyte reabsorption in the proximal tubule (p. 312) is comparable to that of mammals. In the avian proximal tubule, there is also an isoosmotic reabsorption of about 60% of the glomerular filtered fluid. Glucose is also greatly reabsorbed (p. 323) here as in mammals. The loop of Henle serves to concentrate urine. It is only present in mammalian-type nephrons and it is of shorter length in the transitional nephron types. In the thick ascending part of the loop of Henle, secondary active NaCl reabsorption from the tubule lumen (p. 312) into the interstitium occurs, as in mammals. The resulting **increase in osmolality** in the interstitium serves as a **driving force** for **water reabsorption** from the descending part of the loop of Henle and the collecting duct. Similar to the mammalian nephron, a countercurrent principle operates between the ascending part of the loop of Henle and the collecting duct (p. 318). In birds also, osmotically driven water reabsorption depends on the incorporation of **aquaporins** in the membrane of epithelial cells of the collecting duct, which allow the passage of water from the collecting duct lumen to the blood side of the cells. Despite these mechanisms being similar to those of mammals, urinary concentration in birds is not as pronounced as in mammals (**Table 12.4**). Most avian urine is isoosmolar or only slightly hyperosmolar to plasma. Even in strong antidiuresis, birds can only concentrate their urine **to 2 to 3 times the plasma osmolality** (in diuresis, urine can take on values of about 40 mosmol·kg^{-1}). However, comparison of these values between birds and mammals is only valid to a limited extent, since in the bird's kidney hardly any urea is excreted as an osmotically active degradation product (see above).

The incorporation of aquaporins and thus the reabsorption of water in the collecting duct is hormonally stimulated by **AVT**. In addition to AVT, other hormones and mechanisms found in the mammalian kidney also have a role in the kidneys of birds, which also have a **juxtaglomerular apparatus** (**Fig. 12.5**, **Fig. 12.6**). The **renin-angiotensin-aldosterone system** (**Fig. 12.7**) and the atrial natriuretic peptide (p. 314) have comparable roles to those in mammals. However, it should be noted that our knowledge of hormonal regulation of electrolytes in the avian kidney is much more limited than that of mammals.

14.1.3   Intestine and cloaca

The advantages of the comparatively low urine osmolality in the avian kidney become apparent during further concentration in the posterior intestinal segments. After urine formation in the kidneys, it is discharged into the **urodaeum** (the urinary tract) of the **cloaca** (**Fig. 14.1**). From there, urine passes by retro-peristalsis into the **coprodaeum** (faecal space) of the cloaca and then further into the rectum and the appendix. The urine here is especially distributed over the mucosal surface. Urine with very high osmolality would osmotically lead to water loss into the intestinal lumen. Interestingly, retro-peristalsis seems to be inhibited if urine osmolality is too high (> 200 mosmol·kg^{-1} more than the plasma osmolality). Detection of

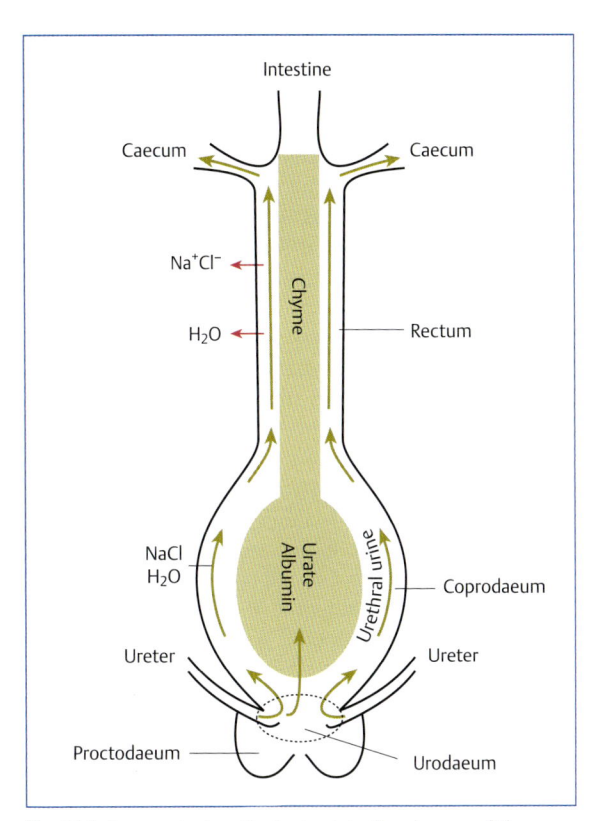

Fig. 14.1 Transport of urethral urine into the cloaca and the posterior intestinal segments. The liquid part of urine flows directly along the wall. NaCl and water are reabsorbed here. The pasty urate-containing part of urine provides nitrogen compounds for microbial protein synthesis. There is no direct mixing with faeces.

urinary osmolality occurs via receptors in the wall of the cloaca.

Sodium and water are reabsorbed from urine by the epithelium of the posterior intestinal segments and in the coprodaeum by means of **epithelial sodium channels** (**ENaC**), promoted by **aldosterone** (for the mechanism see **Fig. 12.11**).

Retro-peristalsis transports not only urine from the mammalian-type nephrons into the intestine, but also urate from the reptilesn-type nephrons (**Fig. 14.1**). Urate is metabolised by bacteria, especially in the caeca, where the nitrogen is then available (p. 459) for bacterial **protein synthesis**.

Urethral urine also contains considerable amounts of albumin which is also metabolised by bacteria to **SCFA**. The SCFA are available to the bird as an energy source. The microbial metabolism of urate and albumin also produces ammonia. After absorption, ammonia passes through the renal portal vein system to the kidney and can be secreted into the proximal tubules. In the tubule lumen, protons can bind to ammonia, so that this recycling effectively contributes to the excretion of acids. This **nitrogen recycling** plays a role especially in avian species that consume little protein in their diet (ch. 16.10.1.5 (p. 459)).

Inner milieu

14.1.4   Salt glands

For avian species in marine habitats that mainly drink **salt water**, or for species in arid areas with little access to drinking water, the concentrating capacity of the kidneys is not sufficient to eliminate excess NaCl without large water losses. In these species, NaCl is excreted through **salt glands** located in a hollow at the base of the beak or near the orbit. The salt gland consists of branched, blind-ending tubules that open into a main duct on both sides. The tubules are lined with a strongly secretory glandular epithelium. The blood vessels are arranged parallel to the tubules, and the blood flow is **countercurrent** to the tubule secretion, which supports the secretion of NaCl (**Fig. 14.2**). Chloride enters the glandular epithelial cells from blood via a **Na$^+$-K$^+$-2Cl$^-$ cotransporter**. Chloride leaves the cell via apical **chloride channels** and thus enters the glandular lumen. K$^+$ ions leave the cell via basolateral **K$^+$ channels** and Na$^+$ ions are pumped out of the cell by a **Na$^+$/K$^+$-ATPase**. The accumulation of sodium in the tubular fluid results from **paracellular permeation**. Here, sodium follows the electrical gradient established by chloride diffusion (**Fig. 14.2**). The secretory activity of the salt gland and its blood flow is positively correlated with the sodium concentration in plasma as well as with extracellular volume. **Acetylcholine** and **vasoactive intestinal peptide** increase secretion, while **noradrenaline** and **adrenaline** inhibit it. In addition, **ANP** increases secretory activity, **angiotensin II** inhibits it (probably indirectly via a reduction in blood flow).

IN A NUTSHELL   !

The bird's kidney produces urine which Is only a little concentrated, and it excretes nitrogen end products as uric acid salts. The cloaca and posterior intestine serve to modify the urine. Excess salt can also be excreted via salt glands in some birds.

14.2   Excretion in reptiles

ESSENTIALS   ✗

The osmoregulatory organs of reptiles include the kidneys, the urinary sac and the salt glands (in marine habitats). An unconcentrated urine containing uric acid is produced by the kidneys. Urine concentration is not possible because there is no loop of Henle in the nephrons. However, urine passes from the cloaca into the urinary sac, where water is reabsorbed. The urinary sac therefore has an important function as a water reservoir. Like birds, various reptile species are also able to output large amounts of NaCl through salt glands on the head.

14.2.1   Kidneys

The reptile kidneys, unlike those of mammals and birds, are relatively simple in structure. There is no division into cortex and medulla. There is also no renal pelvis. Reptile kidneys have **fewer nephrons than mammalian kidneys**. Often, only a few thousand nephrons are present in both

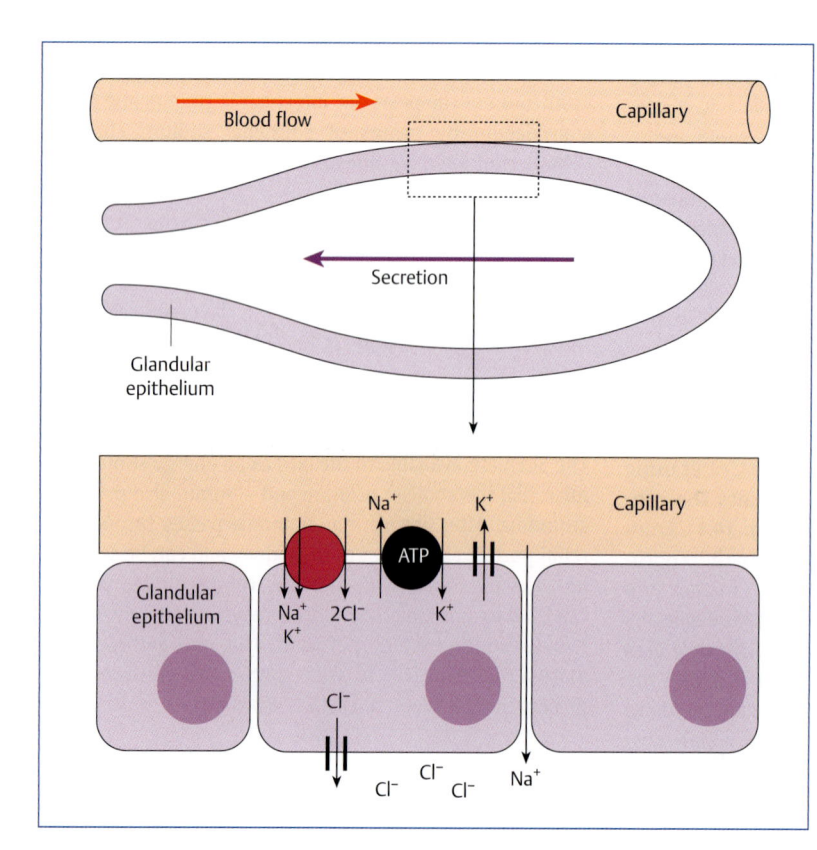

Fig. 14.2 NaCl excretion in salt glands of birds and reptiles and in the rectal gland of elasmobranchs. The opposite direction of blood flow and gland secretion ensures a concentration gradient for NaCl from blood towards gland secretion along the entire contact section.

kidneys together (for comparison, bovine: approx. 4 million) and these lack a loop of Henle. As a result, the kidneys are unable to produce hyperosmolar urine. The glomeruli are also less developed and equipped with fewer capillaries than those of birds.

The **nephrons** of reptiles mirror (p.337) **the "reptile-type nephrons"** of birds in structure and function. Accordingly, **uric acid** (**or urate**) is secreted in the proximal tubule, which then forms complexes with proteins and can be excreted as a white pasty mass. In addition, some aquatic species also produce **ammonia** as the main nitrogenous excretory product (e.g., turtles, crocodiles).

In reptiles, the distal tubule is followed by a so-called **sexual segment**. In all female reptiles and in male turtles, mucus-secreting cells are found here. In male snakes and lizards, the lining cells are flat and filled with mucus outside the mating season. During the mating season, the cells enlarge and produce alkaline phosphatase, phospholipids, glycoproteins, mucoproteins and amino acids. The functions of these secretions have not yet been conclusively defined. It is possible that they form a plug after mating to prevent male rivals from successfully mating, or that the secretions separate seminal fluid and urine during mating. They could also serve as a source of energy for the sperm. The sexual segments are followed by **collecting tubules**, which then converge into the ureter.

The blood supply of reptile kidneys includes a **renal portal venous system**, just as in birds. However, only a few species of reptiles have valves (as in birds (p.337)) and are thus able to direct blood flow either through the renal portal veins or directly to the heart. The renal portal veins supply the kidney with an adequate amount of blood even when there is reduced afferent blood flow to the glomeruli. The afferent blood flow to the kidney and thus glomerular filtration rate is regulated by **AVT**, as in the bird.

14.2.2 Salt glands

Various reptile species in marine habitats excrete excess salt through their **salt glands** in a similar manner to birds. In some lizard species the salt glands are quite comparable to those of birds (**Fig. 14.2**). In addition, some turtle species also have **orbital glands**, snakes have **sublingual** or **premaxillary glands**, and crocodiles have a gland localised in the region of the **tongue** for excreting excess salt.

14.2.3 Urinary sac

Some species of reptiles have a so-called **urinary sac** which is filled with urine from the cloaca. This applies to all turtles and many lizard species, such as the green iguana. Snakes, on the other hand, do not have a urinary sac. In contrast to the urinary bladder, the urinary sac is not an appendix of the urinary tract, but an outpouching – a very thin-walled and extremely variable structure – at the bottom of the **urodaeum**. The urinary sac has a special function in **water balance**, so that it is much more than a storage organ. Water can not only be reabsorbed from the urine released into the cloaca, but can also be drawn into the urinary sac via the cloaca when the animal is in water. From there, water can be transferred into the systemic circulation. Accordingly, surgical removal of the urinary sac could cause problems. Two important **disease processes** can develop in the urinary sac: the formation of **urinary stones** and paralysis with consequent marked expansion of the urinary sac, as a result of severe systemic disorders (kidney failure).

IN A NUTSHELL !

The reptile kidneys are simpler than those of birds and mammals. Urine produced is hardly concentrated, but is modified in the urinary sac. The end products from protein metabolism are urates, which are filtered and secreted in the kidney. Some reptile species also have salt glands.

14.3 Osmoregulation in fish

ESSENTIALS ✖

Fish can live in habitats with different levels of salinity. While some cartilaginous fish are osmoconformers, bony fish are osmoregulators that keep their body osmolality within narrow limits. Depending on whether the ambient osmolality is higher or lower than the body osmolality of the fish, water input or water loss must occur to maintain constant osmolality. The most important osmoregulatory organs are the gills, but the kidneys and the rectal gland are also involved in regulating water and ion balance.

14.3.1 Osmoregulation in aquatic habitats

Depending on the salinity of their habitat, fish face the challenge of living in either a hypo- or a hyperosmolar medium. **Seawater** has an osmolality greater than 1000 mosmol·kg^{-1}, while the osmolality of **freshwater** is only a few mosmol·kg^{-1}.

A basic distinction has to be made between osmoconformers and osmoregulators. In **osmoconformers**, body osmolality corresponds to that of the surrounding medium, while **osmoregulators** actively control osmolality. Bony fish are osmoregulators, while some cartilaginous fish such as sharks and rays are osmoconformers.

However, all fish are **ion regulators**, i.e., even with osmolality adapted to the surrounding water, the ionic composition of body water is not the same as that of seawater and is controlled by the fish.

14.3.2   Osmoregulation in sharks and rays (elasmobranchs)

■ Urea

Most **elasmobranchs** live in marine waters, so they are adapted to an environment with a high salt content. Although they are osmoconformers, they are nevertheless ion regulators. Their body osmolality thus corresponds to the surrounding medium or is slightly higher. The NaCl content of their body water is, however, lower than that of seawater. Instead of NaCl, **urea** and **various methylamines** are the osmotically active components of their body fluids. These solutes are responsible for more than 30% of plasma osmolality, and for more than 50% of the intracellular osmolality.

> **MORE DETAILS**   Maintaining high extra- and intracellular osmolality in elasmobranchs by high concentrations of urea and methylamines has advantages over increasing ion concentrations. Inorganic ions such as Na^+, K^+, Cl^-, and SO_4^{2-} can negatively influence the function of macromolecules. These ions can attach to proteins. If the ion concentration is too high, it can disturb the hydrate shell of proteins and finally lead to their denaturation. Urea and methylamines also have an influence on macromolecules in the intracellular and extracellular space. Urea interferes with hydrophobic interactions and methylamines favour them. However, due to the presence of both urea and methylamines, the net effect of solutes is balanced.

The formation of **urea** occurs mainly in the liver in the ornithine-urea cycle. Synthesis is variable, i.e., it is increased when euryhaline fish move into water with higher salinity. Species such as bull sharks are able to tolerate both seawater and freshwater and switch between water of different salinities around river mouths. An adjustment of intra- and extracellular osmolality thus occurs from changes in urea synthesis rather than from changes in ion concentrations (**Table 14.1**).

Some of the synthesised urea is lost by diffusion through the **gills**. However, this loss is many times less in elasmobranchs than in bony fish. It is not entirely clear why elasmobranchs lose so little urea via the gills. It could be because the basolateral membrane of the gill epithelium contains a lot of **cholesterol**. This hinders the diffusion of urea. The apical membrane is also only slightly permeable to urea. The mucus layer on the gills is probably also responsible for the reduced release. In addition to the inhibition of diffusion, there are active transport mechanisms for urea. In the basolateral membrane there is a **Na⁺/urea exchanger** that transports urea towards blood (**Fig. 14.4**).

In the **kidney**, urea is filtered, but 70–99% of filtered urea is reabsorbed. Compared to the gills, the kidney thus hardly contributes to urea output of fish. Urea recovery in the kidney probably occurs via a **cotransporter** for sodium and urea.

■ NaCl

In contrast to urea, which is conserved in elasmobranchs, Na^+ and Cl^- must be excreted more readily. Although the internal fluid of sharks and rays is usually slightly **hyperosmolar** compared to seawater, the concentration of NaCl is significantly lower than in seawater, so that these ions increasingly enter the body via the gills down a concentration gradient.

The excess NaCl is mainly excreted via the **rectal gland**. This is a finger-shaped gland that arises dorsally in the posterior region of the colon. The glandular tubules are surrounded by numerous capillaries. The three ions, Na^+, K^+ and Cl^- are pumped from blood into the epithelial cells of the glandular tubules by means of a **Na⁺-K⁺-2Cl⁻ cotransporter**. The chloride ions then leave the epithelial cells via apical chloride channels. Although, as in the salt gland of birds and reptiles (p. 340), sodium is first transported basolaterally out of the epithelial cells by the **Na⁺/K⁺-ATPase**, it then follows the negatively charged chloride along a paracellular pathway into the glandular lumen, from where both ions are excreted (**Fig. 14.2**).

> **MORE DETAILS**   In freshwater and brackish water, the adjustment to increased osmotic water absorption is by increased urinary excretion. Reduced urea production and retention, along with decreased retention of Na^+ and Cl^- allows osmolality adjustment to the reduced salinity of the environment. In species that can live in water with varying salinity (e.g., bull sharks), those living in freshwater have lower osmolality than individuals of the same species in seawater. This is mainly due to different intra- and extracellular concentrations of urea and methylamines.

Table 14.1   Concentration (in $mmol \cdot l^{-1}$) of Na^+, Cl^- and urea in blood plasma of various elasmobranchs in salt or fresh water. The actual osmolality of plasma reaches higher values ($> 1000 \, mosmol \cdot kg^{-1}$) than the indicated sum, especially in salt water, because the methylamines are not considered here.

Species	Habitat	Na⁺	Cl⁻	Urea	Total
Atlantic stingray	Salt water	310	300	394	1004
	Freshwater	12	208	196	616
Bull shark	Salt water	289	296	370	955
	Freshwater	208	203	192	603
Spiny Dogfish	Salt water	286	246	351	883
Freshwater stingray	Freshwater	178	146	1.2	325.2

Source: Hammerschlag N. Osmoregulation in elasmobranchs: a review for fish biologists, behaviourists and ecologists. Marine and Freshwater Behaviour and Physiology 2006; 39(3): 209–228

For marine elasmobranchs, salt excretion via the gills does not play a role. Species living in freshwater, on the other hand, take up salt through the gills. The **Na$^+$/K$^+$-ATPase-rich** cells responsible for this are more than twice as numerous in the gill epithelium than in marine species. These cells are also involved in the excretion of acids through the expression of a **Na$^+$/H$^+$ exchanger**. Another cell type with the function of proton conservation in the gill epithelium has an **H$^+$-ATPase in** its basolateral membrane, which pumps protons back into blood. This ATPase has, for example, a five times higher activity in freshwater stingrays than in marine species. Furthermore, these cells have a **Cl$^-$/HCO$_3^-$ exchanger** which transfers bicarbonate into the surrounding water in exchange for Cl$^-$ uptake into the cells.

The excretion of NaCl and water by the **kidneys** can adapt to environmental salinity. This plays a role especially in adjusting to low environmental salinity, when large amounts of highly dilute urine are produced by the kidneys. The **amount of urine** can be increased 20 to 50 times. Although Na$^+$ and Cl$^-$ can be reabsorbed in the tubular system of the kidneys, the kidneys are not able to raise urine osmolality above that of plasma. Thus, renal excretion of excess saline (as the rectal glands can do) is only possible to a very limited extent.

14.3.3 Osmoregulation in bony fish
■ Mechanisms in freshwater fish

Since freshwater has a very low osmolality, the difference between the internal osmolality and that of the environmental water is enormous in freshwater fish. Freshwater fish are therefore at permanent risk of **hyperhydration** and **loss of osmolality**.

Some water can be absorbed through the body surface, but the main entry route is via the **gills**, and this can be as much as 50% of total body water per hour. In contrast, comparatively little water is absorbed by freshwater fish from the gastrointestinal tract.

Any osmotically driven water intake must be compensated for by a corresponding amount of water excretion, which is mainly in **urine**. The kidneys can excrete large amounts (50–150 ml·d^{-1}·kg^{-1} body weight) of highly dilute urine. This is achieved by a **high GFR** and an almost complete reabsorption of NaCl (95% of the filtered amount). The **amount of urine** is regulated by **AVT**. The most important effect of AVT is systemic vasoconstriction, which increases GFR and thus urine production. In bony fish, only the posterior (caudal) part of the kidney is involved in urine production, as the kidneys of bony fish are divided into two functionally distinct regions: The cranial part of the kidneys is a **haematopoietic organ** since fish do not have bone marrow for blood cell production. The caudal part has the typical kidney functions of filtration and secretion.

In addition to continuous water uptake, freshwater fish are also exposed to the risk of continuous **osmolyte loss**. Electrolyte loss through the thin-walled, dense capillary bed of the gills is minimised by tight junctions that are denser than those of saltwater fish. Nevertheless, in order to keep body osmolality constant, freshwater fish must also continuously absorb electrolytes (especially NaCl) via the gills (**Fig. 14.3**) where Na$^+$ and Cl$^-$ uptake from water are independent of each other. For this purpose, there are two different types of mitochondria-rich cells in the gill epithelium, the **chloride cells** and the mitochondria-rich **pavement cells**. There are also mitochondria-poor pavement cells, the role of which in osmoregulation is not fully understood. The chloride cells take up Cl$^-$ in exchange with bicarbonate (**Fig. 14.4**). In the pavement cells, Na$^+$ is absorbed in exchange for H$^+$ ions pumped out of the cell apically by an ATPase. This increases the negative charge of the cell interior, which is constantly maintained by the Na$^+$/K$^+$-ATPase (**Fig. 14.4**). Na$^+$ then enters the cell apically via a Na$^+$ channel. These ion-exchanging cells are located on the primary gill lamellae between the secondary lamellae (**Fig. 11.33**).

■ Mechanisms in saltwater fish

Unlike elasmobranchs living in salt water, marine bony fish are not osmoconformers, but osmoregulators. Their interior fluids thus have significantly lower osmolality than seawater (osmolality of seawater is 3 to 4 times higher than osmolality in the fish). Thus, the osmoregulatory challenge for these fish is to prevent or compensate for **water loss** due to the osmotic gradient from within the body. As with freshwater bony fish, the scales and overlying mucus of skin of saltwater fish make it relatively impermeable to water. Water losses occur mainly through the gills. Compensation for these water losses is by absorption in the alimentary tract of larger quantities of water from drinking salt water. A typical marine fish drinks about **10–20% of its body weight per day**. If the salt content of the water is high, this amount can be increased to 35–40%.

The continuous intake of salt water requires effective mechanisms for eliminating the absorbed ions. However, absorption of these ions is also necessary for the absorption of water. The most important ions for osmoregulation are the **monovalent ions Na$^+$, K$^+$** and **Cl$^-$** and the **divalent ions Mg^{2+}** and **SO$_4^{2-}$**. The monovalent ions are absorbed in large quantities in the **gastrointestinal tract** and provide a driving force for water absorption. Only 20% of the divalent ions are absorbed so that 80% are eliminated in faeces. The excess monovalent ions (especially Na$^+$ and Cl$^-$) are excreted by the **gill epithelium** (Fig. 14.3, Fig. 14.4).

The **kidneys** are not the main organ of electrolyte regulation in saltwater fish. Nevertheless, modification of the primary urine takes place along the tubular system. In saltwater fish, the renal tubule system is highly permeable to water along its entire length. Urine is thus modified by the secretion of divalent ions and the reabsorption of water and NaCl in the tubular system. The osmolality of the glomerular filtrate and urine is the same, at about 400 mosmol·kg^{-1}, but the composition is very different because of these secretion and reabsorption processes. Urine has little organic content and few monovalent ions compared to filtrate. There is also further reabsorption of monovalent ions and water in the bladder. The **amount of urine** finally

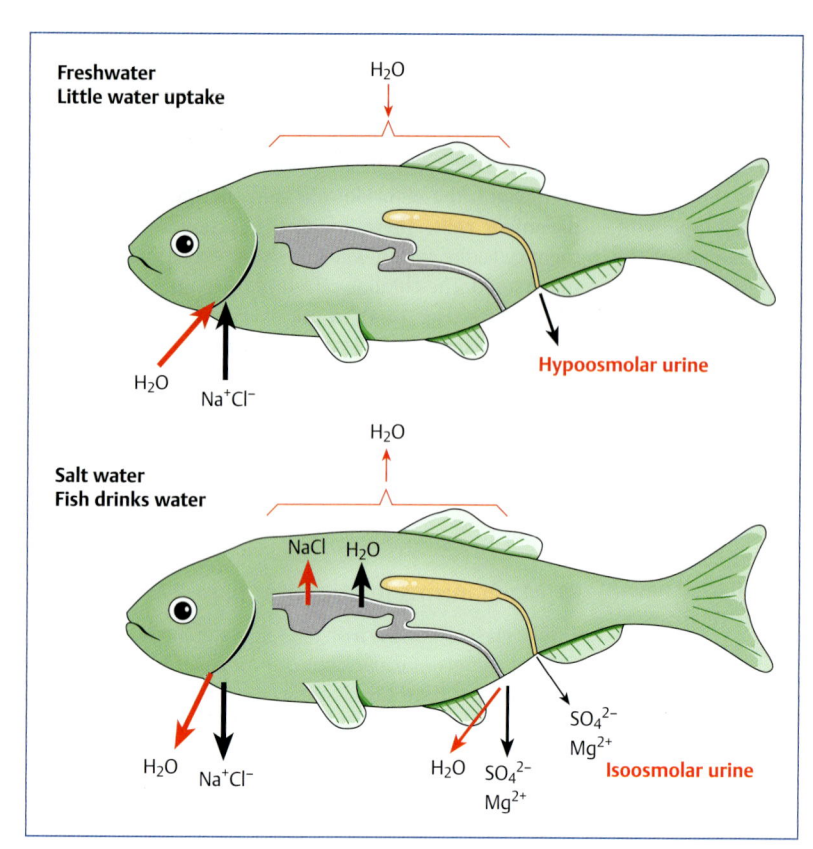

Fig. 14.3 Electrolyte and water movements in bony fish in fresh and salt water. Red arrows show uptake and release that run counter to body osmolality. Black arrows indicate uptake and release of electrolytes and water that stabilise body osmolality.

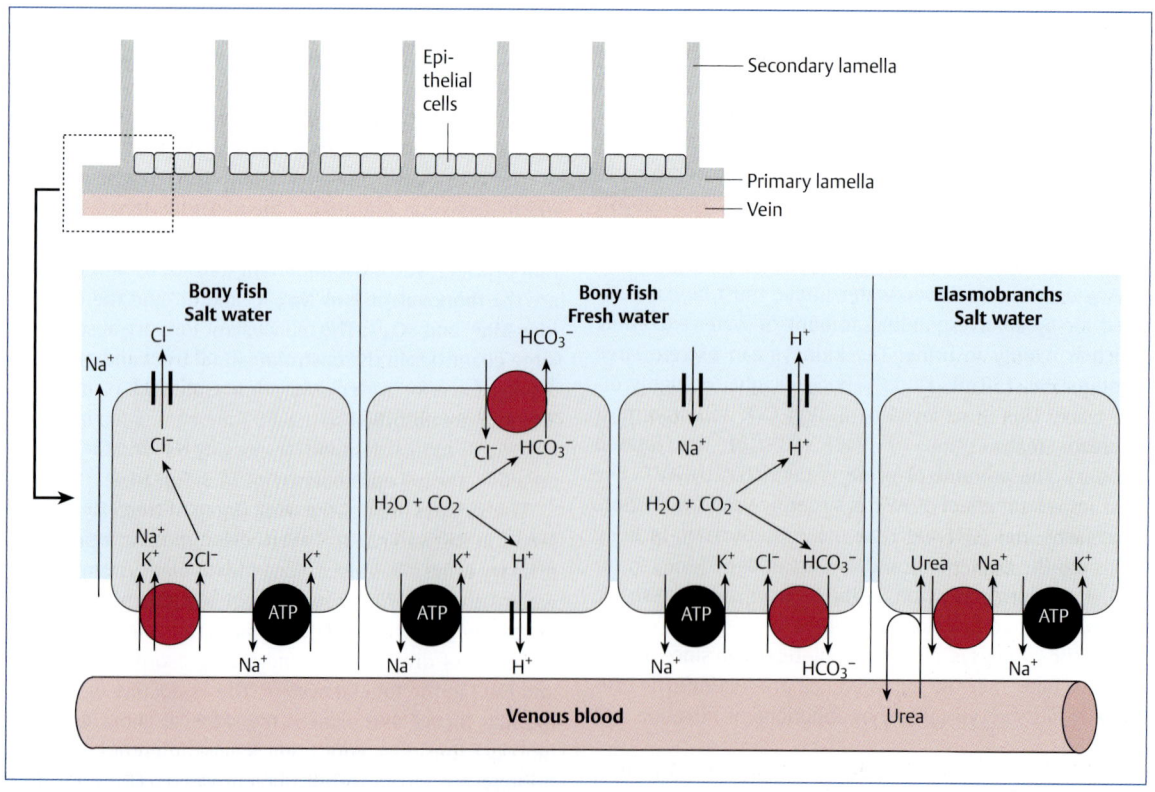

Fig. 14.4 Transport systems in the gill epithelium. The epithelial cells responsible for osmoregulation are located on the primary lamellae between the secondary lamellae. Chloride cells secrete chloride ions when in salt water or absorb chloride ions when in freshwater. Specific pavement cells are responsible for the excretion of protons. Other types of pavement cells are also found in gill epithelium (not shown here). In elasmobranchs, a barrier function of the gill epithelium prevents loss of urea into the surrounding water.

excreted is very small (approx. $8\,\text{ml} \cdot \text{d}^{-1} \cdot \text{kg}^{-1}$ body weight; mammals: see **Table 12.4**).

> **IN A NUTSHELL**   !
>
> Fish are either osmoregulators (bony fish) or osmoconformers (sharks and rays). All fish are ion regulators. Osmoregulation takes place mainly through ion secretion or absorption across the gill epithelium. The kidneys excrete a highly dilute urine in freshwater fish. Excess salt is released through the rectal gland in cartilaginous fish.

Suggested reading

Hammerschlag N. Osmoregulation in elasmobranchs: a review for fish biologists, behaviourists and ecologists. Marine and Freshwater Behaviour and Physiology 2006; 39 (3): 209–228

Moyes CD, Schulte PM. Principles of Animal physiology. Pearson; 2008

O'Malley B. Clinical Anatomy and Physiology in Small Pets, Birds, Reptiles and Amphibians. Munich, Jena: Elsevier Urban & Fischer, 2008

Scanes CG, Dridi S. Sturkie's Avian Physiology. Philadelphia: Elsevier, 2021

15 Acid-base balance

Gotthold Gäbel

15.1 Regulation, buffering and disturbances of pH

> **ESSENTIALS**   ✗
>
> In mammals, the pH of extracellular fluid is maintained within a very narrow range around 7.4 by buffer systems that are adjusted by the kidneys, liver and lungs. An important regulator is the bicarbonate-carbonic acid system. CO_2 is released from the lungs in respiration. HCO_3^- is both conserved and produced by the kidneys. The kidneys are also able to excrete protons. The liver supports the regulatory function of the kidneys. The Henderson-Hasselbalch equation describes the relationship between bicarbonate concentration, partial pressure of CO_2 (p_{CO_2}) and pH. Disorders in acid-base balance can be caused by dysfunction of the regulatory organs, the kidneys, lung and liver. However, excessive losses or overproduction of protons or bicarbonate exceeding the capacity for regulation can also give rise to acid-base imbalances. Deviations in pH downwards or upwards from the normal value are called acidosis or alkalosis. In respiratory disorders, the primary cause of changes to pH is an increase or decrease in p_{CO_2}. In a metabolic (non-respiratory) disorder, the bicarbonate concentration is the main factor that is altered. To diagnose disturbances in acid-base balance, the pH, p_{CO_2}, HCO_3^-concentration and the base excess (BE) in blood can be determined.

15.2 The pH of body fluids

The pH of extracellular fluid in most mammals is in the range of 7.21–7.54 with a mean of about 7.4. Under physiological conditions, fluctuations in pH are extremely small. Even small deviations are associated with systemic disturbances. A drop in pH below 7.0 or an increase above 7.8 leads to severe dysfunction and even death.

The high sensitivity to changes in pH is because of the influence of protons on functional structures, especially proteins, in the membranes or cytosol of cells. Proteins (especially those containing histidine) are characterised by a high sensitivity to changes in pH, since their degree of dissociation depends on the proton concentration. Because proteins are involved in all biochemical functions in an animal, any shift in pH has far-reaching effects. The catalytic action of enzymes is pH-dependent so when the pH decreases the activities of key enzymes of glycolysis and of Na^+/K^+-ATPase are inhibited. The functions of many ion channels are also pH-dependent, which explains the sometimes dramatic effects of acidosis on nerve transmission and on skeletal muscle and heart muscle contraction. In addition to the effects on ion channels in muscle, the interaction between actin and myosin is also modified by pH, so that acidosis usually also leads to vasodilation. DNA replication and cell proliferation are also pH-dependent. Thus, the effect of growth factors is often mediated by an alkaline change in the local pH, i.e., alkalinisation has a growth-promoting effect.

Regulation of H^+ concentration follows the same basic principle as the regulation of other ion concentrations. Therefore, to maintain a constant concentration, H^+ output and H^+ conservation must be in balance. If H^+ output exceeds H^+ generation, there is a net loss of H^+ ions and the increase in pH gives rise to **alkalosis**. Likewise, if H^+ output is less than H^+ generation and pH falls, then **acidosis develops**.

Table 15.1 summarises the mechanisms of **H^+ production** and **H^+ removal**. As can be deduced from the table, the loads from the acidic side usually predominate. Accordingly, the buffer and regulation systems are more efficient in the acidic range than in the alkaline range.

Inner milieu

Table 15.1 H⁺ balance.

Mechanisms of H⁺ production and removal

H⁺ production

1.	**Via CO_2**
	▪ from oxidative metabolism (mainly citrate cycle/respiratory chain) $CO_2 + H_2O \rightarrow H_2CO_3 \rightarrow H^+ + HCO_3^-$
2.	**Via H_2SO_4/H_3PO_4**
	▪ from the oxidative degradation of S- and P-containing amino acids (carnivores!)
3.	**From lactic acid**
	▪ from anaerobic glycolysis
4.	**From fatty acids**
	▪ from lipolysis
5.	**From ketonic acids (acetoacetic acid, β-hydroxybutyric acid)**
	▪ from hepatic and ruminal ketogenesis
6.	**From H⁺ production as a result of buffer loss**
	▪ HCO_3^- excretion via the kidneys
	▪ HCO_3^- loss in faeces (diarrhoea!)
	▪ HCO_3^- "loss" via saliva (ruminants)

H⁺ removal/utilisation

1.	**Via CO_2**
	▪ via breathing $H^+ + HCO_3^- \rightarrow H_2CO_3 \rightarrow CO_2 + H_2O$ $\downarrow$ Lungs
2.	**As H⁺**
	▪ H⁺ excretion via the kidneys
	▪ conversion of organic salts (citrate, aconitate, etc.) into their acids (herbivores!) → consumption of H⁺
	▪ vomiting

When there is a net generation of H⁺, the acids must first be differentiated as either **volatile acids** (as CO_2) or **non-volatile acids** (as H_3PO_4/H_2SO_4).

Quantitatively, most H⁺ ions are produced in **volatile form** as a result of CO_2 production ($CO_2 + H_2O \rightarrow H_2CO_3 \rightarrow H^+ + HCO_3^-$), such as during the decarboxylation of ketonic acids or in the citrate cycle. A 10 kg dog in maintenance metabolism (p. 489) produces about 5000 mmol CO_2 and about 100 mmol non-volatile acids per day. Despite the greater quantity of CO_2 this is not a problem for acid-base regulation under physiological conditions, as CO_2 can normally be removed **quickly** and **effectively** through the **lungs**. More difficult for acid-base regulation are H⁺ ions generated from **non-volatile acids**, such as the oxidation of SH groups of sulphur-containing amino acids (methionine, cysteine) and the hydrolysis of organic phosphoric acids, when protons are released in addition to sulphate and phosphate. Naturally, this type of proton production is increased with the consumption of protein-rich food. This type of proton excess can only be eliminated by the kidneys (p. 326), so carnivores usually excrete acidic urine. If plant food is being consumed, dietary salts of organic acids (citrate, aconitate, fumarate, malate, etc.) are absorbed.

However, these salts must be converted into the corresponding acid, i.e., protonated, before they can be introduced into the catabolic metabolic pathways (oxidative degradation to CO_2). In this way, protons are "consumed" in the overall balance, which must be compensated for by increased bicarbonate excretion by the kidneys. Consequently, herbivores excrete an alkaline, bicarbonate-containing urine.

> **IN A NUTSHELL** !
>
> Acids are produced in animals in both volatile (CO_2) and non-volatile forms. CO_2 production poses hardly any problems for acid-base regulation.

15.3 Regulatory systems

Several control and regulatory systems are available to prevent acidosis/alkalosis:

1. **Buffer systems:** All body fluids contain various types of buffers that are able to bind protons or hydroxyl ions. The bicarbonate/carbonic acid buffer is of particular importance for buffering in biological fluids.
2. **Pulmonary regulation:** If the pH of blood drops and/or p_{CO_2} rises, the respiratory centre is stimulated and ventilation is activated. The bicarbonate/carbonic acid buffer is readjusted by an increased CO_2 release with the exhaled air.
3. **Renal regulation:** Depending on the metabolic situation, the kidney is able to excrete protons or bicarbonate and thus adjust the bicarbonate/carbonic acid buffer in both the alkaline and acid direction.
4. **Hepatic regulation:** The liver produces glutamine, which is metabolised to give NH_3 in the epithelial cells of the renal tubules. Protons can be bound and excreted in the conversion of NH_3 to NH_4^+ in the tubule lumen.

The regulatory systems are described in more detail below.

15.3.1 Buffer systems

If only a few drops of a strong acid (HCl, H_2SO_4) are added to a beaker of pure water, there is complete dissociation into anions and free protons, and the pH falls. When an alkali like potassium hydroxide is added to pure water, alkalisation occurs by the release of OH^- ions. However, if a buffer system is present, the protons or OH^- ions are largely "captured" by the buffering molecules and the pH value changes only slightly. In biological fluids, protection against over-acidification is usually more important than protection against excessive alkalinisation. In the simplest case, **buffer systems** effective in the acidic range comprise a **weak acid** and its **conjugate base**. Buffering in biological fluids, however, is usually through several buffer systems acting simultaneously.

> **IN A NUTSHELL** !
>
> Buffering in the acidic range means that free H⁺ ions are taken up by buffer bases and thus the concentration of free H⁺ ions changes only slightly.

Henderson-Hasselbalch equation

Every acid can dissociate to a certain extent. The stronger the acid, the stronger its tendency to dissociate, i.e., to release protons. Consequently, the fall in pH caused by the acid is also correspondingly increased. Quantitatively, the dissociation tendency is characterised by the **dissociation constant K_a** of an acid or by the **pK_a value ($pK_a = \log K_a$)**. Note that the pK_a value scale is a decadic logarithmic one, i.e., a pK_a value one unit lower means that the acid is ten times stronger. Acids where the pK_a is < 1 are generally referred to as strong acids, while acids with a pK_a value between 1 and 5 are medium strong, and those with a pK_a value above 5 are described as weak acids.

The concentration of free H^+ ions and thus the pH value results from the degree of dissociation of an acid. This can be calculated according to the **Henderson-Hasselbalch equation:**

$$pH = pK_a + \log_{10} \frac{[\text{conjugate base}]}{[\text{acid}]} \tag{15.1}$$

$\log_{10}$: decadic logarithm

In **Fig. 15.1** the relationship between acid-base ratio and pH value, calculated according to the Henderson-Hasselbalch equation, is shown for a bicarbonate/carbonic acid buffer. The degree of change in pH from the addition of an acid or a base depends on the initial value. In the central region of the curve – in the range of the pK_a value – the addition of OH^- or H^+ causes only a slight shift in the ratio of base to acid and thus only a slight change in pH. At the ends of the curve, the corresponding pH value changes are much greater.

For the assessment of a buffer system, the following conclusions can be drawn from the Henderson-Hasselbalch equation:

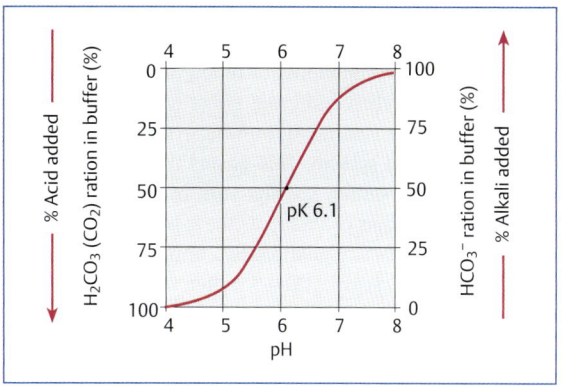

Fig. 15.1 Titration curve for the bicarbonate/carbonic acid (CO_2) buffer. The left y-axis marks the proportion of added H^+ ions and the resulting proportion of H_2CO_3. The right y-axis shows the proportion of OH^- ions added and the resulting proportion of HCO_3^- are plotted.

- The pH of a buffer system is determined by the ratio of conjugate base to acid, not by their absolute concentration.
- The more the pK_a value of an acid is below the set pH value of the solution, the greater the proportion of conjugated bases in this solution.
- If the concentrations of conjugated base and acid are equal, the result is: **$pH = pK_a$** (since log 1 = 0). The **buffer capacity** is **greatest** in this range.

Biological buffer systems

The four most important buffer systems of blood are:
- anionic haemoglobin/haemoglobin
- anionic protein/protein
- hydrogen phosphate/dihydrogen phosphate
- bicarbonate/carbonic acid (CO_2)

Table 15.2 summarises the buffer systems of blood and their localisation, pK_a values and concentrations.

Inner milieu

Table 15.2 Buffer systems of blood.

	Buffer system	Localisation	pK_a value	Concentration in blood plasma (mmol · l^{-1})
Closed systems	Deoxygenated haemoglobin $Hb^- + H^+ \leftrightarrow HHb$	intracellular	8.25	
	Oxygenated haemoglobin $O_2Hb^- + H^+ \leftrightarrow O_2HHb$	intracellular	6.95	
	Proteins $Pr^- + H^+ \leftrightarrow HPr$	intracellular and extracellular	–	24
	Hydrogen phosphate $HPO_4^{2-} + H^+ \leftrightarrow H_2PO_4^-$	intracellular and extracellular	6.8	
Open system	Bicarbonate $HCO_3^- + H^+ \leftrightarrow H_2CO_3 \leftrightarrow H_2O + CO_2$	intracellular and extracellular	6.1	24
			Total	**48**

First of all, a distinction must be made between **open** and **closed systems**.

The buffering components of blood add up to approx. 48 mmol $\cdot$ l^{-1}, but their buffering effect cannot be derived from concentration alone. All non-bicarbonate buffers belong to the **closed system**. This means that the total concentration of the buffer, i.e., the sum of basic and acidic components, remains constant, as these buffer systems are not subject to direct regulation. By contrast, in the bicarbonate/carbonic acid (CO_2) buffer, the CO_2 and HCO_3^- concentrations can be regulated by respiration and by the kidneys, so this is an **open system**.

Anionic haemoglobin/anionic protein buffer

About half of the base concentration in blood consists of proteins (**Table 15.2**). In these proteins, including the globin of haemoglobin, protons are mainly bound to histidine. Among the non-bicarbonate buffers the **haemoglobin/anionic haemoglobin** system occupies a **prominent position**, since it is present intracellularly in high concentration (MCHC > 250 g $\cdot$ l^{-1}; **Table 9.6**). The importance of this system is primarily in buffering protons released during CO_2 uptake by erythrocytes. A special feature here is that the pK$_a$ value of haemoglobin depends on its degree of oxygenation. Deoxygenated haemoglobin (Hb$^-$) has a pK$_a$ value that is more than one unit higher than the oxygenated form (O_2Hb$^-$; **Table 15.2**), i.e., Hb$^-$ (anionic haemoglobin, deoxygenated) can buffer more than 10 times as many protons as O_2Hb$^-$. This means that Hb$^-$ is also more effective in buffering the protons resulting from the metabolic production of CO_2 – a reaction that mainly takes place in tissues, i.e., the location where haemoglobin is being deoxygenated at the same time. Conversely, when Hb is oxygenated in the lungs, protons are released due to the shift in pK$_a$, which in turn promotes the release of CO_2 and its subsequent diffusion into the alveolus. This mechanism is called the **Christiansen-Douglas-Haldane** effect and is described in more detail in ch. 11.5.2 (p. 280). Like haemoglobin in erythrocytes, various intracellular anionic protein buffers act in other cell types. The extracellular proteins in plasma are effective as buffers almost entirely during acidification, with little buffering capacity for alkalinisation, because they are mainly anions at physiological pH (isoelectric points between 4.9 and 6.4).

Dihydrogen phosphate/hydrogen phosphate buffer

Of all buffer systems, the dihydrogen phosphate/hydrogen phosphate system has a **pK$_a$ value** closest to physiological pH (**Table 15.2**). It therefore comes closest to the criteria of an **ideal buffer**. However, due to its **low concentration** in blood plasma (1.5–2 mmol $\cdot$ l^{-1}), the buffering effect is not very high. The $H_2PO_4^-$/HPO_4^{2-} buffer, however, has a greater role in **pH regulation** by the **kidney**. HPO_4^{2-} is filtered in the glomerulus and is then concentrated in the tubules, where the buffering capacity therefore increases. The tubular fluid can then "bind" protons secreted by the tubular cells and excrete (p. 327) them as "titratable acid".

H_2CO_3/CO_2/bicarbonate system

In this system, the concentration of the acidic component, carbonic acid (H_2CO_3), must first be compared to the concentration of the alkaline component, bicarbonate (HCO_3^-). However, it is almost impossible to measure the concentration of H_2CO_3 in biological systems because carbonic acid is quite unstable and splits immediately into CO_2 and water. This process is additionally accelerated in most tissues by the enzyme carbonic anhydrase (**Fig. 15.3** and **Fig. 15.4**). This means that CO_2 concentration in biological fluids is proportional to the H_2CO_3 concentration so that CO_2 instead of H_2CO_3 concentration can be determined in extracellular fluid. The physiological CO_2 concentration of extracellular fluid is on average 1.2 mmol $\cdot$ l^{-1}, where this is physically dissolved as a gas.

> **MORE DETAILS**   Dissolved CO_2 and partial pressure of CO_2 are closely related physically. The solubility coefficient for CO_2 at 37 °C is 0.0304 mmol $\cdot$ mmHg $\cdot$ l^{-1} or 0.228 mmol $\cdot$ kPa$^{-1}\cdot$ l^{-1}. The mean concentration of 1.2 mmol $\cdot$ l^{-1} CO_2 in plasma would thus correspond to a CO_2 partial pressure of 5.3 kPa (= 40 mmHg). In the diagnosis of disorders in acid-base balance, the partial pressure of CO_2 and not its concentration is usually given.

The **pK$_a$ value** of the HCO_3^-/CO_2 system is **6.1** in biological fluids. According to the **Henderson-Hasselbalch equation**, for 1.2 mmol $\cdot$ l^{-1} CO_2 to set the physiological pH of 7.4, the following ratio of HCO_3^- to CO_2 is necessary:

$$7.4 = 6.1 + \log_{10} \frac{24 \text{ mmol} \cdot \text{l}^{-1} HCO_3^-}{1.2 \text{ mmol} \cdot \text{l}^{-1} CO_2} \tag{15.2}$$

From this equation the following conclusions can be drawn:
- the **pK$_a$ value** is relatively **far** from the **physiological pH** value and
- due to the divergence between the pH and pK$_a$ values, the main direction of the concentration ratio of HCO_3^- to CO_2 is towards bicarbonate.

At first glance, these findings **contradict** the conditions set out for an **ideal buffer system**. However, the HCO_3^-/CO_2 system is an **open system** and therefore other criteria have to be applied in assessing this system, as explained in more detail below.

From **Fig. 15.2** it is apparent from the activities of the kidneys and respiration that both acidic and basic components of the HCO_3^-/CO_2 system are subject to regulation. If the relative importance of kidney and respiration are compared, respiration is quantitatively more important for two reasons:
- CO_2 is a **membrane-permeable gas** that **equilibrates** rapidly across cell boundaries. Thus, adjustment of CO_2 concentration can occur very quickly, while adjustment of HCO_3^- concentration in the kidney takes a longer time.
- From the above formula, the quotient of HCO_3^- to CO_2 (which is critical in determining the pH) is very high. This means that a relatively **small shift in CO_2 concentration** (due to increased or decreased respiration) causes a relatively **strong change** in the **quotient** and thus in the **pH value**. It should be noted that this is only possible because the pK$_a$ value of the HCO_3^-/CO_2 buffer

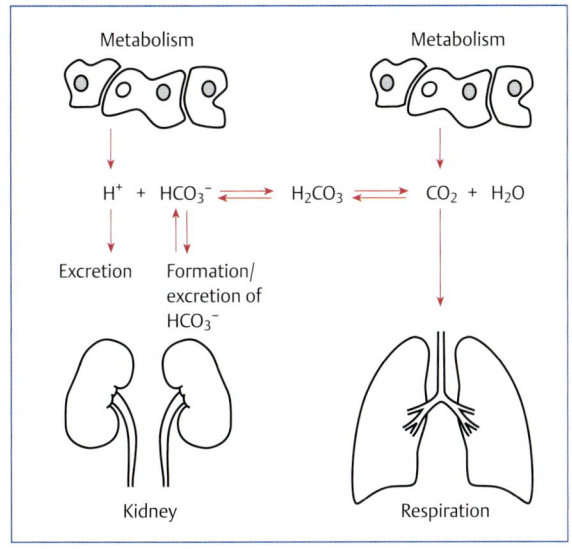

Fig. 15.2 Adjustment of the bicarbonate/carbonic acid (CO_2) buffer by the kidney and by respiratory activity.

does not correspond to an ideal buffer system for extracellular fluid.

The effectiveness of the regulation of the open HCO_3^-/CO_2 system becomes clear when one calculates how an (assumed) closed system would react to an acid load, contrasted with the reaction of an open system. If one assumes that $4\,mmol \cdot l^{-1}$ of lactic acid is released in anaerobic metabolism, the following reactions would take place in a **closed system**:

1. $4\,mmol \cdot l^{-1}$ protons of lactic acid would react with $4\,mmol \cdot l^{-1}$ bicarbonate: $4\,HCO_3^- + 4\,H^+ \rightarrow 4\,H_2CO_3$
2. The ratios in the bicarbonate/CO_2 buffer would shift in the following way:
   - HCO_3^-:
     - before: $24\,mmol \cdot l^{-1}$
     - after: $20\,mmol \cdot l^{-1}$ ($-4\,mmol \cdot l^{-1}$)
   - CO_2 :
     - before: $1.2\,mmol \cdot l^{-1}$
     - after: $5.2\,mmol \cdot l^{-1}$ ($+4\,mmol \cdot l^{-1}$)
3. According to the Henderson-Hasselbalch equation, the pH value would now be as follows:

$$pH = 6.1 + \log_{10}\frac{20\,mmol \cdot l^{-1}\,HCO_3^-}{5.2\,mmol \cdot l^{-1}\,CO_2} = 6.69 \qquad (15.3)$$

Extreme acidosis would be the result.

In an **open system**, however, the CO_2 **is effectively exhaled**. According to the Henderson-Hasselbalch equation, the pH value after CO_2 exhalation is as follows:

$$pH = 6.1 + \log_{10}\frac{20\,mmol \cdot l^{-1}\,HCO_3^-}{1.2\,mmol \cdot l^{-1}\,CO_2} = 7.32 \qquad (15.4)$$

Through the relatively small regulatory intervention on CO_2 concentration, the pH has (almost) returned to its physiological range. The further compensation that follows is described in ch. Pulmonary regulation (p. 349).

The HCO_3^-/CO_2 system is an open system. The CO_2 concentration is adjusted via the respiratory system, the HCO_3^- concentration mainly via the kidneys.

15.3.2 Pulmonary regulation

Pulmonary regulation comes about in two ways:

1. **By variation of blood** p_{CO_2}. If the metabolic production of CO_2 increases, so too does p_{CO_2} in the extracellular fluid. As a result, the pressure gradient of CO_2 from blood to the alveolus lumen increases, and more CO_2 is released by diffusing into the exhaled air. In this way, the altered pressure gradient by the increased p_{CO_2} in blood is sufficient to enable the pH to revert to the normal range, without any change in respiration.
2. **By change in alveolar ventilation**. In addition to the processes described above, the lungs can directly influence the p_{CO_2} in blood. Thus, an increase in p_{CO_2} and/or a decrease in pH stimulates chemosensors in the glomera carotica and medulla oblongata with subsequent activation of the respiratory centre (p. 291). In this way, deviations from the physiological pH can be compensated for by a corresponding change in respiratory activity.

IN A NUTSHELL !

CO_2 is produced metabolically, especially in the citrate cycle, and this is released very effectively in the lungs. The lungs can compensate very well for increases in CO_2 concentration in blood. It is therefore the central organ in the adjustment of plasma pH.

15.3.3 Renal regulation

The exact mechanisms of renal regulation of pH are described in ch. 12.14. In principle, the kidney has the following tasks in regulating the bicarbonate/CO_2 system (**Fig. 15.3**):

1. **Tubular recovery of bicarbonate filtered in the glomerulus**. This process is not regulation in the true sense. The kidney only ensures that no buffer bases are lost. **Fig. 15.3** shows these processes in simplified form (the mechanisms are described in more detail in **Fig. 12.24** and **Fig. 12.25**). The bicarbonate filtered in the glomerulus combines with the secreted protons to form H_2CO_3, which is then split into CO_2 and water catalysed by a lumen oriented carbonic anhydrase. CO_2 diffuses into the cell through the lipid phase of the cell membrane. The intracellular CO_2 is reconverted by an intracellular carbonic anhydrase to H_2CO_3. H_2CO_3 then dissociates into H^+ and bicarbonate and the H^+ is released back into the lumen. The remaining HCO_3^- is transported through the basolateral membrane into blood by various mechanisms.
2. **New formation of bicarbonate**. The kidney is able to form new bicarbonate from CO_2 and thus contribute this HCO_3^- to the buffer system in blood. The production of

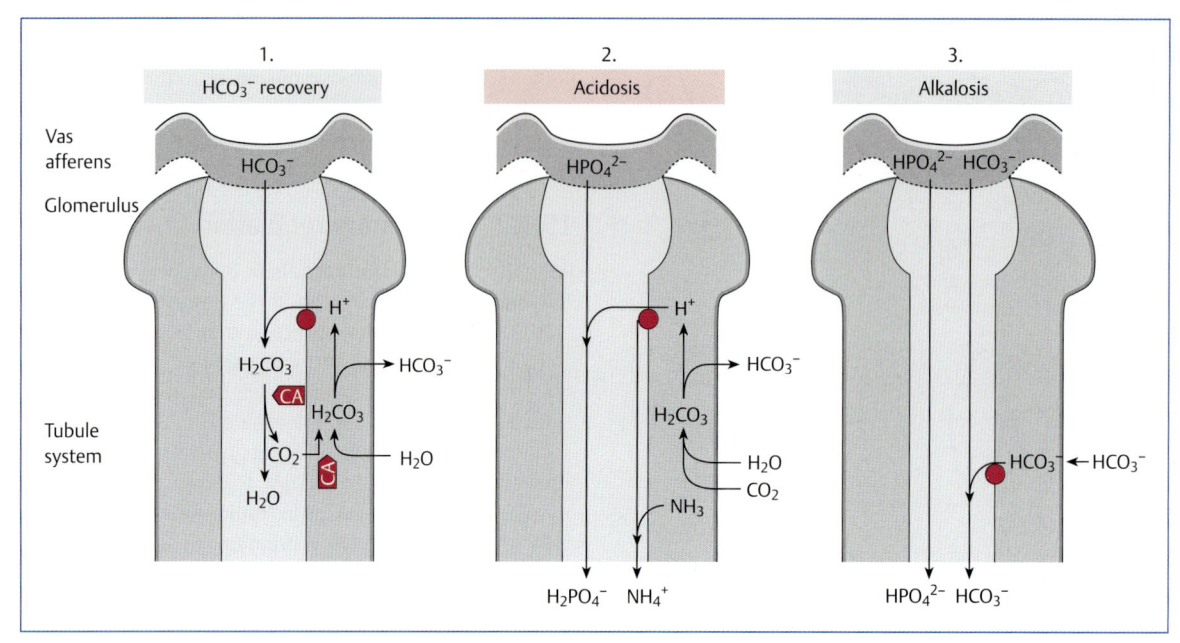

Fig. 15.3 Renal adjustment of the bicarbonate/carbonic acid buffer.
1. Recovery of filtered bicarbonate. The filtered HCO_3^- associates with the secreted H^+ ions and is converted into H_2CO_3, which subsequently dissociates into CO_2 and H_2O. The CO_2 diffuses into the cells, where it is reconverted to H_2CO_3, which dissociates intracellularly into H^+ and HCO_3^-. HCO_3^- is then transferred into blood, and the H^+ ions are secreted.
2. In acidotic stress, the kidney is capable of:
– secreting H^+ as $H_2PO_4^-$ or NH_4^+ which are excreted;
– forming new HCO_3^- which is stoichiometrically always associated with H^+ secretion.
3. When there is an alkalosis, the kidney can excrete HCO_3^-.
CA = carbonic anhydrase.

HCO_3^- occurs inside the cells of the proximal tubule according to the reaction equation:

$$CO_2 + H_2O \rightarrow H_2CO_3 \rightarrow H^+ + HCO_3^-$$

The CO_2 in this conversion can also diffuse into the cell from blood. This process is naturally enhanced if, for example in respiratory acidosis, the p_{CO_2} in blood is elevated. Since protons are produced in the intracellular conversion of CO_2 to HCO_3^-, these must be excreted as titratable acid, i.e., the production of new bicarbonate is only possible in combination with the processes mentioned under point "4" below.

3. **Excretion of bicarbonate**. The processes mentioned under point "2" are activated in metabolic acidosis. When there is a metabolic alkalosis (herbivores!) the kidney is able to excrete bicarbonate. In this way, the total base content of body fluids is reduced.

4. **Secretion of protons**. The epithelial cells of the proximal tubule, the distal tubule and the collecting duct can secrete protons. These serve to recover filtered bicarbonate. In metabolic acidosis, these protons can be "captured" by HPO_4^{2-} and released as $H_2PO_4^-$. Likewise, protons can be "trapped" by NH_3 produced in the tubule cells and excreted in urine as NH_4^+. $H_2PO_4^-$ can be detected analytically in urine as a so-called titratable acid. However, when titrated with NaOH to a pH of 7.0, the protons hardly dissociate (i.e., they are still bound to NH_3) because of the high pK_a value of the NH_3/NH_4^+ system of 9.2. Therefore, NH_4^+ is not determined in this titration procedure. It is referred to as a non-titratable acid.

15.3.4   Hepatic regulation

In the tubules of the kidney, protons are bound to NH_3, which is produced by the epithelial cells from the catabolism of glutamine derived from the liver. In the liver, glutamine is involved in urea synthesis (see ch. 17.4.5 (p.472)). The key enzyme for the release of ammonium from glutamine in the liver is **glutaminase**. Hepatic glutaminase is inhibited in acidic conditions so that less glutamine is catabolised in the liver, and more is released into blood and transported to the kidneys. In this way, the liver is indirectly involved in pH regulation, so that when there is liver failure, disturbances in acid-base balance are also to be expected. The glutamine arriving in the kidney is filtered and reabsorbed by the epithelial cells from the tubular fluid and catabolised as shown in **Fig. 12.25**. In contrast to liver glutaminase, this enzyme in the tubular epithelium of the kidney is stimulated by metabolic acidosis.

> **IN A NUTSHELL**   !
>
> The kidney excretes protons by binding them to buffer bases. Important buffer bases for binding protons are HPO_4^{2-} and NH_3. NH_3 is produced in the epithelial cells of the proximal tubule from glutamine, which comes from the liver.

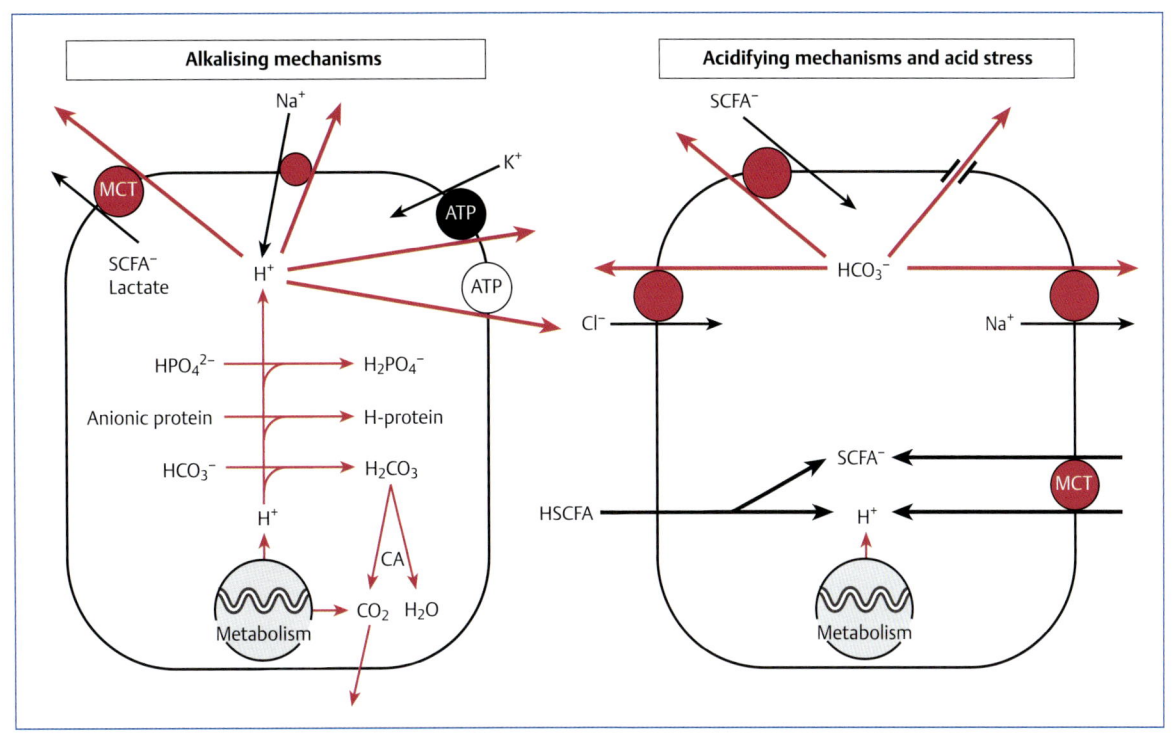

Fig. 15.4 Cellular mechanisms of acid-base regulation.
The figure on the right depicts the acid loads of the cytosol. In addition to the generation of protons and CO_2 from intracellular metabolism, membrane transport mechanisms lead to a loss of bicarbonate and input protons to the intracellular environment. The acidifying mechanisms are essentially those that mediate the vectorial transport of substrates across the cell membrane in polarised, epithelial cells. These mechanisms are described in more detail in other chapters and are only summarised here. The cell counters these acid stresses by various alkalising mechanisms shown in the figure on the left. In addition to intracellular buffer systems (HPO_4^{2-}, anionic protein, and HCO_3^-), transport proteins play a major role in expelling protons - especially the Na^+/H^+ exchanger. The acidifying mechanisms can of course also have a regulating effect in the (rarer) case of an alkalotic load. CA = carbonic anhydrase; $SCFA^-$ = short-chain fatty acid anions (acetate, propionate, butyrate); HSCFA = undissociated SCFA (acetic, propionic, butyric acid).

15.3.5 Speed of acid-base regulation

The **buffer systems** described regulate pH within **seconds**, and **respiration** regulation can restore pH within **minutes**. The **renal** regulatory systems, however, need several **days** to correct the pH. This is mainly due to the fact that metabolic changes are required for alterations in the excretion of $H_2PO_4^-$ and NH_4^+ and these take several days to adapt. It should be emphasised, however, that the non-volatile acids formed during the oxidation of sulphur- and phosphorus-containing amino acids must be excreted via the kidneys. In this case, therefore, stability of the acid-base balance can only be achieved through the activity of the kidneys.

15.4 Regulation of intracellular pH

The mechanisms described so far are aimed at adjusting the pH of extracellular fluid. However, the main requirement for acid-base regulation is inside cells, where metabolism is producing CO_2 and protons.

The intracellular pH is maintained close to 7.1 in most cells. Any stress on intracellular pH comes mainly from acid production (**Fig. 15.4**, right). To counter this acidic load, cells have specific mechanisms to maintain a constant intracellular pH. These include:

- **Buffer systems** such as anionic proteins, anionic haemoglobin (in erythrocytes), bicarbonate and phosphate buffers. Anionic protein and phosphate concentrations are much higher intracellularly than extracellularly (cf. **Table 1.4**, **Fig. 15.4** left), so that their buffering efficacy is greater intracellularly than extracellularly.
- Cell **membrane proteins** that are capable of ejecting protons.

Intracellular protons are transported to the extracellular fluid by membrane transport proteins. It must be emphasised that although these mechanisms initially maintain the intracellular pH, they ultimately impose a strain on the extracellular regulatory systems. Hence, the need to adjust extracellular pH is a consequence of intracellular metabolic processes, but maintaining a stable extracellular pH enables cells to avoid the harmful effect of protons that they are generating.

The effectiveness of the elimination of protons via transport proteins, for example the Na^+/H^+ exchanger, depends on the existence of a concentration gradient for sodium from extracellular to intracellular. The ion gradients are set by the Na^+/K^+-ATPase. A failure of the Na^+/K^+-ATPase, because of a diminished blood supply (ischaemia), would also indirectly cause hyperacidity in tissues, with numerous consequential damages.

The acidifying mechanisms can also have a regulating effect when there is alkaline stress (**Fig. 15.4**).

15.5   Disorders of acid-base balance

15.5.1   Classification

Disorders in acid-base balance are usually not separate diseases, but are consequences or complications of various underlying diseases.

In the maintenance of acid-base balance, a pH of 7.4 is considered to be the physiological value. Deviations from this are acidosis or alkalosis. For values of p_{CO_2}, HCO_3^- and the base excess (BE), standard values of 5.3 kPa CO_2, 24 mmol $\cdot$ l^{-1} HCO_3^- and a BE of 0 are assumed to be physiological. The BE indicates the depletion or generation of bases. Thus, as shown in **Table 15.2**, the total concentration of all buffer bases (bicarbonate and non-bicarbonate) is 48 mmol $\cdot$ l^{-1}. Here, the base excess would be classified as 0 mmol $\cdot$ l^{-1}. Any excess amount over 48 mmol $\cdot$ l^{-1} is called a (positive) base excess, and any shortfall is called a base deficit or a negative base excess. A BE of + 1 would therefore mean that the base concentration is 49 mmol $\cdot$ l^{-1}. This reference value was taken from human medicine, but there are often greater differences in the veterinary reference values depending on the animal species. For example, in cats a BE of −10 (= base deficit) is defined by laboratory manuals as being physiological and can be explained by the protein-rich diet of cats.

Depending on the underlying condition, the disorders are classified as follows:

- respiratory acidosis
- respiratory alkalosis
- non-respiratory (formerly: metabolic) acidosis
- non-respiratory (formerly: metabolic) alkalosis

In **Table 15.3** possible causes of acid-base imbalances are summarised.

Table 15.4 summarises changes in plasma where there are disturbances in acid-base balance and presents possible compensatory mechanisms. The buffer systems (p. 346) serve as the "first line of defence". In order not to deplete these buffers and to restore pH to its physiological range, compensation mechanisms are necessary. In general, metabolic disturbances are mainly compensated by the lungs, and respiratory disturbances by the kidneys.

> **IN A NUTSHELL**   !
>
> Acid-base balance disorders are called respiratory or non-respiratory acidoses or alkaloses, depending on their origin.

15.5.2   Respiratory acidosis

As its name implies, respiratory acidosis is a consequence of **reduced ventilation** or **reduced gas exchange** in the alveoli, either as a result of hypoventilation or a disturbance in diffusion (e.g., due to pulmonary oedema). These underlying conditions result in a reduced CO_2 release, so that the

Table 15.3 Some underlying conditions that can cause acid-base imbalances.

Malfunction	Basic condition
Respiratory acidosis	Hypoventilation (anaesthesia), obstructive airway diseases (asthma, etc.), diffusion disorders (pulmonary oedema)
Respiratory alkalosis	Hyperventilation (in case of oxygen deficiency)
Non-respiratory acidosis	Diarrhoea (loss of bicarbonate), kidney diseases, excessive formation of ketone bodies (diabetes mellitus, "ketosis"), rumen acidosis, lactic acidosis, hyperkalaemia (resulting, among other things, in reduced proton excretion or reduced bicarbonate production in the kidney)
Non-respiratory alkalosis	Vomiting (HCl loss), hypokalaemia (resulting, among other things, in increased proton excretion or increased bicarbonate production in the kidney)

Table 15.4 pH changes in plasma and possible compensations.

Malfunction	Plasma pH	Cause	Compensation
Respiratory acidosis	↓	p_{CO_2} ↑	**Kidney:** H$^+$ excretion ↑ HCO_3^- new-formation ↑
Respiratory alkalosis	↑	p_{CO_2} ↓	**Kidney:** H$^+$ excretion ↓ HCO_3^- excretion ↑
Non-respiratory acidosis	↓	HCO_3^- ↓	**Lungs:** Hyperventilation (p_{CO_2} ↓)
Non-respiratory alkalosis	↑	HCO_3^- ↑	**Lungs:** Hypoventilation (p_{CO_2} ↑)

p_{CO_2} level in blood increases. When the CO_2 concentration increases, the reaction

$$CO_2 \uparrow + H_2O \rightarrow H_2CO_3 \rightarrow H^+ + HCO_3^- \qquad (15.5)$$

shifts to the right, i.e., bicarbonate and protons are produced. The accumulation of protons decreases the pH of extracellular fluid.

The increase in p_{CO_2} and in the H^+ concentration stimulates kidney to produce more HCO_3^- and to increase H^+ excretion. As a result, the HCO_3^- concentration in plasma increases and pH is restored to the physiological range. **Compensation** via **respiration** does **not** take place because of the existing underlying condition of reduced ventilation or reduced gas exchange in the alveoli.

15.5.3 Respiratory alkalosis

Respiratory alkalosis is usually the result of **hyperventilation**. In reversal of the processes in respiratory acidosis, the increased CO_2 exhalation drives the reaction

$$CO_2 \downarrow + H_2O \leftarrow H_2CO_3 \leftarrow H^+ + HCO_3^- \qquad (15.6)$$

to the left. The plasma H^+ and bicarbonate concentrations decrease. Renal compensation (p. 326) (which requires a longer time to adapt) is mediated by reducing the excretion of H^+/NH_4^+ and/or by increasing HCO_3^- excretion. This decreases plasma HCO_3^- concentration so the pH value declines.

15.5.4 Non-respiratory acidosis

Non-respiratory acidosis results either from an increased **production of non-volatile acids** (e.g., in anaerobic glycolysis → lactic acid or in ketosis → β-hydroxybutyric acid, acetoacetic acid), or from excessive excretion of HCO_3^- (e.g., in diarrhoea or kidney failure) and/or from inadequate excretion of protons by the kidneys. The interactions between potassium and acid-base balance play a special role in this context. Acidosis leads to hyperkalaemia which is often associated with acidosis. These interactions are described in more detail in ch. Interactions between potassium and acid-base balance (p. 316).

With the accumulation of protons, the reaction equation

$$H^+ \uparrow + HCO_3^- \rightarrow H_2CO_3 \rightarrow H_2O + CO_2 \qquad (15.7)$$

is driven to the right. HCO_3^- is thus depleted so that plasma pH and bicarbonate concentration decline. This drop in pH stimulates chemosensors to increase respiratory minute volume (**respiratory compensation**) which causes more CO_2 to be released and a drop in p_{CO_2}. In contrast to renal compensation, respiratory compensation occurs very quickly, and respiratory minute volume is increased after only a few minutes. If the kidney is not involved in the disorder that has caused acidosis, it can also participate in the compensation process by the mechanisms described for respiratory acidosis.

15.5.5 Non-respiratory alkalosis

Non-respiratory alkalosis results either from the **absorption** of dietary **alkalis** or from the **increased loss of non-volatile acids** (e.g., during vomiting → HCl loss). The reaction equation

$$H^+ \downarrow + HCO_3^- \leftarrow H_2CO_3 \leftarrow H_2O + CO_2 \qquad (15.8)$$

is driven to the left by proton depletion, plasma pH and bicarbonate concentration rise accordingly. The compensation mechanisms are the reverse of those in non-respiratory acidosis.

> **IN A NUTSHELL** !
>
> Disorders in acid-base balance are caused by
> - insufficient exhalation of CO_2 (respiratory acidosis),
> - unphysiologically increased exhalation of CO_2 (respiratory alkalosis),
> - loss of bicarbonate via the kidneys and/or intestines or increased proton accumulation (non-respiratory acidosis),
> - increased absorption of alkalis in food or increased loss of protons (non-respiratory alkalosis).

15.5.6 Diagnosing acid-base disorders

The following parameters of acid-base status in plasma can be used to assess the pathogenesis (non-respiratory/respiratory) of disturbances in acid-base balance and possible compensations:
- pH
- p_{CO_2} [mmHg or kPa]
- HCO_3^- [mmol·l^{-1}]
- base excess [BE in mmol·l^{-1}], for negative values: base deficit

Blood gas analysers usually measure pH and p_{CO_2} and from these the bicarbonate concentration is calculated according to the Henderson-Hasselbalch equation. This is then called the "actual bicarbonate concentration". The "standard bicarbonate concentration" is also provided. This is the "actual bicarbonate concentration" standardised to a p_{CO_2} of 40 mmHg and complete saturation of haemoglobin with oxygen.

The pH value only provides information about the direction (acidotic or alkalotic) of the disorder. The p_{CO_2} value can be used to assess whether the disorder is respiratory or non-respiratory in nature. The bicarbonate concentration and the BE are parameters for the assessment of non-respiratory disorders.

The procedure for assessing disturbances in acid-base balance from pH, p_{CO_2} and bicarbonate concentration is shown in **Fig. 15.5**. Another criterion is the BE. Changes in bicarbonate concentration usually lead in the same direction to changes in BE.

> **MORE DETAILS** Under physiological and also most pathophysiological conditions, acid-base status can be described sufficiently accurately using the Henderson-Hasselbalch equation. However, in patients with massive hypo- or hyperproteinaemia or hypo- or hyperchloraemia, changes in pH cannot always be satis-

Inner milieu

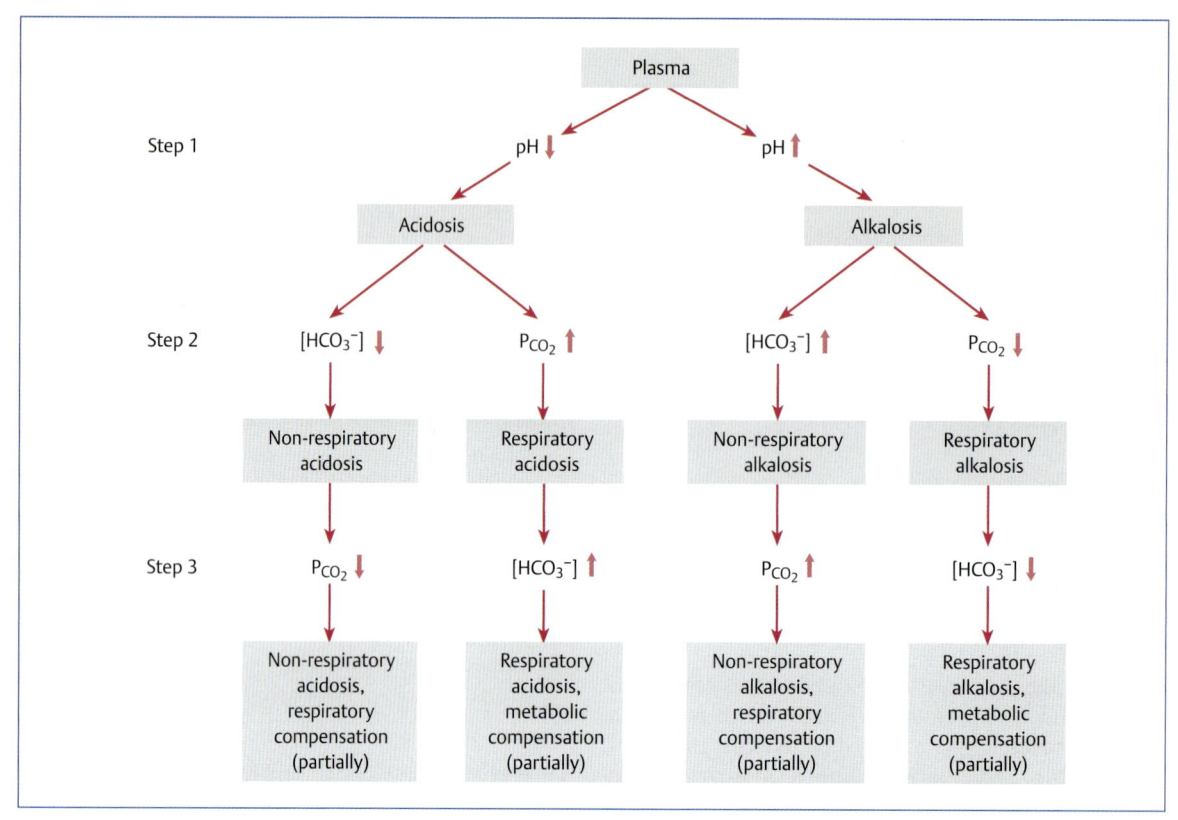

Fig. 15.5 Procedure for assessing disturbances in acid-base balance from pH, p_{CO_2} and HCO_3^- concentration.

factorily interpreted by the Henderson-Hasselbalch model. In addition to pH, bicarbonate concentration, p_{CO_2} and BE, increasing attention is therefore also being directed at the plasma concentration of ions in acid-base diagnostics. Bicarbonate, anionic proteins and bases of the other buffer systems are also charge carriers so the principle of electroneutrality must be maintained with the concentration of anions matching that of cations. Therefore, a shift in the concentration of anions also has an indirect effect on the concentration of buffer bases. For example, if the concentration of chloride increases and the concentration of cations remains constant, the concentration of bicarbonate must decrease in order to maintain electroneutrality. In this way, hyperchloraemia is accompanied by acidosis. To detect such shifts, a total balance of cations and anions in plasma would have to be determined. Under routine conditions, however, it is not practical to measure the plasma concentration of all anions and cations, which is why the term "anion gap" has been introduced in analytics. The "**anion gap**" is a concept to analytically capture the importance of electroneutrality in pH regulation.

The "anion gap" represents the difference between the unmeasured anions and the unmeasured cations and is usually calculated indirectly from the measured concentration of sodium, chloride and bicarbonate:

$$\text{anion gap} = [Na^+] - [HCO_3^-] - [Cl^-] \tag{15.9}$$

$$12 = 144 - 24 - 108 \ (mmol \cdot l^{-1})$$

The cations not measured in this analysis are mainly calcium, magnesium and potassium. The unmeasured anions are albumin, phosphate, sulphate and other organic anions. The "anion gap" increases when the concentration of unmeasured anions is increased or when the concentration of unmeasured cations decreases. In hyperchloraemic non-respiratory acidosis, the "anion gap" remains normal if the concentration of chloride increases at the same rate as the concentration of bicarbonate decreases. If the decrease in the concentration of bicarbonate is not accompa-

nied by an increase in chloride concentration, the concentration of the unmeasured anions also increases, which can be determined by an increase in the calculated anion gap. This analysis can thus be used to make an additional statement about the pathogenesis of **non-respiratory acidosis**. For example, an increased anion gap with normochloraemia is found in acidosis due to diabetes mellitus and lactic acidosis. A hypochloraemic non-respiratory acidosis with increased anion gap can occur in diarrhoea.

The principle of maintaining electroneutrality is further integrated in a model developed by **Stewart** (1983) to further specify the diagnosis of disturbances in acid-base balance. Stewart differentiates between strong ions (e.g., Na^+ and K^+), which are not present as salts, but are completely dissociated, and weak ions (buffer bases such as HCO_3^-). From the calculation of the "**strong ion difference**" (SID = $[Na^+] + [K^+] + [Ca^{2+}] - [Cl^-]$) and the inclusion of the dissociation equilibria of the buffer systems, Stewart's calculations provide a combined quantitative coverage of the electroneutrality variables and those of the Henderson-Hasselbalch equation. It must be emphasised, however, that determination of the Stewart variables is an additional analytical procedure and as with the calculation of the anion gap it only provides a clear diagnosis of metabolic disturbances.

Suggested reading

Akers RM, Denbow DM. Anatomy and Physiology of Domestic Animals. Ames: Blackwell Publishing; 2013

Grogono AW. Acid Base Tutorial: www.acid-base.com

Seifter JL, Chang H-Y. Extracellular acid-base balance and ion transport between body fluid compartments. Physiology 2017; 32: 367–379

Stewart PA. Modern quantitative acid-base chemistry. Can J Physiol Pharmacol 1983; 61: 1444–1461

Nutrition and energy balance

16 Gastrointestinal tract

Jörg R. Aschenbach, Gerhard Breves, Franziska Dengler, Martin Diener, Kristin Elfers, Gotthold Gäbel, Romy Monika Heilmann, Gemma Mazzuoli-Weber, Michael Pees, Helga Pfannkuche, Reiko Rackwitz, Wolfgang von Engelhardt, Siegfried Wolffram

16.1 Food intake and salivary secretion

Gerhard Breves

> **ESSENTIALS** ✖
>
> - Food intake, chewing activity and the onset of the chemical processes of digestion are characterised by large differences when comparing animal species.
> - In the oral cavity, saliva is formed from a mixture of secretions of different compositions from the various salivary glands, the secretion of which is controlled by mechanical and chemical stimuli acting through the autonomic nervous system.
> - In all animal species, saliva has a protective function on the oral mucosa.
> - In ruminants, large amounts of bicarbonate and phosphate are secreted in saliva and act as buffer systems in the forestomachs.
> - Urea secretion via saliva is part of a rumino-hepatic nitrogen circulation.

16.1.1 Food intake, chewing and swallowing

In all domestic mammals, lips, teeth and tongue are the key organs for **food intake**. There are considerable differences in the actual mechanisms of food intake among various animal species. When **horses** are fed from a manger, food intake is firstly by the action of their highly mobile lips. The lips are retracted when grazing to allow the upper and lower incisors to cleave the top of grass leaves from their lower stems. In contrast, the lips of **cattle** and **sheep** are characterised by relatively low mobility. In those animals, small tufts of grass are entwined by their long, slender and mobile tongues and are torn off by movements of the head and neck. When grazing, **pigs** dig the ground

with their proboscis and transport food into the oral cavity mainly by the forward tapering of their lower lip. **Carnivores** use mainly their teeth to ingest food, with the forelimbs often helping to hold the food while eating.

In carnivores, the free and mobile end of the tongue is shaped like a spoon for drinking **liquid**, whereas in all other domestic mammals the suction created by air inspiration and tongue contraction transports liquid into the oral cavity.

The **chewing process** breaks up a piece of food and at the same time moistens it with saliva to convert it into a form that is easier to swallow. The **intensity of chewing** varies between species and is also influenced by the degree of toughness of the food. While carnivores chew ingested feed only to a small extent, herbivores are characterised by a high chewing intensity. In ruminants, the chewing of each bolus is maintained for an average of 60 s. While chewing, the **jaw movements** of carnivores and omnivores are mainly in a vertical direction. In herbivores the jaws move horizontally, so the actual chewing movement is always on one side of the oral cavity. The **swallowing** of the chewed food mixed with saliva is a complex process of **voluntary** and **reflex** movements of individual structures at the start of the alimentary tract. The **voluntary action** is the positioning of the bolus of food approximately halfway between the tongue and the hard palate by movements of the mouth and tongue. In this position, the food stimulates receptors in the epithelial layer at the back of the oral cavity and pharynx. These stimuli generate action potentials which are transmitted to the **swallowing centre** via afferents of various nerves (vagal, glossopharyngeal and trigeminal nerves). The swallowing centre is a group of neurons at the base of the 4th brain ventricle. From this stimulation, the reflex part of swallowing is controlled by motor efferents of the Vth, IXth, Xth, XIth and XIIth cranial nerves. These innervate the tongue, oral cavity, pharynx and laryngeal muscles. At the start of the **reflex** of **swallowing**, the oral cavity is first closed off from the nasopharynx and trachea by raising the soft palate close to the posterior pharyngeal wall and displacing the larynx so that its opening into the pharynx is partially covered. At the same time, the arytenoid cartilages, where the posterior ends of the vocal cords attach, are narrowed by contraction of the laryngeal muscles. In this phase, a brief inhibition of respiration occurs. In the next step, the bolus is transported from the oral cavity to the cranial end of the oesophagus, by contraction of the myohyoideus and hyoglossus muscles. Contraction of the myohyoideus muscle pushes the tongue against the hard palate, and contraction of the hyoglossus muscle pulls it backwards. The reduction in volume of the closed pharyngeal cavity results in a marked increase in intrapharyngeal pressure and a relaxation at the junction between the pharynx and the oesophagus. This region is controlled by a sphincter muscle with a high resting tone, so that relaxation is achieved by inhibiting the tonic contraction. In humans, relaxation of the sphincter begins about 0.2–0.3 s after the onset of the swallowing act and lasts about 0.5–1.2 s. With the pressure gradient in the craniocaudal direction from these processes, the food bolus is transported through the sphincter region and, from the initial relaxation, arrives at the upper end of the oesophagus. From there a peristaltic wave moves caudally accompanied by a contraction of the sphincter region that is stronger than its resting tone and only returns to that resting tone after the bolus has been transported down the oesophagus.

The so-called primary peristaltic wave induced by the swallowing act should be distinguished from a possible secondary peristaltic wave, which can be generated directly by local stimulation of the oesophagus.

These **contractions** are mediated by the muscular parts of the oesophageal wall. In most domestic mammals, the circular and longitudinal muscles of the oesophagus consist of striated muscle fibres. In horses and cats, the caudal parts of the oesophageal wall are formed by smooth muscle cells. The cranial region of the oesophagus is inner-

vated by fibres of the recurrent nerve, and the lower regions by thoracic branches of the vagus. The speed of bolus passage down the oesophagus in dogs is about $5\,cm \cdot s^{-1}$, which gives a total transit time of about 4–5 s.

> ### IN A NUTSHELL !
> The act of swallowing is a very complex, neurologically controlled process of voluntary and involuntary actions.

16.1.2   Salivary secretion

Mixed saliva, which is composed of **serous, mucous** or **seromucous** secretions of the individual salivary glands, is a digestive secretion with multiple functions at the start of the alimentary tract and, in ruminants, in the forestomachs. In mammals, the main salivary glands are the parotid, mandibular (submaxillary) and sublingual glands, each of which are arranged in pairs. Their secretions are supplemented by those of numerous smaller salivary glands (buccal, palatine, pharyngeal, and labial glands). In **Fig. 16.1** the histological structure of a seromucous gland is shown. The terminal end of each gland (acinus) is formed from morphologically different serous and mucous cells. Serous cells have a pyramidal structure, with round nuclei located centrally and dense rough endoplasmic reticulum in the basal region of the cells. Mucous cells, on the other hand, have flattened nuclei located in the basal part of the cell and abundant diffusely distributed secretory granules. The acini cells are partially covered by myoepithelial cells, the so-called basket cells. These are modified contractile epithelial cells with a cytoskeleton of myofilaments of actin and myosin. Gap junctions connect neighbouring myoepithelial cells. The acini are followed by intercalated ducts which are considered the regenerative zone of acinus cells. Intercalated ducts are followed by striated ducts, which are only partially developed in ruminants.

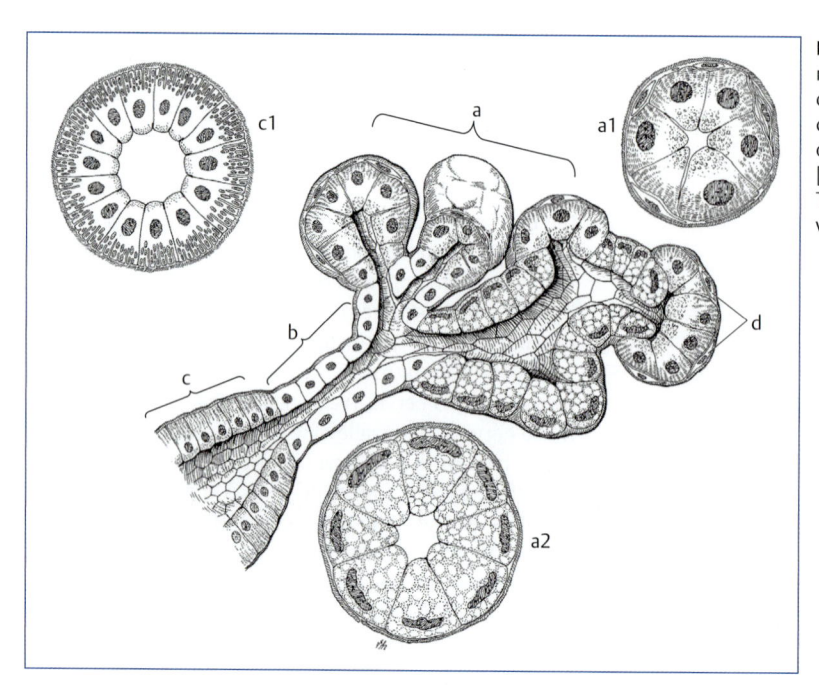

Fig. 16.1 Histological structure of a seromucous gland. **a** Acinus, **a1** Serous acinus cell, **a2** Mucous acinus cell, **b** Intercalated ducts, **c** Striated duct, **c1** Epithelial cells of the striated duct, **d** Myoepithelial cells. [Source: Anatomisches Institut, Stiftung TiHo Hannover. Illustration: Caren-Imme von Stemm]

Functions of saliva

The various functions of saliva can be classified as either **primary** or **secondary digestive functions**. In all mammals, primary digestive functions include protection of the oral mucosa and teeth from dehydration and acidity, facilitation of swallowing by moistening and lubricating the food bolus and, in some species such as humans and pigs, the initiation of enzymatic digestion of carbohydrates. In ruminants, the high secretion rates of phosphate and bicarbonate in saliva provide further physiological digestive functions by regulating rumen pH. Secondary digestive functions of saliva include bactericidal action, temperature regulation in panting animals and, in some species, saliva is part of a behavioural defence measure.

Secretion rate and composition of saliva

Saliva is a colourless, slightly opalescent fluid consisting mainly of H_2O, electrolytes and mucin. Daily salivary secretion is not constant. The pattern of glandular secretion is generally discontinuous, except for the parotid and ventral buccal glands. The data on daily salivary secretion from various studies are only estimates, because of major methodological problems in quantifying output. There are considerable differences between species in the daily volume of salvia produced. While **cats** secrete only about 0.1–0.2 l of saliva daily, the daily saliva volume of **cattle** can be more than 250 l. In the other domestic mammals, the secretion rates range between these extreme values (**Table 16.1**).

On average, about 90% of saliva comes from the parotid and mandibular glands. The other 10% comes equally from the sublingual and other smaller salivary glands (**Table 16.2**).

Table 16.1 Daily saliva volumes in different species.

Species	Saliva volume ($l \cdot d^{-1}$)
Human	1–1.5
Cat	0.1–0.2
Pig	1–1.5
Sheep	6–16
Cattle	60–250
Horse	5–10

In **ruminants**, the salivary glands can be functionally differentiated into two groups. In the first group, the composition of the secretion is largely **isoosmolar** to plasma, regardless of the flow rate, and is characterised by high **bicarbonate** and **phosphate** concentrations. This group includes the parotid and lower buccal glands, which produce a **serous** secretion, and the palatine, buccal and pharyngeal glands, which produce a more mucous secretion. The second group produce a mixed **seromucous secretion** that is **hypoosmolar** to plasma at basal secretion rates. This saliva is characterised by low bicarbonate and high phosphate concentrations, and secretion is stimulated mainly by the intake of food. This group includes the mandibular, labial and sublingual glands, which secrete only a comparatively very small amount of saliva. The mucous properties are provided by the glycoprotein mucin. The physiological significance of these different secretion characteristics is not clear. It is possible that the buffering properties of the serous secretions are of primary importance, whereas the mucous or seromucous secretions have primarily a mucosal protective function.

In **non-ruminants**, at a **basal secretion rate**, the osmolarity of saliva is between 60 and 80 mosmol·l^{-1} (**hypoosmolar**). Saliva contains Na^+, K^+, Cl^-, and HCO_3^- with total concentrations between 10 and 30 mmol·l^{-1} and low $H_2PO_4^-$ concentrations at pH 7.4. **Stimulation** of **secretion** causes the saliva to approach **isoosmolar** values by increasing the concentrations of Na^+, Cl^- and HCO_3^-, with only slight changes in K^+ concentration (**Fig. 16.2**). The mean concentrations of Na^+, K^+, Cl^-, HCO_3^- and phosphate are listed in **Table 16.3**.

In **ruminants, parotid saliva** is approximately **isoosmolar** with a pH of about 8.2, irrespective of flow rate, and with relatively constant concentrations of Na^+, K^+, Cl^-, HCO_3^- and HPO_4^{2-}. The HCO_3^- and HPO_4^{2-} concentrations are several times **higher** than their **concentrations** in **plasma**, with values of about 110 mmol·l^{-1} and 20 mmol·l^{-1} respectively. In contrast, the saliva of the ruminant **mandibular gland** is **hypoosmolar** during basal secretion and has pronounced changes in ion concentrations when stimulated. The increase in HCO_3^- concentration with increasing flow rate may possibly be due to a lower extraction of HCO_3^- during passage through the secretory duct system (**Fig. 16.3**).

Table 16.2 Salivary secretion and the type of secretion from different salivary glands.

Name	Share (%)	Secretion	Special features
Parotid gland	90	Serous	Isoosmolar
Submaxillary (mandibular) glands		Seromucous	Hypoosmolar – isoosmolar
Sublingual glands	5	Seromucous	Hypoosmolar – isoosmolar
Labial glands	5	Seromucous	Hypoosmolar – isoosmolar
Buccal glands		Serous or mucous	Hypoosmolar – isoosmolar or isoosmolar
Paracaruncular glands		Mucous	–
Lingual glands		Serous	"Flushing glands" for the taste buds
Palatal glands		Mucous	Isoosmolar
Pharyngeal glands		Mucous	Isoosmolar

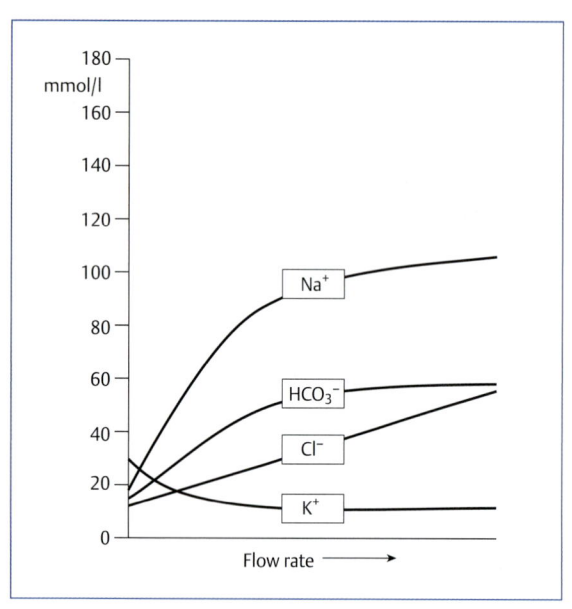

Fig. 16.2 Influence of salivary flow rate on the ionic composition of saliva of the parotid and mandibular glands in dogs; based on data from Reece WO, Erickson HH, Goff IP et al (eds). Duke's Physiology of Domestic Animals. 13th ed., Ames: Wiley-Blackwell, 2015

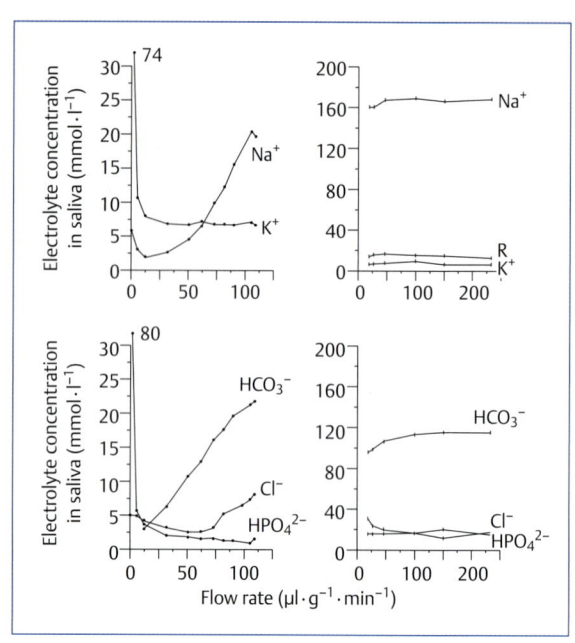

Fig. 16.3 Influence of salivary flow rate on the ionic composition of saliva of the mandibular gland (left) and parotid gland (right) in sheep (note scales on ordinates!). [Source: Cook DJ. Salivary secretions in ruminants. In: von Engelhardt, Leonhard-Marek, Breves, Giesecke (eds.). Ruminant Physiology: Digestion, Metabolism, Growth and Reproduction. Stuttgart: Enke; 1995: 153–170]

Table 16.3 Mean concentrations of Na^+, K^+, Cl^-, HCO_3^- and phosphate ($mmol \cdot l^{-1}$) in non-ruminants under basal and stimulated conditions and in ruminants.

	Non-ruminants		Ruminants
	basal	stimulated	
Na^+	10	100	160
K^+	10	10	5
Cl^-	10	40	15
HCO_3^-	5	60	90–140
Phosphate	Traces	Traces	5–35

Source: Sjaastad ØV, Sand O, Hove K. Physiology of Domestic Animals. 2nd ed., Oslo: Scandinavian Veterinary Press; 2010

In addition to electrolytes, saliva contains various **N-containing compounds**, of which the largest component in ruminants is **urea** at about 80% of these compounds. The urea concentration in saliva of ruminants can be between 50 and 65% of plasma urea concentration. The physiological significance of urea secretion is its rumino-hepatic circulation into the **forestomachs** with subsequent rapid cleavage by microbial urease and utilisation of the resulting ammonia for microbial protein synthesis (**Fig. 16.36**). **Amylases** are salivary proteins in **pigs, rats** and **rabbits**, and a **lipase** is present in the saliva of **calves**. In addition, traces of lysozyme, lactoferrin and immunoglobulins can be detected in saliva.

■ Cellular mechanisms of salivary secretion

The process of saliva production is mainly in two regions of the salivary glands, the **acini**, where **primary saliva** is produced, and also in the **striated** and **excretory ducts**, where **secondary saliva** is formed. In ruminants, the striated ducts are only partially developed.

In comparing ruminants and non-ruminants, considerable differences are sometimes found in the functions of salivary glands and also between different glands. In the following, therefore, essential cellular mechanisms of saliva formation will be compared between the mandibular gland of rats and rabbits and the parotid gland of ruminants.

IN A NUTSHELL   !

The cellular secretion of the components of saliva is mediated by membrane transport processes similar to those demonstrated in other secretory epithelia.

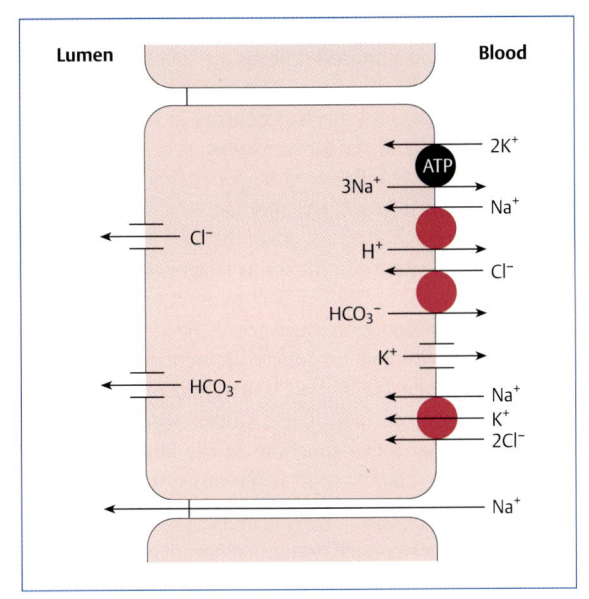

Fig. 16.4 Cellular model of the secretion mechanism of the rat and rabbit mandibular gland; based on data from Cook DJ. Salivary secretions in ruminants. In: von Engelhardt, Leonhard-Marek, Breves, Giesecke (eds.). Ruminant Physiology: Digestion, Metabolism, Growth and Reproduction. Stuttgart: Enke; 1995: 153–170

Secretory mechanisms of the mandibular gland

The cellular mechanisms of saliva formation are shown schematically in **Fig. 16.4**. The basolateral membrane contains Na^+/K^+-ATPase, a Na^+/H^+ and a Cl^-/HCO_3^- antiporter and a Na^+-K^+-$2Cl^-$ symporter. Both the Cl^- absorbed into the cell and intracellularly formed HCO_3^- are discharged through ion channels in the apical membrane, and the resulting negative potential difference is corrected by a transfer of positive charge by paracellular Na^+ transport.

These ion shifts are followed by an osmotic efflux of H_2O. The electrogenic anion flux out of the cell is matched by basolateral K^+ efflux through K^+ channels. These transport processes can be stimulated parasympathetically by **acetylcholine** which increases intracellular Ca^{2+} concentration. The apical Cl^- and HCO_3^- channels and the basolateral K^+ channels are considered the primary targets of these regulatory mechanisms.

The composition of acinar saliva flowing into the **intercalated and striated ducts** can be modified by more ion transport processes and thus becomes secondary saliva. In the collecting ducts, Na^+ and Cl^- are absorbed while K^+ and HCO_3^- are secreted into the secondary saliva. This high **reabsorption of Na^+ and Cl^-** and the low water permeability of the duct epithelium result in the **secondary saliva** in monogastric animals becoming **hypoosmolar** compared to plasma.

Secretion mechanism of the parotid gland in ruminants

In ruminants, important characteristics in the composition of primary saliva formed in the acinus cells of the parotid glands are the **high phosphate** and **bicarbonate concentrations**. The transport mechanisms for these ions are in the basolateral membrane and differ considerably from those in monogastric animals. Furthermore, the transport mechanisms are different between spontaneous, non-stimulated and acetylcholine-stimulated secretion. The cellular models developed for both stimulated and non-stimulated secretion are shown in **Fig. 16.5**. In the non-stimulated cell, the cytosolic $H_2PO_4^-$ concentrations are increased by the basolaterally localised $Na^+/H_2PO_4^-$ cotransporter, which is activated by the Na^+/K^+-ATPase. In addition to this cotransporter, Na^+ is transported into the cell via a Na^+/H^+ antiporter.

Nutrition, energy

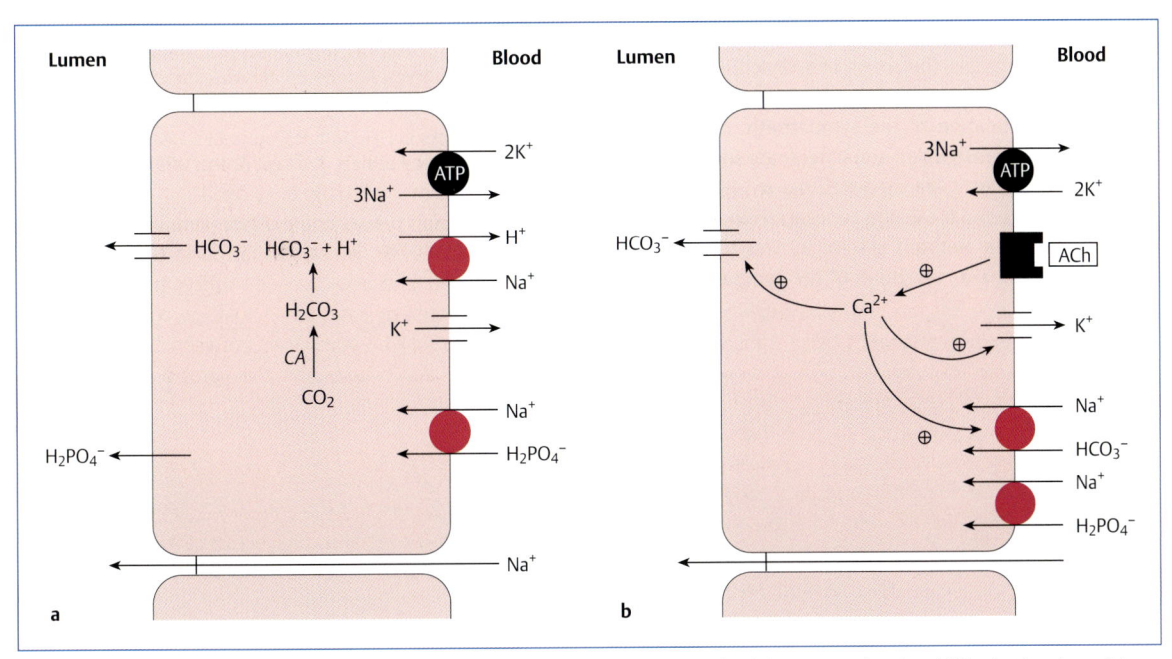

Fig. 16.5 Cellular model of the secretion mechanism of the ovine parotid gland under (**a**) non-stimulated and (**b**) stimulated conditions. Ach = acetylcholine; CA = carbonic anhydrase; based on data from Cook DJ. Salivary secretions in ruminants. In: von Engelhardt, Leonhard-Marek, Breves, Giesecke (eds.). Ruminant Physiology: Digestion, Metabolism, Growth and Reproduction. Stuttgart: Enke; 1995: 153–170

The mechanism of $H_2PO_4^-$ transport when secreted across the luminal membrane has not yet been characterised. Intracellularly formed HCO_3^- is discharged from the cell on the luminal side via an anion channel, which is possibly identical to the Ca^{2+}-activated Cl^- channel. The negative potential difference resulting from HCO_3^- and Cl^- anion discharges is compensated by paracellular Na^+ transport followed by H_2O transport. Intracellularly, the electrogenic anion efflux is compensated by influx of K^+ through basolateral K^+ channels.

During salivary secretion stimulated by **acetylcholine**, i.e. by the parasympathetic nervous system, a basolaterally localised Na^+-HCO_3^-cotransporter is activated by increasing intracellular Ca^{2+} concentration. Change in Ca^{2+} concentration also leads to activation of the Na^+-$H_2PO_4^-$ cotransporter. The efflux of both $H_2PO_4^-$ and HCO_3^- across the luminal membrane and the basolateral K^+ efflux are also mediated by Ca^{2+}-dependent channel activation.

The specific transport processes in saliva secretion in ruminants develop postnatally with the onset of roughage intake and the full development of innervation by the parasympathetic nervous system. The secretion of organic components of saliva, such as glycoproteins, is also by the acinar cells, where the contents of secretory granules are released by exocytosis.

■ Control of salivary secretion

The salivary glands are innervated by **parasympathetic fibres** of the facial and glossopharyngeal nerve and by **sympathetic fibres** originating from the first three thoracic segments. Stimulation of the **parasympathetic** fibres leads to **vasodilation** via muscarinic receptors (M_3) inducing secretion of vasoactive substances (**bradykinin**). Parasympathetic stimulation also causes a large **increase in salivary secretion**, mainly by the parotid gland. In addition to acetylcholine, other neurotransmitters, such as VIP, are also important in regulating salivary secretion. In monogastric and ruminant animals, the action of acetylcholine is mediated by changes in cytosolic Ca^{2+} concentrations as second messenger. Stimulation of the **sympathetic nervous system** causes vasoconstriction and a **decrease in salivary secretion**. These effects are mediated via α_1 receptors and changes in intracellular calcium concentration. Stimulation of the sympathetic nervous system increases the tone of the basket cells via α_1 receptors of the sympathetic effer-

ents and also increases the protein and mucin content of saliva. **Innate** and **acquired reflexes** are involved in the reflex control of saliva secretion. The innate reflexes are controlled by chemo- and mechanosensors in the oral cavity, the oesophagus, and the forestomachs. While the chemosensors are mainly influenced by pH changes in the contents of the forestomach, the mechanosensors are mainly influenced by the fibrous nature of the feed.

Evidence of **acquired reflexes** as triggers of salivary secretion goes back to the classical experiments of **Pavlov**, who gave dogs food after they heard the sound of a bell. After repeated training, he noticed an increase in saliva secretion even when the animals heard the acoustic stimulus without being given food. These studies were the first to demonstrate that reflex functions of the alimentary tract can be influenced by the central nervous system.

MORE DETAILS   Various other hormones possibly control saliva secretion. These include parathyroid hormone, calcitonin and aldosterone as well as gastrointestinal hormones such as gastrin or secretin. They can bring about changes in salivary composition and secretion rate.

Suggested reading

Cook DJ. Salivary Secretion in Ruminants. In: von Engelhardt S, Leonhard-Marek G, Breves G, Giesecke D, eds. Ruminant Physiology: Digestion, Metabolism, Growth and Reproduction. Stuttgart: Enke; 1995: 153–170

Cook DJ, van Lennep EW, Roberts ML, Young JA. Secretion by the Major Salivary Glands. In: Physiology of the Gastrointestinal Tract. 3rd ed. New York: Raven Press; 1994: 1061–1118

Kunzelmann K, Schreiber R, Hadorn HB. Bicarbonate in cystic fibrosis. J Cystic Fibrosis 2017; 16: 653–662

Maekawa M, Beauchemin KA, Christensen DA. Effect of Concentrate Level and Feeding Management on Chewing Activities, Saliva Production, and Ruminal pH of Lactating Dairy Cows. J Dairy Sci 2002; 85: 1165–1175

Proctor GB, Carpenter GH. Regulation of salivary gland function by autonomic nerves. Autonomic Neuroscience: Basic and Clinical 2007; 133: 3–18

Reece WO, Erickson HH, Goff JP, Uemura EE, eds. Duke's Physiology of Domestic Animals. 13th ed. Ames: Wiley-Blackwell; 2015

Sjaastad ØV, Sand O, Hove K. Physiology of Domestic Animals. 2nd ed. Oslo: Scandinavian Veterinary Press; 2010

16.2 Enteric nervous system and innervation of the gastrointestinal tract

Helga Pfannkuche, former collaboration: Michael Schemann

ESSENTIALS ✖

All essential gastrointestinal functions such as secretion and motility are controlled by the autonomic nervous system. This control can be extrinsic or intrinsic in origin. In extrinsic control, the relevant nerve cells are located outside the wall of the gastrointestinal tract. The afferent (sensory) parts of extrinsic innervation are known as vegetative afferents, while efferent nerves are supplied by the parasympathetic and sympathetic systems. A special feature of control of the gastrointestinal tract are intrinsic nerve cells in the gastrointestinal wall. These collectively are referred to as the enteric nervous system which is able to generate reflexes and thus control most intestinal functions independent of extrinsic innervation. The extrinsic nerves have the task of coordinating functions of different regions of the gastrointestinal tract and also of synchronising the various functions of the digestive tract with those of other organ systems.

16.2.1 The enteric nervous system

The **enteric nervous system** is an independent, third part of the autonomic nervous system, along with the sympathetic and parasympathetic nervous systems (p.121). It contains the somata of approximately 100 million enteric nerve cells which is about the same as the total number of nerve cells in the spinal cord. The enteric nervous system is a continuous network within the wall of the entire length of the gastrointestinal tract from the oesophagus to the rectum. It is divided, both anatomically and functionally, into two parts. The **myenteric plexus** is located between the longitudinal and circular muscles, and the **submucosal plexus**, as its name implies, is between the mucosa and the circular muscle. Both plexuses consist of ganglia, containing the somata of the nerve cells, and interganglionic fibre strands, which are the axons of those nerve cells. The **myenteric plexus** mainly controls the activity of the **muscles**. The **submucosal plexus** controls various **mucosal functions** such as **secretion** and **absorption**. Both plexuses play a role in regulating **blood flow** and are interconnected within the enteric nervous system. This communication between nerve cells of the two plexuses on controlling effector functions is by the release of excitatory or inhibitory neurotransmitters (**Table 16.4**; **Fig. 16.7**). There are functionally different cell types in the enteric nervous system which regulate the various functions of the intestine (**Fig. 16.6**). Like the central nervous system, the enteric nervous system also has **sensory neurons**, **interneurons**

Nutrition, energy

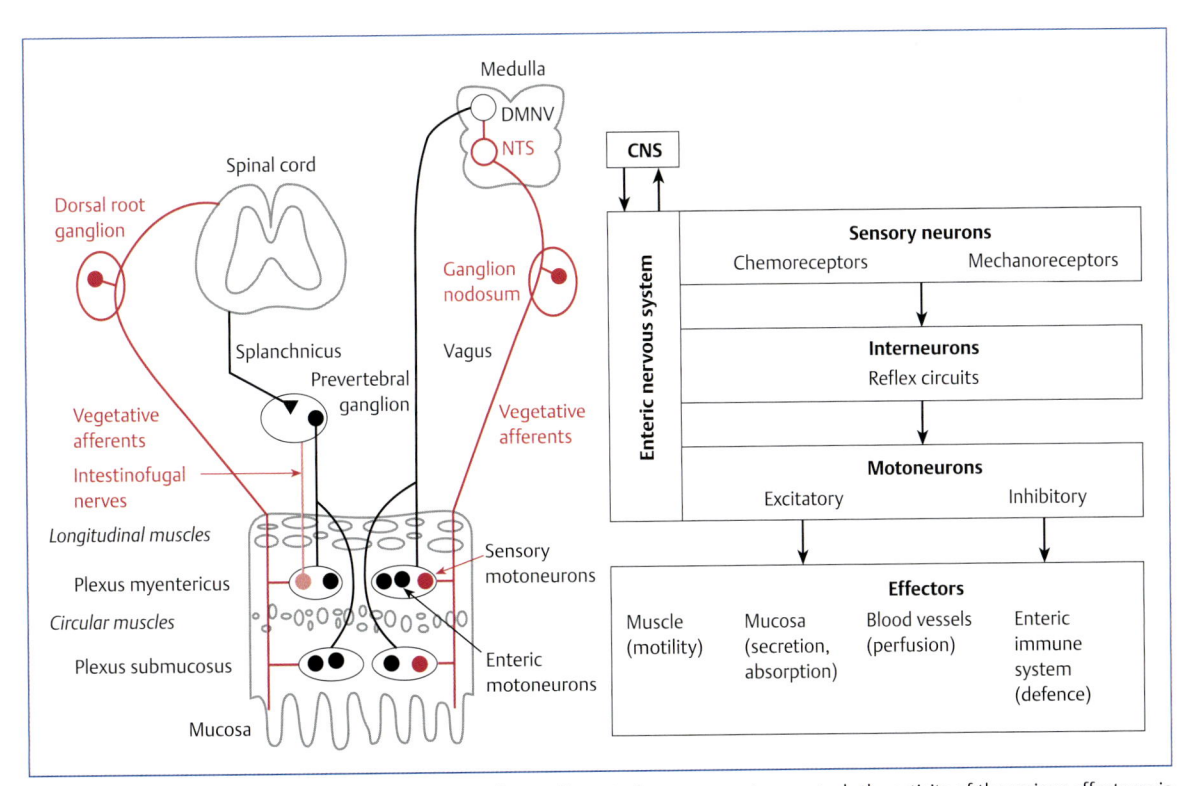

Fig. 16.6 Model of the innervation of the gastrointestinal tract. The enteric nervous system controls the activity of the various effectors via sensory neurons, interneurons and motoneurons. Vegetative afferents run with the sympathetic or parasympathetic nervous system to the central nervous system. In addition, there is an afferent connection through intestinofugal nerves to prevertebral sympathetic ganglia. Efferent feedback takes place via the sympathetic (splanchnic) and parasympathetic nerve (vagus nerve).
DMNV = dorsal motor nucleus of the vagus nerve; NTS = nucleus tractus solitarius.

and **motoneurons**. These neuron types run fixed programmes (reflex circuits) according to the particular stimuli acting in the intestine.

MORE DETAILS

Neurochemical coding

In principle, the enteric nervous system can synthesise almost all of the neurotransmitters that are characteristic of the central nervous system (CNS). For communication within the enteric nervous system and for control of the effector systems, there are about 25 different functional transmitters (**Table 16.4**). The enteric nerve cells usually synthesise not just one transmitter, but a particular mixture of transmitters. Depending on the anatomical region and the animal species, the neurochemical code, i.e. the range of transmitters synthesised by the nerve cells, is characteristic for each cell type. From their different neurochemical codes, 30 different populations of enteric nerve cells have been characterised to date, and these operate as sensory neurons, interneurons or motoneurons.

IN A NUTSHELL !

The enteric nervous system is located within the wall of the entire length of the intestinal tract. It controls all the important functions of the intestine such as motility, absorption and secretion.

■ Control of the musculature

The enteric nervous system regulates the musculature of the intestine within the framework of local reflexes. Nerve cells of the **myenteric plexus** are particularly involved in this. The coordination of different regions of the intestine is under the control of central nervous components (p.366). However, local control of the intestinal musculature by myenteric nerve cells is essential for coordination of intestinal motor function. This is particularly noticeable in patients where part of the myenteric plexus was not properly laid down during foetal development. Such **aganglionosis** is characterised by the absence of nerve cell bodies in one region of the myenteric plexus. This absence of nerve cells causes a marked disturbance in the onward transport of chyme, because of local constriction of the intestinal wall in the aganglionotic region, with resultant build up of intestinal contents on the cranial side of the constriction. This demonstrates one of the basal roles of myenteric neurons: to prevent the smooth musculature of the intestine from immediately and persistently contracting when stretched, which would make the intestinal tube impassable. The musculature of the intestine is thus continuously under **inhibitory nervous control** by the myenteric nerve cells.

MORE DETAILS

Lethal white foals

An aganglionosis in the region of the myenteric plexus leads to massive problems in the transit of chyme in the neonatal period. Such aganglionoses are known both in humans and in domestic mammals. In horses, this is the so-called Lethal White Foal Syndrome. This disease is a genetic defect inherited together with the predisposition for a so-called frame overo spotting pattern. Homozygous foals are not pied, but are completely white and die

of intestinal obstruction within a few days after birth. The Lethal White Foal Syndrome is comparable to certain forms of Hirschsprung's disease in humans.

However, maintaining an inhibitory tone of the musculature is not the only task of the myenteric plexus. If we look at an isolated piece of intestine that is no longer innervated by the sympathetic or parasympathetic nervous system, we can observe that the intestinal contents are moved along by caudally directed **contractions**. This **propulsive peristalsis** can be prevented by blocking the enteric nervous system.

The onward movement of intestinal contents, controlled by the enteric nervous system, is called the **peristaltic reflex**. Propulsive peristalsis and antiperistalsis are described in more detail in the chapter on transport movements (p.389).

The primary trigger of the peristaltic reflex is a stretching of the intestinal wall. This is detected by mechanosensitive myenteric nerve cells, which are excited by an increase in wall tension within the muscle layers and/or by the action of shear forces on the mucosal epithelium.

The activated sensory nerve cells of the myenteric plexus can now excite further nerve cell populations. Two functional groups are prominent here: **muscle motoneurons** and **interneurons**.

Muscle motoneurons innervate the longitudinal and circular muscles. The activation of motoneurons that control the **longitudinal musculature** leads to their contraction, so that the intestinal tube shortens at that point. The control of the **circular muscles** by muscle motoneurons is particularly important for the peristaltic reflex. Throughout the gastrointestinal tract, the muscle motoneurons that control the circular muscles are arranged in a particular pattern in the intestinal wall. The somata are located in the myenteric plexus and the axons extend into the muscles they innervate. Motoneurons that stimulate the muscles, i.e. lead to their contraction, have an axon that extends in a **cranial** direction (**ascending neurons**). Neurons that inhibit the circular muscles have an axon that extends in the **caudal** (=anal) direction (**descending neurons**). This type of axonal arrangement is known as the **polarised projection** of neurons (**Fig. 16.8**). Through these polarised projections, the ascending and descending neurons, after a local stimulus, cause the circular muscles cranially of the stimulus to contract and the muscles caudally of the stimulus to relax. This then leads to a further movement of intestinal contents in the caudal direction.

For this "processing" of the stimulus, only sensory neurons and muscle motoneurons are needed. Nevertheless, there are also a large number of **interneurons** in the myenteric plexus which can perform various functions. The interneurons can reinforce the peristaltic reflex by activating additional muscle motoneurons. In addition, interneurons can prepare circuits with ascending and descending neurons during propulsive peristalsis for the "arrival" of the food mass, so that when the food is advanced, the local circuits are more easily excited and thus onward transport of lumen contents is facilitated.

The control mechanisms described here depend on close communication between the enteric nerve cells and also with the musculature. Enteric nerve cells influence their target tissues through the release of inhibitory and excitatory **neurotransmitters** (**Fig. 16.7**). Like the other parts of the autonomic nervous system (p. 112), enteric nerve cells do not form classical synapses, but instead form **varicosities** in the terminal region of the axon. Nevertheless, the nerve cells that are influenced by other enteric neurons are referred to as postsynaptic nerve cells. Probably the most important transmitter of the excitatory neurons is **acetylcholine**. It is synthesised by sensory neurons, excitatory interneurons and excitatory (ascending) muscle motoneurons. Acetylcholine binds to **muscarinic receptors** on the intestinal muscles (M_3) and to **nicotinic receptors** on enteric nerve cells. Inhibitory (descending) muscle motoneurons in the enteric nervous system often use **nitric oxide (NO)** as a transmitter. In addition to acetylcholine and NO, most enteric neurons synthesise a variety of **cotransmitters**. These are not necessarily released together with the primary transmitter (acetylcholine or NO) when the corresponding nerve cells are activated. Often, a stronger activation of the neuron (through a higher frequency of incoming action potentials) is required for the release of the cotransmitters than for the release of the primary transmitter (e.g. acetylcholine or NO). A cotransmitter in many acetylcholine-synthesising neurons is the neuropeptide **substance P**. Its release from the presynaptic neuron occurs during increased activation. Compared to acetylcholine, substance P triggers a prolonged excitatory postsynaptic potential (EPSP (p. 61)) at the postsynaptic neuron or at the muscles. Another neuropeptide, **vasoactive intestinal peptide (VIP)**, is often found in inhibitory muscle motoneurons together with NO.

Although muscle cells in the intestine have receptors for all the important transmitters of the muscle motoneurons, they do not appear to be the only target for modifying motor function. The **interstitial cells of Cajal** (**Fig. 16.9**) are also influenced by myenteric nerve cells. Thus, the rhythmic **slow waves** at their maximum depolarisation can reach the **threshold** for generating action potentials under the influence of excitatory transmitters. The contractions of the intestinal musculature are therefore often controlled by the interstitial cells of Cajal and therefore follow the rhythm of the slow waves.

The peristaltic reflex is based on an interconnection of sensory nerve cells, muscle motoneurons (and interneurons) found along the full length of the intestine. The process of the peristaltic reflex can be seen as a kind of recall of a stored **movement programme**, similar to programmes in the motor nervous system (p. 130) for locomotion (running, jumping, etc.). In addition to the peristaltic reflex, there are other "programmes" that can be called up according to local conditions in the intestine, for example, a "programme" for the initiation of segmentation contractions (p. 389). An important role for the "decision" between segmentation or **propulsive peristalsis** is played by the modulability of sensory neurons in the enteric nervous system. In addition to the mechanosensitive nerve cells

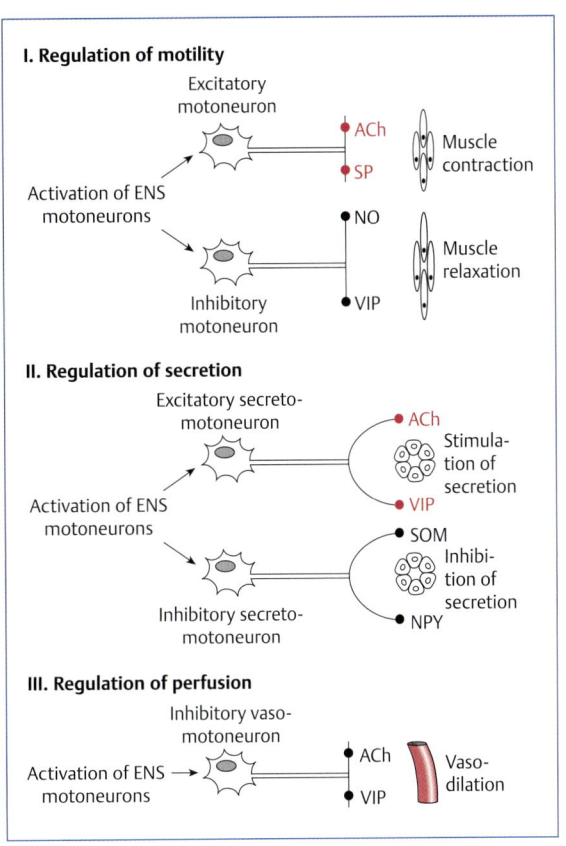

Fig. 16.7 The excitatory and inhibitory effects of the motoneurons, secreto-, and vaso-motoneurons of the enteric nervous system. The motoneurones are in the myenteric plexus, the secreto-motoneurons are in the submucosal plexus, while the vaso-motoneurons are found in both plexuses. Activation of inhibitory or excitatory motoneurons leads to corresponding changes in effector systems such as muscle (**I**), mucosa (**II**) or blood vessels (**III**). Note that motoneurons, even if they secrete identical transmitters, may belong to different populations. Co-localised transmitters often act synergistically, but often have different durations of action.
ACh = acetylcholine; ENS = enteric nervous system; NO = nitric oxide; NPY = neuropeptide Y; SOM = somatostatin; SP = substance P; VIP = vasoactive intestinal peptide.

there are also chemosensitive nerve cells which receive nutrients from the intestinal lumen. These nerve cells are not usually directly excited by nutrients, but by transmitters from **enteroendocrine cells** in the mucosa. In this context, **serotonin (5-HT = 5-hydroxytryptamine)** and **cholecystokinin (CCK)** are particularly important.

The supply of nutrients from the intestinal lumen is essential in determining whether a "segmentation" or a "propulsive peristalsis" programme is initiated. If there is a high level of nutrient supply, the "propulsive peristalsis" programme does not begin, despite a strong mechanical stimulus (stretching of the intestinal wall). Although there is a contraction of the circular musculature at defined points, due to activation of the local muscle motoneurons, a progression of the peristaltic wave, as shown above, is suppressed. A similar situation is conceivable for migrating and stationary contraction groups (p. 389). Inhibition of the onward transport of chyme is probably in response to inhibitory nerve cells becoming activated by secreted me-

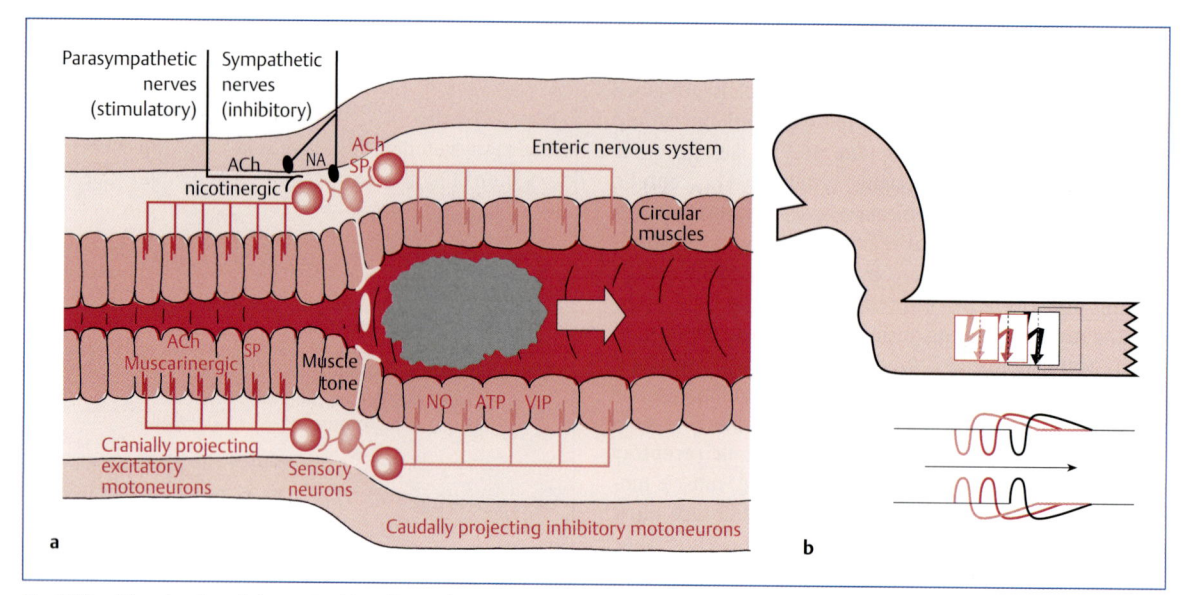

Fig. 16.8 a The circuitry of the peristaltic reflex and its modulation by extrinsic parasympathetic or sympathetic nerves. The peristaltic reflex is based on enteric circuits that are controlled by sympathetic and parasympathetic nerves. The peristaltic reflex is triggered by a bolus that stretches a segment of the intestine, which then increases its tone. The increased wall tension activates a sensory neuron. This activates inhibitory and excitatory muscle motoneurons (for simplicity, interneuron circuitry is not shown). Caudal direction relaxation and cranial direction contraction occur through the polarised projection of the excitatory and inhibitory muscle motoneurons. The axons of the excitatory muscle motoneurons transmit cranially and release acetylcholine (ACh) and substance P (SP). The axons of the inhibitory muscle motoneurons project caudally and secrete nitric oxide (NO) and vasoactive intestinal peptide (VIP).
Reflexes in the enteric nervous system can be modulated by the sympathetic and parasympathetic nervous systems. Activation of the sympathetic nervous system leads to the release of its transmitter noradrenaline (NA) acting presynaptically via α_2 receptors and thus inhibiting the release of acetylcholine. This inhibition exists primarily in the excitatory part of the circuit. Since the activity of the inhibitory neurons remains essentially unchanged, the result is a pronounced inhibition of motor activity. Stimulation of the parasympathetic nervous system leads to the release of its transmitter, acetylcholine (ACh), which activates enteric nerve cells via nicotinic receptors. When excitatory enteric pathways are activated, acetylcholine (ACh) is released from enteric neurons, and muscles then contract.
b Enteric circuits (shown as boxes), consisting of cranially projecting excitatory muscle motoneurons and caudally projecting inhibitory muscle motoneurons, are strung along the gastrointestinal tract like a string of pearls. The components of the circuits are shown in **a**. Sequential activation results in propulsion of the contents in a caudal direction (bottom right, black arrow). The basis of the propulsion is the contraction-relaxation cycle triggered by the peristaltic reflex.

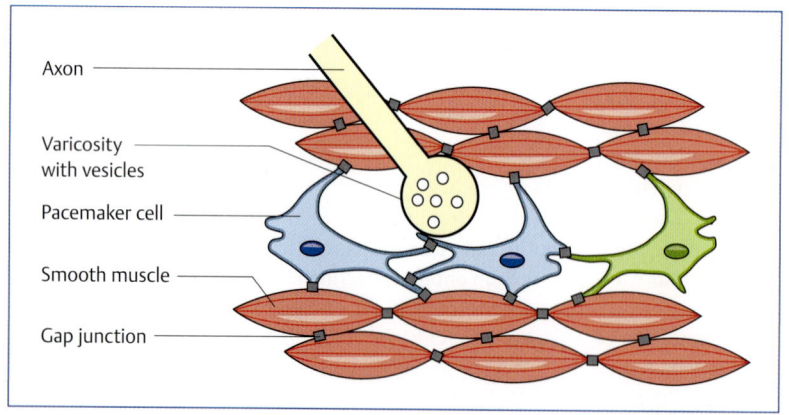

Fig. 16.9 Schematic representation of the interaction between nerve endings of the enteric nervous system, pacemaker cells (Cajal cells and PDGFRα^+ cells; symbolised by different colours) and smooth muscle in the gastrointestinal tract. The pacemaker cells are coupled to each other and to smooth muscle cells by gap junctions. There are also gap junctions between neighbouring smooth muscle cells.

diators (e.g. 5-HT or CCK), which inhibit contraction of the musculature. The coordination between propulsion or mixing of intestinal contents, related to the nutrients being absorbed, prevents intestinal contents from being propelled onwards too rapidly, before sufficient time has elapsed for the digestion and absorption of nutrients. However, if the caloric density of the digesting food is low, then the food mass is propelled onward more rapidly.

MORE DETAILS

Postoperative ileus

For the peristaltic reflex to be triggered, it is crucial that increased wall tension is generated at the site of stretching through reflex-controlled increase in muscle tone. However, pathological **hyperactivity** of the **inhibitory system** can cause relaxation to such an extent that the intestine becomes atonic. In extreme cases, complete paralysis of the intestine occurs, a condition in which the peristaltic reflex can no longer be triggered because the sensors do not register an increase in wall tension even when the intestine is severely stretched. This occurs, for example, in postoperative ileus, where **intestinal atony** is a consequence of disproportionately increased activity of inhibitory enteric nerve cells or an excessively high sympathetic tone. Such an overactivation of the inhibitory systems can be caused by mechanical manipulation of the intestine during surgery. The accompanying activation of the enteric immune system further aggravates the symptoms. In contrast, pathological **hyperactivity** of the **excitatory system** leads to accelerated transport which can contribute to **diarrhoea**.

> **IN A NUTSHELL** !
>
> Nerve cells of the myenteric plexus control the muscles by releasing excitatory and inhibitory neurotransmitters. A polarised arrangement of the nerve cells enables the onward transport of the digesting food mass.

■ Control of epithelial functions

Nerve cells of the **submucosal plexus** are mainly responsible for the control of epithelial functions. These nerve cells innervate the epithelium and also communicate closely with the myenteric nerve cells, which allows motor function, secretion and absorption to be coordinated. The nerve cells that directly innervate the epithelium are called **secreto-motoneurons**. In addition, sensory nerve cells and interneurons are also found in the submucosal plexus, similar to the myenteric plexus, which partly connect the two plexuses. Like the muscle motoneurons, the secreto-motoneurons also control their target tissue (the epithelium) through inhibitory and excitatory neurotransmitters, the most important of which are **acetylcholine** and **VIP**. Both of these are excitatory in the epithelium and have a pro-secretory effect, i.e. they increase the **secretion** of **chloride** into the intestinal lumen and consequently also the secretion of **water**. VIP therefore has a completely different function in the epithelium than in smooth muscles, where it has an important inhibitory role. Acetylcholine and VIP stimulate chloride secretion by different mechanisms. Acetylcholine binds to epithelial cells, mainly at M_3 receptors, which causes an increase in intracellular calcium concentration. In contrast, the binding of VIP to its specific receptors causes an increase in the intracellular cAMP level. In addition to these pro-secretory transmitters, there are also transmitters that inhibit secretion like **neuropeptide Y (NPY)** and **somatostatin**.

Activation of the secreto-motoneurones can be by different mechanisms. An important one of these is the secretion of mediators such as serotonin (5-HT) by enteroendocrine cells in the intestinal epithelium in response to absorbed nutrients. Also mechanical stimuli, such as those triggering the peristaltic reflex, provoke increased secretion in the epithelium. Furthermore, **bacterial** or **viral toxins** and various **inflammatory mediators** can also activate the secreto-motoneurones. Under such pathophysiological conditions, there is a surge in secretion of VIP from the nerve endings, which causes a strong secretory response by the epithelial cells which disperses pathogens in the intestinal lumen.

At the same time as increased secretion, there is also an increase in **local blood supply** to epithelium with intensive metabolic activity. **Vasodilator neurons** in the **submucosal plexus** are responsible for this local **vasodilation**. As with the secreto-motoneurons, there is also a group of vasodilator neurons that use acetylcholine, and another group that use VIP as a neurotransmitter. In addition to this local control of vasomotor function by the enteric nervous system, there is also control of vasomotor function by vegetative afferents (p. 119) in the intestine.

> **IN A NUTSHELL** !
>
> Mucosal functions are controlled by nerve cells in the submucosal plexus. Secretion is stimulated by excitatory secreto-motoneurons, the activity of which is aligned with local motor activity and with blood flow.

■ Neuro-immune interactions

The intestinal epithelium is an animal's largest contact surface with its environment. Consequently, it is also exposed to high levels of ingested antigens. The intestine has a well-developed immune system. This communicates intensively with the enteric nervous system and also with other parts of the autonomic nervous system. Through these communication links, local defence mechanisms can be strengthened, and the intestinal barrier can be maintained even after the penetration of antigens.

Antigens activate cells of the intestinal immune system. These immune cells secrete pro-secretory mediators such as **histamine**, **prostaglandins** or **leukotrienes**, which stimulate epithelial cells directly. These immunological mediators also activate enteric secreto-motoneurons (p. 365) as well as the muscle motoneurons of the myenteric plexus.

The functional significance of these processes lies in the fact that luminal toxins are greatly diluted by antigen-induced stimulation of secretion and pass along the intestinal tract more quickly due to increased motility. The enterotoxic effects of many **bacterial toxins** are by excessive activation of neuro-immune interactions. Thus, it is known that the pro-secretory and motility-increasing effects of **cholera toxin**, *Clostridium difficile* **toxin A**, **heat-stable toxins** of *Escherichia coli* and *Salmonella typhimurium*, are all partly mediated by their interaction with the enteric nervous system. The primary agents of this cascade are, on the one hand, inflammatory mediators released locally by the defence mechanisms. On the other hand, the bacterial enterotoxins also increase cAMP and/or cGMP levels in the tissue, which leads to a massive secretion of serotonin from enterochromaffin cells. Serotonin then activates pro-secretory enteric pathways. See more in ch. „Infectious diarrhoea (p. 447)".

> **IN A NUTSHELL** !
>
> Interactions between the enteric nervous system and the intestinal immune system activate mechanisms that often lead to increased secretion.

Table 16.4 Neuron populations in the gastrointestinal tract.

	Nerve type	Transmitter	Effects
Extrinsic	Parasympathetic nervous system	Acetylcholine	Activation of inhibitory and excitatory enteric nerves via nicotinic receptors
	Sympathetic nervous system	Norepinephrine	1. Presynaptic inhibition of acetylcholine release from enteric neurons (presynaptic α_2 receptors)
			2. Direct postsynaptic inhibition of enteric neurons (postsynaptic α_2 receptors)
	Afferents (extrinsic sensors)	Substance P Calcitonin gene-related peptide	Activation of enteric neurons, increased blood flow, secretion and motility
Intrinsic	Enteric sensory neurons	Acetylcholine	Activation of enteric neurons via nicotinic receptors
		Substance P	Activation of enteric neurons
	Enteric interneurons	Acetylcholine	Activation of enteric neurons via nicotinic receptors
		Substance P	Activation of enteric neurons
		Somatostatin	Inhibition of enteric neurons
	Enteric excitatory muscle motoneurons	Acetylcholine	Activation of the muscle cell via muscarinic receptors
		Substance P	Activation of the muscle cell
	Enteric inhibitory muscle motoneurons	Nitric oxide (NO)	Inhibition of the muscle cell via NO-induced increase in cGMP level
		Vasoactive intestinal peptide	Inhibition of the muscle cell
	Enteric excitatory secreto-motoneurons	Acetylcholine	Activation of the epithelial cell via muscarinic receptors
		Vasoactive intestinal peptide	Activation of the epithelial cell
	Enteric inhibitory secreto-motoneurones	Neuropeptide Y	Inhibition of the epithelial cell
		Somatostatin	
	Enteric vaso-motoneurones	Acetylcholine	Relaxation of blood vessels via muscarinic receptors
		Vasoactive intestinal peptide	Relaxation of the blood vessels

16.2.2 Interactions between central nervous system and enteric nervous system

The enteric nervous system can regulate, locally and independently, the functions of the musculature and the mucosal epithelium in the intestine. However, since the sensory nerve cells of the enteric nervous system only receive information from a small section of the intestine, that system is not able to coordinate the activity of more widely separated regions of the intestine or to adapt the activity of the digestive tract to the situation in the whole animal. These functions are performed by the other parts of the **autonomic nervous system** (sympathetic, parasympathetic, vegetative afferents), which receive information from other organ systems through their connection with the brain. A typical example of higher-level central regulation is the reduced activity of the gastrointestinal tract when there is high sympathetic tone.

■ Vegetative afferents and intestinofugal neurons

Information from the gastrointestinal tract is transmitted to the central nervous system by means of vegetative afferents. Parameters that are received are the luminal concentrations of various nutrients, luminal pH, osmolarity and the degree of wall tension in the gastrointestinal tract. The vegetative afferents (p. 119) run with the vagus nerve or the splanchnic nerve. Those in the vagus nerve are axons of bipolar sensory nerve cells located in the **ganglion nodosum**. The centrally oriented fibres of the bipolar nerve cells run to the **nucleus tractus solitarii** (NTS), where the first interconnection of the "vagal afferents" takes place. Nerve cells of the NTS project to the nearby **dorsal motor nucleus** of the **vagus nerve** (DMNV), where the wiring to efferent vagal fibres occurs.

Another part of the autonomic afferent nerve fibres runs with the sympathetic **splanchnic nerve**. The sensory nerve cells are located in the **posterior root ganglion**. The centrally oriented fibres of the posterior root ganglion terminate in the **spinal cord**. There, the signals are synaptically transmitted further to **thalamic regions**. The efferent motor pathways of these sensory nerve fibres run in the splanchnic nerve.

In addition to the autonomic afferents, there are also sensory neurons in the enteric nervous system, the axons of which pass from the intestine to prevertebral sympathetic ganglia. These nerve cells are called **intestinofugal neurons**. Their particular importance is for reception of mechanical stimuli in the colon and rectum.

There appears to be two ways of perceiving mechanical stimuli in the intestine. One of these is by vegetative afferents and the other is by intestinofugal neurons. However, intestinofugal neurons detect stretching of the intestinal wall in a circular direction and thus pass on information about the filling state of the posterior intestinal segments. Through their synaptic transmission to efferent sympathetic fibres in the prevertebral ganglia, stretching of the intestinal wall leads directly to an increase in sympathetic tone and an inhibition of the intestinal musculature.

The vegetative afferents, on the other hand, perceive the wall tension in the intestine which is influenced by both the degree of filling and by the contraction of the circular muscles. They have a higher stimulus threshold and are also involved in the reception of pain-inducing noxious stimuli in the intestine. From their projections into the central parts of the autonomic nervous system, the autonomic afferents are particularly involved in the circuits for coordinating the activity of different parts of the intestine.

In addition to their sensory, i.e. afferent function, the vegetative afferents also have an **efferent function**. Before the vegetative afferents leave the intestinal wall in the direction of the brain, they form branches within the intestinal wall, so-called **axon collaterals**. If signals are transmitted along the vegetative afferents to the brain, these axon collaterals are also activated and release transmitters locally in the intestinal wall. Thus, these sensory nerve fibres are not governed by a strict one-way principle. Rather, with the help of these axon collaterals, they also take on local efferent functions. This phenomenon is also known as the **axon reflex**. It is not only specific to the gastrointestinal tract, but is also involved in the control of many other organ systems. The substances released locally in the gastrointestinal wall are usually neuropeptides such as **substance P** and **calcitonin gene-related peptide**. Although such **axon reflexes** regulate the activities of all effectors in the intestinal wall, they play a particularly important role in the regulation of **blood flow**. Activation of the efferent function of these afferents leads to increased blood flow and thus allows, for example, the rapid removal of harmful substances.

■ Effects of the parasympathetic nervous system

Activation of the parasympathetic nervous system has a stimulating effect on the activity of the gastrointestinal tract, which is largely innervated parasympathetically via the vagus. However, only a few thousand efferent **vagus fibres** innervate the gastrointestinal tract. This means that there are too few vagus fibres available for direct innervation of the muscles or the mucosa to influence them effectively. The vagus fibres therefore are directed to enteric nerve cells and thus use enteric pathways as intermediate amplifiers (**Fig. 16.8**).

The efferent vagus fibres are cholinergic and on activation release **acetylcholine**, which activates all downstream enteric nerve cells via **cholinergic nicotinic receptors**. **Activation** of the **vagus** leads to increased secretion in the gastrointestinal tract. This can be explained by the vagus fibres responsible for secretion activating enteric circuits having a pro-secretory effect. However, the vagus can have both an excitatory and an inhibitory effect on the activity of the muscles. This differentiated influence on muscle activity is achieved by some vagus fibres activating excitatory nerve cells, while other vagus fibres activate inhibitory nerve cells. The excitatory enteric nerves secrete acetylcholine at the neuromuscular junctions and activate the muscle cells via muscarinic receptors. Inhibition of the musculature is by the release of the transmitters NO or VIP from enteric nerve cells.

Classical examples of parasympathetically mediated reflexes are the **receptive relaxation** of the stomach during filling (inhibitory (p. 382) reflex) or increased acid secretion when it is distended (excitatory (p. 413) reflex). More complex reflexes such as activation of various motor components during **vomiting** are also vagally mediated.

MORE DETAILS

Pathological changes in parasympathetic tone

A pathologically **increased parasympathetic tone** leads to increased motor activity and can trigger spasmodic contractions. Successful treatment of these contractions can in some cases be achieved by blocking muscarinic receptors. However, hypermotor activity often has other primary causes and the elimination of muscarinic mechanisms is a symptomatic rather than a causal treatment.

In addition to its classical role, the parasympathetic nervous system also has **anti-inflammatory actions**. Activation of this **cholinergic-nicotinergic anti-inflammatory signalling pathway** begins with a vagally mediated increased release of acetylcholine, which inhibits the release of pro-inflammatory cytokines from macrophages via nicotinic receptors. It is likely that the enteric nervous system is also involved here as a transmission point between the vagus nerve and macrophages.

A pathologically **low parasympathetic tone** rarely has dramatic consequences in monogastric animals. A total failure of the parasympathetic system can be quickly balanced by the enteric nervous system after a short period of adaptation. In ruminants, on the other hand, the motor activity of the **forestomachs** is very strongly dependent on parasympathetic activation. A lack of vagal tone as a result of functional vagus lesions ("vagus indigestion") leads to more or less pronounced paralysis of the forestomachs. An additional constriction of the sphincters leads to abomasal reflux and an accumulation of contents in the rumen which cannot be transported further because of the atony. Additional inflammatory processes damage visceral afferents which run as extrinsic sensory fibres together with the vagus. As a result, stretch-induced reflexes can no longer be initiated, which further aggravates functional atony. Since the forestomachs of ruminants also have a functionally fully developed enteric nervous system, it is unclear why the enteric nervous system in the ruminant stomach cannot compensate for a failure of extrinsic innervation. The most likely explanation is that enteric reflex circuits, due to their more local projections, are unable to coordinate the motility of distant compartments.

■ Effects of the sympathetic nervous system

Sympathetic nerves usually do not directly influence effectors in the intestinal wall, but use enteric circuits (**Fig. 16.8**). This is especially true for muscle and mucosal activity. In contrast, blood vessels in the gastrointestinal tract are innervated directly by sympathetic fibres. Muscle and mucosal activity are inhibited by activation of sympathetic fibres because the norepinephrine released binds to α_2 receptors on nerves located pre- or postsynaptically.

Presynaptic inhibition (p.63) predominates in the **myenteric plexus**, where **α_2 receptors** are mainly on cholinergic synapses. Activation of these receptors by noradrenaline **inhibits acetylcholine release** at both the **interneuronal synapse** and the **neuromuscular junction** (**Fig. 16.8**). This blocks the activating effect of the excitatory muscle motoneurons, while the activity of the inhibitory muscle motoneurons remains largely unaffected. **Pre- and postsynaptic inhibitory α_2 receptors** in the **submucosal plexus** are responsible for inhibiting secretion. Here, α_2 receptors are also located directly on excitatory **secreto-motoneurons**, which hyperpolarise after receptor activation. These secreto-motoneurons are thereby put into an unexcitable state and no longer release transmitters with a pro-secretory effect.

In addition to the indirect action of the sympathetic nervous system through inhibition of enteric nerve cells, there are also some direct targets for sympathetic fibres in the gastrointestinal tract. Thus, through the binding of noradrenaline to β receptors on the gastric chief cells, pepsinogen secretion (p.414) is stimulated. Furthermore, noradrenaline causes contraction of sphincters in the gastrointestinal tract by binding to α_1 receptors on the smooth muscle cells. Functionally, however, this effect also represents an inhibition, since, for example, the constriction of the pylorus slows down gastric emptying.

> **MORE DETAILS**
>
> **Pathological changes in sympathetic tone**
>
> A pathologically **increased sympathetic tone** leads to strong inhibition of motor activity and secretion. If this inhibition persists over a long period of time, a paralytic ileus can occur, and the gastrointestinal tract becomes atonic. Increased sympathetic tone, along with disturbances in the ENS, is probably one of the causes of **intestinal atony and disturbed peristalsis** in equine **grass sickness**.
>
> The increased sympathetic tone is not responsible for stress-associated symptoms such as **diarrhoea**. The exact mechanisms of these stress-induced changes in the gastrointestinal tract are largely unknown. However, it is suspected that the **intestinal immune system** is involved which, after sensitisation, releases substances that lead to hypersecretion. The sensitisation of the intestinal immune system probably occurs via **vegetative afferent fibres**, which activate immune cells through massive release of their transmitter substances.

> **IN A NUTSHELL** !
>
> The central nervous system receives information from the intestine via vegetative afferents. The activity of different parts of the intestine can be influenced by both the parasympathetic and sympathetic nervous system. This influence is mainly by pre- and postsynaptic modulation of enteric pathways.

Suggested reading

Costa M, Brookes SH. Architecture of enteric neural circuits involved in intestinal motility. Eur Rev med pharmacol Sci 2008; Suppl. 1: 3–19

Wood JD. Enteric nervous system: reflexes, pattern generators and motility. Curr opin gastroenterol 2008; 24: 149–158

16.3 Gastrointestinal motility

16.3.1 General functions and characteristics of the gastrointestinal motor system

Martin Diener, Jörg R. Aschenbach

> **ESSENTIALS**
>
> The motor system of the gastrointestinal tract ensures that nutrients from food are transported in a coordinated manner to the separate, highly specialised regions of the gastrointestinal tract. The food is mixed with secretions of the digestive glands of the stomach and intestine. Undigested and digested nutrients are brought into contact with the gastrointestinal mucosal cells to be absorbed.
>
> In general, motor activity is under intrinsic control of intestinal pacemaker cells, intramural neural circuits and paracrine messengers. However, individual motor functions are mainly under extrinsic control by higher-level regulatory centres, such as control of forestomach motility of ruminants, and defecation and vomiting. The process of defecation removes indigestible food residues while vomiting prevents the absorption of potentially harmful substances from food.

An important task of the gastrointestinal tract is the **movement** of **contents along the gastrointestinal tract (GIT)**. This transport must be well regulated so that sufficient time is available for digestion and absorption processes in different regions of the gastrointestinal tract. Regarding motility, the GIT segments either have a predominant **reservoir function** or they are mainly concerned with the **movement** of **food** along the tract. Reservoirs have various roles supported by slow or mixing motor functions. One role is early **storage** of **larger amounts** of **food** (pregastrically: e.g. forestomachs, crop/ within the stomach: "proximal" part), to allow discontinuous feed intake. A longer stay in such storage structures with good mixing and slightly acidic pH values also promotes **microbial fermentation** (forestomachs, large intestine), whereby fibrous carbohydrates can become a source of nutrients. Furthermore, stationary or slow motor function is important for the absorption of water and electrolytes, to prevent their loss in faeces from the end of the digestive tract.

The aboral ("distal") stomach and the small intestine can be regarded as regions with mainly transport functions

The mean **retention time** of food components in the gastrointestinal tract varies greatly. In general, it is lower for liquids than for solid food components. Carnivores such as dogs, adapted to diets of highly digestible food, have a relatively short gastrointestinal tract, with fast transit times of about one day for solid food (**Table 16.5**). In herbivores, the transit time may be as long as several days and the relative length of the gastrointestinal tract is considerably greater, with either an upstream (forestomachs of ruminants) or downstream (colon of horses or caecum of rabbits) fermentation chamber. From the short transit time in omnivores and carnivores it follows that large meals can be digested and absorbed in about twelve hours, with periods of time when the stomach and small intestine are largely empty. This extensive emptying of the stomach and small intestine depends on powerful cleansing contractions, which either have the character of relatively rapid strong contractions (especially carnivores), completely emptying the stomach and small intestine, or as slowly migrating motor complexes (MMC) starting in the stomach and running distally along the length of the small intestine.

Consequently, a distinction must be made between **digestive motor activity** occurring after food intake and **interdigestive motor activity** occurring during the resting period of digestion. The interdigestive motor activity has a cleansing function to prevent microbial colonisation in the small intestine. Since herbivores feed relatively continuously, there is an overlap of digestive and interdigestive motor functions in the small intestine. The cleansing or emptying of the large intestine is also linked to food intake and is promoted by so-called long reflexes (p.392) as the stomach fills.

> ### IN A NUTSHELL !
>
> In the gastrointestinal tract, there are regions with predominantly a reservoir function and regions with predominantly a transport function, and these differ in their motor activity. The motor patterns are also different between the digestive and interdigestive phases.

Table 16.5 Species differences in the structure of the gastrointestinal tract as well as mean retention time of solid food particles in the entire gastrointestinal tract.

Species	Segment	% of total gastro-intestinal capacity	Ratio body length: length of gastrointestinal tract	Mean retention time of solid particles in the gastrointestinal tract
Horse	Stomach	9	1:12	25 h (hay) 94 h (pellets)
	Small intestine	30		
	Large intestine	61		
Cattle	Forestomach and stomach	71	1:20	55 h (hay)
	Small intestine	18		
	Large intestine	11		
Pig	Stomach	30	1:14	48 h (hay + grain)
	Small intestine	33		
	Large intestine	37		
Dog	Stomach	62	1:6	22 h (canned food)
	Small intestine	23		
	Large intestine	15		
Cat	Stomach	69	1:4	26 h (canned food)
	Small intestine	15		
	Large intestine	16		

Based on data from Argenzio RA. General functions of the gastrointestinal tract and their control. In: Reece WO (ed.). Dukes' Physiology of Domestic Animals. 12th ed. London: Cornell University Press; 2004, 381–390

Nutrition, energy

The smooth muscles of the gastrointestinal tract have a high degree of autonomy. There are so-called pacemaker cells in the stomach and intestinal wall. These are **interstitial cells of Cajal** (**Fig. 16.9**) in close relationship to the smooth muscle cells between the longitudinal and circular muscles in the submucosa. In the Cajal cells, spontaneous oscillations of cytosolic Ca^{2+} concentration occur (see ch.6.3.2 (p.161) and ch. 16.2.1 (p.361)) which act on Ca^{2+}-dependent Cl^- channels to cause oscillations of the membrane potential which spread to neighbouring smooth muscle cells via gap junctions. These pacemaker potentials are also called **slow waves** because of their relatively low frequency. However, they do not trigger any contractions when they alone act on smooth muscles. Only when additional factors such as an excitatory neurotransmitter are present (e.g. acetylcholine), action potentials develop in smooth muscle cells with consequent contractions (**Fig. 6.17**). Cajal cells also mediate some of the action of neurotransmitters released from the myenteric plexus. They have receptors for excitatory and inhibitory neurotransmitters. Accordingly, not only slow waves, but also the potential changes after transmitter action can spread to smooth muscle cells via gap junctions. Like the Cajal cells, the PDGFRα⁺ cells (fibroblast-like cells that express the platelet-derived growth factor receptor α) are also connected to smooth muscle cells via gap junctions and transmit their potential changes to those cells in response to a transmitter stimulus.

Since there is no electrical coupling between the stomach and the small intestine, the slow waves must be re-initiated in the small intestine. Slow waves occur in the stomach with a frequency of about 3–8 min⁻¹, whereas in the proximal small intestine they have a frequency of 10–20 per minute. In the large intestine, their frequency rate is less, with values similar to the stomach. As well as these differences in frequency, there is also a change in the speed at which electrical excitations are transmitted through the functional syncytium of intestinal smooth muscle. Propagation speed is several cm·s⁻¹ in the duodenum and decreases to values around 0.5 cm·s⁻¹ in the ileum, because of increasing electrical resistance (i.e. poorer electrical cell-cell coupling) in the distal intestinal sections. As a result, peristaltic waves (**Fig. 16.8**) propagate much further in the proximal small intestine before they fade in more distal sections. This slows the onward passage of intestinal contents towards the distal region, and the rate of passage adapts to the decreasing volume from progressive absorption of water and nutrients. Slow waves usually only travel a few centimetres before colliding with another slow wave from a neighbouring intestinal segment.

The intrinsic rhythm of the gastrointestinal muscle cells is modulated by the enteric nervous system (p.361), especially by motoneurons of the myenteric plexus. These motoneurons are influenced by the sympathetic and parasympathetic nervous system, whereby the activity of the

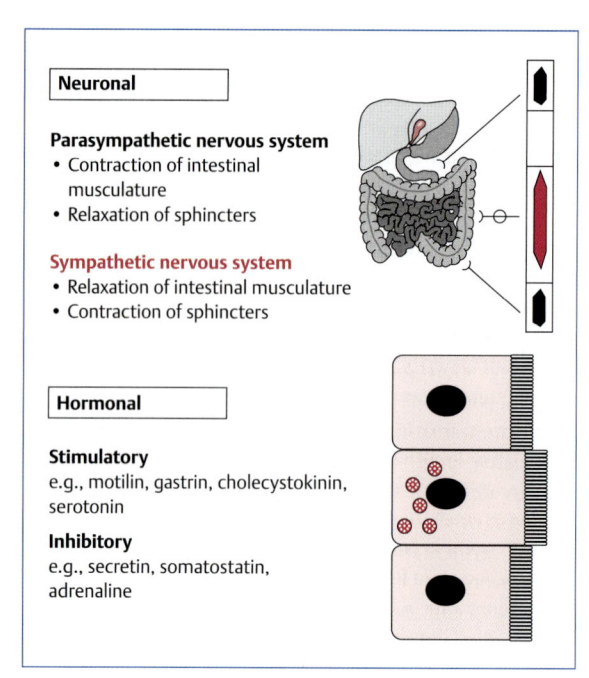

Fig. 16.10 Excitatory and inhibitory influences on intestinal motor function by sympathetic and parasympathetic nervous system and by hormones from enteroendocrine cells.

gastrointestinal tract is adapted to the needs of the whole body (**Fig. 16.10**). The parasympathetic nervous system promotes the activity of the intestinal musculature and increases contractility, i.e. a higher proportion of slow waves are overlaid by action potentials. Sphincters, such as the sphincter ileocaecale, then relax so that onward passage of intestinal contents is maintained. The sympathetic nervous system, in contrast, inhibits the activity of the gastrointestinal musculature when the sphincters are closed, which prevents onwards passage of intestinal contents. Strong sympathetic activations can lead to **intestinal atonia** (i.e. persistent and complete relaxation), since the sympathetic nervous system not only inhibits the enteric motoneurons via α₂ receptors, but also exerts a direct inhibitory influence on the total intestinal musculature via β₂ receptors on the myocytes.

In addition to the autonomic nervous system, a large number of hormones, especially those from enteroendocrine cells, i.e. the hormone-producing cells of the gastrointestinal tract, act on smooth muscles (**Fig. 16.10**).

IN A NUTSHELL   !

The motor function of the gastrointestinal tract is controlled by several regulatory systems: myogenic by pacemaker cells, neuronal by the enteric, sympathetic and parasympathetic nervous systems, and by paracrine and endocrine hormones.

16.3.2 Ruminant forestomach motor function and ingesta passage

Gemma Mazzuoli-Weber, Kristin Elfers;
former collaboration: M. Kaske

ESSENTIALS ✖

The forestomachs of ruminants form a fermentation chamber before the stomach proper. Ruminants have a symbiotic relationship with forestomach microorganisms that have the ability to digest otherwise indigestible cellulose-rich feeds (grasses). This process requires not only a long retention time of feed in the forestomachs, but also a large capacity of this compartment. Digestion of feed is facilitated by intensive rumen motility, regulated by an innate, complex reflex circuit. This motility also serves to homogenously mix the contents of the forestomach which promotes microbial fermentation.

The ingested feed of ruminants is regurgitated for further oral mastication for several hours each day. Regular contraction sequences of the different parts of the reticulum and rumen thoroughly mixes the contents, and the gases of fermentation are released by eructation. After it is mainly digested, the residual feed leaves the rumen through the reticulo-omasal orifice into the omasum and abomasum. The motor function of the reticulum controls the selective retention of particles ("sorting function") for further digestion in the rumen. Regulation of the forestomach motor function is by vagovagal reflexes from a reflex centre in the brain stem. New-born ruminants are functionally monogastric animals because the milk they drink enters the abomasum directly by the reticular groove reflex.

■ Introduction

The digestive strategy of Ruminantia has proven to be very successful in the course of evolution. Representatives of the three most important Ruminantia families Bovidae (e.g. cattle, sheep, goats, antelopes), Cervidae (e.g. roe deer, elk) and Giraffidae (e.g. giraffe, okapi) have colonised almost all climatic regions of the world with a total of 158 species.

During evolution, ruminants have developed a microbial fermentation chamber before the actual stomach, which ensures particularly efficient use of grasses as a feed source. Older grasses are poor quality feed due to their low protein and high fibre content (cellulose, hemicellulose and lignin). This evolutionary adaptation enables ruminants to digest parts of plant food that are largely indigestible by monogastric animals. The anatomical organisation of the gastrointestinal tract of modern ruminants is the result of an evolutionary adaptation to **cellulose-rich feed**. The β-glycosidic bond of glucose monomers in the cellulose molecule cannot be cleaved by mammals because they lack endogenous cellulolytic enzymes. Ruminants have therefore developed a fermentation chamber with the forestomach system (p. 395), in which bacteria, protozoa and fungi break down the feed under anaerobic conditions. The complete **hydrolysis** of the **cell wall components** requires the synergistic interaction of numerous microbial enzymes and proceeds **slowly**. The efficiency of digestion thus depends on the time the ingesta remain exposed to the microorganisms. The superiority of ruminants in the utilisation of cellulose-rich feed, compared to monogastric herbivores, is particularly because of the **long retention time** of ingesta in the forestomach system. Ruminants can thus largely compensate for the disadvantage of the slow degradation of the cell wall components. Microorganisms in the forestomach ecosystem use food ingested by the host and in return supply energy in the form of short-chain fatty acids.

The particular conditions in the forestomachs favour microbial fermentation with bacterial cellulose cleavage enzyme activity being optimal at 39 °C. However, because of high heat generation by fermentation, effective temperature regulation is required. Furthermore, the fall in pH from the acidic products of fermentation (short-chain fatty acids) must be prevented by buffering. This is achieved by buffers in the voluminous saliva produced by ruminants (**Table 16.1**) and by the rapid absorption directly through the rumen mucosa of microbial products, especially acetic, propionic and butyric acids (see ch. Absorption of short-chain fatty acids (p. 401) and ch. Absorption of N-containing compounds (p. 403)). This avoids accumulation of fermentation products, which would severely disturb the ecosystem of the forestomachs.

Foregut motility enables continuous mixing of the ingesta, expulsion of the rumen fermentation gases (especially CO_2, CH_4, and also H_2, H_2S, see ch. Microbial metabolic processes/Carbohydrates (p. 398)), the return of food to the mouth during rumination, and the passage of largely digested particles into the omasum. Motility also promotes the absorption of short-chain fatty acids and the buffering effect of saliva through its homogeneous distribution in the rumen.

IN A NUTSHELL !

The symbiosis of ruminants with microorganisms ensures efficient use of cellulose-rich feed.

■ Functional anatomy of the forestomach system

Anatomically, the forestomachs comprise the **reticulum** (syn. honeycomb), **rumen** (syn. paunch) and **omasum** (syn. manyplies). The **forestomach system** of domestic ruminants is extraordinarily **voluminous** and occupies the entire left abdominal cavity from the diaphragm to the pelvic cavity. The rumen has the largest volume (about 80 % of the total volume of the forestomachs). The reticulum lies cranially in the diaphragmatic dome and its mucosa forms a honeycomb network of quadrangular to hexagonal cells, with small mucosal folds and papillae at their base. These structures are important for segregation processes of the ingesta. The reticulum is separated from the rumen atrium by the rumino-reticular fold. The **reticulum** and **rumen** form a single functional **unit** and are therefore also called the **reticulorumen**.

An important prerequisite for effective microbial fermentation processes is the constant, intensive **mixing** of ingesta in the reticulorumen. Contractions of the smooth muscles of the forestomach wall would not be sufficient for this because of the large volume, so contractions of the rumen pillars, which project as strong muscular ridges into the lumen, enable vigorous mixing of the ingesta in the forestomachs. The rumen is divided into compartments by cranial and caudal rumen pillars, coronal pillars and left and right longitudinal pillars. These compartments are the rumen atrium, dorsal and ventral rumen sac and the ventral and dorsal blind sac. As an adaptation to roughage with often sharp, pointed feed components, the rumen **mucosa** has a **multi-layered, keratinised epithelium**, which histologically shows some similarities to the epidermis of skin. Nevertheless, large quantities of a wide variety of digestion products are absorbed in the reticulorumen, see ch. Absorption of short-chain fatty acids (p. 401), ch. Absorption of N-containing compounds (p. 403) and ch. Transport processes for minerals in the rumen (p. 405). To facilitate this, there is a considerable **increase in mucosal surface area** from numerous **papillae**, especially in the ventral rumen sac and rumen atrium. The blood supply to the highly vascularised forestomach system comes from the coeliac artery. The venous blood first enters the liver via the portal vein and then reaches the caudal vena cava.

The **reticulo-omasal orifice** forms the anatomical barrier in the passage of ingesta out of the reticulorumen into the omasum and is located medially at the level of the rumino-reticular fold where it merges into the rumen atrium. The reticulo-omasal orifice is surrounded by the two muscular ridges of the **reticular groove**, which spiral caudoventrally from the dorsally located cardia. In calves, reflex closure of the reticular groove (p. 379) allows ingested milk to pass directly into the abomasum, bypassing the reticulorumen.

The **omasum** as the third forestomach has a round to oval shape and lies medial to the reticulum in the intrathoracic space of the abdominal cavity. The many, differently sized mucosal folds ("plies") with numerous papillae provide an enormous increase in surface area, indicative of the large volumes of water absorbed in the omasum.

The pear-shaped **abomasum** corresponds to the glandular stomach of monogastric animals and lies mainly ventral to the omasum and in the right side of the abdomen. It communicates with the omasum via a wide-mouthed omaso-abomasal opening. The abomasal mucosa has large folds in the fundus area becoming smaller towards the pylorus. These mucosal folds prevent the reflux of abomasal contents into the omasum during contractions of the abomasal wall.

> ### IN A NUTSHELL   !
>
> The large volume and the clear compartmentalisation of the forestomach system allow a long retention time of feed particles and thus effective microbial digestion of plant fibre. The increase in the mucosal surface area by papillae enables extensive absorption of digestion products from the forestomachs.

■ Reticulum and rumen motor function

The basic pattern of the reticulorumen motor system is characterised by **regular, stereotyped contraction sequences** that travel successively over the different regions of the **reticulum** and **rumen**. A distinction is made between the so-called A-cycles (syn.: primary or complete cycles) and the B-cycles (syn.: secondary or incomplete cycles) (**Fig. 16.11**).

A-cycles spread from cranial to caudal (**Fig. 16.12**). Each A-cycle first begins with a biphasic contraction of the reticulum, which separates coarser feed components from material that has already been broken into small particles. During this first contraction, the reticulum is compressed

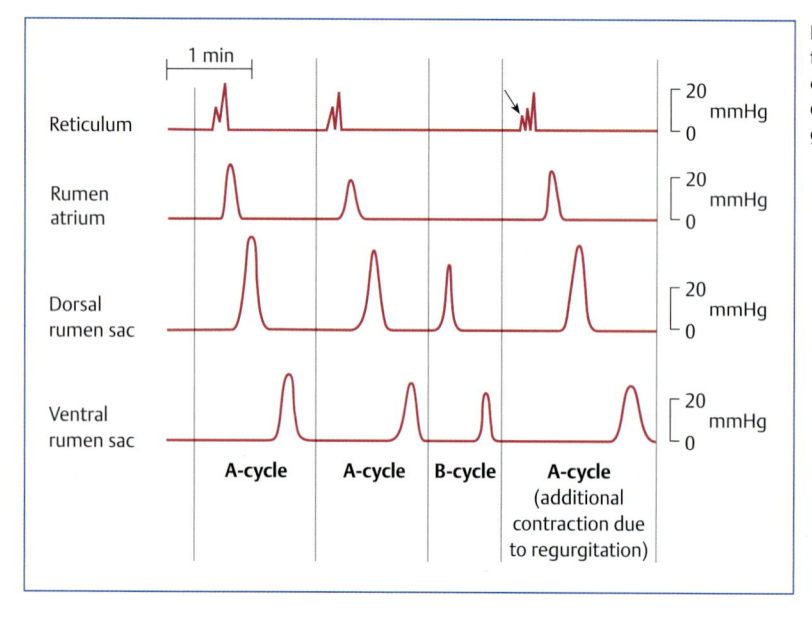

Fig. 16.11 Schematic representation of two A-cycles, one B-cycle and one A-cycle during ruminating with additional (third) contraction of the reticulum due to regurgitation (arrow).

	Time (s)	Sequence of contractions	Schematic drawing	Movement of ingesta
Reticulum First contraction Second contraction	0–2 2–4	The base of the reticulum moves cranio-dorsally; the lumen of the reticulum becomes smaller. After short relaxation, the lumen of the reticulum almost disappears during the second contraction. Opening of the ROO and widening of the omasal canal at maximum of the second reticulum contraction.		Large, light particles get cranio-dorsally; fluid partially flows into rumen atrium. Movement of ingesta into the omasum via ROO
Rumen atrium	6–9	The bottom of the atrium moves dorsally. Reticulum relaxes.		Part of the contents of the forestomach gets back into the relaxed reticulum. Coarse-textured feed is circulated; smaller particles are pressed ventrally; the dorsal gas bubble is pushed cranially (possibly eructation).
Rumen dorsal sac Rumen dorsal blind sac	6–13	Contractions starting cranially and proceeding caudally. At the same time, the pillars of the rumen build a ring and move dorsally.		
Rumen ventral sac Rumen ventral blind sac	20–30	Contractions from cranial to caudal direction; the rumen pillars again contract annularly and move downwards; then the the ventral blind sac contracts.		Fluid with small particles is pressed dorsally and enters the rumen atrium via the cranial rumen pillar.

Fig. 16.12 Individual phases of an A-cycle and effect on the ingesta. ROO = reticulo-omasal orifice. The areas outlined in red are in contraction.

to about half its full size. This is followed by a partial relaxation, immediately after which there is a second reticulum contraction. This is even more powerful than the first and causes the lumen of the reticulum to almost disappear. The contents are squeezed upwards allowing the finely ground and liquid material to flow through the reticulo-omasal orifice, while the coarse material, which has to be chewed again, enters the rumen atrium. This is followed by contraction of the rumen atrium, which leads to a backflow of liquid, largely digested feed via the rumino-reticular fold into the relaxing reticulum. The still coarse, undigested material is pushed by the cranial rumen pillar into the dorsal rumen sac. Now the dorsal rumen sac begins to contract progressively from cranial to caudal. This causes intense mixing of the ingesta. During this process, the rumen pillars form a ring and move dorsally. During the subsequent contractions of the ventral rumen sac and ventral blind sac, the ring of rumen pillars moves ventrally again, allowing fluid to pass cranially through the cranial rumen pillar into the rumen atrium.

B-cycles are also called incomplete cycles, because they do not involve the reticulum or the rumen atrium. They begin with a contraction of the dorsal rumen sac followed by a contraction of the ventral rumen sac (**Fig. 16.11**). During these secondary cycles, the gas phase is pushed dorsally to the cardia, where it reflexively stimulates (p. 379) its release up the oesophagus (eructation).

The rumen contractions and their frequency can be detected by auscultation or palpation in the left paralumbar fossa. A strong crackling sound can be heard, caused by the movement of coarse ingesta particles against the contracting wall of the dorsal rumen sac. In healthy cattle, about three contractions are audible every two minutes, with no discernible difference between A and B cycles. During feed intake, the frequency is almost twice as high. Before feed intake, the ratio between A and B cycles is about 3:1. Immediately after feed intake, each A cycle is usually followed by a B cycle.

> **IN A NUTSHELL** !
>
> The motor system of the reticulum and rumen is characterised by A-cycles and B-cycles. The forestomach motor system enables intensive mixing of the ingesta, the release of rumen gases (eructation), and the regulated onward transport of ingesta from the reticulorumen into the omasum.

Regulation of the reticulorumen motor function

Regulation of the reticulorumen motor function with the largely stereotyped sequences of A and B contractions is controlled by both intrinsic and extrinsic neuronal control mechanisms. Intrinsic neuronal control of motility is through neurons of the myenteric plexus of the enteric

Nutrition, energy

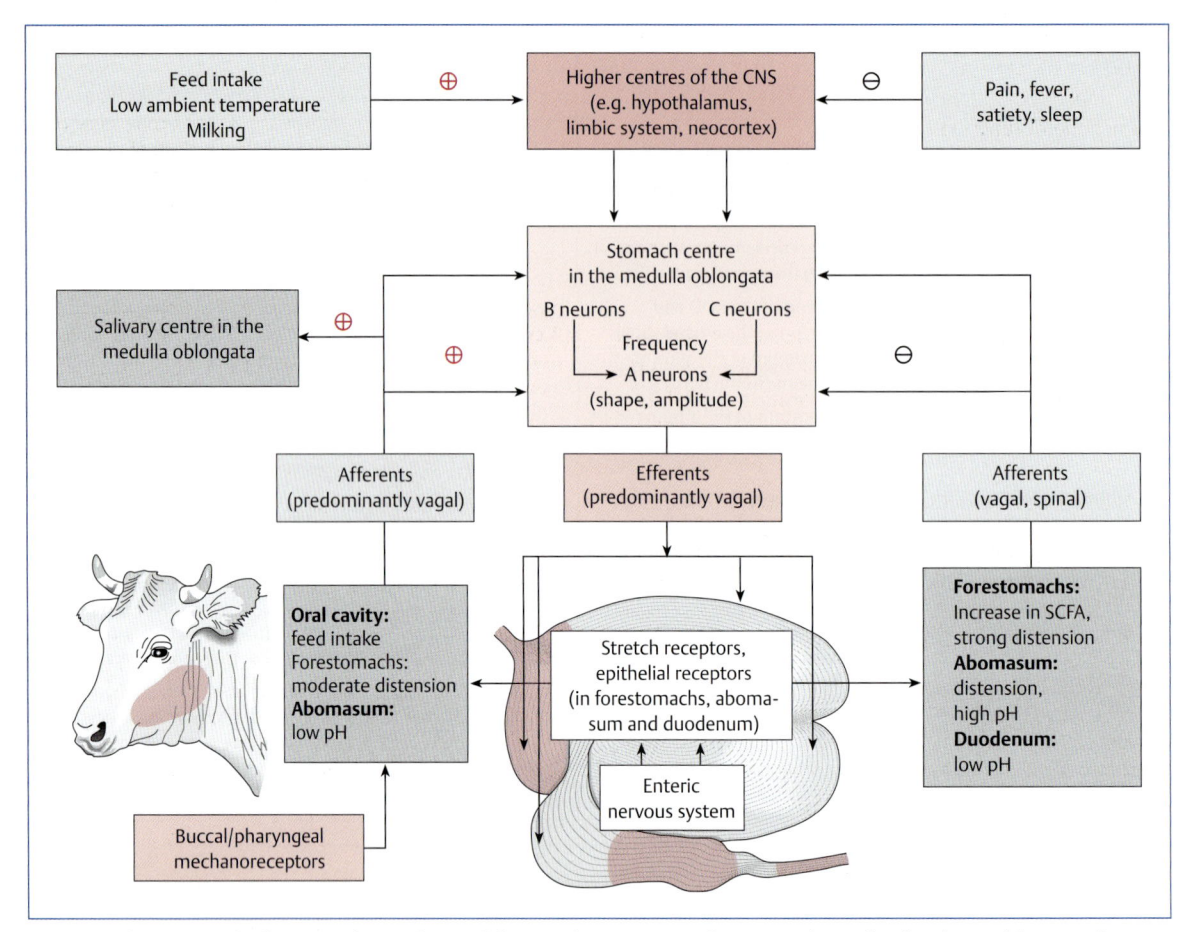

Fig. 16.13 The vagovagal reflex arc in the regulation of the reticulorumen motor function with peripheral and central factors influencing the frequency and amplitude of the contractions. The areas marked in red on the reticulum, abomasum, duodenum and oral cavity are the zones with the highest receptor densities. SCFA = short-chain fatty acids.

nervous system (ENS). These neurons generate specific combinations of excitatory and inhibitory neurotransmitters. However, there is little information about the control of forestomach motility by the ENS. It is thought to have only a modifying influence by local reflex action. The main regulation of reticulorumen motor function is from **extrinsic innervation**. The extrinsic reflex centre is located in the brain stem and vagovagal reflexes are essential in regulating forestomach motor function.

Components of the **reflex arc** which regulates the motor function of the reticulum and rumen are:
- receptors in the oral cavity, in the wall of the forestomachs (especially in the anterior dorsal rumen and in the reticulum), the abomasum and the duodenum,
- afferent nerve fibres that project via the vagus nerve (partly also via the splanchnic nerve),
- a paired, bilateral gastric centre in the medulla oblongata,
- efferent nerve fibres, which run mainly via the vagus nerve,
- innervation of smooth muscle of the forestomach wall.

Receptors in the wall of the reticulum and rumen are the most important for regulating motor function.

Tension receptors are located deep in the smooth musculature. The greatest density of these slow-adapting re-

ceptors is found in the reticulum and in the regions of the cardia, rumino-reticular fold and the cranial rumen pillar (**Fig. 16.13**). These tension receptors respond to passive stretching of the smooth muscle caused by the ingesta as well as by active stretching of the wall during contractions. The field diameter of these receptors is 5–20 mm.

Epithelial receptors are located quite superficially, immediately below the basement membrane of the epithelium, especially in the reticulum and in proximity to the rumen pillars. These receptors adapt rapidly and react to different types of stimuli ("polymodal receptors"). They are mechanosensitive and are thus activated by stretching stimuli, as well as being chemosensitive, responding to changes in the ruminal concentration of short-chain fatty acids.

Both the muscular stretch receptors and the epithelial receptors project via **afferent vagal fibres** to clusters of ganglion cells in the **medulla oblongata** and the **formatio reticularis**. The ratio between afferent and efferent fibres in the vagus nerve is 9:1. It is thus mainly a sensory nerve.

Serosal receptors, activated by stretching of the forestomach wall, have been detected in the serosa, especially at the base of the mesentery. They project mainly via the **splanchnic nerve**. Although no tonic activity can be detected by the splanchnic nerve, the activation of these serosal receptors can potentially have an indirect **inhibitory** effect on the reticulorumen motor system. Bilateral transection of the splanchnic nerve has no effect on reticulorumen motor function.

Reticulorumen motor function is also influenced by vagally innervated mechano- and chemosensitive **epithelial receptors** in the **abomasum** and **duodenum** (**Fig. 16.13**). In addition, **buccal mechanosensors** which project via the trigeminal nerve are involved in the generation of more frequent A-cycles during feed intake.

The **bilateral paired gastric centre** is located in the region of the dorsal motor nucleus of the vagus nerve in the **medulla oblongata**. Here there is **integration** of **inhibitory** and **excitatory signals** from the periphery and from higher centres of the central nervous system (**Fig. 16.13**).

> **MORE DETAILS**   The A and B cycles are initiated by excitations from the gastric centre in the CNS and reach the reticulorumen via efferent vagal fibres. The primary control of the frequency, shape and amplitude of the contraction cycles has not been well defined. It is postulated that so-called A interneurons – located close to the vagal motor neurons – determine the shape and amplitude of the cycles ("inotropic regulation"). These interneurons have no resting discharge frequency. The contraction cycle frequency results from the influence of B- and C-interneurons ("chronotropic function") on A-interneurons. The discharge frequency of the B-interneurons increases progressively, the longer the interval since the last reticulum contraction. In contrast, signals from C-interneurons inhibit the A-interneurons. Several types of A-interneurons seem to be responsible for initiating contraction of the reticulum and dorsal or ventral rumen sac.

The nuclei of parasympathetic neurons, responsible for motor innervation of the forestomachs, are located in the dorsal motor nucleus of the vagus nerve in the CNS and in the nucleus ambiguus of the medulla. The neurites are very long and extend to the visceral ganglia of the abdominal cavity. A distinction is made between the head, neck, thoracic and abdominal segments of the vagal nerve. The short head segment extends to the origin of the cranial laryngeal nerve, the neck segment is formed by the vagus nerve and the cervical sympathetic trunk (vagosympathetic trunk). These two nerves separate again at the level of the thoracic aperture. The left and right vagus nerve run dorsolaterally and divide into a dorsal and a ventral branch. After passing through the oesophageal hiatus, both dorsal branches and both ventral branches join and enter the abdominal cavity dorsally and ventrally of the oesophagus. The **dorsal vagus** innervates the rumen in particular and gives off only a few fibres to the omasum and abomasum. It is therefore also called the "**rumen nerve**". The **ventral vagus**, on the other hand, primarily innervates the **reticulum, omasum** and **abomasum** ("**reticulo-omasal-abomasal nerve**").

MORE DETAILS

Regulation of the B-cycles

The dorsal motor nucleus of the vagus nerve is also involved in the control of the B-cycles, but the excitatory and inhibitory influences are not identical. Thus, experimental stretching of the reticulum leads to an increased frequency of A-cycles, and decreased B-cycle frequency. The B-cycles are therefore considered comparatively autonomous. It is noticeable that especially in cattle the ratio between A- and B-cycles can fluctuate markedly.

Intrinsic innervation

The prominent role of vagovagal reflexes for the reticulorumen motor system becomes clear after experimental cutting of the cervical vagi (vagotomy). Both A and B cycles completely cease and within a few days the animal dies as a result of massive disturbances of ingesta passage. However, if the rumen contents are removed through a rumen fistula and replaced by a nutrient solution, the animals survive a vagotomy. Within about two weeks, tonic activity of the forestomachs is restored by rhythmic discharges of neurons of the enteric nervous system (myenteric plexus). However, regular contraction cycles, comparable to A or B cycles, no longer occur. Such "intrinsic contractions" originate from the discharge of neurons, especially of the myenteric plexus.

Functional stenosis ("Hoflund syndrome")

The central role of the vagus nerve in regulation of reticulorumen motor function is also evident in animals suffering from so-called functional stenosis. The clinical picture arises from damage to the vagus nerve, caused directly, for example, by nails and other sharp metals penetrating the reticulum ("reticulo-peritonitis traumatica") or indirectly by inflammation and abscess formation from such penetration. The result is disturbance in the sorting function of the reticulum, so that coarse feed particles are able to pass into the omasum and abomasum, which disrupts passage of ingesta and can cause obstruction of the pylorus. There is progressive distension of the dorsal and ventral rumen sacs, which can be observed externally as distension of the abdomen in the "papple" shape where the right side looks like half a pear and the left side like half an apple. The disease was first described by the Swedish scientist Sven Axel Hoflund (1906–1979).

> **IN A NUTSHELL**   !
>
> The enteric nervous system has a modulating influence on the reticulorumen motor system through intrinsic tonic contractions.

Peripheral influences on reticulorumen motor function

The forestomach motor system is influenced by the amount, type and texture of the food. **Slight** to **moderate stretching** of the wall of the reticulum is probably the most important stimulus for **activation** of the reticulorumen motor system, in response to signals from the tension receptors. High feed intake thus leads to stronger contractions and increased salivation from simultaneous signals from the salivary centre in the medulla (**Fig. 16.13**). The **intake of roughage** has a more pronounced effect than the intake of concentrated feed. This is not surprising given the larger volume of roughage compared to concentrated feed of the same nutritional value.

In contrast, a strong **(over-)stretching** of the forestomachs, as in ruminal tympany or bloat, **inhibits** reticulorumen motor function. This is probably mediated by massive activation of the mechanosensitive epithelial receptors, whereby their inhibitory influence on motor function is obviously greater than the excitatory influence of the tension receptors.

Chemical stimuli also have an **inhibitory influence** on forestomach motor function by activation of epithelial receptors. The most important chemical stimulus is from short-chain fatty acids, produced by microbial fermentation of carbohydrates in the forestomachs. The receptors react to the **acidity** of the rumen contents. Since the epithelial receptors are about 150 μm below the mucosal surface, they are mainly influenced by highly permeable acids, such as butyric acid, that diffuse quickly through the epithelium. The epithelial receptors are also activated by strong **hypo- and hypertonicity** of the forestomach contents. However, this does not have a significant effect because fluctuations in the osmolarity of the forestomach contents are usually quite small.

The gastric centres in the brain are also excited when **epithelial receptors** in the **abomasum** are activated by low pH of abomasal contents. The vagovagally induced increase in forestomach motor activity thus ensures that the abomasum is always sufficiently filled. In contrast, unphysiological distension of the abomasum and a high pH inhibit forestomach motor function via vagovagal reflexes. Inhibition of motor activity also occurs from activation of serosal receptors that project via the splanchnic nerve. Overfilling of the abomasum is prevented by these two mutually independent sensory pathways.

Finally, epithelial **receptors** in the **duodenum** can lead to inhibition of both abomasal and reticulorumen motor activity when stimulated by low pH or hypo- or hyperosmolarity. Thus, excessively rapid passage of ingesta from the abomasum into the duodenum is prevented.

> **IN A NUTSHELL !**
>
> Moderate stretching of the reticulum wall leads to increased reticulum and rumen motor activity. Severe stretching and high fatty acid concentrations inhibit reticulorumen motor activity. Activation of receptors in the oral cavity, abomasum and duodenum has additional effects.

Influence of higher centres of the CNS on reticulorumen motor function

Inhibition of the reticulorumen motor function by **painful stimuli** results from
- a direct effect on the dorsal nucleus of vagus nerve in the CNS,
- activation of the sympathico-adrenergic system (inhibition of motor activity via the splanchnic nerve),
- reduction or cessation of feed intake ("anorexia"), which often occurs in conjunction with pain (**Fig. 16.13**).

In sick animals with fever, the forestomach motor function is also reduced as a result of direct effects of pyrogens on the dorsal nucleus of vagus nerve and indirect effects of prostaglandins.

> **IN A NUTSHELL !**
>
> Reticulorumen motor function is inhibited by pain and by fever.

■ Motility of the omasum

With regard to the motility of the omasum (**Fig. 16.14**), a distinction must first be made between the motor function of the omasal **canal** and that of the omasal **body**. The motor function of the omasal **canal** is closely **related to the reticulorumen motility**.

The **omasal canal** always widens at the peak of the second reticulum contraction. When the reticulo-omasal orifice is open, ingesta are sucked into the omasum from the lower regions of the reticulum ("**suction phase**"). Immediately afterwards, the reticulo-omasal orifice closes and the omasal canal contracts so that the ingesta are partially squeezed between the omasal lamellae ("**pressure phase**"). This is followed, after a delay of about 10 s, by a slowly increasing cranial to caudal **contraction** of the **omasal body**. The ingesta are thereby pressed out of the omasum towards the wide-lumened abomasal entrance. Immediately before the next biphasic contraction, the omasal body relaxes completely again. The motility of the **omasal body** is

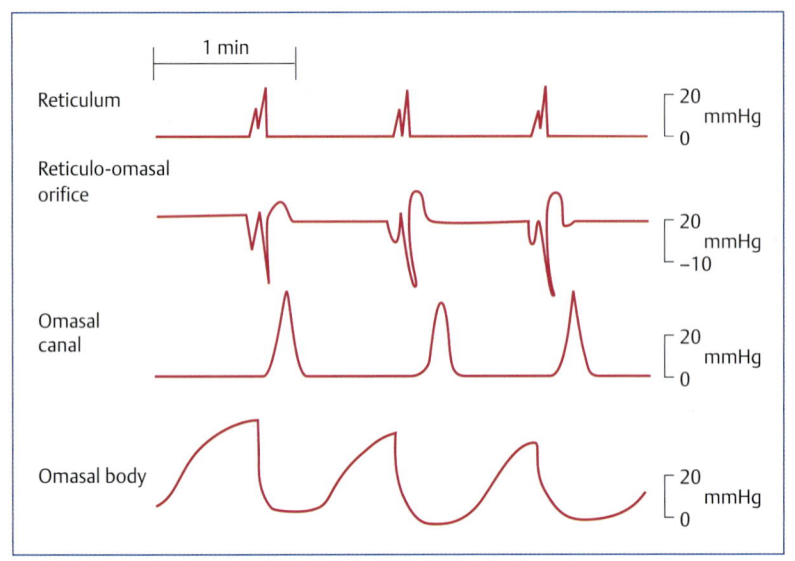

Fig. 16.14 Schematic representation of the connection between reticular and omasal motility. A vacuum is created in the reticulo-omasal orifice during the second reticulum contraction. The resulting suction effect transfers ingesta from the reticulum into the omasum.

not strictly **coordinated** with the **reticulorumen motility**, especially in cattle, where contractions of the omasal body are often absent during several contraction cycles of the reticulorumen.

In contrast to the reticulorumen motility, the **motility of the omasal body** is **mainly regulated locally** ("intrinsic contractions"). After vagotomy or induction of anaesthesia, the motility of the omasal body is almost unaffected, while the reticulorumen motility is suspended. However, the composition and quantity of ingesta from the reticulum, as well as omasal filling, significantly affect motility. During feed intake, as the frequency of biphasic reticulum contractions increases, the duration of each contraction of the omasal body decreases and therefore influx into the omasum is increased.

> **IN A NUTSHELL** !
>
> The omasum functions as a suction-pressure pump. The motility of the omasum is only partially coordinated with the reticulorumen motility and is largely independent of control via the vagus nerve.

■ Functional significance and regulation of ruminating activity

Rumination, which gave the suborder Ruminantia its name, is a basic requirement for the physiological course of digestion in the forestomachs:

- The **crushing** of large feed **particles** by ruminating increases surface area which enables intensive microbial colonisation and digestion of the plant cell contents. This means that ruminating – especially with high intakes of roughage – indirectly affects the extent of microbial fermentation.
- Activation of buccal mechanosensors during rumination **increases salivary secretion**. Chewing activity thus influences the environment in the reticulorumen. The high bicarbonate concentration of saliva counteracts the acid production in the rumen contents (**Fig. 16.15**).
- The decrease in particle size and increase in particle density associated with ruminating greatly affects the rate of **ingesta passage** from the reticulorumen into the omasum.

Rumination is induced by stimulation of epithelial **receptors** in the mucosa of the **reticulum** and **rumen atrium** (**Fig. 16.15**). Adequate stimulus for these receptors is contact of coarse feed particles with the rumen mucosa. Thus, rumination is dependent on the quantity and composition of the feed intake. When fed roughage rations with a high fibre content, the animals ruminate between **eight** and **eleven hours** per day. When fed concentrated feed or finely ground roughage, ruminating activity drops drastically. The epithelial receptors transmit via vagal fibres to the **chewing centre** in the medulla oblongata.

The actual **chewing cycle** begins with **regurgitation** of a bolus of reticulorumen contents into the oral cavity. However, regurgitation is preceded by an additional contraction of the **reticulum** immediately before the biphasic A-cycle contraction of the reticulum ("**regurgitation contraction**", Fig. 16.11). This lifts ingesta from the reticulum and rumen atrium to the cardia, with simultaneous opening of the lower cardia sphincter. At the same time or shortly before the regurgitation contraction, air **inhalation** also occurs with the **soft palate raised**, which prevents the inflow of air entering the airways thus creating negative pressure in the thoracic section of the oesophagus (−25 to −40 mmHg). This causes the bolus to be **aspirated** into the **oesophagus**. A rapid **antiperistaltic oesophageal contraction then** ejects the bolus into the oral cavity. Closing of the epiglottis prevents ingesta from entering the trachea. Unlike in vomiting, contractions of the abdominal muscles and stomach are not involved in regurgitation. In the oral cavity, the bolus is first compressed by movement of the tongue and the liquid released is immediately reswallowed. Each ruminating cycle lasts about one minute, during which time the bolus is chewed with regular jaw movements. The food particles are thus further disintegrated. Saliva secretion is more than doubled during the chewing cycle compared to the resting period. After about 50 jaw movements, the chewing cycle ends with swallowing, and the next cycle begins after a short pause of 5–10 seconds.

For each regurgitation, it is necessary that reticulorumen motor activity (**regurgitation contraction**), respiration (inspiration with **closure** of the **airways**) and the antiperistalsis **activity** of the **oesophagus** are all synchronised. This complex **coordination**, presumably controlled by the **hypothalamus**, is most effective in a state of rest. Ruminating is therefore mainly observed in recumbent, somnolent animals. **Excitement** and **stress** have a strong **inhibitory** effect on rumination. However, if ruminating is experimentally suppressed by fitting tight masks on cows for several hours, rumination immediately starts after removal of the masks, even with severe stress and despite starvation. This illustrates the great importance of superordinate centres of the CNS for the ruminating process.

Pseudo-rumination is an activity in which boluses are regurgitated without being followed by periods of rhythmic chewing movements. Pseudo-rumination is observed mainly when feeding rations with little fibrous material and is considered to be an indication of central control of the ruminating process.

Ruminating always requires a sense of well-being. Pain, fever and stress inhibit ruminating activity. Thus, **ruminating** is a good **indicator** of an animal's **health**.

> **IN A NUTSHELL** !
>
> Ruminating represents an innate, complex, vagovagally controlled reflexive process. With appropriate feeding of roughage, the ingested food is chewed again for about 8 hours a day. Ruminating is an important sign in the assessment of health of a ruminant animal.

Nutrition, energy

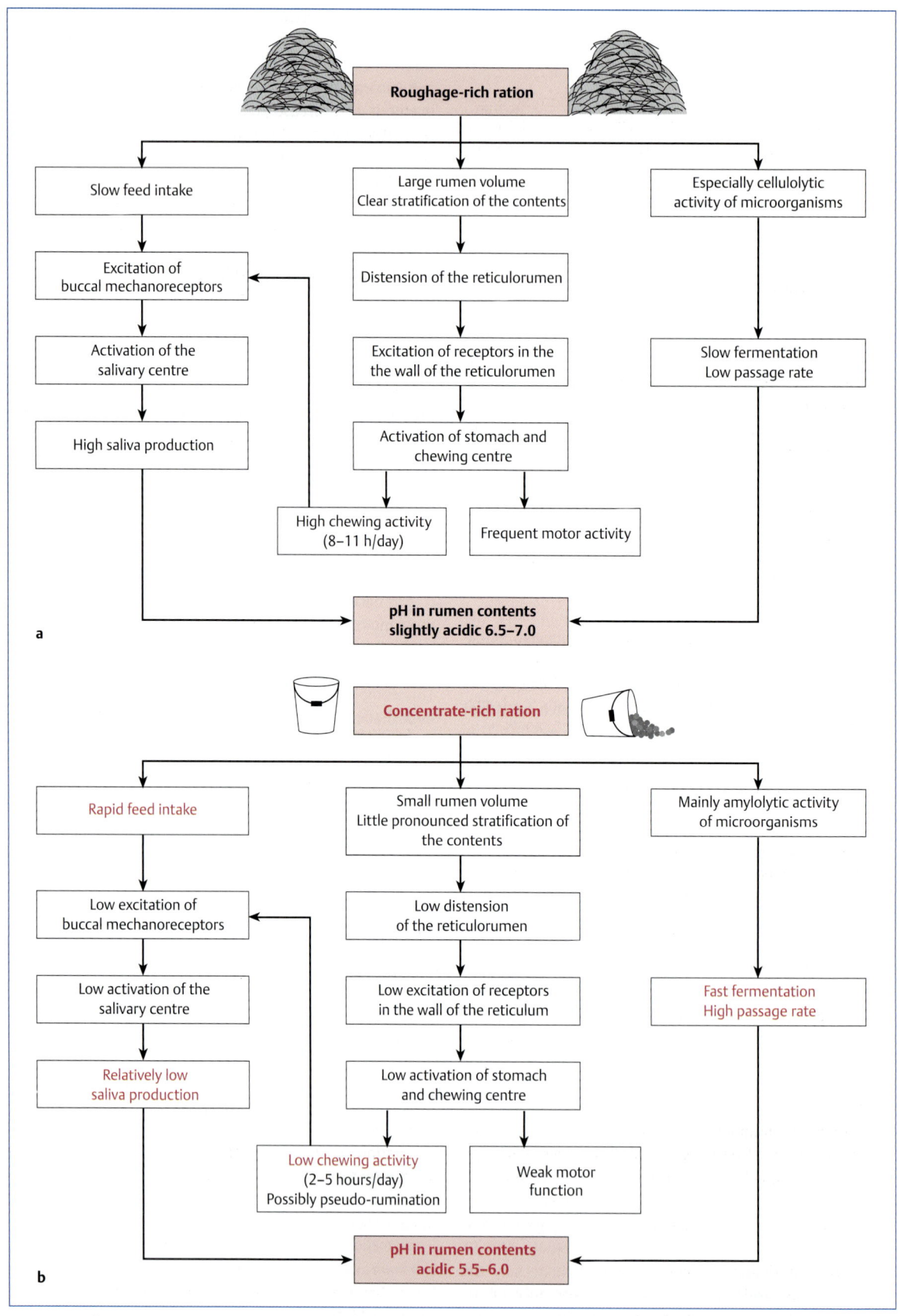

Fig. 16.15 Influence of feeding on the digestive processes in the reticulorumen. **a** Roughage-rich ration. **b** Concentrate-rich ration.

■ Eructation

During microbial fermentation of ingesta in the reticulorumen, gas is produced (formula (16.1)) (mainly carbon dioxide and methane), which collects in a voluminous gas phase in the dorsal rumen sac. Because enormous quantities of gas are generated (500–1500 l per day in cattle), regular release by eructation is essential. This is initiated as a **vagovagal reflex** 1–2 times per minute. The **dorsal rumen sac contracts** during the **B cycle** (only very rarely during the A cycle), which pushes the gas cranially to the **cardia**. Receptors around the cardia are activated so that it opens reflexively, and the gas can then flow into the **oesophagus**. An **antiperistaltic contraction** moves the gas orally. However, the gas is not immediately released to the environment because the nasopharynx is **closed** by the **taut** and raised **soft palate**. The mouth is also closed during eructation, so the **gas** first enters the **lungs**. There, the carbon dioxide is partially absorbed giving rise to temporary hyperventilation by excitation of peripheral chemoreceptors.

MORE DETAILS

Rumen tympany

An unphysiologically large amount of gas accumulating in the rumen is called rumen tympany (bloat). There are two types of rumen tympany, one when there is a failure to release gas produced in normal quantities because of mechanical obstruction (e.g. pharyngeal obstruction by pieces of beet), or by motor or nervous disorders. The second type is **rumen tympany** with **foamy** mixing of the contents resulting from ingestion of forage plants (e.g. fresh rape or lucerne) with components causing fine-bubble foam in the rumen so that the gas trapped in foam cannot be released by eructation.

In both forms, there is an enormous increase in pressure in the rumen and respiratory and circulatory problems can occur within a few hours, mainly due to the cranial protrusion of the diaphragm.

Furthermore, eructation is more difficult when the animal is in a lateral or supine position. This is one of the reasons why surgery in cattle is mostly performed in the standing position under local anaesthesia.

> **IN A NUTSHELL** !
>
> Eructation enables a ruminant to release rumen gases by contraction of the dorsal rumen sac. If eructation is prevented, life-threatening tympany can quickly develop.

■ The reticular groove reflex

The **new-born ruminant** is entirely dependent on milk as a food source for the first weeks of life. The forestomach system is initially small compared to the abomasum, and as it is not yet colonised with microorganisms it is practically functionless. The calf is thus a functional monogastric animal.

For the physiological digestion of milk, especially the coagulation of casein (p.415) under the influence of the enzyme chymosin and hydrochloric acid, it is necessary that milk reaches the abomasum without delay after ingestion. The **reticular groove reflex** enables this. The reflex of spiral rotation of the two folds of the reticulum with si-

multaneous relaxation of the reticulo-omasal orifice and the omasal canal is called the reticular-groove reflex. This reflex thus creates a functional **bypass** between the **oesophagus** and **abomasum**. In non-physiological feeding methods and diseases, calves may experience a complete or partial failure of the reticular groove reflex, so that the milk enters the still poorly developed rumen ("**rumen drinking**"). Due to microbial fermentation of milk in the forestomachs, these calves develop an inflammation of the rumen mucosa (ruminitis) and a possibly serious digestive disorder.

The **triggering** of the **reflex** in new-born ruminants is by activation of chemoreceptors in the oral cavity and pharynx by milk during suckling. Other components of the reflex arc are vagal afferents (via the glossopharyngeal nerve), the medulla oblongata and the dorsal ventral vagal nerve as an efferent reflex pathway. Experimentally, closure of the reticular groove can be prevented by applying local anaesthetics in the mouth, by intravenous injection of atropine or by sectioning vagus branches (vagotomy). Conversely, the reflex can be triggered in lambs and calves by adding copper or sodium salts to the drinker device, even if it does not contain milk. The **reflex** is **conditioned** by other sensory stimuli and the hungrier the animal, the easier it is to trigger. With increasing intake of roughage and progressive development of the forestomach system, the reticular groove reflex eventually disappears.

> **IN A NUTSHELL** !
>
> In young ruminants, the reticular groove reflex causes milk to enter the abomasum directly, bypassing the reticulorumen.

■ Stratification of ingesta in the reticulorumen

Because of different physical characteristics of feed particles (size, shape, density) and by the action of the reticulorumen motor system, a pronounced **stratification** of rumen contents develops in the reticulorumen of healthy domestic ruminants.

With appropriate feed sources, the freshly ingested feed fragments are initially large, and of low density due to air-filled cavities (below $1.0\,\text{g}\cdot\text{ml}^{-1}$). After swallowing, the coarsely chewed feed first enters the rumen atrium and is then pushed dorsally by the reticulorumen motor system to form a dense **layer of coarsely structured feed** in the **dorsal rumen sac**. The gas produced during microbial fermentation accumulates in the dorsal rumen sac above this coarse-textured feed. With rumination, the particle size decreases while the density of the particles increases. The mainly digested particles are thus small and of high density $(1.2–1.4\,\text{g}\cdot\text{ml}^{-1})$, so they gradually sediment into the ventral rumen sac. The **content** of the **ventral rumen sac** is thus characterised by a high proportion of **smaller particles** of **high density**. The ventral rumen sac contains a liquid phase with feed particles of finer structure and denser consistency. With contractions of the ventral rumen sac, these largely digested particles pass into the rumen atrium and then into the reticulum. Through the motility of the reticulum and the omasal canal and orifice, the ingesta pass from the lower part of the reticulum into the omasum.

> **IN A NUTSHELL**   **!**
>
> In normally fed ruminants, the dorsal rumen sac contains mainly coarse, less fragmented ingesta ("rumen fibre mat"), above which is the dorsal gas phase. The contents of the ventral rumen sac and reticulum are relatively liquid.

■ Ingesta passage

The importance of retention time of ingesta in the reticulorumen

The **digestibility** of feed in the reticulorumen is determined by the ratio of its rate of **degradation** and rate of **passage** (**Fig. 16.15**). **Cellulose**, the most important fibrous component of grasses, is a substrate with relatively high potential digestibility, but is **degraded** only **slowly**. Accordingly, the longer the retention time (as a reciprocal value of the rate of passage), the more completely roughage can be fermented by microorganisms in the forestomachs. However, a long retention time can have the disadvantage that relatively few digestion products can be absorbed due to the limited volume of the forestomachs (**Fig. 16.80**). A high feed intake then requires the largest possible volume of the fermentation chamber. Over the course of evolution, as ruminants have adapted to diets rich in cellulose, the **volume** of the **forestomach has increased** more and more and can amount to **20%**, in some species up to more than 30% of body weight.

The degradation rate of a feed or feed ingredient can be estimated by incubating samples in rumen fluid under in vitro conditions ("artificial rumen"). The mean retention time of liquid and feed particles can only be calculated from the kinetics of the faecal excretion of indigestible substances ("markers") in feeding experiments.

Food particles are retained in the reticulorumen much longer (18–72 hours) than liquid (about 12 hours); an observation called **selective retention** of **particles**. However, the retention time of food particles is not uniform, but depends on their density and size. Due to the selective retention of solid particles in the forestomachs, the retention time of particles in the entire gastrointestinal tract of ruminants is considerably longer than that of liquid (**Table 16.5**). In monogastric animals, the retention time of feed particles is much shorter.

> **IN A NUTSHELL**   **!**
>
> The retention time of ingesta in the reticulorumen is determined by the volume of the reticulorumen (pool size), the quantity of feed intake and the rate of its degradation.

Passage of ingesta from the reticulorumen into the omasum

Because of simultaneous timing of the second reticulum contraction and the onward passage of ingesta, the composition of ingesta leaving the reticulorumen is particularly determined by reticulum motor activity. The **segregation processes during reticulum contractions** are mainly based on the different **flotation and sedimentation behaviour** of the ingesta particles. Large, less digested food particles mainly float because of their low density. These particles are thrust dorsocaudally by contractions of the reticulum (**Fig. 16.16**). In contrast, the **density of small**, mainly **digested particles** is relatively **high**, so these particles are more likely to **remain** in the **reticulum** during **reticulum contractions** and can therefore be preferentially aspirated **into** the **omasal canal** at the peak of the second reticulum contraction. Therefore, particles with a size of less than 3 mm are almost exclusively found in the omasum and distal digestive tract. However, **particle size** itself is of **secondary importance**, as the maximum diameter of the reticulo-omasal orifice could also allow passage of larger particles. The key factor determining the particle size is that only small particles are dense enough to remain in the ventral part of the reticulum when it contracts.

This complex relationship between forestomach motility, ingesta passage and physical properties of the food particles results in predominantly largely **digested food particles leaving** the reticulorumen, while **less digested** particles are effectively **retained**.

MORE DETAILS   A pathologically important disturbance of the segregation processes of ingesta in the reticulum is observed in the so-called **foreign body syndrome of cattle**. Due to their less discriminatory feed intake, cattle frequently ingest sharp foreign bodies (nails, screws, wire) with their feed. These lodge in the reticulum after swallowing and, with the strong reticulum contractions, they can perforate the reticulum wall. Local inflammation with connective tissue adhesions between the reticulum and the abdominal wall then rapidly develops (**"reticuloperitonitis traumatica"**). The motility of the reticulum is then more or less restricted, so that segregation of particles is no longer effective. Large food particles can then leave the reticulorumen despite their low density, so that a significantly increased proportion of large food particles are typically found in faeces of affected animals. In some cases, disturbances of the abomaso-duodenal ingesta passage also occur. The composition of the material discharged from the reticulum thus also seems to have an essential

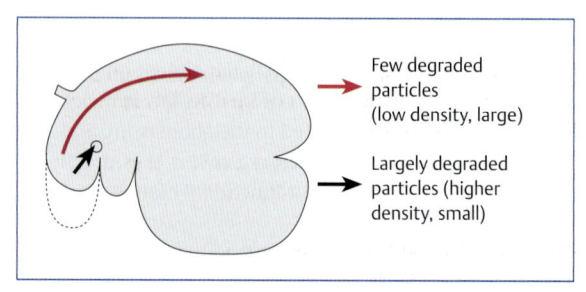

Few degraded particles (low density, large)

Largely degraded particles (higher density, small)

Fig. 16.16 Segregation processes of ingesta particles because of their different flotation and sedimentation characteristics during reticulum contractions. The passage of ingesta into the omasum almost only occurs at the peak of the second reticulum contraction. The shape of the reticulum when relaxed is shown by dashed lines.

role in normal abomasal emptying. Disturbances of ingesta passage in reticuloperitonitis traumatica can also be caused by foreign body-related damage to the vagus branches.

A preventive measure in many cattle farms is the introduction of cage magnets into the reticulum, which bind ingested metallic foreign objects and thus prevent perforation of the wall. Such magnets are introduced orally with the help of special applicators.

> **IN A NUTSHELL** !
>
> The passage of ingesta through the reticulo-omasal orifice into the omasum occurs almost entirely at the peak of the second reticulum contraction. The reticulum motility segregates the different particles of the ingesta, allowing dense, largely digested, small food particles to leave the reticulorumen, while less digested particles are retained mainly because of their low density.

Ingesta passage in the distal digestive tract

The **retention time** of ingesta in the **omasum** is short at 0.5–3 hours. As in the reticulorumen, particles are retained longer than liquid. The ingesta then enters the abomasum almost continuously. In contrast to monogastrics, the inflowing ingesta in ruminants (under physiological conditions) consists only of fluid, microorganisms and small particles. The transpyloric passage of ingesta into the duodenum takes place in spurts or "**gushes**" (approx. ten per hour). The average **retention time** of the ingesta in the **abomasum** is less than one hour, during which time there is a substantial increase in volume from abomasal **secretions**. Uniform **consistency** and low **viscosity** are important requirements for the onward passage of abomasal contents into the duodenum. Ingesta propulsion along the length of the small and large intestine is effected by peristaltic intestinal contractions. Passage time is about 15 hours.

> **IN A NUTSHELL** !
>
> Fluid and particles pass through the gastrointestinal tract distal to the reticulum in about 18 hours.

■ Suggested reading

Grovum WL, Gonzahlez JS. Control of salivation and motility of the reticulorumen by the brain in sheep. In: Cronjé PB, ed. Ruminant Physiology: Digestion, Metabolism, Growth and Reproduction. Oxon: CABI Publishing; 2000: 41–58.

Harding R, Leek BF. The effects of peripheral and central nervous influences on gastric centre neuronal activity in sheep. J Physiol 1972; 225 (2): 309–338

Harding R, Leek BF. The locations and activities of medullary neurones associated with ruminant forestomach motility. J Physiol 1971; 219 (3): 587–610

IWF Knowledge and Media, Nonnenstieg 72, Göttingen; 1980: https://av.tib.eu/media/9235

Kennedy PM, Murphy MR. The nutritional implications of differential passage of particles through the ruminant alimentary tract. Nutr Res Rev 1988; 1: 189–208

Poncet C. The outflow of particles from the reticulorumen. In: Jouany JP, ed. Rumen Microbial Metabolism and Ruminant Digestion. Paris: INRA Editions; 1991: 297–322

Ruckebusch Y. Gastrointestinal motor functions in ruminants. In: Schultz SG, Wood JD, Rauner BB, eds. Handbook of Physiology. New York: Oxford University Press; 1989: 1225–1282

16.3.3 Motility of the monogastric stomach and the ruminant abomasum

Martin Diener, Jörg R. Aschenbach

> **ESSENTIALS**
>
> The motility of the monogastric stomach can be divided into that of a cranial "stomach reservoir" and that of a caudal "stomach pump". The cranial stomach reservoir has a comparatively thin musculature which, controlled neuronally, either contracts tonically or relaxes. The more powerful musculature of the caudal "stomach pump" shows phasic peristaltic contractile waves, which mix and fragment the food particles and gradually release finely divided food particles into the small intestine.

■ Functions of the gastric motor system

The stomach is not only an important **storage organ** that allows the intake of large meals. It is also the first compartment for **digestion** by the body's own enzymes. The stomach also has a significant role in the mechanical **disruption** of **food**. This facilitates digestion by increasing the surface area of food particles to increase access of digestive enzymes. Stomach motility also regulates the rate of **delivery** of **stomach contents** to the small intestine. The particles that leave the stomach as digested food pulp or chyme (Greek: chymos = juice; Latin: digesta) are usually less than 1 mm in size. Larger particles are retained by the pyloric sphincter muscle that constricts the stomach outlet.

■ Morphological and functional structure of the stomach

Anatomically, the stomach is divided into a protruding base (fundus) next to the oesophageal entrance to the stomach (cardia), a more or less elongated body of the stomach (corpus) and the pyloric cavity (antrum pyloricum) proximal to the outlet of the stomach, the pyloric canal (canalis pyloricus) (**Fig. 16.17**).

> **MORE DETAILS** The name fundus is misleading in many respects. Firstly, this part of the stomach is not located ventrally as the name suggests, but dorsally. In addition, the distinction between fundus and corpus does not correspond to the functional division of the stomach, both in terms of motility and secretory functions. In most animals, most of the fundus glands are not in the fundus, but in the gastric corpus. In horses, the actual "gastric fundus" is completely free of fundus glands and has a cutaneous-like mucosa (**Fig. 16.42**).

Nutrition, energy

The stomach is linked to the oesophagus cranially and with the duodenum caudally. A sphincter controls the flow from the oesophagus into the stomach and another sphincter from the stomach into the duodenum. The sphincter at the junction of the oesophagus (sphincter cardiae) is not a morphologically distinct muscle and cannot be distinguished from the muscles of the oesophagus or those of the stomach. It is therefore a functional sphincter. The pyloric sphincter is different. It can also be described morphologically as an independent sphincter muscle with particularly well-developed circular muscles. The musculature of the stomach – like that of the rest of the gastrointestinal tract – consists of an inner circular and an outer longitudinal muscle layer. Over the entire stomach, the circular musculature is the strongest muscle layer. In addition, there is a third, oblique muscle layer, which is, however, only well developed in the region of the lesser curvature and the cardia. It lies on the inside of the circular muscle layer. In contrast to the caudal region of the stomach, the cranial region has much weaker musculature.

With regard to their mechanical and electrical properties, two different regions can be distinguished in the stomach, namely the cranial and caudal halves of the stomach The cranial half has more of a storage function, whereas the caudal half contributes to the onward transport, mixing and fragmenting of the food mass. Accordingly, the cranial part of the stomach has more tonic, i.e. sustained contractions, while the caudal stomach has more phasic, i.e. short, but powerful contractions. These different types of contractions are the result of different electrical characteristics of the muscle cells. The cell membranes of the muscle cells in the cranial gastric regions are slightly depolarised, but still negative. These membrane potentials are very stable and show little fluctuation. Accordingly, myogenic control by pacemaker cells, which is very pronounced in all other sections of the gastrointestinal tract, plays only a subordinate role in the cranial stomach. Towards the pylorus, the membrane potentials increase in magnitude, i.e. the membrane potential becomes more negative. In addition, pacemaker cells now acquire a greater influence. Slow waves occur, which initiate phasic motor activity as rhythmic, spontaneous discharges (**Fig. 16.17**).

■ Motility of the cranial stomach

The slightly depolarised resting membrane potential of the smooth muscle cells in the cranial part of the stomach is close to the threshold potential at which the opening of voltage dependent Ca^{2+} channels is triggered. Accordingly, the musculature of the cranial half of the stomach has a permanent resting tone. However, since no action potentials are triggered, these contractions are tonic, i.e. a more or less constant muscle tension develops. Only very rarely are phasic contractions found in the cranial stomach region, i.e. contractions with rhythmically fluctuating amplitude. The volume of the cranial stomach is regulated by the strength of these tonic contractions. Relaxation of the cranial part of the stomach is necessary for the entry of more food, which is why this part of the stomach is called a **"stomach store"**. Nevertheless, the tone of this cranial stomach determines the internal pressure in the entire stomach and thus also its rate of emptying. Only when the cranial stomach generates sufficient internal pressure, can the peristaltic (pumping) movements of the caudal part of the stomach ("gastric pump" (p. 384)) propel the chyme into the duodenum. Accordingly, signals that indicate a high nutrient concentration in the duodenum (e.g. cholecysto-

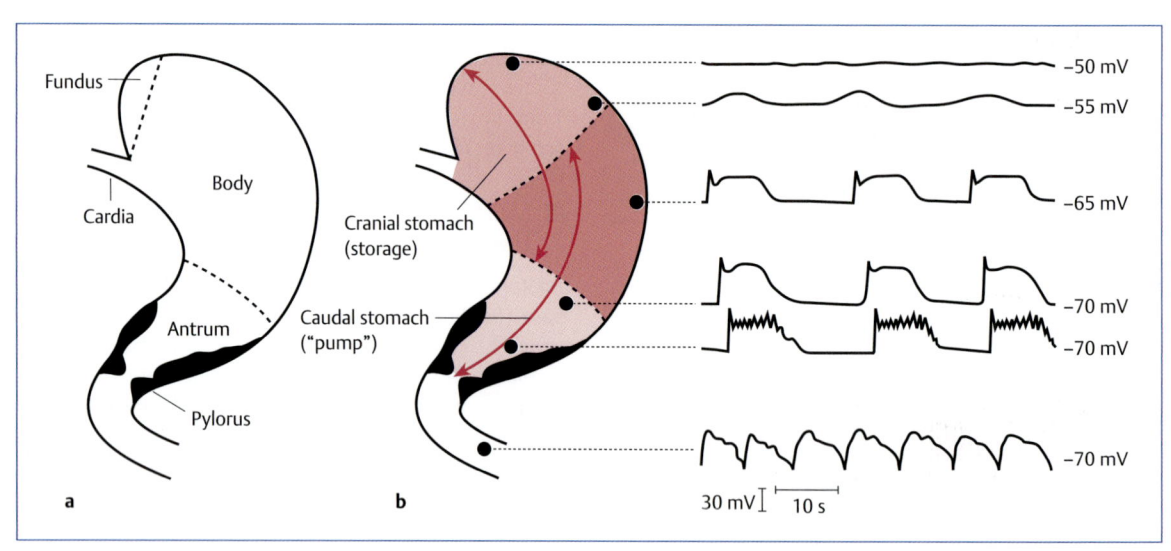

Fig. 16.17 Morphological and functional division of the stomach.
a Morphologically, the stomach is divided into fundus, body, and pyloric antrum.
b A distinction is made between motility in the cranial part of the stomach which has a predominantly storage function, and motility in the caudal part which has a mixing, fragmenting and transporting function. Both parts of the stomach merge smoothly into one another. The membrane potentials of the muscle cells in the cranial stomach are continuously slightly depolarised and mediate the tonic tension of this part of the stomach via a tonic Ca^{2+} influx. The membrane potentials of the muscle cells of the caudal stomach are intermittently depolarised, which leads to phasic contractions through superimposed Ca^{2+} action potentials. The pylorus acts as an electrical insulator. Therefore, the phasic intermittent fluctuations of the muscle membrane potential in the duodenum are independent of the intermittent fluctuations of the muscle membrane potential in the stomach and occur with about three times the frequency.

kinin, secretin), inhibit gastric emptying by inducing relaxation of the musculature of the stomach store (so-called feedback relaxation (p.384)).

Contraction and relaxation of the cranial half of the stomach are subject to distinct **neuronal control** by the enteric nervous system (p.361). Excitatory neurons increase muscle tone and inhibitory neurons decrease it. An important excitatory neurotransmitter in the stomach is acetylcholine, and an inhibitory transmitter is vasoactive intestinal peptide (VIP). Other inhibitory neurotransmitters are adrenaline, noradrenaline, dopamine and nitric oxide (NO). Numerous **hormones complement** the nervous control, usually not by influencing motor function directly, but indirectly via modulation of neuronal activity. This subordinate modulating effect is also the reason why hormones such as gastrin and cholecystokinin have a relaxing effect on the cranial stomach, while they promote contractions of the caudal part of the stomach. Motilin, on the other hand, promotes contractions in both parts of the stomach and secretin inhibits contractions in both parts. The strong neuronal control of motility of the cranial stomach can be impressively demonstrated by two reflexes that physiologically occur during food intake. These are receptive and adaptive relaxations. When the pharyngeal mucosa is mechanically stimulated or the oesophagus is stretched as occurs, when a mouthful of food is swallowed, **reflex relaxation** of the **gastric fundus** occurs, which is called **receptive relaxation**.

The basis of receptive relaxation can be explained by pressure changes in the individual sections of the oesophagus and stomach. The oesophagus (from its intrathoracic transit) is normally slightly under-pressured (Fig. 16.18). When a bolus of food is peristaltically transported towards the stomach, the pressure in the oesophagus increases due to the annular contraction of the musculature. The oesophageal sphincter, on the other hand, relaxes to allow the passage of food into the stomach. At the same time, however, the pressure in the stomach also decreases: the cranial part of the stomach relaxes to "make room" for the additional food. This relaxation starts even before the food bolus has reached the stomach. If experimentally, the va-

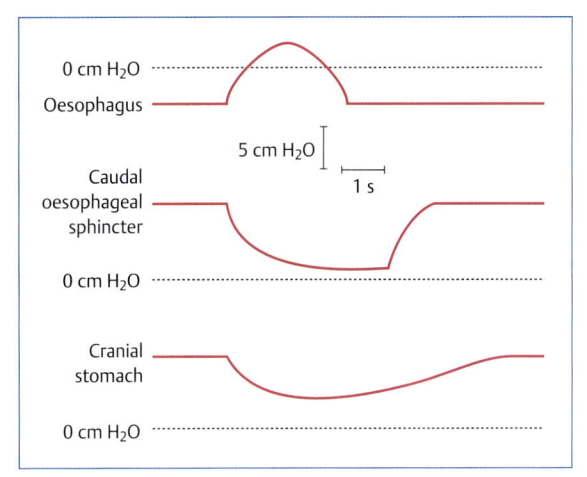

Fig. 16.18 Pressure changes in the oesophagus in the region of the caudal oesophageal sphincter and the cranial part of the stomach during the act of swallowing. The cranial part of the stomach relaxes reflexively before a peristaltic wave from the oesophagus reaches the stomach (receptive relaxation).

gus nerve is sectioned, the oesophageal sphincter and the cranial stomach do not relax. Hence this relaxation is a reflex, mediated by the vagus nerve. Since the afferent parts that transmit the information from the mechanosensors to the brain and the efferent fibres that trigger the gastric relaxation both run in the vagus, this is a **vagovagal reflex**.

Adaptive relaxation is another reflex that supports the oral stomach's task of acting as a food reservoir. It is a reflexively triggered relaxation as the stomach fills. This is particularly pronounced in carnivores, as they kill prey at irregular intervals in the wild and then consume large amounts of food in a very short time.

Adaptive relaxation can be studied experimentally by inserting a balloon probe into the stomach via an oral catheter and measuring the pressure inside the stomach as a function of stomach filling (Fig. 16.19). Despite increasing filling of the stomach through the balloon catheter, the pressure inside the stomach increases only moderately due to reflex relaxation of the stomach wall. The reason for this is that gastric distension is registered by mechanosen-

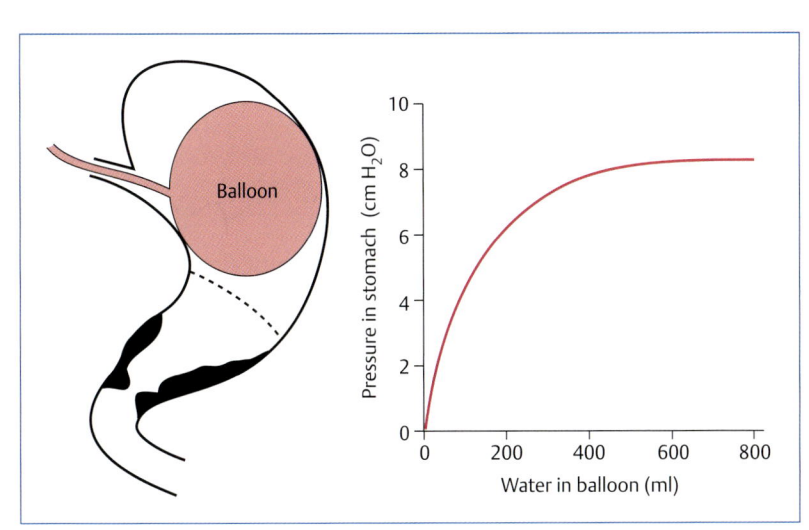

Fig. 16.19 Pressure changes in the stomach during expansion. If the stomach is experimentally filled by means of a balloon catheter, the pressure increases initially as the balloon begins to inflate. Then, pressure inside the stomach increases only moderately, although the stomach continues to be filled. This is in response to reflex relaxation of the stomach wall (adaptive relaxation).

Nutrition, energy

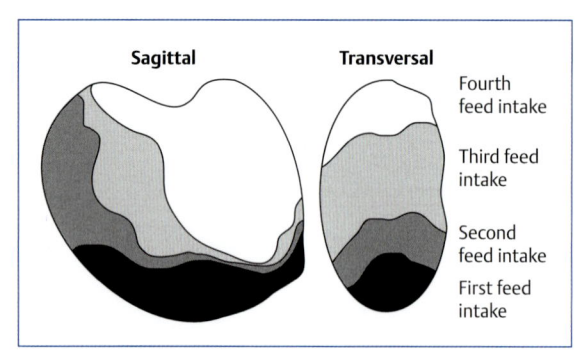

Fig. 16.20 Typical superimposition of stomach contents in a horse from four successive feed intakes, labelled with different dyes.

sors in the stomach wall and reflex inhibitory motoneurons are activated. These trigger muscle relaxation. The result is a decrease in wall tension, so that the pressure remains constant or increases only slightly with further stretching. This reflex is also vagovagally mediated.

Relaxation of the cranial part of the stomach during food intake results in **overlapping** of new food with that already present in this part of the stomach. Only in the caudal part of the stomach is there a mixing of the solid components (**Fig. 16.20**). Liquid entering from the oesophagus, on the other hand, can flow past this food mass in the cranial stomach.

> **MORE DETAILS**   The layering of the stomach contents protects the (stretched) cranial stomach from excessive acidification by gastric acid. Disturbances of this stratification from a lack of solid feed (e.g. shot or liquid feeding in pigs) or excessive physical stress (e.g. in racehorses when HCl "spills" from the glandular part of the stomach into the pars proventricularis) favour the development of gastric ulcers.

> **IN A NUTSHELL** !
>
> The oral stomach has a storage function. Its motor function is largely neuronally controlled. It relaxes reflexively during food intake.

■ Motility of caudal part of the stomach

In contrast to the cranial half of the stomach, the muscle cells of the caudal stomach have higher membrane potentials (**Fig. 16.17**). These are more negative the further in the caudal direction they are measured. Thus, values of approx. $-55\,mV$ are found in the cranial part of the gastric body, $-65\,mV$ in the caudal part and $-70\,mV$ in the pyloric antrum. The muscle cells in the caudal half of the stomach, in contrast to those in the cranial stomach, exhibit spontaneous oscillations of membrane potential, initiated as slow waves (p. 370) by pacemaker cells. It is important for the mechanical action of the stomach that the amplitude of these slow waves increases caudally. The increase is ensured since the resting membrane potential is becoming more negative in the caudal direction. In association with a wall thickness that also increases caudally, the force of the contractions towards the pylorus increases.

However, not every pacemaker potential triggers action potentials. Inhibitory nerves reduce the probability of action potentials and thus of contractions during a slow wave, while excitatory nerves increase the chance of contractions. The activity of the excitatory neurons is regulated by the hormones motilin, gastrin and cholecystokinin, while secretin enhances the inhibitory neuronal influence (see next section). The **speed** of **propagation** of slow waves also increases towards the pylorus. It is about $0.5\,cm \cdot s^{-1}$ in the gastric corpus, but $4\,cm \cdot s^{-1}$ in the caudal part of the antrum, i.e. slow waves propagate in a 20 cm long corpus in a medium-sized dog in 40 seconds, while in a 4 cm long antrum they propagate in one second.

When the slow wave reaches the threshold potential for opening voltage-dependent Ca^{2+} channels, it generates an action potential and thus a contraction. This results in a **peristaltic wave**, i.e., an annular constriction of the hollow organ that starts at about the middle of the corpus at the greater curvature and spreads caudally (**Fig. 16.21**). In the first phase, the contraction wave moves from the corpus to the antrum and pushes the stomach contents forward (**phase** of **propulsion**). When the progressively stronger constricting contraction wave reaches the middle antrum, the gastric contents are thoroughly mixed and a small amount of the chyme (especially liquid and small-particle portions) are flushed through the opened pylorus into the duodenum (**phase** of **mixing and emptying**). In the antrum, the speed of electrical propagation then progressively increases. As a result, the contraction wave partly overtakes the propelled food mass. Because of this, the electrical excitation reaches the pylorus before the contraction wave. It initiates a contraction there and thus closure of the sphincter. The bulk of the food is therefore propelled back into the corpus of the stomach following this contraction wave. In this phase, the contraction force in the antrum is so strong that practically the entire antrum is compressed. Solid food components grind together and are crushed (**phase** of **fragmentation and retropulsion**).

Since the pylorus closes before the food mass has reached it, solid components can only leave the stomach when they are greatly fragmented. Liquids, on the other hand, enter the small intestine relatively quickly.

> **IN A NUTSHELL** !
>
> The caudal region of the stomach acts as a "stomach pump" and ensures complete mixing of the contents as well as the release of liquid and highly fragmented solid components into the small intestine.

■ Stomach filling and emptying

In most animals, there are still remnants of previous meals in the stomach when food is consumed. If there is still food in the stomach, it is mixed with the new intake in the stomach corpus (**Fig. 16.20**). Liquid, on the other hand, can flow past this residual food mass, especially around the gastric small curvature. In contrast to solid food components, it also reaches the small intestine much more quickly.

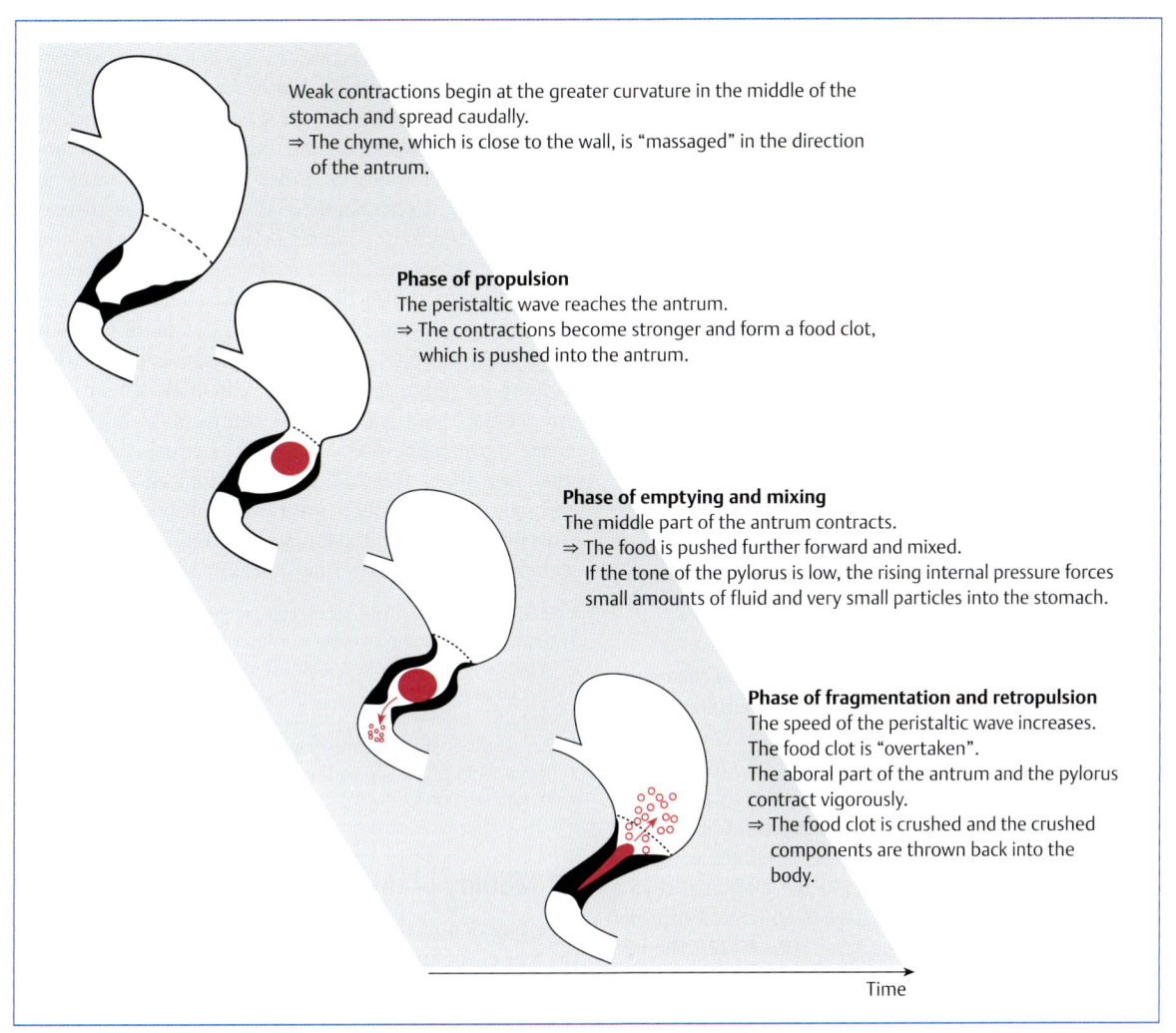

Weak contractions begin at the greater curvature in the middle of the stomach and spread caudally.
⇒ The chyme, which is close to the wall, is "massaged" in the direction of the antrum.

Phase of propulsion
The peristaltic wave reaches the antrum.
⇒ The contractions become stronger and form a food clot, which is pushed into the antrum.

Phase of emptying and mixing
The middle part of the antrum contracts.
⇒ The food is pushed further forward and mixed.
   If the tone of the pylorus is low, the rising internal pressure forces small amounts of fluid and very small particles into the stomach.

Phase of fragmentation and retropulsion
The speed of the peristaltic wave increases.
The food clot is "overtaken".
The aboral part of the antrum and the pylorus contract vigorously.
⇒ The food clot is crushed and the crushed components are thrown back into the body.

Time

Fig. 16.21 Course of a peristaltic wave in the stomach. It begins with a ring-shaped constriction in the middle of the stomach, which spreads caudally. Because of the increased speed of conduction of electrical currents across the gap junctions, the excitation wave overtakes the food bolus so some of the stomach contents are forced back into the body of the stomach. Only a small portion of the food enters the duodenum, the larger part is propelled back into the body of the stomach (retropulsion).

This is especially true for herbivores. In carnivores in the wild which kill prey sporadically, the stomach may be completely emptied between meals.

The pylorus is a barrier which regulates the onward passage of gastric contents into the duodenum. Anatomically, the pyloric lumen is strongly constricted by a thickening of the pyloric mucosa. The strong circular muscles also close the pylorus completely during the time of highest transpyloric pressure (retropulsion phase). This passage obstruction ensures that only a small proportion of the food in the stomach enters the small intestine with each contraction. This prevents the small intestine from being overloaded. Dilation of the pylorus is controlled by nerves and hormones mostly in the opposite direction to the motor function of the cranial part of the stomach, i.e. relaxation of the cranial stomach is usually coupled with increased tone of the pylorus.

The speed of gastric emptying is continuously adapting to the digestive and absorptive capacities of the small intestine. High nutrient concentrations in the duodenum or ileum inhibit hydrochloric acid secretion and emptying of

the stomach as a so-called **duodenal** or **ileal brake**. The effect on motility is called **feedback relaxation** of the proximal stomach. Sensors in the duodenum detect changes in pH, osmolarity and the presence of nutrients in the intestinal lumen. Acidic contents or an increase in osmolarity in the duodenum inhibit gastric emptying. Glucose, amino acids, peptides and especially fats in the duodenum, as well as glucose and fatty acids in the ileum also have an inhibitory effect on gastric emptying. Thus, fatty foods can "lie in the stomach for a long time" (**Fig. 16.22**). An accumulation of gastric acidity or material to be digested in the small intestine thus causes less food to be released from the stomach.

Different neuronal and humoral control systems play a role in mediating the reflex inhibition of gastric emptying. Parasympathetic fibres from the vagus nerve promote gastric emptying into the duodenum, while sympathetic fibres from the coeliac ganglion inhibit it. Secretin is released from S-cells in the duodenum in response to acidic duodenal pH and nutrient-rich chyme, and cholecystokinin is secreted by special enteroendocrine cells, the I-cells,

In the duodenum there are:
1. pH sensors
2. Osmosensors
3. Chemosensors   sensing   – Carbohydrates
                            – Fats
                            – Peptides, amino acids

Excitation of these sensors leads to the inhibition of the gastric motor function.
Function: Avoiding overloading the small intestine.

Stimulation of gastric motor function:
Acetylcholine, motilin   (whole stomach)
Gastrin, cholecystokinin   (caudal stomach only)

Inhibition of gastric motor function:
Adrenaline, noradrenaline, secretin   (whole stomach)
Gastrin, cholecystokinin   (cranial stomach only)

Fig. 16.22 Gastroduodenal feedback mechanisms. Hormones that have an inhibitory effect in the cranial stomach and a stimulating effect in the caudal stomach promote the mixing of stomach contents without emptying. The hormones printed in red are released from the duodenum.

in the duodenum when osmolarity is high and the chyme is rich in amino acids or fats. These two hormones from the duodenum play a role in relaxation of the cranial stomach and in delaying gastric emptying. Motilin from duodenal M-cells enhances contraction of both cranial and caudal parts of the stomach, and thereby promotes gastric emptying. The secretion of motilin is stimulated when free fatty acids and bile acids remain in the duodenal chyme, after amino acids and glucose have been largely absorbed and fats enzymatically broken down (**Fig. 16.22**). The ileal brake is primarily activated by peptide YY (in the case of high-fat chyme) and the glucagon-like peptide-1 (GLP-1, in glucose-rich chyme).

Even when the stomach is completely empty, its motility does not cease. In an empty stomach, there are periods when there are no contractions and periods with weak contractions. These weak contractions often do not reach

the antrum. There are also regular periods when particularly strong motility occurs. This cyclical motor pattern is known as the **migrating motor complex (MMC)**. It is called migrating because it spreads from the stomach over the entire small intestine. In contrast to the pattern of digestive gastric motility described so far, the migrating motor complex is characteristic of interdigestive (between meals) gastric motor function. Since it occurs (in omnivores and carnivores) in the fasting state, it is also referred to as "hunger contractions". The cycles last about 90 to 120 minutes. Overall, several phases can be distinguished (**Fig. 16.23**). In phase I, the stomach shows practically no activity. In phase II, pacemaker potentials spread across the stomach and lead to weak contractions. In phase III, these movements intensify into very strong contractions that last about five minutes. The stomach contracts so strongly that its lumen practically collapses completely. This produces the sound known as a stomach growl due to compression of residual fluid and air in the stomach.

MORE DETAILS   The strong contractions of phase III of the migrating motor complex have an important physiological function. In phase III, the pylorus is open. Thus, these contractions ensure that large particles are "cleaned out" of the stomach. Only in this way can larger particles that cannot be further fragmented by the gastric motor system be emptied from the stomach. These movements propagate to the small intestine. Motilin is involved in triggering phase III.

■ Motility of the abomasum in ruminants

The function of the abomasum in ruminants corresponds to that of the monogastric stomach, and it is generally assumed that its motor function is also similar to that of the monogastric stomach. For example, peristaltic waves are also observed in the abomasum, but phase III contractions are absent, although they do occur in the ruminant small intestine. In the adult ruminant there is no stratification of the abomasal contents, as there is a more or less continuous inflow of forestomach contents into the abomasum.

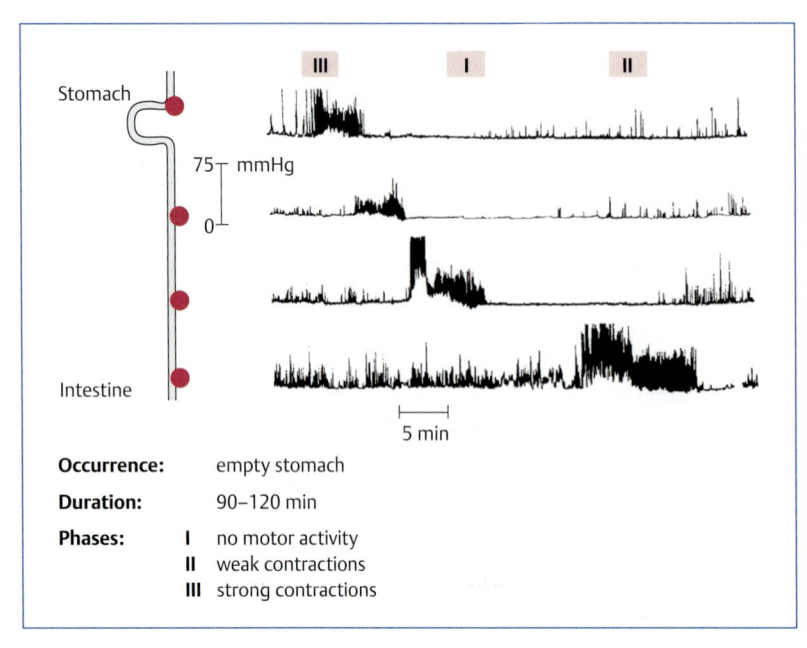

Fig. 16.23 The migrating motor complex. Pressure probes were used to measure the pressure in the lumen of the stomach and at various positions in the small intestine (red filled circles). The three phases of the migrating motor complex can be seen, which spread in a cranial to caudal direction, resulting in a phase delay between proximal and more distal parts of the intestine.

Stomach

75 ┬ mmHg

0 ┴

Intestine

├─┤
5 min

Occurrence: empty stomach

Duration: 90–120 min

Phases: I   no motor activity
              II   weak contractions
              III strong contractions

A clinically significant disease of ruminants is the so-called **displacement** of the **abomasum**. It occurs with genetic predisposition mainly in Holstein-Friesian cows after calving. In addition to changes in anatomical arrangement of the alimentary tract after calving, increased gas production and hypomotility of the abomasum are the critical pathogenetic factors. The abomasum, which fills with gas, usually moves to the left between the rumen and the abdominal wall. However, it can also rise to the right, in which case the abomasum often rotates. The displacement of the abomasum obstructs the flow of food and causes the contents of the abomasum to return into the forestomachs (internal vomiting resulting in hypochloraemic alkalosis).

MORE DETAILS   Feed which is low in fibre and of high-energy density promotes abomasal displacement not only because of reduced rumen filling, but also through increased accumulation of gas and short-chain fatty acids in the abomasum. The high content of short-chain fatty acids, together with the Ca^{2+} concentration in blood, which often drops postpartum, lead to hypomotility of the abomasum. Hypomotility is intensified by inhibitory neuronal circuits when bloating begins. Animals with abomasal displacement show abomasal atony, i.e. reduced muscle tone, characterised by increased activity of inhibitory (nitrergic) neurons and reduced responsiveness to acetylcholine. In addition to surgical treatment, the administration of erythromycin has become established therapy. Although erythromycin was originally developed as an antibiotic, it also stimulates motilin receptors and thus counteracts gastric atony.

■ Vomiting

Vomiting is the retrograde emptying of the contents of the stomach up the oesophagus into the oral cavity. Vomiting is relatively common in carnivores and omnivores, but only rarely in herbivores. In horses in particular, vomiting is almost impossible because the caudal oesophageal sphincter has a very strong tone, and the oesophagus opens into the horse's stomach at a steep angle, so that if the stomach is very full, the oesophagus is compressed by the pressure of the stomach contents. In the horse, therefore, if the stomach is overloaded, rupture of the stomach is more likely to occur than vomiting.

A variety of stimuli can trigger vomiting (**Fig. 16.24**). These include mechanical stimuli from the throat and chemical or mechanical stimuli from the stomach or small intestine. Also, excessive stimulation of the vestibular organ as well as hormonal imbalances (pregnancy) can also trigger vomiting. All these processes lead to an excitation of a particular region in the brain stem (medulla oblongata), the **vomiting centre**. A signal is transmitted to the vomiting centre via the 7th–10th cranial nerves. In addition, there is a so-called **chemosensitive trigger zone** in the area postrema in the rhomboid fossa of the 4th cerebral ventricle in the brain stem. It reacts to disturbances of the "internal milieu", for example in uraemia from renal insufficiency, or to particular pharmacological agents inducing vomiting. The function of vomiting is to stop the absorption of harmful substances from the gastrointestinal tract by immediately emptying the stomach.

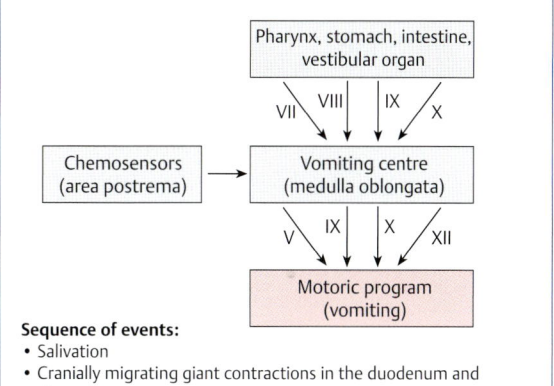

Sequence of events:
- Salivation
- Cranially migrating giant contractions in the duodenum and stomach
- Inspiration with closed glottis (gagging) → thoracic negative pressure becoming more negative
- Relaxation of the cranial oesophageal sphincter and aspiration of stomach contents into the oesophagus
- Expiration with closed glottis, including abdominal squeeze; increase in pressure in the thorax leads to transfer of the oesophageal content into the oral cavity

Fig. 16.24 The vomiting reflex. The Roman numerals indicate the cranial nerves involved (V: trigeminal nerve; VII: facial nerve; VIII: vestibulocochlear nerve; IX: glossopharyngeal nerve; X: vagus nerve; XII: hypoglossal nerve).

Vomiting is a relatively complex process that is accompanied by strong parasympathetic stimulation. This involves an increased production of saliva which facilitates the expulsion of vomited material and protects the oral cavity from irritation by gastric acid. Orally migrating giant contractions then begin in the duodenum and stomach. Bile is often flushed into the stomach, which increases the urge to vomit by irritating the gastric mucosa. Repeated inspiratory movements of the diaphragm with the glottis closed, gagging, creates negative pressure in the thoracic cavity. The caudal oesophageal sphincter relaxes, and the stomach contents are propelled into the oesophagus by thoracic negative pressure. The retching finally ends with a violent contraction of all expiratory muscles, especially the abdominal muscles, with the glottis closed. This creates a sudden increase in pressure in the oesophagus and stomach, forcing oesophageal and stomach contents into the oral cavity. By lifting the soft palate, the nasal cavity is closed to the pharynx, preventing vomit from entering the nose.

MORE DETAILS   Dogs and cats in particular often ingest spoiled food, poisons or large amounts of hair, which they can only get rid of effectively by vomiting. This protective reflex should not be routinely suppressed with medication. If, on the other hand, one is sure that the vomiting was triggered by irritation of the organ of equilibrium (motion sickness), a drug therapy can be helpful. This is aimed at reducing parasympathetic tone and inhibiting central histamine receptors (H_1). Chemical stimuli to vomit from the area postrema act via receptors for dopamine (D_2), serotonin ($5-HT_3$) and substance P (NK_1) and can be inhibited by appropriate antagonists.

IN A NUTSHELL   !

Vomiting is a protective reflex with the aim of removing potentially harmful substances from the gastrointestinal tract before there has been any significant absorption.

Nutrition, energy

16.3.4 Motility of the small and large intestine

Martin Diener, Jörg R. Aschenbach

ESSENTIALS ✗

Motility of the intestine is defined by various types of contraction of intestinal musculature. The purpose of this motility is to mix the chyme with secretions from the pancreas and with bile and to bring the nutrient products of digestion into contact with the absorbing epithelia. In addition, the chyme must be propelled caudally quite quickly, at rates determined by the various digestive processes. With powerful cleansing contractions of the small intestine, microbial colonisation of the alimentary tract is thereby largely limited to the large intestine. Finally, large intestine motility supports fermentative digestion and serves to excrete indigestible food components.

■ Intestinal motility and digestion

The intestine has both storage and transport functions, which are supported by appropriate motility. The **storage function** is particularly pronounced in different segments of the large intestine and enables the lengthy process of fermentative digestion of plant fibres by bacterial enzymes and the reabsorption of water. The **transport function** allows sequential nutrient absorption in various specialised intestinal segments, limits microbial colonisation as far as possible to the large intestine, and ultimately also serves to excrete undigested food components and fermentation gases. The third important task is the mixing of **intestinal contents**. In the small intestine, the mixing of the food mass with pancreatic enzymes and the fat-emulsifying components of bile is particularly important for optimal digestion. In the large intestine, the microorganisms must continuously be brought into new contact with digestible substrate. Fourthly, **nutrients** are **brought to the brush border membrane** by intestinal motor activity. This initiates the membranous phase of enzymatic digestion (small intestine only) and finally the absorption of small molecules produced during digestion (small and large intestine).

IN A NUTSHELL !

The intestinal motor system has four different tasks, which include storage, transport and thorough mixing of the chyme, as well as bringing absorbable nutrients to the epithelial surface.

■ Morphological and functional basics of intestinal motility

The small intestine is where most of the digestion and absorption of nutrients takes place. In order for the food components to be broken down and then absorbed, they must come into contact with secreted enzymes or those on the brush border membrane of the small intestinal epi-

thelial cells. A number of contractile structures ensure the constant mixing of intestinal contents. These include the muscular layer of the intestinal wall, the **tunica muscularis**, which consists of an outer longitudinal muscle layer and an inner circular muscle layer (**Fig. 16.25**). Between the two muscle layers lies the myenteric plexus, the nerve plexus of the enteric nervous system, which innervates the circular and longitudinal muscle layers. A single contraction of the circular muscles constricts the intestinal lumen, whereas a single contraction of the longitudinal muscles produces a peristaltic movement. In addition to these characteristic contractions, the circular musculature has the important task of withstanding intestinal dilatation, while the longitudinal musculature adapts to shearing forces. The musculature of the small and large intestine, like that of the stomach, has regions where the circular muscle is particularly pronounced to form sphincters. There is the sphincter ileocaecale at the junction of the ileum and the caecum, and the internal and external anal sphincters. The latter, however, does not contain any smooth muscle cells, but consists of striated muscle. These sphincters regulate the passage of the intestinal contents from the ileum into the caecum or for defecation (p. 393).

In addition to the main muscle layer, there is also a thinner **muscularis mucosae** directly below the mucosal epithelium, with an outer longitudinal and an inner circular muscle layer with muscle fibres extending into the villi. Around the crypts or in the villi there is an interconnected system of myofibroblasts, i.e. connective tissue cells which contain contractile actin- and myosin fibres. The myofibro-

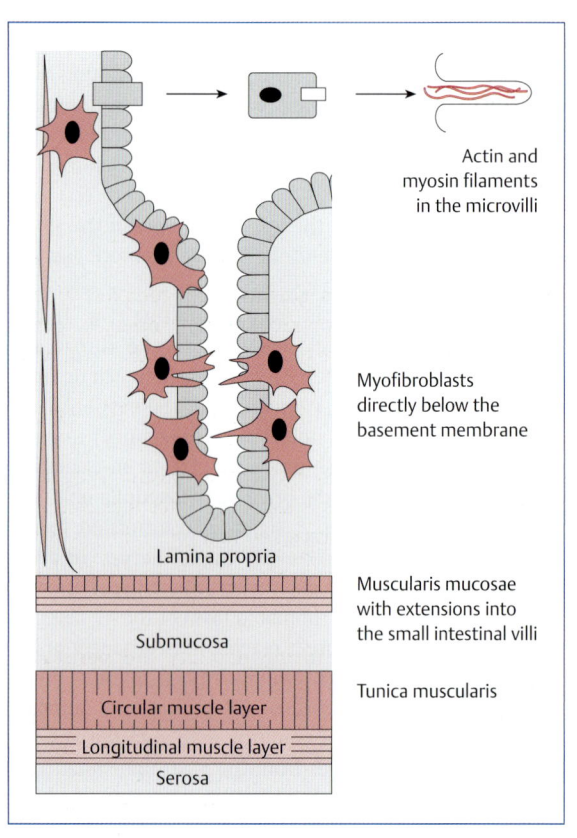

Actin and myosin filaments in the microvilli

Myofibroblasts directly below the basement membrane

Lamina propria

Muscularis mucosae with extensions into the small intestinal villi

Submucosa

Tunica muscularis

Circular muscle layer

Longitudinal muscle layer

Serosa

Fig. 16.25 Contractile structures in the intestinal wall.

blasts sit below the collagen fibres of the lamina basalis, to which the epithelial cells attach. The myofibroblasts surround each crypt as a contractile envelope and additionally form a contractile core in the villi of the small intestine. The muscularis mucosae and myofibroblasts give the individual villi motility which assists mixing of the adjacent food mass, and as a so-called **villus pump**, promotes the transit of absorbed water from the connective tissue of the lamina propria into lymphatic vessels (p. 207). The myofibroblasts surrounding the crypts probably also support their secretory function by expressing fluid from interstitium into the crypt lumen.

> **MORE DETAILS**   The lowest level of the contractile elements of the small and large intestine are actin and myosin filaments in the **microvilli**, the protrusions of the brush border membrane of the epithelial cells. These filaments consist of bundles of about 20 individual fibres. They perform fine movement of the microvilli. Interaction of the actin and myosin filaments in the epithelial cells always occurs when the Ca^{2+} concentration in the cytosol of these cells increases.

> **IN A NUTSHELL**   !
>
> Intestinal motor function is mainly caused by contractions of smooth muscle of the tunica muscularis. In addition, smooth muscle cells of the lamina muscularis mucosae, subepithelial myofibroblasts and actin filaments in microvilli of the intestinal epithelial cells support absorption and secretion functions of the intestinal epithelium.

■ Patterns of small intestinal motility

The contraction phases of the small intestine are either mixing movements or propulsion movements, but the different functions can rarely be completely separated from each other.

Mixing motility

Contractions with the primary purpose of mixing the food take the form of groups of contractions in segments. In these **segmentations**, there are contractions of the circular muscle layer in adjacent segments, often completely closing the lumen. These contractions only occur in short lengths of the musculature (in dogs approx. 0.5–1 cm) with more or less wide, non-contracting spaces in between. This results in a series of constrictions, like a string of pearls, along the intestinal tube. Segmentation contractions are stationary, i.e. they remain in the same intestinal segment and do not migrate. This kneads the intestinal contents and delays the onward passage so that more time is available for digestion and absorption. Segmentation contractions in the small intestine are particularly prominent with protein-rich chyme.

The second form of mixing motility are **peristaltic waves** propagated over very short distances that do not lead to any significant forward movement of intestinal contents. The intestinal contents are compressed briefly, and then again as the intestinal segment relaxes. Since this process happens over and over again at the same intestinal segment, these are called **contraction groups**. They can

continue for quite some time in the same region of the proximal small intestine as so-called stationary contraction groups. Typically, however, they progress slowly in a caudal direction as so-called migrating contraction groups which are particularly noticeable after ingestion of high-fat food.

Propulsion motility

Contractions that have the primary function of propelling chyme onwards are peristalsis/antiperistalsis, giant contractions, and phase III of the activity of the motor system between meals. The **peristaltic reflex** is the most common and best-known form of contraction for propulsion of small intestinal chyme. It was described in detail in the chapter on muscle control (p. 362). The caudal migration direction of this contraction sequence is illustrated in **Fig. 16.26**. Peristaltic waves are initiated by stretching of the intestinal wall. On the cranial side of the site of stretching, the circular muscle layer contracts, named **ascending contraction**, while on the caudal side of the stretched region there is **relaxation of the circular muscle layer**, named **descending relaxation**. This descending relaxation creates space for the food mass to advance under the force of the ascending contraction. Relaxation and contraction describe the behaviour of the circular muscle layer of the tunica muscularis, which is intrinsically controlled by the myenteric plexus. The peristaltic contractions of the small intestine in dogs and pigs have a maximum frequency of approx. $17\,min^{-1}$ and a decreasing speed of propagation from the duodenum (approx. $8\,cm \cdot s^{-1}$) to the ileum (approx. $0.5\,cm \cdot s^{-1}$). **Antiperistalsis**, i.e. cranially directed waves, are very rarely observed in the small intestine and can be classified as a pathological form of contraction in this GIT compartment (**Fig. 16.27**).

Control of small intestinal motility has already been briefly described (**Fig. 16.10**) and is similar to control of motility in the caudal part of the stomach (**Fig. 16.22**). Neuronal control and its modulation by sympathetic and parasympathetic nerves predominate. Strong sympathetic or parasympathetic activation or weakness of the cholinergic system, which often occurs postoperatively, can completely block the onward propulsion of chyme, resulting in functional intestinal obstruction (ileus). Clinically, it is important to distinguish between paralytic ileus and spastic ileus. In paralytic ileus, parasympathomimetics are used for treatment and in spastic ileus parasympatholytics are therapeutically effective. Motilin, gastrin, cholecystokinin and serotonin promote propulsion motility, whereas secretin and somatostatin inhibit peristalsis.

Caudally migrating giant contractions, formerly also called mass movements, are contraction sequences intrinsically connected by the enteric nervous system, but they are also often triggered by extrinsic signals. They differ from peristaltic waves in that they occur without slow waves of the Cajal cells and are more powerful and progress more slowly (approx. $0.5\,cm \cdot s^{-1}$). The intestinal lumen is completely closed, and the entire contents of the intestine are pushed forward over longer distances. In the pig's ileum, giant contractions occur as part of the diges-

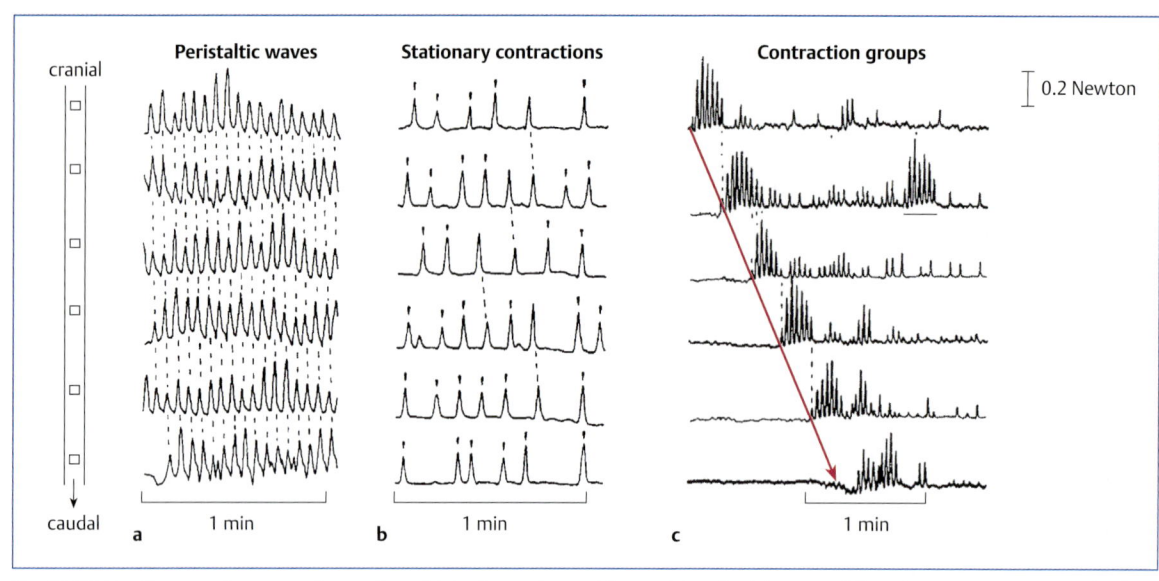

Fig. 16.26 The three most common forms of small intestine motor activity are (**a**) peristaltic waves, (**b**) stationary contractions in the form of segmentations, and (**c**) contraction groups. Contraction groups are either slowly migrating caudally (first red arrow) or are stationary. The squares in the intestinal segment represent sensory probes. The dashed lines connect peristaltically propagated contractions. Experimentally, peristaltic waves can be triggered by simple stretch stimuli (e.g. by nutrient-free buffer solutions), while a chyme containing glucose and amino acids tends to cause segmentations. Chyme containing long-chain fatty acids tends to initiate groups of contractions that remain mainly stationary.

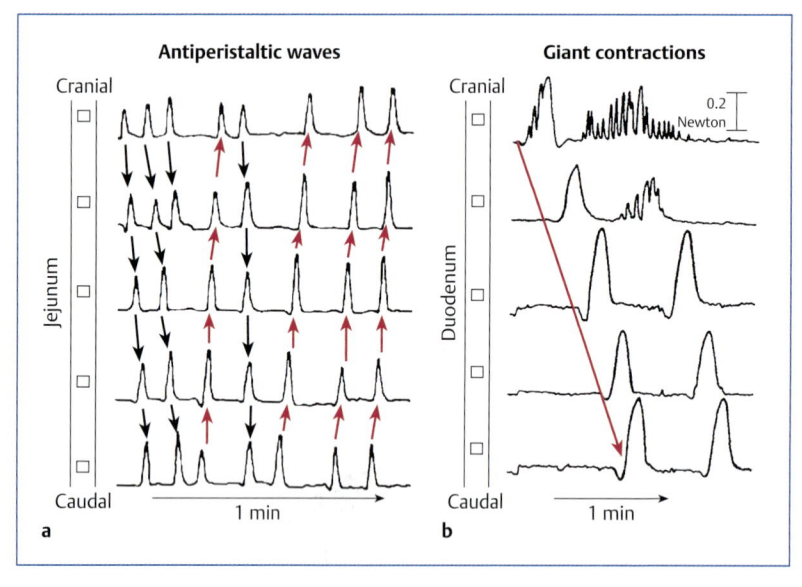

Fig. 16.27 (**a**) Antiperistaltic waves and (**b**) giant contractions are pathological forms of contraction of the proximal intestinal segments. Experimentally, such disorders can be induced in dogs by removing the gastrin-producing cells in the pyloric region (distal gastrectomy). The arrows in (**a**) mark peristaltic (black arrows) and antiperistaltic waves (red arrows). The red arrow in (**b**) marks the caudal spread of the contraction wave.

tive motor system. In the ileum of dogs, cats and horses, caudally migrating giant contractions also have the function of a cleansing motor system between meals, and these giant contractions complement the high-frequency peristaltic waves of **phase III** of the Migrating Motor Complex (p. 392) in their effect. Otherwise, caudal direction giant contractions of the small intestine are typically seen in diarrhoea and cause the rapid emptying of the intestine (**Fig. 16.27**).

MORE DETAILS   Caudally migrating giant contractions can be caused by various bacterial toxins (e.g. enterotoxins of *Escherichia coli*, cholera toxin) or by irritating substances (e.g. castor oil). They contribute particularly to the symptom complex of diarrhoea and play a role in **intestinal cleansing in intestinal infec-**

tions. After initial inhibition of intestinal motor activity at the onset of diarrhoea, giant contractions then develop in the small and large intestine. In extreme cases, the entire intestine can empty almost completely within a few minutes. **Cranially migrating giant contractions**, on the other hand, precede the act of vomiting (p. 387).

In most species, the papillae-like ileocaecal orifice is characterised by a thickening of the ileum's circular muscles. This **ileocaecal sphincter** prevents reflux of the contents of the large intestine into the ileum. It normally has a relatively high pressure of about 20 mmHg. In humans, it can withstand pressures of up to 40 mmHg. In horses, the occlusion is further enhanced by a submucosal venous plexus.

The contraction state of the ileocaecal sphincter is regulated by the filling state of neighbouring segments of the small intestine. Stretching of the ileum triggers relaxation of the sphincter so that contents of the ileum can flow into the large intestine. An increase in pressure in the caecum or colon, on the other hand, triggers an increase in sphincter tone to prevent reflux into the ileum. Also, severe irritation of the caecum due to inflammation leads to a closure of the sphincter, which interrupts the onward transport of the food mass.

In most species, the contents of the small intestine enter the ascending colon due to the orientation of the orifice and subsequently reach the caecum by antiperistaltic movements. In contrast to the small intestine, antiperistaltic waves are physiological in the large intestine and occur mainly in the proximal colon of ruminants, rodents and cats. In contrast, peristaltic waves always predominate in the distal colon. The **alternating peristaltic and antiperistaltic waves** of the proximal colon and caecum have a low frequency (in sheep and rabbits approx. 1–2 min⁻¹) and are low strength constrictions. They therefore serve primarily to mix and to maintain a long retention time of the residual food mass. This promotes bacterial colonisation and fermentation, especially in herbivorous and omnivorous species. It also allows structural plant carbohydrates to be utilised, which otherwise would not have nutritional value as animals do not have endogenous cellulolytic enzymes (p. 438).

In many species of animals, **haustra (semilunar folds)** contribute to a long retention time and intensive mixing of the contents of the large intestine. Haustra-separated intestinal parts are very common and well-developed in herbivores with extensive digestion in the large intestine. In so-called **caecum fermenters** (e.g. guinea pigs, rabbits), haustra are mainly in the voluminous caecum, whereas in so-called **colon fermenters** (e.g. horse, rhinoceros, elephant) haustra are additionally and predominantly present in the colon.

The haustra are bulges in the intestinal wall oriented along thickened longitudinal muscles, the taenia (ligamentous strips). The haustra are not permanent structures, but develop and disappear through local contraction or relaxation of a thickened circular muscle that separates two haustra, or by contraction and relaxation of each haustrum. With each of these so-called **haustral movements**, a special form of segmentation motility, the intestinal contents are mixed. Even with the weak constrictions caused by peristaltic and antiperistaltic waves, the haustra still promote mixing because the intestinal contents churn across these irregular structures. A special feature of the rabbit colon is the cranial "rolling" movement of the haustra, in which liquid contents in particular are propelled back into the caecum one haustra at a time after a peristaltic caecum-colon contraction. The haustra also act as a trap for fermentation gases. This allows the gases to be transported as small bubbles instead of collecting in one large gas bubble.

If there is no haustration (e.g. in carnivores) or if haustration decreases or is lost in more anal sections of the

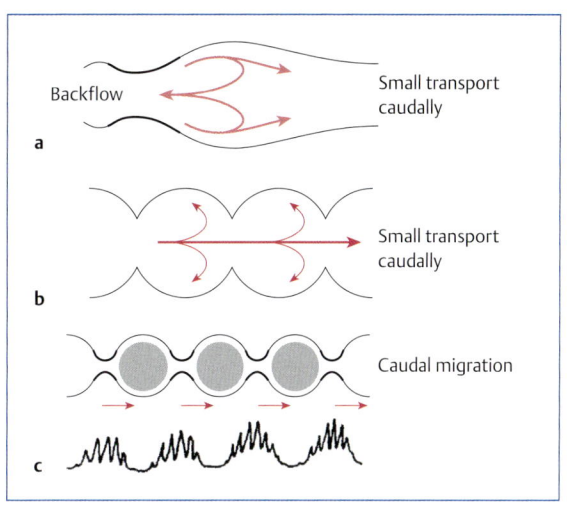

Fig. 16.28 With the exception of giant contractions, motility of the large intestine generally contributes both to mixing and onward propulsion of intestinal contents.
a Peristaltic wave at the non-haustrated large intestine: Peristaltic waves, because of their low constrictive force, glide over the intestinal contents in the non-haustrated large intestine. At the central constriction ring, there is a resultant backflow and simultaneous mixing of contents.
b Peristaltic wave at the haustrated large intestine: At the haustrated large intestine, peristaltic waves cause less of a central flow and more of a churning movement of the contents across the haustra.
c Caudally migrating segmentation contractions: Segmentation contraction are often migratory in the large intestine. The food residue is mixed and formed into faecal balls or pellets while being slowly propelled. Recorded pressure curves show the segmentation contractions gradually increase, with superimposed groups of phasic contractions. This contraction pattern is called colonic motor complexes.

large intestine, haustration movements are replaced by classical **segmentation motility**. In contrast to the small intestine, segmentation movements in the large intestine do not occur briefly in different regions, but are prolonged and migrate anally. In horses and dogs, they are therefore also called **colonic motor complexes**. However, these must not be equated with the migrating motor complex of the small intestine, which is predominantly peristaltic in character and is not synchronised in time with the colonic motor complexes. In the colon of some animal species, such migrating constrictions, like a string of pearls and with simultaneous dehydration of the intestinal contents, can lead to the formation of characteristic **faecal balls** (horse) or **faecal pellets** (sheep, goat, rodent).

The migrating segmentation contractions as well as the peristaltic waves of the large intestine contribute to both the mixing and onward transport of the intestinal contents (Fig. 16.28).

Giant contractions occur physiologically in the colon of some animals. In humans, dogs and cats they occur about two or three times a day. They can start at different points in the colon and then progress as a powerful contraction wave towards the rectum. During each giant contraction, the intestinal contents can be moved about ⅓ of the length of the colon. These giant contractions are often triggered

Nutrition, energy

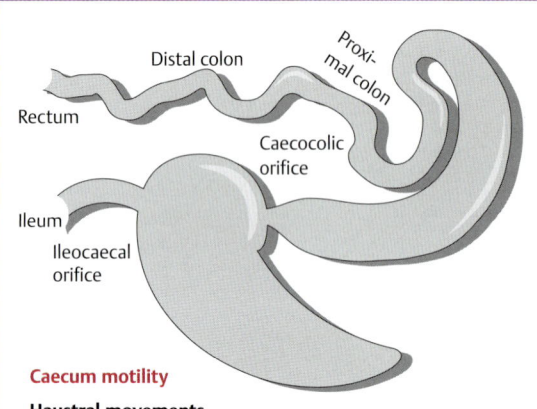

Caecum motility

Haustral movements
stationary constrictions of the circular muscles
→ back and forth movement of the caecum
  content between the haustra
→ mixing of the caecal content

Antiperistalsis
running from the caecum base to the apex of the caecum
→ mixing and prolonging the retention time

Peristalsis
running from the caecum apex to the base of the caecum
→ dilatation of the caecum base
→ contraction of the caecum base
→ emptying into the proximal colon through
  the caecocolic orifice

Fig. 16.29 Special features of the equine caecum. Because of a particular anatomical structure, the ileal contents in the horse directly enter the caecum through the ileocaecal orifice. The caecum is also closed to the colon by a narrow caecocolic orifice and thus forms a more or less closed fermentation chamber. Haustra movements, antiperistalsis and peristalsis all contribute to intensive mixing of the caecal contents. At the start of a peristaltic wave, the increase in pressure in the caecum propels caecal contents into the ascending colon. After further fermentation in the ascending colon, solid faecal balls are finally formed in the descending colon by migrating segmentation contractions and by dehydration of the faecal mass.

by gastric distension during food intake and the prandial/postprandial nutrient detection or hormone secretion in the stomach (gastrin) and duodenum (cholecystokinin). This is called the **gastrocolic reflex** and leads to rapid rectal filling and an urge to defecate.

MORE DETAILS   There are a number of species-specific differences in the motor pattern of the large intestine. In the **horse**, the contents of the ileum do not pass directly into the proximal colon, but rather into the caecal pouch that developed originally from the colon. As a second special feature, the caecocolic orifice, i.e. the connection between the caecum and the colon, is closed in the horse by a mucosal fold and a sphincter, so that the contents from the ileum remain in the caecum for some time before being further fermented in the proximal colon. In the caecum base, gas is produced by fermentation which causes stretching of the caecal wall and stretch sensors then stimulate a contraction. This triggers a migratory contraction wave that runs antiperistaltically to the apex of the caecum (**Fig. 16.29**). Peristaltic waves occur in the equine caecum approximately every three to five minutes and spread from the apex along the body of the caecum, forcing caecal contents towards and through the caecocolic orifice into the ventral region of the ascending colon. At the point of transition from the ventral to the dorsal region of the ascending

colon (pelvic flexure), the lumen becomes considerably narrower, so that the onward moving digesta exerts increasing pressure and shear forces on the intestinal wall at this point. Accordingly, the pelvic flexure is the main origin of the colonic motor complexes as well as of contraction waves which propagate as peristaltic waves towards the anus and as antiperistaltic waves towards the caecocolic orifice. This enables coarse particles to be preferentially transported in a cranial direction and smaller particles preferentially in an anal direction, resulting in a size separation of mainly digested and less digested contents. Such antiperistalsis before the pelvic flexure can provoke the development of **constipation** (intestinal blockage), which can become life-threatening.

In **rabbits**, the rolling movements of the haustra are of great importance for returning liquid colonic contents into the caecum and thereby favour the formation of **hard faecal pellets** by caudally migrating segmentation contractions. During the soft faeces phase, the cranial directed haustra movements are suppressed and faeces movement through the colon is accelerated by giant contractions. At the same time, with low plasma aldosterone level, Na^+ and fluid absorption in the distal colon is inhibited, so that **soft faeces** are formed. This is rich in nutrients and microbial products and is collected from the anus and eaten by these coprophagous animals.

In sheep, the formation of soft faeces also occurs during grazing. In this process, the caudally migrating segmentation contractions are increasingly replaced by peristaltic waves and giant contractions. As a result, large soft faecal balls are deposited instead of small hard faecal pellets.

> **IN A NUTSHELL**   !
>
> Segmentations in the colon are responsible for the formation of the characteristic faecal pellets of horses, sheep, goats or rodents.

■ Coordinated motility patterns of different gastrointestinal segments

The motility of individual sections of the gastrointestinal tract does not proceed independently of each other, but in a coordinated manner, with food intake in particular acting as a timer. In addition, there are (so-called "long") reflexes which influence the motor patterns in a more distant section via stretching stimuli and by detection of nutrients in the lumen. The **enterogastric reflexes** as **duodenal and ileal brakes**, inhibit gastric emptying during nutrient loading of the small intestine. The **gastrocolic reflex** has already been discussed in the chapter on large intestine motor function (p. 389). As the stomach fills up and the small intestine begins to flood with nutrients, it reflexively leads to colonic emptying and thus to the urge to defecate. This makes room for newly ingested food. The **gastroileal reflex** functions in a similar way, where increasing filling of the stomach initiates an ileal contraction, which propels the contents of the small intestine into the large intestine. In ruminants, this reflex is absent because of the continuous flow of food material from the forestomachs into the abomasum and then into the small intestine. Hence, in ruminants, ileal emptying is mainly independent of stomach filling.

A particularly distinct coordinated motility pattern of the stomach and small intestine is the **migrating motor**

Sequence
- In carnivorous and omnivorous species after prolonged fasting (approx. 6 h after meal)
- In herbivorous species phase III also in the fed state (approx. every 90 min)

Three phases
- Phase I   no significant contraction
- Phase II   irregular contractions
- Phase III   strong contractions in the form of peristaltic waves; progression from cranial to caudal

Function
- Forward movement of intestinal contents in phases II and III
- "Cleaning function" of phase III

Fig. 16.30 Properties of the migrating motor complex. For the time course see Fig. 16.23.

complex **(MMC)**. The MMC is also called the interdigestive (between meals) motor complex in carnivorous and omnivorous species. In dogs, for example, the MMC develops after about six hours of fasting. Up to that time, the basal types of motility predominate. This pattern is also seen in pigs when fed only once a day. The situation is different in herbivorous species or in pigs that are fed ad libitum when the MMC largely overlaps the digestive motility patterns.

A migrating motor complex recurs on average every 70–120 minutes. It can be divided into three different phases (**Fig. 16.23**, **Fig. 16.30**). Phase I is a period without significant contractile activity. In phase II, segmentation contractions occur irregularly as well as individual peristaltic waves, by which some of the contents of the small intestine are propelled into the large intestine. Phase III finally consists of high frequency, relatively long peristaltic waves. The length of time of each phase at any one point in the intestine in dogs is approx. 60 minutes for phase I, approx. 15 minutes for phase II and 5–8 minutes for phase III. The phases then migrate with decreasing speed over the entire small intestine. In dogs, the migration speed decreases from 6.5 cm·min⁻¹ in the duodenum to 1.7 cm·min⁻¹ in the ileum. When phase III reaches the ileum, a new interdigestive cycle is triggered at the stomach and duodenum if fasting continues. However, two interdigestive cycles can also run through the intestine at the same time. In pigs in particular, it is common for the next phase III to begin at the stomach and duodenum before the previous one has reached the terminal ileum. In the cat, instead of phase III in the interdigestive period, giant contractions occur.

The individual phases have different functions. During phase II, residual intestinal contents are mixed again and individual boluses are propelled forward by peristalsis. Phase III with its strong contractions has a "cleaning effect" and ensures that the last remnants in the intestine are transported distally. Any disturbance of phase III contractions allows colonisation of the small intestine with colon bacteria.

MORE DETAILS The migrating motor complex begins at the stomach (**Fig. 16.23**). However, there is no transition of the signal from the stomach to the duodenum, but the complex is triggered simultaneously in both the stomach and the duodenum. The hormone **motilin** promotes strong contractions during the migrat-

ing motor complex. An increase in the concentration of motilin in plasma can be detected during phase III and, conversely, phase III contractions can be provoked by motilin administration. The release of motilin, which is secreted at approximately 2-hour intervals during fasting, is often followed or superimposed by a release of the peptide hormone **ghrelin** from the empty stomach. Ghrelin stimulates appetite (**Fig. 22.3**), so that emptying of the stomach and small intestine is indirectly linked to an increased **feeling of hunger**. The saying "My stomach is growling" describes precisely this feeling of hunger. Rats and mice produce neither motilin nor motilin receptors. In these animals, phase III-like contractions are probably promoted directly by ghrelin.

IN A NUTSHELL   !

"Long reflexes" coordinate the motor function of individual sections of the gastrointestinal tract depending on food intake and progress of digestion. After food has been digested, the stomach and small intestine are emptied by migrating motor complexes.

■ Defecation

A final and important task of the motility of the gastrointestinal tract is the excretion of non-digestible food components by the act of defecation. While the formation of faeces is a continuous process, defecation is periodic and can also be initiated voluntarily.

Closure of the rectum is by two **sphincters**, the smooth muscle **internal anal sphincter** and the **external anal sphincter** of striated muscle which can therefore be voluntarily controlled (**Fig. 16.31**). Distension of the rectum reflexively induces an urge to defecate. Faeces in the rectum stimulate stretch sensors in the rectal mucosa and in the musculature. This stimulates enteric neurons of the myenteric plexus, which initiate peristaltic colonic waves (**rectocolic reflex**). This drives more colon contents into the rectum as well as causing the inner anal sphincter to relax during the peristaltic reflex. This increases pressure on the external anal sphincter and the consciously perceived stretching of the anal region is transmitted via the pudendal nerve to motor neurons in the sacral spinal cord, which cause the external, striated anal sphincter to contract. Since this process is repeated several times due to intermittent filling of the rectum, these reflex sequences are also called **phasic rectosphincteric reflexes**. (This kind of rhythmic "pumping" of the anal sphincter can also be observed in cattle after rectal examinations if the sensors in the rectum and anus have been very strongly stimulated by the examiner).

The information about the stretching of the rectum is communicated to a superordinate centre, the **defecation centre in the medulla oblongata**. With the inclusion of further information from other regions of the brain, the defecation centre makes the final decision whether to give in to the urge to defecate and whether defecation should be initiated. If defecation is decided to take place, the motor neurons for the external sphincter in the sacral medulla are inhibited from this centre and the external sphincter relaxes. In herbivores (horses, ruminants), this is usually sufficient to initiate defecation. In animals that defecate less frequently (carnivores, pigs), an intensive abdominal

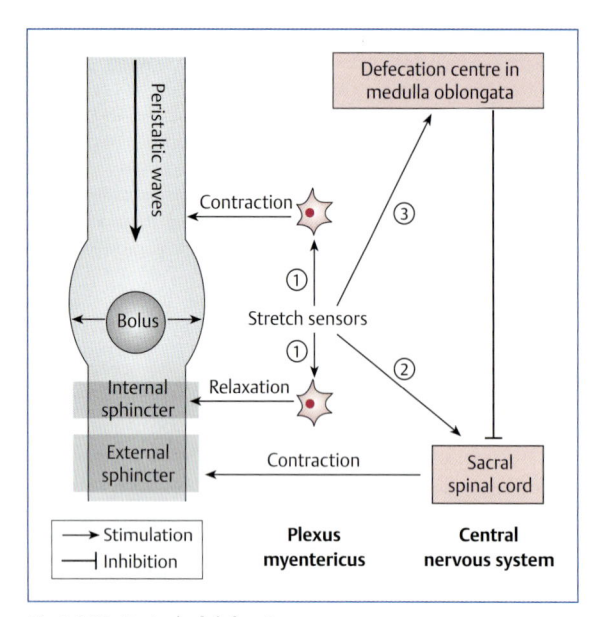

Fig. 16.31 Control of defecation.
1: Excitation of stretch sensors triggers the ascending contraction and descending relaxation.
2: Stimulation of motor neurons in the sacral spinal cord is responsible for closure of the external anal sphincter.
3: The defecation centre, which is informed by the stretching of the rectum, ultimately decides whether defecation is to be initiated or not.

squeeze is usually also necessary (defecation with curved back).

The number of defecations per day depends on the amount of faeces to be excreted. In animals that eat highly digestible food, such as dogs, faeces are normally defecated 1–2 times a day. In cattle, which usually ingest low digestibility food, defecation occurs 10–16 times a day.

> MORE DETAILS   **Atresia ani** (imperforate anus) is a common, hereditary anomaly in pigs and leads to death in male piglets in the first days of life. Female animals can be saved by diverting faeces to the vagina via a surgically created fistula. The animals then defecate (without arbitrary control) via the vagina.

IN A NUTSHELL   !

Defecation is controlled and influenced voluntarily by a complex interaction of the autonomic and somatic nervous systems.

■ Suggested reading

Argenzio RA. General functions of the gastrointestinal tract and their control. In: Reece WO, ed. Dukes' physiology of domestic animals, 12th ed. London: Cornell University Press; 2004, 381–390

Hansen MB. Neurohumoral control of gastrointestinal motility. Physiol Res 2003; 52: 1–30

Komuro T. Three-dimensional observation of the fibroblast-like cells associated with the rat myenteric plexus, with special reference to the interstitial cells of Cajal. Cell Tissue Res 1989; 225: 343–351

Sanders KM, Koh SD, Ward SM. Interstitial cells of Cajal as pacemakers in the gastrointestinal tract. Annu Rev Physiol 2006; 68: 307–343

Schneider S, Wright CM, Heuckeroth RO. Unexpected roles for the second brain: enteric nervous system as master regulator of bowel function. Annu Rev Physiol 2019; 81: 235–259

16.4   Forestomachs

16.4.1   Development of the forestomachs

Gerhard Breves

ESSENTIALS

– Ruminants are functionally born as "monogastric" animals. The small forestomachs initially have no significant digestive function.
– The development of the forestomachs begins with the ingestion of fibrous feed (e.g. hay), the establishment of microbial colonies of bacteria, protozoa and fungi and the resulting fermentation of the feed in the reticulorumen.
– Luminal factors such as short-chain fatty acids as well as hormones such as insulin, IGF-1 (insulin-like growth factor) and EGF (epidermal growth factor) contribute significantly to the development of the forestomachs.

The three forestomachs, the reticulum, rumen, and omasum, as well as the abomasum all develop from a common anlage and can already be distinguished embryonically. Thus, although all (forestomach/stomach) compartments are present at birth, the typical proportions in size of these organs in an adult ruminant are not yet established in newborn ruminants. At **birth**, the **abomasum** is the main compartment, accounting for **55–60%** of the volume of total **stomach system**. Furthermore, the relative weight of the total stomach system (forestomachs + abomasum) as a proportion of the weight of the total alimentary tract is only slightly more than 20%. These weight ratios change considerably, both within the forestomach compartments and the forestomach system relative to the entire alimentary tract, within a few months after birth when newborn lambs or calves are consuming raw fibre-rich feed. Important **stimuli** for the increase in weight and volume of the forestomachs, the growth of papillae, and keratinisation of the epithelium are the short-chain fatty acids produced by the onset of **fermentation** of the **fibrous feed**. Furthermore, growth factors such as insulin, IGF-1 (insulin-like growth factor), and EGF (epidermal growth factor) play a role. After completion of these adaptation processes to the ruminant-appropriate feed, the **forestomachs** account for about **80–90%** of the weight of all stomach compartments, and the four stomachs together account for about 50% of the total weight of the gastrointestinal tract. These relative numbers do not indicate the absolute increase in size. In the adult ruminant, the forestomach system fills practically the entire left half of the abdominal cavity. The volume in the reticulorumen corresponds on average to 25% of body weight, i.e. 10–18 l in small ruminants and over 150 l in high milk yielding cows.

MORE DETAILS **Development** of the forestomach system can be considerably **delayed** if calves to be fattened are only offered liquid feed (milk or milk replacer). Under such feeding regimes, not only is there no stimulus for the development of the forestomach but behavioural problems may also occur. Lick addiction may occur leading to the ingestion of hair and, as a consequence, to the formation of bezoars in the rumen. Bezoars are round solid aggregates of mainly undigested material. If they consist mainly of hair, they are known as trichobezoars. Their presence in the rumen can lead to harmful effects on digestion. The continued feeding of newborn ruminants with liquid feed must therefore be critically evaluated and not just in terms of nutritional physiology.

IN A NUTSHELL

The postnatal development of the forestomachs is critically determined by feeding practice. The intake of crude fibre initiates fermentation in the forestomachs and thus their development.

16.4.2 Digestion and absorption in the forestomachs

Gerhard Breves, Reiko Rackwitz

ESSENTIALS

- The reticulum, rumen and omasum are known as the forestomachs, in which microbial populations of bacteria, protozoa and fungi become established after birth and contribute significantly to total digestion of feed.
- Microbial enzymes can digest nutrients that could not be made available to the host animal through the body's own digestive processes. In addition to microbial fermentation, the synthesis of microbial cell mass and thus above all of microbial protein as well as water-soluble vitamins are important nutritional contributions of microbial fermentation.
- The composition of the microbial population is influenced by diet.
- The fibrous components of the feed provide optimal environmental conditions for microorganisms in the forestomachs by stimulating salivary secretion and reticulorumen motility.
- Considerable quantities of short-chain fatty acids, ammonia and electrolytes can be absorbed across the forestomach epithelium.

The digestion of feed in the forestomachs of ruminants is determined by microbial colonisation. The microorganisms form an ecosystem within the forestomach compartments that contributes significantly to the digestive physiology of the host animal, both qualitatively and quantitatively. The relationship between the host animal and the microorganisms is symbiotic as each of these provides a service that benefits the other. The **services** provided **by the host animal** to the microorganisms include maintenance of a favourable temperature, the provision of substrate from food and endogenous secretions, and the maintenance of a flow equilibrium through saliva secretion and fluid or particle turnover. In return, the **services** provided **by the micro-**

organisms to the host animal are the supply of high-quality nutrients from feed components that could not be obtained from the host's own digestion processes alone.

One of the most important fermentation activities is microbial anaerobic degradation of plant cell wall components such as cellulose and other long-chain polysaccharides to produce short-chain fatty acids which the host animal can use. Other physiologically important microbial functions are the production of essential and non-essential amino acids in microbial protein and water-soluble vitamins. In addition, some microorganisms are able to detoxify potentially toxic substances such as nitrites, phytoestrogens, and plant and fungal toxins.

IN A NUTSHELL

The microorganisms of the ruminant forestomachs live in symbiosis with the host animal and make important qualitative and quantitative contributions to nutrient supply by their degradative and metabolic processing of feed.

■ Microorganisms in the forestomachs

The microorganisms in the forestomachs are **bacteria, protozoa** and **fungi** of which many species have been taxonomically, morphologically and biochemically characterised. A complete analysis of the microbial community and in particular how it is influenced by exogenous factors such as changes in feeding is not yet available. The majority of the microorganisms are bacteria and protozoa, each of which represents approx. 10% of the total microbial biomass forming functional microbiological communities or consortia. Foregut bacteria are essential for basic metabolic activities. There are many metabolic interactions between microorganisms, especially through their mutual provision and utilisation of metabolic products of digestion. Changes in feed supply can bring about changes in the composition of these communities with considerable consequences for the health and productivity of the host animal.

Bacteria

Bacterial colonisation of the developing forestomachs begins immediately after birth. It occurs mainly through contact with other animals and the environment as well as through feed. During the first few weeks of life, the density of the bacterial population in the forestomachs gradually increases. In adult animals, the typical **bacterial density** is between $10^9 \cdot ml^{-1}$ and $10^{11} \cdot ml^{-1}$. The spherical bacteria are between 1 and 10 μm in diameter, and the rod-shaped bacteria are about 5 μm in length. The bacterial population consists **predominantly** of **anaerobic** bacteria. Obligate and facultative **aerobic** bacteria represent only a **small part** of the total bacterial population at about $10^4 \cdot ml^{-1}$. In **Table 16.6** and **Table 16.7** some important representatives of gram-positive and gram-negative bacteria and their shape, preferred substrates and metabolic products are listed. However, bacteria outlined in the Tables represent only a small part of the total bacterial population. In the lumen contents of the forestomachs, there are three different regions where bacteria grow: in the liquid, in close association with the epithelium, and on the surface of feed particles. About **70–80%** of bacteria are on the **surface of feed particles** or associated with the **rumen epithelium**. In addition to the adhesion of bacteria to surfaces, so-called consortia can form from groups of morphologically and biochemically different bacteria. For the binding of bacteria to each other and to surfaces, extracellular structures such as mucopolysaccharides and glycoproteins are required. Among the various bacterial groups in the forestomach system, the mucosa-associated bacteria in particular are thought to have the function of keeping the O_2 partial pressure low by utilising oxygen, thus maintaining anaerobic conditions in the forestomachs. Oxygen can be introduced into the forestomach system through drinking and feeding as well as, to a certain extent, through the forestomach epithelium. In forestomach metabolism, reducing and oxidising reactions take place at the same time. The redox potential is the electron transfer potential and is defined as the electrical voltage generated in a redox system by electron movement from an electron donor (reducing agent) to an electron recipient (oxidising agent). The redox potential of a redox coupling characterises its reducing or oxidising effect in aqueous solution. The more positive the potential of an element the greater its oxidising capacity and the more negative the potential the greater the reducing capacity of an element. Since the reducing power of the redox system is predominant in the forestomach, **redox potentials** are measured over the range of −250 to −300 mV. This emphasises the prevailing anaerobic environment in the forestomachs. The negative redox potential in the rumen is responsible for carbohydrates only being metabolised to short-chain fatty acids and not completely to CO_2 and H_2O. Hence the chemical energy of the short-chain fatty acids is available to the host animal.

Table 16.6 Examples of gram-positive bacteria in the forestomachs.

Species	Shape	Preferred substrates	End products
Ruminococcus albus	Spherical	Cellulose, xylan	Formate, acetate, ethanol, H_2, CO_2
Ruminococcus flavefaciens	Spherical	Cellulose, xylan	Formate, acetate, succinate, H_2
Streptococcus bovis	Spherical	Starch, soluble sugars, succinate, protein	Formate, acetate, lactate, ethanol, CO_2
Lachnospira multiparus	Rod-shaped	Pectin, protein, starch	Formate, acetate, lactate, H_2, CO_2
Eubacterium ruminantium	Rod-shaped	Soluble sugars	Formate, butyrate, lactate, CO_2
Lactobacillus ruminis	Rod-shaped	Soluble sugars	Lactate
Lactobacillus vitulinus	Rod-shaped	Soluble sugars	Lactate
Clostridium spp.	Rod-shaped	Cellulose, protein	Formate, acetate, butyrate, ethanol, H_2, CO_2

based on data from Stewart CS. The rumen bacteria. In: Jouany JP (ed.). Rumen microbial metabolism and ruminant digestion. Paris: INRA Editions; 1991: 15–26

Table 16.7 Examples of gram-negative bacteria in the forestomachs.

Species	Shape	Preferred substrates	End products
Bacteroides ruminicola	Rod-shaped	Hemicellulose, pectin, xylan	Formate, propionate, acetate, NH_4^+
Bacteroides amylophilus	Rod-shaped	Starch, pectin, protein	Formate, acetate, succinate
Bacteroides succinogenes	Rod-shaped	Cellulose, starch	Formate, acetate, succinate
Selemonas ruminantium	Crescent	Starch, soluble sugars, glycerol, protein	Acetate, lactate, propionate, H_2, CO_2
Butyrivibrio fibrisolvens	Rod-shaped	Cellulose, xylan	Formate, acetate, lactate, butyrate, ethanol, H_2, CO_2
Anaerovirio lipolytica	Rod-shaped	Lactate, glycerol, fat	Acetate, propionate, succinate
Wolinella succinogenes	Arched	H_2	Succinate, CO_2
Treponema bryantii	Spiral	Pectin, soluble sugars, fat	Formate, acetate, lactate, succinate, ethanol
Megasphaera elsdenii	Spherical	Soluble sugars, lactate	Acetate, propionate, butyrate, valerate, caproate, H_2, CO_2
Succinimonas amylolytica	Spherical-stick-shaped	Starch, dextrin	Acetate, succinate

based on data from Stewart CS. The rumen bacteria. In: Jouany JP (ed.). Rumen microbial metabolism and ruminant digestion. Paris: INRA Editions; 1991: 15–26

The qualitative and quantitative **composition** of the **bacterial flora** is mainly determined by the **feed components**. For example, changing from a raw fibre-rich feed source to a starch-rich ration can cause a decline in the population of cellulolytic bacteria and a simultaneous growth of amylolytic bacteria and streptococci, lactobacilli and lactate-utilising bacteria. In addition to these effects of dietary change, the anaerobic conditions in the forestomachs and the rate of breakdown of feed components are other factors affecting the activity and composition of the bacterial flora. Genetic characteristics of the host animal also influence the activity and diversity of the bacterial flora although the mechanism of this has not yet been precisely characterised. In the past, about 300–400 different species were assumed to be present in the forestomachs. Now, estimates of the bacterial population from molecular genetic studies indicate that there are more than 3000 species, many of which, however, have not yet been clearly taxonomically and biochemically defined. This high diversity of species contrasts with a marked redundancy in their functions (**Table 16.6** and **Table 16.7**).

Archaea

Another physiologically important group of microorganisms are the various species of **Archaea** (*Methanobacteriaceae*, *Methanococcaceae* and others). Colonisation with these strictly anaerobic microorganisms is already occurring a few days after birth, and they eventually reach a density of between 10^8 and $10^9 \cdot ml^{-1}$. The feature they have in common is the production of **methane** with lesser amounts of CO_2 and H_2, which keeps the H_2 partial pressure in the forestomach fluid low. This prevents a too negative redox potential and thus ultimately a limit on the formation of ethanol and lactate during fermentation.

IN A NUTSHELL   !

Bacteria are predominantly found on the surface of feed particles and on the rumen epithelium. The composition of the bacterial flora is mainly determined by the nature of the feed supply. O_2-utilising bacteria maintain anaerobic conditions and a negative redox potential. Methane producers control the H_2 partial pressure. These two factors determine the balance of chemical reactions in the forestomach contents.

Protozoa

In addition to bacteria, the obligate or facultative **anaerobic protozoa** with different species of **ciliates** and **flagellates** form a further group of forestomach microorganisms. The colonisation of the forestomachs with protozoa also begins postnatally by direct contact between animals. The **ciliates** are found in the rumen fluid in concentrations between 10^5 and 10^8 cells $\cdot ml^{-1}$. Because of their length of approx. 20–200 µm, they make up about half of the microbial biomass in the rumen. The genera *Isotricha* and *Dasytricha*, belonging to the family *Isotrichidae* and *Dasytricha*, have cilia over their entire cell surface. Species of the genera *Entodinium* and *Diplodinium*, belonging to the family *Ophryoscolecidae* are non-ciliated. Microscopic examination of ciliates often reveals ovoid granules of amylopectin in the cytoplasm next to cell organelles. Depending on the composition of the feed, these granules can make up a considerable part of the ciliate dry matter. The **flagellates** in rumen fluid represent a relatively small part of the protozoan biomass. The few flagellate species so far determined are small in size, ranging from 4 to 14 µm in width, with a concentration of between 10^3 and 10^4 cells $\cdot ml^{-1}$ rumen fluid. Compared to bacteria, the density of protozoa in rumen fluid is highly variable. The most important factors affecting the number of protozoa are the amount of concentrate in the ration, the frequency of meals and various physicochemical factors.

IN A NUTSHELL   !

The colonisation of the forestomachs with protozoa occurs through contact with other animals. Although protozoa are outnumbered by bacteria, they also account for half of the microbial biomass in the forestomachs because of their large size. Reduction or elimination of the protozoa does not cause any fundamental impairment of metabolic processes in the forestomach contents.

Specific digestive physiological functions of protozoa

1. Involvement in **microbial forestomach digestion**. Since protozoa possess carbohydrate-, protein- and fat-cleaving enzymes, they are also significantly involved in intraruminal nutrient degradation. Like bacteria, **protozoa** are also characterised by marked differences in **substrate specificity**. While the species of the genera *Isotricha* and *Dasytricha* prefer to act on soluble carbohydrates and either ferment them or store them as amylopectin, those of the genus *Diplodinium* prefer to degrade fragments of plant cell walls. All protozoa obtain N-containing nutrients by ingesting small food particles, bacteria, fungi and other protozoa. The **storage capacity of easily fermentable carbohydrates** is also an effective protective mechanism to reduce the risk of rumen acidosis (p. 408). Thus, the gradual change from a raw fibre-rich to a starch-rich ration leads to an increase in the protozoan population and thus to a higher storage capacity of carbohydrates in the rumen biomass. If the ration is changed too quickly, the temporary drastic fall in pH and the increase in osmolarity can lead to a considerable reduction in the protozoan population (defaunation).

2. Provision of **fermentation products**. The fermentation products provided by the protozoa to the host organism include acetate, butyrate and lactate. The CO_2 and H_2 they produce is partially converted to methane by archaea. After their passage from the forestomach system, the protozoa can be digested chemically and enzymatically in the abomasum/small intestine and thus provide additional **protein of high biological value**. However, it should be noted that protozoa, just like feed particles

Nutrition, energy

and the bacteria adhering to them, can be selectively retained in the forestomach system and thus their protein would not all be available to the host.

3. **Detoxification reactions**. Because of their numerous hydrolytic and reducing enzymes, toxic feed components can be neutralised by protozoa. This includes the already long known reduction of nitrite groups of organic compounds to amines. This also explains the lower sensitivity of protozoa to pesticides and various antibiotics compared to bacteria.

4. Formation of poorly absorbable **heavy metal compounds**. Uptake and digestion of insoluble proteins by protozoa lead to an increased supply of peptides and amino acids for bacterial metabolism. This increases the production of sulphides, which bind with copper, forming insoluble copper sulphide compounds with low absorbability. Another possibility is the formation of copper chelates which also have low absorbability. In this way, protozoa can reduce the risk of copper intoxication; however, they can also contribute to the development of copper deficiency when copper supply is low and molybdenum intake is high. Very large amounts of copper sulphate cause the death of protozoa.

5. **Regulation** of the **bacterial population** and the concentration of degradation products. The ability of protozoa to ingest bacteria can reduce and regulate the concentration of bacteria in the forestomach fluid. The digestion of bacteria by the protozoa increases the supply of organic and inorganic breakdown products in the rumen fluid and can thus improve the growth efficiency of the remaining bacteria. Some protozoa may also help to keep the O_2 partial pressure low and thus to maintain anaerobic conditions.

> **IN A NUTSHELL** !
>
> Protozoa meet their nutrient requirements by ingesting feed particles, bacteria, fungi and other protozoa, thereby also regulating the size of the bacterial population. They can store easily fermentable carbohydrates and thus reduce the risk of rumen acidosis. Digestion of protozoa in the abomasum/small intestine provides biologically high-quality protein. Protozoal metabolism can limit toxicity of plant toxins and heavy metals.

Fungi

All fungi identified in the forestomachs are **obligate anaerobes** with a narrow temperature optimum between 33 °C and 41 °C. They can be found as zoospores in the rumen fluid and in their sporangium vegetative form in close association with plant particles. Colonisation begins in the first days of life; in adult ruminants, concentrations in the rumen fluid range between 10^4 and 10^5 zoospores · ml^{-1}. The density of the fungal population increases with the crude fibre content of the ration. The highest concentrations of the fungal population are present about twelve hours after feeding. The species found in the rumen belong to the genera *Neocallimastix, Piromyces, Orpinomyces, Caecomyces, Anaeromyces* and *Cyllamyces*. Various functions in forestomach metabolism are attributed to the fungi. Through primary colonisation and hyphal growth, the cell walls of plant components are penetrated. This facilitates bacterial colonisation and plant cell wall degradation. In addition, they also contribute biochemically to microbial forestomach metabolism. They can metabolise a wide range of soluble carbohydrates and plant polysaccharides. This results in end products similar to those produced during carbohydrate fermentation by bacteria and protozoa. Proteolytic properties have been demonstrated for several fungal species. Like protozoa, they are considered non-essential for microbial forestomach metabolism.

■ Microbial metabolic processes in the forestomachs and absorption of the end products

Quantitatively and qualitatively, the **bacteria** perform the **predominant part of microbial metabolism** in the forestomachs.

Carbohydrates

In ruminant nutrition, the term "**crude fibre**" is often used to characterise the least degradable fraction of the feed. This is **not** a biochemically **uniform group** of nutrients but is the insoluble residue of forage plants. The composition of crude fibre is determined by the extraction methods used to analyse it. In a narrow sense, the term "crude fibre" is considered to be the structural components of **cell wall constituents** of plants, defined as three layers, the middle lamella and the primary and secondary cell wall. These are **pectins, hemicelluloses, cellulose, lignin, wax, cutin** and **suberin**.

The **pectins** are the main component of the middle lamella and, together with the hemicelluloses, are an essential part of the primary walls. The most important pectins are α-D-1,4-polygalacturonan and rhamnogalacturonan, which consist respectively of D-galacturonic acid, L-rhamnose, L-arabinose and D-galactose. The **hemicelluloses** are also mixed polymers with a high xylose content, as well as L-arabinose, D-galactose, D-mannose, D-glucose, D-glucuronic acid and 4-O-methyl-glucuronic acid as further components. They can be connected to cellulose via hydrogen bonds. The hemicelluloses are important for the flexibility and plasticity of the plant cell walls. Their content decreases significantly in the secondary cell wall. The total content of hemicelluloses is determined by each plant species.

Cellulose is a high molecular weight glucose polymer of **cellobiose subunits** linked together in **β-D-1,4-glycosidic** bonds. Cellulose is a major component of the secondary cell wall and is responsible for its strength and toughness. **Lignin** is incorporated in all cell wall layers as the **plant ages** and is a mixed polymer of phenylpropane compounds, coniferyl, p-coumaryl and sinapyl alcohol. **Waxes**, **suberin** and **cutin** are polymers of long-chain alcohols, oxygenated fatty acids and aromatic compounds. They can be constituents of the cuticle or function as tertiary coatings.

The cell wall components are to be distinguished from the plant **cell internal components** which consist of **proteins, nucleic acids, carbohydrates, lipids, lipoids, vitamins** and **minerals**. Antinutritive or toxic substances can also be found in some plants.

Evaluation of the digestibility of plant components is based on the extent to which these components can be digested by the body's own or microbially produced enzymes and can thus be utilised by the host animal. Cell constituents are usually degraded by an animal's endogenous enzymes, whereas microbially formed enzymes are required for degradation of most of the cell wall components.

Of all cell wall components, **lignin** is characterised by the **lowest microbial degradability**. Since lignin can form various bonds with potentially degradable cell wall components, various technological treatment processes are used to try to loosen these bonds in order to achieve a higher utilisation of lignified plant components.

A prerequisite for the microbial degradation of cell wall components is the colonisation of the fibre components by microorganisms. The **ability** to **colonise** has been demonstrated for bacteria, protozoa and fungi. It occurs mainly through openings in the plant epidermis or through leaf stomata. Bacterial colonisation is facilitated by fungi.

Numerous studies on isolated strains of microorganisms have demonstrated their ability to produce **enzymes** that **degrade cell wall components**. The majority of the enzymes are exoenzymes of bacterial or protozoal origin. However, some of the hydrolytic enzymes originate from fungi. In **Table 16.8** relevant enzymes for the degradation of cellulose, hemicellulose and pectin are listed.

Table 16.8 Cellulose-, hemicellulose- and pectin-cleaving enzymes.

Substrate	Enzyme
Cellulose	Endo-1–4-β-glucanase
	Cellobiohydrolase
	β-glucosidase
Hemicelluloses	L-arabinase
	D-galactanase
	D-mannase
	D-xylanase
	β-Xylosidase
	β-glucosidase
	α-L-arabinofuranosidase
Pectin	Esterases
	Hydrolases

The monomers formed by hydrolysis of plant cell wall components, after uptake into bacteria, are further metabolised by **anaerobic glycolysis** (Embden-Meyerhof pathway) or by the **pentose-phosphate cycle**. Pyruvate is the central intermediate product of microbial **carbohydrate metabolism**. However, because it is rapidly converted to **short-chain fatty acids** (**SCFA = acetate, propionate** and **butyrate**, also known as "**volatile fatty acids, VFA**") and **rumen gases**, pyruvate is practically undetectable in rumen fluid. The degradation of high molecular weight carbohydrates via glycolysis and the pentose-phosphate pathway to pyruvate is shown schematically in **Fig. 16.32**. There are

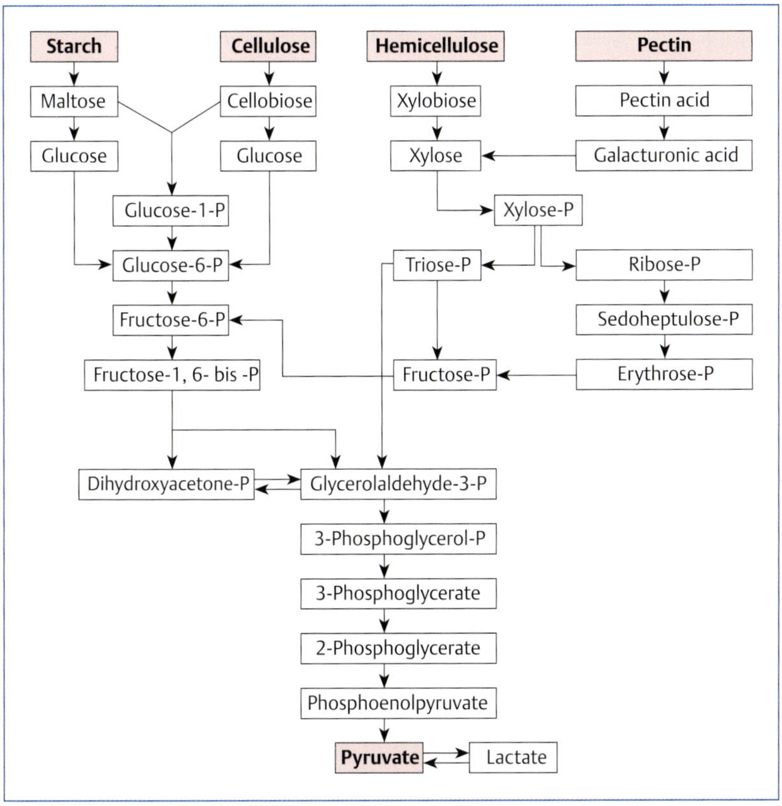

Fig. 16.32 Degradation of carbohydrates to pyruvate.

Nutrition, energy

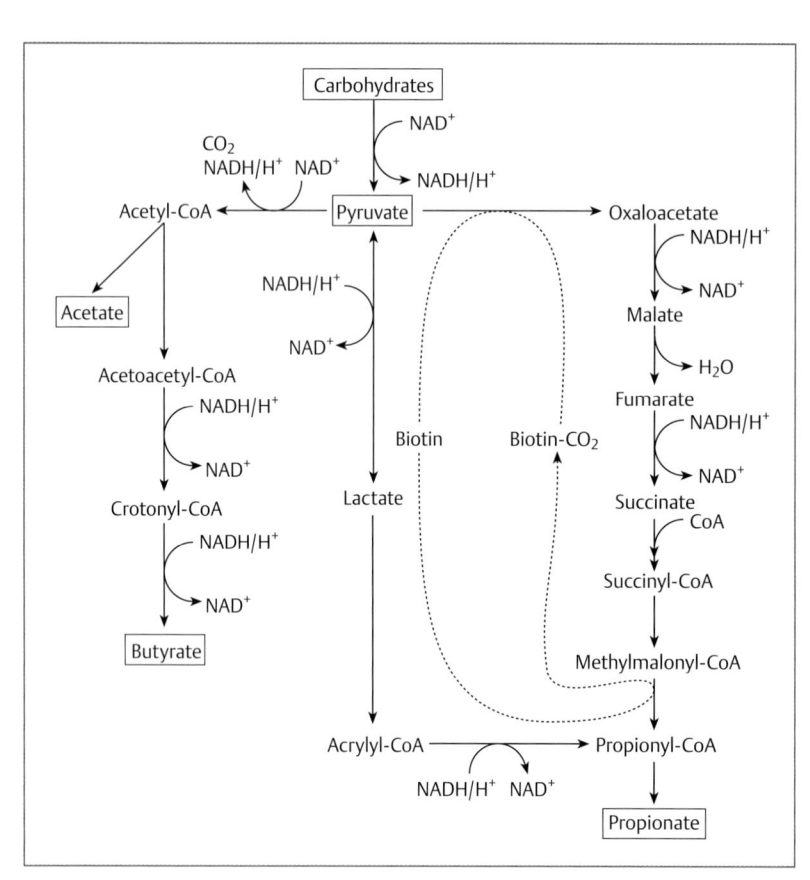

Fig. 16.33 Formation of short-chain fatty acids from pyruvate.

individual enzymatic degradation pathways for starch, cellulose, hemicelluloses and pectin, which ultimately all lead to the formation of dihydroxyacetone-P and glycerolaldehyde-3-P, from which pyruvate is formed in further metabolic steps. Starting from **pyruvate**, the short-chain fatty acids and rumen gases can be formed by various metabolic pathways which include hydrogen-releasing and hydrogen-consuming reaction steps. Thus, in the synthesis of propionate and butyrate, NAD⁺ is regenerated while NAD⁺ is consumed in the synthesis of acetate. Quantitatively, the regeneration of NAD⁺ is the predominant pathway. The various biochemical degradation pathways are distributed throughout numerous bacterial species. The most important steps are shown in **Fig. 16.33**. The short-chain fatty acids can be formed in different molar proportions. Acetate always predominates, followed by propionate and butyrate. Important factors influencing their molar proportions are the type and amount of carbohydrates ingested and the physical structure of the feed. For example, a starch-rich diet leads to a reduction in acetate and an increase in propionate production. The butyrate content remains relatively unchanged, but it can be increased if the feed is finely ground before ingestion.

The influence of the carbohydrate source on the molar SCFA fractions is explained in **Table 16.9**. The **SCFA concentrations** in rumen fluid are not constant and fluctuate between 60 and 180 mmol·l⁻¹, mainly determined by the type and amount of feed consumed. Thus, SCFA concentrations rise within 1–3 hours after feed intake and then fall again. If there is a high content of easily digestible carbohydrates in the ration, the rapid increase in SCFA concentrations can lead to a drastic fall in pH of rumen fluid, which

can be partially offset by limiting the supply of such carbohydrates. A persistent marked fall in pH in rumen fluid can give rise to the clinical syndrome of rumen acidosis (p. 408). Besides acetate, propionate and butyrate, valerate and the branched-chain fatty acids isobutyrate and isovalerate are also formed in small quantities. It is not possible to determine fermentation intensity from SCFA concentrations in the forestomach fluid, as these are influenced not only by their production rate, but also by the volume of rumen fluid, their rate of absorption across the forestomach wall and the onward rate of passage of digesta towards the abomasum. Determination of fermentation intensity requires direct measurement of **SCFA production rates** using labelled short-chain fatty acids. In sheep, with a feed intake of between 600 and 900 g dry matter (DM), the total SCFA production rates are between 3 and 6 mol·d⁻¹. For high-producing cows a daily SCFA production rate of about 125 mol is assumed at a feed intake of 25 kg DM per day. Ingested carbohydrates are broken down to varying degrees in the forestomachs. Factors that affect the rate of digestion are the type of carbohydrate, the level of feed intake and the rate of passage out of the reticulorumen. Thus, the degradation of cell wall components in the rumen decreases with higher feed intake and/or higher passage rate. For some years now, maize starch has been specifically used in ruminant rations because it is less degraded in the rumen compared to other starch sources. Maize starch therefore increases the passage of unfermented starch into the small intestine (bypass starch). In this way, a part of the carbohydrate digestion can be shifted to the small intestine.

Table 16.9 Percentages of molar SCFA concentrations (%) in ruminal fluid as a function of the carbohydrate composition of the ration.

SCFA	Cellulose-rich (hay)	Starch-rich concentrate
Acetate	60–70	40–50
Propionate	15–20	30–40
Butyrate	10–15	10–15

During microbial metabolism processes, **rumen gases** are formed of which approx. 40–70% is CO_2 and 20–40% is **methane** as quantitatively the most important gases. Methane is a climate-relevant gas that makes a substantial contribution to the global greenhouse effect. Traces of O_2, H_2, H_2S and CO can occur in the rumen gas. Nitrogen (N_2) and part of the O_2 originate from atmospheric air and are not considered fermentation gases. CO_2 is produced from bicarbonate secreted with saliva or via the rumen wall, by decarboxylation of pyruvate, by oxidative decarboxylation of amino acids and by cleavage of urea. Reducing equivalents (H_2) required to form CH_4 from CO_2 are produced during glycolysis in the pentose-phosphate pathway due to decarboxylation of pyruvate, and during amino acid degradation. Methane formation by individual species of archaea occurs in close cooperation with bacteria, protozoa and fungi and is a stepwise reduction of CO_2 using the reduction equivalents

$$CO_2 + 4\,H_2 \rightarrow CH_4 + 2\,H_2O \qquad (16.1)$$

The **formation of methane** means considerable **losses of feed energy** which can range between 2 and 18% of gross energy intake (**Fig. 16.34**). The daily gas formation is a function of feed intake, feed composition and diversity of the microbial population and is therefore subject to considerable fluctuations. In relation to dry matter intake, methane production ranges between 10 and $40\,g \cdot (kg\ DM)^{-1}$. This corresponds to a volume of $14–56\,l \cdot (kg\ dry\ matter)^{-1}$ or about 560 l methane at a feed intake of 25 kg dry matter per day. Methane must be released by eructation (p. 379) as it is not significantly absorbed by the forestomach mucosa. Since methane exhalation from ruminants contributes significantly to global methane emissions, numerous experimental approaches have been tested to reduce methane formation. Globally, annual methane release into the atmosphere was estimated to be about 600 million tonnes in 2017, of which about 30% is believed to come from agriculture. The contribution of ruminants is estimated to be about 11–17% of global methane release.

MORE DETAILS Various factors limit the extent to which plant cell wall components can be quantitatively digested by microbes. These include, above all, the strength and integrity of the plant epidermis, which form an effective protection against colonisation by microorganisms. Furthermore, the degradability is determined by the structure of polysaccharides. Although it has been shown that there are no significant differences between the degradability of amorphous and crystalline cellulose, the degree of lignification of the plant material affects the rate of cellulose digestion. The low porosity of lignified cell walls prevents the free

$$31\ C_6H_{12}O_6 + 62\ H_2O \longrightarrow 62\ CH_3COOH + 62\ CO_2 + 124\ (2H)$$
$$11\ C_6H_{12}O_6 + 22\ (2H) \longrightarrow 22\ CH_3CH_2COOH + 22\ H_2O$$
$$16\ C_6H_{12}O_6 \longrightarrow 16\ CH_3CH_2CH_2COOH + 32\ CO_2 + 32\ (2H)$$
$$58\ C_6H_{12}O_6 + 40\ H_2O \longrightarrow 62\ CH_3COOH + 22\ CH_3CH_2COOH + 16\ CH_3CH_2CH_2COOH + 94\ CO_2 + 134\ (2H)$$
$$134\ (2H) + 33.5\ CO_2 \longrightarrow 33.5\ CH_4 + 67\ H_2O$$

$$58\ Hexose \longrightarrow 62\ Acetic\ acid + 22\ Propionic\ acid + 16\ Butyric\ acid + 33.5\ Methane + 60.5\ Carbon\ dioxide + 27\ Water$$
$$163.1\ MJ \longrightarrow 54.4\ MJ + 33.8\ MJ + 34.9\ MJ + 29.4\ MJ + 0\ MJ + 0\ MJ + 10.6\ MJ\ Heat$$

Fig. 16.34 Stoichiometry of the fermentation of carbohydrates in the rumen, based on 100 mol SCFA as the end product.

diffusion of cellulolytic enzymes, so that microbial degradation can only take place on the cell surface. Therefore, microbial degradability decreases with increasing lignin content.

IN A NUTSHELL !

The plant cell wall consists of pectins, hemicelluloses, cellulose and lignin. These substances can only be degraded by microbially produced enzymes. The central intermediate product of degradation is pyruvate, from which the short-chain fatty acids (SCFA = acetate, propionate and butyrate) as well as the rumen gases CO_2 and CH_4 are produced. The type of feed determines SCFA production. Methane formation means a loss of feed energy.

Absorption of short-chain fatty acids

The concentrations of short-chain fatty acids in forestomach fluid are determined by their rate of production, volume of distribution, their rate of absorption across the forestomach wall, and the outflow rate towards the abomasum. Removal of SCFA from the forestomachs is essential as accumulation of these end products in the rumen fluid leads to an undesirable fall in pH and an increase in osmotic pressure. **Effective absorption** of SCFA prevents their accumulation. In this process, 50–85% of SCFA produced in the forestomachs is absorbed directly across the forestomach wall. Since the undissociated SCFA are lipophilic, they can diffuse across the cell membrane into the cytoplasm of forestomach epithelium (**Fig. 16.35**). They dissociate intracellularly and thus increase the intracellular proton concentration, which can be moderated by intracellular buffering or by ejection of H^+ by Na^+/H^+ exchangers (NHE) in the apical and basolateral cell membranes. Ionic transport after dissociation of protons from of the carboxyl group has been demonstrated as a further step in the absorption mechanism for SCFA. Since SCFA when dissociated are hydrophilic, membrane transport proteins are required to export the ionised SCFA out of the cells. This mechanism consists of an $SCFA^-/HCO_3^-$ antiporter. It has been shown

Nutrition, energy

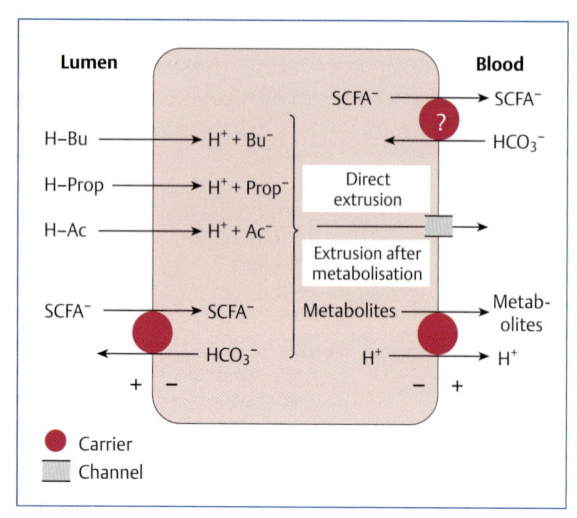

Lumen **Blood**

SCFA⁻ ──────→ SCFA⁻
?
H–Bu ──────→ H⁺ + Bu⁻   ←────── HCO₃⁻
H–Prop ─────→ H⁺ + Prop⁻   **Direct
                           extrusion**
H–Ac ───────→ H⁺ + Ac⁻
                           **Extrusion after
                           metabolisation**
SCFA⁻ ──────→ SCFA⁻   **Metabolites** ──────→ Metab-
         ←─── HCO₃⁻   H⁺ ──────→ H⁺   olites
          + –   – +

● Carrier
▨ Channel

Fig. 16.35 The transcellular transport of SCFA through the rumen epithelium can take place in dissociated and undissociated form.

that the stimulation of SCFA absorption by a low pH in the forestomach fluid is mainly due to the HCO_3^- gradient across the mucosal cell membrane and not to the pH gradient itself. The release of HCO_3^- into the lumen during SCFA absorption contributes significantly to the buffering of the forestomach fluid. No exact numbers are available on the quantitative proportions of ionic and non-ionic transport. With a $pK_a \approx 4.8$, the SCFA are, according to the Henderson-Hasselbalch equation (p. 347), mainly dissociated in the physiological pH range of forestomach fluid.

IN A NUTSHELL   **!**

Short-chain fatty acids (SCFA) are absorbed either when undissociated (non-ionic diffusion) or as anions (SCFA⁻/ HCO_3^- exchanger). The SCFA-coupled secretion of HCO_3^- is an essential factor in buffering the forestomach fluid.

In absorption studies of SCFA, it has been repeatedly observed that the amount of SCFA absorbed by the mucosal cells is greater than the amount released basolaterally. The three most important short-chain fatty acids can be **metabolised intraepithelially**. The extent of this metabolism varies greatly (butyrate >> propionate > acetate). Up to 90% of **butyrate** taken up by the cells is metabolised to the ketone bodies **acetoacetate** and **β-hydroxybutyrate**. **Propionate** is partially converted to **lactate** while **acetate** is not metabolised at all or only to a **small** extent into ketone bodies. All SCFA can be metabolised to CO_2 in the mucosal cells, thereby providing energy (ATP) for cell turnover and active transport mechanisms. The transport of Na^+, Mg^{2+} and Ca^{2+} is stimulated by SCFA. No conclusive experimental results are yet available on the mechanisms of basolateral export of SCFA from rumen mucosal cells. The proven anion conductivity could allow efflux of SCFA anions, driven by the electrical gradient across the membrane (cell interior negative). The monocarboxylate transporter (MCT) enables the transport of both SCFA and their metabolites

(cotransport of acetoacetate or lactate with protons) out of the epithelial cell (**Fig. 16.35**).

> **MORE DETAILS** Because SCFA are important for the health and productivity of ruminants, the mechanisms of their absorption across the forestomach wall are being intensively investigated. A very complex picture is emerging. For example, there appears to be another MCT on the luminal side of the epithelium that mediates the proton-coupled uptake of SCFA into the epithelium. There is also evidence for the involvement of a cotransport of SCFA anions and Na^+ in the uptake. Furthermore, the functionality of the SCFA⁻/HCO_3^- antiport is realised by several different proteins with specific substrate affinities. This complexity ensures and regulates the supply of energy substrates and structural components to ruminants under different feeding conditions.

Proteins and non-protein N-containing compounds

The N-containing compounds in feed are **proteins** and **non-protein N (NPN) compounds** (free amino acids, nitrate, uric acid and urea). In addition to these exogenous sources, endogenous secretion processes contribute to the N supply of the forestomach microorganisms. These include secretion of **mucoproteins** and urea in saliva, as well as urea permeation across the **forestomach wall**, and N release from exfoliation of epithelial cells.

Digestion of **proteins** is by microbial proteases to oligopeptides, dipeptides and amino acids. Most of these **proteases** come from **bacteria**, but protozoa and fungi can also contribute to proteolytic activity. In addition to microbial proteases, proteases of plant origin also contribute to protein degradation and are significant in the high ruminal degradability of protein from fresh grass. The extent of ruminal protein digestion is variable and is determined by protein solubility, protein secondary and tertiary structure, and the proportion of disulphide bridges. Depending on the source of protein, between 30 and 70% of total feed protein is degraded in the rumen although up to 100% of protein from fresh grass can be degraded intraruminally. Various plant constituents, such as tannins (polyphenols), or chemical treatment processes can reduce protein degradation by reducing protein solubility and thus protect feed proteins from microbial degradation. If feed proteins are to be fed directly to the ruminant, they must be technically "packaged" during feed production and thus **protected** from microbial degradation ("**protected protein**"). Smaller peptides and amino acids can be taken up by microorganisms and degraded intracellularly to ammonia and carboxylic acids to be used for the **synthesis of microbial protein** (**Fig. 16.36**). With a pK_a value of 9.25, 99.9% of **ammonia** in rumen fluid at a pH of 6.25 is NH_4^+ and only 0.1% is present as NH_3. NPN compounds are also degraded by enzymes of microbial origin. The main end products are NH_4^+, CO_2 and, depending on the substrate, organic acids.

Ammonia produced by microorganisms is released into rumen fluid, and its concentration and pool size are determined by the rate of assimilation by microorganisms, absorption across the rumen wall and outflow into the lower digestive tract.

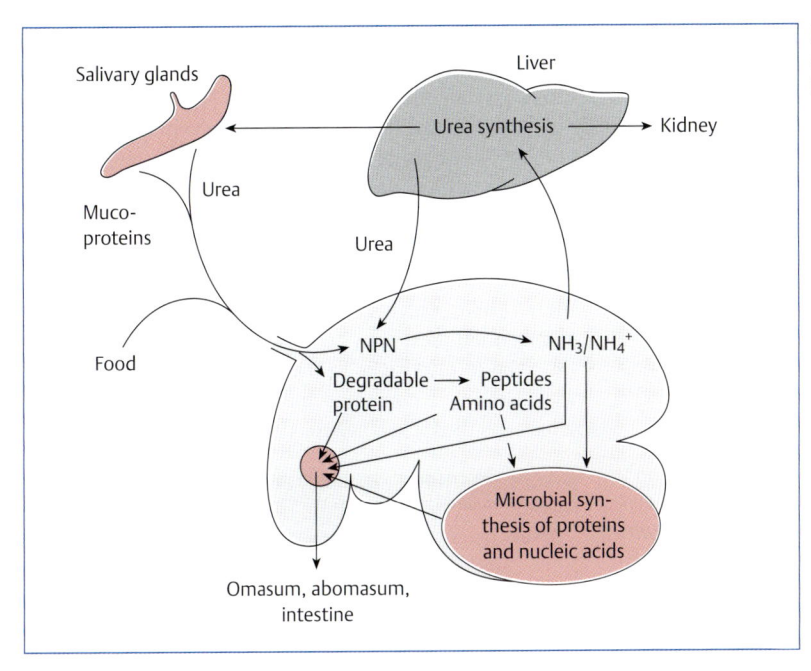

Fig. 16.36 Conversion of N-containing compounds in the forestomachs; rumino-hepatic circulation.

MORE DETAILS The NH_4^+ assimilation by microorganisms represents the first and quantitatively most important step in microbial protein synthesis. Depending on the feed, 40–95% of bacterial protein can originate from NH_4^+ in rumen fluid, with the rest coming from amino acids and peptides. For NH_4^+ assimilation, two systems have been demonstrated. Under the influence of NADP-dependent glutamate dehydrogenase utilising ATP, glutamate is formed from NH_4^+ and α-ketoglutarate, and glutamine is formed from NH_4^+ and glutamate. Glutamine and glutamate are substrates for other amino acid synthesis pathways.

Microbial **protein synthesis** from NPN compounds is the most important aspect of rumen microbial metabolism, along with fermentation of cell wall components. If there is sufficient supply of N, microbial protein synthesis is largely determined by **energy supply**. The average synthesis rate is 10 g protein·MJ^{-1} metabolizable energy.

There is a continuous **recirculation of urea** into and out of the rumen by **rumino-hepatic circulation**. After absorption of NH_3/NH_4^+ across the **rumen wall** and transport to the liver in portal blood, **urea** is synthesised ("ammonia detoxification"). Urea leaves the liver via the hepatic vein and, after passing through the pulmonary circulation, is taken up from arterial blood by **salivary glands** and the **forestomach wall** and secreted into the forestomach where **microbial urease** converts urea into NH_4^+ and CO_2. The amount of urea secreted by the salivary glands and its concentration in mixed saliva is about 65% of that in plasma. Quantitatively, urea secretion across the rumen mucosa is a more important source than that from saliva.

IN A NUTSHELL   !

From 30–100% of feed protein is degraded in the rumen, mainly by bacteria. The end product is ammonia, which is used for the synthesis of microbial protein or, after ruminal absorption, is converted to urea in the liver. Urea reaches the forestomachs again by secretion of the salivary glands and across the forestomach wall (rumino-hepatic circulation), so that urea nitrogen is again available for microbial protein synthesis. The ruminant digests microorganisms and microbial protein in the abomasum and small intestine. Peptides and amino acids products from microbial protein are then absorbed by the small intestinal epithelium.

Absorption of N-containing compounds

Ammonia

Depending on protein or NPN supply from feed and intra-ruminal protein turnover, the ammonia concentrations in the forestomach fluid can be extremely variable ranging from 3 to 15 mmol·l^{-1}. Since the ammonia concentration in blood (100–200 μmol·l^{-1}) is considerably lower because of its potential toxicity, there is a concentration gradient from the lumen to blood and thus the possibility of passive absorption by diffusion. As with SCFA uptake, special mechanisms are required for transport across rumen epithelium. At rumen fluid pH of 5.5–7.0, only a very small proportion of ammonia is present as NH_3 (<1%), which is readily **lipid-soluble** and can therefore easily pass through the epithelium in this form. This mechanism of absorption is important with high ammonia concentrations and high pH values (>7.0) in rumen fluid. The increased ammonia absorption under these circumstances may exceed the detoxification capacity of the liver, so that there is a risk of ammonia poisoning.

Nutrition, energy

However, ammonia is also absorbed when the pH is < 7.0 and when NH_3 is in very low concentrations. Absorption of NH_4^+ is also possible although NH_4^+ cannot diffuse freely through epithelial membranes like NH_3 due to its low lipid solubility. The absorption of NH_4^+ into the epithelial cell probably occurs through cation channels present in the apical membrane (**Fig. 16.38**).

> **IN A NUTSHELL**   !
>
> Ammonia is mainly absorbed in the lipid-soluble form as NH_3 (pH > 7.0), but also some NH_4^+ (pH < 7.0) can be absorbed.

Urea

Urea passes across rumen epithelium by **diffusion** down a concentration gradient from blood to the lumen and with the aid of urea transport proteins (urea transporter B = UT-B) in the rumen epithelium. There it is immediately cleaved by microbial urease. The concentration gradient for urea from plasma to the contents of the forestomach is thus always maintained. However, the transport rate of urea can vary considerably, and ruminal NH_4^+ concentration seems to be important in affecting the rate of transport. High ammonium concentrations inhibit diffusion of urea from plasma into the rumen in a way that is not yet known. This dependence on ammonium concentration makes physiological sense because microbial protein synthesis requires an influx of urea to maintain adequate concentration of NH_4^+. However, if NH_4^+ concentration is sufficient for microbial protein synthesis, then further influx of nitrogen compounds is not necessary. This regulation of urea recycling has important practical consequences. With a **low-protein diet** and thus low NH_4^+ concentrations, up to more than **90%** of the total urea produced in the body can be **recycled** into the forestomachs and **reused**. The remaining amount (< 10%) is excreted in urine. However, recirculation is of **little importance** when **protein-rich feeds** are consumed, which lead to high NH_4^+ concentrations in rumen fluid. Under these circumstances, most of the urea produced is excreted by the kidneys and milk (**Fig. 16.37**).

The absorption of NH_4^+ and urea recirculation are opposite transport processes of nitrogenous substances through the rumen epithelium: NH_4^+ is absorbed, and urea-N diffuses into the forestomach contents. The net balance of this nitrogen passage is of practical importance. At low protein intakes and with sufficient energy supply, and thus high microbial metabolism, urea entry diffusion is the main nitrogenous flux across the rumen epithelium. There is thus a **net gain of nitrogen**, used for microbial protein synthesis, within the forestomach system. However, this situation is only rarely found in cows with high milk yields that are fed protein-rich feed to maintain milk production. The ammonia concentration is then often very high in the rumen fluid, which favours absorption. Under these circumstances, there can be a **net absorption of nitrogen** from the forestomachs in the form of NH_4^+. Excess NH_4^+ then has to be converted into urea (p.472) in the liver which can thus stress hepatic metabolism.

> **IN A NUTSHELL**   !
>
> Under practical feeding conditions, the amount of ammonia absorbed should, as far as possible, not exceed the amount of urea entering the forestomachs. Hence ruminal nitrogen balance should be close to zero.

Amino acids and peptides

The digestion of proteins by microorganisms releases large amounts of peptides and amino acids products. The absorption of amino acids or peptides is quantitatively of little significance because their concentrations in rumen fluid are very low ($\mu mol \cdot l^{-1}$).

Fat

In most plant-based feeds, the fat content is low, at less than $50 g \cdot kg^{-1}$ dry matter. Exceptions are oilseeds, which have significantly higher fat content. Considerable amount of fat can be **hydrolysed** in the rumen by **microbial enzymes**. The most important of these bacterial and protozoal enzymes are lipases and phospholipases which completely cleave fatty acids from triacylglycerols. Most long-chain unsaturated **fatty acids** released are then **hydrogenated** resulting in transfatty acids and conjugated linoleic acids (CLA). Milk fat-lowering effects have been demonstrated for various CLA isomers. The component glycerol and galactose in the feed fat can be microbially converted to SCFA. Long-chain fatty acids can be incorporated into microorganisms as phospholipid or sterol ester, structural

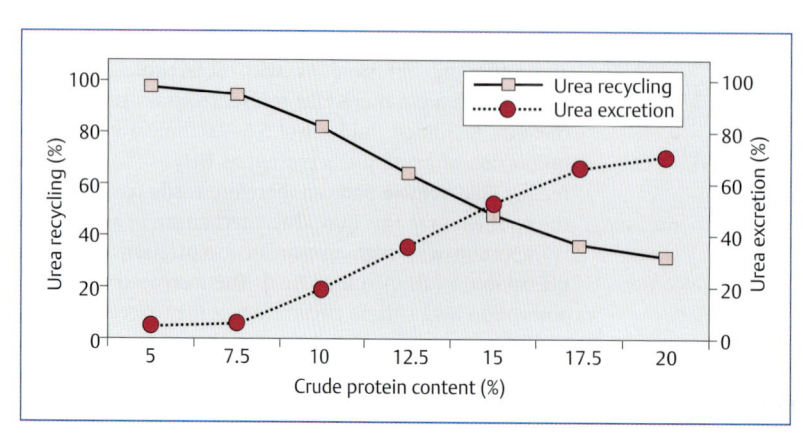

Fig. 16.37 Urea recycling into the gastrointestinal tract and urea excretion in urine and milk depends on the crude protein content of the feed. At low crude protein intake, almost all urea passes into the gastrointestinal tract with only small amounts being excreted in urine and milk; based on data from Reynolds CK, Kristensen NB. Nitrogen recycling through the gut and the nitrogen economy of ruminants: A asynchronous symbiosis. J Anim Sci 2008; 86: E293–E305

components of the microbial cell mass. Native feed fats can cause considerable reduction in microbial growth. This effect which mainly affects cellulolytic bacteria increases with increasing amounts of polyunsaturated fatty acids in the feed and can be inhibited by divalent cations such as Ca^{2+}. Very few long-chain fatty acids cross the forestomach epithelium. They are mainly absorbed in the small intestine.

> **IN A NUTSHELL**   !
>
> Fats can be hydrolysed in the rumen. Subsequently, the unsaturated fatty acids are largely hydrogenated. Glycerol can be microbially converted to SCFA. Too high a content of feed fat can significantly reduce microbial growth.

Vitamins

Forestomach microbial synthesis of vitamins can be a significant source of these essential micronutrients for the host animal. These include the water-soluble **vitamin C** and **B-complex vitamins** and fat-soluble **vitamin K**. In calves and lambs, with incomplete development of the forestomach system, all vitamins must be supplied in the diet. In some circumstances, thiamine (B_1) or cobalamin (B_{12}) deficiencies can develop in adult ruminants. Thiamine deficiencies in growing animals can be caused by sudden increased intake of carbohydrate-rich feed, or from bacterial thiaminases. Cobalamin deficiency can result from insufficient supply of cobalt. There is no significant absorption of vitamins across the forestomach wall.

■ Transport processes for minerals and water in the rumen

Sodium

The high secretion of sodium in saliva ($> 500\,g$ sodium per day in a cow) raises the question of possible absorption mechanisms for this mineral in the forestomachs. However, since the concentration of sodium in blood (140–$145\,mmol \cdot l^{-1}$) is always higher than that in the forestomach fluid, transepithelial sodium transport from lumen side (= mucosal/apical side) to blood side (= serosal/basolateral side) must occur against a **chemical gradient**. At the same time, the transepithelial potential difference is 20–$60\,mV$ (serosal side positive), so Na^+ must also be transported across the epithelium against an **electrical gradient**. Transport against an **electrochemical gradient** requires active, i.e. energy-consuming transport mechanisms.

All studies so far support the assumption of two uptake mechanisms for sodium: **electrogenic** and **electroneutral** sodium transport (**Fig. 16.38**). Sodium enters rumen epithelial cells through an apical **channel**. A concentration gradient (e.g. ruminal 30–$100\,mmol \cdot l^{-1}$ sodium, intracellular 8–$15\,mmol \cdot l^{-1}$) and an electrical gradient (cell interior negative) both facilitate this uptake of sodium. The apical channel is activated by depolarisation of the **potential difference** at the apical membrane. It is therefore not the ENaC as in the kidney and colon (**Fig. 12.1**). Na^+ is pumped

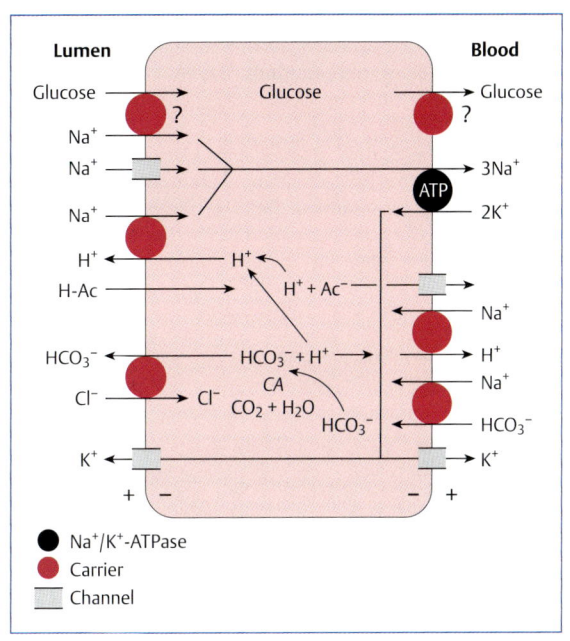

Fig. 16.38 Uptake of Na^+ across the ruminal mucosa cell membrane can take place via an apical channel and a Na^+/H^+ exchanger. The efflux of Na^+ through the basolateral membrane is by the action of a Na^+/K^+-ATPase. K^+ can re-enter the cell by a membrane potassium channel. Only a small amount of potassium leaves the epithelial cell via a channel in the apical membrane which determines the potential difference of this membrane, PD_a. The Na^+-HCO_3^- cotransporter in the basolateral membrane and the Na^+/H^+ exchangers in the apical and basolateral membranes are important mechanisms in the regulation of intracellular pH and transcellular HCO_3^- transport. Luminal uptake of Cl^- is facilitated by an anion exchanger (Cl^-/HCO_3^-). The intracellular supply of H^+ and HCO_3^- for the cation and anion exchanger is by carbonic anhydrase (CA) action producing H_2CO_3 from H_2O and CO_2.

out basolaterally by a Na^+/K^+-ATPase (serial action of the apical channel and Na^+/K^+-ATPase; **Fig. 16.38**). In this way, a positive charge is transported through the epithelium as a sodium ion. This process is therefore electrogenic transport.

In addition to the electrogenic mechanism, a second, **electroneutral mechanism** is also present. The uptake of sodium into rumen epithelial cells is mediated by a **Na^+/H^+** exchanger (NHE type 3), which enables sodium uptake in exchange for the output of protons (**Fig. 16.38**). For the Na^+/H^+ exchanger, only the chemical gradient of these two ions is the driving force, so transepithelial sodium transport requires a continuous supply of protons from within the epithelial cells by the action of **carbonic anhydrase** ($H_2O + CO_2 \leftrightarrow H_2CO_3 \leftrightarrow H^+ + HCO_3^-$). Protons are also released after the uptake of undissociated SCFA into the cytosol.

MORE DETAILS The physiological significance of two parallel transport systems for sodium across reticulorumen epithelium can be deduced from the kinetic data of each system. For electrogenic sodium transport there is a low Michaelis constant, K_m, and a low V_{max}, but for the NHE-mediated, electroneutral transport, significantly higher values apply for K_m and V_{max} (K_m = half saturation of the transport system, V_{max} = maximum transport capacity). This results in a realistic balance between the two, with **electrogenic** sodium transport from rumen fluid into blood occurring mainly at **low rumen sodium concentrations** (< 20 mmol · l^{-1}) while **electroneutral** transport is active at **higher ruminal sodium concentrations**. This ensures that sodium is absorbed over the full physiological range of sodium concentrations in the forestomach fluid.

The electrochemical Na$^+$ gradient at the luminal membrane can be used for another Na$^+$ facilitated transport process. This is the Na$^+$-coupled glucose transport (SGLT 1 = sodium-glucose-linked transport), which has been demonstrated in the forestomach epithelium. However, since glucose concentration in rumen fluid is usually very low, there is no quantitative significance of this transport mechanism in vivo.

> ### IN A NUTSHELL !
>
> Two luminal uptake mechanisms for sodium, electrogenic and electroneutral, working in parallel, in combination with the Na$^+$/K$^+$-ATPase in the basolateral membrane, allow ruminal sodium absorption over the full physiological range of sodium concentrations in rumen fluid. Any physiological significance of Na$^+$-coupled glucose transport (SGLT 1) has not been determined.

Chloride

Chloride transport from lumen to blood is closely coupled to Na$^+$ electroneutral transport This relationship results from the use of the dissociation products of H_2CO_3: H$^+$ and HCO$_3$$^-$. The transport of protons by the Na$^+$/H$^+$ exchanger (NHE) is associated with the transport of HCO$_3$$^-$ by an **anion exchanger** in the apical membrane of reticulorumen epithelial cells (**Fig. 16.38**). The anion exchanger transfers HCO$_3$$^-$ to the lumen in exchange for the uptake of chloride. Little is known about the basolateral delivery of chloride. An anion channel detected in isolated rumen epithelial cells could explain this function.

Potassium

Potassium can be **absorbed** from the rumen or **secreted** into the lumen. At low luminal potassium concentrations of 4 or 5 mmol · l^{-1} there is always a very low net secretion of potassium into the lumen. This process is explained in **Fig. 16.38**. The Na$^+$/K$^+$-ATPase pumps out three sodium ions and, in exchange, transports two potassium ions into the cell. This potassium must then leave the cell to avoid excess intracellular accumulation. In gastrointestinal epithelia, this release is mostly through a **channel** in the **basolateral membrane** (**Fig. 16.38**, **Fig. 16.39**). In the rumen epithelium, there is an additional potassium channel in the **apical membrane** (**Fig. 16.38**, **Fig. 16.39**), through which small amounts of potassium are secreted into the lumen, so that net transport of potassium from the serosal side into the lumen is observed. Under in vivo conditions, ruminal potassium concentrations show very large fluctuations, which are mainly due to the potassium content of the feed. With increasing potassium content in the feed or increasing potassium inflow in saliva (when there is Na$^+$ deficiency), the potassium concentration in rumen fluid increases linearly and can reach more than 100 mmol · l^{-1}.

This considerably exceeds the plasma concentration of 4–5 mmol · l^{-1}, so this large concentration gradient favours absorption. In all in vivo experiments, a linear relationship was observed between ruminal potassium concentration and rate of potassium absorption. A passive mechanism can be assumed, the properties of which have not yet been conclusively clarified.

MORE DETAILS

Potassium and potential difference

High ruminal potassium concentrations cause important electrophysiological changes in rumen epithelial cells. The transepithelial electrical potential difference of rumen epithelium, PD$_T$, increases linearly with the logarithmic rumen potassium concentration. This relationship can be explained by the function of the potassium channel in the apical membrane (**Fig. 16.38**). The electrical **potential difference** of the apical membrane, PD$_a$, is essentially determined by the **potassium gradient** between luminal and intracellular compartments and is about −40 mV (cell interior negative). Any increase in luminal potassium concentration causes a decrease in the outflow of K$^+$ from the cell through the apical membrane and therefore leads to depolarisation of PD$_a$. Since PD$_T$ = PD$_a$ − PD$_b$ (PD$_b$ = potential difference of the basolateral membrane, is about −60 mV), a depolarisation of PD$_a$ results in an increase of PD$_T$. The wide variation in PD$_T$ between + 20 and + 60 mV (serosal side positive) is mainly related to differences in luminal potassium concentration.

> ### IN A NUTSHELL !
>
> The potassium concentration in the rumen fluid has a significant effect on electrical potential difference of PD$_a$ and thus also of PD$_T$. The change in these electrical potential differences is of great importance in understanding epithelial electrophysiology and thus, among other things, for ruminal magnesium transport.

Magnesium

The special interest in mechanisms of ruminal magnesium transport is because the pathogenesis of **hypomagnesemia** (**grass tetany**) of ruminants is in many cases due to insufficient Mg^{2+} absorption (p. 409) from the forestomachs. Mg^{2+} is **only** absorbed actively in the **forestomachs**. There is no significant net absorption of Mg^{2+} in the other regions of the alimentary tract.

Two luminal uptake mechanisms have been described for Mg^{2+} (**Fig. 16.39**). In one of these, Mg^{2+} is absorbed passively through a membrane channel, a process largely determined by the potential difference of the apical membrane, PD$_a$, and is thus called **potential-dependent Mg^{2+} transport**. The second uptake mechanism is **potential-independent** and thus is electroneutral. It is very likely that potential-independent Mg^{2+} transport takes place in co-transport with two monovalent anions, probably Cl$^-$ (**Fig. 16.39**).

The release of Mg^{2+} out of cells through the basolateral membrane is by a Na$^+$/Mg^{2+} exchanger. The Na$^+$ taken up in this process is then removed from the cell by the Na$^+$/K$^+$-ATPase, i.e. transepithelial Mg^{2+} transport can be described as secondary active.

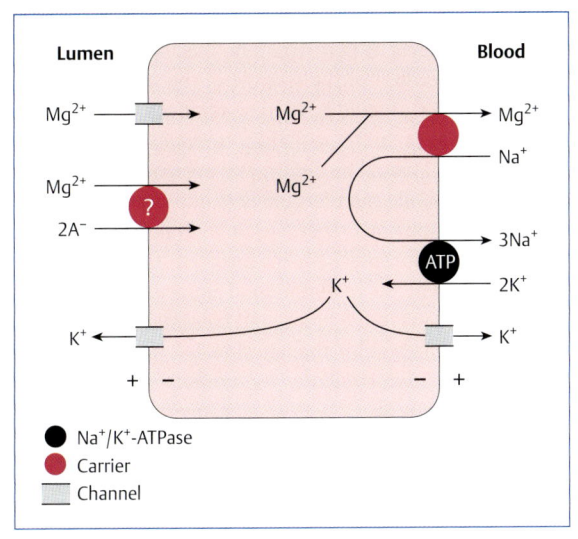

Fig. 16.39 Ruminal Mg^{2+} transport. The two uptake mechanisms across the luminal membrane enable effective Mg^{2+} absorption at low and high Mg^{2+} concentrations in rumen fluid. The basolateral output of Mg^{2+} is by a Na^+/Mg^{2+} exchanger. The Na^+ taken into the cell in exchange for this Mg^{2+} output is then pumped out by the Na^+/K^+-ATPase. The uptake of Mg^{2+} from rumen fluid is thus a secondary active process.

MORE DETAILS   The existence of two luminal uptake mechanisms for Mg^{2+} leads, as with Na^+, to the question of their physiological significance. Since Mg^{2+} absorption from the forestomachs is essential in maintaining normal blood magnesium concentration, the ruminal Mg^{2+} transport mechanisms, especially at very low Mg^{2+} concentrations ($1\,mmol \cdot l^{-1}$ or less), must still enable sufficient Mg^{2+} absorption. This can be achieved by the **potential-dependent** Mg^{2+} transport process using the electrical gradient of the PD_a. By this mechanism, continuous Mg^{2+} uptake is possible even when luminal Mg^{2+} concentration is equal to or slightly less than intracellular Mg^{2+} concentration of 0.5–$1\,mmol \cdot l^{-1}$. Mg^{2+} uptake by **electroneutral cotransport** is determined solely by the concentration gradients of the two transported ions, Mg^{2+} and Cl^-. High Mg^{2+} concentrations in the rumen therefore facilitate Mg^{2+} absorption using this transport mechanism, which is not directly influenced by K^+ concentration as it is independent of PD_a as a driving force (p. 406).

IN A NUTSHELL   !

The absorption of Mg^{2+} from the forestomachs is essential for adequate magnesium supply of ruminants. Disturbances in this process can result in hypomagnesemia and possibly also tetany (hypomagnesaemic grass tetany). Prophylaxis of grass tetany is possible through supplementary feeding of magnesium to increase ruminal Mg^{2+} concentrations.

Calcium

For sheep, goats and cattle, there is evidence that Ca^{2+} can be actively absorbed from the rumen, but little is known about the transport mechanism. This also applies to the control of rumen Ca^{2+} transport by calcitriol. It is possible that a $Ca^{2+}/2H^+$ exchanger is involved in luminal Ca^{2+} uptake stimulated by SCFA in rumen fluid. There are so far no reliable data on the mechanisms of basolateral output of Ca^{2+} (possibly a Na^+/Ca^{2+} exchanger and/or a Ca^{2+}-ATPase).

MORE DETAILS   Little is known about the physiological significance of ruminal Ca^{2+} transport in calcium homeostasis of ruminants. Experiments indicate that absorption of Ca^{2+} from the forestomachs could be of nutritional-physiological significance at high Ca^{2+} intakes.

Phosphate

The high phosphate content in saliva and the large saliva volumes lead to high phosphate concentrations of 10–$15\,mmol \cdot l^{-1}$ in rumen fluid, which contribute to buffering and far exceed plasma concentrations of 2–$3\,mmol \cdot l^{-1}$. This concentration gradient between rumen fluid and plasma is amplified by a transepithelial potential difference of 20–60 mV (serosal side positive), which provides a significant electrochemical driving force for passive absorption of this anion. Current data supports an assumption of diffusion (passive), which is most likely paracellular, but **quantitatively small**.

Water

The contents of the reticulorumen is about 10–15% of body weight and is mainly water (about 90% of the weight). Osmolality of forestomach fluid is slightly **hypoosmolar** (260–$280\,mosm \cdot kg^{-1}$) **before feeding**. From fermentation after **feed intake**, there can be significant increases in osmolality of **$> 400\,mosm \cdot kg^{-1}$**. These differences in osmotic pressure must be regarded as a major cause of water movement, despite insufficient knowledge of the mechanisms and passageways of water transport through the rumen epithelium. It is possible that there are water transport channels (aquaporins) in the epithelial cells. Hypoosmolar contents of the forestomach favour water absorption which can be observed up to an osmolality of $340\,mosm \cdot kg^{-1}$. Thus, under normal feeding conditions, the prerequisite for low water absorption should apply during most of the day. Further increases in osmotic pressure ($> 340\,mosm \cdot kg^{-1}$) in the fluid of the forestomach contents cause a net transport of water from blood into the rumen. This is very common in high milk yield cows. With a net influx of water into the rumen, there is increased outflow of forestomach contents from the reticulorumen into the omasum.

IN A NUTSHELL   !

Water transport through the rumen epithelium follows the laws of osmosis. Mechanisms such as water channels or other passageways (trans/paracellular) are not known.

■ Transport mechanisms in the omasum

Knowledge of the transport mechanisms in the omasum is limited compared to the numerous studies which have revealed these processes across rumen epithelium. Nevertheless, some information is available.

In in vivo studies, the passage of forestomach contents from the reticulorumen into the omasum was compared with the outflow from the omasum into the abomasum. The difference between these two indicate either net absorption or net secretion. From these findings, it is apparent that the omasum is an important organ for the **absorption of water, sodium, potassium, HCO₃⁻ and SCFA**. In small ruminants, absorption rates of 10–20% (based on the amount of fluid entering the omasum) have been found, and in cattle 40–50% is absorbed. The significance of these percentages is apparent when considering the amounts of fluid that flow into the omasum each day of 15–25 l in small ruminants, and up to 200 l or more in cows.

In the omasum epithelium, Na^+ is absorbed by electrogenic and electroneutral transport mechanisms (NHE) (**Fig. 16.40**). In addition, there is also electroneutral Na^+-Cl^- cotransport. Absorption of Mg^{2+} has also been demonstrated, but its quantitative significance is very low. SCFA are probably absorbed across the apical membrane of omasum epithelial cells exclusively in the undissociated form. Dissociation in the epithelial cell would release H^+ and activation of NHE3.

However, a significant and **physiologically** important **difference** to the rumen epithelium applies to Cl^- and HCO_3^- transport: In all in vivo experiments, a **net secretion of Cl^-** and **absorption of HCO_3^-** was observed. This HCO_3^- absorption is certainly advantageous because entry of

HCO_3^- into the acidity of the abomasum would have undesirable side effects as CO_2 would be released immediately from HCO_3^- because of the low pH in the abomasum (pH 2–3) and this CO_2 would have to be removed. Furthermore HCO_3^- acts as a buffer, so that correspondingly larger amounts of HCl would be required to overcome this buffering capacity. While the physiological importance of HCO_3^- absorption is obvious, there is only limited knowledge about the transport mechanisms involved. The findings are best explained by the assumption of anion exchangers (Cl^-/HCO_3^- exchanger) in the apical and basolateral membrane. Of particular interest for the apical HCO_3^- uptake is a Na^+-Cl^- cotransport, which allows the uptake of Cl^-, which in turn is recycled by the Cl^-/HCO_3^- exchanger (**Fig. 16.40**).

> ### IN A NUTSHELL ❗
>
> The transport mechanisms for known and important absorption functions for water and electrolytes by the omasum have been described. Of particular physiological importance are the absorption of HCO_3^- and SCFA. Because of their buffering effect, both would require increased HCl secretion or lead to CO_2 release from HCO_3^- in the abomasum.

16.4.3 Pathophysiology

Gerhard Breves, Reiko Rackwitz

■ Rumen acidosis

The pH of forestomach fluid of 5.5–7.0 results from interactions between the rate of SCFA production and SCFA removal by absorption and outflow towards the abomasum. Furthermore, intraruminal pH is influenced by the buffering capacity by saliva and by HCO_3^- secreted by rumen epithelium (**Fig. 16.35, Fig. 16.38**). This balance is always endangered when the feed contains large amounts of **easily fermentable carbohydrates (starch)**, thus increasing the production of SCFA while decreasing buffering capacity because of a lower rate of saliva secretion. Under these circumstances, the concentration of SCFA can increase rapidly ($> 130 \, mmol \cdot l^{-1}$), with consequent fall in pH. Effective buffering by saliva does not occur if the carbohydrate-rich feed has a low fibrous content so that rumination decreases and consequently salivary secretion is reduced (**Fig. 16.15**). The **accumulation of SCFA** in the forestomach fluid and the decrease of **pH < 5.5** can lead to considerable disturbances in the barrier and transport functions of forestomach epithelium. A decrease in pH is associated with an increase in the undissociated fraction of SCFA. The pK_a value of SCFA is 4.8, i.e. at this pH value 50% of the SCFA is present in dissociated and 50% in undissociated forms. Since the SCFA are lipophilic when undissociated, they are rapidly absorbed into the epithelial cells. In the cell, rapid dissociation of SCFA (99%) then occurs at a pH of about 7.0, imposing a load of protons on the epithelial cells. To avoid intracellular acidosis, the Na^+/H^+ exchanger in the luminal membrane is activated to **remove** these **protons** from the

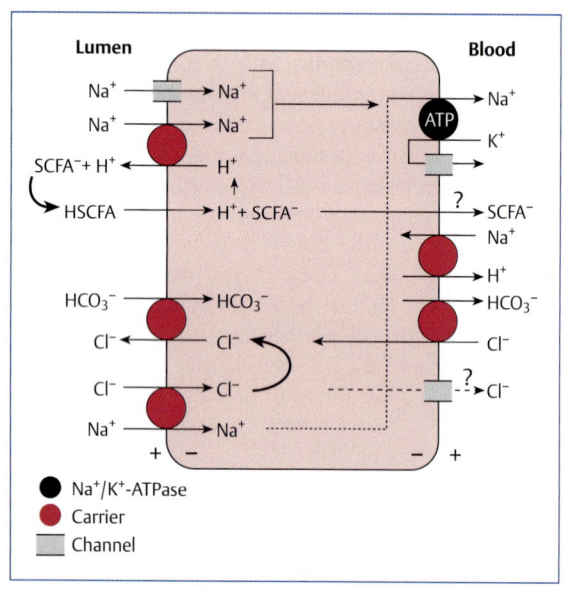

Fig. 16.40 Schematic representation of the transport mechanisms detected so far in the omasum epithelium. The anion exchangers in the apical and basolateral membranes (Cl^-/HCO_3^-) enable the transport of Cl^- or HCO_3^- with corresponding ion gradient directions indicated by arrows. Absorption of HCO_3^- (HCO_3^- concentration: mucosal > serosal) and the secretion of Cl^- (Cl^- concentration: serosal > mucosal) is shown. The parallel transport of undissociated SCFA and HCO_3^- requires effective regulation of intracellular pH. It is assumed that the apical Na^+/H^+ exchanger contributes significantly to the transport out of H^+ from absorbed SCFA. Intracellular pH can be influenced by a number of transport mechanisms (HSCFA; Na^+/H^+ exchanger; Na^+-Cl^- cotransport (indirectly); anion exchanger and carbonic anhydrase [not shown]), which in turn can alter the transport of HCO_3^-.

cell and release them into the **rumen lumen**. The protons are also buffered by other intracellular mechanisms such as carbonic anhydrase, as well as by basolateral uptake of $NaHCO_3$. Sodium taken up by the luminal Na^+/H^+ exchanger and the basolateral Na^+-HCO_3^- cotransport is removed from the cell basolaterally by Na^+/K^+-ATPase (**Fig. 16.38**). Furthermore, the basolateral monocarboxylate fatty acid transporter can assist in removal of H^+ (**Fig. 16.35**).

MORE DETAILS   The **pathogenesis** of disturbance of epithelial functions in **acidosis** begins with the increased uptake of undissociated SCFA. As a result the load of protons in the cells exceeds the capacity of the Na^+/H^+ exchanger and intracellular buffer systems (**Fig. 16.41**: uptake of protons (1) > removal (3) + buffering (2; HPx = unknown buffer systems), so that intracellular acidosis occurs which, among other things, also leads to inhibition of the Na^+/K^+-ATPase (4). As a result, the increased Na^+ taken up into the cell can no longer be transported out and the basolateral Na^+-HCO_3^- cotransport is also disturbed (**Fig. 16.38**). The intracellular accumulation of Na^+ can lead to cell swelling and, from the altered gradients for Na^+, a decreased activity of the Na^+/H^+ exchanger and the basolateral $NaHCO_3$ cotransport, which in turn leads to reduced removal of protons and reduced proton buffering. Consequently, intracellular acidosis is further exacerbated, which can lead to cell damage and **cell lysis**, which explains the epithelial lesions observed in this disease.

If acute acidosis persists, a change in the microbial community can significantly alter the usual fermentation pattern of acetate, propionate and butyrate production occurring at normal pH values. A persistently low pH favours the growth of **lactate-forming microorganisms** so that lactate concentration increases and that of SCFA decreases. This has two negative consequences: **Lactate** is a stronger acid (**pK_a 3.8**) than **SCFA** (**pK_a 4.8**) and is only **absorbed** to a **small extent** from the forestomachs with intact epithelium. The resulting luminal accumulation of lactate causes an increase in osmotic pressure with a consequent **water influx** into the forestomachs and further deterioration of the **barrier** and **transport functions** of the epithelium. However, the negative effects of forestomach acidosis are not limited to epithelial function. Forestomach motility is also inhibited and the acid-base balance of the animal is disturbed.

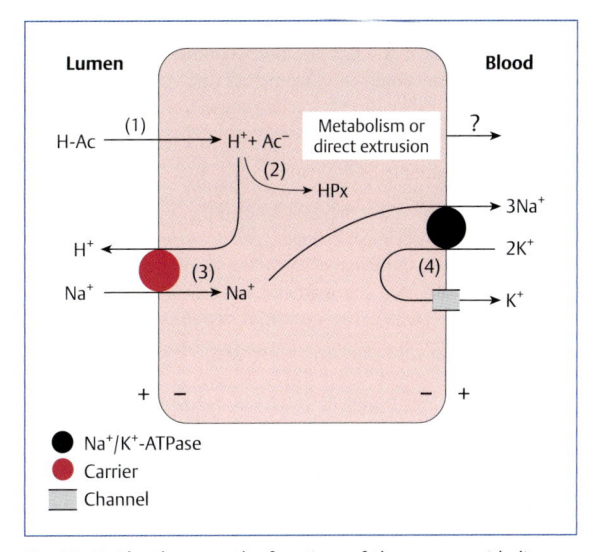

Fig. 16.41 The threat to the functions of the rumen epithelium – barrier and transport – from increased luminal uptake of undissociated SCFA (1). The intracellular release of protons can lead to an overload of the possible compensatory mechanisms (e.g. removal via Na^+/H^+ exchangers (3) or buffering (2); HPx = unknown buffer systems), so that intracellular acidosis is induced with the possibility of cell damage or lysis. The Na^+/K^+-ATPase is also inhibited at low pH (4).

crobial protein, as the relatively low carbohydrate content is providing too little energy and carbon structures for protein synthesis. The high **pK value** of **ammonia** causes an increasingly alkaline rumen environment. This inhibits microbial fermentation and, with increasing pH, the degree of ionisation of Ca^{2+} and Mg^{2+} decreases and thus their rate of absorption.

■ Rumen tympany

Certain plant feeds promote a foamy fermentation and thus **rumen tympany (bloat)**. Foamy fermentation is thought to be caused by a stable dispersion of small feed particles, especially chloroplast membranes. The gases formed during microbial fermentation are trapped in these particles in the form of tiny bubbles. This prevents them from coalescing into the gas phase in the dorsal rumen sac and then being released by eructation. The gas formed remains in the forestomachs and quickly leads to life-threatening distension of the rumen.

■ Disorders of Mg^{2+} absorption

Disturbances in Mg^{2+} absorption from the ruminant forestomach have been known for many years and are of great importance in the pathogenesis of hypomagnesaemic **grass tetany**. The forestomach is practically the only region of the ruminant alimentary tract where Mg^{2+} is absorbed, so disturbances in Mg^{2+} absorption in this section of the digestive tract are not compensated by absorption in the intestine. A reduction in Mg^{2+} absorption in the forestomachs is therefore associated with increased excretion of Mg^{2+} in faeces. **Potassium concentration** in rumen fluid is of great importance for Mg^{2+} absorption, as an **increase** always causes a decrease in Mg^{2+} absorption.

IN A NUTSHELL   **!**

Acute and especially chronic acidosis of the forestomachs (possibly also systemic) is a widespread problem in the practical feeding of high-producing cows. The cause is always an imbalance between the amount of SCFA produced by fermentation and the buffer capacity of the forestomach fluid. As a consequence, there are disturbances of the epithelial barrier and transport functions as well as the danger of a general metabolic acidosis. Subacute rumen acidosis (SARA) with a ruminal pH < 5.5 for several hours per day is becoming increasingly important. Clinical signs include reduced feed intake and non-specific abnormalities such as lameness or diarrhoea.

■ Rumen alkalosis

An imbalance between protein and carbohydrate content of the feed with a relatively high supply of nitrogenous compounds favours the development of **rumen alkalosis**. In this situation, ammonia produced during proteolytic degradation is greater than can be incorporated into mi-

MORE DETAILS The electrophysiological consequences of an increase in potassium concentration on rumen epithelium are well known. The potential difference of the apical membrane, PD_a, is determined by the intracellular and extracellular potassium concentrations (**Fig. 16.39** potassium channel in the apical membrane). High ruminal potassium concentrations always cause a **depolarisation** of PD_a with a consequent increase in PD_T ($PD_T = PD_a - PD_b$). These intraepithelial (PD_a) and transepithelial (PD_T) electrophysiological changes lead to a reduction in Mg^{2+} absorption due to reduction of PD_a as the absorption driving force for Mg^{2+} uptake into the epithelial cell (mechanisms of Mg^{2+} transport; **Fig. 16.39**). The **potential-dependent** Mg^{2+} **transport** is therefore also referred to as **potassium-sensitive transport**.

The negative relationship between the level of potassium intake with the feed and the apparent availability of Mg^{2+} in feed can be explained by the electrophysiological laws. The negative effect of potassium is particularly pronounced when Mg^{2+} intake is low. There are two transport mechanisms for Mg^{2+} across the apical membrane of epithelial cells, which enables effective Mg^{2+} uptake when Mg^{2+} concentration in the forestomach fluid fluctuates. However, at low Mg^{2+} concentrations ($< 1\,mmol \cdot l^{-1}$) in the lumen, Mg^{2+} uptake through the apical membrane is only possible by potential-dependent Mg^{2+} transport, which is negatively influenced by the potassium-dependent changes of PD_a. This pronounced negative effect of high potassium concentrations on Mg^{2+} transport (at low Mg^{2+} concentrations) can be countered by increasing the Mg^{2+} content of the feed. Although this does not influence the absolute effect of potassium on potential-dependent Mg^{2+} transport, the potential-independent Mg^{2+} transport becomes dominant because of the high luminal Mg^{2+} concentration. With higher Mg^{2+} intake the effects of potassium are lower, so potential-independent **Mg^{2+} transport is** therefore also called **potassium-insensitive absorption**. Since PD_T (blood side positive) is increased by the ruminal K^+ concentration depolarising PD_a, the resulting potential difference is a passively acting driving force for ions and thus also for the passive Mg^{2+} reverse transport through the rumen epithelium paracellularly from blood into the rumen lumen. However, this is not of great importance for Mg^{2+} homeostasis because its paracellular permeability is low.

IN A NUTSHELL !

The essential requirement of ruminal Mg^{2+} absorption becomes apparent when this absorption is disturbed by high K^+ intakes in feed. Knowledge of Mg^{2+} transport mechanisms provides explanations for how disturbance of this transport develops, and for the effectiveness of increased Mg^{2+} intake for **prophylaxis** of **grass tetany**.

Suggested reading

Abdoun K, Stumpff F, Martens H. Ammonia and urea transport across the rumen epithelium: a review. Anim Health Rev 2006; 7: 1–17

Allen MS. Relationship between fermentation acid production in the rumen and the requirement for physically effective fibre. J Dairy Sci 1997; 80: 1447–1462

Aschenbach JR, Penner GB, Stumpff F, Gäbel G. Ruminant Nutrition Symposium: Role of fermentation acid absorption in the regulation of ruminal pH. J Anim Sci 2011; 89: 1092–1107

Baaske L, Gäbel G, Dengler F. Ruminal epithelium: a checkpoint for cattle health. J Dairy Res 2020; 87(3): 322–329

Baldwin RE, McLeod KR, Klotz JL et al. Rumen development, intestinal growth and hepatic metabolism in the pre- and post-weaning ruminant. J Dairy Sci 2004; 87: E55-E65

Gäbel G, Aschenbach JR, Müller F. Transfer of energy substrates across the rumen epithelium. Implications and limitations. Anim Health Rev 2002; 3: 15–30

Gäbel G, Martens H. Transport of Na and Cl across forestomach epithelium: Mechanism and interactions with short-chain fatty acids. In: Tsuda T, Sasaki Y, Kawashima R, eds. Physiological Aspects of Digestion and Metabolism in Ruminants. San Diego: Academic Press; 1991: 129–151

Gäbel G, Sehestedt J. SCFA transport in the forestomach of ruminants. Comp Biochem Physiol 1997; 118A: 367–374

Jouany JP, ed. Rumen microbial metabolism and ruminant digestion. Paris: INRA Editions; 1991

Leonhard-Marek S, Stumpff F, Martens H. Transport of cations and anions across forestomach epithelia: conclusions from in vitro studies. Animal 2010; 4(7): 1037–1056

Martens H, Schweigel M. Pathophysiology of grass tetany and other hypomagnesemias. Implications for clinical management. Vet Clin North Am Food Anim Pract 2000; 16: 339–368

Meng QX, Ren LP, Cao ZJ, eds. Proceedings of the 7th International Symposium on the Nutrition of Herbivores. Beijing: China Agricultural University Press; 2007

Nocek JE. Bovine acidosis: implication of laminitis. J Dairy Sci 1997; 80: 1005–1028

Plaizier JC, Krause DO, Gozho GN et al. Subacute ruminal acidosis in dairy cows: the physiological causes, incidence, and consequences. Vet J 2008; 176: 21–31

Reynolds CK, Kristensen NB. Nitrogen recycling through the gut and the nitrogen economy of ruminants: A asynchronous symbiosis. J Anim Sci 2008; 86: E293-E305

Rowe JB. Rumen acidosis. Anim Nutri Austr 1999; 12: 61–68

Schröder B, Breves G. Mechanisms and regulation of calcium absorption from the gastrointestinal tract in pigs and ruminants: comparative aspects with special emphasis on hypocalcemia in dairy cows. Anim Health Rev 2007; 7: 31–41

Sejrsen K, Hvelplund T, Nielsen MO, eds. Ruminant Physiology: Digestion, metabolism and impact of nutrition on gene expression, immunology and stress. Wageningen, Netherlands: Academic Publishers; 2006

Stevens CE, Hume ID. Contributions of microbes in vertebrate gastrointestinal tract to production and conservation of nutrients. Phys Rev 1998; 78: 393–427

Stewart CS. The rumen bacteria. In Jouany JP, ed. Rumen microbial metabolism and ruminant digestion. Paris: INRA Editions; 1991: 15–26

Stumpff F. A look at the smelly side of physiology: transport of short-chain fatty acids. Pflüg Arch 2018; 470: 571–598

von Engelhardt W, Leonhard-Marek S, Breves G Giesecke D, eds. Ruminant Physiology: Digestion, Metabolism, Growth and Reproduction. Stuttgart: Enke; 1995

Weiss WP. Macromineral digestion by lactating cows: factors affecting digestibility of magnesium. J Dairy Sci 2004; 87: 2167–2171

16.5   Monogastric stomach

Siegfried Wolffram

ESSENTIALS   ✖

The monogastric stomach has a variety of functions, among which is acting as a food store, thus allowing discontinuous food intake in humans and animals. Gastric emptying of ingested food, mixed with saliva and gastric juice as "food pulp" (chyme), into the small intestine at a relatively constant rate is under precise regulation by the duodenum. The actual volume of chyme is less important than its energy density in the rate of gastric emptying. This regulatory mechanism ensures that the digestive and absorption capacity of the small intestine is not overtaxed. The storage function of the stomach and the regulation of gastric emptying (p. 381) have already been described in detail. The stomach also has some limited function in the digestion of proteins and triacylglycerols.

The secretory functions of the gastric mucosa and their regulation, as well as the digestive and protective functions of these secretions, the microbial activity in the stomach, and the absorption capability of the mucosa are described below.

16.5.1   Secretory functions

Three glandular regions can be distinguished in the gastric mucosa: the **glandular regions** of the **cardia**, **fundus** and **pylorus** (**Fig. 16.42**). In the horse, rat and hamster, and to a lesser extent in the pig, there is a large region of **cutaneous mucosa** without glands at the junction of the oesophagus and stomach (= cardia) (**Fig. 16.42**).

With the exception of the pig, where the stomach has a relatively large cardiac gland region adjoining the region of cutaneous mucosa, in the stomach of other monogastric domestic animals there is only a narrow cardiac gland region adjoining the cutaneous mucosa at the cardia. The distal fundus and pylorus gland regions are prominent in all domestic animals (**Fig. 16.42**). All the gastric glands are tubular glands opening into gastric pits.

The function of the fundus glands is thus mostly for secretion of HCl and enzymes. The function of the cardiac and pyloric glands is mainly to secrete mucus and bicarbonate.

The total secretion volume per day is 0.2–0.5 l in dogs, 2–3 l in pigs, 6–8 l in horses, and 1–2 l in humans. These (and the following) volume numbers are only estimates, as exact quantification is not possible.

■ Secretion of the fundus glands

The fundus glands consist of **mucus cells** (foveolar cells = neck cells), **parietal cells (oxyntic cells)** and **chief cells (peptic cells)** (**Fig. 16.43**). All these cells arise from stem cells in the "neck region" of the glands and are constantly replaced by new cells.

The mucus (neck) cells secrete mucus like the surface epithelium lining the **gastric pits (faveolae)**. The parietal cells secrete hydrochloric acid (HCl), while the chief cells secrete enzymes, especially pepsinogen.

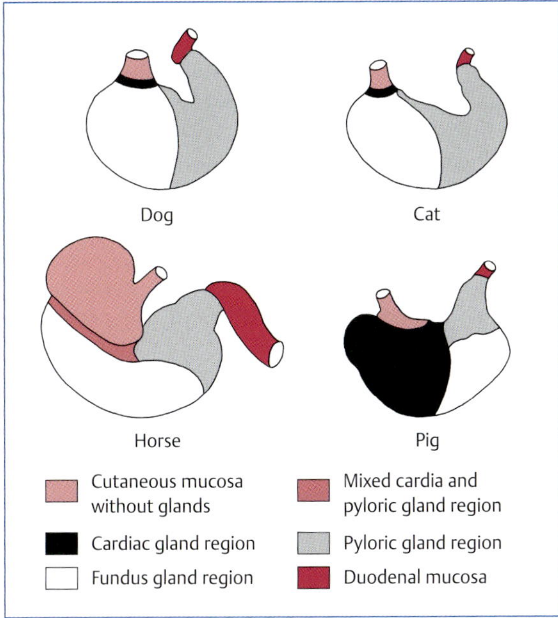

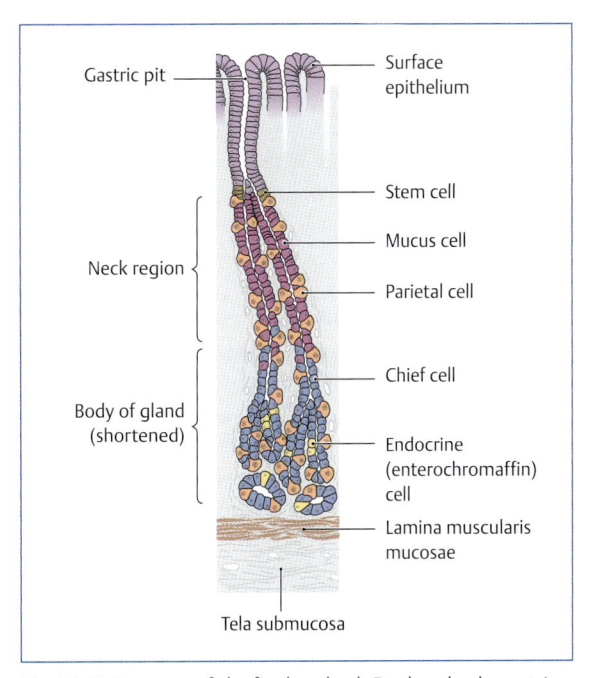

Fig. 16.42 The different regions of gastric mucosa in monogastric domestic animals. With the exception of the region with cutaneous mucosa, the gastric mucosa contains tubular glands. The fundus glands produce hydrochloric acid, enzymes and mucus, while the cardia and pyloric glands mainly secrete mucus and bicarbonate, forming a gel like mucous barrier.

Fig. 16.43 Structure of the fundus gland. Fundus glands contain four different cell types: The secretion of hydrochloric acid is by parietal cells. The chief cells produce digestive enzymes, and the mucus cells produce "gastric mucus". At the base of the glands, there are isolated endocrine (enterochromaffin) cells that secrete gastrointestinal peptide hormones. [Source: Schünke M, Schulte E, Schumacher U. Prometheus LernAtlas der Anatomie – Innere Organe. Illustrated by K. Wesker and M. Voll. Stuttgart: Thieme; 2015]

Nutrition, energy

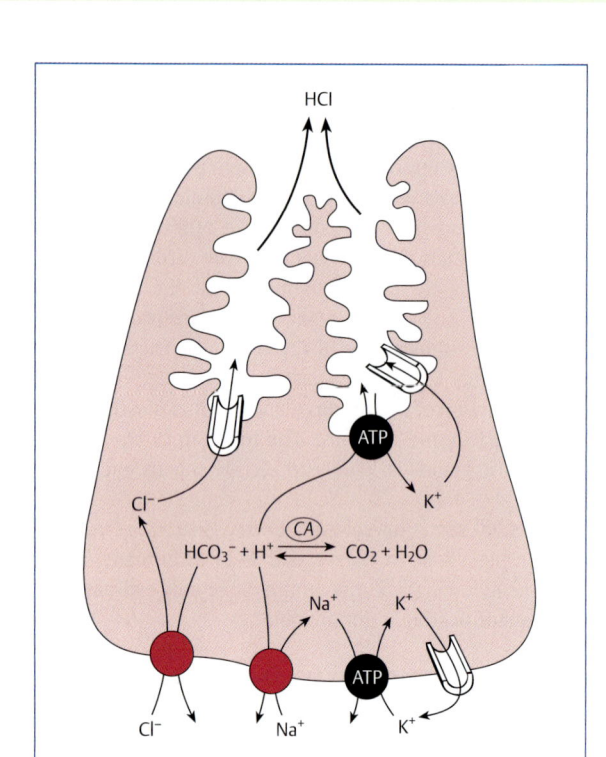

HCl

Cl⁻

$HCO_3^- + H^+ \rightleftharpoons CO_2 + H_2O$

CA

ATP

K⁺

Na⁺   K⁺

ATP

Cl⁻   Na⁺   K⁺

Fig. 16.44 Mechanism of HCl secretion by parietal cells. Activation causes fusion of intracellular membranes (canaliculi) with the outer cell membrane and thus greatly increases surface area. H^+ and HCO_3^- are produced by carbonic anhydrase (CA). Protons enter the glandular lumen by active transport, and HCO_3^- is released into blood in exchange for Cl⁻ which enters the glandular lumen via Cl⁻ channels.

HCl secretion of the parietal cells

The parietal cells have many intracellular **canaliculi**, the membrane of which corresponds functionally to the apical (lumen-facing) membrane of the cells (**Fig. 16.44**). When the parietal cells are activated by various stimuli, the ends of the canaliculi partly fuse with the apical membrane so that its lumen opens to the glandular lumen. In this way, the surface area of the apical membrane, and thus the secretion rate, is increased.

Mechanism of HCl secretion

An **H^+/K^+-ATPase** in the apical membrane of parietal cells transports H^+ against a 10^6-fold concentration gradient into the gland lumen and simultaneously, in exchange, K^+ into the cell. The energy required for this is provided by ATP. **K^+ and Cl⁻ channels** in the apical membrane enable K^+ and Cl⁻ to exit the cell down concentration gradients. K^+ is then reabsorbed into the cell by the H^+/K^+-ATPase, while Cl⁻ enters the gastric lumen together with H^+ (**Fig. 16.44**).

The intracellular generation of H^+ for secretion is promoted by **carbonic anhydrase** (CA):

$$CO_2 + H_2O \overset{CA}{\leftrightarrow} H_2CO_3 \leftrightarrow H^+ + HCO_3^- \qquad (16.2)$$

The CO_2 is derived from oxidative metabolism in the mucosal cells. The HCO_3^- generated exits the cells by a **Cl⁻/ HCO₃⁻ exchanger** in the basolateral ("blood side") membrane, and Cl⁻ is taken up in exchange. The basolateral membrane also contains a Na^+/K^+-ATPase (Na^+/K^+ pump)

and a Na^+/H^+ exchanger. The Na^+/H^+ exchanger eliminates excess protons when secretory activity of parietal cells is low. The Na^+/K^+-ATPase, which pumps Na^+ out of the cell and K^+ into the cell, maintains transmembrane Na^+ and K^+ gradients and thus the membrane potential of approx. −50 mV (inside negative), which drives the Cl⁻ outflow through the Cl⁻ channels of the apical membrane.

The mucosal cells also secrete **intrinsic factor**, a glycoprotein that forms a complex with **vitamin B_{12}**, which, together with haptocorrins (vitamin B_{12}-binding proteins of saliva), is crucial for vitamin B_{12} absorption in the ileum.

> ### IN A NUTSHELL   !
>
> In parietal cells of the gastric fundus glands, HCl is secreted as H^+ from the action of K^+/H^+-ATPase and as Cl⁻ through Cl⁻ channels, with resulting acidification of stomach contents.

Enzyme secretion of the chief cells

Pepsinogen, the inactive precursor of the endopeptidase **pepsin**, is synthesised on ribosomes of the chief cells. Pepsinogen is then packaged by the Golgi apparatus into membrane-enveloped secretory granules that migrate to the apical membrane. The release of pepsinogen into the glandular lumen occurs by **exocytosis**, where the secretory granule membrane fuses with the apical membrane of the chief cells.

The constant transport of membrane material as small vesicles, from the apical membrane back to the Golgi apparatus, prevents cell surface area increasing from exocytosis. Both migration of secretory granules to the apical membrane and the vesicular return of membrane material to the Golgi apparatus take place through the cytoskeleton.

In **dairy calves** and **suckling lambs**, and also to a limited extent in early postnatal life of other domestic mammals, the chief cells of the fundus glands of the abomasum mainly produce the inactive **precursor (prochymosin = prorennin)** of **chymosin=rennin** instead of pepsinogen, secreted by exocytosis.

Following secretion, both pepsinogen and prochymosin are activated by cleavage of several peptide chains by the low pH of the fundus gland secretion (pH 1) to **pepsin** and **chymosin**.

In addition to superficial epithelial cells, chief cells in monogastric animals also secrete a **gastric lipase** in an active form, which corresponds to the lingual lipase in calves and lambs. In the lower third of the fundus glands of the abomasum, where the chief cells are mainly located, the enzyme **lysozyme**, which attacks bacterial cell walls, is also secreted and assists in digestion of bacteria from the rumen.

> ### IN A NUTSHELL   !
>
> Digestive enzymes produced in the chief cells of the fundus glands are stored in secretory granules and released into the gastric lumen by exocytosis.

■ Secretion of the cardia and pyloric glands

The cells of the cardia and pyloric glands mainly correspond to the mucus cells of the fundus glands and, like the superficial epithelial cells, secrete **mucus** by **exocytosis**. Mucus consists of large-molecular weight **glycoproteins (mucins)**, present in cells as secretory granules. Mucus is also secreted along with HCO_3, through a **Cl^-/HCO_3^- exchanger** in the apical membrane. This results in the formation of a secretion granule in the 0.5–1 mm thick mucus layer overlying the gastric mucosa, which ensures **neutral pH conditions on the epithelial surface** despite the acidic pH of the gastric contents (pH 1–4).

> **MORE DETAILS** Especially in pigs (fattening pigs, breeding sows), but also in horses, stomach ulcers often occur (gastric ulcers). The pathogenesis of gastric ulcers (p. 416) in pigs and horses is very complex and not yet fully understood. However, the integrity of the mucus layer on the gastric mucosa is of particular importance for the protection of the gastric mucosa. Changes in this mucus layer (e.g. as a result of very low pH, or increase in the viscosity of the mucins, or possible loss of the mucus layer) lead to a partial to complete loss of the protective function. In horses, gastric ulcers often also occur in the pars proventricularis (glandless, cutaneous mucosa).

> **IN A NUTSHELL**   !
>
> Mucus, together with bicarbonate, is secreted into the gastric lumen especially from the cardia and pyloric glands to protect the epithelium.

16.5.2 Regulation of gastric secretion

■ Regulation of HCl secretion

The secretion of HCl by the gastrointestinal cells is regulated by **nerves, hormones** and **paracrine** substances (e.g. histamine). Food intake causes release of acetylcholine from postganglionic parasympathetic neurons, which innervate, among other things, the parietal cells. **Acetylcholine** stimulates HCl secretion via muscarinic receptors in the cell membrane. Diacylglycerol and inositol triphosphate (IP_3), produced by phospholipase action on membrane phospholipid, are released into the cytoplasm and act as second messengers to cause fusion of intracellular canaliculi with the apical membrane of parietal cells and thus HCl secretion.

Gastrin produced by **endocrine cell** (**G cells**) of the **pyloric glands** is released into blood and stimulates gastrin receptors on the membrane of parietal cells and initiates production of the same second messengers (diacylglycerol and inositol triphosphate) which stimulate HCl secretion. Gastrin secretion into blood is also indirectly stimulated by the intake of food or by the presence of food in the stomach. The stimulators of gastrin secretion are amino acids and peptides produced during protein digestion, which already begins in the stomach, as well as by **gastrin-releasing peptide** (**GRP**), released as a transmitter by certain postganglionic parasympathetic neurons in the stomach wall (**Fig. 16.45**).

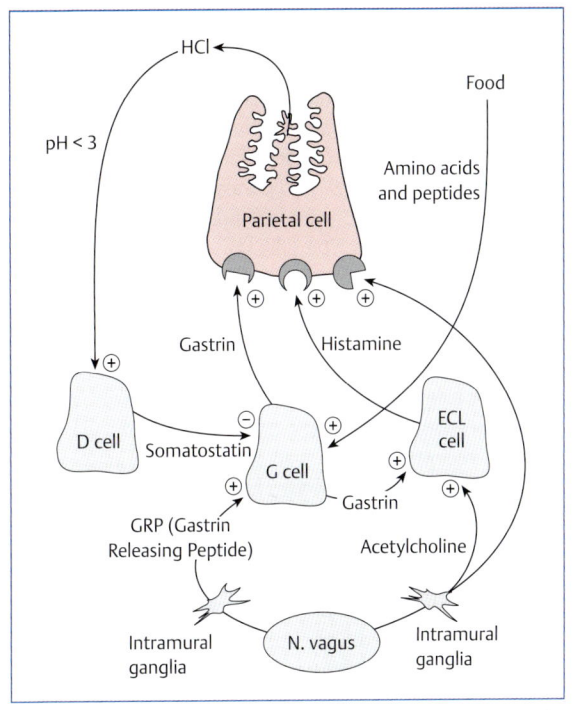

Fig. 16.45 Nervous and hormonal regulation of HCl secretion in the parietal cells. The gastrointestinal hormone gastrin, produced by G cells in the pyloric region, plays a central role in stimulating hydrochloric acid secretion. The secretion of gastrin is stimulated by both luminal factors and the vagus nerve (transmitters: acetylcholine and GRP). The action of gastrin is largely due to the release of paracrine histamine from ECL (enterochromaffin-like) cells. Inhibition of HCl secretion is autoregulated by gastric pH. A drop in pH leads to increased release of somatostatin by D cells and a paracrine inhibition of gastrin secretion.

Gastrin secretion is indirectly inhibited by lowering the **pH** of the gastric contents. Since gastrin causes gastric pH to fall by stimulating HCl secretion, this is a **negative feedback loop**, mediated by the peptide **somatostatin**. Somatostatin is released by **D-cells** located near the endocrine **G-cells**, when gastric pH is lowered. Then somatostatin inhibits gastrin secretion from G-cells by a paracrine pathway (**Fig. 16.45**).

Histamine-producing cells resembling enterochromaffin-like cells (ECL cells) are often found in the interstitium near the parietal cells. The release of histamine by these cells is stimulated by **gastrin** and by **acetylcholine**, the transmitter of parasympathetic neurons. Histamine, the amine of the amino acid histidine, also stimulates HCl secretion of parietal cells by H_2 **receptors**, with cAMP as a second messenger.

The various stimuli that promote HCl secretion potentiate each other in their effects on the parietal cells. Potentiation is when two simultaneously acting stimuli have a greater effect than the sum of their individual actions. This applies to the stimulating effect of gastrin and histamine on HCl secretion and explains why HCl secretion is regulated by several food intake-dependent stimuli.

Nutrition, energy

■ Regulation of enzyme secretion

Enzyme secretion by the chief cells of the fundus glands is controlled by both neural and hormonal factors (**Fig. 16.46**). The nervous stimulation of secretion with feed intake is mediated by **acetylcholine**, the most important transmitter of postganglionic **parasympathetic** neurones, and by **noradrenaline**, the transmitter of postganglionic **sympathetic** neurones. The effect of acetylcholine induces the second messengers diacylglycerol and inositol triphosphate as in parietal cells. Inositol triphosphate causes the release of Ca^{2+} from endoplasmic reticulum. The consequent increased intracellular Ca^{2+} concentration plays an important role in the exocytotic secretion of enzymes.

Noradrenaline stimulates enzyme secretion via **β-adrenergic receptors** on the cell membrane to activate adenylate cyclase which increases intracellular concentration of the second messenger cAMP which promotes exocytosis and thus enzyme secretion by phosphorylation of specific proteins.

The gastrointestinal hormones **cholecystokinin (CCK)** and **secretin** also stimulate enzyme secretion via the second messengers diacylglycerol and inositol triphosphate (by CCK) and cAMP (by secretin). The release of these hormones into blood from endocrine cells of the proximal small intestine is also stimulated by feed intake-related stimuli (CCK: amino acids and fatty acids in the duodenal lumen; secretin: low pH in the duodenum).

■ Regulation of mucus and bicarbonate secretion

Mucus secretion is much less affected by food intake than are secretion of hydrochloric acid and enzymes. Stimulation of mucus secretion is by **acetylcholine**, the transmitter of the parasympathetic nervous system, and by **prostaglandin E**, produced from arachidonic acid after it is released from membrane phospholipids by phospholipase A_2. For acetylcholine, the second messenger system is diacylglycerol and inositol triphosphate, while for prostaglandin E the second messenger is cAMP. **Low pH** in the stomach is the most important stimulus for mucus secretion, and via a vagovagal reflex, activates acetylcholine release from parasympathetic neurons in the stomach wall which promotes the formation of prostaglandin E.

Non-steroidal anti-inflammatory drugs, such as **acetylsalicylic acid**, inhibit prostaglandin formation and thus limit mucus secretion and its protective action on the gastric mucosa. **Glucocorticoids** (adrenocortical hormones), which act as stress hormones, also have a similar effect in high concentrations. Gastric HCO_3^- secretion is mainly regulated in the same way as mucus secretion.

> **IN A NUTSHELL**   !
>
> The secretion of HCl, enzymes and mucus is stimulated in the stomach by the parasympathetic nervous system and by gastrointestinal hormones, in response to food intake.

■ Dependence of gastric secretory activity on feed intake

Food intake is a strong stimulus for HCl and enzyme secretion, but less so for secretion of mucus and HCO_3^-. Gastric juice secretion is stimulated by smell and taste and by **anticipation of eating** even before any food reaches the stomach. The anticipatory, **cephalic phase** of the **gastric juice release** can be influenced by learning processes (**Pavlovian conditioning**) and is controlled by the CNS, mainly via the vagus nerve. The trigger for gastric juice secretion during the cephalic phase is predominantly the neurally increased **gastrin secretion**.

The **gastric phase** of gastric juice secretion is reflexively induced by **distension** of the **stomach** after food ingestion (vagovagal reflex), as well as by **amino acids** and **peptides** from partial digestion of food protein (pepsin action!). From both stimuli, there is an increased release of **gastrin** and thus increased HCl secretion. **Gastric distension** also stimulates the **parasympathetic nervous system** to increase enzyme secretion.

To a lesser extent, gastric juice secretion is also stimulated from the proximal small intestine by mechanical and chemical (amino acids) stimuli associated with feed intake (**intestinal phase**). However, details of these mechanisms are not yet known.

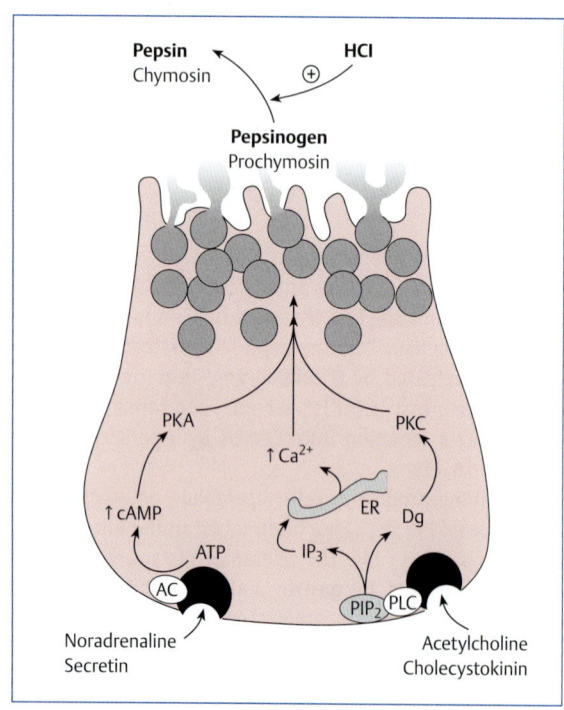

Fig. 16.46 Neural and hormonal regulation of pepsinogen (prochymosin) secretion by chief cells. In addition to the neurotransmitters acetylcholine (parasympathetic) and noradrenaline (sympathetic), the gastrointestinal peptide hormones secretin and cholecystokinin from duodenal mucosa also play a role. Signal transduction is via second messengers cAMP and Ca^{2+}. Activation of the chief cells causes secretion of pepsinogen and prochymosin by exocytosis. These proenzymes are activated by HCl in the gastric lumen to pepsin and chymosin, respectively.
AC = adenylate cyclase; Dg = diacylglycerol; ER = endoplasmic reticulum; IP$_3$ = inositol triphosphate; PIP$_2$ = phosphatidylinositol diphosphate; PKA = protein kinase A; PKC = protein kinase C; PLC = phospholipase C.

With a high secretion rate, the H⁺ concentration of gastric juice increases greatly, while that of Na^+ is markedly decreased. This is because when gastric juice secretion is stimulated, HCl secretion increases disproportionately compared to other secretions, which contain Na^+ as the main cation. The already high Cl^- concentration increases only slightly, as the other secretions also contain a lot of chloride.

16.5.3 Role of gastric secretions

◼ Hydrochloric acid

The **low pH** of stomach contents (pH 1–4) from secretion of HCl **kills** many **microorganisms** ingested with food. In ruminants, the rumen microorganisms that enter the abomasum with the rumen contents are killed by the low pH. However, some species of bacteria colonise and multiply in the mucus layer lining the stomach, such as *Helicobacter pylori*, a spiral bacterium that can cause inflammation and ulcers in the mucosa of the stomach and duodenum in humans. Similar microorganisms are also found in the stomach of dogs and cats. By producing **urease**, which generates NH_3 and CO_2 from urea diffusing from blood into the stomach, *Helicobacter pylori* is able to create neutral pH conditions in its environment and thus survive in the stomach.

As well as its **bactericidal effect**, the low pH of stomach contents **activates pepsinogen** to **pepsin** and **prochymosin** to **chymosin** by cleavage of short peptide chains.

◼ Pepsin

Pepsin functions as an **endopeptidase** (pH optimum: pH 1–3), which mainly cleaves peptide bonds of dietary protein with aromatic amino acids to produce small peptides and amino acids. Mucus is not attacked by pepsin.

◼ Chymosin (rennin)

The milk protein **casein** is a phosphoprotein in high concentrations in the milk of ruminants (cow's milk: approx. 2.5% of dry matter). It consists of several subunits that are coupled to each other via calcium phosphate bridges. One of these subunits is **kappa(κ)-casein** with a hydrophobic and a hydrophilic structure. It acts as a solubiliser for the other hydrophobic casein components. The hydrophilic part of κ-casein is a glycopeptide (M = 8000) with many acidic amino acids as well as hydroxy-amino acids.

Chymosin cleaves off the glycopeptide by hydrolysis of a **peptide** bond between phenylalanine and methionine, so that the remaining hydrophobic κ-casein part (= para-κ-casein, M = 20000) precipitates together with the remaining **casein complex**.

With casein precipitation (rennet coagulation) in the **calf's stomach** the **emptying of the stomach is delayed**. This prevents overload of the digestive and absorption capacities of the small intestine. Diarrhoea may occur if casein precipitation is prevented. This is of particular importance in very young animals in the first weeks of life, as the production and secretion of digestive enzymes of the exocrine pancreas is not yet fully developed.

Chymosin is also used for casein precipitation in cheese production. Nowadays, instead of chymosin from the abomasum of calves, it is obtained from genetically engineered microorganisms.

◼ Lysozyme

The lysozyme secreted in the **abomasum** of **ruminants** is, unlike other lysozymes, effective at low pH and is not attacked by pepsin. It is probably involved in the digestion of a peptidoglycan (murein) of the cell wall of **rumen bacteria**. Lysozyme is not found in the gastric juice of monogastric domestic animals.

◼ Gastric lipase

Gastric lipase (pH optimum 3.0–7.0) of monogastric domestic animals cleaves **triacylglycerols** in the acidic environment of the stomach, analogous to the lingual lipase of calves and lambs, to produce **diacylglycerols and free fatty acids**. In this process, **medium-chain fatty acids** (relatively often found in milk fat) and **unsaturated long-chain fatty acids** are preferentially split off. In young dogs, it was found that 50–60% of milk fat is digested in the stomach, in a similar manner to calves, where fat in gastric contents is digested by lingual lipase. Gastric lipase is highly resistant to the proteolytic activity of pepsin.

◼ Intrinsic factor

Intrinsic factor is a glycoprotein that, together with the haptocorrins, is required for the intestinal absorption of **vitamin B₁₂ (cobalamin)**. This vitamin forms a complex with intrinsic factor, to enable binding to a specific receptor on the apical membrane of **epithelial cells** in the ileum and subsequent uptake into those cells. After gastrectomy, vitamin B₁₂ absorption is therefore inhibited resulting in anaemia, as vitamin B₁₂ has an important role in red blood cell production.

◼ Mucus

The 0.5–1 mm thick **mucus layer** lining the stomach **serves to protect** the gastric mucosa from mechanical trauma and from the H⁺ ions in the lumen. The secretion of bicarbonate by the mucus-secreting cells ensures neutral pH conditions under the mucus layer.

> **IN A NUTSHELL** !
>
> The low pH of gastric contents has a bactericidal effect and activates pepsinogen and prochymosin to pepsin and chymosin. A bicarbonate-containing mucus layer prevents damage to the stomach lining. Protein and fat digestion already begins in the stomach.

16.5.4   Microbial activity in the stomach

In the proximal part of the stomach, considerable microbial activity has been detected in **pigs** and **horses**. Thus, an increase in concentration of **short-chain fatty acids** (up to approx. 40 mmol·l⁻¹) and **lactic acid** (up to 50 mmol·l⁻¹) can be observed after feeding. In this region of the stomach, the pH is relatively high after feeding (pH 4–6), so that bacteria are able to colonise the stomach and convert some carbohydrates to short-chain fatty acids (acetic acid, propionic acid, butyric acid) and lactic acid. Short-chain fatty acids in combination with a low pH value can cause **gastric ulcers** in **pigs**, especially in the cutaneous mucosa region. In the pathogenesis of gastric ulcers, damage to the mucous layer lining the stomach is a critical factor, along with factors related to feed composition as well as the effects of stress. The frequent occurrence of gastric ulcers in **horses** has also been reported. Whether short-chain fatty acids also play a role in this is an open question. As in pigs, stress certainly has a role in the development of gastric ulcers in horses.

16.5.5   Absorption functions of the stomach

Weak acids, such as **short-chain fatty acids**, are **effectively absorbed in the stomach** because they are mainly undissociated at the low pH. Undissociated short-chain fatty acids are relatively lipid-soluble and can therefore quickly pass through the lipid matrix of the cell membrane. In the cytosol of the gastric epithelium, dissociation of the short-chain fatty acids can lead to acidification, which in extreme cases can cause epithelial damage.

Suggested reading

Chang EB, Sitrin MD, Block DD. Gastrointestinal, Hepatobiliary and Nutritional Physiology. Philadelphia: Lippincott-Raven; 1996

Guilford WG, Center SA, Strombeck DR et al. Strombeck's Small Animal Gastroenterology. 3rd ed. Philadelphia: W. B. Saunders; 1996

Ito S. Functional Gastric Morphology. In: Johnson LR, ed. Physiology of the Gastrointestinal Tract. Vol. 1. New York: Raven Press; 1981: 517–550.

Johnson LR, ed. Physiology of the Gastrointestinal Tract. Vol 1. and 2. 5th ed. London: Elsevier Academic Press; 2012

16.6   Functions of the small intestine and its accessory organs

Siegfried Wolffram

> **ESSENTIALS**
>
> In the small intestine, food is digested by secreted enzymes and the products of digestion are absorbed (e.g. monosaccharides, amino acids and di- and tripeptides, fatty acids, fat- and water-soluble vitamins, etc.).
>
> Approx. ⅔ of electrolyte and water absorption from the entire length of the gastrointestinal tract occurs in the small intestine under physiological conditions.
>
> Furthermore, the small intestine has an important immunological function as a protective "barrier" (p. 247) against noxious components of food.
>
> The motor function of the small intestine (p. 388) has already been discussed. Hence, only the secretory functions of the small intestine and pancreas, digestion in the small intestine and absorption of nutrients will be considered in this section. The secretion of bile by the liver is outlined in ch. 17.3.1 (p. 466). Here, only the function of the gallbladder and the importance of bile in fat digestion are discussed.

16.6.1   Secretions of the small intestine

The secretory processes in the small intestine include mucus and bicarbonate secretion by Brunner's glands, bicarbonate secretion by duodenal epithelium, mucus secretion by goblet cells interspersed between intestinal mucosal cells, and Cl⁻ secretion by glandulae intestinales (crypts of Lieberkühn).

■ Secretion of Brunner's glands

Brunner's glands are tubulo-alveolar glands in the submucosa with excretory ducts opening into the duodenum. They secrete **mucus** and **bicarbonate** and thus contribute to **protecting the duodenal mucosa** from the acidic gastric contents that enter the duodenum. As in the stomach, mucus secretion occurs by exocytosis, while bicarbonate secretion is mediated by a Cl⁻/HCO₃⁻ exchanger. Cl⁻ is probably reabsorbed, partly through a Cl⁻ channel in the apical cell membrane. The secretion of Brunner's glands is **stimulated** by the **parasympathetic** nervous system and **inhibited** by the **sympathetic nervous** system.

■ Bicarbonate secretion of the duodenal epithelium

HCO_3^- secretion by the duodenal mucosa is both transcellular and paracellular. Transcellular secretion is by Na^+-HCO_3^- transport into the cells across the basolateral membrane of the villous epithelium and a Cl^-/HCO_3^- exchanger in the apical membrane. There is also an anion channel, permeable to HCO_3^- and Cl^-, in the apical membrane. The secreted HCO_3^- is partly that which enters cells by Na^+-HCO_3^- cotransport and partly that produced by intracellular carbonic anhydrase. The H⁺ produced in the process is discharged via a Na⁺/H⁺ exchanger across the basolateral membrane.

Duodenal HCO_3^- **secretion** assists in **neutralising HCl** and is stimulated by the low pH of the duodenal contents via a **vagovagal reflex** and also by locally produced **prostaglandin E**. The **sympathetic nervous system** inhibits HCO_3^- secretion.

■ Mucus secretion of goblet cells

Goblet cells differ from epithelial cells of small intestinal villi and crypts by containing numerous mucus-filled secretory granules. The number of goblet cells increases in the small intestine from proximal to distal. Most goblet cells are found in the large intestine.

Mucus secretion occurs through a special type of **exocytosis** (collective exocytosis), whereby all stored secretory granules are emptied together. The storage of secretory granules is confined to the so-called theca, an apical cytoplasmic compartment bounded by microtubules and intermediate filaments.

Mucus secretion is stimulated by **acetylcholine** and **prostaglandin E**. Acetylcholine is released as a transmitter by neurons of the enteric nervous system in response to luminal mechanical and chemical stimuli. Prostaglandin production is also stimulated by luminal chemical stimuli (e.g. low pH). Some **bacterial toxins** (e.g. toxins of *Esche-*

richia coli, cholera toxin) also promote mucus secretion. When the small intestine is colonised with parasites, an increase in number of goblet cells and thus in mucus secretion has also been observed.

The epithelium of the small intestine is covered by a **mucus layer** about 0.5 mm thick, which has a **protective function** against mechanical, chemical (low pH, proteases) and noxious agents from bacteria, parasites, and viruses.

■ Functions of the crypts of Lieberkühn

The mucosal invaginations at the base of intestinal villi are called **crypts of Lieberkühn** (**Fig. 16.47**). In contrast to the cylindrical epithelium of the small intestine villi, the crypt epithelium consists of cubic cells with numerous **mitoses**. There are also **goblet cells, Paneth cells** (secreting lysozyme) and **endocrine cells**, secreting **intestinal hormones** into the bloodstream.

The crypts not only have secretory functions, but they are also the site of **epithelial cell replication**. The new cells from cell division migrate to the tips of the villi within

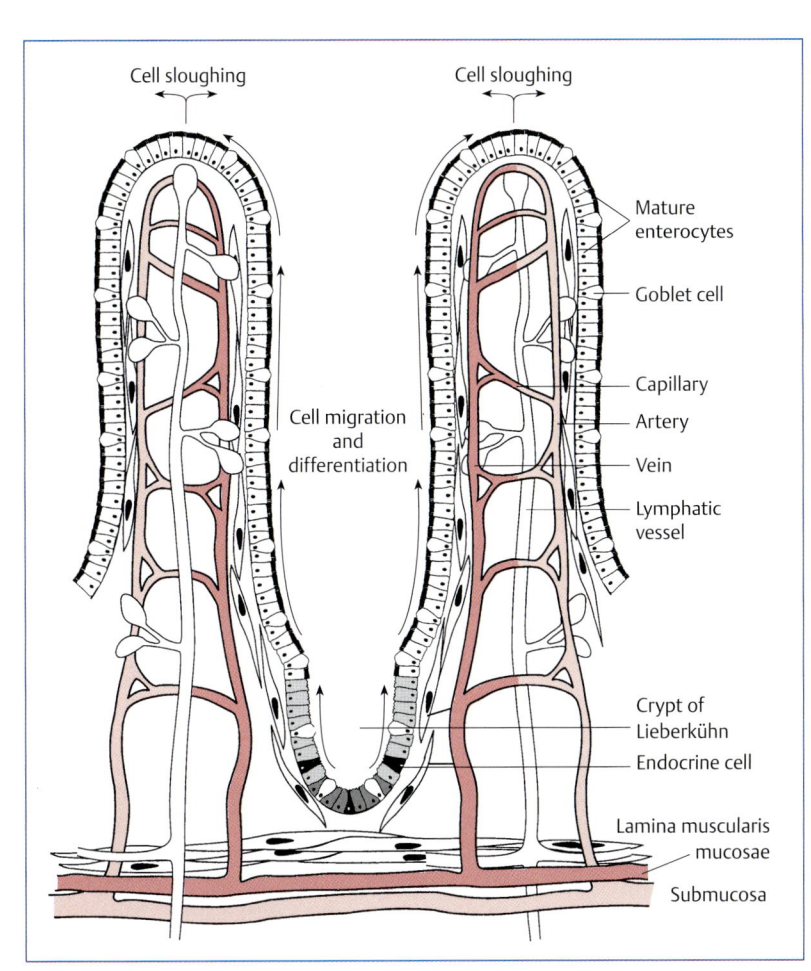

Cell sloughing

Cell sloughing

Cell migration and differentiation

Mature enterocytes

Goblet cell

Capillary

Artery

Vein

Lymphatic vessel

Crypt of Lieberkühn

Endocrine cell

Lamina muscularis mucosae

Submucosa

Fig. 16.47 Schematic representation of the intestinal villi and crypts of Lieberkühn. At the base and between the finger-shaped protrusions of the mucosal villi, are the crypts of Lieberkühn as invaginations of the mucosa. Regeneration of intestinal epithelium (every 2–3 days) is by continuous cell division in the crypts. The immature crypt cells differentiate into mature enterocytes with digestive and absorptive functions during their migration to the villous tip where they are finally expelled into the intestinal lumen. Capillaries and lymphatic vessels run in the villous stroma.

Nutrition, energy

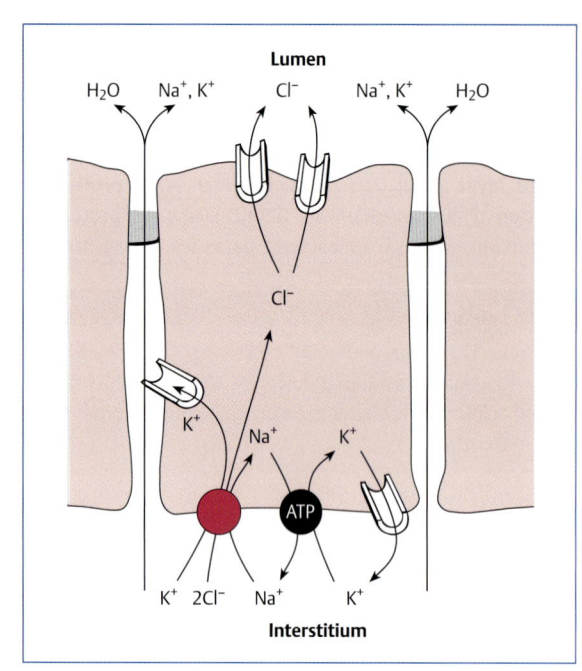

Fig. 16.48 Cl⁻ secretion in the crypts of Lieberkühn. Crypts of Lieberkühn produce intestinal secretions. Crypt cells actively secrete Cl⁻ after its uptake from blood together with Na⁺ and K⁺ ions. Cl⁻ flows down an electrochemical gradient through Cl⁻ channels into the crypt lumen, while Na⁺ and K⁺ exit the cells across the basolateral membrane. To maintain electroneutrality, Cl⁻ secretion is followed by paracellular diffusion of Na⁺ and K⁺ ions and by water from an osmotic gradient. Infections with some pathogenic bacteria can strongly stimulate secretion by producing enterotoxins which cause secretory diarrhoea.

three days and slough off there into the lumen. During this **migration**, they **differentiate** into cylindrical cells with mechanisms to absorb nutrients from the intestinal lumen. The crypt epithelium mainly has a secretory function.

The crypt epithelium secretes Cl⁻ (**Fig. 16.48**) which enters the cells against an electrical potential gradient by a **Na⁺-K⁺-2Cl⁻ cotransport** across the basolateral membrane, driven by the transmembrane electrochemical Na⁺ gradient, and then "downhill" through a Cl⁻ channel in the apical membrane into the crypt lumen. The Na⁺ that enters the cell with the cotransporter is pumped out of the cell by the Na⁺/K⁺-ATPase in the basolateral membrane, consuming energy (ATP) to maintain the transmembrane Na⁺ gradient. K⁺ re-enters the cells through K⁺ channels in the basolateral membrane. Cl⁻, which is actively secreted in this way, is followed by Na⁺ and to a lesser extent K⁺ by paracellular diffusion through the zonulae occludentes (tight junctions), so that NaCl and KCl are transferred into the lumen to maintain electroneutrality. Water then follows osmotically. An estimated 0.5–1 l of fluid is secreted per day in a medium-sized dog. The secretion of Cl⁻ is stimulated by (parasympathetic) neurons of the **submucosal plexus**, which release **acetylcholine** and sometimes **VIP** (vasoactive intestinal peptide) as transmitters. Both transmitters act using Ca²⁺ (acetylcholine) and cAMP (VIP) as **second messengers** to increase Cl⁻ secretion. The secretory process is linked mainly with food intake so as to increase the fluidity of chyme (= intestinal contents) and thus promote

digestion and absorption of nutrients. Local reflexes of the intestinal nervous system, as well as **vagovagal reflexes**, are triggered by dilatation stretching of the intestine.

Toxins of bacterial **diarrhoeal pathogens** (e.g. **enterotoxins** of *Escherichia coli*, cholera toxin) can massively stimulate Cl⁻ secretion resulting in secretory diarrhoea (p. 445). Toxin receptors on crypt cells activate second messenger systems (e.g. cGMP in the case of heat-stable coli enterotoxin) and cause Cl⁻ channels to open. Bacterial pathogens are a major cause of diarrhoea, especially in young animals.

> **MORE DETAILS** In many species (not in dogs, cats, and pigs!), so-called **Paneth cells** with eosinophilic granules at the base of the crypts secrete lysozyme and defensin-like peptides. Lysozyme digests peptidoglycans (murein) in the cell wall of many bacteria. Defensins damage bacterial cell walls by forming pores and thus, like lysozyme, have a bactericidal effect. Both lysozyme and defensin are protective against bacterial toxicity on intestinal mucosa.

> **IN A NUTSHELL**   !
>
> The watery intestinal secretion comes from crypts of Lieberkühn. Infections with intestinal pathogenic bacteria produce enterotoxins which strongly stimulate secretion and thus cause a secretory diarrhoea.

16.6.2 Exocrine pancreas

The **exocrine pancreas** is a compound tubulo-alveolar gland with acini and a complex **duct system** lined with cubic cells (**Fig. 16.50**). Pancreatic secretion enters the duodenum via the excretory duct (ductus pancreaticus). The acinar cells have the typical appearance of protein-producing and -secreting cells, with distinct rough endoplasmic reticulum, large **Golgi apparatus** and numerous **secretory granules**. Many acini also contain some cells that resemble duct cells (centroacinar cells). Cells lining the ducts have only a sparse endoplasmic reticulum and no secretory granules. They are specialised in the secretion of a **bicarbonate-rich** electrolyte solution, while the acinar cells, with the exception of the centroacinar cells, mainly secrete **digestive enzymes**.

In humans, 1–2 l of pancreatic juice are secreted per day, but the precise quantities in domestic animal species are not known. It can be assumed that dogs produce 0.2–0.4 l, pigs 1–2 l and cattle 10–15 l of pancreatic juice per day. In contrast, much **more pancreatic juice** is secreted in **horses** (30–35 l·d⁻¹). As these volumes have not been measured in domestic animals, the numbers are estimates.

The flow rate of pancreatic juice in monogastric animals is highly dependent on feeding activity, and this generally also affects its electrolyte composition and pH. With increasing flow rate, the HCO₃⁻ concentration increases (up to 140 mmol·l⁻¹), while the Cl⁻ concentration decreases with increasing flow rate (to 25 mmol·l⁻¹). The Na⁺ and K⁺ concentrations are independent of the flow rate and mainly correspond to their plasma concentrations. In the horse, the HCO₃⁻ concentration hardly changes with flow rate and is always lower (approx. 60 mmol·l⁻¹) than the Cl⁻ concentration (approx. 90 mmol·l⁻¹).

The increase in the HCO_3^- concentration of pancreatic juice with increased flow rate seen in most monogastric animals reflects the disproportionate increase of the **HCO_3^--rich duct cell secretion** compared to the **enzyme-rich acinar secretion**. In the horse, on the other hand, both secretions seem to increase proportionally. This explains why the electrolyte composition of horse pancreatic juice hardly changes with changes in flow rate.

■ Electrolyte and water secretion

Electrolytes and water are secreted both by **duct** and **acinar cells**. However, the duct cells are generally dominant in these secretory activities. The **acinar cells** secrete an electrolyte solution with a **plasma-like** composition, analogous to the secretion of the primary saliva. Cl^- mainly enters the lumen through a Cl^- channel on the apical cell membrane, with Na^+ and K^+ following paracellularly through the zonulae occludentes, to maintain electroneutrality. The uptake of Cl^- through the basolateral membrane of crypt cells (**Fig. 16.48**) is by a **Na^+-K^+-2Cl^- cotransporter** driven by the transmembrane Na^+ gradient. The Na^+ and K^+ that enter cells by this mechanism are then discharged by the Na^+/K^+ pump and K^+ channels in the basolateral membrane. Activation of these Cl^- and K^+ channels can thus stimulate electrolyte secretion and, by osmosis, water secretion.

In contrast to the Cl^--rich secretion of the acinar cells, the secretion of the **duct cells** is HCO_3^--rich and therefore alkaline. The **HCO_3^- secretion** of the duct cells depends in particular on cytoplasmic **carbonic anhydrase**, on a Cl^-/HCO_3^- exchanger in the apical membrane (functionally coupled to a Cl^- channel), and on a Na^+/H^+ exchanger in the basolateral membrane. This secretion process is driven by the Na^+/K^+-ATPase and is responsible for maintaining transmembrane electrochemical Na^+ gradient. Na^+ and K^+ passively follow the secreted HCO_3^- by paracellular diffusion. Water is osmotically transferred into the ductal system. **Fig. 16.49** illustrates the secretion mechanism of the duct cells.

■ Secretion of digestive enzymes

Digestive enzymes, some inactive, some active, are secreted by exocytosis from the **acinar cells** of the pancreas. The secretion of inactive proenzymes protects the pancreas from self-digestion.

- **Peptidases** (inactive): trypsinogen, chymotrypsinogen, proelastase, procarboxypeptidase A, procarboxypeptidase B
- **Nucleases** (active): ribonuclease, deoxyribonuclease
- **Amylase** (α-amylase; active)
- **Lipases:** lipase (active), procolipase (inactive), prophospholipase A_2 (inactive), cholesterol esterase (active)

The secretory or zymogen granules of the acinar cells contain a mixture of these enzymes. The pattern of enzymes synthesised and secreted by the pancreas adapts to the **diet composition** in monogastrics over a period of several days. For example, starch-rich food causes an increase in amylase secreted by the pancreas, while fat- or protein-rich food leads to an increase in lipases or peptidases.

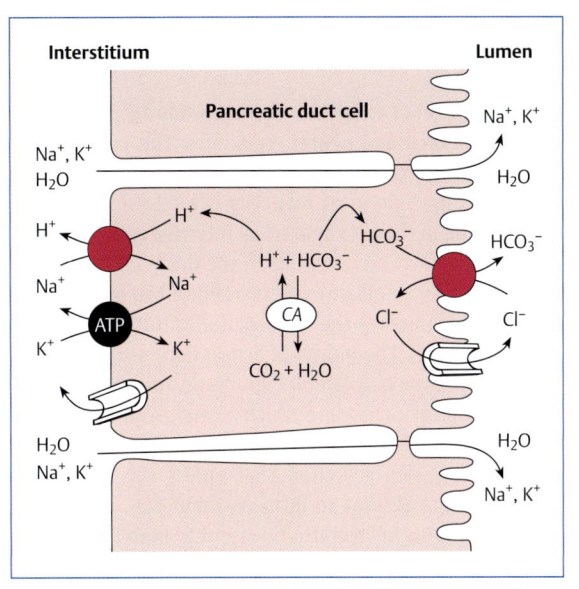

Fig. 16.49 : HCO_3^- secretion in the cells of the pancreatic ducts. These cells produce most of the bicarbonate-rich pancreatic secretion. Bicarbonate is produced by intracellular carbonic anhydrase (CA) and is released into the pancreatic ducts by a Cl^-/HCO_3^- exchanger. To maintain electroneutrality, the Cl^- is followed by paracellular diffusion of Na^+ and K^+ ions and water, in response to osmotic changes.

The acinar cells of **ruminant pancreas** secrete much more nucleases than monogastric species. These nucleases assist in digesting the large quantity of nucleic acids entering the small intestine from rumen microorganisms. In **horses**, the pancreas secretion contains relatively little amylase, because the horse evolved as a grass-eater and grass contains little starch. In ruminants, on the other hand, the composition of the ration has a clear influence on the amylase activity in the small intestine. If the feed contains a large amount of so-called rumen-stable starch (e.g. untreated maize starch), this is well digested in the small intestine by the increased secretion of pancreatic amylase.

Activation of the **pancreatic enzymes**, secreted in inactive form, only occurs after they reach the lumen of the **small intestine**. In this process, the enzyme **enteropeptidase** (enterokinase) in the brush-border membrane activates **trypsinogen** by splitting off a hexapeptide to form **trypsin**. Trypsin then activates the remaining trypsinogen by **autocatalysis** so that all trypsin becomes active. The other pancreatic enzymes secreted in inactive form are also activated by trypsin by means of peptide cleavage. A trypsin inhibitor is also secreted with the pancreatic digestive enzymes, which prevents the activation of trypsin while still in the pancreas.

IN A NUTSHELL   !

The exocrine pancreas is a compound tubulo-alveolar gland in which the cells of the ductal system secrete a NaHCO₃-rich solution, while the cells of the acini secrete digestive enzymes in a NaCl-rich solution which flows into the intestinal lumen.

■ Regulation of secretion

Duct cells

The production of a NaHCO₃-rich secretion by duct cells is under hormonal and neural regulation. The peptide hormone secretin induces secretion. Secretin release into blood by endocrine intestinal cells is induced by the low pH of chyme in the proximal small intestine (gastric acid!). Secretin then acts on receptors in the duct cell membrane and stimulates adenylate cyclase and thus the formation of cAMP, which initiates the release of a NaHCO₃-rich secretion (**Fig. 16.50**). The points of action here are the Na⁺/H⁺ exchanger on the basolateral membrane and the Cl⁻ channel of the apical membrane which promotes the intracellular formation of HCO₃⁻ (**Fig. 16.49**).

The HCO₃⁻-rich secretion that enters the duodenum neutralises the H⁺ ions to form H₂O and CO₂, so that the low pH stimulus for secretin release into blood is then diminished. The **parasympathetic nervous system** also stimulates secretion by the duct cells through activation of VIP-ergic neurons. The action of **VIP** is also mediated via cAMP.

Acinar cells

The secretion of the acinar cells (enzymes, NaCl-rich secretion) is regulated by the intestinal hormone **cholecystokinin (CCK)** as well as by the **parasympathetic nervous system** (transmitter: acetylcholine) (**Fig. 16.50**). CCK and acetylcholine exert their effects respectively via **CCK receptors** and by **muscarinic cholinergic receptors** on the cell membrane. Activation of these receptors causes the in-

tracellular release of the second messengers inositol triphosphate and diacylglycerol. Inositol triphosphate then increases intracellular Ca²⁺ concentration by opening Ca²⁺ channels to release Ca²⁺ stores in endoplasmic reticulum. Ca²⁺ and diacylglycerol together then activate a protein kinase (protein kinase C), which, by phosphorylating proteins, stimulates exocytosis and Cl⁻ secretion.

CCK release by endocrine cells of the proximal small intestine into the bloodstream is stimulated particularly by the products of protein and fat digestion (amino acids and fatty acids).

■ Stimulation of pancreatic secretion by food intake

Stimuli related to food intake (smell, taste, gastric distension, low pH in the duodenum, protein and fat digestion products in the small intestine) all strongly stimulate pancreatic secretion in **monogastrics**.

Depending on the site of action of the stimuli, there are cephalic, gastric and intestinal phases of pancreatic secretion.

The **cephalic phase** of secretion is induced by the smell and taste of food as well as by chewing-related tactile stimuli. It is mediated by parasympathetic fibres of the vagus nerve. The **gastric phase** of secretion is based on the stretching of the stomach wall by the ingestion of food, which via a vagovagal reflex increases the secretion of the pancreas. In quantitative terms, the most important phase of increased pancreatic secretion related to food intake is the **intestinal phase**. This is when there is increased secretion of the intestinal hormones, secretin and CCK into blood. The stimuli for this increased hormonal secretion are the fall in pH in the duodenal contents (secretin) or the accumulation of the products of protein and fat digestion (CCK) in the small intestinal lumen.

In **ruminants**, the increase in pancreatic secretion with the ingestion of a "meal" is much less pronounced than in monogastrics. This is probably because the food first enters the forestomach system and therefore a pronounced gastric and intestinal phase of pancreatic secretion does not immediately occur.

■ Pancreatic secretion disorders

MORE DETAILS Impairment of the secretion of the exocrine pancreas **(pancreatic insufficiency)** is relatively common, especially in **dogs**. The cause is often a chronic inflammation of the pancreas (chronic pancreatitis), which results from repeated acute inflammations. Acini in particular are destroyed by auto-digestion and replaced by connective tissue. The causes of pancreatitis are largely unknown. In a few cases, pancreatic insufficiency in dogs can also be congenital.

Pancreatic insufficiency manifests itself after extensive destruction of the acini leading to maldigestion, mainly affecting fat and protein digestion, followed by an **increased fat excretion** in faeces (steatorrhoea). Undigested protein excretion is also increased. Dogs with severe pancreatic insufficiency become anorexic as a result of the reduced nutrient supply caused by **maldigestion**, even with increased food intake. The addition of pancreatic enzyme extracts to food can at least partially compensate for the lack of those enzymes in affected animals.

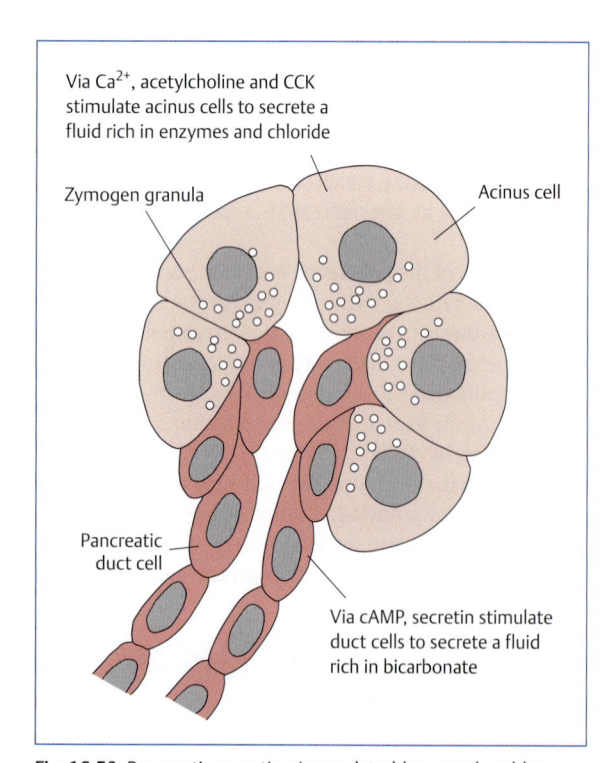

Via Ca²⁺, acetylcholine and CCK stimulate acinus cells to secrete a fluid rich in enzymes and chloride

Zymogen granula

Acinus cell

Pancreatic duct cell

Via cAMP, secretin stimulate duct cells to secrete a fluid rich in bicarbonate

Fig. 16.50 Pancreatic secretion is regulated by neural and hormonal factors. Acetylcholine as a transmitter of the parasympathetic nervous system and the peptide hormones secretin and cholecystokinin secreted by the duodenal mucosa play a role.

> **IN A NUTSHELL**   !
>
> Stimulation of pancreatic juice secretion by food intake is both by the parasympathetic nervous system (transmitter acetylcholine) and by the gastrointestinal hormones, secretin and cholecystokinin, produced by the duodenal mucosa.

16.6.3 Bile secretion and gallbladder function

Bile is formed (p. 466) in **liver cells** and the epithelial cells of the hepatic bile ducts ($NaHCO_3$ secretion, analogous to the duct cells of the pancreas), and is stored in the **gallbladder** where electrolytes and water are reabsorbed. Bile formed in the liver thus has a different composition to that in the gallbladder (**Table 16.10**). In species without a gallbladder (e.g. horse, camel, rat, pigeon), the liver bile passes directly into the proximal small intestine via the choledochal duct.

The amount of bile entering the small intestine per day via the **choledochal duct** is 0.5–1 l in humans and pigs, 0.1–0.2 l in dogs, 0.5–0.7 l in sheep, 3–5 l in cattle and 7–10 l in horses. As with the information on secretion by the stomach and pancreas, these volume numbers are also estimates.

Table 16.10 Composition of bile (carnivores).

Parameter	Liver bile (mmol·l⁻¹)	Gall bladder bile (mmol·l⁻¹)
Conjugated bile acids[1]	35	300
Bile pigments[2]	1	5
Phospholipids[3]	2	15
Cholesterol	2	10
Na^+	165	280
K^+	5	10
Ca^{2+}	2.5	12
Cl^-	90	15
HCO_3^-	45	10
pH	8.2	6.5

[1] Mainly tauro- and glycocholic acid and tauro- and glycocheno deoxycholic acid.
[2] Mainly bilirubin diglucuronide
[3] Mainly lecithin

■ Concentration of bile in the gallbladder

Concentration of the **organic components of bile** (conjugated bile acids, bile pigments, phospholipids, cholesterol) in the gallbladder takes place through the reabsorption of water. For this, water osmotically follows the reabsorption of Na^+ and Cl^-. There is no absorption or secretion of organic components by the gallbladder epithelium.

Na^+ is absorbed into the epithelial cells of the gallbladder through a Na^+/H^+ exchanger and Cl^- through a Cl^-/HCO_3^- exchanger in the apical membrane. Na^+ is dis-

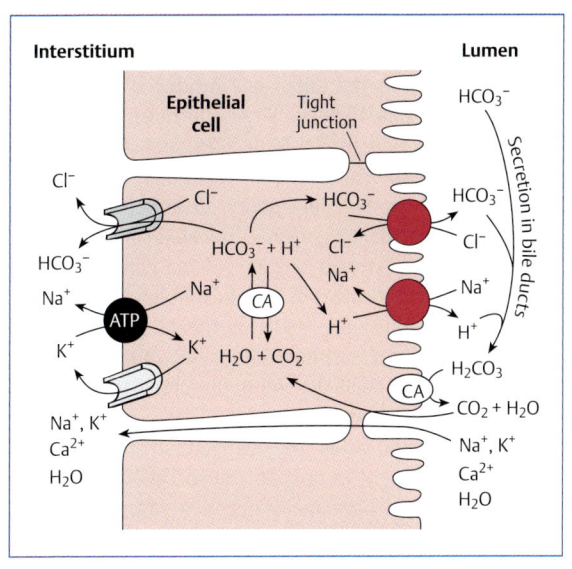

Fig. 16.51 Electrolyte and water reabsorption by the gallbladder epithelium. In the gallbladder, net reabsorption of water concentrates the organic components of bile. The osmotically induced water reabsorption is driven by the reabsorption of NaCl. Na^+ and Cl^- are reabsorbed in exchange for H^+ and HCO_3^- (intracellular carbonic anhydrase [CA] reaction) from the lumen into the epithelium and then transported across the BLM via the Na^+/K^+ pump or by an anion channel into blood. Together with the water flow, some electrolytes are also absorbed paracellularly.

charged through the basolateral membrane by the Na^+/K^+ pump and Cl^- through an anion channel, which is also permeable to HCO_3^- (**Fig. 16.51**).

The reabsorption of Na^+ and Cl^- into blood leads to a local increase in osmolarity in the intercellular spaces, which are sealed off from the gallbladder lumen by zonulae occludentes (tight junctions). The increased osmolarity in the intercellular space causes **water reabsorption** down a local osmotic gradient (**Fig. 16.64**). The removal of HCO_3^- from gallbladder bile is linked to the secretion of H^+ by the Na^+/H^+ exchanger. Secreted H^+ at the epithelial membrane combines with HCO_3^- to form H_2CO_3, which decomposes into CO_2 and H_2O (catalysed by a membrane-bound form of carbonic anhydrase). With its high lipid solubility, CO_2 diffuses into the epithelium where **carbonic anhydrase (CA)** converts it into HCO_3^- and H^+ ($CO_2 + H_2O \overset{CA}{\leftrightarrow} H_2CO_3 \to H^+ + HCO_3^-$). H^+ then passes into the lumen via the Na^+/H^+ exchanger, while HCO_3^- leaves the epithelial cell partly via the anion channel of the basolateral membrane into blood, and partly via the Cl^-/HCO_3^- exchanger in the apical membrane into the lumen of the gallbladder (**Fig. 16.51**). Thus, HCO_3^- absorption depends on the Na^+/H^+ exchanger of the apical membrane, carbonic anhydrase, and the anion channel in the basolateral membrane.

A 5–10 times higher concentration, compared to liver bile, of bile acids, bile pigments, phospholipids (lecithin) and cholesterol is found in gallbladder bile of carnivores, poultry and humans, but is only 2–3 times higher in other domestic animal species. The concentration of bile in the gallbladder is caused by water reabsorption driven by electrolyte reabsorption. The organic components of bile are hardly reabsorbed at all in the gallbladder. Despite the high

concentration of bile acids and other organic components (Table 16.10), the bile of the gallbladder has almost the same osmolarity as the initial bile produced in the liver. This is because bile acids are largely in micelles and thus have little osmotic activity. Molecules such as **bile acids** and **phospholipids** which have a **hydrophilic** and a **hydrophobic end** are called **detergents**. In aqueous solution, they form molecular aggregates (**micelles**) in which the hydrophobic end (steroid skeleton of the conjugated bile acids or fatty acid residues of the phospholipids) forms the core and the hydrophilic end (taurine or glycine of the conjugated bile acids or phosphate group of the phospholipids) forms the shell. Hydrophobic cholesterol is also partly incorporated into the core.

Conjugated bile acids are relatively strong acids and are therefore present as anions. The so-called **mixed bile acid micelles** thus have many negative charges on their outside representing **polyanions** that are able to **bind** and thus immobilise **cations** according to their valence. This largely explains the high concentrations of cations (Na^+, K^+, Ca^{2+}) in the bile of the gallbladder (**Table 16.10**) and their relatively low osmotic activity.

The osmotic activity of Na^+ and Ca^{2+} in the gallbladder corresponds to concentrations of about $145\,mmol \cdot l^{-1}$ (Na^+) and $1.5\,mmol \cdot l^{-1}$ (Ca^{2+}), respectively. The low concentration of inorganic anions (Cl^-, HCO_3^-) in the gallbladder bile is due to the fact that the conjugated bile acids are not completely dissolved in micelles and are thus partially present as "free" anions.

MORE DETAILS   In **domestic animals, gallstones** occur relatively **rarely** compared to humans. In humans, gallstones consist mainly of cholesterol, which has limited micellar solubility, whereas in domestic animals, gallstones consist mainly of Ca^{2+} bilirubinate. Gallstone formation in domestic animals is often preceded by bacterial infections of the gallbladder, which hydrolyses bilirubin diglucuronide to bilirubin and glucuronic acid. The poorly soluble Ca^{2+} salt of bilirubin then precipitates.

> **IN A NUTSHELL**   !
>
> The bile formed in the liver is stored in the gallbladder. The reabsorption of NaCl leads to a net reabsorption of water and thus to a concentration of the organic components of bile (conjugated bile acids, bile pigments, phospholipids, cholesterol).

■ Filling and emptying the gallbladder

In the fasting state, the ductus choledochus is closed at the junction with the duodenum by contraction of the smooth circular musculature (sphincter of Oddi), especially in dogs and cats as well as in humans, so that bile secreted by the liver reaches the gallbladder from the ductus hepaticus via the ductus cysticus instead of entering the duodenum via the ductus choledochus. In ruminants and pigs, the tonus of the sphincter of Oddi is relatively low, so that bile is stored and concentrated less efficiently in the gallbladder. In horses, due to the absence of the gallbladder, bile enters the duodenum more or less continuously.

As already mentioned in the regulation of pancreatic secretion, the cleavage products of fat and protein diges-

tion in the small intestine cause the release of the intestinal hormone **cholecystokinin**, which triggers contraction of the smooth muscles of the gallbladder as well as the relaxation of the sphincter of Oddi and thus the **emptying** of the gallbladder following feeding. The concentrated bile from the gallbladder is thus transferred to the proximal small intestine to promote fat digestion (p.429). Feeding-induced emptying of the gallbladder is also stimulated by the reflex release of **acetylcholine** by postganglionic parasympathetic neurons, which has a contractile effect on the smooth muscles of the gallbladder.

> **IN A NUTSHELL**   !
>
> Pulse-like emptying of the gallbladder is induced by food intake, whereby the hormone cholecystokinin, which is increasingly released in the proximal small intestine, causes contraction of the smooth muscles of the gallbladder as well as relaxation of the circular muscles of the ductus choledochus at the junction with the duodenum (sphincter of Oddi).

16.6.4   Digestion and absorption of carbohydrates

Starch (and glycogen), sucrose and lactose from food are digested by enzymes in the small intestine from **pancreatic juice (amylase)** and the **small intestinal epithelium (di- and oligosaccharidases)**. Structural carbohydrates such as cellulose, hemicellulose and pectin, which are components of the plant cell wall, are not attacked by these enzymes. They are mainly broken down by microbial enzymes in the large intestine (p.439) or, in the case of ruminants, in the forestomach system (p.398), to short-chain fatty acids (acetic acid, propionic acid, butyric acid). In the small intestine, this microbial degradation of carbohydrates plays only a minor role.

■ Starch digestion

Starch consists of glucose units linked by 1,4-α-glycosidic and 1,6-α-glycosidic bonds. The fraction of starch consisting only of unbranched spiral chains of 1,4-α-glycosidically linked glucose units is **amylose** (50–2000 glucose units). The branched-chain fraction consisting of 1,4- and 1,6-α-glycosidically linked glucose units (the branching occurs through the 1,6-α-glycosidic bond) is **amylopectin** (2000–200000 glucose units). Amylopectin makes up 70–80% of starch. Starch is mainly stored as granules in grains (cereals) and tubers (potatoes) as a reserve carbohydrate.

Glycogen in liver and muscles is a reserve carbohydrate ("animal starch") and largely corresponds in structure to that of amylopectin with more branching.

Starch digestion is more effective after mechanical (milling) or thermal (boiling) destruction of the internal structure of the starch granules than without such pretreatment. With these treatments, amylase from pancreatic juice and saliva can better attach to the starch molecules. The main site of starch digestion is the **proximal third** of the **small intestine**, since the activity of pancreatic amylase and of the brush border membrane enzymes involved in starch digestion (glucoamylase, α-dextrinase, saccharase) is highest in this section of the intestine.

Amylase is only able to **hydrolytically** cleave the 1,4-α-glycosidic bonds of **starch**, with the final fragments being **maltose, maltotriose** and **α-dextrins** (**Fig. 16.52**). α-Dextrins are branched-chain oligosaccharides with at least one 1,6-α-glycosidic bond and several 1,4-α-glycosidic bonds, which cannot be cleaved by amylase which is blocked by the proximity of chain branching at the 1,6-α-glycosidic bond.

The products of amylase digestion are then further broken down by oligo- or disaccharidases located in the apical membrane of small intestinal epithelial cells. These include **glucoamylase** (maltase), **α-dextrinase** (isomaltase) and **saccharase**.

> **MORE DETAILS** Glucoamylase and saccharase break down glucose by hydrolysis of 1,4-α-glycosidic bonds. Glucoamylase acts on large starch fragments, while saccharase mainly breaks down sucrose, maltose and maltotriose. α-Dextrinase cleaves the 1,6-α-glycosidic bonds of α-dextrins, the fragments of which are then further hydrolysed to glucose by glucoamylase and saccharase.

In contrast to the 1,4-α- and 1,6-α-glycosidic bonds of starch, the **1,4-β-glycosidic bonds** of **cellulose**, the most important plant skeletal carbohydrate, which also consists of many glucose units, can**not be** hydrolytically **cleaved** by amylase and oligo- and disaccharidases in the brush bor-

der membrane of intestinal mucosal cells. However, cellulose and other fibrous carbohydrates (hemicellulose, pectin) can be **anaerobically digested and metabolised by microorganisms** to short-chain fatty acids in the forestomach of ruminants or in the large intestine.

■ Digestion of lactose and sucrose

Lactose (milk sugar) is a disaccharide consisting of a glucose and a galactose molecule linked by a 1,4-β-glycosidic bond. Lactose is converted into glucose and galactose by the **brush border membrane** enzyme **lactase**. **Sucrose** (beet or cane sugar), a 1,2-α-glycosidic bound disaccharide, is hydrolysed to glucose and fructose by the brush border membrane enzyme **saccharase**, which is also able to cleave maltose and maltotriose.

■ Postnatal development of carbohydrate digestion

In early postnatal life, **lactase activity** in the small intestine is **high** in all domestic mammals. The highest activity at 1–3 weeks of age then drops, more or less rapidly, with weaning from the dam (**Fig. 16.53**). This drop is genetically programmed and can only be slightly delayed by prolonged feeding of milk.

The activities of **other enzymes** of carbohydrate digestion (amylase, glucoamylase, saccharase, α-dextrinase) are **low** during the **infant phase**. Their activity increases

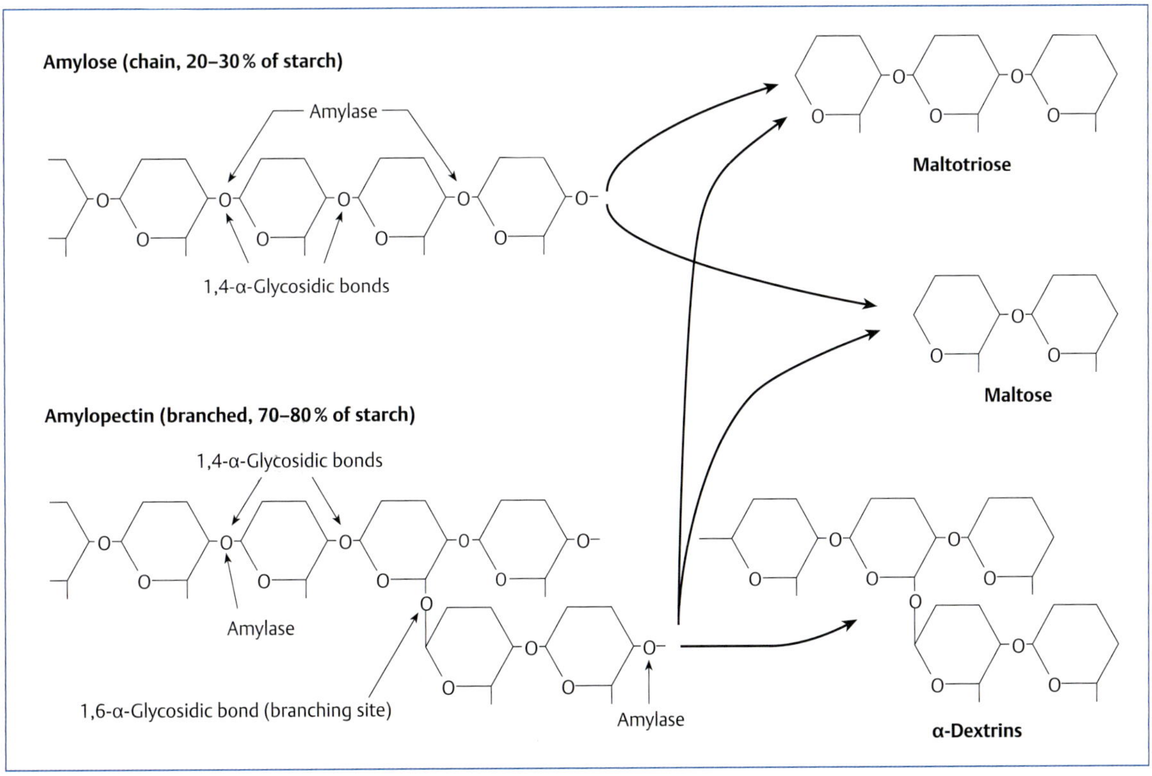

Amylose (chain, 20–30 % of starch)

Amylase

1,4-α-Glycosidic bonds

Maltotriose

Maltose

Amylopectin (branched, 70–80 % of starch)

1,4-α-Glycosidic bonds

Amylase

1,6-α-Glycosidic bond (branching site)

Amylase

α-Dextrins

Fig. 16.52 Intraluminal digestion of starch by amylase. Starch is first broken down by amylase in the intestinal lumen into di- or trimeric units (maltose, maltotriose). Since amylase can only cleave 1,4-α-glycosidic bonds, branched glucose oligomers (α-dextrins) containing a 1,6-α-glycosidic bond (branching site) are also formed during the digestion of amylopectin. However, the starch cleavage products formed by amylase can only be absorbed after degradation to monomeric glucose units by disaccharidases in the brush border membrane of epithelial cells.

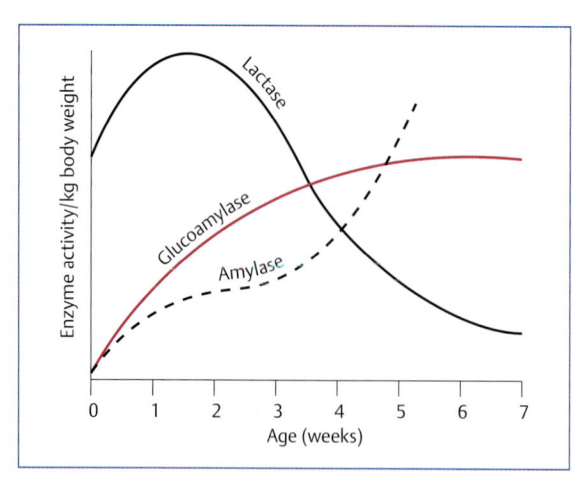

Fig. 16.53 Developmental change in the activity of some enzymes of carbohydrate digestion in piglets. During the infant phase, the luminal membrane of the small intestine has a high level of lactase activity, which ensures the breakdown of lactose. With the intake of solid feed with increasing age, lactase activity decreases, and the activities of amylase and disaccharidases (glucoamylase) increase. These age-dependent changes in carbohydrate-digesting enzymes are essentially genetically programmed and can only be slightly influenced by prolonged feeding of milk.

sharply at the age of 4–6 weeks and, with the exception of the horse, reaches adult levels at approx. 2–3 months of age (horse: approx. one year). These developmental changes in enzymes of carbohydrate digestion reflect the developmental changes in the mode of feeding. For example, piglets at the age of 2–5 weeks, when given the opportunity, will increasingly consume solid supplementary feed containing mainly starch (cereals) as a carbohydrate, in addition to lactose in their mother's milk. From the 3rd-5th week after birth, piglets are usually separated from the mother sow (weaning of piglets) and thenceforth fed a starch-rich diet.

■ Species differences

There are considerable species differences in carbohydrate digestion. Starch digestion in the small intestine is relatively limited in obligate carnivores such as the **cat**, but **not strongly limited** in the more omnivorous **dog**. The same applies to the **horse**, in which relatively **little amylase** reaches the small intestine in pancreatic juice. This can probably be explained from an evolutionary-biological point of view of horses being grass-eaters. Grass contains hardly any starch, so that during evolution there was probably no selection pressure for effective starch digestion.

Starch digestion in the small intestine in **pigs** and also in **chickens** is very **effective**. A special feature in **birds** is the **absence of lactase** in the brush border membrane of the small intestinal epithelium. Since in **ruminants** carbohydrates are mainly microbially degraded to short-chain fatty acids in the forestomach, a **low activity** of the enzymes of carbohydrate digestion (amylase, glucoamylase, α-dextrinase, saccharase) in the small intestine of ruminants is understandable. However, a considerable proportion of starch may not be microbially degraded in the rumen ("rumen-stable starch"), e.g., if maize starch is fed.

The same applies if large quantities of starch are fed. Starch is, however, subsequently digested relatively well in the small intestine (p.422) mediated by the induction of carbohydrate degrading enzymes.

If the digestive capacity for carbohydrates in the small intestine is exceeded, this is often, at least partially, compensated by increased microbial degradation of carbohydrates to short-chain fatty acids in the large intestine. Furthermore, the enzymes of carbohydrate digestion are able to adapt to a limited extent, within approximately three days, to a long-term increase in starch intake.

■ Carbohydrate digestion disorders

MORE DETAILS   It is not uncommon for humans and cats to develop **lactose intolerance** after infancy. This is because of genetically determined marked decline in lactase activity in the brush border membrane of the small intestine epithelium. The consumption of quantities of milk or lactose often leads to **diarrhoea** as the lactose that is not digested in the small intestine is only partially broken down microbially in the large intestine. Furthermore, the microbial degradation of lactose produces acetic acid, propionic acid and butyric acid as well as a relatively large amount of lactic acid, with limited absorption in the large intestine and leads to osmotic diarrhoea (p.445).

In the quite frequent occurrence of intestinal epithelial damage by viruses, carbohydrate digestion is impaired along with other digestive processes from the diminished activity of membrane enzymes (lactase, saccharase, glucoamylase, α-dextrinase), with consequent diarrhoea.

> **IN A NUTSHELL**   !
>
> The complete digestion of starch cleaves it into glucose units. Oligomers (maltose, maltotriose, α-dextrins) are formed by amylase in the intestinal lumen, which are broken down into absorbable glucose units by brush membrane disaccharidases.

■ Absorption of monosaccharides

The monosaccharides produced in the small intestine by the digestion of starch, lactose and sucrose (glucose, galactose, fructose) are absorbed into epithelial cells through the brush border membrane (BBM) and leave through the basolateral (antiluminal) membrane (BLM). They then enter capillaries and travel via the portal vein first to the liver and then partly to the caudal vena cava. To a small extent, glucose and fructose are metabolised during absorption in the epithelium of the small intestine to lactate, which also appears in the portal blood.

Transport of glucose through the brush border membrane (BBM)

The uptake of glucose and galactose by the BBM into the epithelial cell is by carrier-mediated **Na+ cotransport** (secondary active transport) against a concentration gradient.

MORE DETAILS   The expression of the Na+-dependent glucose carrier in the small intestine is induced, among other things, by the presence of glucose in the small intestine. This was shown in ruminants where only a low activity of this transporter is present when feed rich in crude fibre is being consumed. However, if starch or glucose enters the small intestine in larger quantities, such as with rations rich in concentrated feed, there is increased expression of this transport mechanism.

The glucose carrier (SGLT 1) has two binding sites for Na^+ and one binding site for glucose. The attachment of Na^+ to its binding sites is a prerequisite for the binding of glucose to the carrier (**Fig. 16.54**). Na^+ thus increases the **affinity** of the **carrier** for glucose and simultaneously energises the transmembrane transport of glucose due to the **electrochemical Na^+ gradient** across the BBM (**Fig. 16.54**). To maintain a low Na^+ concentration in the epithelial cell ($15\,mmol \cdot l^{-1}$), Na^+ is then actively pumped out across the basolateral membrane by the Na^+/K^+-ATPase. The K^+ thereby taken up into the cell recirculates through K^+ channels of the BLM. Opening of these channels is modulated by the activity of the Na^+/K^+-ATPase.

MORE DETAILS   In addition to glucose and galactose, some non-metabolizable monosaccharides, for example α-methyl-glucoside and 3–0-methylglucose, also have an affinity for the Na^+-glucose cotransporter of the brush border membrane. The pentose xylose also has a slight affinity for this cotransporter. The increase and time course of xylose concentration in blood after oral xylose administration are used as a clinical test to assess absorption disorders in the small intestine.

The Na^+-dependent uptake of glucose across the brush border membrane into epithelial cells is a saturable process, i.e. as glucose concentration increases, the glucose uptake rate gradually levels off and finally reaches a **maximum value** (V_{max}). The glucose concentration at which the glucose transport rate reaches the half-maximum value corresponds to the K_m value (**Michaelis constant)** of the Na^+-glucose cotransporter. The K_m value is inversely proportional to the affinity ($1/K_m$) of glucose for the glucose carrier. The K_m value for glucose is approx. $0.3\,mmol \cdot l^{-1}$ and is thus relatively low (high-affinity carrier). There is some dispute as to whether there is also in the small intestine a low-affinity glucose carrier (higher K_m value) with one binding site for Na^+, analogous to that in the proximal renal tubule (p.323), in addition to the high-affinity glucose carrier with two binding sites for Na^+.

MORE DETAILS   It has been found that at high glucose concentrations in the small intestine (e.g. after a starch-rich meal) Na^+-independent glucose carriers (GLUT2) are also transiently incorporated into the brush border membrane, so that glucose can be absorbed down a concentration gradient from the intestinal lumen into blood. However, the physiological significance of this mechanism is still controversial.

Transport of glucose through the basolateral membrane (BLM)

Discharge of glucose, accumulated in epithelial cells of the small intestinal villi through the BLM into the interstitium (villous stroma), is "downhill" through a **Na^+-independent glucose carrier** (**facilitated diffusion**; Fig. 16.54). This is also a saturable process (K_m for glucose: $20\,mmol \cdot l^{-1}$). The glucose carrier of the BLM (GLUT2) has an affinity for glucose, galactose and fructose and is thus also capable of ex-

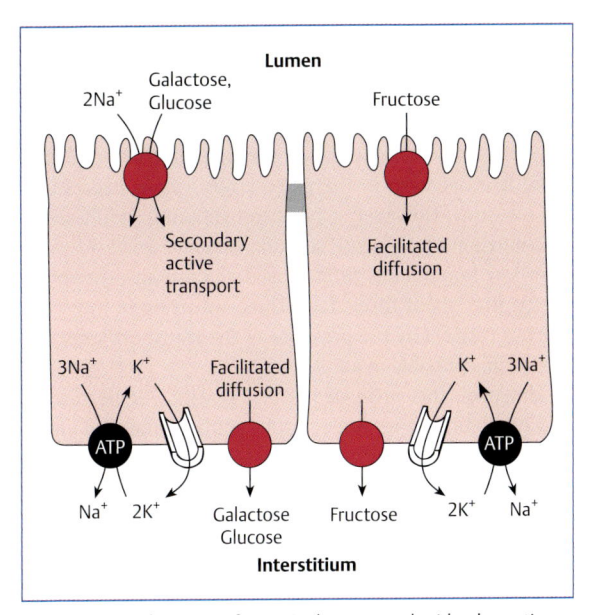

Fig. 16.54 Mechanisms of intestinal monosaccharide absorption. Glucose, galactose and fructose are mainly absorbed transcellularly. The uptake of glucose and galactose across the brush border membrane is by a Na^+ cotransporter (SGLT 1). Fructose is absorbed by facilitated diffusion (GLUT5) into the epithelium. Glucose, galactose and fructose are then transported into blood by facilitated diffusion (GLUT2) through the basolateral membrane of epithelial cells.

pelling the latter two monosaccharides from the epithelial cell.

However, GLUT2 functions in both directions, so that when there is no glucose to be absorbed from the intestinal lumen (e.g. in feed deprivation, and also in the large intestine), glucose is taken up from blood by the glucose carrier of the BLM to supply energy to the intestinal epithelium.

Fructose absorption

Fructose is taken up from the small intestinal lumen by a different carrier (GLUT5) by downhill **facilitated diffusion** into the epithelial cells of the intestinal villi and then passes by the glucose carrier of the BLM (GLUT2) into the interstitium (**Fig. 16.54**). Fructose absorption is thus a **passive process**.

Regulation of monosaccharide absorption

Analogous to adaptation of the enzymes of carbohydrate digestion, the mechanisms of intestinal monosaccharide absorption can also adapt to carbohydrate-rich diets. With such diets, the transport rate for glucose and fructose through the BBM and BLM increases within about three days. Furthermore, glucose transport via the BLM can be activated within 30 minutes by an increase in the blood glucose concentration.

The very **low** intestinal **glucose absorption capacity** of **adult ruminants**. In adult ruminants, carbohydrates in feed have already been degraded to short-chain fatty acids by microbial activity in the forestomach (p.398). In **dairy calves** and **lambs**, on the other hand, which ingest a considerable amount of lactose in their milk, which is broken down into glucose and galactose in the small intestine, **monosaccharides** are **effectively** absorbed. Obviously, during the development of the forestomach, which in cattle is physiologically completed at the age of three months, there is a decrease in the glucose absorption capacity of the intestine. However. it has been shown in adult sheep that infusion of a glucose solution into the small intestine for a few hours leads to increased glucose absorption capacity after about three days. Thus, induction of intestinal glucose carriers by the presence of the transport substrate also seems possible in adult ruminants.

However, this principle, which is valid for herbivores and omnivores, does not seem to apply to obligate carnivores such as the cat, since the transport capacity of the Na$^+$-glucose cotransport of the brush border membrane is relatively high in cats despite the physiologically low digestible carbohydrate intake in food.

Monosaccharide absorption disorders

MORE DETAILS   When the epithelium of the villi of the small intestine is damaged, by viruses or bacteria, monosaccharide absorption as well as the absorption of other nutrients is impaired. This is still the case even after the epithelial defects have been repaired by rapid "replenishment" of newly formed epithelial cells from the crypts, as these are often functionally not yet mature cells. Only the upper half of the small intestinal villi has fully mature epithelial cells capable of all absorptive functions. When larger epithelial defects are repaired, the entire villus of the small intestine may still be temporarily covered by immature epithelial cells (crypt cells), and the villi are often shortened and thickened (**villous atrophy**).

> **IN A NUTSHELL**   !
>
> While glucose and galactose are transported "uphill" through the brush border membrane into the small intestinal epithelial cells by Na$^+$ cotransport, fructose enters the cell from the intestinal lumen by facilitated diffusion. Exit through the BLM of the epithelial cell is also by facilitated diffusion.

16.6.5   Digestion and absorption of proteins

Protein digestion takes place mainly in the small intestine, but begins in the stomach. Absorbable end products of protein digestion are short-chain peptides (mainly di- and tripeptides) and amino acids. The end products are absorbed by the small intestinal epithelium mainly by tertiary (peptides) or secondary (amino acids) active transport systems. It is assumed that peptide absorption from the intestinal lumen is quantitatively more important than amino acid absorption.

■ Protein digestion

The **peptidases** of the **gastric** and **pancreatic secretions** and the and the enzymes located in the **BBM** of the **small intestinal epithelium** are summarised in Table 16.11. They are divided into endopeptidases, exopeptidases and peptidases with special functions according to their points of action.

Table 16.11 Peptidases involved in protein digestion in the gastrointestinal tract.

Enzymes	Function	Fission products
Endopeptidases		
Pepsin (stomach)[1]	Cleavage of peptide bonds with aromatic AA[4]	Peptides (AA)[6]
Trypsin (pancreas)[2]	Cleavage of peptide bonds with basic AA	Peptides (AA)
Chymotrypsin (pancreas)[2]	Cleavage of peptide bonds with aromatic AA incl. tryptophan	Peptides (AA)
Elastase (pancreas)[2]	Cleavage of peptide bonds with neutral AA without ring system	Peptides (AA)
Exopeptidases		
Carboxypeptidase A (pancreas)[2]	Cleavage of peptide bonds with C-terminal AA	AA, peptides
Carboxypeptidase B (pancreas)[2]	Cleavage of peptide bonds with C-terminal basic AA	AA, peptides
Carboxypeptidase (BBM)[3]	Cleavage of peptide bonds with C-terminal AA	AA, peptides
Aminopeptidase (BBM)	Cleavage of peptide bonds with N-terminal AA	AA, peptides
Other peptidases		
γ-Glutamyl transpeptidase (BBM)	Splitting off glutamic acid of the tripeptide glutathione[5]	AA, dipeptide
Dipeptidyl peptidase (BBM)	Cleavage of proline-containing dipeptides from peptides	Dipeptides, peptides
Dipeptidases (BBM)	Cleavage of certain dipeptides	AA

[1, 2] Secretion in the stomach or pancreas as inactive proenzymes
[3] BBM = Brush border membrane
[4] AA = amino acid(s)
[5] Glutathione consists of glutamic acid, glycine and cysteine and enters the small intestine via food and bile.
[6] Small amounts

Endopeptidases cleave peptide bonds by hydrolysis, in the mid-regions of proteins, while **exopeptidases** cleave terminal amino acids of protein molecules. Depending on whether a terminal amino acid (AA) with a free carboxyl group (C-terminal AA) or with a free amino group (N-terminal AA) is cleaved off by the exopeptidase in question, it is referred to as a **carboxypeptidase** or an **aminopeptidase**.

Endopeptidases are **pepsin**, secreted by the chief cells of the fundus glands of the stomach as pepsinogen, and also **trypsin, chymotrypsin** and **elastase**, which enter the duodenum in pancreatic juice as inactive proenzymes (trypsinogen, chymotrypsinogen, proelastase). The carboxypeptidases A and B also enter the duodenum in inactive form (procarboxypeptidase A and B) in pancreatic juice.

Activation of pancreatic peptidases, as already discussed in ch. Exocrine pancreas (p. 418), takes place in the small intestine by the BBM enzyme enteropeptidase (trypsinogen → trypsin) as well as by trypsin (trypsinogen → trypsin, chymotrypsinogen → chymotrypsin, proelastase → elastase), each by splitting off a peptide.

In addition to the above-mentioned peptidases of the stomach or pancreas, various BBM peptidases (aminopeptidase, carboxypeptidase, γ-glutamyltranspeptidase, dipeptidyl peptidase, dipeptidase) are involved in protein digestion. The functions of the individual peptidases are listed in **Table 16.11**. They generally have a more or less specific affinity for particular peptide bonds.

The digestion of food proteins **begins** in the **stomach**, where they are first denatured in the acidic environment (denaturation = loss of secondary and tertiary structure of the proteins). The acidic pH favours the proteolytic action of **pepsin** (**pH optimum: 1–3**) to produce peptides and AA. Pepsin not only attacks peptide bonds in the mid-regions of proteins, but can also, to a small extent, cleave off terminal AA. Since the pH of the intestinal contents in the duodenum proximal to the entry of the pancreatic duct is acidic, pepsin is still effective in the duodenum. In quantitative terms, however, pepsin does not seem to be very significant for overall protein digestion, since protein digestion is not significantly diminished by loss of pepsin production in the stomach (e.g. after removal of the stomach). Apparently, the endopeptidases of the pancreas are able to compensate for the loss of pepsin.

The endo- and exopeptidases that enter the small intestine in **pancreatic juice** as proenzymes hydrolyse, after activation, dietary proteins to oligopeptides (maximum seven amino acids) and individual AA. The peptidases of the BBM break down the oligopeptides to di- and tripeptides and AA, so that di- and tripeptides as well as AA are produced as **absorbable end products** of protein digestion in the small intestine. About twice as much AA are absorbed as di- and tripeptides than are absorbed as individual free AA.

In addition to dietary proteins, the digestive tract also digests **endogenous proteins**. These mainly enter the lumen of the small intestine in gastrointestinal secretions (mucins, enzymes) and as **epithelial cells** exfoliated from the tips of villi. The amount of endogenous protein entering the intestine per day is equal to the amount of food protein per day (15% protein based on dry matter)! Mucins and digestive enzymes are digested mainly in the ileum and large intestine by bacterial peptidases, while the rest of endogenous protein is digested in the small intestine.

> **IN A NUTSHELL** !
>
> Endopeptidases of the stomach and pancreas, exopeptidases of the pancreas and the brush border membrane (BBM) of the small intestine epithelium as well as other BBM peptidases are involved in protein digestion. The end products of protein digestion that can be absorbed are amino acids and di- and tripeptides.

■ Amino acid absorption

Neutral amino acids (e.g. alanine, serine, cysteine, leucine), acidic AA (glutamic acid, aspartic acid), basic AA (lysine, arginine, cystine), imino acids (proline) and β-AA (taurine, β-alanine) are taken up into the small intestinal epithelial cell by individual **Na^+ cotransport systems** located in the BBM. There is also a Na^+-independent carrier that exchanges basic AA for intracellularly accumulated neutral AA (**Fig. 16.55**). The imino acid, proline, as well as some short-chain AA (glycine, alanine) are taken across the BBM by an H^+ cotransport system, analogous to that for the absorption of di- and tripeptides. The molecular structure and arrangement in the BBM of the Na^+-dependent car-

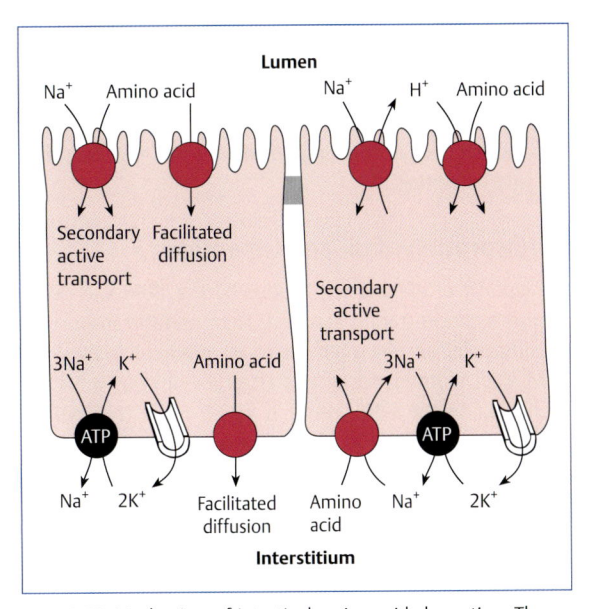

Fig. 16.55 Mechanism of intestinal amino acid absorption. The uptake of AA across the BBM is "uphill" by means of five Na^+-dependent and two H^+-dependent cotransport systems. For basic AA, there is an additional Na^+-independent system (facilitated diffusion). The exit through the BLM into the interstitium is "downhill" by facilitated diffusion, and several transporters are also involved here. In addition, Na^+-dependent transport systems for AA are also present in the BLM, which supply the epithelium with AA from blood. The uptake (BBM) or release (BLM) of basic AA against intracellularly accumulated neutral AA is not shown because of limited space.

Nutrition, energy

riers for AA resemble the Na^+-dependent glucose carrier of the BBM. The "uphill transport" of AA across the BBM is therefore energised by the transmembrane electrochemical Na^+ gradient (**secondary active transport**) so that AA accumulate in the cytoplasm of epithelial cells (**Fig. 16.55**). The Na^+ gradient is maintained, as for active glucose transport, by the Na^+/K^+ pump in the BLM. As for Na^+-glucose cotransport, the Na^+-dependent AA carriers in the BBM must first bind Na^+ before AA can attach to their binding sites. Na^+ thus increases substrate affinity of the BBM carriers. The Na^+-dependent AA carriers have either one Na^+ binding site (applies for carrier of neutral AA, iminoacid carrier, carrier of basic AA) or two Na^+ binding sites (applies for carrier for acidic or β-AA). If several AA have an affinity for a particular carrier, they compete for its AA binding site and therefore inhibit each other competitively during transport through the BBM.

The exit of AA from the epithelial cell through the BLM into the interstitium is "downhill" by carrier-mediated **facilitated diffusion** (**Fig. 16.55**). There are separate carriers for different AA groups (carriers for neutral, acidic or basic AA). Like the uptake across the BBM, basic AA are exchanged at the BLM for Na^+-dependent uptake of neutral AA from blood.

There are also additional Na^+-dependent AA carriers in the BLM through which the epithelial cells are supplied with AA for their own protein synthesis as well as to supply energy when no AA are being absorbed from the intestinal lumen. This applies particularly to crypt cells and to hindgut epithelium, since the BBM of those cells does not have any Na^+-dependent AA carriers. However, the BLM of epithelium of the small intestinal villi does have Na^+-dependent AA carriers. These cells are mainly dependent on the incorporation of the AA glutamine across the BLM, since **glutamine**, along with ketone bodies, are the most important **energy-providing substrates** for epithelium of the small intestine.

■ Absorption of di- and tripeptides

The uptake of di- and tripeptides by the BBM can occur against a concentration gradient. This "uphill transport" is energised by an electrochemical **H^+ gradient** across the BBM. The maintenance of this H^+ gradient is by a Na^+/H^+ exchanger in the BBM, through which H^+ is transported out of the cell against an electrochemical gradient and Na^+ enters the cell down an electrochemical gradient (**Fig. 16.56**). The Na^+ gradient energises the "uphill export" of protons, which acidify the surface of the BBM (acidic microclimate). Peptide transport through the BBM is thus indirectly dependent on Na^+. The molecular structure of the **H^+-peptide cotransporter** was recently elucidated.

MORE DETAILS The peptide carrier also transports some **antibiotics** which have a peptide bond (e.g. cephalosporins and penicillin). In the small intestinal epithelial cell, the di- and tripeptides taken up by the BBM are mainly hydrolysed by cytoplasmic di- and tripeptidases to free AA, which pass through the BLM by facilitated diffusion into the interstitium, see ch. Absorption of amino acids (p. 427). However, a peptide carrier is also present in

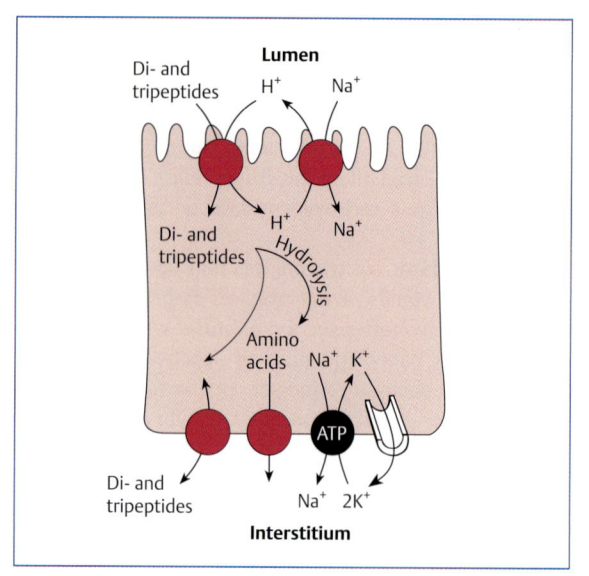

Fig. 16.56 Mechanism of intestinal di- and tripeptide absorption. The "uphill transport" of di- and tripeptides through the BBM is driven by an H^+ gradient into the cell, generated by a Na^+/H^+ exchanger in the BBM. After intracellular hydrolysis, the amino acids produced from di- and tripeptides leave the cell as free amino acids by specific transport systems in the BLM. To a small extent, intact di- and tripeptides can also be discharged by means of a peptide transporter in the BLM.

the BLM which, in contrast to the peptide carrier of the BBM, is not electrogenic. It functions in both directions, and di- and tripeptides can thus be discharged through this carrier to enter the portal blood.

■ Protein absorption in the new-born

New-borns can only produce small amounts of **immunoglobulins (antibodies)** against infectious agents as their immune system is not yet mature. They are therefore dependent on the immunoglobulins (p. 252) produced by the mother. Transfer of maternal immunoglobulins to the foetus in the uterus is across the placenta, and to the newborn in ingested colostrum (p. 604) (= milk with a high immunoglobulin content produced immediately before and after birth, **Fig. 25.3**). Species differences are listed in **Table 16.12**.

In early postnatal life, **intestinal absorption** of **immunoglobulins** as well as other proteins is by **endocytosis** (BBM) and **exocytosis** (BLM). Proteins are transported in vesicles from the BBM to the BLM, where several endocytosis vesicles fuse to form larger vesicles. During transcellular transport, vesicles can associate with lysosomes near the nucleus (phagolysosomes). When this happens, proteins in the vesicles are digested by lysosomal peptidases. In species like guinea pigs and rabbits, that are unable to absorb intact immunoglobulins postnatally, proteins taken up by endocytosis through the BBM into the small intestinal epithelial cells are completely digested in phagolysosomes.

Table 16.12 Transfer of immunoglobulins from mother to foetus or new-born.

Species	Transfer mode		Period of absorption of immunoglobulins
	Intrauterine	**With colostrum**	
Horse	–	+ + +	24 hours
Pig	–	+ + +	36 hours
Cattle, sheep, goat	–	+ + +	24 hours
Dog, Cat	+	+ +	1–2 days
Rat, Mouse	+	+ +	16–20 days
Human	+ + +	(+)	–
Guinea pig	+ + +	–	–
Rabbit	+ + +	–	–

+ slight, + + moderate, + + + intensive

After **exocytosis**, the immunoglobulins as well as other proteins are transported away mainly in lymphatic capillaries as they are too large to enter blood capillaries through the tightly linked endothelium.

> **MORE DETAILS** Some absorbed proteins (M < 70000 Da) are excreted in urine (proteinuria of new-borns). However, this does not apply to immunoglobulins with molecular weights above 150,000 Da.

A **trypsin inhibitor** in **colostrum** and the relatively low secretion of gastric acid and pepsinogen in new-borns ensures that digestion of immunoglobulins in colostrum is limited during the **first days of life**.

The mechanisms for the termination of intact protein absorption, one to two days after birth, (exception: rat; **Table 16.12**) are not definitively known.

> **IN A NUTSHELL** !
>
> Amino acids are taken up by several Na$^+$ cotransport systems in the BBM "uphill" against a concentration gradient into enterocytes. The amino acids exit these cells by facilitated diffusion at the BLM. The di- and tripeptides are absorbed by H$^+$ cotransport.

■ Digestion of nucleoproteins and nucleic acids

The nucleoproteins and free nucleic acids (ribonucleic acid = **RNA;** deoxyribonucleic acid = **DNA**) are digested in the gastrointestinal tract by peptidases of the stomach, pancreas and BBM into AA and oligopeptides (protein portion of the nucleoproteins). **Endonucleases in pancreatic juice** (ribonuclease, deoxyribonuclease), and **exonucleases, mononucleotidases, N-glycosidase** and **nucleoside phosphorylase** in the **BBM** digest nucleic acids to nucleosides, purine and pyrimidine bases, pentoses (ribose and deoxyribose) and ribose-1-phosphate (nucleic acids). Ribose-1-phosphate is digested by alkaline phosphatase of the BBM to ribose and phosphate.

The digestion of the nucleic acids is shown in **Fig. 16.57**.

Nucleic acid digestion is of particular importance in **ruminants** as large amounts of nucleic acid enters the small intestine from rumen microorganisms. This probably explains why many more nucleases are secreted by the pancreas in ruminants than in monogastrics.

■ Absorption of nucleic acid cleavage products

Purine- and pyrimidine bases (e.g. guanine, uracil) are taken up by a **Na$^+$-dependent carrier** in the BBM into the small intestinal epithelial cell. Purine bases are partly metabolised intracellularly (xanthine → uric acid). Pyrimidine bases appear to pass through the small intestinal epithelium largely unchanged. **Nucleosides** are also actively transported by **Na$^+$-dependent carriers** through the BBM into the epithelial cell where to a small extent they are substrates for local nucleic acid synthesis, but are mainly hydrolysed to pentoses and pyrimidine or purine bases.

> **IN A NUTSHELL** !
>
> Nucleic acids are degraded to nucleosides, purine and pyrimidine bases, pentoses and phosphate by the nucleases of the pancreas and enzymes in the BBM. The nucleosides and the purine and pyrimidine bases are absorbed by separate Na$^+$ cotransport systems in the BBM.

16.6.6 Digestion and absorption of fats

The most important dietary lipids are triacylglycerols, phospholipids (predominantly lecithin) and cholesterol (esters), but triacylglycerols are the main lipids in food.

■ Digestion of triacylglycerols

The digestion of triacylglycerols already begins in the stomach by **gastric** or **lingual lipase** (pH optimum: 3–7), which hydrolyse triacylglycerols to diacylglycerols, monoacylglycerols and fatty acids. In this process, mainly medium-chain and unsaturated long-chain terminal fatty acids are cleaved from triacylglycerols. The gastric and lingual lipases are still active in the duodenum due to the intraluminal acidic environment. However, intragastric lipolysis is only significant in the digestion of dietary fats in new-borns or during the first weeks of life. In older or adult animals, lipolysis takes place mainly in the small intestine.

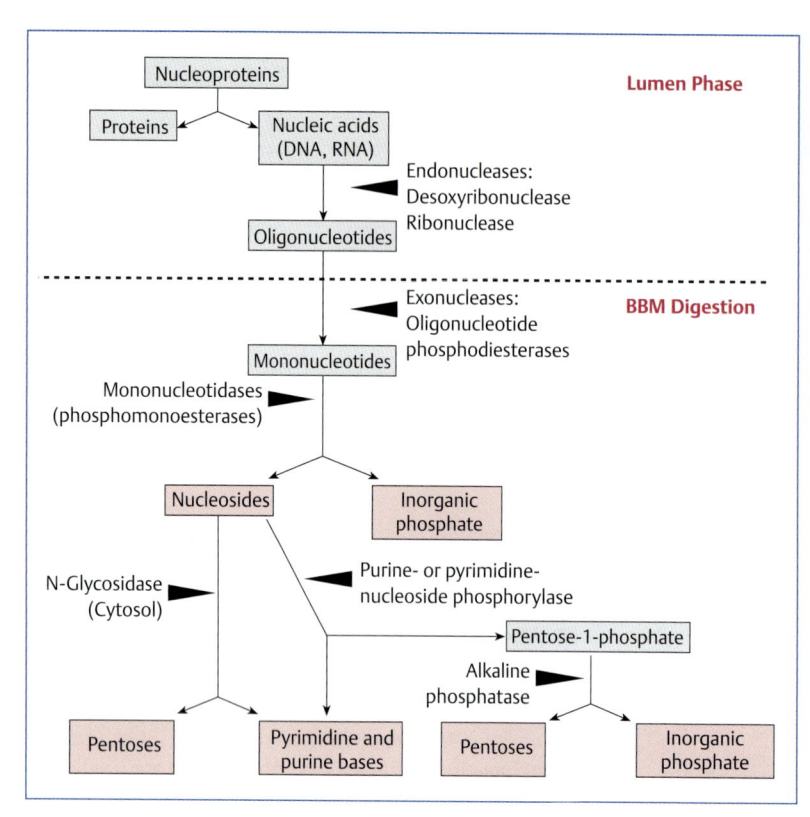

Fig. 16.57 Digestion of nucleic acids. In the small intestine, nucleic acids are first cleaved into oligonucleotides (lumen phase) by enzymes of the pancreas (endonucleases). Subsequently, enzymes of the BBM (exonucleases, mononucleotidases, N-glycosidases, alkaline phosphatase) further degrade the oligonucleotides into mononucleotides and mononucleosides, and then to pentoses, purine and pyrimidine bases, and inorganic phosphate. Both purine and pyrimidine bases as well as their nucleosides, pentoses and inorganic phosphate are absorbed across the BBM into the small intestine epithelial cells by specific individual mechanisms.

Distal to the entry of the pancreatic duct into the duodenum, triacylglycerol digestion is continued by **pancreatic lipase**, which hydrolyses di- and triacylglycerols to β-monoacylglycerols (with medium chain fatty acid) and individual fatty acids.

However, this process is dependent on the presence of **colipase** which enters the small intestine in pancreatic juice as **procolipase**. Procolipase is activated by **trypsin** which cleaves off a pentapeptide (= enterostatin) to produce active colipase. The activity of lipase requires **conjugated bile acids** in the intestinal lumen. Conjugated bile acids (tauro- and glycocholic acid as well as tauro- and glycochenodeoxycholic acid) are **detergents** and **emulsify** the water-insoluble triacylglycerols in the small intestinal lumen. The conjugated bile acids form a monomolecular layer on the surface of the triacylglycerol droplets, whereby the hydrophobic pole of the conjugated bile acids faces the triacylglycerols, and the hydrophilic pole faces the aqueous medium (**Fig. 16.58**). The greater the quantity of conjugated bile acids in the small intestinal lumen, the smaller the triacylglycerol droplets become and the larger their total surface area (many small spheres have a larger surface area than one large sphere with the same volume). **Lecithin** that enters the small intestine in bile (**phosphatidylcholine**) is also a detergent and therefore supports the emulsifying effect of the bile acids. The **increase in surface area** of triacylglycerol droplets caused by emulsification favours the action of lipase since lipase can act only on the surface of the lipid droplets (oil-water interface)

(**Fig. 16.58**). Colipase acts as a placeholder for lipase on the surface of the triacylglycerol droplets and prevents its inactivation by bile acids. Monoacylglycerols and fatty acids produced during the hydrolysis of triacylglycerols by lipase are also detergents and thus also support the emulsification of triacylglycerols.

Monoacylglycerols and **fatty acids** are **poorly soluble** in the aqueous milieu of the small intestinal lumen. Under these conditions, they form **mixed micelles** with conjugated bile acids as detergents. These molecular aggregates in which the hydrophobic part (e.g. hydrocarbon chain of the fatty acids) is directed centrally and the hydrophilic part (e.g. COOH group of the fatty acids) is directed outwards (**Fig. 16.58**). The mixed micelles in the small intestine have a diameter of approx. 3–5 nm, while emulsion globules have a diameter of 100–1000 nm.

Conjugated bile acids are thus important for the emulsification of triacylglycerols as well as the **solubilisation** of the **cleavage products** (micelle formation) of triacylglycerol digestion. Solubilisation is a prerequisite for the absorption of fatty acids and monoacylglycerols.

> **IN A NUTSHELL** !
>
> Triacylglycerols are digested in the stomach and small intestine by acid-stable gastric or lingual lipase and by pancreatic lipase. Free fatty acids and monoacylglycerols are the main absorbable cleavage products.

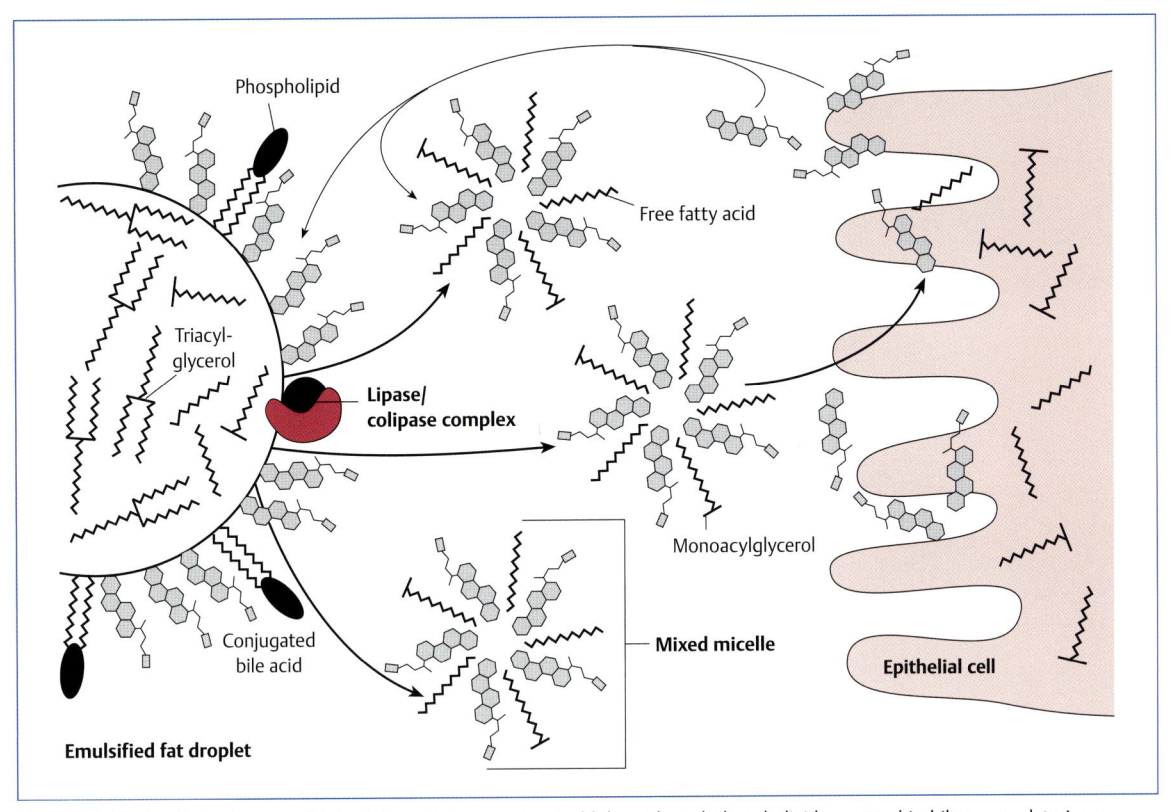

Fig. 16.58 Intraluminal digestion of triacylglycerols. The conjugated bile acids and phospholipids secreted in bile accumulate in a monomolecular layer around the fat droplets from the stomach causing emulsification. At the water-oil interface, the lipase/colipase complex cleaves triacylglycerols into free fatty acids and β-monoglycerols. These are integrated into mixed bile acid micelles and thus dissolved in the aqueous environment. The micelles disintegrate at the brush border membrane of the epithelium. The cleavage products of lipolysis are absorbed in the duodenum, while the bile acids remain in the small intestine lumen and are subsequently reabsorbed in the ileum.

■ Absorption of fatty acids and monoacylglycerols

Fatty acids and monoacylglycerols in the small intestinal lumen in micellar solution diffuse through the BBM of cells in the villous epithelium in the **proximal half of the small intestine** assisted by specific proteins (see below). With an **acidic microclimate** created by the Na^+/H^+ exchanger in the BBMs at the epithelial surface, fatty acids are **undissociated**. Diffusion through the BBM is therefore enhanced because of their higher **lipid solubility** compared to dissociated fatty acids. Although there is evidence for various BBM-related proteins (fatty acid translocase (FAT/CD 36), fatty acid transport protein (FATP4)) or cytosolic proteins (fatty acid binding proteins (FABP)), the exact functions of these proteins in intestinal lipid absorption, especially in farm and companion animals, are not yet fully understood. **Conjugated bile acids**, with low pK_a (pK_a of taurocholic acid: 2.5), are hardly present in the undissociated form. Consequently, their uptake into the epithelium of the jejunum by **diffusion** is **low**. They are only absorbed in the **ileum** by Na^+-dependent secondary active transport. This favours the emulsification and solubilisation function of conjugated bile acids in the jejunum. In the cytoplasm of the **small intestinal epithelium**, the monoacylglycerols and fatty acids taken up across the BBM are metabolised via two pathways to form **triacylglycerols** again: the α-glycer-

ol phosphate pathway and the **monoacylglycerol pathway** (**Fig. 16.59**).

MORE DETAILS The α-glycerol phosphate required for the α-glycerol phosphate pathway is mainly produced by reduction of dihydroxyacetone phosphate, a metabolite of glycolysis. To combine with α-glycerol phosphate or monoacylglycerols, the fatty acids must first be activated by linking with coenzyme A (CoASH) using the energy of ATP.

Triacylglycerols formed inside the enterocytes are coated by a phospholipid layer and by apolipoprotein molecules formed in the epithelial cells. Via a precursor (PCTV = Pre-Chylomicron Transport Vesicle), **chylomicrons** are formed in the endoplasmic reticulum (diameter: 50–400 nm; **Fig. 16.60**). FAT/CD 36, playing a role in the transport of fatty acids and cholesterol, is also involved in the formation of chylomicrons. In addition to triacylglycerols, the chylomicrons, which are categorised as triacylglycerol-rich lipoproteins, also contain fatty acid esters of cholesterol as well as fat-soluble vitamins and provitamins (vitamin A, carotenes, vitamin E, vitamin D, vitamin K) and other fat-soluble substances.

In the Golgi apparatus, several chylomicrons are enveloped by a membrane. In this form, the chylomicrons are transported via the cytoskeleton to the BLM, where they are discharged by **exocytosis** into the interstitium and then pass mainly into the **lymphatic capillaries**. Therefore,

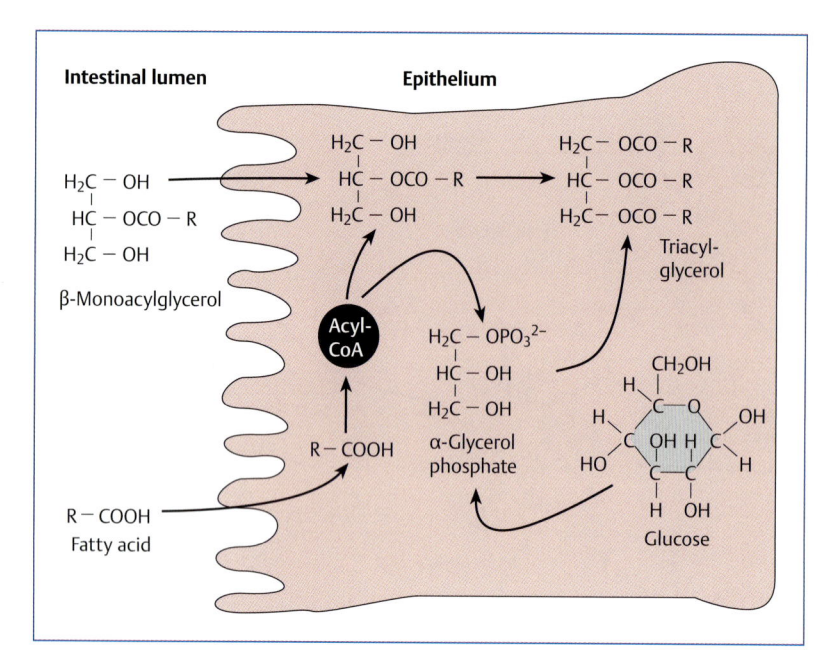

Fig. 16.59 Intracellular resynthesis of triacylglycerols in small intestinal epithelial cells. After the uptake of long-chain free fatty acids, they are activated to form acyl-CoA with subsequent esterification to triacylglycerols. The β-monoacylglycerol or α-glycerol phosphate required for this comes from the luminal lipolysis of triacylglycerols or from intracellular glycolysis.

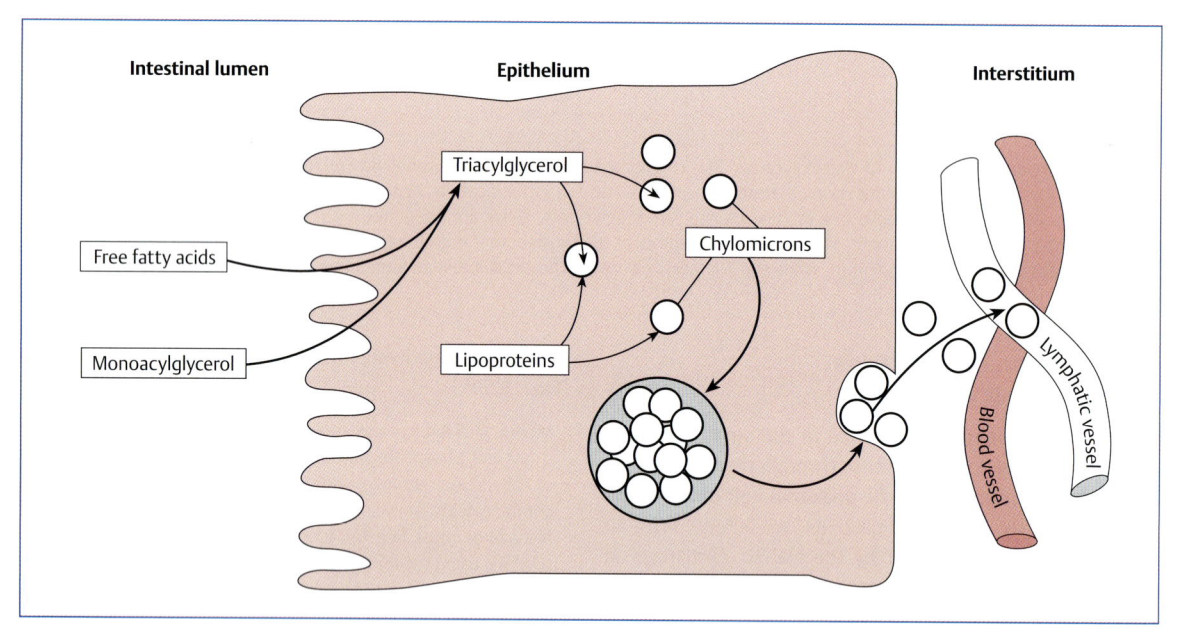

Fig. 16.60 Formation, transport and exocytosis of chylomicrons. Chylomicrons consist mainly of triacylglycerols and carry apolipoproteins on the outside. In the Golgi apparatus, several chylomicrons are enveloped by a common membrane. After release by exocytosis, the chylomicrons are transported in the lymphatic system.

only a few chylomicrons appear in the portal blood. During exocytosis, only the membrane surrounding the aggregate of chylomicrons fuses with the BLM (**Fig. 16.60**).

Short- and **medium-chain fatty acids** (up to twelve C atoms) are little incorporated into triacylglycerols in the epithelium of the small intestine. They leave the epithelial cell via the BLM and enter the blood capillaries and thus the portal blood.

■ Digestion and absorption of phospholipids

The most important dietary phospholipid is phosphatidyl-choline (lecithin). Considerable amounts of this phospholipid also enter the small intestine in bile.

Phosphatidylcholine is converted into lysophosphatide by **phospholipase A_2** by cleavage of the mid-position fatty acid. Phospholipase A_2 enters the small intestine in **pancreatic juice** as an inactive **proenzyme** and is activated by **trypsin**. Lysophosphatide enters the epithelial cell by diffusion and is reconverted to phosphatidylcholine by re-esterification with a fatty acid. Phosphatidylcholine is required in epithelial cells to form the lipoprotein shell of **chylomicrons** and thus enters the lymphatic capillaries with the chylomicrons and finally the vena cava.

Little is known about the digestion and absorption of other phospholipids ingested in food.

■ Cholesterol absorption

Cholesterol is mainly found in feedstuffs of animal origin. Cholesterol also enters the small intestine in bile. About 15% of cholesterol in food is esterified with fatty acids. Cholesterol ester is cleaved in the lumen of the small intestine by pancreatic cholesterol esterase. Cholesterol enters the epithelial cell by carrier-mediated **facilitated diffusion** and is incorporated into **chylomicrons** re-esterified with fatty acids. Both uptake from the intestinal lumen and incorporation into chylomicrons appear to involve FAT/CD 36. Cholesterol can be synthesised in the crypt cells. The main site of cholesterol synthesis, however, is the liver.

■ Bile acid reabsorption

As already briefly mentioned in section 16.6.3 (p. 421), bile acids conjugated with taurine or glycine are absorbed against an electrochemical gradient across the BBM of villous epithelial cells of the **ileum** by a **Na^+ cotransporter** specific for conjugated bile acids. Conjugated bile acids are discharged through the BLM via an anion exchanger into the interstitium in exchange for bicarbonate and are then transported to the liver via the portal blood. The bile acids are taken up by the liver cells and secreted back into the bile ducts. There is thus an enterohepatic circulation for **conjugated bile acids** (Fig. 16.61). In the jejunum, conjugated bile acids are absorbed to a limited extent by diffusion.

The **conjugated bile acids** pass through the **intestinal tract 5–10 times** per day. Only about 3–4% of conjugated bile acids that enter the small intestine in bile pass into the large intestine, where they are deconjugated by bacteria and absorbed in this form to a small extent by diffusion. In the liver, reconjugation with taurine or glycine then takes place. However, most of the bile acids that reach the large intestine and are deconjugated there are excreted in faeces. This loss is compensated for by hepatic synthesis of bile acids (p. 466) from cholesterol. The bile acids excreted in faeces can thus be regarded as the sole excretion products of cholesterol metabolism.

■ Disturbances in fat digestion and absorption

MORE DETAILS   With a high-fat diet, disorders of fat digestion or fat absorption manifest themselves as an increased output of fat in faeces, called **steatorrhoea**. This can develop from lipase deficiency in the quite common exocrine pancreas insufficiency in **dogs**. Steatorrhoea also results from impaired fat absorption in diarrhoea of **suckling piglets**, caused by virus-induced damage to the epithelium of the intestinal villi. This steatorrhoea, which often occurs even without diarrhoea, is promoted by the high fat content (7%) of sow's milk. Steatorrhoea is often characterised by clay-like faeces. Since the large intestine is not able to absorb the products of fat digestion, any lipid that passes into the large intestine because of disorders in fat digestion or absorption is almost completely excreted in faeces.

> **IN A NUTSHELL**   **!**
>
> Free fatty acids and monoacylglycerols enter epithelial cells in the jejunum by diffusion and with the participation of specific proteins, where they are re-esterified to triacylglycerols. Together with apolipoproteins, they form chylomicrons which, after exocytosis, pass into the lymph capillaries.

16.6.7 Absorption of minerals and trace elements

■ Absorption of Na^+ and Cl^-

The Na^+ and Cl^- ions from ingested food as well as from secretions into the digestive tract (saliva, gastric secretions, small intestinal secretions, pancreatic secretions, bile) are absorbed in the **small intestine** with an efficiency of about **60–70%**. Na^+ is mainly absorbed through the **Na^+ cotransport systems** for glucose (p. 424) and amino acids (p. 427) (Fig. 16.62). Through these and other (less quantitatively important) Na^+ cotransport systems, Na^+ passes down a concentration gradient through the BBM into the epithelial cells of the small intestinal villi and is pumped out by a Na^+/K^+ pump through the BLM into the interstitium (Fig. 16.62). As positive electrically charged Na^+ passes through the epithelium (**electrogenic Na^+ absorption**), a transepithelial electrical potential difference of approx. 5 mV builds up (serosal side of the epithelium positive). This **potential difference** induces the **diffusion** of Cl^- through the zonulae occludentes (tight junctions) into the intercellular spaces and the interstitium. The denser the zonulae occludentes, the greater the transepithelial potential difference caused by electrogenic Na^+ absorption. This explains why the transepithelial potential difference is greater in the ileum (denser zonulae occludentes!) than in the proximal jejunum.

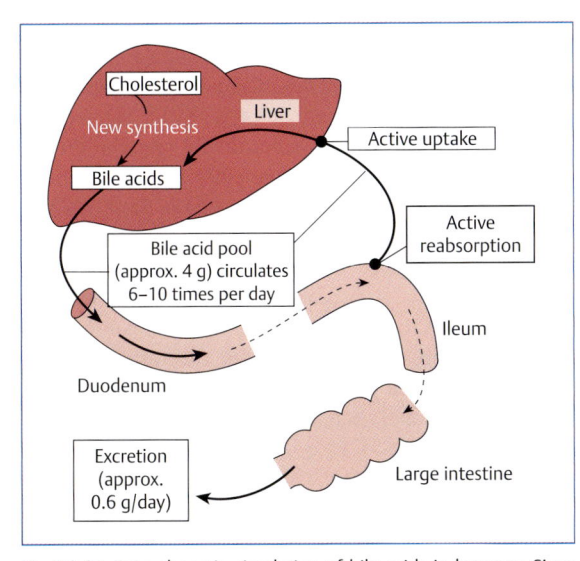

Fig. 16.61 Enterohepatic circulation of bile acids in humans. Since the bile acid pool of the liver is only about 4 g, bile acids have to recirculate several times a day during the digestion of dietary fats. Both absorption from the ileum and uptake from portal blood into liver cells are by secondary active transport. The unavoidable intestinal losses of bile acids during enterohepatic recirculation are compensated for by new synthesis from cholesterol.

Nutrition, energy

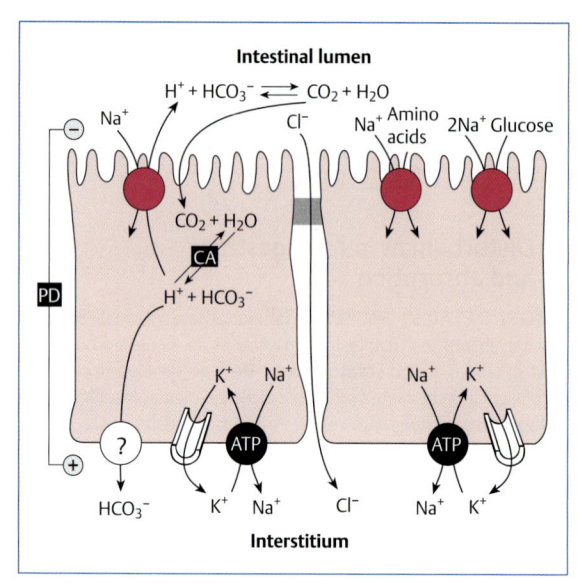

Fig. 16.62 Mechanisms of Na^+, Cl^- and HCO_3^- absorption in the small intestine. Na^+ is transported through the BBM by secondary active transport systems (e.g. glucose and amino acid transporters) and by a Na^+/H^+ exchanger. At the BLM, Na^+ is transported into the interstitium by a Na^+/K^+ pump. The partial electrogenic transport of Na^+ (e.g. Na^+-glucose cotransport, Na^+/K^+ pump) establishes a transepithelial electrical potential (PD) difference that drives Cl^- paracellular uptake from the intestinal lumen into the interstitium. H^+ secreted into the lumen via the Na^+/H^+ exchanger can react at the epithelial surface with HCO_3^- to form CO_2, which is converted intracellularly by carbonic anhydrase (CA) again into HCO_3^-. HCO_3^- then enters the interstitium through the BLM by a mechanism that is not yet precisely known.

In addition to electrogenic Na^+ absorption, there is **electroneutral Na^+ absorption** in the jejunum by a **Na^+/H^+ exchanger** in the BBM. The H^+ exported across the BBM by the exchanger reacts in the intestinal lumen partly with HCO_3^- to form H_2CO_3. Carbonic acid is cleaved to CO_2 and H_2O. The CO_2 enters the epithelial cell by diffusion and is again converted into carbonic acid by carbonic anhydrase. After dissociation of carbonic acid into protons and bicarbonate, the HCO_3^- leaves the epithelial cell "downhill" through the BLM, while H^+ is discharged again through the Na^+/H^+ exchanger of the BBM. Na^+ is pumped into the interstitium by the Na^+/K^+ pump of the BLM. The Na^+/H^+ exchanger of the BBM thus mediates, among other things, the absorption of $NaHCO_3$ (**Fig. 16.62**).

In the distal jejunum and ileum, in addition to the Na^+/H^+ exchanger, there is a **Cl^-/HCO_3^- exchanger**, so that NaCl is absorbed transcellularly in these intestinal segments. The exit of Cl^- through the BLM takes place through Cl^- channels, while Na^+ is transported out of the epithelial cell by the Na^+/K^+ pump of the BLM.

The extensive **absorption of water** in the small intestine (in pigs about ten litres per day; **Fig. 16.63**) is coupled osmotically to the absorption of **electrolytes** (especially Na^+ and Cl^-), although there is generally no osmotic gradient between the contents of the small intestine and the portal blood. Rather, trans- and paracellular water absorption appears to be driven by a **local osmotic gradient** existing between the intercellular space and the small intes-

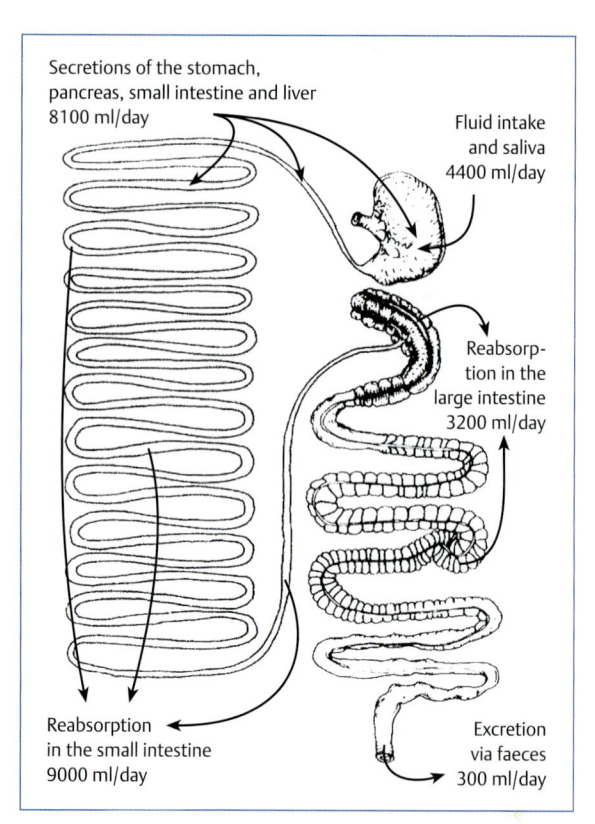

Fig. 16.63 Water balance in the gastrointestinal tract of the pig.

tinal lumen. Particularly, from the absorption of Na^+ and Cl^- (incl. HCO_3^-, glucose, amino acids, etc.), there is a local **increase in osmolarity** in the **intercellular space**, which induces water uptake from the intestinal lumen into the intercellular space (**Fig. 16.64**), from where it passes into the villous stroma down a hydrostatic pressure gradient and then enters the capillaries.

Since the zonulae occludentes are partially permeable to electrolytes, paracellular water absorption enhances Na^+ and Cl^- absorption. This phenomenon is called convection or **solvent drag** (entrainment of solutes by the water flow). Solvent drag reduces the amount of ATP required for Na^+ absorption in the small intestine since only transcellular Na^+ absorption is directly dependent on the Na^+/K^+-ATPase of the BLM and thus on the requirement for ATP. In addition to the described paracellular downstream flow of water, some water is absorbed transcellularly. Na^+ cotransport systems of the BBM (e.g. glucose carriers) also transport water into cells together with the respective substrate, as well as a possible role of aquaporins (proteins functioning as water channels) in the BBM and BLM.

■ Absorption of K^+

K^+, which enters the small intestine from food and digestive tract secretions, is mainly absorbed in the small intestine. Because of the high permeability of K^+ through the zonulae occludentes, paracellular absorption occurs mainly through **solvent drag**.

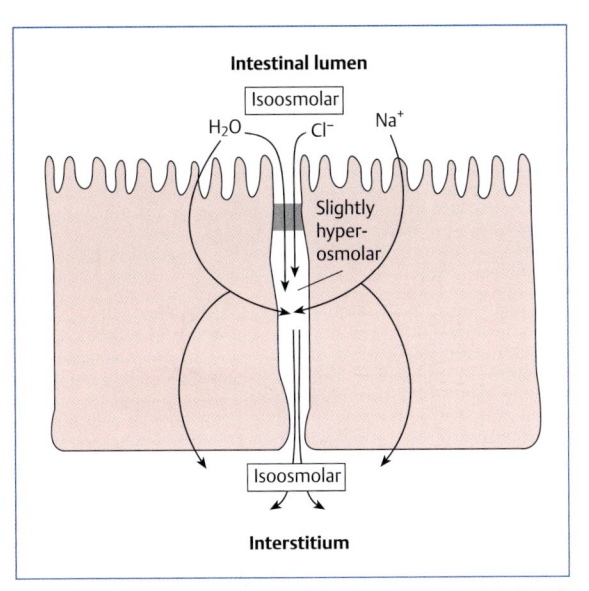

Fig. 16.64 Water absorption in the small intestine. Particularly with absorption of Na^+ and Cl^-, there is a slight increase in osmolarity (local osmotic gradient) in the intercellular space which allows para- and transcellular flow of water from the intestinal lumen. The transfer of fluid into the interstitium and blood capillaries occurs down a hydrostatic gradient.

> **IN A NUTSHELL** !
>
> In the small intestine, 60–70% of the Na^+, Cl^- and water from food and gastrointestinal secretions are absorbed. While Na^+ is partly absorbed by active transcellular transport, the absorption of Cl^-, K^+ and Mg^{2+} in the small intestine is by a passive paracellular pathway.

■ Ca^{2+} absorption

Ca^{2+} is absorbed in the **duodenum** and **proximal jejunum** by **active transport**. In the distal jejunum and ileum, Ca^{2+} is even secreted paracellularly into the intestinal lumen, with the transepithelial potential difference (serosa side positive) acting as the driving force. The acidic environment in the duodenum favours the ionisation of Ca^{2+} salts and thus the absorption of Ca^{2+}. Food ingredients that reduce the solubility of Ca^{2+} by forming insoluble Ca^{2+} salts impair Ca^{2+} absorption. These include, among others, **oxalic acid** (e.g. contained in beet leaves) and **phytic acid** (phosphate ester of the hexavalent alcohol inositol), which occurs mainly in cereals.

The mechanism of active and secondary active Ca^{2+} absorption is shown in **Fig. 16.65**. Ca^{2+} enters the **cytoplasm** down a steep electrochemical gradient through **Ca^{2+} channels** of the **BBM** as the concentration of free Ca^{2+} in the cytoplasm of the villous epithelium is very low (< 1 $\mu mol \cdot l^{-1}$). In the cytoplasm, Ca^{2+} is largely reversibly bound to a **Ca^{2+}-binding protein (calbindin)** and is transported in this form to the BLM, through which Ca^{2+} is exported from the cell by a **Ca^{2+} pump (= Ca^{2+}-ATPase)** and a **Na^+/Ca^{2+} exchanger** driven by the transmembrane Na^+ gradient (stoichiometry: 3 Na^+ : 1 Ca^{2+}).

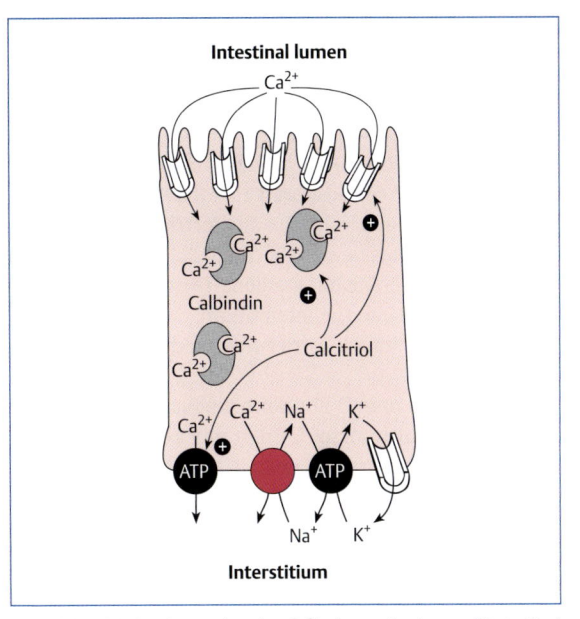

Fig. 16.65 Mechanisms of active Ca^{2+} absorption in small intestinal epithelial cells. The active, transcellular absorption of Ca^{2+} is regulated by calcitriol and includes influx through Ca^{2+} channels in the BBM, intracellular buffering by binding to calbindin as well as the "uphill transport" across the BLM by a Ca^{2+}-ATPase and a Na^+/Ca^{2+} exchanger.

The efficiency of active Ca^{2+} absorption depends on the Ca^{2+} and phosphate supply in food as well as on the Ca^{2+} requirement, which is higher during growth, lactation, and egg laying (chicken). In these cases, the production of **1,25-$(OH)_2$ D_3 (vitamin D hormone = calcitriol)** in the kidney (p. 328) is increased. This hormone promotes the incorporation of Ca^{2+} channels into the BBM as well as the incorporation of Ca^{2+} pumps into the BLM. It also stimulates the formation of calbindin. In this way, Ca^{2+} absorption is increased (**Fig. 16.65**).

> **IN A NUTSHELL** !
>
> When there is a dietary Ca^{2+} deficiency or an increased demand for Ca^{2+}, active calcitriol-dependent absorption of Ca^{2+} takes place in the duodenum.

■ Mg^{2+} absorption

In contrast to **ruminants**, where Mg^{2+} absorption (p. 406) is mainly in the **forestomach** (Fig. 16.39), Mg^{2+} is absorbed in the **small and large intestine in monogastric animals**. In the proximal small intestine, most Mg^{2+} is absorbed by paracellular solvent drag. In the distal small intestine, as well as in the colon, Mg^{2+} can be absorbed transcellularly by active transport mechanisms. However, details of the mechanism have not been clarified. In most domestic animal monogastric species (exception: horse), the net absorption of Mg^{2+} in the small intestine seems to be quantitatively of minor importance. Absorption in the large intestine seems to be more important.

■ Phosphate absorption

Inorganic phosphate is absorbed transcellularly by active transport in the small intestine, especially in the jejunum. In this process, dihydrogen phosphate and hydrogen phosphate ($H_2PO_4^-$ and HPO_4^{2-}) are absorbed into the villous epithelium by **Na⁺ cotransport** across the BBM. The driving force for this transport against an electrical gradient (the inside of the BBM is negatively charged!) is thus provided by the transmembrane Na⁺ gradient. The exit of phosphate through the BLM into the interstitium, on the other hand, seems to occur through carrier-mediated facilitated diffusion.

The active vitamin D hormone produced in the kidney, $1,25\text{-}(OH)_2D_3$ (calcitriol (p. 322)), stimulates phosphate absorption by incorporating more Na⁺-phosphate cotransporters into the BBM. The increased phosphate absorption in **monogastrics** in calcium and phosphorus deficiency is in response to increased production of $1,25\text{-}(OH)_2D_3$. In **ruminants**, calcium deficiency has a similar effect, whereas phosphorus deficiency does not increase Na⁺-dependent phosphate absorption in the jejunum by increased production of $1,25\text{-}(OH)_2D_3$ because phosphorus deficiency in ruminants does not cause increased formation of $1,25\text{-}(OH)_2D_3$.

The absorption of phosphorus from **phytic acid** (cereals!) and its salts (both fractions together = phytin) requires the release of phosphate by bacterial phytase or by phytase from plant feeds. In ruminants, the phosphate of phytin is almost completely released by rumen bacterial phytase and is absorbed in the small intestine. In monogastric animals, phytin-P is only partially available for absorption (approx. 50% from wheat, barley and rye, and approx. 20% from maize and oats). The utilisation of phytin-P can be improved by adding phytase to the feed.

IN A NUTSHELL   !

The absorption of phosphate (HPO_4^{2-}, $H_2PO_4^-$) takes place through Na⁺ cotransport.

■ Absorption of trace elements

Iron absorption

In food, **iron** is mainly in the trivalent form. The low pH of the stomach and duodenal contents favours the **dissolution of iron salts and complexes** and thus the absorption of iron in the duodenum. Since **only Fe²⁺ is actively absorbed**, the reduction of Fe³⁺ to Fe²⁺ is necessary. Vitamin C, cysteine (mainly from protein digestion) and the cysteine-containing tripeptide glutathione, which enters the small intestine in bile, favour this reduction.

An enzymatic **reduction** of iron occurs at the BBM where **duodenal cytochrome B** (**DcytB**) acts as a membrane-bound **iron reductase**. Fe²⁺ then enters the epithelial cell together with H⁺ "downhill" via a BBM **transporter for divalent cations** (**DMT1**). Intracellular Fe²⁺, which is protein-bound (binding proteins not yet identified in detail), forms the so-called **labile iron pool** (Fig. 16.66). During **carrier-mediated extrusion** from the epithelial cell at

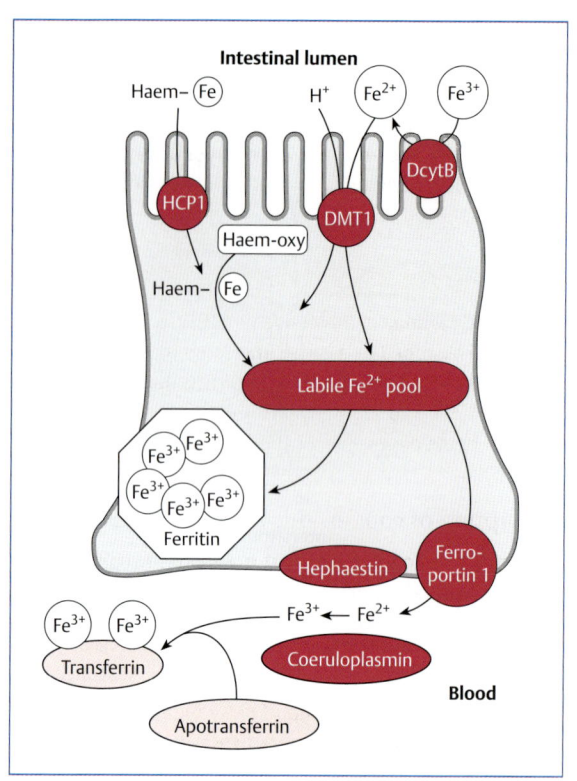

Fig. 16.66 Model of intestinal iron absorption. Fe³⁺ from food is reduced to Fe²⁺ by the BBM ferroxidase DcytB (duodenal cytochrome B) and transported through the BBM by the divalent cation transporter DMT1. Intact haem is taken up across the BBM by a haem carrier protein (HCP1) and degraded intracellularly by haem oxygenase (haem oxy) to release Fe²⁺. From the cytosolic Fe²⁺ pool (= labile Fe²⁺ pool), Fe²⁺ is transported through the BLM by ferroportin 1. Fe³⁺ is generated by hephaestin (present in the BLM) or by coeruloplasmin in blood. Fe³⁺ circulates in blood as transferrin after binding to apotransferrin. Depending on the iron status of an animal, a variable amount of cytosolic iron remains in the enterocytes as Fe³⁺ bound to ferritin.

the basolateral membrane by **ferroportin 1**, Fe²⁺ is oxidised to Fe³⁺ by **hephaestin**, a membrane-bound **Cu-containing ferroxidase** and by the Cu-containing ferroxidase **coeruloplasmin**, which circulates in blood. In the circulation, Fe³⁺ is bound to the plasma protein **transferrin** (Fig. 16.66). From the oxidation of Fe²⁺ to Fe³⁺ during or immediately after extrusion across the BLM, a concentration gradient is maintained for the egress of Fe²⁺. Also, during the transfer through the epithelial cell, Fe²⁺ can be partially oxidised to Fe³⁺ and in this form can be bound to the protein **apoferritin** to form **ferritin** (Fig. 16.66). The iron bound as ferritin then re-enters the intestinal lumen when the epithelial cells are shed at the tips of the villi (life span: 2–3 days) and is almost completely excreted in faeces. In the **regulation of intestinal iron absorption**, depending on the iron status of an animal, the peptide hormone **hepcidin**, produced in the liver, plays a central role. An increase in hepcidin leads to decreased iron absorption because of a lower density of ferroportin 1 in the BLM. In iron deficiency the efficiency of iron absorption increases considerably with increased expression of ferroportin 1, DMT1 and a decrease in the ferritin content of the enterocytes. Normally, only about 10% of the dietary inorganic iron is absorbed. However, iron in the form of **haem** (**myoglobin, haemoglobin**) is much better absorbed across the BBM by a **haem carrier protein (HCP1**, also involved in the transport of folate). The enzyme **haem oxygenase** then releases Fe^{2+} from the haem and it enters the labile iron pool of the enterocytes (**Fig. 16.66**).

> **IN A NUTSHELL** !
>
> During absorption in the duodenum, Fe^{3+} is reduced to Fe^{2+} and absorbed by a carrier-mediated mechanism across the BBM. During carrier-mediated output across the BLM, Fe^{2+} is oxidised by ferroxidases to Fe^{3+} and bound to the plasma protein transferrin.

Absorption of copper, zinc and manganese

Absorption of **copper**, **zinc** and **manganese** mainly occurs in the **proximal small intestine**. The absorption mechanisms are similar to the mechanism of iron absorption ("downhill transport" through the BBM into epithelial cells, partial binding to cytoplasmic storage and transport proteins, export through the BLM by means of an energy-dependent, saturable transport process). The cytoplasmic storage protein is **metallothionein**, a small cysteine-rich protein with a particular affinity for zinc and copper, and little affinity for manganese. The inhibitory effect of a high dietary zinc intake on copper absorption seems to be from the induction of metallothionein in the small intestinal epithelial cells. Metallothionein binds more copper as well as zinc and thus reduces the export of copper across the BLM. Zinc and manganese absorption is inhibited by excess calcium, so that a competition of these cations for common transport mechanisms can be assumed.

Usually, about 20% of copper ingested in feed is absorbed. For zinc and manganese, the respective values are about 50% and less than 5%. When the intake is low or when the demand for these trace elements increases, such as during growth, the efficiency of absorption increases.

> **IN A NUTSHELL** !
>
> The absorption mechanisms for copper, zinc and manganese correspond to those for Fe^{2+}.

Absorption of iodine, selenium, and molybdenum

About 90% of i**odide** (I^-) secreted in saliva and gastric juice is absorbed in the small intestine. Iodide uses the absorption mechanisms for chloride, especially the Cl^-/HCO_3^- exchanger of the BBM and the anion channel of the BLM. Furthermore, the zonulae occludentes are partially permeable to iodide, so that the transepithelial potential difference (blood side positive) as well as water absorption (solvent drag!) both contribute to iodide absorption.

Selenium (Se) is absorbed in the small intestine as effectively as iodine. Se is mainly absorbed as **selenomethionine** in food proteins in place of the sulphur-containing

amino acid, methionine. To a much lesser extent, Se is also present in food protein as selenocysteine. Selenocysteine is only found in the active centre of selenium-containing enzymes. The absorption of both selenium-containing amino acids, in which the sulphur of methionine and cysteine is replaced by selenium, takes place by the Na^+-dependent absorption mechanism for neutral amino acids (amino acid absorption (p. 427)). Particularly in selenium deficient areas, selenium is added to the feed as inorganic selenite (SeO_3^{2-}) or selenate (SeO_4^{2-}) or as organic selenomethionine in selenium-enriched yeast. **Selenite** is reduced to selenide (SeH^-) in the small intestine by cysteine and glutathione and is effectively absorbed in this form, while **selenate** is absorbed in the distal small intestine, like sulphate, by Na^+ cotransport. Sulphate and selenate compete for the same transport mechanism. In ruminants, selenium absorption is only about half as effective as in monogastric animals (absorption of about 40% of the selenium ingested in the feed). Because of the reductive environment of the forestomach system, partially water-insoluble elemental selenium is formed from various selenium compounds. Elemental selenium is hardly absorbed.

Molybdate (MoO_4^{2-}), the most important molybdenum compound in feed, is also very effectively absorbed. The efflux of the anions SO_4^{2-}, SeO_4^{2-}, MoO_4^{2-} through the BLM probably occurs passively, with the membrane potential (outside positive) favouring the transfer of anions from the epithelial cell into the interstitium.

> **IN A NUTSHELL** !
>
> While both inorganic and organic sources of selenium are effectively absorbed in monogastric species (70–90%), the efficiency of selenium absorption in ruminants is only about 40% due to the reduction of selenium to insoluble compounds by microbial activity in the rumen.

16.6.8 Microbial activity in the small intestine

Like all segments of the gastrointestinal tract, the small intestine is also colonised by microorganisms that are predominantly anaerobic with some facultative aerobic bacteria. Generally, the **number of bacteria** in the intestinal contents increases from proximal to distal. However, rapid transit of chyme in the duodenum and jejunum prevents bacterial proliferation. Consequently, the number of microorganisms in the duodenum and jejunum is relatively low compared to the large intestine, at about $10^6 \cdot 10^7$ bacteria per gram of intestinal content. In contrast, up to 10^9 bacteria per gram of content can be found in the ileum. The denser microbial colonisation in the **ileum** is also reflected in the concentrations of **short-chain fatty acids** (approx. $8–10\,mmol \cdot l^{-1}$, in horses and pigs up to about $50\,mmol \cdot l^{-1}$) and lactic acid (up to $20\,mmol \cdot l^{-1}$) as fermentation products. However, microbial activity in the small intestine generally has no role in nutrient digestion.

Suggested reading

Barrett KE, Donowitz M,eds. Gastrointestinal Transport: Molecular Physiology. San Diego: Academic Press; 2001

Chang EB, Sitrin MD, Block DD. Gastrointestinal, Hepatobiliary and Nutritional Physiology. Philadelphia: Lippincott-Raven; 1996

Guilford WG, Center SA, Strombeck DR et al. Strombeck's Small Animal Gastroenterology. 3rd ed. Philadelphia: W. B. Saunders; 1996

Johnson LR, ed. Physiology of the Gastrointestinal Tract. Vol 1. and 2. 5th ed. London: Elsevier Academic Press; 2012

O'Dell BL, Sunde RA, eds. Handbook of Nutritionally Essential Mineral Elements. New York: Marcel Dekker; 1997

16.7   Large intestine

Gerhard Breves

ESSENTIALS   ✕

- Despite considerable species differences in the anatomy of the large intestine, this part of the digestive tract fulfils a number of functions that apply to all animal species.
- Important functions are microbial degradation of organic matter, microbial synthesis of certain compounds and absorption of short-chain fatty acids as end products of microbial metabolism.
- The epithelial transport of short-chain fatty acids, electrolytes and water is a physiologically important transport function of the hindgut epithelium.
- The large intestine also serves for chyme storage and regulation of faecal quantity and composition.
- With these functions, the large intestine can be regarded as a part of the digestive system with complex influences on overall metabolism, which are primarily mediated by microbial metabolic activities.
- Diarrhoea can be caused by changes in secretory functions of the large intestine epithelium.

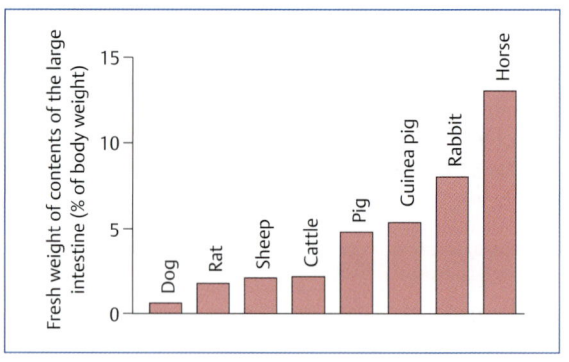

Fig. 16.67 Fresh weight of contents of the large intestine as a% of body weight in different species. [Source: von Engelhardt W, Rechkemmer G. The physiological effects of short-chain fatty acids in the hindgut. In: Wallace G, Bell L (eds.). Fibre in Human and Animal Nutrition. Wellington: Royal Society of New Zealand, Bulletin 20; 1983: 149–155]

16.7.1   Volume and digesta passage

Due to considerable animal species differences in the macroscopic anatomy of the large intestine, there are many differences between species in the volume of this organ as well as the transport rate and thus the residence time of the digesta. In humans and carnivores, the **wet weight** of the contents of the **large intestine** is only about 1% of body weight. In rats and ruminants, the wet weight values are about 2% of body weight. The content of the large intestine is even greater in pigs (5% of body weight), rabbits (8%) and horses (13%) **Fig. 16.67**. These are average values. In horses in particular, this proportion can be significantly higher, depending on the body mass and the diet.

There are considerable differences in the daily **passage rate of digesta** into the large intestine between individuals of the same species and between species. The passage rate in pigs is between 4 and $61 \cdot d^{-1}$, in small ruminants between 2 and $8.5 l \cdot d^{-1}$, in ponies about $20 l \cdot d^{-1}$. The large variation within a species is mainly determined by the type and amount of feed consumed. Large intestine motility (p. 392) also influences the passage rate. The average residence time of contents in the large intestine is considerably longer than in the small intestine which favours microbial colonisation. Anatomically, the haustra contribute to the long residence time and mixing of contents of the large intestine. Haustra are differently developed in the caecum and colon in different species.

16.7.2   Microbial metabolism

The gastrointestinal tract of mammals is colonised by microorganisms immediately after birth. These include bacteria, protozoa and fungi. Besides the forestomach system of ruminants, the large intestine of all domestic mammals is the main site of **microbial colonisation**. The bacterial density in the large intestine can be even higher than in the forestomachs, with values between 10^{10} and 10^{12} colony-forming units per g of large intestine content. As in the forestomachs (p. 395), microbial diversity in the contents of the large intestine is extraordinarily high. The most common bacteria include various species of the genera *Bacteroides, Fusobacterium, Streptococcus, Eubacterium, Ruminococcus, Lactobacillus* and *Treponema* as well as coliform bacteria such as *Escherichia coli*. Like the forestomachs, there are three main sites in the large intestine where the **bacterial population** is distributed: the **liquid phase**, the **digestive particles** and the **region near the wall**. To maintain large intestinal flora and its metabolic functions, the following conditions are required:

1. neutralisation of acidic end products of microbial metabolism,
2. adequate residence time of digesta in the large intestine,
3. dilution of metabolic waste products in the liquid phase of the large intestine contents,
4. absorption of end products of microbial metabolism.

As in the forestomach system, the **buffer systems** in large intestine are mainly HCO_3^- and $H_2PO_4^-/HPO_4^{2-}$. The HCO_3^- buffer comes mainly from secretions in different parts of the intestinal tract, while phosphate is mainly of dietary origin. In **pigs** and **horses**, HCO_3^- is the main buffer system, while in **carnivores** the phosphate buffer system predominates. The pH of the large intestinal contents is slightly acidic, ranging between 6 and 7. In contrast to microorganisms in the forestomachs, which mainly use ingested feed components as metabolic substrates, the microorganisms in the large intestine have a complex mixture of available substrates from two different sources. Most **substrates** reach the large intestine in the liquid phase from the terminal ileum and are those food components that have **not** been **digested** or have only been **partly digested** in the proximal stomach and small intestine. The other substrate supply for microbial metabolism is of **endogenous origin** as secretions or exfoliated epithelia of the intestinal tract.

IN A NUTSHELL !

Microbial metabolism in the large intestine is by a microbial population similar to that in the forestomachs of ruminants.

■ Microbial carbohydrate metabolism

Carbohydrate fermentation, under **anaerobic conditions**, is an important source of carbon and energy for microflora of the large intestine and at the same time is a limiting factor for maintenance and growth of the flora. Carbohydrate fermentation also provides energy for the host animal from the production of short-chain fatty acids, see ch. Microbial metabolic processes in the forestomachs and absorption of the end products (p. 398). Carbohydrates that are microbially degradable in the large intestine consist mainly of cell wall components of plant origin that cannot be degraded by the body's own enzymes. These include all polysaccharides with β-glycosidic bonds such as **cellulose** and **non-cellulose polysaccharides** such as **hemicelluloses**, **pectin**, **inulin** and also **guar**, a polysaccharide consisting of D-galactose and D-mannose. Low-molecular carbohydrates such as mono-, di- or trisaccharides and polysac-

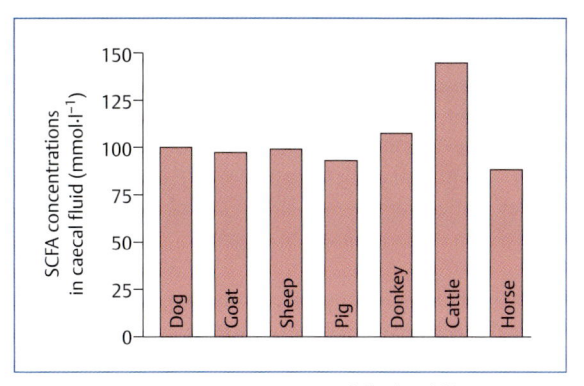

Fig. 16.68 SCFA concentrations in caecal fluid in different species. SCFA = short-chain fatty acids. [Source: von Engelhardt W, Rechkemmer G. The physiological effects of short-chain fatty acids in the hindgut. In: Wallace G, Bell L (eds.). Fibre in Human and Animal Nutrition. Wellington: Royal Society of New Zealand, Bulletin 20; 1983: 149–155]

charides with an α-glycosidic bond such as starch can also reach the large intestine when the capacity of the carbohydrate digesting enzymes in the small intestine is exceeded. The **glycoprotein mucin** from the epithelium and carbohydrates from exfoliated cells are microbially fermentable endogenous substrates.

There are many **similarities** in carbohydrate fermentation between the **large intestine** and the **forestomachs**. Short-chain fatty acids (SCFA) acetate, propionate and butyrate are the most important end products of anaerobic carbohydrate fermentation in the large intestine (**Fig. 16.32, Fig. 16.33**). At the pH of the lumen contents of the large intestine and with pK_a of approx. 4.8, the SCFA are about 99% dissociated and only about 1% are undissociated acids. In all domestic mammals, SCFA are quantitatively the most important anions in the large intestine contents, their concentrations being about $100\,mmol \cdot l^{-1}$ in caecal or colonic fluid with molecular proportions of about 65% acetate, 25% propionate and 10% butyrate. The fermentation pattern can be modified to a limited extent by changing the feed composition. For example, when feeding starchy rations, the acetate-propionate ratio in the large intestine can be reduced. Both the **SCFA concentrations** and the molar ratios are of a similar order of magnitude as in the forestomach fluid (**Table 16.9, Fig. 16.68**). Carbohydrate fermentation also produces small amounts of formate, valerate and lactate. From the degradation of various amino acids (valine, leucine, isoleucine) the branched-chain fatty acids isobutyrate, isovalerate and 2-methylbutyrate are formed. During microbial carbohydrate fermentation, CO_2 and H_2 are also produced as **fermentation gases**. H_2 in the large intestine contents is kept low by H_2 oxidising microorganisms. However, methane production as a percentage of fermented organic matter is significantly lower in the large intestine than that in the forestomachs. Reductive **acetogenesis** has been identified as an additional metabolism specific to the large intestine, a process not yet demonstrated for the forestomachs. Reductive acetogenesis is the following reaction:

$$4H_2 + 2HCO_3^- + 2H^+ \rightarrow CH_3COO^- + H^+ + 4H_2O \qquad (16.3)$$

The formation of **acetate** from **H₂** instead of methane not only reduces methane output, but also improves the yield of useful fermentation metabolites, by increasing the supply of acetate for the host animal.

Sulphate- and nitrate-reducing microorganisms are further H_2 -consuming microorganisms, the quantitative significance of which depends on the availability of sulphate or nitrate in the large intestine contents.

■ Microbial metabolism of proteins and N-containing compounds

Although the mechanisms of protein metabolism in the large intestine have been less extensively studied than the corresponding processes in the forestomachs (p. 402), similar metabolic pathways are assumed. N-turnover in the large intestine results from the action of different microbial enzymes such as proteases, deaminases, decarboxylases and ureases. Keto acids, amines, CO_2 and the common end product ammonia, are products of protein degradation. **Ammonia** is also the most important nitrogen source for the synthesis of microbial amino acids and thus for **microbial protein synthesis** in the large intestine. The ammonia pool in the large intestine is mainly determined by the intake of food N components. It can also be influenced from urea secretion in the small and large intestine, with subsequent urea cleavage by urease. The main **limitation** for protein synthesis by microorganisms in the large intestine is **energy supply**. Thus, raw fibre intake is of central importance for microbial growth. With sufficient energy supply, the efficiency of microbial growth in the large intestine is similar to that in the forestomachs. With absorption of ammonia and secretion of urea by the hindgut epithelium, the large intestine is part of the nitrogenous enterohepatic circulation (Fig. 16.36).

> **MORE DETAILS** In recent years, the ability of microorganisms to synthesise potentially toxic substances has gained particular interest in human medicine related to various diseases of the large intestine. These include a range of enzyme activities, and also the synthesis of nitrosamines from secondary amines by nitrate-reducing bacteria.

■ Microbial metabolism of fats, steroids, and bile acids

Only small amounts of dietary fats and long-chain fatty acids reach the large intestine, as they are mainly digested in the proximal small intestine. Nevertheless, fats can be substrates for microbial lipases and long-chain fatty acids can be transformed by cis-trans isomerisation and subsequent hydrogenation or hydration. Since no significant fat absorption takes place in the large intestine, any remaining fats and long-chain fatty acids are excreted in faeces.

> **MORE DETAILS** Natural and synthetic steroids conjugated with sulphate or glucuronate can be excreted into the small intestine with bile. In the large intestine, the steroids are deconjugated by microbial sulphatases and glucuronidases and metabolised by redox reactions, hydroxylations, dehydroxylations and dehydrogenations.

The quantitatively most important **primary bile acids**, cholic acid and chenodeoxycholic acid, can be **microbially deconjugated** in the large intestine, dehydroxylated to form secondary bile acids, oxidised or aromatised. **Faecal colour** is mainly determined by the degradation products of **bile pigments** and by **dietary components**.

Because of the high ileal absorption capacity for bile acids, the amount reaching the large intestine is normally low. Secretion of bile acids is stimulated by high-fat diets, and this can lead to more bile acids passing into the large intestine if the ileal absorption capacity is exceeded.

■ Microbial vitamin synthesis

Large intestine microorganisms can synthesise vitamins of the **B group** and **vitamin K** as in the forestomachs. The rate of synthesis of these vitamins is related to the extent of microbial growth and thus on the availability of energy and nitrogen in the large intestine. Due to the **low absorption capacity** of the large intestine epithelium for vitamins, the utilisation of these metabolic products is only important in animals with caecotrophy (p. 442).

> **IN A NUTSHELL** !
> The biochemistry of microbial hindgut metabolism is very similar to that in the forestomach of ruminants.

16.7.3 Absorption and secretion

The large intestine has an important function in **absorbing water** and **electrolytes** as well as **SCFA**. With a few exceptions, there is **no absorption of carbohydrates** or **amino acids** in the large intestine. Water from food must be absorbed and also that from secretions of the gastrointestinal tract, the volume of which is several times greater than that of ingested water. For example, in addition to about 2 l of water ingested daily with food, humans must also reabsorb about 7 l of fluid per day from gastrointestinal secretions. Most of this **fluid (70–90%)** is absorbed in the **small intestine**, the remaining **10–30%** in the **large intestine**. Water absorption is driven by active Na⁺ transport, which creates an osmotic gradient (Fig. 16.69). Depending on the functional state of the large intestine, however, the mucosa of the large intestine is also able to actively secrete electrolytes into the intestinal lumen, which are then followed osmotically by water. It was assumed that absorption and secretion take place in different cells, with secretion restricted to young, proliferating cells in the depths of the crypts, and absorption only by differentiated epithelial cells. However, more recent studies have shown that some cells in the large intestinal mucosa can both secrete and absorb.

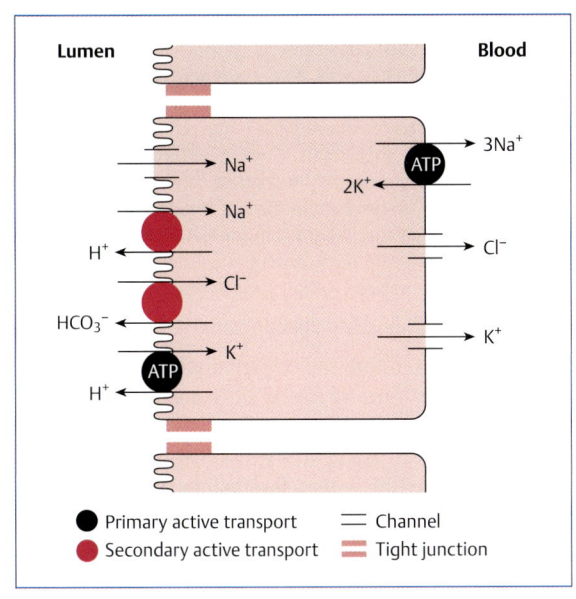

Fig. 16.69 Possible mechanisms of absorption of Na⁺, Cl⁻ and K⁺ in colonic epithelial cells.

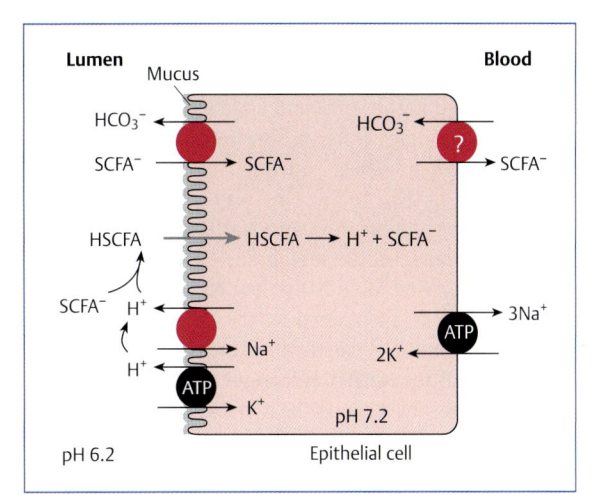

Fig. 16.70 Cellular mechanisms of short-chain fatty acid (SCFA) absorption in the large intestine.

Absorption of organic ions

Microbial fermentation in the large intestine is similar to fermentation by the complex microbial diversity in the forestomachs of ruminants. It ensures that structural carbohydrates such as **cellulose** or hemicelluloses, which cannot be broken down by the body's own enzymes, are converted into **short-chain fatty acids**. Depending on the species, a large proportion of nutritional energy supply can be obtained from the oxidation of short-chain fatty acids produced in the large intestine. Thus, depending on the type of feed, about 15–30% of energy comes from large intestine SCFA in pigs, about 30% in horses, 30–40% in rabbits, 6–9% in humans and about 7% in dogs.

> **IN A NUTSHELL** !
>
> The production and absorption of SCFA in the large intestine makes a contribution to energy metabolism that varies with species.

Short-chain fatty acids can be absorbed very well by the intestinal epithelium (**Fig. 16.70**). They are weak acids and are therefore about 99% dissociated, i.e. ionic in the neutral to slightly acidic pH of hindgut contents. Acetate, propionate and butyrate anions are therefore substrates to be taken up by the epithelial cells. There are two different uptake mechanisms for short-chain fatty acids in the large intestine. Because short-chain fatty acids are relatively lipophilic, i.e. fat-soluble compounds, they easily penetrate the cell membrane, provided they are **not dissociated**, i.e. provided they do not carry a charge. The conversion of short-chain fatty acids into their non-dissociated, uncharged form is facilitated by an acidic compartment, the so-called **acidic microclimate** on the surface of the **brush border**

membrane. Epithelial cells of the large intestine actively secrete protons via the Na⁺/H⁺ exchanger which accumulate in the mucus layer on the brush border membrane. In the immediate vicinity of the membrane, the accumulation of protons facilitates the conversion of fatty acid anions to **non-dissociated, lipophilic fatty acids** which can then **pass through** the cell membrane relatively **freely**. The intracellular pH is more alkaline than the acidic microclimate which causes the absorbed short-chain fatty acids to dissociate inside the cell. The concentration gradient of the free acid from the microclimate into the cell is thus maintained, and the short-chain fatty acids can continue to flow into the cell.

In addition to this diffusion, facilitated by the pH in close proximity to the membrane, cells of the large intestine have also developed special transport mechanisms for the uptake of short-chain fatty acids. Thus, an **anion exchanger** was detected in the brush border membrane, which transports **short-chain fatty acids** into the cell in exchange for HCO₃⁻. Short-chain fatty acids are then released into blood across the basolateral membrane by as yet unknown mechanisms. In some species, an anion exchanger is also responsible for this. The quantitative significance of these exchangers for the absorption of short-chain fatty acids is still unclear, although it is estimated that they account for up to 50% of total SCFA transport. Short-chain fatty acids are also the most important substrates for supplying energy to the hindgut epithelium. They are thus also an important **trophic factor** for the **mucosa** and they stimulate Na⁺ absorption.

> **IN A NUTSHELL** !
>
> While the function of the large intestine was previously only regarded to be electrolyte and water absorption, the caecum and upper colon in particular are now known to have essential microbial digestive processes.

■ Absorption of inorganic ions

Sodium is quantitatively the most important ion to be actively absorbed in the small and large intestine. Na^+ transport also determines **water absorption**. There are a number of different transport pathways for Na^+, especially in the distal colon (**Fig. 16.69**). One way to absorb Na^+ is to exchange it for protons through a **Na^+/H^+ exchanger** in the apical membrane, i.e. the membrane facing the intestinal lumen. The driving force is the low Na^+ concentration in the cell, which is maintained by the Na^+/K^+ pump in the basolateral membrane, i.e. the membrane facing the interstitial tissue. If the **Na^+/H^+ exchanger** were to act alone in the membrane, there would be a net loss of protons from the cytoplasm. With the loss of protons, the cytosol would become more alkaline. To avoid alkalinisation, the **Na^+/H^+ exchanger** is usually associated with a Cl^-/HCO_3^- exchanger which maintains a constant cytoplasmic pH. The second mechanism for transcellular absorption of Na^+ in the large intestine is through **Na^+ channels** in the **apical membrane**. This is **electrogenic Na^+ transport**, as there is a net charge transport of positively charged ions from the lumen through the epithelium to the blood. The sodium channels in the large intestine correspond to those in the collecting tube of the renal nephron (ENaC; **Fig. 12.11**) and can be controlled in the same way by aldosterone. When there is a **Na^+ deficiency**, the adrenal cortex secretes more **aldosterone**, which stimulates the incorporation of Na^+ channels into the brush border membrane and thus promotes increased Na^+ absorption in the distal colon. This is probably achieved by both incorporating preformed Na^+ channels from membrane vesicles and de novo synthesis of Na^+ channels. Plasma aldosterone concentration is strongly dependent on the Na^+ content of the diet and it partly shows a **circadian rhythm**. Lagomorphs and rodents excrete two different types of faeces. During the day, **hard**, low water content, bean-shaped **faeces** are produced, while at night a higher water content, **soft faeces** are produced, which are ingested as **caecotrophs** by caecotrophic animals. These faecal phases correlate with diurnal fluctuations in plasma aldosterone concentration. In the hard faeces phase, aldosterone concentration is high, and in the soft faeces phase it is low. The reason for the different water content in faeces is the change in Na^+ transport by aldosterone. Aldosterone causes an increased opening of existing channels and the installation of additional Na^+ channels in the brush border membrane. These can very efficiently take up Na^+ from the lumen, along with a considerable amount of water which then results in hard faeces. If, in contrast, the number of Na^+ channels or the proportion of opened Na^+ channels is low, more fluid remains in the large intestine lumen and the faeces are soft.

> **IN A NUTSHELL** !
>
> Aldosterone-dependent Na^+ absorption via Na^+ channels is an important regulatory function of the hindgut epithelium.

MORE DETAILS The proportion of Na^+ channels and the Na^+/H^+ exchangers in Na^+ absorption shows clear species differences and also regional differences along the length of the large intestine. In **humans**, **pigs** and **rabbits**, Na^+ absorption in the distal colon is through Na^+ channels, while in the proximal colon it is by means of Na^+/H^+ exchangers. Sodium absorption via Na^+/H^+ exchangers is electroneutral, in contrast to absorption through Na^+ channels. In species such as the **rat**, when aldosterone levels are low, exchange mechanisms absorb Na^+ in the distal colon. When plasma aldosterone concentration rises, the exchange mechanisms are replaced by Na^+ channels resulting in an increase in Na^+ absorption.

The Na^+ ions taken into the cell are discharged **basolaterally** to the interstitium by the Na^+/K^+ pump in exchange for K^+. This process transports Na^+ and K^+ ions against their respective chemical gradients, with energy provided by cleavage of ATP. This is therefore mainly an active transport process. Entry of Na^+ from the hindgut lumen into the cell interior is down a concentration gradient since Na^+ concentration in the cytoplasm is kept low by the activity of the Na^+/K^+ pump. This is why the Na^+/H^+ exchanger is referred to as secondary active transport. When Na^+ flows into the cytosol via Na^+ channels, the membrane potential, i.e. the negative charge on the inside of the membrane, is an additional driving force for uptake of Na^+ ions from the intestinal lumen. Because of its higher driving force and faster rate of transport, absorption of Na^+ through Na^+ channels is considerably greater than absorption by Na^+/H^+ exchangers.

Cl^- is also actively absorbed in the large intestine (**Fig. 16.69**). Active, transcellular **Cl^- absorption** is mediated by a **Cl^-/HCO_3^- exchanger** in the **apical** membrane. This works in close association with the Na^+/H^+ exchanger in the apical membrane. It is also a secondary active transport process as the active step is the Na^+/K^+ pump. Because of the Na^+ gradient generated by the pump, the Na^+/H^+ exchanger transports protons out of the cell. This increases the cytoplasmic pH which is the driving force for Cl^- uptake into the cell in exchange for HCO_3^-. From HCO_3^- secretion, intracellular pH returns to normal. The Cl^- ions leave the cell basolaterally via mechanisms that have so far not been well characterised. In tissues where Na^+ is primarily absorbed via Na^+ channels, Cl^- ions follow passively through the tight junctions and the intercellular space to maintain electroneutrality.

In contrast to the small intestine, where K^+ only passes passively through the mucosa via the intercellular space, the large intestine has transcellular mechanisms for **K^+ transport** (**Fig. 16.69**, **Fig. 16.71**). A **K^+/H^+ pump** in the apical membrane has a major role in active **K^+ absorption** in the large intestine. This pump transports K^+ ions into the cell interior against its concentration gradient, using energy from ATP, and in return it removes protons. A **similar transport mechanism** in the **gastric mucosa is** involved in the secretion of hydrochloric acid. The absorbed K^+ ions leave the cell via basolateral K^+ channels.

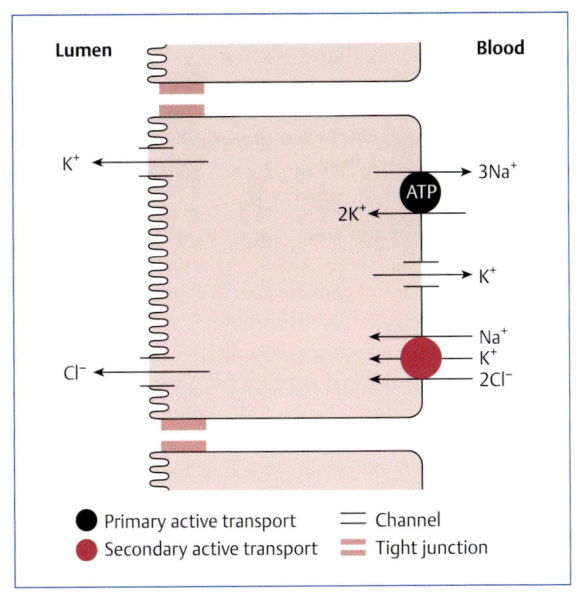

Fig. 16.71 Mechanisms of secretion of K^+ and Cl^- in colonic epithelial cells.

■ Secretion of inorganic ions

The quantitatively most significant ion to be actively secreted by the hindgut mucosa is Cl^-. **Cl^- secretion** is under neural control initiated by stretching of the intestinal wall. However, it also is important under pathophysiological conditions, such as when **bacterial toxins** or **inflammatory mediators** cause an unphysiologically strong activation of secretion and thus lead to diarrhoea (p. 447). The energy for Cl^- secretion is ultimately from the activity of the Na^+/K^+ pump in the basolateral cell membrane (**Fig. 16.71**). This actively transports three Na^+ ions out of the cell, with an ATP cleavage, in exchange for two K^+ ions. As a result, there is considerable accumulation of K^+ in the cell compared to the extracellular fluid. Since the cells simultaneously have K^+ channels in the basolateral membrane, a K^+ diffusion potential builds up. The membrane potential of such crypt cells, in the range of -70 mV to -50 mV (cell interior negative), is mainly determined by the K^+ conductivity. In addition, the crypt cells possess a Na^+-K^+-$2Cl^-$ cotransporter in the basolateral membrane. This transports Na^+, K^+ and Cl^- together into the cell in a ratio of 1:1:2. The driving force for the entry of Cl^- is the Na^+ gradient, which is maintained by the activity of the Na^+/K^+ pump. Thus, there is a secondary active transport mechanism that accumulates Cl^- beyond its electrochemical equilibrium in the crypt cell. **Cl^- channels** are located in the apical membrane. When more of these channels open, and/or more Cl^- channels are incorporated into the membrane, Cl^- ions flow down the electrochemical gradient out of the cell into the crypt lumen. Thus Cl^- is secreted. The **main driving force** for the outflow of Cl^- ions is the **membrane potential**. Na^+ ions passively follow through the intercellular space to maintain electroneutrality, and the osmotic changes caused by the secreted NaCl causes water also to follow.

In the large intestine (as well as in the duodenum and ileum) there is also **HCO_3^- secretion**. Bicarbonate is re-

leased into the intestinal lumen via the **Cl^-/HCO_3^-** and **SCFA/HCO_3^- exchangers** (**Fig. 16.69**). Bicarbonate is formed from metabolically produced CO_2, which is converted to carbonic acid by intracellular carbonic anhydrase. The carbonic acid then rapidly dissociates to H^+ and HCO_3^- which are then exported out of the cell by the Na^+/H^+ exchanger or the Cl^-/HCO_3^- and SCFA/HCO_3^- exchanger.

Potassium ions are not only actively absorbed by the hindgut epithelium (**Fig. 16.69**), but they are also **actively secreted** (**Fig. 16.71**). The direction of **K^+ transport** in the large intestine depends on the state of potassium balance. Under normal conditions, there is usually a net secretion of K^+. To achieve this, K^+ ions are taken up basolaterally by the epithelial cell Na^+/K^+ pump or by the Na^+-K^+-Cl^- cotransporter. Their release from the cell into the intestinal lumen then takes place through K^+ channels in the apical membrane.

■ Water transport

There is no active transport system for water in the whole animal. Water can only flow passively along osmotic gradients established by substrate transport. Due to the active absorption mainly of Na^+ and Cl^-, which are quantitatively the most significant ions in the food mass, the interstitial spaces become hyperosmolar with respect to the intestinal lumen. This osmotic gradient drives a flow of water from the intestinal lumen into the interstitium of the mucosa, so water can be absorbed both transcellularly and paracellularly, i.e. through the tight junctions and the **intercellular spaces** (**Fig. 16.64**). In sheep, rabbits and rats, osmolarity in the intercellular spaces can rise to values of up to 800–1200 mosmol·l^{-1}, whereas in cattle it can only rise to about 350 mosmol·l^{-1}. The degree to which the contents of the large intestine can be dehydrated varies by species. Water uptake in the large intestine of cattle is only weakly performed.

IN A NUTSHELL !

The cellular mechanisms of absorption and secretion of inorganic ions by the large intestine epithelium are mainly similar to those in the small intestine. In addition, an apical K^+/H^+ pump is present in the large intestine.

■ Intra- and extracellular regulation of electrolyte transport

Cl^- secretion in epithelial cells is mainly regulated by three **intracellular second messenger systems**, i.e. the **cAMP, cGMP** and **Ca^{2+} signalling pathways** (**Fig. 16.72**). These have different targets. **cAMP** directly promotes Cl^- secretion by triggering the opening of Cl^- channels in the brush border membrane. The mechanism is phosphorylation of apical Cl^- channels by cAMP-dependent protein kinase A. An increase in the intracellular **cGMP** concentration has the same effect. Here, too, a protein kinase mediates the phosphorylation of apical Cl^- channels. **Intracellular Ca^{2+}** has a different mechanism of action. An increase in intracellular Ca^{2+} concentration leads mainly to the opening of basolat-

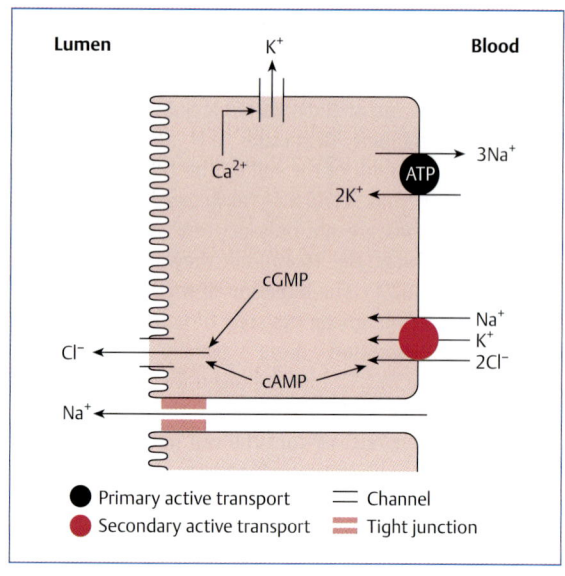

Fig. 16.72 Intracellular regulation of Cl⁻ secretion in colonic epithelial cells.

eral K^+ channels. This brings the membrane potential closer to the equilibrium potential of the K^+ ions and hyperpolarises the cell membrane. This increases the driving force for the exit of the negatively charged Cl^- ions from the cell. Cl^- secretion is thus indirectly stimulated. In parallel with these effects, all three signalling chains inhibit NaCl absorption, but this inhibition is limited to electroneutral NaCl transport via Na^+/H^+ and Cl^-/HCO_3^- exchanger. Electrogenic Na^+ transport via Na^+ channels is not inhibited.

Water passively follows secreted electrolytes osmotically. The secretion of crypt cells throughout the gastrointestinal tract has an important physiological role in the onward transport of intestinal contents, which these secretions promote as a flushing effect.

MORE DETAILS If crypt cell secretion is activated to an unphysiological extent, there can be a many-fold increase in secretion volume, which clinically results in diarrhoea (p. 445). A misdirected activation of Cl⁻ secretion can occur, when a bacterial toxin, the heat-stable **toxin** of *Escherichia coli*, stimulates guanylate cyclase and thus increases intracellular cGMP concentration. Cholera toxin has a similar effect, causing long-term activation of adenylate cyclase and increased cAMP production by a change in G-proteins.

Examples of extracellular messengers that act on electrolyte transport in the colon:

- Secretory messenger substances (**Fig. 16.74, Fig. 16.75, Fig. 16.76, Fig. 16.77, Fig. 16.78**)
  - effect via stimulation of the **cAMP pathway:**
    - vasoactive intestinal peptide (VIP), prostaglandin E_2
    - cholera toxin, heat-labile toxin of *Escherichia coli* (LT)
  - effect via stimulation of the **cGMP pathway:**
    - guanylin
    - heat-stable toxin of *Escherichia coli* (ST)
  - effect via stimulation of the
    Ca^{2+}-/protein kinase C pathway:
    - acetylcholine, serotonin, substance P

- Proabsorptive messengers
  - somatostatin, neuropeptide Y, adrenaline, noradrenaline

The large intestine has a special function in **water** and **electrolyte balance**. The large intestine provides the last opportunity to influence the composition of faeces. Because of this, ion transport in the large intestine is precisely **regulated** by the enteric nervous system plexuses in the intestinal wall. Nerve cells of the **enteric nervous system** release a series of transmitters that promote secretion and simultaneously inhibit absorption. The most quantitatively significant secretory transmitters are **acetylcholine** and **vasoactive intestinal peptide (VIP)** which exert their effect by stimulating Ca^{2+} and cAMP pathways in epithelial cells. Other transmitters of the enteric and sympathetic nervous system such as **somatostatin**, **neuropeptide Y** or **noradrenaline** promote absorption while simultaneously inhibiting secretion. In addition to neurotransmitters, a variety of paracrine substances released by immunological processes such as antigen-antibody reactions, or in inflammation also influence ion transport.

MORE DETAILS In contrast to ruminants, where fermentation takes place before the small intestine in the forestomachs, the **bacterial proteins** or **vitamins** synthesised in the large intestine **cannot be used** by the host animal, as there is no significant protein or vitamin absorption in the large intestine. However, animals such as the **rabbit** partially ingest their **soft faeces** (caecotrophic animals (p. 442)), so that the proteins or vitamins synthesised by bacteria in the caecum can enter the small intestine and be absorbed there.

IN A NUTSHELL   !

In the epithelium of the large intestine, unlike in the small intestine, there is no transport mechanism for amino acids or for monosaccharides.

Suggested reading

Binder HJ, Cummings J, Soergel KH, eds. Short chain fatty acids. Amsterdam: Kluwer Academic Press; 1994

Binder HJ, Sandle GJ. Electrolyte transport in the mammalian colon. In: Johnson LR, ed. Physiology of the gastrointestinal tract. 3rd ed. New York: Raven Press; 1994: 2133–2171

Clauss W. Segmental heterogeneity and regulation of electrolyte transport in the rabbit !arge intestine. In: Clauss W, ed. Ion transport in vertebrate colon. Adv Camp Environ Physiol 1993; 16: 95–112.

Jovany JP, ed. Rumen microbial metabolism and ruminant digestion. Paris: INRA Editions; 1991

Kunzelmann K, Mall M. Electrolyte transport in the mammalian colon: mechanisms and implications for disease. Physiol Rev 2002; 82: 245–289

Stevens CE, Hume ID. Comparative physiology of the vertebrate digestive system. 2nd ed. Cambridge: Cambridge University Press; 1995

16.8 Pathophysiology of diarrhoea

Franziska Dengler, Gotthold Gäbel,
Romy Monika Heilmann

Diarrhoea is defined as an increased volume of faeces and/ or frequency of defecation and is usually associated with an increased faecal water loss. A variety of diseases are associated with this clinical sign, and diarrhoea as such is not a primary disease. Rather, it is an important mechanism to defend and remove noxious agents. However, excessive diarrhoea can lead to serious disturbances of homeostasis and marked fluid and electrolyte imbalances (p. 329) as well as acid-base imbalances (p. 345). Administration of specific treatment to address the triggering noxious agent is not always possible; thus, symptomatic treatment of the diarrhoea often remains the only treatment option. An inappropriate approach to treatment, however, may cause an aggravation of the diarrhoea. Therefore, a thorough understanding of the underlying pathophysiological mechanisms of diarrhoea is important to arrive at the correct (and ideally targeted) treatment plan.

ESSENTIALS ✖

Large amounts of water are shifted daily throughout the gastrointestinal tract. The amount of fluid ingested with food and water presents only a fraction of the total fluid volume, which is complemented by the fraction originating from the secretion of saliva, gastric juice, pancreatic juice, bile, and extensive secretory processes along the intestines. Physiologically, water is reabsorbed along the entire gastrointestinal tract but the colon can compensate considerably for fluid losses occurring further proximal in the gastrointestinal tract to prevent the development of diarrhoea (Fig. 16.63).

Movement of water across the intestinal epithelium is primarily a passive process following the movement of several substances. The principle driving force for **water absorption** is the **absorption of cations**, especially Na^+. In contrast, **water secretion** typically follows the **secretion of anions**, particularly Cl^- and HCO_3^-. Hence, depending on the underlying mechanisms two main types of diarrhoea are distinguished: **osmotic** and **secretory diarrhoea**. In clinical practice, however, a mixture of both mechanisms is often encountered, rendering this subclassification a diagnostic tool (Table 16.13). In addition, **intestinal motility** plays an important role in the development of diarrhoea.

IN A NUTSHELL !

The main consequences of persistent diarrhoea are the loss of water and electrolytes (clinically detected as **dehydration**), acid-base imbalances (usually causing a **metabolic acidosis**) and energy deficit from malabsorption of nutrients (**hypoglycaemia**). Especially in very young animals, these factors can quickly lead to fatal outcomes. Therefore, diarrhoea should raise concern particularly in young animals.

16.8.1 Secretory diarrhoea

Secretory diarrhoea results from **increased secretion**, particularly of Cl^- and also HCO_3^-. This leads to an increased accumulation of water in the intestinal lumen, exceeding the capacity for water reabsorption and resulting in an increased loss of water in the faeces. This mechanism is often referred to as "self-cleansing" to flush out potentially harmful substances from the intestinal lumen.

16.8.2 Osmotic diarrhoea

Osmotic diarrhoea results from an **increased osmotic gradient** from the intestinal lumen to the subepithelial tissue of the intestinal wall. This is caused by the accumulation of large amounts of non-absorbable, osmotically active substances (e.g., sugar polymers) in the intestinal lumen.

16.8.3 Mechanisms

The mechanisms regulating intestinal fluid and electrolyte reabsorption are redundant, and the pathomechanisms of diarrhoea development are similar, if not the same, for the different aetiologies. Enterocytes, enteric nervous system (ENS, see ch. 16.2 (p. 361)), gut-associated lymphatic tissue (GALT, see ch. 10.4.2 (p. 252)), and systemic influences, including the autonomic nervous system or endocrine regulation (i.e., hormones), form a complex network to maintain the balance between activating and inhibiting processes.

■ Nutrient absorption

Absorption of nutrients occurs mainly, but not exclusively, by the differentiated enterocytes at the villus tips (**Fig. 16.47**) in symport with Na^+ (e.g., via the Na^+-dependent glucose transporter SGLT1, see **Fig. 16.54** and **Fig. 16.73**). These processes concurrently draw water osmotically from the intestinal lumen. Diseases causing insufficient nutrient absorption also limit the osmotically-driven absorption of water. Basic requirements for effective nutrient absorption are the presence and function of **nutrient transporters** and the presence and **activity of digestive enzymes**. Maldigestion (p. 449) occurs when one or more of these essential components are deficient or completely absent, the underlying causes of which will be discussed in more detail below.

■ Transepithelial transporters

Secretory diarrhoea is mainly caused by an increased secretion of **chloride**, which is primarily mediated by the chloride channel CFTR (cystic fibrosis transmembrane regulator). Secretion of HCO_3^- via CFTR is also possible (**Fig. 16.73**). This secretory mechanism can be significantly increased by noxious stimuli such as infectious agents or toxins. Other anion exchangers, such as DRA (down-regulated in adenoma), can also contribute to increased intestinal secretion. Beyond the secretion of anions, an increased incorporation of K^+ channels in the apical membrane of enterocytes can further cause increased secretion.

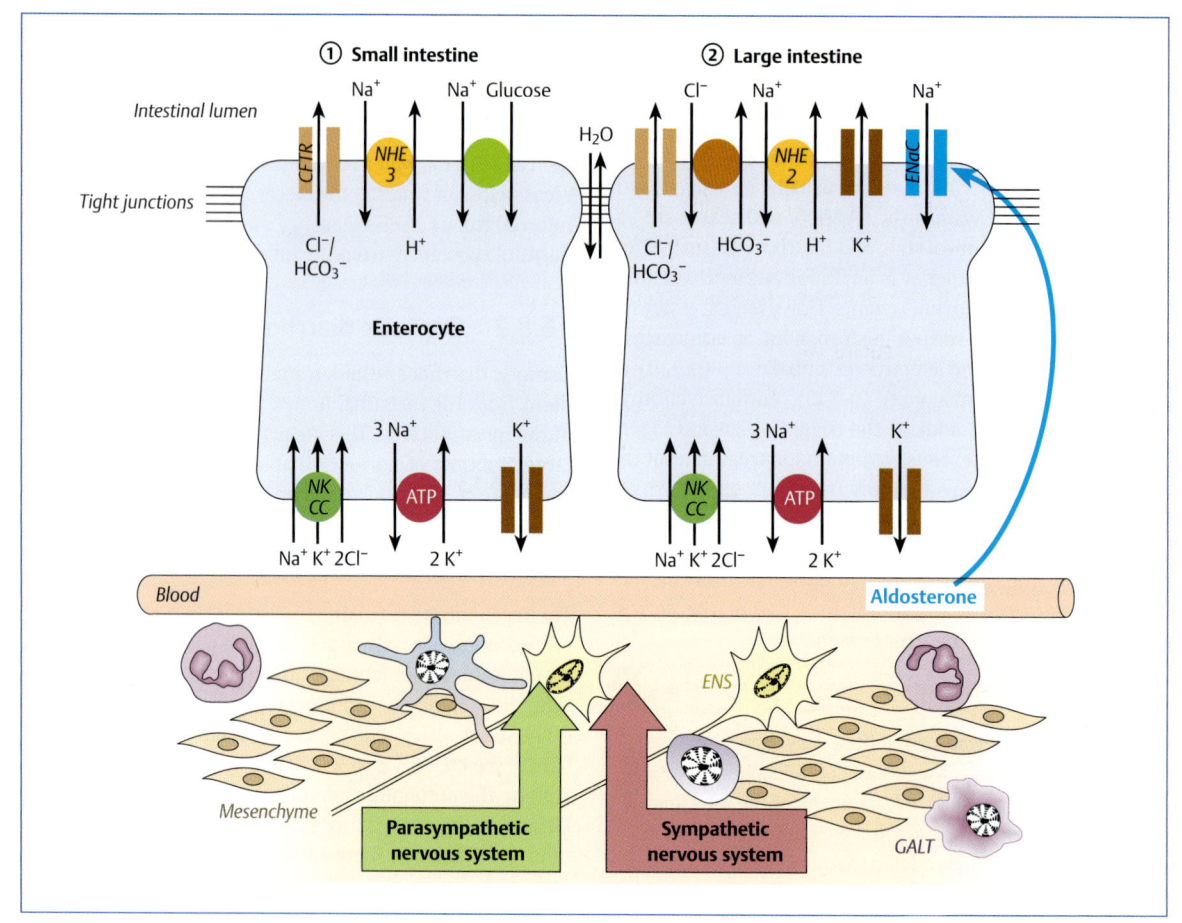

Fig. 16.73 Physiological secretory and absorptive processes in the small and large intestines, which play an important role in the development of diarrhoea. CFTR = cystic fibrosis transmembrane regulator, NHE = Na$^+$/H$^+$ exchanger, NKCC = Na$^+$-K$^+$-Cl$^-$ cotransporter, ENaC = epithelial sodium channel.

Another important transport mechanism involved in the development of diarrhoea is the NHE3 (Na$^+$/H$^+$ exchanger-3). Na$^+$ absorption and the osmotically driven water uptake in the small intestine critically depend on this ion exchanger. An impaired function of this ion exchange mechanism will invariably lead to diarrhoea.

In the large intestine, sodium is also absorbed through a Na$^+$ channel (ENaC, epithelial sodium channel), which is regulated by aldosterone (p. 442). This transporter can be dysregulated with disease (e.g., with chronic intestinal inflammation), contributing to the diarrhoea.

■ Intracellular mechanisms

Intracellular mediators that modulate secretory and absorptive processes are cAMP (cyclic adenosine monophosphate) and – to a lesser extent – cGMP (cyclic guanosine monophosphate) and intracellular calcium concentration ($[Ca^{2+}]_i$). As an example, CFTR activity is regulated by endogenous mediators (e.g., neurotransmitters of the ENS) as well as by exogenous agents (e.g., toxins) via cAMP-mediated phosphorylation. Another pathomechanism involves the cAMP-mediated inhibition of NHE3. The net effect of the reduced absorption of sodium and increased secretion of chloride is an increased loss of water. The concurrent ac-

cumulation of H$^+$ within the cytoplasm of the enterocytes, together with the loss of HCO$_3^-$, cause a metabolic acidosis.

MORE DETAILS NHE3 is primarily expressed in the enterocytes of the small intestine, whereas the NHE2 isoform is localized to the large intestine. NHE2 is cAMP-insensitive, which secures water absorption via this transporter in the large intestine despite elevated cAMP levels.

■ Intestinal motility

Similar to the regulation of intestinal absorption and secretion, intestinal motility is also modulated by higher-order centres. Both an increase or decrease in intestinal motility (i.e., faster intestinal passage or less mixing of ingesta) can reduce the volume of water being absorbed and increase faecal water loss. Examples include the diarrhoea seen with irritable bowel syndrome (IBS), endocrine diseases such as hyperthyroidism, or side effects of several medications (e.g., the chemotherapeutic vincristine). Especially an activation of ENS motoneurons by inflammatory mediators or bacterial toxins results in increased motility (hypermotility).

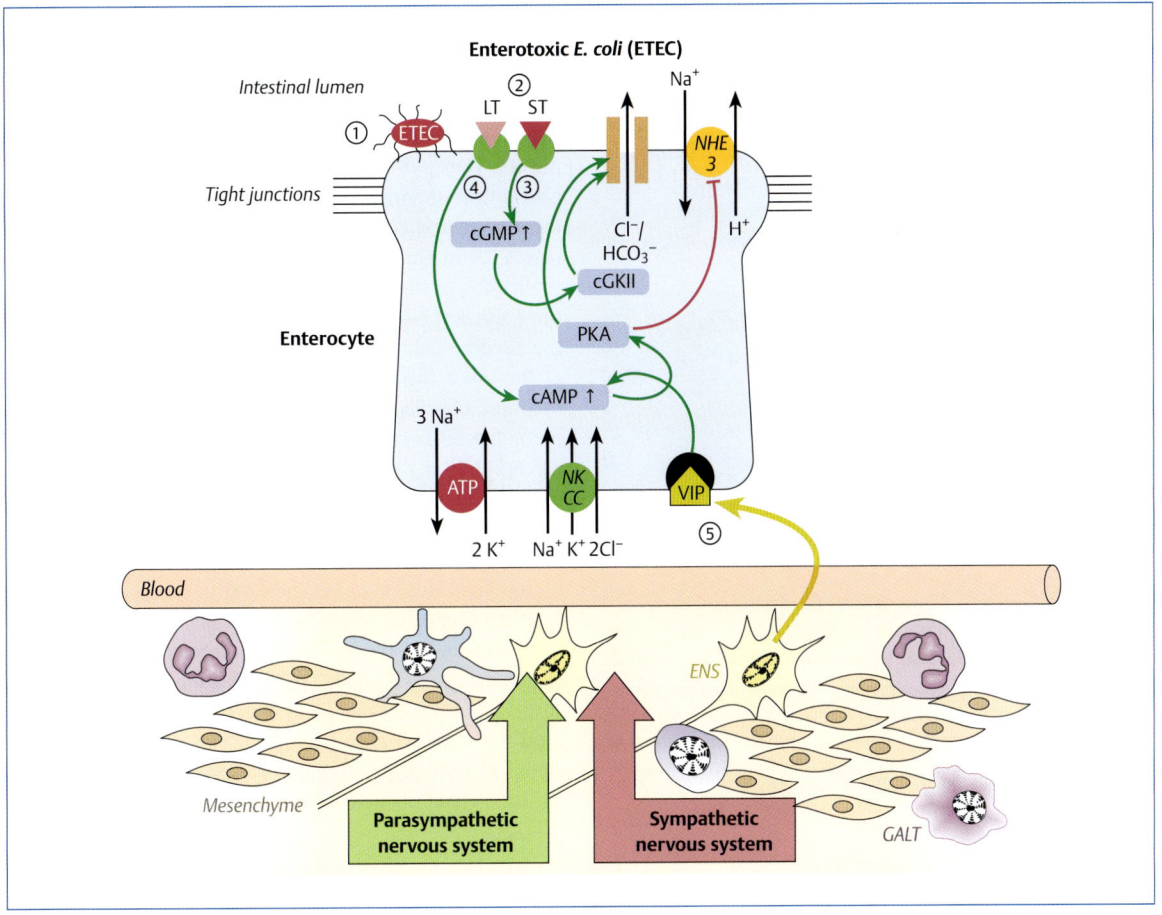

Fig. 16.74 Mechanisms of diarrhoea induction by enterotoxic *E. coli* (ETEC) infections. LT = heat-labile toxin, ST = heat-stable toxin, VIP = vasoactive intestinal peptide. See **Fig. 16.73** for the remainder of the key. Mechanisms are explained in the text.

16.8.4 Infectious diarrhoea

The three main mechanisms of bacterial and viral pathogens causing diarrhoea are illustrated in **Fig. 16.74**, **Fig. 16.75**, **Fig. 16.76**, and **Fig. 16.77**. Some pathogens (e.g., *Clostridium difficile*) disturb the tight junctions of the enterocytes and disrupt the epithelial barrier function. Furthermore, some bacteria and viruses attach to the epithelial surface or subepithelial structures, preventing them from being flushed out with the movement of the ingesta. In addition, pathogens may produce a range of different toxins. To counteract the colonization of pathogens, the intestinal secretion is increased to eliminate the infectious organisms with the increased passage of watery faeces.

> **IN A NUTSHELL**   !
>
> Acute diarrheal disease is common, particularly in young animals. This condition is mostly due to infectious aetiologies.

■ Diarrhoea absent morphological lesions of the intestinal mucosa

Infections with enterotoxic *Escherichia* (*E.*) *coli* (**ETEC**) or *Vibrio cholerae* illustrate the strategies of microbial attachment and toxin formation. ETEC- or cholera-associated diarrhoea are classical examples of secretory diarrhoea. ETEC typically does not cause structural changes, and the barrier function of the intestinal epithelium remains intact. Diarrhoea primarily results from the increased intestinal secretion that is induced by the toxins.

Fig. 16.74 depicts the mechanisms of ETEC-induced diarrhoea (numbers refer to the circled numbers in **Fig. 16.74**): ① ETEC bind to the epithelial cell surface via bacterial fimbriae. ② ETEC can produce a heat-labile toxin (LT) and a heat-stable toxin (ST). ③ ST increases intracellular levels of cGMP, which activates the CFTR. ④ LT (similar to the cholera toxin) binds to a G-protein-coupled receptor, which activates adenylate cyclase and increases intracellular levels of cAMP. This activates protein kinase A (PKA), phosphorylating and increasing the activity of CFTR and decreasing NHE3 activity. ⑤ ST also leads to ENS activation by an as-of-yet unknown mechanism, further increasing the cAMP-mediated intestinal secretion.

■ Diarrhoea associated with morphological intestinal lesions

Viral and parasitic infections primarily, but not exclusively, cause destruction of the apical enterocyte membrane, enterocyte shedding, and flattening of the intestinal villi. This leads to a reduced intestinal surface area available for absorptive processes and impairment of important transport mechanisms (**Fig. 16.75**), resulting in maldigestion and os-

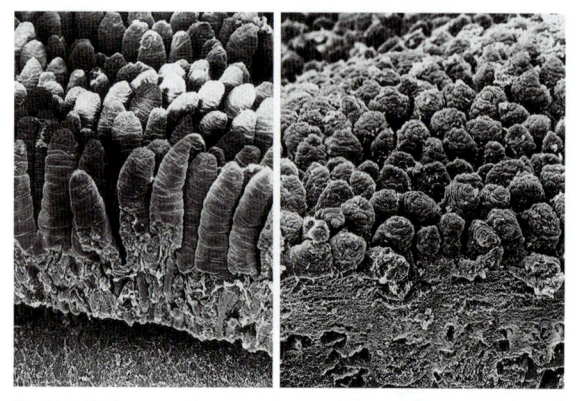

Fig. 16.75 Electron microscopy image of the small intestine of a calf. Left image: healthy small intestine, right image: intestinal surface after infection with rota-/coronavirus, showing atrophy of the intestinal villi and loss of absorptive surface area. [Source: Hofmann W, Farbatlas Rinderkrankheiten. Stuttgart: Eugen Ulmer; 2007]

motic diarrhoea (p. 449). Examples are infections with **rotaviruses**, **coronaviruses**, or **parvoviruses** and infections with ***Cryptosporidium parvum*** or other protozoa.

Coinfection with **rotaviruses** and **coronaviruses** is a common problem in young animals, such as calves and piglets. These viruses penetrate the enterocytes to replicate intracellularly, which damages the brush border membrane and compromises essential absorptive mechanisms (① in **Fig. 16.76**, **malabsorption**). The intracellular replication of the virus causes cell death, desquamation of the epithelium and shortening of the intestinal villi. Given the predominantly absorptive capacity of the enterocytes at the villus tips, this leads to disturbances in water absorption. **Giardia** sp. can have a similar effect on intestinal epithelial cells. The rotavirus toxin, NSP4 (non-structural glycoprotein 4), additionally inhibits the translocation of disaccharidases to the brush border membrane (②) by increasing $[Ca^{2+}]_i$, resulting in **maldigestion**. Furthermore, the (presumed) activation of the ENS increases intestinal secretion as illustrated in **Fig. 16.74** (③).

With ***Cryptosporidium parvum*** infection, replication of the parasite and the production of oocysts also destroys the enterocytes (① in **Fig. 16.77**), leading to a reduced absorptive surface area and loss of active transporters for Na^+ (and thus water) absorption. Proteins released from the sloughed enterocytes further draw water osmotically into the intestinal lumen. In addition, activation of the GALT in-

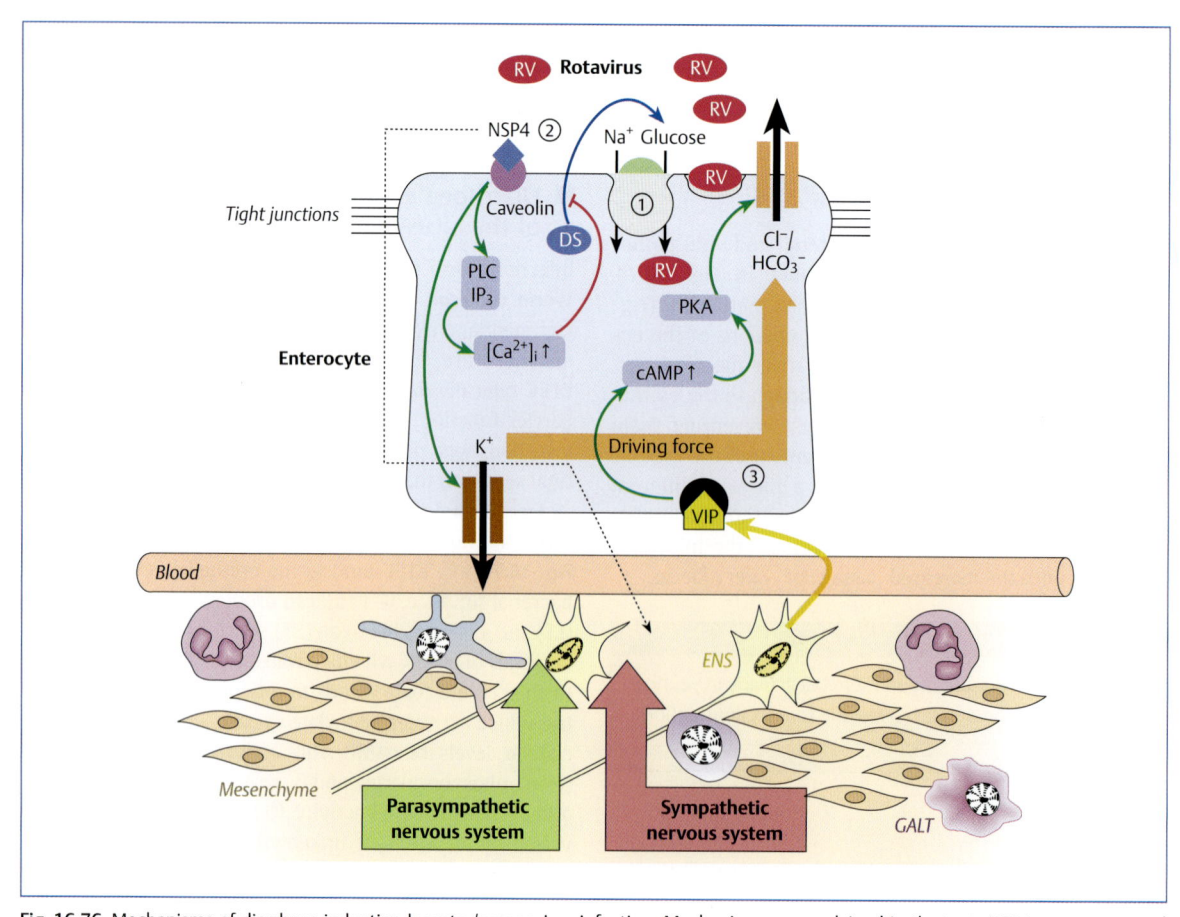

Fig. 16.76 Mechanisms of diarrhoea induction by rota-/coronavirus infection. Mechanisms are explained in the text. NSP4 = non-structural protein 4, DS = disaccharidases, RV = rotaviruses, PLC = phospholipase C, IP3 = inositol-1,4,5-triphosphate. See **Fig. 16.73** for the remainder of the key.

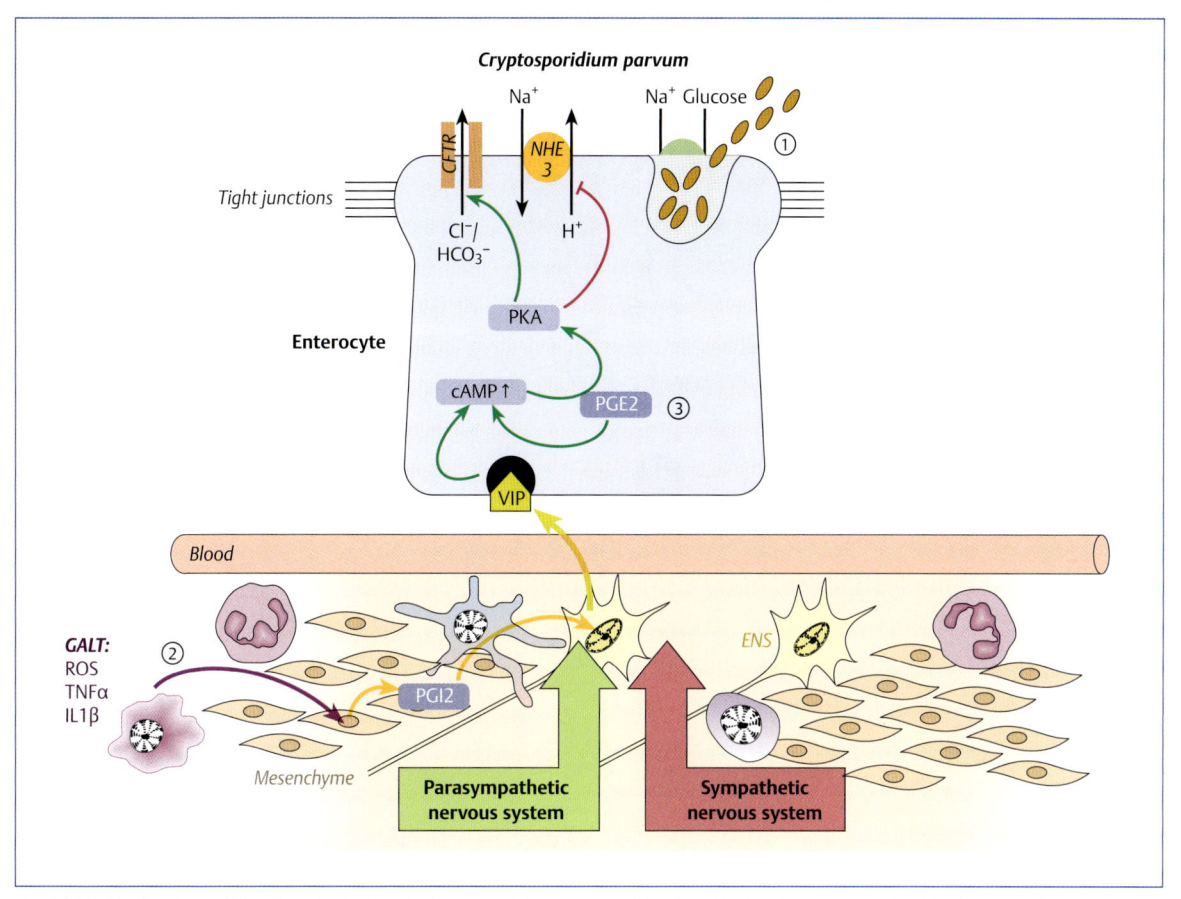

Fig. 16.77 Mechanisms of diarrhoea induction by *Cryptosporidium parvum* infection. Mechanisms are explained in the text. ROS = reactive O_2 species, TNFα = tumour necrosis factor-α, IL 1β = interleukin 1 β, PGE2 (I2) = prostaglandin E2 (I2). See **Fig. 16.73** for the remainder of the key.

duces the formation of mucosal PGI2 via inflammatory cytokines and other mediators. This activates secretory motoneurons (②). Concurrently PGE2 production in the enterocytes further stimulates the cAMP-mediated intestinal secretion (③).

16.8.5   Non-infectious diarrhoea

Beyond infectious causes, there are many non-infectious aetiologies that can cause or contribute to diarrhoea (**Table 16.13**). This section covers pathomechanisms of diseases that are commonly seen in veterinary practice.

■ Chronic idiopathic inflammatory bowel disease

In recent years, the importance of the inflammatory response of the GALT – with essentially the same key players induced by pathogens – has been increasingly recognized in the onset of chronic diarrhoea. Chronic **inflammatory bowel disease (IBD)** is an idiopathic non-infectious condition in humans and has become an increasingly recognized problem also in dogs and cats, where it is referred to as **chronic inflammatory enteropathy (CIE)** (**Fig. 16.78** and **Fig. 16.79**). In IBD and CIE, both secretory and osmotic processes contribute to the development of diarrhoea. If the small intestine is predominantly or exclusively af-

fected, the disease can occasionally (particularly in cats) occur without significant (or any) diarrhoea because of the large absorptive reserve capacity of the large intestine.

In IBD, the GALT is activated (① in **Fig. 16.78**) leading to an imbalance between absorptive and secretory processes. In addition, inflammatory mediators contribute to the break-down of the intestinal barrier by changing the expression of tight junction proteins (②).

■ Maldigestion

Maldigestion can result from various causes and leads or contributes to osmotic diarrhoea. Enzymatic digestion of nutrients within the intestinal lumen is critical (p. 422). If these digestive processes are impaired, disaccharides cannot be absorbed because carbohydrate absorption requires their break-down to monomers (e.g., glucose or fructose). Deficient disaccharidase activity in the brush border membrane therefore leads to (osmotic) diarrhoea. An example is the condition called "lactose intolerance" in people, which results from a genetically determined deficiency in the activity of small intestinal lactase or a decrease in its activity during adolescence. Adult dogs and cats generally also have low lactase activities in the small intestinal brush border, and this may be associated with an intolerance to milk or dairy products in these species. However, the activity of other disaccharidases in the brush border membrane

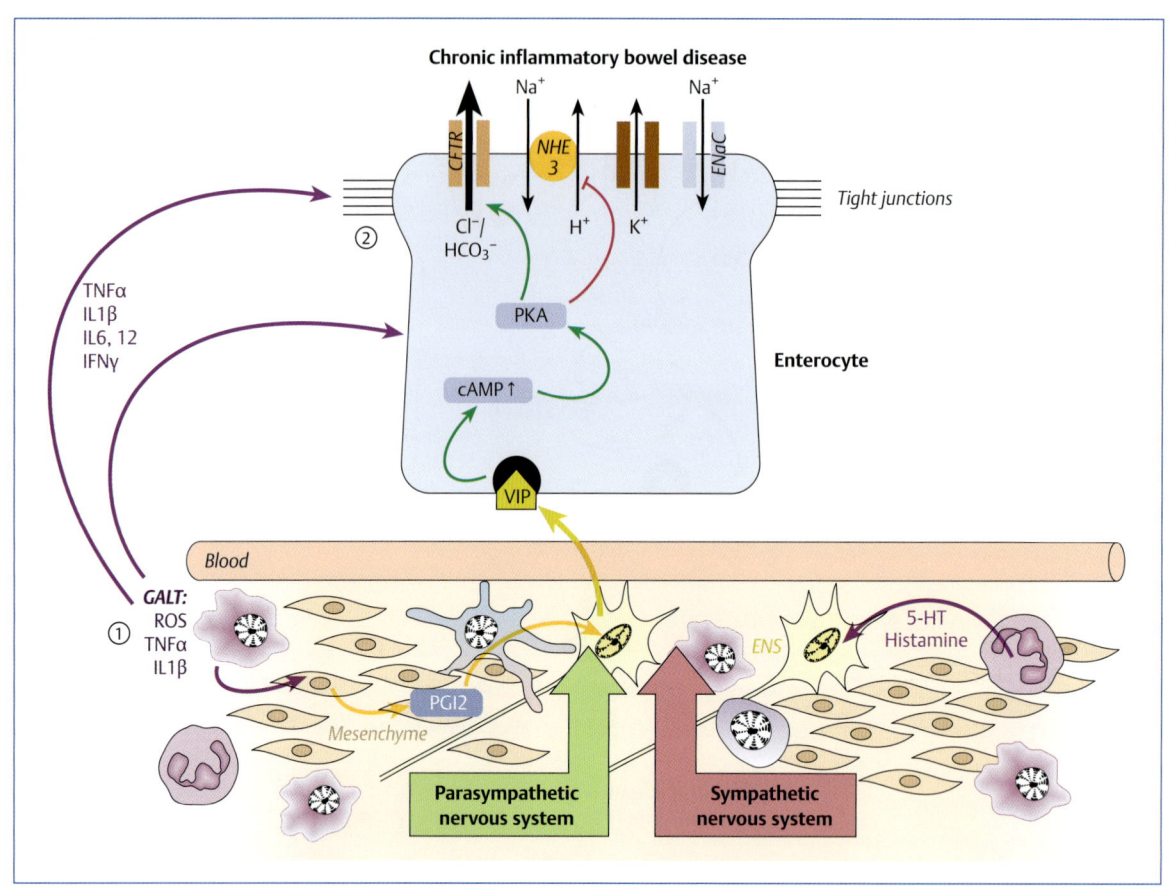

Fig. 16.78 Mechanisms of diarrhoea development in chronic idiopathic inflammatory bowel disease. Mechanisms are explained in the text. IFNγ = interferon γ, 5-HT = 5-hydroxytryptamine (serotonin). See **Fig. 16.73** for the remainder of the key.

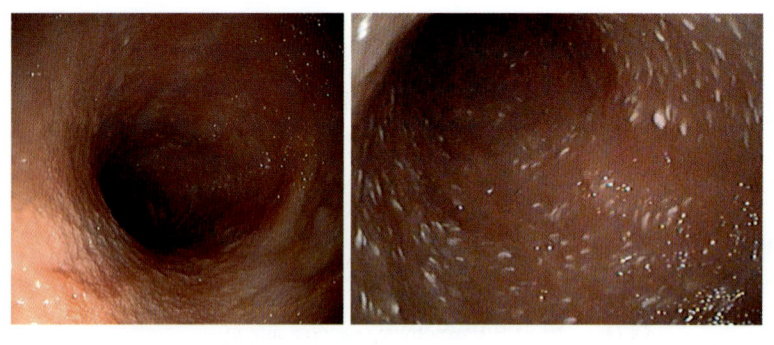

Fig. 16.79 Endoscopic views of the duodenum in dogs with chronic inflammatory enteropathy (idiopathic inflammatory bowel disease). Left image: increased mucosal redness (erythema) and granularity resulting from mucosal inflammation, right image: patchy mucosal erythema due to mucosal inflammation and multifocal white stipples reflecting dilated lymphatic ducts (lymphangiectasia). [Source: Prof. Dr. Romy Heilmann, Kleintierklinik, Universität Leipzig]

may also be impaired. For example, rotavirus infections disrupt the transfer of these enzymes to the enterocyte membrane resulting in carbohydrate maldigestion (**Fig. 16.75**).

Diseases of the liver/biliary tract or exocrine pancreas can severely impair the digestion of macronutrients. Consequently, disorders affecting the production and/or secretion of bile acids (e.g., insufficient liver function or biliary obstruction) or the production and/or release of pancreatic enzymes (e.g., exocrine pancreatic insufficiency) lead to reduced fat digestion and increased fat excretion, along with fat-soluble vitamins, in faeces (**steatorrhea**). **Pancreatitis** (inflammation of the pancreas) is particularly common in dogs and cats and, in addition to the systemic effects of prematurely activated pancreatic enzymes, can be associated with a reduced secretion of pancreatic enzymes

and thus reduced luminal and intestinal brush border enzyme activity. Pancreatic enzymes can be added to the food to treat exocrine pancreatic insufficiency.

Premature shedding of differentiated enterocytes (e.g., in parvovirus enteritis or cryptosporidiosis) also limits the uptake of simple sugars and/or amino acids due to the loss of transport capacities.

16.8.6 Aetiological classification of diarrhoea

In addition to the mechanisms detailed above, diarrhoea can also be classified according to the underlying clinical aetiology (**Table 16.13**) or primary location within the gastrointestinal tract (**Table 16.14**).

Table 16.13 Common causes, pathophysiologic mechanisms, and therapeutic approaches of diarrhoea in animals.

Aetiology	Primary mechanisms	Therapeutic approach
Vascular: Dilation of the intestinal lymphatics, mesenteric ischaemia ("intestinal infarction")	O, M	Dietary and (as needed) symptomatic/medical treatment
Inflammatory: Pancreatitis, food intolerance/allergy	O, M	Elimination diet, anti-inflammatory treatment (if indicated)
Endocrine: Hyperthyroidism, adrenocortical insufficiency	S, M	Medical treatment aiming at the primary condition (antithyroid medication, adrenocortical hormone supplementation)
Toxic: Feed toxins, poisonous plants, adverse drug effects	S, M, O	Elimination of the underlying cause, symptomatic treatment
Congenital: Portosystemic (liver) shunt	O	Surgical shunt occlusion and/or medical treatment
Alimentary: Abrupt dietary change, dietary indiscretion	O	Elimination of the underlying cause, easily digestible (gastrointestinal) diet or elimination diet
Metabolic: Impaired function (insufficiency) of the liver, kidneys, or exocrine pancreas	S, O, M	Medical and dietary therapy, specific treatment depending on the underlying condition
Mechanical: Intestinal foreign body or intussusception	M	Surgical intervention
Infectious: • Bacterial pathogens (**Fig. 16.74**)	S, M	Antibiotics, if indicated pro-/prebiotics or synbiotics
• Viral agents (**Fig. 16.75**, **Fig. 16.76**)	S	Symptomatic treatment, if indicated pro-/prebiotics or synbiotics
• Parasitic causes (**Fig. 16.77**)	S, O	Anthelmintics, antiprotozoal drugs
• Fungi or yeast organisms	S, O	Symptomatic treatment, antifungal medications (if indicated)
Idiopathic: Chronic inflammatory enteropathy (CIE) (**Fig. 16.78, Fig. 16.79**)	S, O, M	Elimination diet, anti-inflammatory/immuno-suppressive drugs (if indicated)
Neoplastic: Lymphosarcoma, mast cell tumour	O, M	Chemotherapy and/or surgery
Neurologic: Irritable bowel syndrome (IBS), stress/anxiety/agitation	M	Symptomatic treatment, stress avoidance or reduction/relieve
Degenerative: Idiopathic megacolon	M	Medical and dietary therapy

S = secretory, O = osmotic, M = motility-associated.

Table 16.14 Clinical criteria to categorise diarrhoea based on the primarily affected site within the gastrointestinal tract.

Characteristic	Small intestinal diarrhoea	Large intestinal diarrhoea
Frequency of defecation	Ø to ↑	↑ ↑
Straining to defecate (tenesmus)	Ø	↑ to ↑ ↑
Faecal volume (per defecation)	↑ to ↑ ↑	Ø to ↓
Other stool abnormalities	Digested blood (melaena), watery faeces, undigested material	Fresh blood (haematochezia), mucus
Body weight	Ø to ↓ ↓	Ø

Ø normal or absent; ↑ slightly increased; ↑ ↑ markedly increased; ↓ reduced; ↓ ↓ markedly reduced

Table 16.15 Composition of an oral rehydration solution recommended by the WHO.

Ingredient	Concentration (mmol · l^{-1})	Mechanism of action
NaCl	45	Electrolyte replacement
KCl	20	Electrolyte replacement
Trisodium citrate	10	Compensation of acidosis
Glucose	75	Energy supply, increased intestinal absorption

16.8.7 Therapeutic approach

Diarrhoea is often self-limiting and, as detailed above, is a physiologic mechanism to eliminate harmful agents or substances. Therefore, supportive (symptomatic) treatment will be sufficient in some cases. Rapid and aggressive treatment is indicated if life-threatening complications are imminent or have already developed. Symptomatic treatment primarily aims to correct dehydration (up to 20% of body mass!, might result in shock), acidosis, electrolyte imbalances, and the energy deficit rather than specifically addressing the causes of the diarrhoea, which can vary considerably (**Table 16.13**).

Research efforts have led to the development of optimized oral **rehydration solutions**. These **formulas** can be cost-effective and efficient treatments to reduce the net water loss, lowering the risk of cardiovascular failure. Essential characteristics of the currently recommended oral rehydration solutions are a mild hypoosmolality and high concentrations of glucose and in some cases amino acids (promoting water reabsorption via Na$^+$symport, see **Fig. 16.73**). A buffering agent, usually NaHCO$_3$, is included to correct acidosis.

Instead of NaHCO$_3$, the WHO (World Health Organization) recommends sodium citrate or acetate to be added, which is because oral rehydration solutions were originally developed to treat cholera infections (**Table 16.15**). These bacteria benefit from an alkaline intestinal microenvironment, making excessive buffering counterproductive in these cases. Most commercially available oral rehydration solutions are composed as specified by the WHO. Resistant starch, which is metabolised to short-chain fatty acids (SCFA) in the large intestine and increases water absorption concurrent with SCFA absorption, can also be added for diseases that affect primarily the small intestine (**Fig. 16.70**).

Depending on the severity of dehydration, intravenous fluid administration may be indicated. In addition to 0.9% NaCl (physiologic saline) solution or balanced crystalloid solutions (e.g., lactated Ringer's or acetate Ringer's solution), HCO$_3$⁻- or glucose-containing solutions may be used (if indicated) for refractory acidosis (i.e., marked acidosis not responding to symptomatic treatment alone) or with existing or impending hypoglycaemia.

The use of adsorbent medications, which can decrease the faecal water content (e.g., activated charcoal, kaolin), should be carefully considered as the resulting improvement in faecal consistency is merely a cosmetic effect. However, such treatments (e.g., adding psyllium husks to the food) can also have positive effects on the intestinal mucosa and benefit the intestinal regeneration.

Finally, the role of maintaining a healthy gastrointestinal **microbiome** is becoming increasingly evident. In line with this, antibiotic treatments are also increasingly questioned in diarrheic conditions. Their combination or replacement with the administration of **pre- or probiotics (or synbiotics)** to reduce intestinal dysbiosis and diarrhoea or restore intestinal normobiosis may be beneficial. Faecal material transplantation (FMT) – essentially the transfer of a "faecal bacterial culture" from a healthy animal harbouring a healthy intestinal microbiome – has also shown benefit in the treatment of free faecal water as well as acute and chronic diarrheic conditions in horses and dogs.

Suggested reading

Anbazhagan AN, Priyamvada S, Alrefai WA, et al. Pathophysiology of IBD associated diarrhea. Tissues Barriers 2018; 6: e1463897.

Foster DM, Smith GW. Pathophysiology of diarrhea in calves. Vet Clin Food Anim 2009; 25: 13–36. doi: 10.1016/j.cvfa.2008.10.013

Jones SL, Blikslager AT. Role of the Enteric Nervous System in the Pathophysiology of Secretory Diarrhea. J Vet Intern Med 2002; 16: 222–228.

Magalhães D, Cabral JM, Soares-da-Silva P, et al. Role of epithelial ion transports in inflammatory bowel disease. Am J Physiol Gastrointest Liver Physiol 2016; 310: G460-G476. doi:10.1152/ajpgi.00369.2015

Priyamvada S, Gomes R, Gill RK, et al. Mechanisms underlying dysregulation of electrolyte absorption in IBD associated diarrhea. Inflamm Bowel Dis 2015; 21: 2926–2935.

16.9 Comparison of digestion in forestomach and large intestine

Wolfgang von Engelhardt

> **ESSENTIALS**
>
> Herbivores can digest by microbial degradation in large **fermentation chambers**. By such means, herbivores can also digest plant substances that cannot be digested by the body's own enzymes.
> - In **foregut fermenters**, the fermentation chambers are located before the small intestine. In **hindgut fermenters**, the fermentation chambers are located after the small intestine.
> - Comparison of the advantages and disadvantages of microbial digestion in the forestomachs and in the large intestine are considered.

Domestic ruminants belonging to the suborder **Ruminantia**, have large **forestomachs**. Camels and llamas, belonging to the family Camelidae, also have large forestomachs and they also ruminate. Camelidae have evolved quite independently from the Ruminantia as they are phylogenetically much older. In addition to the ruminant foregut fermenters, there are other non-ruminant foregut fermenters that belong to various systematic taxa, for example, kangaroos, hippos, sloths, colobus monkeys.

Species that use microbial digestion in the **large intestine** can be divided into two groups. One group are those species where microbial digestion is mainly in the caecum (**caecum fermenters**), for example hamsters, guinea pigs, beavers, voles, capybaras, rabbits, chinchillas, koalas. In other animals, the colon is the more important and also a larger fermentation chamber (**colon fermenters**), e.g. horses, elephants, rhinos, wombats, many species of monkeys, pigs). The size of the large intestine (p. 438) varies greatly between animal species (**Fig. 16.67**). For example, in horses and elephants, the large intestine content is about 13% of body weight. These large intestinal fermentation chambers thus account for a considerable proportion of the entire digestive tract.

16.9.1 Cellulose digestion in foregut and hindgut fermenters

Cellulose and other **cell wall components** of plants cannot be degraded by endogenous enzymes. In the fermentation chambers of herbivores, microorganisms produce enzymes that can **cleave β-glycosidic bonds**, see ch. Carbohydrates (p. 398). The microorganisms in the large intestine are mainly similar to those in the forestomachs (see ch. 16.7.2 (p. 438)). Microbial hydrolytic cleavage of large cellulose molecules is a comparatively **slow process**. The efficiency of degradation therefore depends on how long the food remains in the fermentation chambers. The **extent of cellulose digestion** in the forestomachs or in the large intestine is therefore closely correlated with the **retention time** of the food mass in those compartments. Since domestic ruminants can **selectively** (compared to the liquid) **retain feed particles** in the forestomachs for a relatively long time. Because of this long retention time (p. 380) in the forestomachs, efficient degradation of plant structural substances can be achieved. In goats, the selective retention of feed particles in the rumen is somewhat less developed than in sheep. Goats are therefore less efficient in breaking down poorly digestible feed in the forestomachs than cattle and sheep. In **hindgut fermenters** with a large intestine volume approximately equal to that of the forestomachs, cellulose digestion is significantly lower than in sheep and cattle due to the **shorter retention time** of the digesta.

> **IN A NUTSHELL**
>
> In the forestomachs, cellulose and hemicelluloses are better digested than in the large intestine.

16.9.2 Advantages and disadvantages of foregut and hindgut fermentation when feeding grass of different quality

When fed medium and **good quality** grass, **domestic ruminants** are **superior** to horses in terms of **cellulose digestion** because of the long selective retention time of forage particles in the forestomachs (**Fig. 16.80 a**). However, this is different when **poor quality** grass is fed (**Fig. 16.80 b**). Then, because of the **long retention time** of such forage in the forestomachs, **ruminants** cannot ingest sufficient quantities of poor quality forage to meet their nutritional requirements. The long retention time of feed in the forestomachs limits the quantity of feed that can be ingested by ruminants. In **horses**, feed intake is not limited in this way. Equidae can increase the intake of poor quality feed by **increasing** the **rate of passage** through the gastrointestinal tract and still obtain sufficient nutrients from that large quantity during digestion in the small and large intestine.

Nutrition, energy

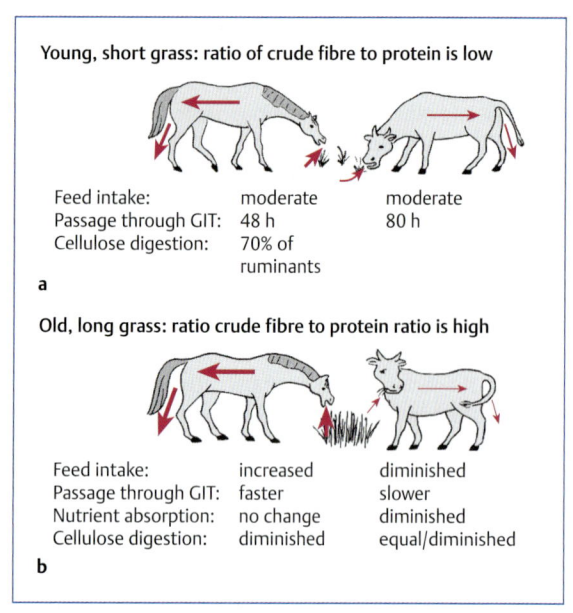

Fig. 16.80 There are significant differences in feed intake strategy between horses and cattle when given poorly digestible, low quality old grass or good quality young grass. With good quality grass or hay, ruminants are superior to equids (including zebras) in terms of cellulose digestion efficiency (a). However, equids can survive better on low quality forage than ruminants because equids are able to increase feed intake and rate of passage through the gastrointestinal tract (GIT). Although the digestibility of cellulose is reduced, equids may still be able to obtain sufficient nutrients from the overall larger feed quantity (b). Because of the long retention time of feed in the forestomachs, the amount of feed that can be ingested is limited in ruminants. [Source: Van Soest P J, Dierenfeld E S, Conclin N L Digestive Strategies and Limitations in Ruminants In: von Engelhardt, Leonhard-Marek, Breves, Giesecke eds. Ruminan Physiology: Digestion, Metbolism, Growth and Reproduction. Stuttgart: Enke 1995 581–600]

MORE DETAILS   In the large grass savannas of Africa, these **advantages of equids** can often be observed during periods in the dry seasons when only poor vegetation is available. While zebras are then usually still in astonishingly good nutritional condition, the predominantly grass-eating ruminants are often severely emaciated. During the long dry seasons, carcasses of ruminants are often seen in the savannas.

16.9.3   Digestion of easily digestible carbohydrates, feed protein and fat in forestomach and large intestine

Microorganisms in the forestomachs and large intestine metabolise monosaccharides, disaccharides and polysaccharides into short-chain fatty acids. The short-chain fatty acids are rapidly absorbed by mechanisms in the large intestine epithelium similar to those in the forestomachs. The short-chain fatty acids are an essential source of energy for the animal (see ch. 16.4.2 (p.395) and ch. 16.7.2 (p.438)). Since ruminants, depending on ration composition, convert carbohydrates in feed to short-chain fatty acids to a considerable extent in their forestomachs, they must therefore obtain the glucose for endogenous metabolism by glucogenesis from propionate, from glucogenic

amino acids, from lactate/pyruvate, or from glycerol (see gluconeogenesis (p.469) and **Fig. 17.5**). High-quality protein is also microbially degraded in the forestomachs. From protein degradation, the ammonia as well as the amino acids can be used for microbial protein synthesis. However, the ammonia formed during degradation is mainly absorbed in the forestomachs and must be detoxified in the body; see the sections on absorption of N-containing compounds (p.403) and urea synthesis (p.472). Microbial degradation of high-quality carbohydrates and high-quality feed protein are major disadvantages of forestomach fermentation.

In contrast, hindgut fermenters can readily break down easily digestible carbohydrates and also digestible protein in the stomach and small intestine and absorb the resulting monosaccharides and amino acids or dipeptides, see ch.s Digestion of proteins (p.426), Absorption of amino acids (p.427), and Absorption of di- and tripeptides (p.428). Only those carbohydrates and proteins that cannot be digested in the small intestine enter the large intestine where they can be microbially degraded and metabolised.

Fats are also split by microbial lipases in the forestomachs. The unsaturated fatty acids that are released can then be partially hydrogenated to form saturated fatty acids, especially stearic acid. Only a small part of this stearic acid can later be converted into oleic acid by desaturases in the small intestine and elsewhere in the body. Long-chain fatty acids are absorbed in the small intestine, see ch. Fats (p.404) and ch. Digestion and absorption of fats (p.429). Body fat in ruminants therefore contains mainly saturated and only small amounts of unsaturated fatty acids.

In hindgut fermenters, ingested triacylglycerols are broken down in the small intestine. The unsaturated fatty acids in the feed fat are largely retained and incorporated into body fat. In contrast to the forestomach fermenters, the fatty acid profile of body fat in monogastric animals therefore largely corresponds to the fat composition of the feed.

> **IN A NUTSHELL** !
>
> Easily digestible carbohydrates, high-quality proteins and unsaturated fatty acids are broken down or converted in the forestomachs with a considerable loss. Hindgut fermenters, on the other hand, can digest and absorb these readily digestible nutrients in the small intestine.
>
> Therefore, hindgut fermenters can use high-quality nutrients contained in the feed more efficiently than foregut fermenters.

16.9.4   Body mass of foregut and hindgut fermenters

The **basal metabolic rate** per kg body weight decreases with increasing body mass (**Fig. 19.5**). The relatively **high energy requirements** of very small animals cannot be met by the slow breakdown of cell wall components alone. **Small herbivores cannot afford** the wasteful degradation and microbial metabolism in a **forestomach system**. **Very small herbivores** (hamster, guinea pig, chinchilla) can therefore **only** be **hindgut fermenters**. As non-forestomach animals, they must obtain sufficient energy from food in the small intestine to supply their relatively high energy requirements, after which they can also microbially break down plant fibrous material in the large intestine.

IN A NUTSHELL   !

Very small herbivores cannot obtain enough energy from foregut fermentation.

MORE DETAILS   Some herbivores with a body weight of just over 4–5 kg are nevertheless ruminants. These **small ruminants** have adapted their grazing behaviour to meet their high energy requirements. Such small ruminants include tragulids, muntjac, small duiker, dikdik and also roe deer. When feeding, these small ruminants mainly choose easily digestible fruits, flowers and leaves, which can be broken down relatively quickly in the forestomachs. These ruminants are therefore also called **concentrate selectors**. Some larger ruminants have also evolved as concentrate selectors (e.g. gerenuk, and giraffe). They use ecological niches that are not or only slightly accessible to other animals. In these concentrate selectors, the **volume of the forestomach is** significantly **smaller** in relation to body weight, and the **retention times** are **shorter** than in the predominantly grass-eating ruminants, see ch. Microbial metabolism of proteins and N-containing compounds (p. 440) and ch. Proteins and NPN-containing compounds (p. 402).

16.9.5   Microbial protein synthesis and utilisation of the protein formed

In ch. 16.4.2 (p. 395) and ch. 16.7.2 (p. 438), it was pointed out that in the forestomachs and also in the large intestine the microorganisms produce high-quality **microbial protein**. This **protein** from the **forestomachs** reaches the abomasum and **small intestine** where it is **digested** to amino acids (p. 427) and di- and tri-peptides (p. 428) which are then **absorbed**.

In synthesising protein, microorganisms can also use non-protein nitrogen (p. 402) (NPN), especially ammonia (**Fig. 16.36**). On **low-protein diets** with **sufficient energy content**, up to 80% of the urea produced in the body can be recirculated into the forestomachs in saliva and, after cleavage to ammonia by microbial urease, be used for microbial protein synthesis. It could be assumed that this use of urea is a general benefit of foregut fermentation. However, this is **only** an **advantage** a. if ruminants are fed just the **maintenance requirements** (p. 489), b. if milk yield is very low and c. if the feed provides enough energy for microbial metabolism.

In **high-producing animals**, **urea circulation** into the forestomachs is even a **disadvantage**. High-producing animals can only be productive if they are fed sufficient amounts of high-quality, relatively easily digestible, and protein-rich feed. With such a high protein intake, the ammonia concentration in the forestomachs becomes very high and is increased even more by the recirculating urea.

The extensive ammonia absorption from the forestomachs and its subsequent conversion to urea in the liver (p. 472) is an **additional metabolic burden** for high-producing animals.

IN A NUTSHELL   !

Foregut fermenters can utilise poor quality feed proteins and non-protein nitrogen to synthesise high quality microbial protein. However, this is only an advantage over hindgut fermenters if ruminants are not fed more than their maintenance requirements. For a high-yielding cow, the recirculation of urea into the forestomachs is an additional metabolic burden.

Microbial protein produced in the large intestine is also of high quality. However, it cannot be utilised by most hindgut fermenters, as there are no mechanisms for absorption of amino acids by the large intestine mucosa, see ch. 16.7.3. Hence, microbial protein formed in the large intestine is excreted in faeces, while ammonia from protein degradation is absorbed and converted to urea in the liver.

Lagomorph animals (rabbits, hares, pikas) have developed a strategy that enables them to use the protein produced in the large intestine. These animals, by continuous weak antiperistaltic motor activity in the proximal colon, can propel **microorganisms** and **water** back into the **caecum**, see ch. on large intestine motor function (p. 392). As a result, much **microbial protein** is present in the caecal contents of rabbits. In the large intestine, the food particles have a relatively short retention time and are rapidly transported to the anus. Although **cellulose digestion** by rabbits is consequently quite **poor**, these animals have the **advantage** of being able to **use** a large part of the **microbial protein** produced in the caecum. About once a day, some of the caecal contents are transported through the colon by rapid peristalsis. In the proximal colon, the viscous caecal contents are packed into small pellets with a mucus en-

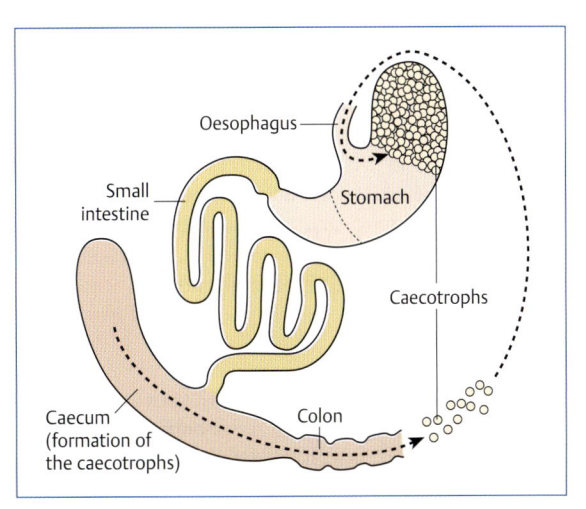

Fig. 16.81 Caecotrophs formed in the caecum of rabbits are usually discharged once a day as soft faeces, eaten directly from the anus, temporarily stored in the stomach, and then digested in the small intestine.

Nutrition, energy

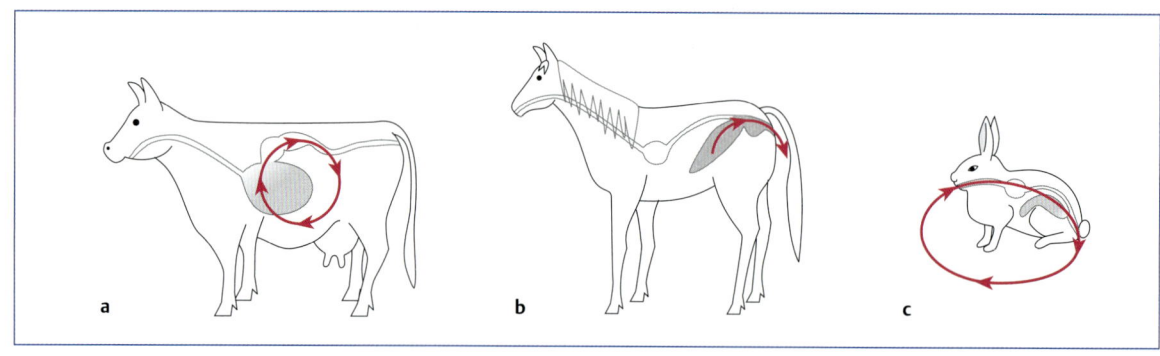

Fig. 16.82 Utilisation of microbial protein produced by one forestomach fermenter and two hindgut fermenters. **a** Microbial protein formed in the forestomachs can be degraded in the small intestine where the amino acids can be absorbed. Part of the end product of endogenous protein metabolism, urea, is secreted into the forestomachs and can be used there for microbial protein synthesis. **b** Most hindgut fermenters cannot use the microbial protein formed in the large intestine and it is excreted in faeces. **c** Rabbits can ingest the microbial protein enriched caecal contents per os (caecotrophy) and then digest this in the small intestine.

velope, which protects against digestion during passage through the colon. The composition of these pellets is quite different from the hard **faecal pellets**, and are called **soft faeces** or **caecotrophs**. The caecotrophs, which are rich in protein and also Vit. K and Vit. B_{12}, are sucked by the rabbits from the anus, mostly in the very early morning hours. The caecotrophs packed in the mucus coat are temporarily stored in the stomach (**Fig. 16.81**). In the small intestine, they are then digested and the amino acids and other nutrients are absorbed. Caecotrophy is not the same as coprophagy which is the eating of faeces in general, whereas caecotrophy refers to the ingestion of only the soft caecal contents.

> **IN A NUTSHELL**   **!**
>
> Hindgut fermenters usually cannot use the microbial protein formed. An exception is caecotrophy of lagomorphs.

Fig. 16.82 shows a comparison and summary of the utilisation of the microbial protein produced in the body in forestomach digestion and two different types of large intestine digestion. The utilisation of the high-quality microbial protein is very different. In ruminants, microbial protein produced in the forestomachs is digested in the small intestine where the amino acids are absorbed. Most large intestine digestors cannot use microbial protein from the large intestine and it is excreted in faeces. A special strategy has been developed by rabbits, which consume caecal contents (caecotrophy) and are thus able, by digestion in the small intestine, to use a significant proportion of the microbial protein formed in the large intestine.

Suggested reading

Hörnicke H, Björnhag G. Coprophagy and related strategies for digesta utilization. In: Ruckebusch Y, Thivend P, eds. Digestive Physiology and Metabolism in Ruminants. Westport: AVI Publishing; 1980: 707–730

Kay RN, von Engelhardt W, White RG. The digestive Physiology of wild Ruminants. In: Ruckebusch Y, Thivend P, eds. Digestive Physiology and Metabolism in Ruminants. Westport: AVI Publishing; 1980: 743–761

Stevens CE, Hume ID. Comparative Physiology of the Vertebrate Digestive System. Cambridge: Cambridge University Press; 1995

van Soest PJ, Dierenfeld ES, Conklin NL. Digestive strategies and limitations of ruminants. In: von Engelhardt W, Leonhard-Marek S, Breves G, Giesecke D, eds. Ruminant Physiology: Digestion, Metabolism, Growth and Reproduction. Stuttgart: Enke; 1995: 581–600

16.10   Digestion in birds and reptiles

Michael Pees, Helga Pfannkuche

> **ESSENTIALS**   **✗**
>
> The avian gastrointestinal tract has the same general functions as that of mammals. Bird-specific features in the proximal part of the digestive tract are the beak for crushing and ingesting food, the crop, which serves both for food storage and for feeding of young, and two stomach compartments, the glandular stomach and gizzard. The caecum is involved in recycling nitrogen from uric acid.
>
> Digestion in reptiles is very much dependent on environmental temperature. At the appropriate ambient temperature, herbivorous reptiles continuously eat food. In carnivorous reptiles, especially snakes, the activity of the digestive tract varies greatly with food intake. The use of venoms in snakes not only serves to kill the prey, but also initiates the digestive process, which can last for days to weeks.

16.10.1   Digestion in birds
■ The role of the beak

The avian digestive tract (**Fig. 16.83**) must meet two challenges. One is that its weight must not be too great as this might impair the bird's ability to fly. The other challenge is that avian digestion must be very efficient because of the very high energy requirements for flying. To meet these requirements the avian digestive system is characterised by short transit times and high secretion and absorption

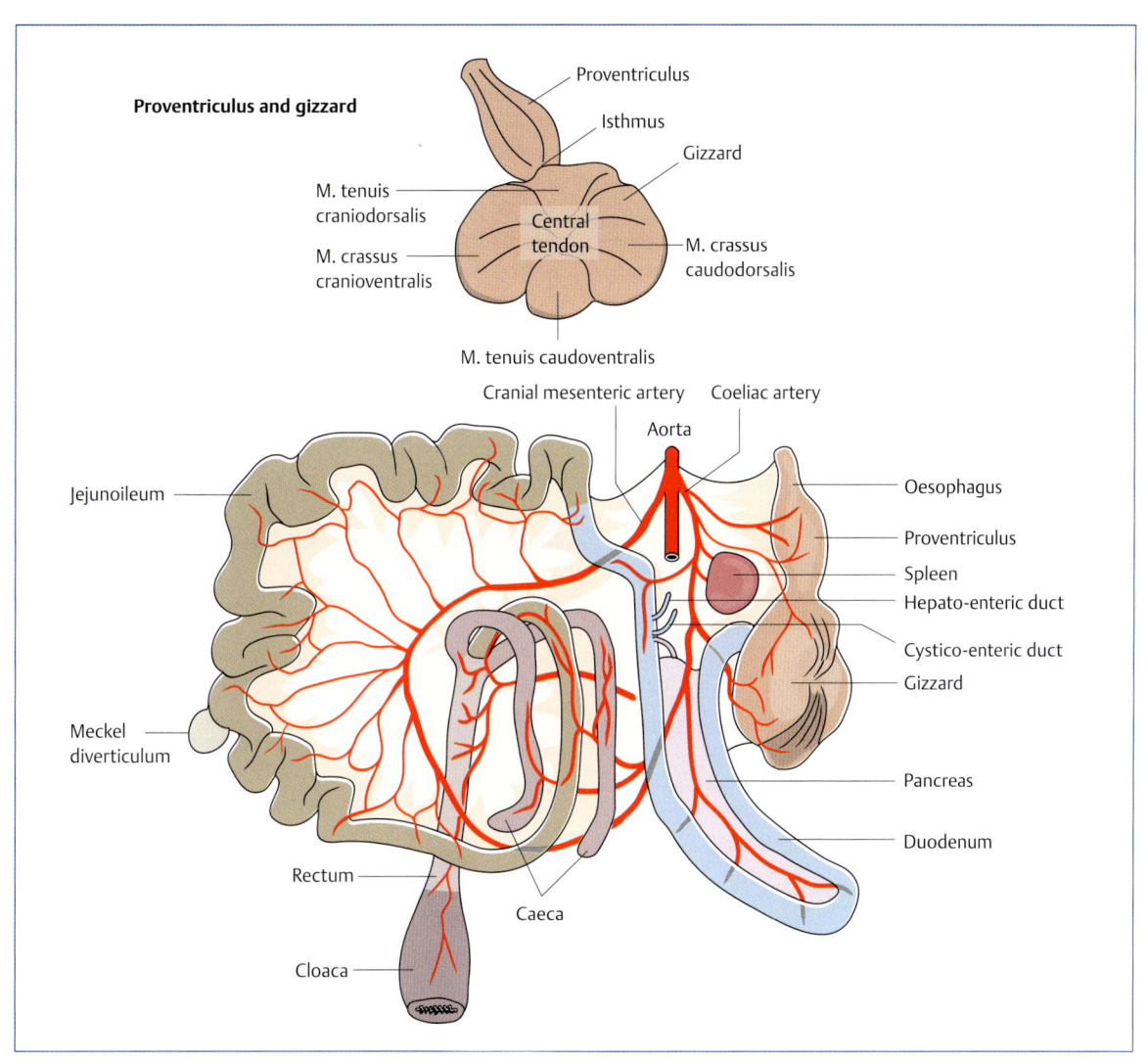

Proventriculus and gizzard

Proventriculus

Isthmus

Gizzard

M. tenuis craniodorsalis

Central tendon

M. crassus cranioventralis

M. crassus caudodorsalis

M. tenuis caudoventralis

Cranial mesenteric artery   Coeliac artery

Aorta

Jejunoileum

Oesophagus

Proventriculus

Spleen

Hepato-enteric duct

Cystico-enteric duct

Gizzard

Meckel diverticulum

Pancreas

Duodenum

Rectum

Caeca

Cloaca

Fig. 16.83 Structure of the digestive system in the domestic chicken.

rates compared to those processes in mammals. At the same time, most avian species depend on frequent feeding to meet their energy needs.

Weight reduction of the digestive tract begins at the very beginning of the digestive tract with the beak. This is a light-weight, but highly sensitive and efficient tool for food intake. Although the beak is partly a substitute for teeth, the ingested food cannot be crushed to the same extent as chewing can in mammals. A soft palate is absent in birds. A hard palate is present, but there is an open connection between the mouth and the nasal cavity, the **choanal cleft**. Under physiological conditions, the choanal cleft is closed reflexively when liquid or solid food is ingested. This closure is not guaranteed in the anaesthetised bird, which must be taken into account when administering substances into the crop. The tongue is essential as an organ of touch and for the transport of food, but its importance as an organ of taste is less significant. The importance of the tongue in food intake differs between the various avian species. In water-fowl the tongue is muscular with horn-like lamellae or projections formed on the surface to help hold food and transport it to the oesophagus.

Parrots also have a very muscular tongue with which they can bring soft food and also liquids into the mouth.

The **act of swallowing** is partially assisted in the bird by raising and lowering the head so that gravity assists the passage of liquid or solid food into the oesophagus.

In birds, the **oesophagus** is on the right side of the neck, which must be considered when administering medication or food into the crop. Since food is swallowed unchewed, the oesophagus of the bird has a larger volume than that of mammals. Peristaltic or antiperistaltic movements of the oesophageal muscles can transport food towards the crop and stomach as well as towards the beak cavity. The latter plays a role particularly in the feeding of offspring.

■ Crop

Another special feature of the avian digestive system is the crop (ingluvies) as a diverticulum of the oesophagus. A distinction is made between storage crops and secretory crops (especially in pigeons). In domestic poultry, the crop is functionally a **storage organ** in which ingested feed remains before later processing. The use of the crop as a feed store depends on the state of filling of the gizzard. Filling of the crop with more food only begins when the gizzard is at least partially filled. The storage of food in the crop and its subsequent emptying helps to sustain digestive and absorptive functions in distal regions of the digestive tract during periods of high or no food intake. Food is released in small portions from the crop to the middle and lower digestive tract resulting in better feed utilisation. Enzyme digestion of food can also begin in the crop with local amylase activity. However, since largely uncrushed food collects in the crop, the enzymatic activity here is not nearly as efficient as in the small intestine. Because of its location cranial to the stomach and small intestine, the crop mucosa does not contribute substantially to the absorption of nutrients. Nevertheless, some absorption of amino acids, sugars and vitamins from the crop has been observed. The absorption of pharmaceuticals after administration into the crop is also of clinical relevance.

The **secretory crop** in pigeons supplies young hatchling birds with food. This functional specialisation of the crop begins during the breeding season when the crop epithelium begins to produce **crop milk**. This is a white, semi-solid secretion containing about 74% water, 12% proteins, 9% fats and 1.4% ash. There is no carbohydrate or calcium in crop milk.

> MORE DETAILS   Tip: Relatively large amounts of food, such as 20 ml/kg bw, can be administered into the crop of ornamental birds. However, the crop is a very thin-walled organ, so such food input must be done very carefully and under proper constraint of the bird, as crop perforation can happen quickly and is often not immediately detected. Food that is too hot can also cause perforation by damaging the sensitive crop wall.

■ Stomach

The stomach of a bird is divided into two parts, a **glandular stomach**, the **proventriculus**, and the **gizzard** (ventriculus muscularis). The gizzard joins the glandular stomach caudally and is connected to it by a narrow **isthmus**. The separation between the two compartments is particularly clear in herbivorous species, where food digestion is much more complex. In carnivorous species, the distinction is less clear, and the isthmus is also less pronounced. The glandular stomach has the same function as the monogastric stomach in mammals, i.e. hydrochloric acid and pepsinogen are secreted there. The secretion rates in the glandular stomach of birds are many times greater than those in the monogastric stomach of mammals. This is related to the faster rate of transit through the gastrointestinal tract of birds compared to mammals (i.e., higher secretion rates could speed up the digestive process to compensate for the shorter transit time). In broilers, the retention time of solid food in the two stomach compartments is just over half an hour, and in the entire small intestine and the final regions of the intestine about three hours each.

Hydrochloric acid and pepsinogen secretion is particularly important in fish-catching and carnivorous bird species, i.e. in animals with a high protein intake. In those species, however, the food also has a relatively long retention time in the glandular stomach (sometimes several days). This long retention time is necessary to ensure denaturation and digestion of the non-macerated, protein-rich food. While protein-rich food is being digested in the glandular stomach, some of the contents are continuously passing into the small intestine.

The low pH of the glandular stomach also protects against colonisation of the distal gastrointestinal tract by pathogenic microorganisms.

After storage and digestion in the glandular stomach, the food passes into the gizzard. There is no secretion of digestive enzymes in the gizzard, but the enzymatic digestion of proteins, which began in the acidic environment of the glandular stomach, continues here to some extent, as the luminal pH is not significantly increased until the contents mix with pancreatic secretion in the small intestine. The main function of the gizzard is the mechanical comminution of ingested food. For this purpose, depending on the species, stomach stones (**grit**) are present in the lumen. The gizzard also has a koilin lining layer, produced by the epithelial cells. This has an abrasive action on food particles. Grit is particularly important in granivorous species such as domestic poultry that do not fragment food during ingestion.

Motility of the gizzard is particularly well developed in granivores. The stomach wall consists of four muscle regions (**Fig. 16.83**). The two thinner muscle parts (mm. tenuis craniodorsalis and caudoventralis) are mainly concerned with propelling the gizzard contents into the duodenum. While these two muscles are contracting, the isthmus is closed, and the pylorus is open. As in mammals, well-fragmented food enters the small intestine during the emptying phase. The pylorus then closes again, the isthmus opens, and the contents of the gizzard are pushed back into the glandular stomach by contraction of the thick muscle regions (mm. crassus cranoventralis and caudodorsalis). Part of the contents remain in the gizzard and are further broken down there. The motility cycle ends with the contraction of the glandular stomach and the subsequent transport of chyme into the gizzard.

In carnivorous avian species, where the gizzards are less developed, this motility cycle is not so pronounced. Here, essentially peristaltic waves transport the contents of the glandular stomach through the gizzard into the small intestine.

In addition to these relatively simple transport processes, the **pelleting** of indigestible material such as fur and feathers by high-frequency, powerful contractions of the gizzard is pronounced in carnivorous species. These pellets are ultimately transported into the oesophagus and towards the beak by antiperistaltic waves.

As in mammals, **motility** is under **neurological control** with inhibition of motility by the sympathetic nervous system and promotion of contractions by parasympathetic action. Nerve cells of the enteric nervous system also seem to play a role in this. Damage to the myenteric plexus leads to a marked reduction in contractions. A clinically relevant example is in infection of nerve plexus by bornavirus in parrots, the consequence of which is a lack of contractility and subsequently dilatation of the glandular stomach. This has given the disease the name of proventricular dilatation disease. Dilatation can be seen radiographically.

■ Small intestine

The main site of digestion and absorption is the small intestine, as in mammals. Anatomically, the different regions of the small intestine are not as well differentiated in birds as in mammals. The avian small intestine is thus divided into **duodenum** and **jejunoileum**. The profile of enzymes, expressed or secreted by the small intestinal epithelium and pancreas is comparable to that of mammals. However, lactase is not produced, so digestion of lactose in the small intestine is not possible in birds. The breakdown of fats, carbohydrates and proteins by pancreatic enzymes is comparable to that in mammals. Consequently, an insufficiency of the exocrine pancreas in birds also manifests itself with similar symptoms as steatorrhoea in dogs (p. 449). The secretion rate of digestive enzymes is higher in the fasting bird than in the mammal. Thus, in contrast to the crop (with its comparatively low amylase activity), starch digestion in the small intestine is highly efficient. This is due both to the higher secretion rate of amylase compared to mammals such as pigs and humans and to the high activity of avian amylase which is about three times higher in broilers than in weaned piglets.

Absorption of the digestion products is also very efficient in birds, not because of higher efficiency of membrane transport proteins compared to other animal classes, but because many essential nutrients in birds, especially glucose, seem to cross the intestinal barrier mainly via the paracellular route.

This efficient absorption of nutrients compensates for the significantly smaller absorptive surface area due to the short intestinal length compared to mammals. The shorter length and lower mass of the gastrointestinal tract helps to keep its weight low in flight-capable avian species. However, there are differences between species in terms of gut length. Carnivores, insectivores and frugivores have relatively short intestines. Herbivorous species, including grain-eaters, have longer intestines.

■ Caecum, rectum and cloaca

The small intestine connects to the two **caeca** and also to the **rectum** and **cloaca**. The twin caeca have various functions. Water, electrolytes and short-chain fatty acids are absorbed there. The latter are produced by microbial conversion of carbohydrates that are difficult to digest by endogenous enzymes. However, this microbial fermentation is substantially less than that in typical mammalian hindgut fermentation (horses/rabbits) (ch. 16.7.2 (p. 438)). The caecum, and thus its digestive processes, are also not well developed in all bird species. Parrots and many pigeons have no caecum, and in many passerine birds the caecum is only rudimentary. This is probably explained by the fact that many bird species forego an efficient conversion of cellulose (which requires a voluminous caecum) in favour of their ability to fly.

A further function of the caeca is in nitrogen recycling. In birds, the uric acid released into the cloaca enters the caeca through antiperistaltic waves and is there available to the resident microorganisms for the production of protein and the corresponding build-up of amino acids (ch. 14.1.3 (p. 463)).

> **IN A NUTSHELL**   **!**
>
> Digestion in birds is similar to that of mammals, but even more efficient. Special features of avian digestion are food storage in the crop, comminution in the gizzard and nitrogen recycling by reflux of uric acid from the cloaca into the rectum.

16.10.2 Digestion in reptiles

■ Food intake and teeth

An essential feature that distinguishes the digestive activity of reptiles from that of birds and mammals is their ectothermic lifestyle. As a result, the energy requirements of reptiles vary greatly according to the ambient temperature. Their food intake and the activities of their alimentary tract adapt to these requirements.

The technique of feeding and the teeth structure varies with reptile species. **Turtles**, both herbivorous and omnivorous or carnivorous, do not have teeth, but break up their food with the help of their continuously growing cornified beak. Deformities of the jaws and beak (congenital, due to deficiency diseases or trauma) have significant consequences for the functionality of the beak, as well as its regular wear.

Crocodiles, lizards and snakes have **teeth**, but they differ in various ways from each other and in the case of lizard and snakes from those of mammals (**Fig. 16.84**).

The teeth of **crocodiles** are similar to those of mammals. They are anchored in the jaw but lack a surrounding periodontium. This type of tooth is called a **thekodont** and is only found in crocodiles.

The teeth of **lizards** can be classified as acrodont or pleurodont. They serve both to grasp prey or plant food and to crush it. **Acrodont teeth** are found in chameleons or agamas. These are relatively simple, conically shaped teeth that are fixed on the biting edge of the upper and lower jaw. In contrast to pleurodont teeth, acrodont teeth are not replaced. **Pleurodont teeth** are also rather simple in their structure. They are fixed to the jawbone in such a way that the labial side of the bone partially covers the teeth, while the lingual side is lower. Pleurodont teeth are continuously replaced throughout life and are found mainly in iguanas and monitor lizards. However, there are also many species in which the tooth forms are mixed, and in which rostral teeth can be replaced.

MORE DETAILS   Dental problems such as periodontitis occur especially with acrodont teeth. Also tooth wear in older animals (agamas, chameleons) can leave only tooth stumps or even only the bone bars remaining.

Nutrition, energy

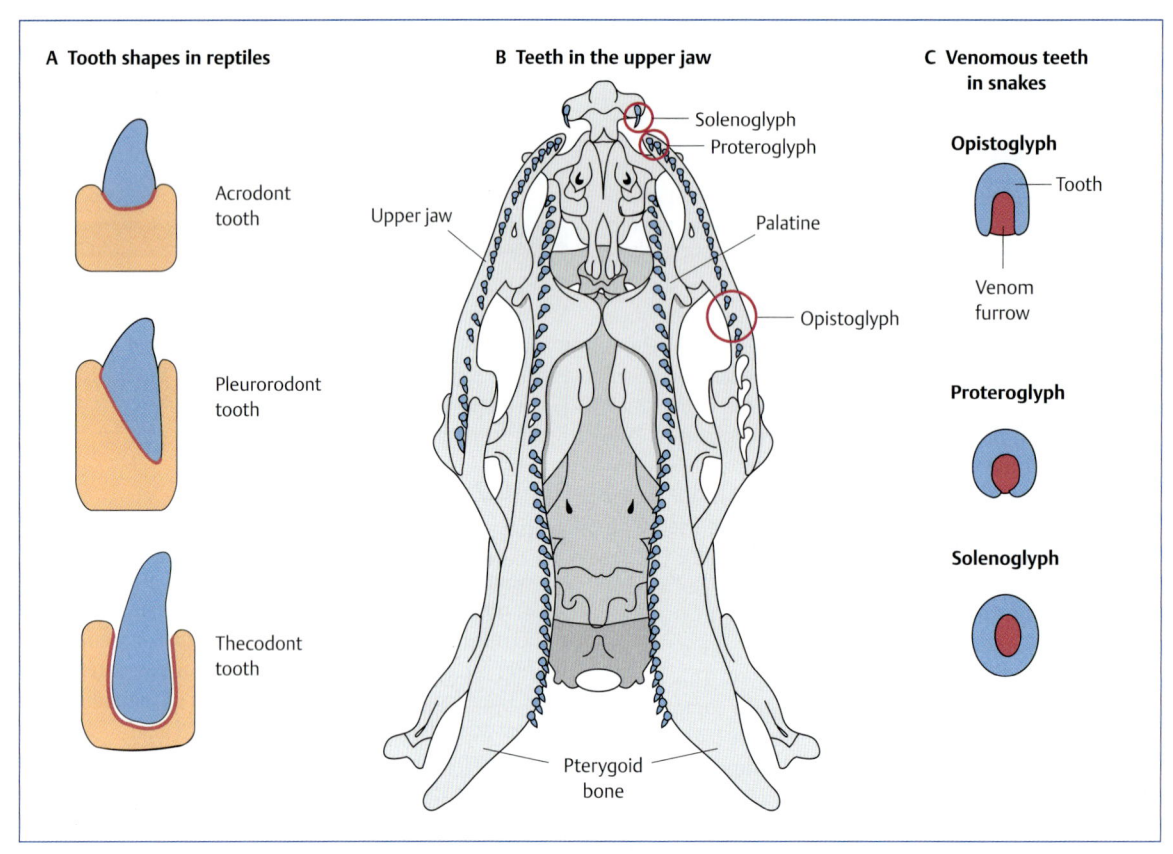

A Tooth shapes in reptiles

Acrodont tooth

Pleurorodont tooth

Thecodont tooth

B Teeth in the upper jaw

Solenoglyph

Proteroglyph

Upper jaw

Palatine

Opistoglyph

Pterygoid bone

C Venomous teeth in snakes

Opistoglyph

Tooth

Venom furrow

Proteroglyph

Solenoglyph

Fig. 16.84
A Reptiles can have different tooth shapes. The teeth are either superficially attached to the jaw (acrodont and pleurodont teeth) or sunk into bone pockets (thecodont teeth). The tooth attachment is shown schematically in red.
B Snakes have four rows of teeth in the upper jaw. The red circles mark the positions where the venomous teeth are located in different venom snakes.
C To introduce the venom into the prey, the venomous teeth have either a furrow or a central channel.

Snakes, like some lizards, have **pleurodont teeth**. However, snakes do not use teeth to cut up food, as they swallow their prey whole. Snake teeth thus essentially serve to fix the food in place and are therefore oriented caudally. Snakes have four rows of teeth in the upper jaw and two rows of teeth in the lower jaw.

There are **venomous species** of **snakes** as well as a few venomous **lizard species**. The **venom glands** in both families are **modified salivary glands** located in the region of the jaws. In lizards (*Heloderma* spp.), the sublingual glands are responsible for venom production. In snakes, venom is produced by modified labial glands.

The teeth of poisonous snakes are a special feature. Here the different snake species can be divided into three groups (Fig. 16.84):

- **Opisthoglyphs** have fangs located in the posterior pharynx. These teeth are enlarged and have a furrow along which the venom is directed into the prey during the swallowing act. An example is the mangrove snake (*Boiga dendrophila*). Opistoglyphs are mostly harmless and only relatively weakly poisonous.
- **Proteroglyphs** on the other hand, are often highly venomous. Their fangs are located in the front of the mouth. They are also enlarged and furrowed and serve to fix the prey as well as to inject the poison. Cobras (*Naja*), mam-

bas (*Dendroaspis*), kraits (*Bungarus*), taipans (*Oxyuranus*), coral snakes (*Micrurus*) and sea snakes belong to the proteroglyphs.

- **Solenoglyphs** also have the fangs in the front of the mouth. However, these are movable and equipped with a thin tube for introducing the venom into the prey. The fangs can fold into the mouth when not in use. In this state, introduction of venom into the tooth is interrupted as the duct leading to it is compressed. When the mouth is opened, the fangs fold forward and the supply duct between the venom glands and the fangs opens. Because solenoglyphs can open their mouths extremely wide (almost 180 degrees), they can also attack large prey. Rattlesnakes (*Crotalus*) are typical examples of solenoglyphs.

Snake venoms have a variety of actions. Venom composition differs between species and sometimes also between animals of the same species, but of different ages. Usually, venom is a mixture of different toxins. Many of these mixtures contain neurotoxic components that often have an effect on cholinergic neurotransmission (p. 148). The effect here can be either a postsynaptic inhibition of acetylcholine action (α-bungarotoxin, cobratoxin, κ-bungarotoxin) or a presynaptic inhibition (β-bungarotoxin, crotoxin, taipoxin) or enhancement of acetylcholine release (dendrotoxin). Ultimately, these **neurotoxic components** lead to paralysis of the prey animal. Other significant effects are irreversible depolarisation of cardiac muscle cells by **cardiotoxins** and the induction of haemorrhage. The latter can occur both through vascular damage by so-called **haemorrhagins** and by initiating disseminated intravascular coagulopathy (p.240). Essential components of snake venoms are always a range of **enzymes**. These can be partly responsible for the effects mentioned, but also lead to **necrosis** of the musculature and initiate tissue **digestion** in various ways. In this respect, venom injection and distribution into the live prey is a component of nutritional strategy for many venomous snake species.

The **swallowing** of the prey as a whole is a challenge for the snake's digestive system, as even large prey can be ingested without first being crushed. The prey is always ingested head first. The snake's mouth can also handle large prey because the upper and lower jaws are only connected by connective tissue. By alternately using both halves of the jaws, the jaws are pushed over the prey. During the act of swallowing and transporting the food towards the stomach, it is not so much the musculature of the **oesophagus** that plays a role, but the rhythmic contraction of the entire surrounding musculature in the front part of the body. The prey is thus pushed inward, piece by piece, internal organs such as the heart are suspended so flexibly that they can be displaced by the intake of a prey animal.

Especially large prey does not necessarily enter the stomach completely during the swallowing process. The transition between the wide-lumen oesophagus and the stomach is not closed by a cardia. The oesophagus can already start to digest the animal being consumed. It serves as a reservoir from which the food gradually slides into the small-lumened, but extremely flexible stomach. During this process, considerable displacement of the stomach and especially the intestinal tract occurs with each meal, and there is adaptation of the heart activity and blood circulation to this sudden, extremely increased oxygen demand (p.216).

■ Stomach

The stomach in reptiles is of simple construction and secretes pepsinogen and hydrochloric acid just like the stomach of mammals and the glandular stomach of birds. In carnivorous reptiles in particular, acid production and thus intragastric pH can fluctuate greatly depending on food intake. For many reptiles, an intragastric pH of 2–2.5 is normal, although the pH can rise to 7 during the resting phase in snakes and then drop rapidly to a value of 2 as prey is ingested.

In carnivorous snakes, the stomach is the least clearly differentiated from the oesophagus and duodenum, and the cardia is barely developed. Therefore, snakes also often vomit their prey, especially if external factors are stressful to the reptile (e.g. noise, other animals, sudden changes in climate, especially temperature). The stomach of snakes is atrophic, strongly pleated and very small in the resting state but expands to the maximum with the ingestion of prey. Through remodelling processes, the stomach and in-

testinal mucosa prepare for digestion in a very short time. In contrast, herbivorous reptiles feed daily and depend on a continuously working gastrointestinal tract, which only remodels itself during longer periods of physiological rest (hibernation). In crocodiles, part of the stomach is highly muscular and lined with a keratinised epithelium to break down food. The animal also ingests stones to aid digestion by grinding the gut contents.

■ Intestine

The intestinal tract fulfils the same essential functions as in mammals and birds. In general, the gastrointestinal tract of carnivorous species is shorter and the transit time of contents is faster. In herbivorous species, distal fermentation chambers (colon or caecum) are present and food digestion and absorption can take a considerable time of several weeks. Especially in herbivorous turtles, the colon can be very voluminous as a fermentation chamber and the food is subjected to longer fermentative processes there. Of clinical relevance in tortoises is the transition to the descending colon, where there is a constriction that only allows appropriately digested and fragmented food to pass. At this point, especially when stones and foreign bodies are ingested, but also due to excessive water absorption from the intestinal contents, disturbances in onward transport often occur, which lead to intestinal stasis and constipation. This constriction is then often visible radiologically (**Fig. 16.85**).

The **cloaca** in reptiles as in birds is divided into several anatomical-functional regions. The **coprodaeum** is the region where faeces are formed. The **urodaeum** is where the ureters and possibly the **oviduct** enter, and the terminal

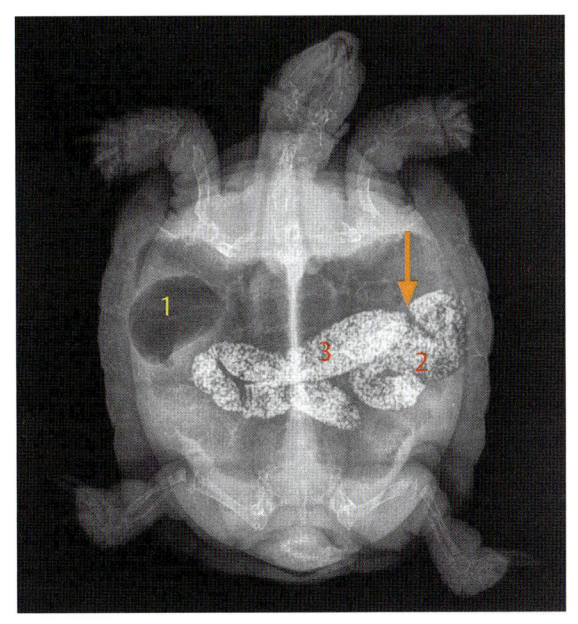

Fig. 16.85 X-ray of a tortoise with constipation in the colon after ingestion of numerous stones (**1** stomach, **2** ascending colon, **3** transverse colon). The cause of the stone ingestion is probably a chronic calcium deficiency, which is also evident in the bone calcification (arrow, constriction). [Source: Prof. Dr. Michael Pees, Klinik für Heimtiere, Reptilien und Vögel, Stiftung TiHo Hannover]

Nutrition, energy

region is the **proctodaeum**. The cloacal mucosa plays an important role in water absorption, especially in species living in dry climates, both for absorbing residual water from faeces and urine and also for direct absorption of external water through the cloacal opening. Some species, especially turtles, but also many lizards have developed a urinary sac as a protrusion of the cloaca – this is also of great importance in water balance (for water storage and also for absorption of water into the circulating blood). Finally, the cloacal mucosa also has a function of absorbing oxygen from water in aquatic species, especially when oxygen demand is reduced. In some reptile species, scent glands are located in the cloaca. Finally, male animals have paired (snakes, lizards, located behind the cloaca) or unpaired (turtles, crocodiles, intracloacal) copulatory organs, which exit the cloaca when filled with lymph and conduct the semen in channels.

■ Liver and pancreas

The liver is comparatively large in reptiles and varies greatly in shape depending on the species. In snakes, it is elongated, and the gall bladder is caudal to the liver in the abdominal cavity. Biliverdin is the main metabolic product of bile. The pancreas is attached to the duodenum and is also differently developed but similar in function to that of mammals.

■ Digestive peculiarities in reptiles

In general, the energy demand of reptiles is lower than that of mammals. However, both energy demand and energy intake (through food intake and conversion of food into metabolisable energy) greatly depend on the body temperature of reptiles. Therefore, these animals seek an environment with a temperature range that allows them to maintain a preferred body temperature. That temperature is in the range of mammalian body temperature, i.e. over 35 °C, depending on the species. Not only do the activities of these animals depend on this internal body temperature, but at the same time the digestive activity (mechanical as well as enzymatic) is directly dependent on body temperature. These activities are significantly reduced when internal body temperature is below 15 °C and they come to a standstill at temperatures below about 7 °C.

> **MORE DETAILS** An optimal body temperature is essential not only for well-being, but also for the functioning of the immune system and digestion. A reduction in temperature by 10 °C means a halving of metabolic activity with correspondingly dramatic

consequences for the reptile. Their preferred temperature is above 30 °C, so keeping the animals at room temperature (without providing "hotspots", i.e. heat islands above 40 °C to raise body temperature) inevitably leads to health problems.

The frequency of **food intake** depends on the type of food. In **herbivorous species**, the precrushing of food is essential when biting off plant material (a crushing chewing method as in many mammals is not found in reptiles.). Like mammals, the food of herbivorous reptiles must also contain sufficient fibrous components to be digested in the colon. As this is a lengthy process, feed intake is relatively continuous to ensure that the microbial population for fermentative processing is maintained. In **carnivorous species**, and especially in snakes, the digestive physiology is designed for intermittent peak performance with long resting phases. Thus, after ingestion of the prey, the digestive tract increases enormously in size (by about 100%), and the heart also enlarges greatly. After digestion is complete, the whole system undergoes involution to a resting mode, which can then last for months.

In **insectivorous reptiles**, digestion of the exoskeleton is a particular challenge. In many species, special enzymes are secreted by the stomach and pancreas to break down chitin into acetylglucosamines.

> **IN A NUTSHELL**   !
>
> The energy and thus food requirements of reptiles are greatly dependent on ambient temperature. This also applies to the internal body temperature for digestive processes to function. Food intake and digestion differ considerably between species. Herbivorous reptiles tend to eat continuously, whereas carnivores such as snakes take very long breaks between episodes of feeding.

Suggested reading

Moyes CD, Schulte PM. Principles of Animal physiology. Pearson; 2008

O'Malley B. Clinical Anatomy and Physiology of Exotic Species: Structure and Function of Mammals, Birds, Reptiles and Amphibians. Balliere Tindall; 2005

Scanes CG, Dridi S. Sturkie's Avian Physiology. Philadelphia: Elsevier; 2021

Starck J, Beese K. Structural flexibility of the small intestine and liver of garter snakes in response to feeding and fasting. The Journal of experimental biology 2002; 205: 1377–1388

17   Physiological functions of the liver

Herbert Fuhrmann, Axel Schöniger, Hans-Peter Sallmann

17.1   Role of the liver

ESSENTIALS   ✖

As part of the digestive tract, the liver is a large paren-chymatous organ in the abdominal cavity. It is directly or indirectly involved in most of the metabolic activities throughout the body. Blood is supplied by the nutrient-rich portal vein and also by the hepatic artery. The liver thus has a central role in metabolism of absorbed nu-trients both in storing incoming substrates and synthesis-ing important metabolites such as glucose and lipids. These substrates for whole body energy supply, and also vitamins and trace elements, can be released from the liv-er in a controlled manner. The liver is thus important for energy metabolism and glucose homeostasis of the whole animal. It also produces ketone bodies, lipoproteins and almost all plasma proteins as well as the bile necessary for fat digestion. In addition, the liver breaks down haem and detoxifies toxic metabolic products such as NH_3 (gluta-mate-glutamine cycle, urea cycle), endobiotics and xeno-biotics (biotransformations).

17.2   Role of the liver in body metabolism and functions of different hepatic cells

The liver is of endodermal origin and develops during on-togeny into one of the large parenchymatous organs in do-mestic animals and humans. Through the portal vein sys-tem the liver is in close contact with the gastrointestinal tract (**Fig. 17.1**). Monomeric and low-molecular-weight nutrients as well as major and trace inorganic elements, vi-tamins, pharmaceuticals and xenobiotics absorbed from the intestinal chyme, and not transported by the lymphatic system (thoracic duct), first reach the liver after absorp-tion. In addition to these substances supplied in portal blood, the liver also utilises other metabolites from its ar-terial supply. The liver therefore has a central role in whole body metabolism.

IN A NUTSHELL   !

The liver is the central organ of metabolism. It mainly metabolises low-molecular weight nutrients, pharma-ceuticals and xenobiotics that are absorbed from chyme and are delivered to it in portal vein blood.

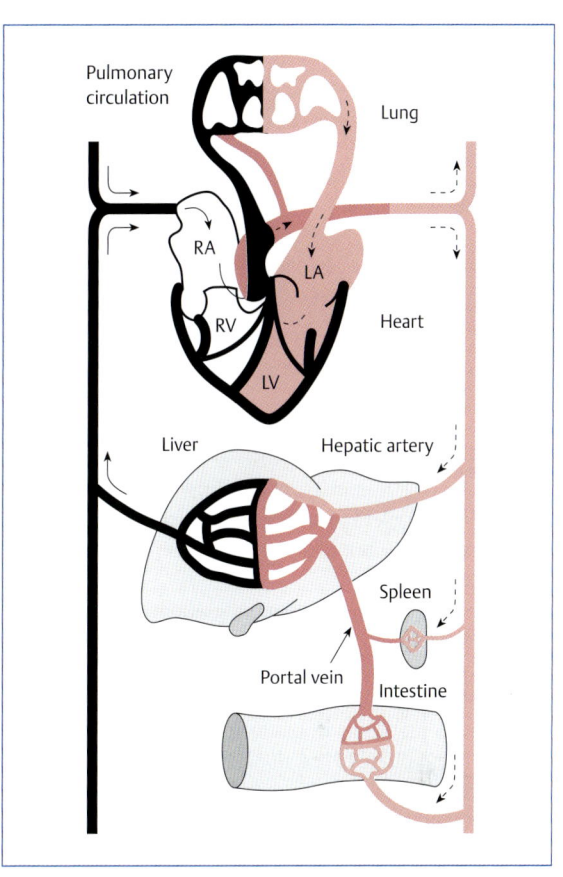

Fig. 17.1 The position of the liver in blood circulation. LA = left atrium; RA = right atrium; LV = left ventricle; RV = right ventricle.

17.2.1   Histological structure of the liver

The physiological functions of the liver are reflected in its microarchitecture, blood supply and bile secretion. Blood from the portal vein (⅔ to ¾ of the total inflow), enriched with nutrients, metabolites and non-nutritional sub-stances from food and the oxygen-rich blood of the a. hepatica enter the sinus zone at the base of the liver aci-nus (**portal triad**). The blood then flows past the **hepato-cellular plates** and out through the **central vein** (Fig. 17.2). The relative proportions of the two inflows are regulated by adenosine. Total blood inflow is controlled by both nervous (sympathetic) and humoral factors (endothelin, NO). The outflow of bile is in the direction of the acinus.

Most hepatic metabolism is performed in parenchymal cells (**hepatocytes**), which make up 60–70% of the cell population of the liver. Their important metabolic func-tions are:

Nutrition, energy

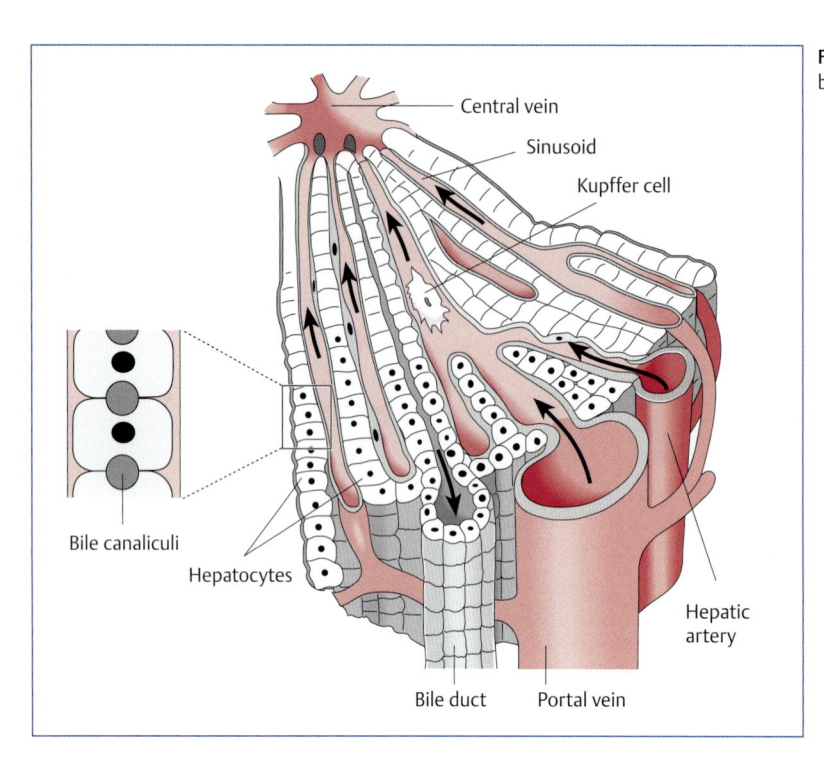

Fig. 17.2 The hepatocellular plate as a basic morphological and functional unit.

Labels in figure: Central vein; Sinusoid; Kupffer cell; Bile canaliculi; Hepatocytes; Hepatic artery; Bile duct; Portal vein

- Partial or complete **metabolism of nutrients** (glycolysis; fatty acid oxidation; complete oxidation of substrates to CO_2 and H_2O),
- **Synthesis** of **energy supplying metabolites** and **proteins** (gluconeogenesis, ketogenesis, and glycogen, lipid and lipoprotein synthesis),
- **Detoxification** (ammonia fixation; urea formation and glutamine metabolism; biotransformation with phase I, phase II and phase III reactions),
- **Bile acid synthesis**, bile formation and excretion.

The liver's role in secreting proteins and lipoproteins into plasma, and the components of bile (bile acids and bile pigments) into the bile duct system characterise the liver as a secreting gland.

> **IN A NUTSHELL** !
>
> Microarchitecture, blood supply, innervation and bile flow determine the metabolic function of the liver. The most important metabolic processes are in the parenchymal cells or hepatocytes.

Although the parenchymal cells appear histologically to be homogeneous, they show pronounced heterogeneity in their metabolic functions. Histochemical and retroportal perfusion studies, and microdissection all indicate that the metabolic pathways differ according to the microcirculation in the liver acinus in the **periportal** or in the **perivenous hepatocytes**. In Table 17.1, important functions of the liver and their location zone are listed. Gluconeogenesis, amino acid metabolism and fatty acid oxidation take place in the periportal region, while glycolysis, lipogenesis and some glycogen synthesis are mainly in perivenous hepatocytes.

An important support of the high metabolic activity in the periportal zone is the union of the nutrient-rich portal blood flow with the oxygen-rich arterial blood of the a. hepatica at the base of the hepatic acinus (**Fig. 17.2**). The high O_2 partial pressure, the abundant supply of nutrients and also the influx of hormones in the periportal region increase the activity of enzymes of **gluconeogenesis**, mitochondrial oxidation processes and synthesis of cholesterol and bile acids. The main perivenous metabolic pathways of **glycolysis** and **lipogenesis** are largely independent of oxygen supply and depend primarily on the perivenous supply of glucose.

The periportal location of the antioxidative enzyme, glutathione peroxidase, is beneficial because oxidative stress to liver cells is most likely in this region because of high oxygen concentrations. In contrast, the mostly oxygen-independent conversions of **biotransformation** (phase II reaction) such as glucuronidation and glutathione conjugation are mainly in the perivenous zone of the liver.

> **IN A NUTSHELL** !
>
> The metabolic functions of the liver are largely in defined zones. The metabolic processes of gluconeogenesis, urea synthesis and oxidation are located periportally, while glycolysis, fatty acid synthesis and glutamine synthesis predominate perivenously.

Table 17.1 Important functions of the liver in the periportal (**pp**) and perivenous (**pv**) zones.

Key metabolic activities	Metabolic processes
Carbohydrate metabolism	Gluconeogenesis (pp), glycogen synthesis, glycogenolysis, glycolysis (pv), fructose and galactose utilisation
Amino acid and protein metabolism	Degradation of amino acids, urea synthesis (pp), synthesis of glutamine (pv), creatine, glutathione, plasma proteins (coagulation factors, factors of fibrinolysis, transport proteins, apolipoproteins)
Lipid metabolism	Fatty acid oxidation (pp), ketogenesis (pp), biosynthesis of cholesterol (pp) synthesis of fatty acids (pv), triacylglycerols and phospholipids, synthesis and degradation of lipoproteins, ketogenesis
Storage functions	Glycogen and lipid storage, storage of fat-soluble vitamins (retinol: stellate cells), cobalamin, folic acid, copper, iron (iron homeostasis)
Synthesis and secretion of bile acids (pp), bile formation	–
Erythrocyte degradation	–
Biotransformation	Detoxification, inactivation, bioactivation of drugs, conversion into water-soluble/reactive compounds, excretion of endogenous (bilirubin, steroid, thyroid hormones) and exogenous substances (drugs)
Synthesis of hormones and mediators	IGF-1, IGF-2, erythropoietin, thrombopoietin, angiotensinogen, 25-hydroxylation of calciferol, conversion of T4 to T3
Defence functions	Synthesis of complement factors, acute phase proteins, phagocytosis (Kupffer cells), NK activity (pit cells)

17.2.2 Cell types

In addition to the large proportion of metabolically active hepatocytes, there are two other cell types in the liver, representing up to 30% of all cells. These are **endothelial cells** and **Kupffer cells** which make up the patchy single-layer endothelial wall (**discontinuous endothelium; Fig. 8.16**), separating the sinusoidal space of the sinusoidal capillaries from the perisinusoidal space (= Dissé space) directly connected to the parenchymal cells. In the sinusoidal capillaries there are intercellular gaps with a width of 0.6–3 μm, which also have a basement membrane. These gaps allow the passage of solutes (e.g. glucose, amino acids) and macromolecules (e.g. proteins) as well as molecular aggregates (e.g. lipoproteins), but not blood cells. The Kupffer cells can be regarded as sedentary macrophages They fulfil immunological functions in the liver. They remove corpuscular antigens from portal blood by phagocytosis, thus preventing their entry into the liver parenchyma. Kupffer cells comprise about 50% of total vascular endothelium, indicating their functional importance, and they represent the largest macrophage subpopulation of the animal. Their arrangement in the periportal region of the hepatic acinus is of particular importance because of the large number of foreign particles and old erythrocytes in the adjacent portal blood. The arrangement of Kupffer cells also complies with the zoning structure of the liver.

Stellate (Ito) cells and pit cells account for no more than 5% of the total cell population of the liver. Both cell types are localised in the Dissé space. **Stellate cells** synthesise collagen and laminin as components of the extracellular matrix. They have a special function of storing a large proportion of the total fat-soluble vitamin A in the body. They

are also classified as modified adipocytes. **Pit cells** are similar to Kupffer cells and act as "**natural killer cells**", protecting against viral infections and metastasising tumour cells.

17.2.3 Regulation of liver function

> **IN A NUTSHELL** !
>
> The regulation of liver functions is very complex, with both nervous and humoral agents (metabolites, hormones) being important regulators.

The efferent **nervous regulators** from the hypothalamus transmit sympathetic signals, which cause release of metabolites from the liver into the circulation. Parasympathetic signals suppress the release of these hepatic products. Afferent nerves in the hepatic branch of the vagus nerve and also spinal afferent nerves carry information about metabolites and hormones to the hypothalamus. Since complete denervation of the liver, as occurs with transplantation of this organ, does not lead to liver dysfunction, the neurological influence on liver function is of secondary importance.

The importance of hormonal regulation is certainly the most significant influence on liver cell function, as they have a multitude of membrane hormone receptors, including those for glucagon, insulin, somatotropic hormone, antidiuretic hormone (perivenous), and various growth factors. Intracellular receptors also have important roles. Activator protein-1 and nuclear factor-κB are crucial for the role of the liver in inflammatory processes. Transcription is likewise influenced by carbohydrate and sterol regulatory element binding proteins. From the steroid hor-

Nutrition, energy

mone receptor family, the liver X receptor, the constitutive androstane receptor, the pregnane X receptor and farnesoid X receptor as well as the peroxisome proliferator-activated receptor-α with their different ligands (fatty acids, bile salts, steroid hormones, oxosterols, etc.) are of great importance.

17.3   The contribution of the liver to intestinal digestion

Through the formation of bile, the liver has a significant role in intestinal fat digestion. The bile secreted by the liver is stored and concentrated in the gallbladder. Exceptions include the horse, camel, deer, rat and pigeon, which all lack a gall bladder. The most important components of bile, making up approx. 10%, are bile acids and bile pigments. Bile acids (p. 421) are necessary for lipid absorption in the small intestine, and regulate absorption of dietary cholesterol and de novo synthesis of cholesterol.

17.3.1   Synthesis and function of bile acids

The most important bile acids are **glycocholic** and **taurocholic acids**. They are synthesised from cholesterol in liver cells. First, cholesterol is hydroxylated, hydrogenated and a C3 fragment is cleaved off, resulting in chenodeoxycholic acid. A further hydroxylation then produces cholic acid (**Fig. 17.3**). The resulting acids have a pK_a value of 5. They are activated with coenzyme A and ATP and react with the amino acids glycine or taurine to form the effective bile acids, with pK_a values of 2–3. Conjugation with amino acids is functionally of great importance, as only in this way can optimal dissociation, and thus an **emulsifying action**, occur at pH 7–8 in the small intestine. In the gallbladder, bile acids, together with phosphatidylcholine, solubilise cholesterol in bile.

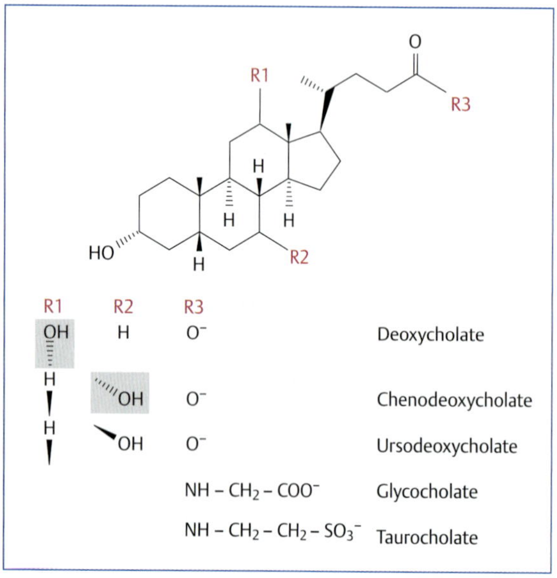

MORE DETAILS   **Ursodeoxycholic acid** is of medical importance and is found in the bile of bears (ursus = lat. bear). The chemical difference to chenodeoxycholic acid is small; the hydroxyl group on the 7th C-atom is in the α-position. In ancient China, dried bear bile has been used in the treatment of liver disorders. In recent decades, this bile acid, which can now be synthesised, has found its way into the treatment of liver diseases. Ursodeoxycholic acid is used, among other things, to dissolve gallstones due to its cholesterol-lowering effect.

A disturbed composition of bile due to faulty function of the liver can lead to the precipitation of cholesterol, so that **gallstones (white stones)** develop. They sometimes also contain bile pigments and Ca^{2+} salts of long-chain fatty acids (yellow and black stones). This metabolic disturbance, frequently observed in humans, occurs rather rarely in domestic animals. In small animals such aggregations in the gall bladder are mainly in the form of a sludge.

> **IN A NUTSHELL**   !
>
> Bile acids are synthesised from cholesterol. When conjugated with glycine or taurine bile acids are effective detergents.

The functions of conjugated bile acids in fat digestion and fatty acid absorption in the small intestine are discussed in ch. 16.6.3 (p. 421) and ch. 16.6.6 (p. 429). The conjugated bile acids, after having fulfilled their tasks in fat digestion and absorption, are mainly reabsorbed (p. 433) in the ileum by a Na^+ cotransporter. A small amount of conjugated bile acids enters the large intestine, where they undergo microbial deconjugation. The bile acids are partly absorbed by diffusion in the large intestine, but mostly excreted in faeces. After reabsorption in the ileum, bile acids return to the liver in portal blood, where they are taken up into hepatocytes by Na^+ cotransport (conjugated bile acids) or by diffusion (deconjugated bile acids) and then, mainly through an ATP-dependent bile acid transporter, are again secreted into the bile canaliculi.

> **IN A NUTSHELL**   !
>
> Bile acids are essential for fat digestion, as they participate in intestinal micelle formation and activation of pancreatic lipase. They are reabsorbed from the ileum and undergo a distinct enterohepatic circulation.

17.3.2   Regulation of bile formation and secretion

Regulation of bile production in the liver is a complex process in which the concentration of bile acids in the portal vein blood and the hormone **secretin** influence the secretion rate. Contraction of the gallbladder to empty bile into the duodenum is regulated by **cholecystokinin** (CCK), an intestinal hormone produced in the mucosa of the small intestine.

R1	R2	R3	
OH	H	O^-	Deoxycholate
H	OH	O^-	Chenodeoxycholate
H	OH	O^-	Ursodeoxycholate
		$NH - CH_2 - COO^-$	Glycocholate
		$NH - CH_2 - CH_2 - SO_3^-$	Taurocholate

Fig. 17.3 Structure of bile acids.

17.4 The liver in intermediary metabolism

The liver is in constant exchange of metabolites with other organs. To understand liver physiology, the basic biochemical conversions of intermediary metabolism must be considered. Details of the metabolic processes in hepatocytes and other liver cells can be found in biochemistry textbooks.

17.4.1 Fat synthesis

In addition to adipose tissue, the liver is also capable of synthesising fatty acids and triacylglycerols, but there are considerable differences between animal species. In herbivores, carnivores, and pigs, adipose tissue is the main site of fat synthesis, whereas in poultry, rodents and humans, fat is mainly synthesised in the liver. In addition to NADPH, hepatic fat synthesis uses glucose as substrate, while fatty acid biosynthesis in adipocytes uses either acetate (herbivores) or glucose (dog, pig) as the initial substrate.

After glycolytic degradation of glucose, entry into the fatty acid synthesis pathway is via acetate or acetyl-CoA. Herbivores with forestomachs produce acetate by anaerobic fermentation of ingested plant material. The subsequent steps of fatty acid and triacylglycerol biosynthesis are the same in all species and in both liver and adipose tissue. The cytoplasmic fatty acid synthase multienzyme complex consists of two identical polypeptide chains (approx. 540 kD) and has several catalytic subunits at which the fatty acid molecule is formed. The first product released from the complex is usually palmitic acid with 16 C atoms. Nutritional factors and also various elongases and desaturases determine the range of fatty acids in triacylglycerols. The triacylglycerols themselves are formed by stepwise linking of fatty acids, starting with the central carbon of glycerol.

While the triacylglycerols synthesised in adipose tissue are initially deposited in their site of formation as energy reserves, those that are synthesised in the liver are exported in special lipoproteins.

17.4.2 Synthesis and function of lipoproteins

Synthesis, function and transport of lipoproteins are illustrated in **Fig. 17.4**. Transport of hydrophobic lipids in the aqueous milieu of plasma requires the assistance of particular proteins. For **free fatty acids** this is **albumin** with 6–8 binding sites per protein molecule. Albumin-fatty acid complexes are formed by non-covalent binding of fatty acids. These complexes are particularly important when fatty acids are released from triacylglycerols by hormone-sensitive lipase (HL) in adipose tissue in response to starvation or energy deficiency.

All other lipids are transported in specific **lipoproteins** synthesised in the liver and in the intestinal mucosa. These lipoproteins have micellar structures. There are four lipoprotein classes (**Table 17.2**), defined by their densities, the proportion of different lipid components, protein content, and the properties of the **apolipoproteins**, which except for apolipoprotein A and B48, are synthesised exclusively in the liver. These proteins are both structural components and ligands for receptors or activators of lipid metabolism enzymes.

Dietary fat consists mainly of triacylglycerols, which after emulsification by bile acids and cleavage of fatty acids by pancreatic lipase are absorbed by enterocytes, and then re-esterified with glycerol (**Fig. 16.59**) This triacylglycerol in enterocytes is assembled, along with cholesterol, phospholipids and apolipoprotein B48, into **chylomicrons** and finally exported across the basolateral membrane into the lymphatic thoracic duct, and then into the general circulation.

> ### IN A NUTSHELL !
> The problem of transporting complex water-insoluble lipids in blood is solved by forming micellar-like lipoproteins.

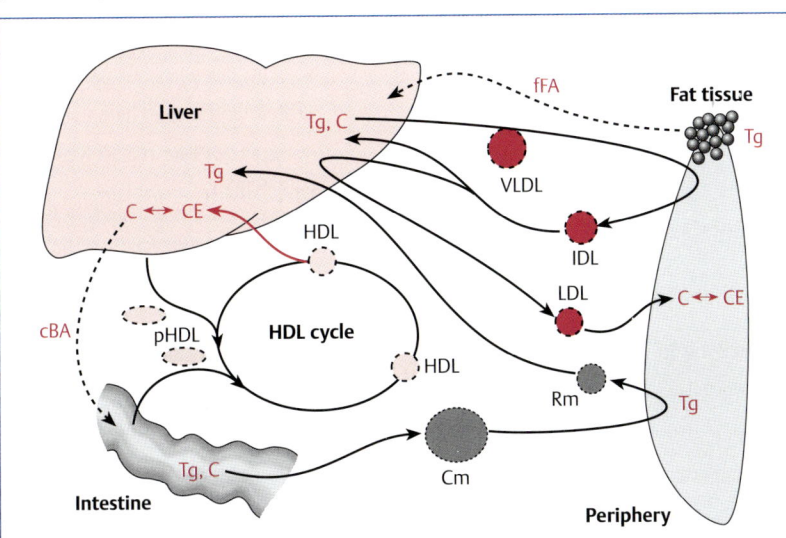

Fig. 17.4 The liver as the central site of lipid and lipoprotein metabolism. Cm: chylomicrons; Rm: chylomicron remnants; VLDL: very low-density lipoproteins; IDL: intermediate-density lipoproteins; LDL: low-density lipoproteins; HDL: high-density lipoproteins; pHDL: primary HDL; C: cholesterol; CE: cholesterol esters; cBA: conjugated bile acids; fFA: free fatty acids; Tg: triacylglycerols.

Nutrition, energy

The **chylomicrons** synthesised in the small intestinal epithelium consist of up to 95% triacylglycerols stabilised by apolipoprotein B48. The **very-low-density lipoproteins** (**VLDL**) contain about 50% triacylglycerols and about equal amounts of cholesterol, phospholipids and proteins. The **low-density lipoproteins** (**LDL**) consist largely of cholesterol (up to 50%), while the **high-density lipoproteins** (**HDL**) are composed of approximately equal parts protein and lipid (**Table 17.2**).

On arrival in capillaries, chylomicrons incorporate apolipoproteins C and E. They are then the substrate for lipoprotein lipase of endothelial cells in adipose tissue and striated muscle. Lipoprotein lipase cleaves triacylglycerols into glycerol and free fatty acids which are then mainly absorbed into fat and muscle cells. During this process, chylomicrons become smaller and are now cholesterol-rich chylomicron remnants which are taken up by liver cells by a chylomicron remnant receptor on the surface of hepatocytes.

> ### IN A NUTSHELL   !
>
> Chylomicrons transport dietary fats mainly to adipose tissue, skeletal muscle and the liver.

Very low-density lipoproteins (**VLDL**), in contrast to postprandial chylomicrons, are produced continuously by the liver and intestine. They are produced by incorporating apolipoprotein B100 (ApoB100), triacylglycerols (Tg), cholesterol esters and phospholipids. ApoB100 is first linked with microsomal triacylglycerol transfer protein in the rough endoplasmic reticulum to form Tg-poor VLDL. These are converted to Tg-rich VLDL depending on the availability of lipid droplets in the cytosol.

Mature VLDL take up apolipoproteins C and E of HDL after secretion from liver cells into blood. Their further fate is similar to that of chylomicrons. In peripheral tissues, triacylglycerols are cleaved into glycerol and free fatty acids, most of which are taken up by cells in those tissues. The resulting IDLs are to a lesser extent absorbed directly by the liver via the LDL receptor. However, they are primarily a substrate for hepatic triacylglycerol lipase. The action of this lipase causes the particles to diminish into **LDL**. LDL contain apolipoprotein B100, are rich in cholesterol esters, and are recognised and internalised by the LDL receptor in cells of the peripheral tissues. This also enables cholesterol entry into the cells of blood vessel walls.

High-density lipoproteins (**HDL**) are the most abundant lipoproteins in many mammals. Apolipoprotein A1-rich primary HDLs (pHDLs) are secreted by the liver and small intestine and stabilised by the uptake of cholesterol and phospholipids. These disc-shaped particles take up additional cholesterol in the blood and in peripheral tissues. Cholesterol is converted by the action of the plasma enzyme lecithin-cholesterol acyltransferase into **cholesterol esters**. Due to their hydrophobicity, these esters move from the outer phospholipid bilayer to the lipid interior of the HDL, forming spherical particles (HDL_3). This creates a concentration gradient from the surface to the interior that allows further uptake of cholesterol from peripheral tissues (HDL cycle).

In addition, this gradient enables **cholesterol ester transfer protein** (CETP) to deliver cholesterol to chylomicrons, VLDL and LDL in exchange for triacylglycerols.

MORE DETAILS   In dogs, HDL_3 continues to take up cholesterol in addition to ApoE in peripheral tissues. The resulting HDL_1 are removed from the circulation by receptors for LDL and chylomicron remnants in the liver. In small horses (Shetland ponies) and donkeys, the triacylglycerols formed in the liver are released in such large quantities as VLDL during energy deficiency, that hyperlipidaemia results.

CETP could not be detected in equids. Here, the HDL cholesterol esters are transferred to LDL, which are then absorbed by the liver. Most other domestic animal species (ruminants, pigs, carnivores) also lack CETP activity. Remarkably, species with CETP (human, monkey, rabbit, hamster, poultry) also show susceptibility to atherosclerosis. Species differences in the proportions of lipoproteins in plasma are shown in **Table 17.3**.

Table 17.2 Main functions of the lipoprotein classes.

Class	Diameter (nm)	Composition Tg/Pl/tC/Protein (%)	Main apo-lipoproteins	Functions
Chylomicrons	up to 1000	85/8/5/2	B48	Transport of dietary lipids, but of little importance in herbivores
VLDL	30–80	50/18/23/9	B100	Transport of liver triacylglycerols in ruminants/ Transport of dietary lipids in birds/ Transport of liver lipids to the ovary
LDL	20	7/22/48/23	B100	Cholesterol transport to the peripheral tissues
HDL	5–15	4/22/18/56	A1, A2, D	Reverse cholesterol transport to the liver/ Provision of apolipoproteins

In chylomicrons, VLDL and HDL, the apolipoproteins C1, C2, C3 and E are also present.
tC = total cholesterol; Pl = phospholipids; Tg = triacylglycerols

Table 17.3 Lipoproteins (mg · l⁻¹ plasma) in food deprived animals.

Lipoproteins	Dog	Cat	Pig	Cattle	Horse	Chicken
VLDL	400	100	550	100	700[1]	600/35000[2]
LDL	500	700	2400	2000	500	1200/2000[2]
HDL$_1$	100	–	–	–	–	–
HDL$_{2,3}$	3500	2700	1500	3400	2200	3600/600[2]

[1] VLDL significantly higher in Shetland ponies; [2] laying chicken.

> **IN A NUTSHELL** !
>
> Very-low-density lipoproteins (VLDL) are responsible for the transport of lipids from the liver to peripheral tissues. Low-density lipoproteins (LDL) mainly transport cholesterol to those tissues. High-density lipoproteins (HDL) transport cholesterol from the periphery to the liver and provide apolipoproteins. VLDL and free fatty acids are important in the development of steatosis.

MORE DETAILS

Steatosis (fatty liver)

This metabolic disorder is due either to abnormal metabolism of triacylglycerols or to overloaded fat transport processes. It occurs in humans, and also in dairy cows, ponies, cats and poultry. Causes are linked to generalised obesity, visceral obesity, lack of exercise, bacterial and parasitic infections, insulin resistance, and rapid weight loss. In the dairy cow, pony and cat, it is assumed that energy deficiency (stress, starvation, high milk yield in the cow) provokes increased lipolysis in adipose tissue, which delivers large quantities of released fatty acids to the liver. There, despite increased β-oxidation of these fatty acids, lipid droplets continue to accumulate in the hepatocytes. Lipid droplets are found in most cells. They consist of a core of neutral lipids surrounded by a phospholipid monolayer integrated with proteins, including those of the perilipin family. Lipid droplets are characterised by Tg synthesis as well as degradation by lipases (lipolysis). The extent of these processes reflects the metabolic state of the whole animal and the availability of energy supplying substrates.

The phase of **lipomobilisation** in cows at the time of **calving** is of great pathophysiological importance. The fatty liver (**hepatosteatosis**) that develops during this transitional period is an important metabolic disorder that can have considerable consequences for fertility. The mobilisation of body fat when there is a negative energy balance, and the resulting increase in plasma concentration of free fatty acids (**NEFA**) are key factors associated with fertility disorders. It is plausible that well-fed cows that are oversupplied with energy during their dry period are particularly susceptible to hepatosteatosis. There is an accumulation of Tg in hepatocytes with simultaneous low secretion of lipoprotein (**VLDL**) from the liver. Recent experiments in dairy cows showed that NEFA particularly induce perilipin 5 expression, which promotes lipid synthesis and inhibits **VLDL assembly**, thus inducing **hepatosteatosis**.

There are also physiological conditions associated with steatosis of the liver. American elk bulls completely stop eating for a fortnight during the mating season. The rumen is then almost empty and the liver shows all the signs of typical fatty degeneration, which, however, does not cause any permanent damage.

In fatty liver syndrome in laying hens, other metabolic pathways are involved in its pathogenesis. The high level of hepatic lipid synthesis in hens, lack of exercise especially in cage reared birds, high oestrogen levels and intensive supply of carbohydrates (high maize content in diets) cause an extremely high rate of triacyl-

glycerol synthesis in the liver. The maximum laying performance of more than 300 eggs per year requires a high oestrogen level and a supply of 5 g of ovarian lipids from endogenous synthesis per egg yolk produced. Despite high rates of VLDL formation, if triacylglycerol synthesis is high, the large amount of fat produced cannot all be removed from the liver, which leads to fatty degeneration.

17.4.3 Gluconeogenesis

Gluconeogenesis is the synthesis of glucose from non-carbohydrate precursors and is a central process of glucose homeostasis. It ensures the maintenance of a constant blood glucose level when there is a limited food supply, in dietary carbohydrate deficiency, and also postprandially. This maintenance of blood glucose concentration is necessary because the brain and erythrocytes are almost completely dependent on glucose as an energy source, and the amount of stored glycogen is very limited.

■ Pathway of gluconeogenesis

The metabolic pathway of gluconeogenesis (**Fig. 17.5**) is only present in liver parenchyma and in the renal cortex. Because of this, hepatocytes produce 80–85% of glucose coming from gluconeogenesis. The main precursor substrates are **glucogenic amino acids**, **lactate**, **glycerol** and **propionate**. These low-molecular weight substrates are supplied to the liver in high concentrations in portal blood and in the hepatic artery, so that gluconeogenesis takes place mainly in the periportal region, partly in the cytoplasm and partly in mitochondria. The final step of gluconeogenesis is the action of glucose-6-phosphatase in the endoplasmic reticulum.

> **IN A NUTSHELL** !
>
> The endogenous synthesis of glucose occurs in liver tissue (~80%) and in the renal cortex (~20%) from glucogenic, non-carbohydrate precursors with at least three C atoms.

MORE DETAILS Glucose synthesis in the liver and kidney is basically the reversal of glycolysis (glucose degradation). Because three enzymatic steps in the degradative pathway show strongly negative changes in free enthalpy (up to −30 KJ · mol⁻¹) at in vivo substrate concentrations, reverse reactions for gluconeogenesis are not possible with these enzymes. The conversion of glucose to glucose-6-phosphate by glucokinase and of fructose-6-phosphate to fructose-1,6-bis-phosphate by phosphofructokinase as well as the step from pyruvate to phosphoenolpyruvate (PEP) catalysed by pyruvate kinase are therefore irreversible reactions.

Nutrition, energy

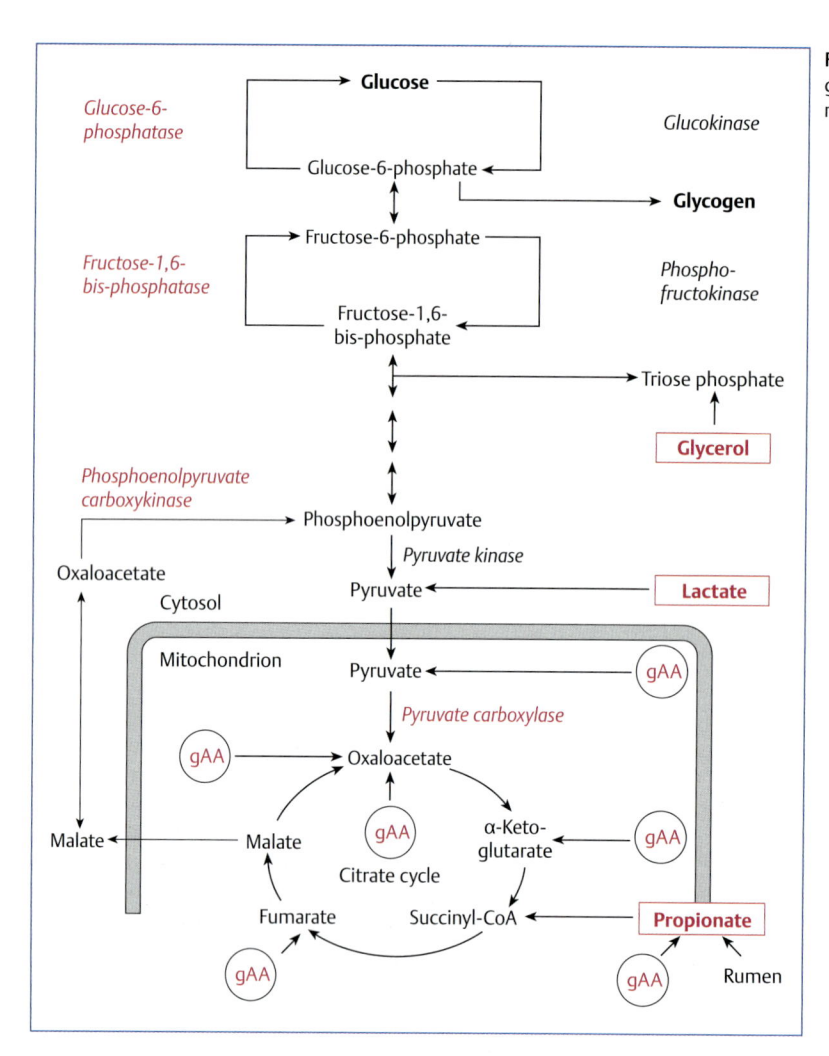

Fig. 17.5 Gluconeogenesis and glycolysis. gAA = glucogenic amino acids; substrates marked in red serve as glucose precursors.

Bypassing this reaction sequence ("bypass") in the opposing gluconeogenesis pathway is established through the action of two phosphatases: glucose-6-phosphatase and fructose-1,6-bis-phosphatase. Both enzymes release phosphate from phosphorylated substrates. On the other hand, bypassing the pyruvate kinase reaction first requires pyruvate to enter the mitochondrion and be carboxylated to oxaloacetate. After hydrogenation to malate, this substrate passes from mitochondria into the cytosol (malate-aspartate shuttle). Cytoplasmic malate dehydrogenase then converts malate to oxaloacetate which is then converted to phosphoenolpyruvate (PEP) by phosphoenolpyruvate carboxykinase (PEPCK) and guanosine triphosphate (GTP) with the release of CO_2.

> **IN A NUTSHELL**　　　　　　　　　　　!
>
> The reaction sequence of gluconeogenesis is in principle a reversal of glycolysis. However, three enzyme steps in glycolysis must be bypassed by specific gluconeogenic enzymes to overcome negative free enthalpy.

The most important precursor substrates for gluconeogenesis in cytoplasm are glycerol at the triose phosphate stage, lactate, and glucogenic amino acids in the synthesis of pyruvate. In the mitochondrial citrate cycle, glucogenic amino acids and propionate enter the gluconeogenesis sequence.

■ Regulation of gluconeogenesis

The regulation of gluconeogenesis is mainly determined by the availability of substrates and occurs reciprocally to glycolysis in monogastric animals. With adequate food intake and a plentiful supply of absorbed glucose, glycolysis and glycogen storage are the main carbohydrate metabolising steps in the liver, so there is no need for gluconeogenesis to maintain glucose homeostasis. In the postabsorptive state after food intake, or when there is a dietary carbohydrate deficiency (starvation), glucose utilisation (glycolysis) and glycogen synthesis are reduced, and glycogenolysis and gluconeogenesis are increased to maintain a constant blood glucose level. The precursor substrates for gluconeogenesis come from catabolic pathways of proteolysis and lipolysis, which are both activated.

The metabolic hormones **insulin** and **glucagon** are regulators of these two opposing carbohydrate metabolic pathways. While insulin promotes the utilisation of glucose in the liver by glycolysis, glucagon activates gluconeogenesis at the fructose phosphate level, which simultaneously counteracts the glycolysis-promoting effect of insulin. Glucagon increases the activity of fructose-1,6-bis-phosphatase via a **cAMP**-induced lowering of the level of fructose-2,6-bis-phosphate, and thus simultaneously reduces the conversion rate of phosphofructokinase.

Gluconeogenesis and glycolysis are reciprocally regulated as bypass reactions. Insulin and glucagon are the main regulators of these metabolic pathways.

At times of increased demand for glucose, hormones of the adrenal medulla also contribute to maintenance of glucose homeostasis. **Adrenaline** and **noradrenaline** activate glycogenolysis and lipolysis via the second messenger cAMP. They thus also counteract the effects of insulin and promote gluconeogenesis, which contributes to the increase in blood glucose levels. **Glucocorticoids** also promote glucose production in the liver, in particular by activating proteolysis to supply glucogenic amino acids.

■ Special features of ruminants

The special features of digestive physiology of **ruminants** have considerable significance for their hepatic carbohydrate metabolism. Almost all carbohydrates (p. 398) ingested with food are broken down in the rumen by bacteria and protozoa into **short-chain fatty acids**. Ruminants thus absorb only small amounts of dietary glucose. The glucose circulating in blood and stored in glycogen as well as that incorporated into lactose in milk is therefore almost exclusively derived from gluconeogenesis. This means that a metabolic-physiological challenge applies particularly for high-lactating cows and pregnant sheep. These animals meet the continuously high glucose demand by intensive continuous gluconeogenesis. Up to 65% of the glucose produced is derived from **propionate** generated by rumen bacteria. Thus, the voluminous forestomach system ensures a steady supply of glucose through a continuous flow of gluconeogenic precursors to the liver. In addition, more than half of the butyric acid also produced in the rumen is converted into hydroxybutyric acid (p. 401) in the rumen wall. This facilitates gluconeogenesis because hydroxybutyric acid, unlike butyric acid, promotes glucose synthesis from propionate.

The regulating metabolic hormones act in the same way in ruminants as in monogastric animals. Nevertheless, their role has not yet been satisfactorily explained in relation to hepatic carbohydrate metabolism. It is assumed that in regulation of glycolysis and gluconeogenesis, it is not so much the absolute levels of these hormone that are important, but rather the ratio of insulin to glucagon. All studies to date indicate that in cattle, glucagon is much more important than insulin in controlling carbohydrate metabolism. Ruminants do not use glucose for fatty acid synthesis. Instead, they use acetate and hydroxybutyrate as substrates. This allows glucose utilisation in the liver to be kept low.

Glucose uptake into the **udder tissue** and into the **uterus** is insulin-independent. A low insulin level regulates the distribution of substrates in favour of the mammary gland or the foetus. At the same time, however, this increases the risk of increased **ketogenesis** in the liver.

MORE DETAILS Catecholamines and glucocorticoids act in the same way in ruminants as in well-studied laboratory rodents and humans and stimulate gluconeogenesis. Also, growth hormone (GH) blood level increases in early lactation, and seems to act also to stimulate gluconeogenesis. It is not clear whether growth hormone directly affects gluconeogenesis or whether its effect on blood glucose levels comes from inhibiting peripheral utilisation of glucose. On the other hand, by increasing lipolysis, STH helps to supply the various organs with an alternative energy source of fatty acids and ketone bodies.

The special features of digestive physiology of ruminants result in very low availability of glucose for intestinal absorption. Endogenous glucose production by gluconeogenesis is therefore the main source of glucose in the circulation. The most important substrate (approx. 60%) for continuous gluconeogenesis is bacterially produced propionate.

17.4.4 Ketogenesis in liver metabolism during energy deficiency

Starvation means a lack of energy for higher animals. There is also a risk of energy deficiency when there are increased requirements during **pregnancy** (particularly for twin pregnancies in small ruminants) or in **lactation (dairy cows)**. These states make particular high demands on energy metabolism (p. 615). If adaptability of intermediate metabolism is defective in these situations, ketosis can develop in humans, ruminants and rodents.

In energy deficiency, the level of insulin and other lipolytic hormones decreases, which allows especially catecholamines, glucagon and glucocorticoids to exert their effects on gluconeogenesis. This is associated with activation of lipolysis in adipose tissue, so that free fatty acid (NEFA) concentration in plasma increases considerably and these are then absorbed by the liver. In the cytosol of hepatic cells, acyl-CoA increases in response. This, as well as the glucagon excess and the reduced insulin action, causes a decrease in the malonyl-CoA concentration, which in turn activates carnitine acyltransferase I. As a result, in ruminants, but also in humans and rats, there is an increased transfer of fatty acids into mitochondria. Ketone bodies are then formed from acetyl-CoA, produced in large quantities during the increased β-oxidation of fatty acids. Acetyl-CoA cannot be completely utilised by the citrate cycle because of a relative lack of oxaloacetate.

The liver is the main site of intramitochondrial ketogenesis. The starting point is the condensation of 3 **acetyl-CoA** to β-hydroxy-β-methyl-glutaryl-CoA with acetoacetyl-CoA as an intermediate. This is followed by the cleavage of acetyl-CoA, so that acetoacetate is formed. **Acetoacetate** can be reduced in a NADH-dependent reaction to **β-hydroxybutyrate**, or it can spontaneously be decarboxylated to produce **acetone**. Thus, the fatty acids released by lipolysis are converted into water-soluble, easily transportable and oxidisable forms. Ketone bodies are released into blood in a varying ratio of β-hydroxybutyrate to acetoacetate according to species (rat 2:1, human 3:1, ruminant 10:1).

The ketone bodies can be **utilised** by **heart** and **skeletal muscles, kidney cortex** and **central nervous system** (exception: ruminants) to at least partially replace glucose as an energy source. In the mammary gland, β-hydroxybutyrate is the most important supplier of carbon (approx. 50%) for fatty acid biosynthesis, along with acetate. In the all these tissues, the oxidation rate initially increases in proportion to the plasma level. If further utilisation is no longer possible, ketone bodies are excreted by the kidney, mammary gland, skin and into respiratory air. If the buffer capacity is exceeded, metabolic acidosis may develop.

For ruminants, ketone body formation is initially an essential metabolic process for processing acetyl-CoA, which can no longer be utilised in the citrate cycle. In addition, the excess fatty acids in the liver are re-esterified to triacyglycerols. This reaction in domestic animals takes place mainly in species that have only a slight tendency to ketogenesis (cat, horse, pig). What all animal species have in common is that a fatty liver can develop in prolonged energy deficiency.

> **IN A NUTSHELL**   !
>
> Ketone bodies are formed in carbohydrate deficiency and in starvation when there is an excess of acetyl-CoA that cannot be utilised in the citrate cycle. The main site of ketogenesis is the liver. Ruminants also synthesise β-hydroxybutyric acid in the rumen wall.

17.4.5   Urea synthesis

Ammonia is a cell poison even in low concentrations. In the liver, there is a complex system for removal of ammonium ions. One of these is **perivenous NH₃ fixation** by producing **glutamine** from **glutamate** by glutamine synthetase. The concentration of free NH_3 is determined by perivenous mitochondrial glutamate dehydrogenase (**Fig. 17.6**). Furthermore, the **release of NH₃ from glutamine** occurs **periportally** with mitochondrial glutaminase. This is the same site (in **mammals**) where the subsequent synthesis of urea is located. In birds and reptiles, uric acid is the NH_3 detoxification product.

Urea is synthesised only in the liver by enzymes of the urea cycle. The nitrogen atoms of urea are supplied directly by ammonia or by the amino acid aspartate. The reaction sequence starts with the intramitochondrial synthesis of **carbamoyl phosphate** from free ammonia, bicarbonate and 2 ATP by carbamoyl phosphate synthetase. This is the rate-determining step of the total synthesis, with N-acetylglutamate being the allosteric activator. The concentration of this effector is in turn closely correlated with the glutamate level in the liver.

In the following, carbamoyl phosphate reacts with ornithine to form citrulline which enters the cytosol via a specific transport protein. The argininosuccinate synthetase catalyses the ATP-dependent combination of citrulline and **aspartate** to form **argininosuccinate**, which is converted into arginine with cleavage of fumarate. The amino acid **arginine** is hydrolytically converted to urea along with ornithine which returns to the mitochondria by a specific transport mechanism, to reinitiate another turn of the urea cycle.

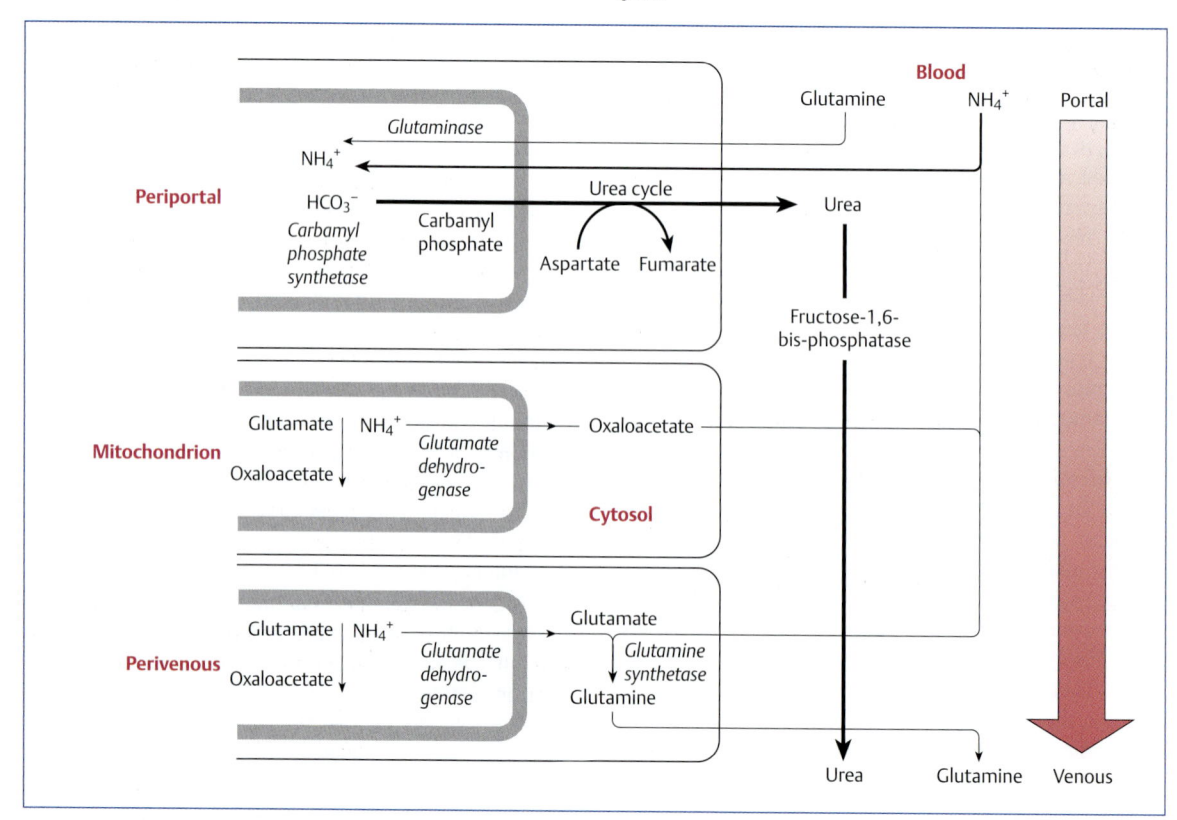

Fig. 17.6 Zonal metabolism of glutamine and ammonium in the liver.

Urea as a non-toxic and water-soluble substance is formed from the nitrogen of free NH_3 and aspartate in combination with HCO_3^-. The pathway is located partly in the mitochondria and partly in the cytosol.

In the perivenous hepatocytes, any remaining ammonia is detoxified by incorporation into glutamate via glutamine synthetase with energy supplied by ATP. Thus, hepatic glutamine balance is regulated by **periportal glutaminase** and the strictly **perivenous glutamine synthetase**. Because this intercellular glutamine cycle requires ATP, it is also energy demanding.

Both systems of ammonia detoxification are not only involved in NH_3 homeostasis, but also in control of acid-base balance (p. 350). In acidosis, inhibition of pH-sensitive glutaminase leads to a decrease in urea synthesis. This also limits the consumption of bicarbonate. At the same time, glutamine synthetase activity is increased, so that detoxification of NH_3 in the liver is still ensured (**Fig. 17.6**). In the renal tubules, NH_3 can be released from **glutamine** and excreted as NH_4^+ which is important for renal regulation of acid-base balance.

MORE DETAILS In the kidney, urea is excreted as a polar, uncharged molecule. However, a variable proportion enters the gastrointestinal tract via saliva or directly across the intestinal mucosa (**Fig. 16.36**, **Fig. 16.37**) and is available again for intestinal absorption (urea recycling). The higher urea recycling of herbivores compared to omnivores is related to the special needs of these species. In horses, urea recycling is between $\frac{1}{3}$ and $\frac{2}{3}$ depending on the protein content of the ration. In cattle, around $\frac{2}{3}$ of urea is excreted by the kidneys and $\frac{1}{3}$ enters the rumen and the small intestine. This ratio is reversed in sheep. The large intestine as an entry point for urea does not seem to play a major role in domestic animals. Herbivores thus benefit from urea recycling from blood to the intestine, which allows them to survive on low quantity and low-quality dietary protein. The forestomach fermenting species are evolutionarily so successful because nitrogen from urea recycling into the rumen can be used to form microbial protein. Although nitrogen recycled in the small intestine is converted into microbial protein in the large intestine, it cannot be recovered by most animals, with the exception of caecotrophic animals (p. 442).

17.4.6 The role of the liver in the metabolism of fat-soluble vitamins

The liver plays a special role in maintaining supply of the fat-soluble vitamins A, D, E and K, as they are preferentially stored and functionally metabolised in this organ.

Hepatic parenchyma is rich in **vitamin A**. Here, retinyl esters are converted by hydrolysis into retinol. Retinol is then secreted into blood bound to retinol-binding protein and to transthyretin to be transported to its target cells, where it is taken up by receptor-mediated endocytosis. In these cells, retinol is either converted to retinaldehyde (visual process; **Fig. 3.25**) or oxidised to retinoic acid. Through isomerisation, all-trans-retinoate is rearranged to 9-cis-retinoate. Both compounds control growth and development of cells and tissues by regulation of gene expression. Excess retinol in the liver is oxidised to 4-oxo retinoic acid by a cytochrome P-450-enzyme and is then glucuronidated and excreted via the kidney.

Vitamin D is the generic term for biologically active calciferols. A distinction is made between ergocalciferol (vitamin D_2) of fungal origin and cholecalciferol (vitamin D_3), which is present in animal tissues. Vitamin D is not a vitamin in the true sense of the word, since the alimentary supply is only relevant in the case of insufficient endogenous synthesis by solar UV irradiation of skin. The actual biologically active substance, calcitriol (1,25-dihydroxy-cholecalciferol), is a steroid hormone. Both ingested and endogenous cholecalciferol are transported in blood bound to a vitamin D-binding protein (DBP) to the liver, where it is converted by mitochondrial hydroxylases to 25-OH-cholecalciferol. This is bound to DBP, transported to the kidneys where it is hydroxylated again to calcitriol. Vitamin D and its metabolites are mainly excreted in bile and only to a small extent by the kidneys. Calcitriol acts synergistically in cells with retinoates and other hormones in calcium metabolism and in the regulation of gene expression of cell proliferation and maturation (p. 549).

Vitamin E is a collective term for all tocopherol and tocotrienol derivatives that exhibit biological activity of the naturally occurring RRR-alpha-tocopherol. Since most of the absorbed α-tocopherol is transported in the lymphatic system and incorporated into lipoproteins, there is a high correlation between α-tocopherol concentration and total lipid in plasma. Transport into cells and cell membranes is mediated by lipoprotein lipase and an alpha-tocopherol binding protein. Catabolic elimination is predominantly in the liver. The effects of tocopherols are manifold, and their mechanism is not yet fully understood. In addition to its antioxidant effect, there are also anti-inflammatory and immunomodulatory effects. Tocopherol requirement is strongly related to the quantity of dietary polyunsaturated fatty acids that are consumed.

Vitamin K or phylloquinone is also a fat-soluble vitamin. It has important roles in blood clotting and bone metabolism, among other things. The key function of phylloquinone is in enzymatic gamma carboxylation of glutamyl residues in particular proteins. Vitamin K is involved in the synthesis of various blood clotting factors (p. 236) in the liver, especially prothrombin. Furthermore, vitamin K is involved in calcium metabolism and bone formation via osteocalcin.

17.5   Contribution of the liver to detoxification

Many harmful endobiotics and xenobiotics are enzymically detoxified by hepatic metabolism and are subsequently eliminated (biotransformation). These are mostly lipophilic substances that are readily absorbed in the gastrointestinal tract but cannot be excreted sufficiently by the kidneys or in bile, because of their physicochemical properties of poor water solubility and being bound to proteins. These noxious substances include xenobiotics (e.g. drugs, feed ingredients, environmental chemicals) and also endogenous compounds that cannot be further metabolised such as steroids and bilirubin.

Biotransformation of these substances takes place in three successive phases. In the first two phases, they are chemically modified and undergo conjugation reactions which convert lipophilic substances into water-soluble compounds and thus make them more readily able to be excreted. In the third phase, these modified compounds are excreted by active transport processes. Various factors can influence these biotransformation processes such as age, gender, species, comedication, health status and environmental factors. If biotransformation is insufficient, endo- and xenobiotics accumulate in an animal (bioaccumulation), which can lead to adverse effects on health. Model calculations have shown that some xenobiotics (e.g. dioxin derivatives) would take years to be excreted, if no biotransformation occurs.

The underlying enzymatic reactions of biotransformation usually also change the pharmacodynamic properties of a substance. Thus, the metabolite produced from a substance (e.g. medicinal product) is usually less effective but sometimes more effective than the parent substance itself.

Besides the liver, other tissues (e.g. lung, kidney, intestine, skin) are also capable of biotransformation. However, the biotransformation capacity is considerably lower than that of the liver. This emphasis on biotransformation in the liver makes physiological sense, since the majority of food substances/xenobiotics absorbed in the intestine reach the liver directly via the portal vein (cf. first-pass effect).

17.5.1   Biotransformation by chemical modification

In phase I of biotransformation, the substances to be detoxified are chemically modified mainly by **oxidation, reduction** or **hydrolytic cleavage**. These enzymically catalysed transformations expose or introduce polar functional groups (e.g. -OH, -SH, -NH$_2$, -COOH) in the molecule, which increase water solubility and usually also cause a loss of bioactivity. For a few substances, however, these reactions can produce pharmacologically active or toxic/carcinogenic metabolites (bioactivation). A well-known example of this is the oxidation of biologically inactive aflatoxin B1, which leads to the formation of a potent mutagenic and carcinogenic epoxide.

Phase I of biotransformation is also referred to as **functionalisation** because the chemical modifications enable the product to subsequently be linked to endogenous substrates in phase II. Hence, phase I metabolites can be regarded as substrates for phase II reactions. Only a small proportion of endobiotics and xenobiotics are sufficiently hydrophilic after phase I biotransformation to be excreted.

Phase I reactions are mainly catalysed by oxidoreductases, including alcohol dehydrogenases, aldehyde dehydrogenases and mixed-function monooxygenases. The latter are **cytochrome P450 enzymes** (CYP enzymes), which have a central role in detoxification. CYP enzymes form a "superfamily" of haem-containing isoenzymes, with the CYP1, CYP2 and CYP3 families being quantitatively most important. Over 90% of these CYP enzymes are located in hepatocytes, where they are mostly anchored in endoplasmic reticulum and the microsomes derived from the endoplasmic reticulum. A characteristic of CYP enzymes is that they sometimes have very broad and partially overlapping substrate specificities.

In their function as monooxygenases, CYP enzymes catalyse the insertion of an oxygen atom into a substrate molecule, by which process a large number of pharmaceuticals and toxic substrates are dealkylated or hydroxylated. This oxygenation reaction is summarised as follows:

$$R–H+O_2+NADPH+H^+ \ \rightarrow \ R–OH+H_2O+NADP^+ \qquad (17.1)$$

Here, after the formation of an enzyme-substrate complex, two electrons of NADPH are needed to cleave the bond in the oxygen molecule, whereby one oxygen atom is split off as water and the remaining oxygen atom is transferred to the substrate together with a proton.

In many reactions catalysed by CYP enzymes, **reactive oxygen species** (e.g. **superoxide**) can be released, which in turn can initiate the complex processes of lipid peroxidation and thus contribute to "oxidative stress". Various antioxidant enzymes, in high concentrations in hepatocytes, are able to directly inactivate these reactive oxygen species as well as other reactive substances produced during lipid peroxidation. Important such enzymes are glutathione peroxidases, glutathione S-transferases, epoxide hydrolases and superoxide dismutases.

> **IN A NUTSHELL**   **!**
>
> Chemical modification of **xenobiotics, pharmaceuticals** and **endobiotics** in hepatocytes in phase I of biotransformation increases their reactivity and mostly results in their inactivation.

17.5.2   Biotransformation through conjugation

The phase I chemical modification is usually followed by an enzymatic coupling reaction. This **phase II** biotransformation is therefore called **conjugation**. Here, polar, negatively charged endogenous substrates are covalently bound to the functional groups introduced in phase I, so that water solubility and thus the capability for excretion of the resulting conjugates via the kidney is significantly enhanced. The quantitatively most important reaction is **glu-**

curonidation, in which activated glucuronic acid (UDP-glucuronic acid) is transferred to the phase I metabolite with the formation of an ether (R–O-R') or an ester bond (R–COO-R').

Phenols and alcohols are converted into O-glucuronides (= R–O-glucuronic acid) by microsomal UDP-glucuronosyltransferases (UGT):

UDP-glucuronic acid + R–OH
$\rightarrow$ UDP + R–O-glucuronic acid + H_2O (17.2)

Aromatic or branched-chain aliphatic acids, including **bilirubin**, can be excreted in bile as ester glucuronides or diglucuronides.

UDP-glucuronic acid +R–COOH
$\rightarrow$ UDP + R–C-OO-glucuronic acid + H_2O (17.3)

Other phase II reactions include sulphation of substrates by sulphotransferases or their conjugation with amino acids (especially glycine and glutamine) by amino acid N-acyltransferases. Also of importance are glutathione-S-transferases, which catalyse conjugation with glutathione (a tripeptide), as well as N-acetyltransferases, by means of which substrates are conjugated with acetyl groups.

The conjugates formed in phase II are then excreted in bile into the intestine or via blood by the kidney.

In neonates and young animals, the activity of the biotransforming enzyme systems (monooxygenases, glucuronosyltransferases) is low. They are therefore much more sensitive to many drugs than adult animals, which has a direct influence on the duration of action and the side effect profile. In cats, the ability to glucuronidate xenobiotics is very limited (**glucuronidation weakness**), as they do not express some UGTs.

> **IN A NUTSHELL**   !
>
> Detoxification of lipophilic endobiotics and xenobiotics takes place in the liver. These compounds are chemically modified and then conjugated with other molecules to increase their water solubility and thus their capability for excretion.

17.5.3 Excretion of endobiotics and xenobiotics

In **phase III** of biotransformation, the phase II conjugates are eliminated by renal or biliary **excretion**. Other excretion routes via the lungs, skin, saliva and tear fluid are only of minor significance. The molecular weight of a conjugate is the main determinant of its route of excretion. This molecular weight threshold is about 300–500 Dalton for biliary excretion, depending on the species, which must be taken into account in pharmacotherapy. Smaller molecules are mainly excreted by the kidney. Water solubility also affects the route of excretion. Various transport mechanisms (efflux transporters) are expressed in hepatocytes of which ATP-binding cassettes (ABC transporters) have a central role. These ATP-linked transporters are a superfamily of transmembrane proteins with a nucleotide-binding site. Their function is to eject detoxified conjugates from hepatocytes into sinusoidal blood or into bile. These are mainly active transport processes, with the necessary energy being provided by ATP hydrolysis. Important ABC transporters are the multidrug resistance protein-1, the multidrug resistance-associated protein-2 and the breast cancer resistance protein.

> **IN A NUTSHELL**   !
>
> Transport processes are crucial in the elimination of an endobiotic or xenobiotic substance. Besides absorption, distribution and metabolism, elimination with ATP-dependent efflux transporters is of particular importance. Excretion is then renal or biliary into urine or faeces. Excretion via the intestine may however result in an enterohepatic recirculation.

17.5.4 Formation of bile pigments

The most important bile pigments are **bilirubin** and **biliverdin**. They are formed when haem is broken down in the reticuloendothelial cells of the liver, spleen and bone marrow. **Haem** belongs to a family of metalloporphyrins which, in addition to haemoglobin and myoglobin, are also found in catalase, cytochromes and peroxidases. The enzymes for haem biosynthesis are present in every cell; and these enzymes in hepatocytes have especially high activities.

The first product of haem degradation is biliverdin, formed by the action of a microsomal haem oxygenase. In the second step, cytosolic bilirubin reductase acts on biliverdin to produce bilirubin. This enzyme is not present in birds, reptiles and nutria, so that the bile of such animals has a greenish colour. Bilirubin is transported to the liver as a lipophilic substance bound to **albumin**. Here it is coupled to glucuronic acid to form a diglucuronide, which is excreted in bile as a water-soluble compound or, to a lesser extent, passes in blood to be excreted by the kidneys (**Fig. 17.7**). In the **large intestine** bilirubin is converted to colourless compounds stercobilinogen and urobilinogen. After oxidation with oxygen or by dehydrogenation, **urobilin and stercobilin** are formed, the latter causing the normal colour of faeces. Various degradation products of bilirubin are partly absorbed in the intestine. They then re-enter the liver (**enterohepatic circulation, Fig. 17.7**). Bile pigments have no physiological significance for digestion. However, they have a pronounced antioxidant effect.

> **MORE DETAILS** Increased concentrations of bile pigments (especially bilirubin) in tissues and blood serum causes yellow discoloured skin and mucous membranes. This metabolic disorder in humans and domestic animals is called icterus and is the result of increased formation of bilirubin either from a high rate of haemolysis (e.g. disintegration and dissolution of large haematomas) which exceeds hepatic degradation and excretion capacities, or it is caused by disturbance of hepatic metabolism itself or bile output disorders (cholangitis, bile duct tumours).

Nutrition, energy

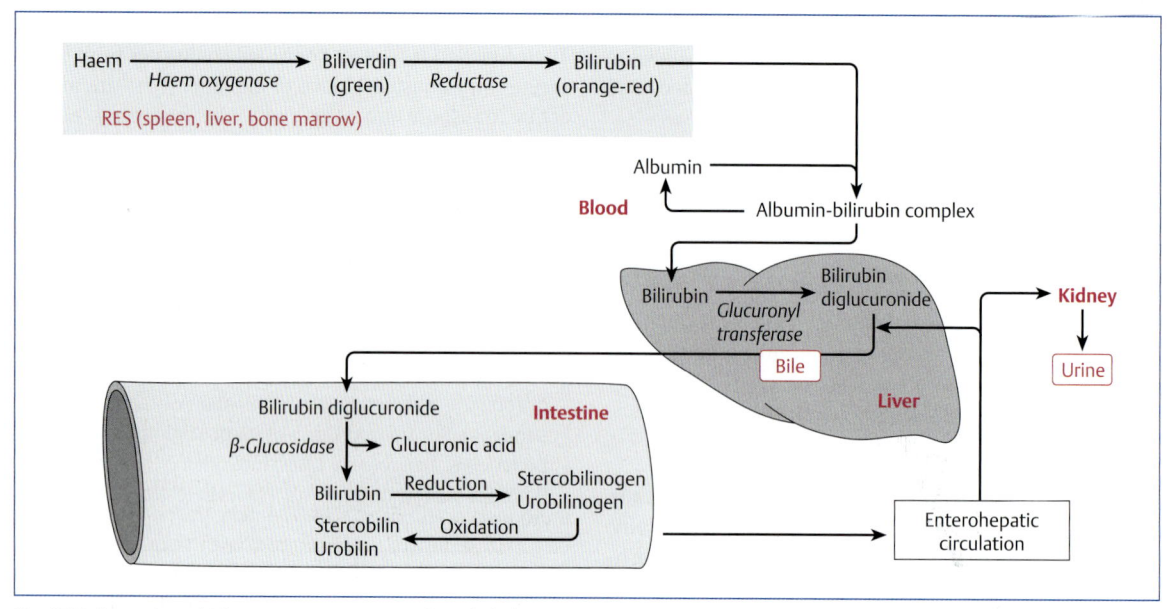

Fig. 17.7 Formation of bile pigments. RES = reticuloendothelial system.

Suggested reading

Anderson N, Borlak J. Molecular mechanisms and therapeutic targets in steatosis and steatohepatitis. Pharmacol Rev 2008; 60: 311–357

Bauer JE. Lipoprotein-mediated transport of dietary and synthesized lipids and lipid abnormalities of dogs and cats. J Am Vet Med Assoc 2004; 224: 668–675

Bergen WG, Mersmann HJ. Comparative aspects of lipid metabolism: impact on contemporary research and use of animal models. J Nutr 2005; 135: 2499–2502

Boyer TD, Manns MP, Sanyal AJ. Zakim and Boyer's Hepatology. Philadelphia: Saunders Elsevier; 2012

Fink-Gremmels J. Implications of hepatic cytochrome P450-related biotransformation processes in veterinary sciences. Eur J Pharmacol 2008; 585: 502–509

Ginsberg HN, Taskinen MR. New insights into the regulation of lipoprotein metabolism: studies in procaryocytes, eukaryocytes, rodents, pigs, and people. Curr Opin Lipidol 1997; 8: 127–130

Guarino MP, Cocca S, Altomare A et al. Ursodeoxycholic acid therapy in gallbladder disease, a story not yet completed. World J Gastroenterol 2013; 19: 5029–5034

Holmes RS, Vandeberg JL, Cox LA. Vertebrate hepatic lipase genes and proteins: a review supported by bioinformatic studies. Open Access Bioinformatics 2011(3); 85–95

Ileri-Buyukoglu T, Guldur T. Dyslipoproteinemias and their clinical importance in several species of domestic animals. J Am Vet Med Assoc 2005; 227: 1746–1751

Jia H, Li X, Liu G et al. Perilipin 5 promotes hepatic steatosis in dairy cows through increasing lipid synthesis and decreasing very low density lipoprotein assembly. J Dairy Sci 2019; 102: 833–845

Lapierre H, Lobley GE. Nitrogen recycling in the ruminant: a review. J Dairy Sci 2001; 84: E223-E236

Maldonado EN, Casanave EB, Aveldano MI. Major plasma lipids and fatty acids in four HDL mammals. Comp Biochem Physiol A Mol Integr Physiol 2002; 132: 297–303.

Toutain PL, Ferran A, Bousquet-Mélou A. Species differences in pharmacokinetics and pharmacodynamics. Handb Exp Pharmacol 2010; 199: 19–48

18 Physiological role of adipose tissue

Korinna Huber

18.1 Morphology and function

ESSENTIALS ✖

White adipose tissue is far more than just a store for energy in the form of fat! Adipose tissue is jointly with liver responsible for the metabolic health of humans and other animals. The following main tasks can be attributed to this metabolically active and adaptable tissue:

- **regulation of energy balance** by providing chemical energy in times of deficiency and storing energy in the form of fat in times of surplus,
- **release of endocrine messengers** to influence feed intake, energy balance and fertility,
- **involvement in the innate non-specific immune system** through secretion of adipocytokines and other factors influencing inflammation,
- **mechanical protection and thermal insulation** through various depots on mechanically stressed parts of the body, subcutaneously and internally.

18.1.1 Structure of adipose tissue

There are **white, brown** and **beige adipose tissues**, with **white adipose tissue** making up the **largest proportion**. **Brown adipose tissue** has this colour because of numerous mitochondria in brown adipocytes as well as plentiful capillaries. Its role is to generate heat (p. 499) rapidly, especially in hibernating species. **Beige adipose tissue** consists of white adipose cells that transform into brown-like cells and is distributed within white adipose tissue. The mechanism that controls this transformation is still largely unknown, however, this ability to transform white cells to beige cells is likely to contribute significantly to the **metabolic flexibility** of adipose tissue. Fat deposits in cells that are not fat cells (hepatocellular fat, intramyocellular fat) must be distinguished from the clearly delineated adipose tissues.

White adipose tissue develops during late embryogenesis from the mesoderm and is a special form of reticular connective tissue. Like all connective tissue, it contains both mobile and fixed cells. The main part of the fixed cells are mature fat cells (**adipocytes**) with their typical single fat vacuole. These cells can vary greatly in number and size in each adipose tissue depot (**Fig. 18.1**). The other cells in white adipose tissue are **preadipocytes** (= progenitor cells of mature adipocytes), mesenchymal multipotent stem cells, endothelial cells, endothelial progenitor cells and connective tissue cells. The mobile cells include migrated macrophages and lymphocytes. Differentiation, growth and metabolic activity of the fixed cells in adipose tissue are closely linked to the development of adequate capillary beds, to supply and remove substrates, endocrine signals and cytokines. The preadipocyte population, enables adipose tissues to grow hyperplastically (= increase in **adipocyte number**). Preadipocytes can differentiate into mature adipocytes, a process known as **adipogenesis**. The hypertrophic growth of adipocytes (= increase in **cell size**) is not like that of other cells like muscle cells, because adipocyte hypertrophy is mainly based on enlargement of the fat vacuole by increasing storage of fat. This allows the fat cell to increase its volume by a factor of 2000. Adipose tissue can make up 2–70% of body mass and is thus the tissue with the highest mass variability. Fatty tissue can be found in many parts of the body. A distinction is made between **subcutaneous** (located in the subcutis), **intramuscular** (located between the muscle fibres) and **visceral** adipose tis-

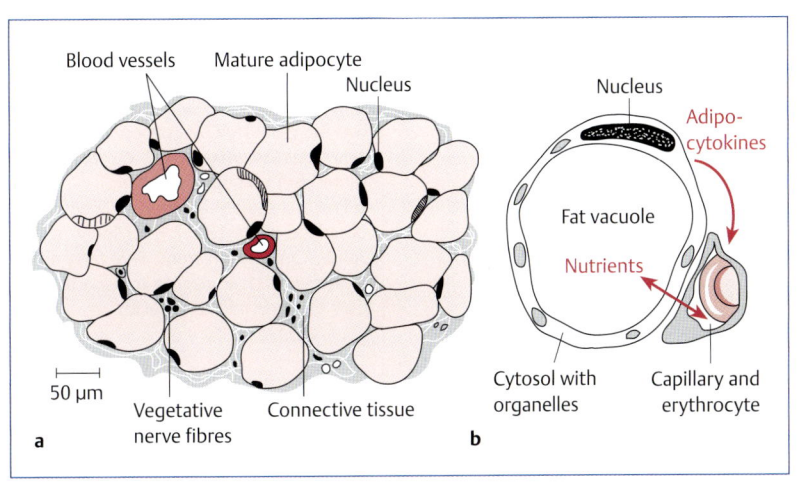

Fig. 18.1 a Histological structure of white adipose tissue. The typical fat vacuole (**b**) completely fills the interior of the cell (signet ring structure), the cytoplasm is only a narrow fringe.
b White fat cell with adjacent capillary: Secretion of hormones into the capillaries and storage and release of substrates.

Figure labels (a): Blood vessels · Mature adipocyte · Nucleus · 50 µm · Vegetative nerve fibres · Connective tissue

Figure labels (b): Nucleus · Adipo-cytokines · Fat vacuole · Nutrients · Cytosol with organelles · Capillary and erythrocyte

Nutrition, energy

sue (found in the body cavities and on the internal organs). Pathophysiologically, in humans and also in many animal species, visceral adipose tissue in the abdominal cavity, when it grows substantially, has greater importance than subcutaneous adipose tissue because of its particular metabolic and secretory properties.

18.1.2   Protective function

An important function of adipose tissue is the mechanical protection of exposed areas on the body surface and the shock protection of internal and external organs. In addition, white adipose tissue serves as thermal insulation, especially for animals in cold regions of the world.

18.1.3   Physiological function

The physiological functions of adipose tissue are far more extensive than just **storing chemical energy** derived from **food**. Flexible adaptation of adipose tissue metabolism (p. 478) to anabolic and catabolic situations enables an animal to adapt to periods with low food intake. Meeting energy requirements at times of starvation in winter or during illness is the physiological role of adipose tissue. However, the intermittent growth and shrinkage of adipose tissues is often not very pronounced with modern feeding practice, especially for companion animals (dogs, cats, horses, rodents). A continuous steady (over)supply of food with simultaneous lack of exercise often leads to obesity and associated diseases. In addition to storing food energy, adipose tissue modulates a host of other functions through secretion of hormones called adipocytokines (p. 479). Adipose tissues influence a number of other processes such as the quantity of food intake, glucose and fat homeostasis and the processes underlying reproduction and lactation. Adipose tissue also participates in the body's innate immune response. Migrated and resident macro-

phages in adipose tissue, along with adipocyte production of **pro-inflammatory adipocytokines**, are involved in the inflammatory status of an animal (p. 482).

18.2   Metabolic activities of adipose tissue

Adipose tissue metabolism responds to both anabolic and catabolic signals, which can be endocrine, neurological or metabolic. Visceral adipose tissue reacts much more strongly to these signals than subcutaneous adipose tissue. Metabolic processes in storage of energy compounds (**lipogenesis**) and release of energy compounds (**lipolysis**) are finely tuned to each other through a multitude of regulatory processes, operating continuously in adipose tissues. These metabolic processes thus influence the entire balance of energy input and energy utilisation in an animal. However, little is known about these processes in most domestic animals, so that the metabolic pathways presented mainly reflect the situations known for humans and laboratory rodents.

18.2.1   Lipolysis

Lipolysis is the **hydrolytic cleavage of triacylglycerols** stored in the fat vacuole of adipocytes, as a sequence of enzymatic cleavage processes. **Adipose tissue triacylglycerol lipase** (ATGL) catalyses diacylglycerol production by splitting off a single fatty acid. Diacylglycerols are then substrates for **hormone-sensitive lipase** (HSL), which produces monoacylglycerols. These in turn are cleaved by **monoacylglycerol lipase** (MGL) and partly also by HSL into individual long-chain fatty acids (LCFA) and glycerol (**Fig. 18.2 a**). For all these lipase reactions, the enzymes are operating at the fat/water interface of the fat droplets, made possible by the fat droplet-associated envelope protein, **perilipin**. Se-

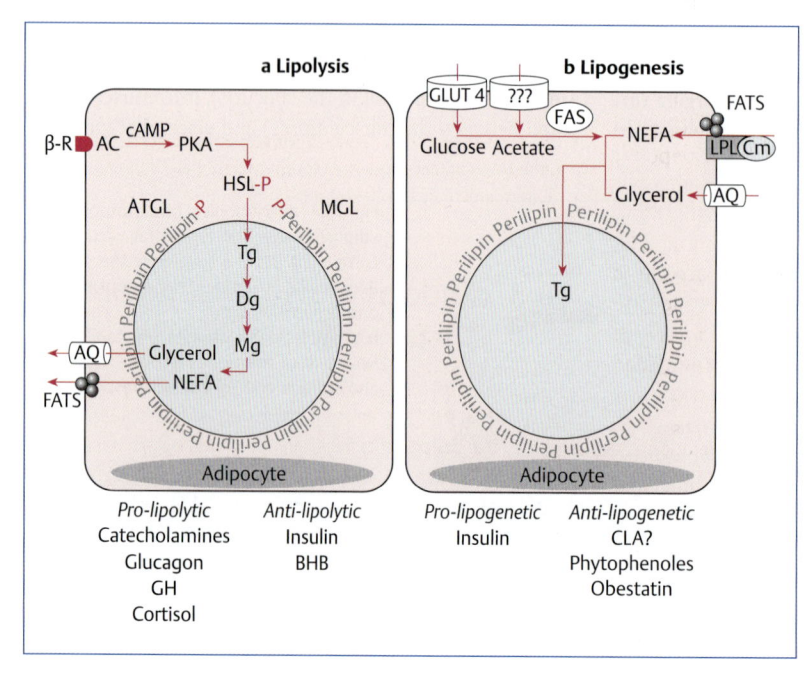

Fig. 18.2 a Processes and regulation of lipolysis. Shown is the β-adrenergic stimulation sequence of lipolysis, which is described in more detail in ch. 18.2.1 (p. 478) (β-R: β-adrenergic receptor; AC: adenylate cyclase; cAMP: cyclic adenosine monophosphate; PKA: protein kinase A; HSL: hormone-sensitive lipase; ATGL: adipose tissue triacylglycerol lipase; MGL: monoacylglycerol lipase; Tg/Dg/Mg: tri-/di-/monoacylglycerols; NEFA: non-esterified fatty acids; AQ: Aquaporin; FATS: fatty acid transport system; GH: growth hormone; BHB: β-hydroxybutyrate).
b Processes and regulation of lipogenesis described in ch. 18.2.2 (LPL: lipoprotein lipase; Cm: chylomicrons; FAS: fatty acid synthase; GLUT4: glucose transporter 4; CLA: conjugated linoleic acid).

cretion of free fatty acids into capillaries occurs by simple diffusion and possibly with the assistance of specific LCFA transporters. The majority of LCFA are then immediately bound to albumin in blood, with a small proportion as free or non-esterified fatty acids (FFA or NEFA). The glycerol released from lipolysis passes out of fat cells through water channels (aquaporins).

Regulation of lipolysis is mainly by neurological and endocrine signals (**Fig. 18.2 a**). Catecholamines from sympathetic nerve endings (noradrenaline) and from the adrenal gland (adrenaline) activate lipolysis via β receptors. The signalling pathway of this activation is shown in **Fig. 18.2 a**. Activated protein kinase A (PKA) phosphorylates HSL and perilipin. This makes the lipid droplet surface accessible to lipolytic enzymes and increases HSL activity. In addition, glucagon, glucocorticoids and growth hormone (GH) promote lipolysis. Catecholamines have an anti-lipolytic effect via α_2 receptors, and insulin acts via the insulin receptor by inhibiting PKA-dependent activation. Prostaglandins (PGE_2) and metabolites such as β-hydroxybutyrate also inhibit lipolysis.

18.2.2 Triacylglycerol synthesis and lipogenesis

The triacylglycerols of adipose tissues are synthesised from fatty acids derived from the following sources:
- from **triacylglycerols** of chylomicrons, which are absorbed in the intestine,
- from **lipoproteins** (VLDL), which are secreted by the liver into blood,
- from the **synthesis** of **LCFA** from acetate, originating in the forestomachs (p. 398) and large intestine (p. 439) and from glucose absorbed in the intestine.

When chylomicrons and lipoproteins reach adipose tissue in blood, lipoprotein lipase on the plasma membrane of adipocytes cleaves the transported triacylglycerols to release free fatty acids which then enter the fat cells where they are re-esterified with activated glycerol (**Fig. 18.2 b**). Passage of fatty acids through the plasma membrane of adipocytes is facilitated by LCFA transporters already mentioned in the chapter on lipolysis (p. 478). The fatty acid profile in triacylglycerols of white adipose tissue depends to some extent on the animal species, on where the adipose tissue is located, and to a large extent on the fatty acid composition of dietary fat. The new synthesis of LCFA from non-fat precursors such as glucose and acetate is called **lipogenesis**. A central enzyme in lipogenesis is fatty acid synthase (FAS), which produces medium-chain length fatty acids (mainly palmitic acid), which are then extended to form LCFA. This new synthesis is very energy-intensive, i.e. in addition to the precursors acetate and glucose, ATP and reduction equivalents in the form of $NADPH_2$ are also required. Lipogenesis is a process used by all animal species to store excess dietary energy as fat. Lipogenesis in non-lactating ruminants, horses, pigs and carnivores occurs mainly in adipose tissue. Lactating animals also synthesise fatty acids (milk fat) in the mammary gland. In birds and humans, lipogenesis occurs mainly in the liver.

Rodents have an equally high capacity for lipogenesis in both liver and adipose tissue. On their standard diets, ruminants, horses and carnivores use mainly acetate for lipogenesis, while pigs, birds and humans use mainly excess glucose for lipogenesis. Three LCFA molecules are esterified with an activated glycerol to form a triacylglycerol which is stored in the cytoplasmic lipid vacuole. LCFA released by lipolysis can also be immediately re-esterified, a process that contributes to the fine regulation of LCFA release. Glycerol is taken up by aquaporins or resynthesised in the cell from glucose during glyceroneogenesis. For lipogenesis in adipose tissue of ruminants, uptake of glucose into adipocytes is necessary in addition to acetate.

Insulin is the most important regulatory hormone for lipogenesis. After food intake, both the uptake of glucose into adipocytes by the insulin-sensitive glucose transporter (GLUT4) and the uptake of fatty acids by the fatty acid transport system is stimulated. Additionally, new synthesis of fatty acids is accelerated by increased expression of the FAS.

MORE DETAILS

Pathophysiology of adipose tissue metabolism

An imbalance between energy intake and output with extreme enlargement of fat tissue (obesity) is responsible for the pathogenesis of some diseases in humans and animals. Excessive energy intake or unbalanced intake of certain nutrients, in combination with insufficient energy expenditure by physical activity, leads to increased fat accumulation, obesity. Consequences can be increased blood pressure, systemic inflammation, atherosclerosis and insulin resistance with disturbances in glucose balance (hyperglycaemia, hyperinsulinaemia) and fat balance (hyperlipidaemia, hepatosteatosis, hyperleptinaemia). An increased tendency to laminitis is observed in obese, insulin-resistant horses, and obese cats may develop a condition similar to type II diabetes in humans. In dairy cows, especially those that become obese ante partum, peripartum diseases such as mastitis, metritis, laminitis and ketosis are thought to be caused by disturbed adipose tissue metabolism. The massive lipo-mobilisation in adipose tissues during postpartum negative energy balance is held responsible for this. Obese ponies also develop massive lipo-mobilisation during periods of negative energy balance, resulting in pathological hyperlipidaemia. Since several obesity-associated diseases often occur simultaneously, this constellation in humans and animals is called the "metabolic syndrome". An inadequate amount of adipose tissue in the body (**lipodystrophy**) can also have pathophysiological consequences for metabolic health because of the lack of control by adipocytokines.

18.3 Endocrine signals of adipose tissue – adipocytokines

Numerous endocrine signals from adipose tissue control many metabolic processes in animals and humans. These signals, the **adipocytokines**, are particularly important for metabolic control of substrate distribution throughout the body. One of the most important variables influenced by adipose tissue activity is **insulin sensitivity (IS)**. A tissue is insulin sensitive if its cells are responsive to insulin. This manifests itself in increased uptake of glucose into muscle and adipose tissue cells after a meal. Adaptive variation in

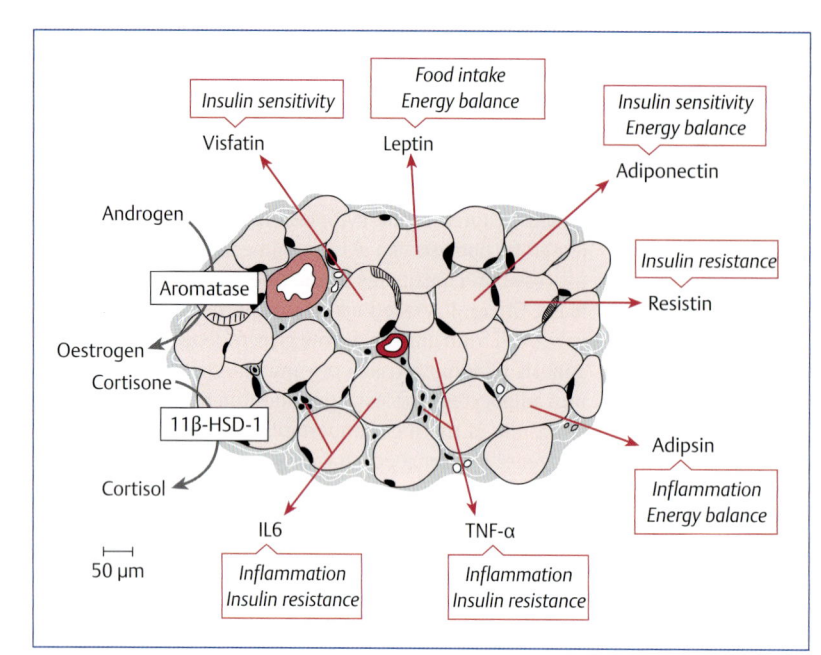

Fig. 18.3 Adipose tissue produces an abundance of adipocytokines that help maintain energy balance and thus control the metabolic activities of an animal. Only a selection of the best-known adipocytokines is shown. IL-6 = interleukin-6; TNF-α = tumour necrosis factor-alpha; 11β-HSD-1 = beta-hydroxysteroid dehydrogenase 1.

the IS of individual tissues is an important mechanism for changes in substrate distribution. For example, at the onset of lactation, a reduction in the IS of muscle and adipose tissue redirects glucose to the mammary gland. A pathophysiological deterioration in insulin sensitivity is termed **insulin resistance (IR)**. This is a metabolic state that can be pro-inflammatory. Variation in IS, the development of IR and associated metabolic diseases are all responses to particular adipocytokines, especially in obese animals and humans. **Fig. 18.3** shows an overview of the best-known adipocytokines with their main functions. The influence of adipocytokines in the control of food intake (p. 519), energy balance (p. 483), reproduction (p. 553) as well as systemic inflammation and immunity (p. 244) will be presented in more detail in the following sections. From this it should become clear that adipose tissue with its adipocytokines is essential in maintaining energy homeostasis. However, "too much" or "too little" body fat can also have negative consequences.

18.3.1 Influence on food intake

The most important adipocytokine in regulating food intake is **leptin**. The main effects of this hormone are mediated via specific leptin receptors in nuclei of the hypothalamus (nucleus arcuatus, dorso- and ventromedial nuclei) which results in a reduction in food intake. Leptin reduces the secretion of the neurotransmitter NPY and thus has an appetite-suppressing (**anorexigenic**) effect in many mammalian species. Leptin also alters the **palatability** of food and thus its attractiveness for consumption. The sensitivity of sweet-taste sensors on the tongue in humans and rats is reduced by leptin. These processes are part of a **lipostatic** (fat tissue-based) **regulation of food intake**. When adipose tissue grows, it secretes more leptin, thus limiting its further growth. Conversely, lower leptin levels in thin animals cause an increase in food intake. In obese animals, central

leptin resistance can develop, leading to a disturbance in food intake behaviour. Despite compensatory hyperleptinaemia, extremely high food intakes, **hyperphagia**, can develop.

18.3.2 Influence on energy balance

Leptin promotes energy utilisation and sympathetic tone, so that basal metabolic rate (p. 489) and thermogenesis (p. 499) both increase. Leptin stimulates lipolysis in adipose tissue, as well as in all other tissues, so that adipose tissue growth is autocrine inhibited. The increased β-oxidation of free fatty acids reduces their cellular concentrations and thus improves the insulin sensitivity of many tissues. Regulation of leptin secretion, in addition to its local control in adipose tissue by insulin, which promotes leptin secretion, is also through the negative effect of leptin in the pancreas where it inhibits insulin secretion (**adipoinsular axis**). This adipoinsular axis significantly controls energy balance via central and peripheral mechanisms. Another important adipocytokine in regulation of energy balance, **adiponectin**, is secreted in large quantities into blood by adipocytes. This hormone stimulates peripheral insulin sensitivity by promoting β-oxidation of free fatty acids and thus stabilises insulin action in liver and muscles. Adiponectin blood concentration is reduced in obese and diabetic (type 2 diabetes) humans and rodents. The insulin resistance that occurs in these states is also promoted by **resistin**, **adipsin**, **TNF-α** and **interleukin-6** (IL-6). These adipocytokines (p. 482), also called pro-inflammatory hormones, are present in high concentrations in blood in obesity and type 2 diabetes.

Because of the presence of relevant enzymes, adipose tissue is also able to produce and secrete classical hormones such as **cortisol** and **oestrogen** from precursor molecules. The effect of oestrogen is mainly for the promotion of subcutaneous fat storage. Androgens as well as cortisol, on the other hand, predominantly promote visceral fat storage and favour the secretion of adipocytokines, which have a negative effect on insulin sensitivity.

18.3.3   Influence on reproduction

Reproduction is one of the physiological processes that consumes the most energy. A close coupling of reproduction to metabolism is therefore essential. When there is metabolic stress there are consequences for fertility in both female and male animals. A reduction in fertility in metabolic stress is a physiological protective reaction for survival of the animal itself. This manifests itself as delayed onset of sexual maturity, in prolonged anoestrus phases and poor conception rates, especially with artificial insemination. The mechanisms underlying this depression of fertility are not yet well understood.

In the **metabolic regulation of reproduction**, central signalling pathways in the **hypothalamus** are involved. These pathways are also responsible for regulating feed intake (**Fig. 18.4**). In addition to insulin and ghrelin, a hormone from gastric epithelium, the adipocytokine **leptin** is important in mammals in coordinating metabolism with the processes of reproduction. At physiological states of adequately filled adipose tissue depots, leptin centrally inhibits food intake (p.480). It also acts on the hypothalamic-pituitary-gonadal axis and stimulates pulsatile gonadotropin (GnRH)/luteinising hormone (LH) secretion.

> **MORE DETAILS**   The mechanism of the leptin effect on GnRH neurons has not yet been sufficiently clarified. Presumably, this leptin effect is achieved indirectly via modulation of hypothalamic transmitters (NPY, AgRP, MSH). These transmitters act in an as yet unexplained way on kisspeptin (Kiss1) neurons, which act directly on the GnRH-forming cells and modulate the pulsatile GnRH release.

The gonadotropic axis is thus able to react to an undersupply of energy from food intake, and also to an oversupply of dietary energy. This indicates that fertility can be directly controlled by metabolic signals. Lactation is a special physiological state of energy deficiency in which, above all, there must be an increased intake of food energy and other nutrients which are then distributed to the mammary gland. Metabolic regulation of reproduction is responsible

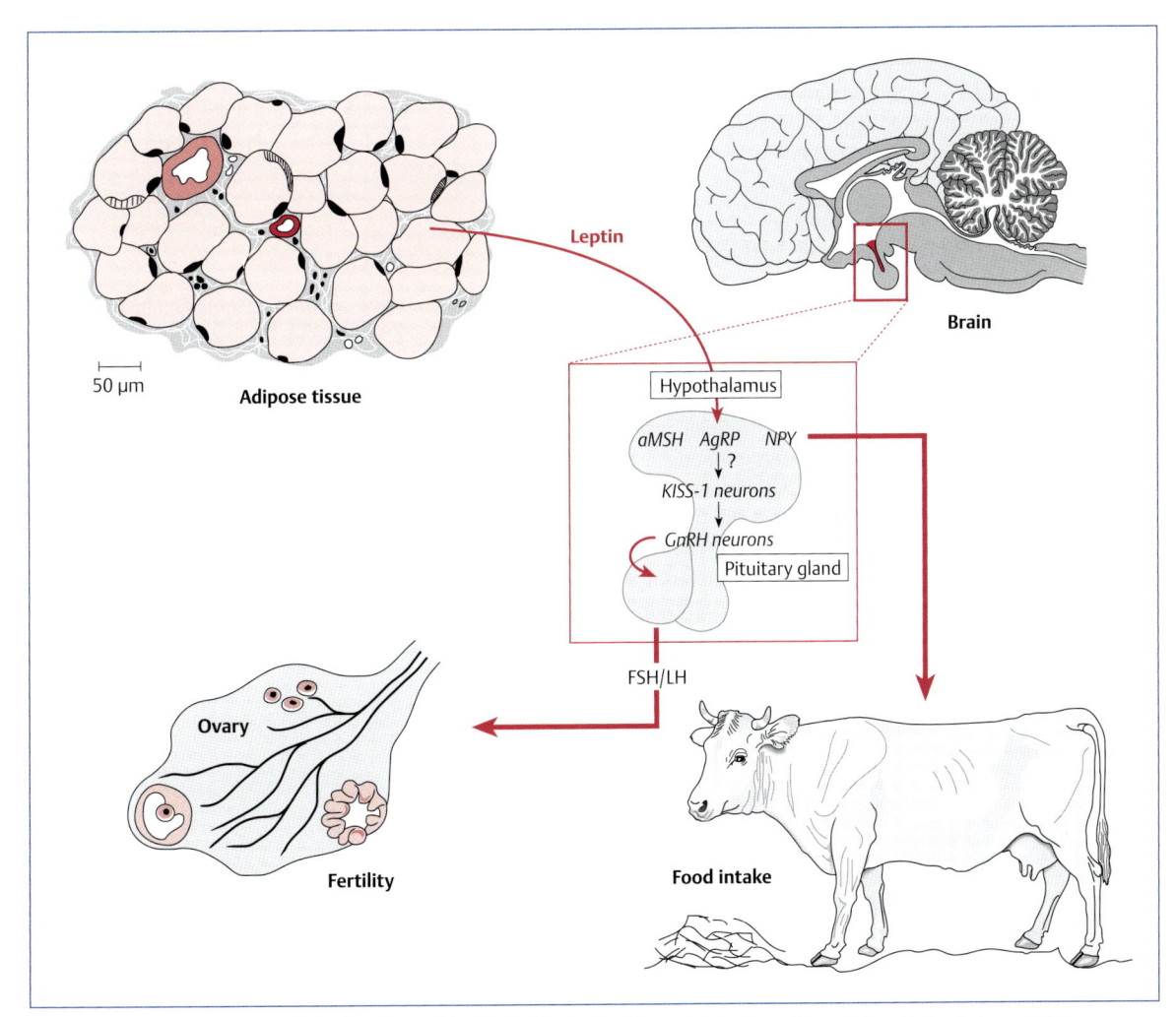

Fig. 18.4 Metabolic regulation of food intake and fertility by leptin. Leptin modulates the release of hypothalamic transmitters (NPY = anorexigenic neuropeptide Y; AgRP = anorexigenic Agouti-related peptide; αMSH = anorexigenic α-melanocyte-stimulating hormone) that influence KISS-1 neurons. These KISS-1 neurons are possible "translators" of metabolic signals into the language of reproduction (GnRH = gonadotropin-releasing hormone; FSH = follicle-stimulating hormone; LH = luteinising hormone).

for suppressing pulsatile GnRH release from the hypothalamus during lactation, thus preventing the ovary from performing its cyclic functions. At the same time, because leptin secretion is low, there is increased secretion of neuropeptide Y (NPY) from the hypothalamus, promoted by the low leptin levels This stimulates food intake, which is able to compensate for the outflow of energy in milk. If this adaptation fails, there is both a negative energy balance (e.g. in dairy cows in early lactation) and also a considerable decline in fertility.

Fertility disorders involving this central leptin-mediated regulatory level can also be triggered by excessive physical exercise in humans (relative lack of energy for reproduction) or by **hypophagia** (reduced food intake and thus negative energy balance). In obese animals and humans, fertility disorders also frequently occur from central leptin resistance and a pro-inflammatory state that develop.

In addition to these central effects, leptin also acts peripherally directly on the gonads in female and male animals, and leptin receptors are found on ovaries and testes. High concentrations of leptin appear to be partly responsible for the development of ovarian cysts in pigs, cattle and humans, thereby further impairing fertility. The reason for this is inhibition of oestrogen production in the follicle by leptin which disturbs ovarian function, so that normal follicle development is impaired. The multifactorial polycystic ovarian syndrome (PCOS) is a common cause of infertility in obese women.

18.3.4 Influence on systemic inflammation and immunity

Adipose tissue actively participates in inflammatory processes by not only responding to **pro-inflammatory signals** but also by secreting such signals itself, which exacerbates the inflammatory situation. For example, toll-like receptors on adipocytes bind bacterial lipopolysaccharides and thus increase local insulin resistance and inflammation. Tumour necrosis factor-α in blood activates the transcription factor NFκB (nuclear-factor-kappa B) pathway, especially in hypertrophied adipocytes, promoting inflammation and also insulin resistance and hyperlipidaemia. Dietary factors such as fatty acids can also cause pro-inflammatory reactions in adipose tissue. However, adipose tissue cells themselves also secrete TNF-α and other inflammatory factors (interleukins, complement factors, adipsin, immune cell-attracting factors such as MCP-1 and MIP1-α). These trigger **autocrine** and **paracrine** mechanisms that increase insulin resistance in adipose tissue and **endocrine secretions** from adipocytes promote insulin resistance in muscle and liver and a systemic inflammatory situation. Leptin and adiponectin are also involved in an inflammatory situation by modulating the secretion of pro-inflammatory adipocytokines. In addition, the inflammatory situation is influenced by interactions between adipocytes and resident or migrated immune cells (macrophages, lymphocytes) via paracrine signalling pathways.

In principle, inflammation is part of the innate immune system (p. 246) and serves as a defence. However, any dysfunction, particularly of visceral adipose tissue, can promote a chronic pro-inflammatory state that is itself a disease process. Even in acquired, cellular immunity, adipocytokines such as leptin have an influence by promoting the proliferation and activation of T cells.

IN A NUTSHELL   !

Adipose tissue is more than an energy store; it generates endocrine signals, the adipocytokines, and thus contributes to metabolic control of the whole animal. This maintains metabolic health, fertility and overall physiological performance. In addition, adipocytokines play an important role in non-specific innate defence and also acquired cellular immunity.

Suggested reading

Fantuzzi G. Adipose tissue, adipokines, and inflammation. J Allergy Clin Immunol 2005; 115: 91–919

Kahn CR, Wang G, Lee KY. Altered adipose tissue and adipocyte function in the pathogenesis of metabolic syndrome. J Clin Invest 2019; 129: 3990–4000

Kolditz CL, Langin D. Adipose tissue lipolysis. Curr Opin Clin Nutr Metabol Care 2010; 13: 377–381

Navarro VM, Kaiser UB. Metabolic influences on neuroendocrine regulation of reproduction. Curr Opin Endocrinol Diabetes Obes 2013; 20: 335–341

Sanchez-Garrido MA, Tena-Sempere M. Metabolic control of puberty: Roles of leptin and kisspeptins. Hormones and Behavior 2013; 64: 187–194

19   Energy balance

Joachim Roth, Gotthold Gäbel

19.1   Energy demand and energy turnover

ESSENTIALS   ✖

Every living organism is dependent on the regular and demand-driven supply of exogenous energy sources via feed, to maintain its internal functions and to perform physical work or produce metabolic products such as in growth, and for milk or egg production. At the cellular level, the way that chemical energy is used is from the incorporation and release of phosphate in ATP.

In the ingested feed, carbohydrates, fats and, under certain conditions, proteins, supply the energy to meet the physiological demand. These nutrients are converted into ATP in various metabolic pathways. During ATP formation and in its use in cell metabolism, a significant proportion of energy is converted into heat. Part of the energy in the feed is lost also in faeces, urine or in fermentation gases without being available to the organism for ATP production.

The basal turnover of energy in an animal's body is referred to as the **basal metabolic rate (BMR)** and can be measured in mammals under defined conditions such as at rest, after feeding and in a thermoneutral environment. In mammals, BMR increases with increasing body mass. An approximate estimation of BMR can be determined by measuring oxygen consumption (indirect calorimetry). At the **maintenance metabolic rate**, an animal has a steady energy expenditure. In addition to the energy required for basal metabolism, additional energy is needed in a thermoneutral environment, to obtain food, for the processes of digestion, and for total body muscular activity. This additional energy is defined as the energy of production, and is the quantity of energy that is required over and above the maintenance energy requirement, in order to perform physical work or for metabolic synthesis.

19.2   Introduction

Animals need energy to maintain their structure, for general body metabolism, to perform external work, and to synthesize various chemical products. A living organism is an open system in which any change in total energy utilisation is balanced by the exchange of energy with its environment.

The energy-requiring processes in an animal include **life-sustaining functions** such as cardiac, respiratory and digestive activity, **transport processes across cell mem-**branes, and also the **biosynthesis of the body's own molecular structures**. Additional energy is required for **growth**, and for various **metabolic syntheses** such as milk, wool or egg production and also for **pregnancy** in reproduction.

Therefore, a supply of energy-providing nutrients is needed, corresponding to the animal's energy expenditure. If energy utilisation is **balanced**, the supply of energy-providing substances is equivalent to the energy expenditure of the animal. In a **positive energy balance**, the energy intake is greater than the energy expenditure, which leads to an increase in body weight. In a **negative energy balance**, such as when the output of an energy containing product like milk, is greater than the amount of energy input from feed, there is mobilisation of the body's energy stores, with a resulting decrease in body mass.

Energy is supplied as chemical energy from ingested feed. **Adenosine triphosphate (ATP)** is the immediately available energy carrier of each cell. In order for ATP to be produced, nutrients must first be digested, and the products after absorption, enter further catabolic pathways in the various tissues and organs. Energy can be stored as fat and also as carbohydrate (glycogen). After absorption, the amino acids of digested feed proteins are primarily used for the synthesis of the body's own protein, but they can also be used for energy production, see ch. on gluconeogenesis (p. 469). For example, in carnivores there is a considerable increase in excretion of nitrogen in urine after eating meat, which indicates an increased use of dietary-derived amino acids as a source of energy.

In the organism, energy-providing substrates are oxidatively degraded with the utilisation of oxygen (O_2). The energy released in this process is used to generate energy-rich phosphate bonds (**Fig. 19.1**). **ATP is** produced in this process. Other energy-rich compounds such as creatine phosphate (p. 157) may also, to a limited extent, be produced directly from ATP (ch. 7.4 (p. 180)) ATP provides the energy for **biosynthetic pathways**, **active transport processes** across cell membranes and **muscle contraction**. During the **hydrolysis of ATP to ADP and P_i**, approx. **30 kJ · mol^{-1}** of chemical energy is released. However, the cellular store of ATP and other molecules with energy-rich phosphate bonds is limited, and would only meet energy demand for a very short time, even under resting conditions. ATP must therefore be continuously generated and made available through the oxidative degradation of substrates (**Fig. 19.1**) (see ch. Energy metabolism of the working muscle (p. 617)).

Nutrition, energy

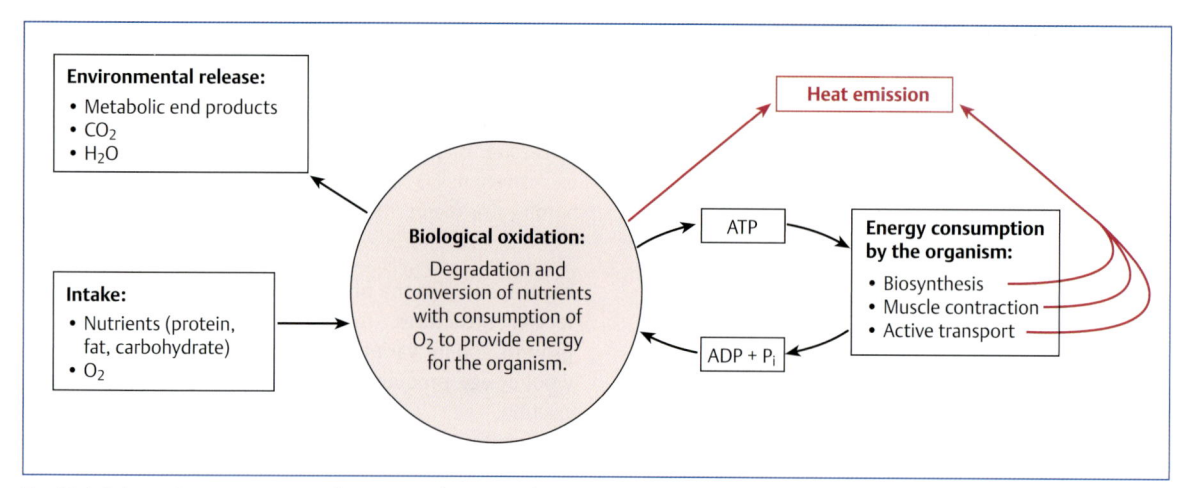

Fig. 19.1 Schematic representation of energy production and consumption in the animal.

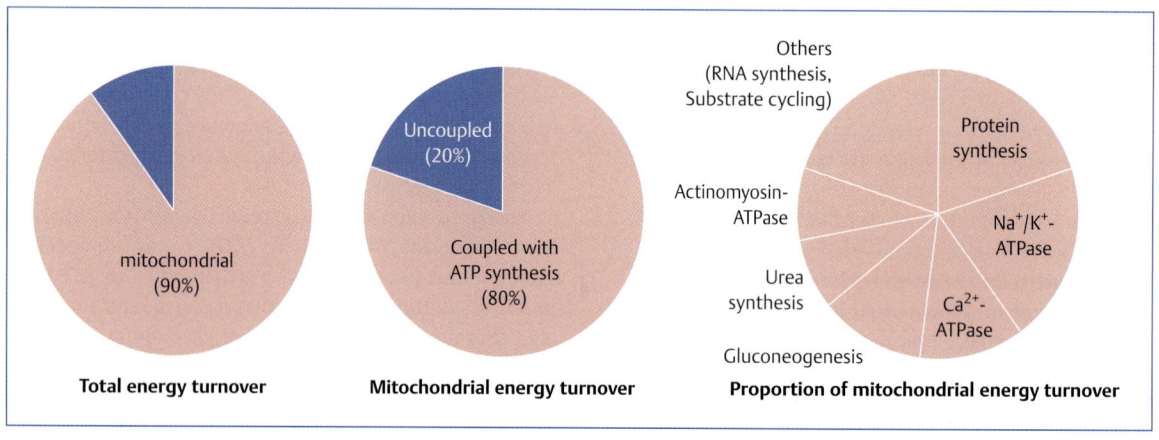

Fig. 19.2 Proportion of total energy expenditure in different cellular processes.

MORE DETAILS   On examining the different cellular processes consuming energy, the following pattern emerges (**Fig. 19.2**): 90% of the available energy is used for mitochondrial processes. The remaining 10% is used by processes in the cytoskeleton or the Golgi apparatus. Of the 90% mitochondrial energy utilisation, approx. 80% is needed for the synthesis of ATP, while the remaining 10% is lost through so-called proton leaks. The ATP produced is used for energy-consuming processes of protein synthesis, membrane active transport, gluconeogenesis, urea synthesis, etc.

Under aerobic conditions, oxidation of 1 mol glucose can produce 36–38 moles of ATP. Under anaerobic conditions glucose degradation produces lactate, and only 2 mol ATP are formed. In the oxidation of long-chain fatty acids such as palmitic or stearic acid, approx. 140 mol ATP are produced per mol, depending on the chain length. The processes of energy production in organs and tissues, need to be distinguished from the energy production of bacteria, protozoa and fungi in the gastrointestinal tract. In the ruminant forestomachs and in the large intestine, microbial fermentation of carbohydrates takes place in a largely anaerobic environment. Under those conditions, carbohydrates are converted into short-chain fatty acids: acetate, propionate and butyrate (see ch. Microbial metabolism in the forestomachs (p. 398) and large intestine (p. 438). The microorganisms use only about 6–7% of the energy con-

tained in the carbohydrates for their own energy requirements. In the rumen and in the large intestine the short-chain fatty acids are absorbed and on complete oxidation of a mol each of acetate, propionate and butyrate 10, 18 and 28 mol ATP are produced, respectively

The efficiency of the energy transformation as shown in **Fig. 19.1** is about 50%, i.e., only about half of this energy can be used for the production of ATP. The remaining 50% is released as heat. Energy released during the hydrolysis of ATP can be converted into mechanical energy for muscle work. However, only half of the energy, at most, that is released during the hydrolysis of ATP can be converted into mechanical energy. The other half is released as heat. The efficiency of energy utilisation for mechanical work is only 25% at best. Energy loss also occurs in the biosynthesis of the body's own tissues. In a resting state (without external work and without major synthesis and storage processes), and basic metabolic conditions (p. 489), almost all the energy being used by an animal is ultimately released as heat.

Therefore, the amount of heat being produced, is a measure of the animal's energy metabolism. Study of an animal's **energy balance** can be done by direct or indirect **measurement** of **heat output** (**calorimetry**).

Nutrition, energy

> **IN A NUTSHELL**   **!**
>
> Animal metabolic processing oxidatively breaks down the nutrients obtained from food. In this process, ATP is produced as a direct energy carrier that is essential for life. A by-product of oxidation is heat.

MORE DETAILS   The standard basic unit for measurement of thermal or electrical energy, is defined as the Joule (J). Depending on the amount of energy, the decimal multiples k (kilo) or M (mega) are used:

1 MJ = 1000 kJ = 1000000 J

In the past, the amount of heat was expressed by the unit of a calorie. One calorie is the amount of energy required to raise the temperature of 1 g of water by 1 °C. The following conversion applies: 1 calorie = 4.187 J. From a physical point of view, the energy turnover is a power (heat energy per time) and is therefore expressed in the unit Watt (W = J · s^{-1}).

19.3   Energy content of nutrients

19.3.1   Measurement of the energy content of nutrients

The principle for measuring the **energy content** of **nutrients, feedstuffs, other oxidisable substances**, faecal and urinary excretions, and fermentation gases, is the measurement of the heat released during the combustion of each of these. The measurement is carried out in a **combustion or bomb calorimeter**. The substance to be burnt is placed in a metal cylinder surrounded by a water jacket. An insulating outer vessel prevents any external heat loss. The substance is completely burnt in pure oxygen under high pressure (O_2 excess). The **heat of combustion** released in this process increases temperature of the surrounding water, which is measured with a precise thermometer. The heating of 1 kg H_2O by 1 °C corresponds to a heat energy of 4.187 kJ (equivalent to 1 kilocalorie). The thermal energy determined in this way, when a substance burns completely, is called the **physical calorific value** or the **gross energy** of the substance.

19.3.2   Physical calorific values of nutrients

With a bomb calorimeter, you can determine how much energy is released by complete combustion of 1 g of carbohydrate, fat, or protein. For example, the complete combustion to CO_2 and H_2O of **glucose** ($C_6 H_{12} O_6$) and other **monosaccharides** with the same molecular formula releases the same quantity of energy of **15.6 kJ · g^{-1}**. The most important dietary carbohydrates (starch, cellulose) are **polysaccharides**: macromolecules consisting of glycosidically linked glucose units where the **physical calorific value** (due to the energy in the glycosidic bonds) is higher than that of monosaccharides, i.e. slightly above **17 kJ · g^{-1}**.

The most important dietary fats are **triacylglycerols** which make up about 90% of the lipids in a diet. They are esters of **glycerol**, each containing three fatty acids of different chain lengths and degrees of saturation. The **physical calorific value** of **fats**, which can also be completely burnt to CO_2 and H_2O, is about **39 kJ · g^{-1}**.

Since **proteins** contain nitrogen and sulphur in addition to carbon, hydrogen and oxygen, they cannot be burned exclusively to CO_2 and H_2O. Combustion of proteins in the bomb calorimeter, therefore additionally leads to variable amounts of N_2 and SO_2. The average **physical calorific value of proteins** is about **23 kJ · g^{-1}**.

19.3.3   Physiological calorific value

Carbohydrates and **fats** are completely oxidised in an animal (just as in the bomb calorimeter) to CO_2 and H_2O, albeit by different chemical reaction pathways. This means that these two nutrients release the same amount of heat energy during their oxidative degradation in an organism as in a bomb calorimeter (Hess's law of the independence of the energy difference between the initial and final product from the number of chemical reactions involved). For **carbohydrates** and **fats**, the **physiological calorific value** therefore corresponds approximately to the physical calorific value determined in the bomb calorimeter.

The combustion of **proteins** in a bomb calorimeter, leads to different end products than their catabolism in living animals. In animals, **ammonia, urea** (mammals) or **uric acid** (birds, reptiles) are formed, and these each have significant calorific values. Their energy content must therefore be subtracted from the calorific value of the protein utilised by an animal. The **physiological calorific value** of **proteins**, at approx. **18 kJ · g^{-1}**, is therefore significantly lower than the physical calorific value or gross energy content.

> **IN A NUTSHELL**   **!**
>
> Carbohydrates and fats can be completely oxidised in the organism to CO_2 and H_2O as in the bomb calorimeter. Their physiological calorific value therefore corresponds to the physical calorific value, or gross energy content. In addition to CO_2 and H_2O, the oxidative degradation of proteins in an animal, also produces N-containing end products which still contain chemical energy which is not available to the animal. The physiological calorific value of protein is therefore always lower than the physical calorific value.

19.3.4   Food as a source of energy

The energy content determined with a bomb calorimeter is referred to as the **gross energy** and corresponds to the physical calorific value (**Fig. 19.3**). However, not all the energy contained in the feed is fully available to the animal.

Thus, from the gross energy content of food, the chemical energy in **faeces** of animals must be subtracted, to determine the proportion of food energy that has been absorbed via the digestive tract. That portion of feed energy is called **digestible energy**. Another part of the feed energy is lost in urine and as methane released by ruminants (p.401) and large intestine digesters (p.439). If this part of

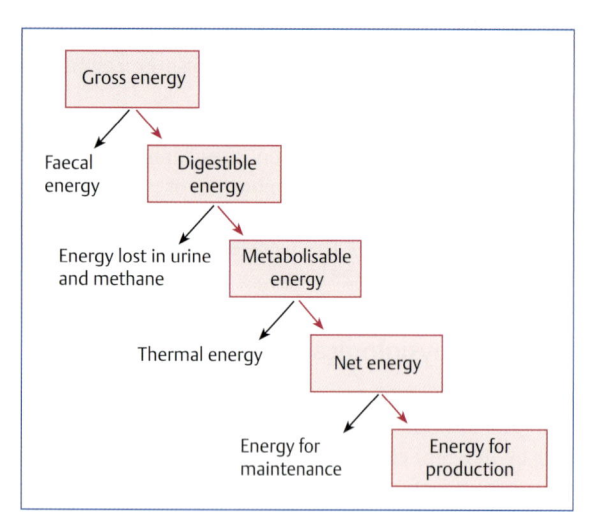

Fig. 19.3 Diagram of the energy stages during digestion and conversion in an animal.

digestible energy is subtracted, the remaining energy obtained from food is the **convertible or metabolisable energy**. When chemical energy is transferred into ATP which is then used in some metabolic process, some energy is released as heat (**Fig. 19.1**). The remaining energy is the **net energy** which can be used for maintenance (p. 489) or for **work** and biosynthesis (p. 490) of animal products. To determine the net energy content of a feed, complex experiments and analyses are necessary, especially because the "energy losses" vary greatly depending on the nature of the feed. The physical composition of the feed alone strongly influences the "energy losses" from the muscle action in chewing and from gastrointestinal motility. Feed for horses is assessed according to its digestible energy content; feed for cattle, small ruminants, pigs, poultry, dogs, cats and fish is assessed according to its convertible energy (metabolisable energy) content.

> **IN A NUTSHELL** !
>
> During the utilisation of feed by an animal, energy losses occur in faeces, urine, in fermentation gases and as heat. The animal can only use a part (net energy) of the energy of the feed consumed (gross energy) for maintenance and for production.

19.4 Measurement of energy metabolism

The energy metabolism of an animal can be determined by measuring the heat released (**direct calorimetry**) or by measuring the gas exchange of CO_2 and O_2 (**indirect calorimetry**).

19.4.1 Direct calorimetry

At rest, no external work is done by an animal. All of the energy transformations in the body are converted into heat, apart from that portion stored in the increased body mass during growth. In endothermic animals, this generated heat must be continuously released to the environment to maintain a constant body core temperature (**heat generation equals heat** release (p. 495)). Thus, the **resting energy turnover** in endothermic animals can be determined by **measuring the amount of heat** released to the outside. This procedure is called **direct calorimetry** and is carried out in an **animal calorimeter**.

> **MORE DETAILS** In the **ice calorimeter**, first used by Lavoisier, the experimental animal is placed in a closed container with air supply and exhaust. This container lies within a layer of ice (or a mixture of ice and water), which in turn is surrounded by an insulating outer container. The weight of ice that melts over time is then measured, to determine the heat emission from the animal. The specific heat of fusion ($334\,kJ \cdot [g\,H_2O]^{-1}$) can then be used to calculate the heat released. Since this method can only be used to measure at $0\,°C$, an alternative has been developed, where the animal is placed in a thermally insulated **chamber** with **controlled temperature**. The heat emitted by the animal is transferred via the ventilation flow or to a system through which water flows. The heat released by the animal can be calculated as the product of the amount of air or water flowing through and the temperature difference between the incoming and outgoing air (or water). Because of this considerable technical complexity, direct calorimetry is rarely used for studies on animals and humans.

19.4.2 Indirect calorimetry

In **indirect calorimetry**, the energy metabolism of an animal is calculated from its gas exchange, i.e., primarily from the **consumption of O_2**. This method assumes that **no anaerobic energy production** takes place during the time of measurement. As a first estimate of energy turnover, measurement of O_2 consumption is quite sufficient. For a more precise determination of energy metabolism and also to record the metabolised substrates, the respiratory quotient (RQ) is calculated, from both, O_2 consumption and CO_2 output. With the RQ (p. 488), energy metabolism of a test animal can be precisely determined from its measured O_2 consumption. The conversion is done with the help of the caloric equivalent (p. 487), which in turn has a different value depending on the RQ.

O_2 consumption can be measured in a **closed** spirometric **system** filled with O_2 (**Fig. 11.8**) or in an airtight chamber. The metabolic end product CO_2 can be adsorbed on soda lime (mixture of $Ca(OH)_2$ and $NaOH$) and H_2O can be bound to silica gel. Under these conditions, the **decrease** in the **amount of gas** in the chamber (or in the spirometer bell) corresponds to the **O_2 consumption of** the animal.

In the more commonly used **open system**, fresh air is pumped at a constant rate through the chamber containing the test animal. The O_2 and CO_2 contents of the air flowing into and out of the chamber are continuously recorded by **gas analysis** (Fig. 19.4). From the air flow through the chamber measured with a gas meter and gas analyser, the **O_2 consumption** and **CO_2 production** of the animal under investigation can be determined.

Alternatively, the amount of inspiratory air with a constant O_2 and CO_2 content can be measured with a gas meter or a pneumotachograph (**Fig. 11.9**). Samples of expira-

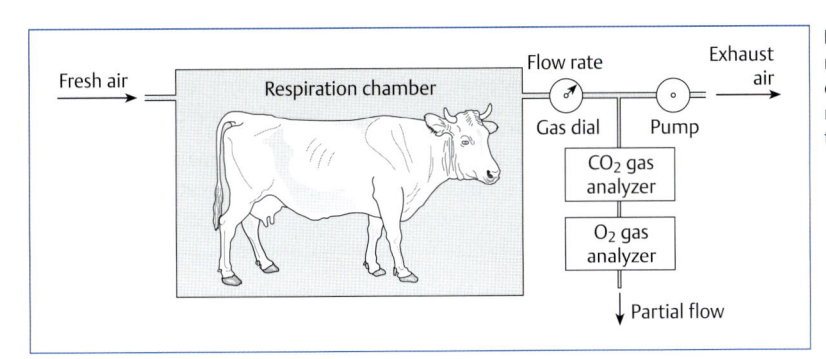

Fig. 19.4 Determination of the energy metabolism of animals from their gas exchange by indirect calorimetry in a respiration chamber with an open ventilation system.

tory air can be collected in a gas-tight bag (**Douglas bag**) and the O_2 and CO_2 contents in the collected expiratory air determined. In free galloping horses, O_2 consumption can also be measured using a pneumotachograph and O_2 sensors in the expired air.

■ The caloric equivalent

During the combustion of 1 mol glucose (180 g; **Table 19.1**) in a bomb calorimeter 2808 kJ of energy (= 15.6 $[kJ \cdot g^{-1}] \cdot$ 180 g) is released, with the consumption of 6 mol O_2, to produce 6 mol CO_2 and 6 mol H_2O as end products. The same amount of energy is released during the oxidative degradation of glucose in an animal, because the same end products are produced. As 1 mol O_2 corresponds to a gas volume of 22.4 litres, 134 litres of O_2 are consumed during combustion or biological oxidation of 1 mol glucose. The equation of this reaction is therefore:

Thus, per litre of consumed O_2, a quantity of heat of 21 kJ is released during the **combustion of glucose** (2808 kJ/134 l O_2). The amount of energy released per litre of consumed O_2 during the oxidative degradation of nutrients is called the **caloric equivalent**.

A corresponding reaction equation (**Table 19.2**) can be obtained for the combustion/biological oxidation of a fatty acid (palmitic acid, a saturated C_{16} fatty acid).

Thus, per litre of consumed O_2, a quantity of heat of 19.4 kJ is released during the combustion of **palmitic acid** (9984 kJ/515 l O_2). The caloric equivalent for the complete **oxidation of fats** is lower than the corresponding value for the combustion of carbohydrates, as more O_2 must be used for the oxidative degradation of fat.

As already mentioned in the chapter on the energy content of nutrients (p. 485), the stoichiometry in the biological **oxidation of proteins** is more complicated, since in addition to CO_2 and H_2O, N-containing compounds (e.g. urea) are also formed. This is exemplified by the degradative oxidation of the amino acid **alanine** (**Table 19.3**) in mammals.

Table 19.1 Combustion of glucose.

1 mol $C_6H_{12}O_6$	+	6 mol O_2	→	6 mol H_2O	+	6 mol CO_2	+	2808 kJ
180 g glucose (15.6 kJ · g⁻¹)		134 l O_2		Respiratory water		134 l CO_2		heat released

Table 19.2 Combustion of palmitic acid.

1 mol $C_{16}H_{32}O_2$	+	23 mol O_2	→	16 mol H_2O	+	16 mol CO_2	+	9984 kJ
256 g palmitic acid (39 kJ · g⁻¹)		515 l O_2		Respiratory water		358 l CO_2		heat released

Table 19.3 Oxidation of alanine.

2 mol CH₃CH-NH₂-COOH	+	6 mol O_2	→	5 mol H_2O	+	5 mol CO_2	+	2723 kJ + 1 mol $CO(NH_2)_2$ (urea)
178 g alanine (15.3 kJ · g⁻¹)		134 l O_2		Respiratory water		112 l CO_2		amount of heat released plus the energy contained in the urea

Table 19.4 Caloric equivalent and RQ.

Substrate	Caloric equivalent $(kJ \cdot [l\ O_2]^{-1})$	Respiratory quotient (mol CO_2 /mol O_2)
Carbohydrates	21,0	1,0
Fat	19,5	0,7
Mixed combustion (⅓ carbohydrates to ⅔ fat)	20,0	0,8

Thus, per litre of O_2 consumed, a quantity of heat of 20.3 kJ is released during the biological oxidation of alanine (2723 kJ/134 l O_2). The energy content of the urea produced is not available to the animal. On average, the caloric equivalent for proteins converted for energy production is approx. $19\ kJ \cdot (l\ O_2)^{-1}$. It should also be noted that in most mammals (exception: carnivores) proteins and amino acids are only used to a small extent as a source of energy (see ch. Physiological functions of the liver (p. 463). Thus, in protein turnover in humans under physiological conditions, only about 12–15% of total energy of the amino acids is available for general energy use.

■ The respiratory quotient (RQ)

A direct measure of whether an animal is obtaining the energy it needs is mainly from the oxidation of carbohydrate or fat is provided by the **respiratory quotient (RQ)**. The **RQ** is defined as the **ratio** of **released CO_2 to consumed O_2**. Since 6 moles of CO_2 are released and 6 moles of O_2 are consumed during metabolic **oxidation of glucose** (see. Table 19.1), the **RQ is 1.0** (6 mol CO_2 /6 mol O_2). For the biological oxidation of **palmitic acid**, on the other hand, the **RQ is 0.7** (16 mol CO_2 /23 mol O_2; see Table 19.2). From the measured RQ as obtained from the gas analysis (**Fig. 19.4**), one can thus calculate the current ratio of fat to carbohydrate of the substrates being oxidised in an animal. If the RQ is closer to 0.7, fat is the main substrate being oxidatively degraded. If the RQ is closer to 1.0, carbohydrate oxidation dominates. In this way, the RQ can be used to directly infer the proportion of metabolised substrates.

The largely constant protein turnover is not taken into account here and can also be neglected in most animal species (exception: carnivores) because of its relatively low proportion of available energy. To determine the exact amount of protein that is used in energy metabolism, the excretion of nitrogenous substances (urea) in urine would have to be measured. Theoretically, with only **protein** being used as a source of energy (which is never the case under physiological conditions), the **RQ** would have a value of about **0.8**.

Each RQ measured by gas analysis (from 0.7–1.0) corresponds to a caloric equivalent value (from 19.5 to 21 kJ $\cdot$ $[l O_2]^{-1}$) depending on the fat to carbohydrate ratio of the oxidatively metabolised substrates (**Table 19.4**).

The RQ can give an erroneous result if the amount of CO_2 produced in metabolism differs from the amount of CO_2 released in respired gasses, during the same period. For this reason, in ruminants, where CO_2 released from the rumen via eructation mixes with the expiratory air, a slightly too high RQ is always measured in the respiratory chamber, from the point of view of intermediate metabolism.

MORE DETAILS   The informative value of the RQ about the composition of the oxidised substrates can be lost due to deviation of respiration from the normal state or due to nutrient conversion. In **hyperventilation**, where there is increased alveolar ventilation beyond metabolic needs, CO_2 is increasingly exhaled from blood and tissue stores, and appears in increased amounts in the expired air (p. 268). Since blood and tissue do not have significantly increased storage capacities for O_2, the measured O_2 consumption remains mainly constant during hyperventilation. Therefore, the **RQ** determined from the composition of respiratory gases, immediately increases to values **above 1.0** during **hyperventilation**.

Substrate conversion also leads to a deviation of the RQ from the current metabolic state. With high carbohydrate intake (“**carbohydrate fattening**, an animal converts **carbohydrate into fatty acids**. Glucose is only metabolised to acetyl-CoA which then goes directly into fatty acid synthesis. Thus, fewer reduction equivalents are produced (NADH/H[+]; FAD-H$_2$). Therefore, there is less oxidative phosphorylation compared to when glucose is completely oxidised. Hence, less O_2 is consumed and the **RQ rises significantly** above the value **1.0**. In **fattening geese** and **pigs** RQ may rise **up to 1.6**).

RQ values below 0.7 can occur during **food restriction**, and also in negative energy balance from severe carbohydrate deficiency or from **impaired carbohydrate utilisation**, as in diabetes mellitus. Under these circumstances, there is a deficit of oxaloacetic acid to enable acetyl-CoA from fat breakdown, to enter the citric acid cycle. The acetyl-CoA is then converted into **ketone bodies** (β-hydroxybutyrate, acetoacetate, acetone). Thus, carbon from the metabolism of fat is only partially oxidised to CO_2, so that the RQ falls below the value for complete metabolic oxidation of fat (0.7).

> **IN A NUTSHELL**   !
>
> The respiratory quotient (RQ) is the quantity of CO_2 released divided by the quantity of O_2 consumed. Under physiological conditions the RQ varies between 0.7 (pure fat oxidation) and 1.0 (pure carbohydrate oxidation).

■ Calculation of energy conversion from O_2 consumption and caloric equivalent

Energy expenditure is the **product** of **O_2 consumption** and **caloric equivalent**. Although according to the previous explanations the value of the caloric equivalent depends on the composition of the nutrients being oxidised (19.5–21 kJ $\cdot$ $[l O_2]^{-1}$), for practical purposes it is usually sufficient to assume a **caloric equivalent** of **20** kJ $\cdot$ $(l O_2)^{-1}$ and multiply this value by the measured O_2 consumption.

MORE DETAILS

Example calculations for indirect calorimetry

A 0.5 kg **guinea pig** is placed in a respiration chamber through which a constant flow of $2 l \cdot min^{-1}$ air passes. The air flowing into the chamber contains 20.9% O_2; the air flowing out of the chamber contains 20.4% O_2. This means that the guinea pig continuously "takes" 0.5% O_2 from the air flowing through the chamber. 0.5% of $2 l \cdot min^{-1}$ corresponds to an O_2 consumption of $0.01 l$ $O_2 \cdot min^{-1}$. Assuming a caloric equivalent of $20 kJ \cdot (l\,O_2)^{-1}$ results in the following energy turnover (E):

$$E = 0.01 l\,O_2 \cdot min^{-1} \cdot 20 kJ \cdot (l\,O_2)^{-1} = \mathbf{0.2\,kJ \cdot min^{-1}}$$
$$= 3.33 J \cdot s^{-1} = 3.33 W \qquad (19.1)$$

For a 70 kg **person**, an O_2 consumption of $0.25 l\,O_2 \cdot min^{-1}$ is measured under resting conditions. For this person, the energy metabolism is calculated as follows:

$$E = 0.25 l\,O_2 \cdot min^{-1} \cdot 20 kJ \cdot (l\,O_2)^{-1} = \mathbf{5\,kJ \cdot min^{-1}}$$
$$= 83.33 J \cdot s^{-1} = 83.33 W \qquad (19.2)$$

Thus, although the much larger human has a much higher energy metabolism in absolute terms than the guinea pig, the situation is different in relation to each kg of body mass:

Guinea pig: $6.7\,W \cdot kg^{-1}$ and human: $1.2\,W \cdot kg^{-1}$, see ch. on energy metabolism and body size (p. 490).

> ## IN A NUTSHELL !
>
> The energy metabolism of an animal can be determined by direct calorimetry (measurement of heat release) or indirect calorimetry (product of the measured O_2 consumption and the caloric equivalent).

19.5 Influences on energy metabolism

The energy metabolism of animals is variable and is under the influence of numerous factors. In adult animals that do not perform any work or synthesis, the level of energy metabolism is primarily determined by **body mass** and the **body surface** area. Animal species, age, sex, ambient temperature, activity status and hormone status are other factors which affect energy turnover. After the intake of **food** (postprandial thermogenesis = "calorigenic effect of food".) and during **physical activity**, as well as during **pregnancy**, energy metabolism is increased. In farm animals with high productivity in the form of growth, milk or egg production, a high proportion of energy metabolism is directed to these production activities.

19.5.1 Basal metabolic rate

Energy metabolism, in an awake, resting animal, in a postabsorptive phase from feeding, and under thermoneutral conditions is called **basal metabolic rate**. Under these standardised conditions, comparisons can be made between different animal species or between animals of the same species, with regard to their energy turnover rate. The basal metabolic rate corresponds to the energy required to maintain vital bodily functions: heat production to maintain constant core body temperature, and also the functions of respiration, cardiovascular system, basal muscle tone, etc.

The **postabsorptive state** required to determine the basal metabolic rate can be explained by the so-called **specific-dynamic effect** of the ingested food. Thus, energy metabolism increases immediately after feed intake. This cannot be explained by the motor, secretory and resorptive digestive activity alone, as the effect is much more pronounced with protein intake than after intake of comparable amounts of other nutrients. This energy loss is due to the strong stimulation of the utilisation of amino acids from food protein. The time of food abstinence necessary for basal metabolic rate measurement depends on the speed of food passage.

> ## IN A NUTSHELL !
>
> The **specific dynamic effect** of the food is the increase of the energy turnover immediately after food intake. Proteins stimulate the downstream protein metabolism, so the specific dynamic effect is higher for proteins than for carbohydrates and fats.

To minimise the energy consumption required for thermoregulation (p. 494) the basal metabolic rate must be measured in a **thermoneutral environment**. This is specific to each species. Below the thermoneutral temperature range, thermoregulatory metabolism increases in endothermic animals. Above the thermoneutral zone, energy expenditure for heat release must increase, by increased respiratory, sweat gland and circulatory activity.

The state of **physical rest** required to measure the basal metabolic rate is only maintained by animals for a short period of time, as spontaneous physical activity occurs regularly. Because of this spontaneous activity, which cannot be switched off, the measurement of animal energy metabolism always contains a more or less pronounced motor component.

19.5.2 Maintenance turnover

At the cellular level, the **maintenance metabolic rate is** the energy that a cell needs to maintain its structure, and thus its basic functionality. At the level of the whole animal, the maintenance metabolic rate goes beyond the basal metabolic rate to a limited extent. In **addition** to the basal metabolic rate, the animal needs energy for vital processes such as the **activities of food intake** and **digestion**. The energy for necessary moderate exercise is also included in the maintenance metabolic rate. If the animal is in maintenance metabolism, neither weight gain nor weight loss occurs. In practice, supplements are often given above the maintenance requirement, if the animal's environment is below the thermoneutral range.

19.5.3   Power metabolism

For specific performances, the animal requires additional energy over and above the maintenance metabolic rate. The **performance metabolism** is the energy required in addition to that for the basal metabolic rate, to be able to perform other activities. In human medicine, the term "**work metabolism**" is used for this. However, only a fraction of the energy, additional to that for basal or metabolic maintenance, can be used for physically defined external work. The greater part of this energy is converted into heat (**Fig. 19.1**). Thus, in humans and animals (e.g. draft **horses**), an efficiency higher than 25% is rarely achieved. This means that for any defined physical work, at least 4 times the amount of energy required for the basic or resting metabolic rate, must be provided. The maximum metabolic rate (p.621) that can be achieved for short periods of time during vigorous physical activity reaches values that are 4-fold (rodents),10-fold (dogs) or even 35-fold (camel or horse at a forced gallop) above the basal metabolic rate.

In addition to intense muscle work, much of the energy from consumed nutrients, is transformed into different products, such as body protein or fat in domestic adult animals. In veterinary medicine, energy transformation is of great importance and a great metabolic challenge in modern high-producing dairy cows (p.601), high performance egg-laying hens (**Table 19.6**) and for the rapid growth rates of young pigs and chickens. For example, in a dairy cow with a milk yield of $40 \cdot d^{-1}$ the energy utilisation increases to almost 5 times the rate for maintenance (**Table 19.5**). It should be emphasised that these increases are continuous, whereas such increases are sporadic in animals used for sport and only occur for a short time during muscle exertion.

A balanced energy state is one in which the net energy supplied through food (**Fig. 19.3**) equals actual energy utilisation. If more energy is required, the body's own energy reserves must be broken down and oxidised to subsidise the energy supply from food. In this situation, there is a **negative energy balance**. This phenomenon occurs not only when there is a **lack of food**, but also in **high-performance cows** in the early phase of lactation (p.615), and in special situations such as during hibernation (p.509).

> **IN A NUTSHELL** !
>
> The basal metabolic rate is measured at physical rest, in a nutritional postabsorptive state, and at thermoneutral ambient temperature. Basal metabolic rate allows intra- and interspecies comparison of energy turnover. The energy metabolism that exceeds the maintenance requirement during physical work or production (growth, eggs, milk, gestation), is called power metabolism.

19.6   Energy metabolism and body size

Since every living cell must constantly utilise energy in order to maintain its functions and to undertake specific tasks, the energy turnover of the entire organism depends on its body mass. The basal metabolic rate of large animals is therefore higher in absolute terms than that of smaller animals. However, **large animals** have a **lower basal metabolic rate** per kg of **body mass**, than **small animals** (**Fig. 19.5** calculation example in ch. 19.4.2 (p.486)).

Table 19.5 Energy requirement in net energy lactation (NEL) and dry matter intake required for this for a dairy cow (650 kg) at different milk yields.

Milk yield (l/day)*	Energy requirement NEL (MJ/day)	% of the maintenance requirement	Dry mass intake (kg/day)**
0 = maintenance	38	100	6
20	104	273	15
40	170	447	25
60	232	610	34

* each with 4% fat; ** at 6.8 MJ/kg dry matter of the feed. Source: Kamphues J et al. Supplemente zu Vorlesungen und Übungen in der Tierernährung. 12th ed., Alfeld-Hannover: M. u. H. Schaper; 2014. Loeffler et al. Anatomie und Physiologie der Haustiere. utb GmbH; 2018

Table 19.6 Convertible energy requirements of laying hens (2 kg body mass) in different housing systems and at different performance levels.

Laying performance (egg mass/day) [g]	Energy requirement (MJ/day) for floor husbandry	Energy requirement (MJ/day) for free-range husbandry
0 = maintenance	0,89	0,93
50	1,37	1,41
65	1,52	1,56

Source: Society for Nutritional Physiology (GfE). Recommendations for the energy and nutrient supply of laying hens and broilers. Frankfurt/Main: DLG-Verlag; 1999. Loeffler et al. Anatomie und Physiologie der Haustiere. utb GmbH; 2018

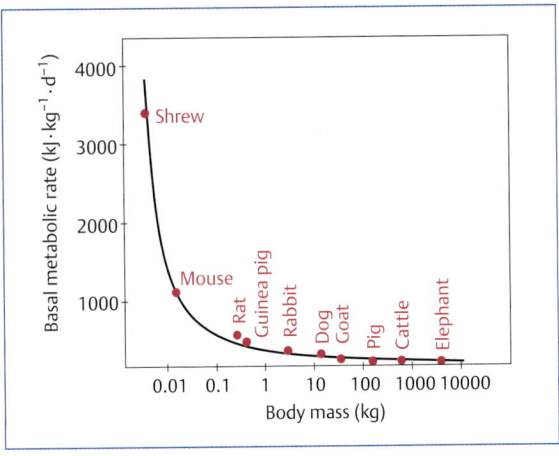

Fig. 19.5 Basal metabolic rate as a function of body mass of different sized mammals in 24 hours (semi-logarithmic representation); based on data from Wieser W. Bioenergetics. Stuttgart: Thieme; 1986

> **IN A NUTSHELL**   !
>
> The basal metabolic rate is lower in small animals in absolute terms, but higher in relative terms (per kg body mass) than in large animals.

The fact that the energy metabolism (basal metabolic rate) does not increase proportionally with increasing body mass has long been proven, among others by Max Kleiber. Accordingly, there is an allometric rather than an isometric relationship between body mass (M) and energy metabolism (MR = metabolic rate), which follows an exponential equation:

$$MR = a \cdot M^n \tag{19.3}$$

For n = 1, basal metabolic rate would be directly proportional to body mass. A hypothesis put forward by Max Rubner stated that the allometric relationship between body mass and basal metabolic rate was due to the size of the relative body surface area (so-called surface area theory). In this case, one would have to assume a value of n = ⅔ for the exponent, since the surface area of a three-dimensional body corresponds to the "⅔-power" of its volume and thus its mass. In fact, it is the ratio of **body surface area** to **body mass** that is of most importance. This is shown by the example of a cube with edge length a (**Fig. 19.6**).

> **MORE DETAILS**   If the edge length is 1, the volume of the cube is $1^3 = 1$ and the total surface area is $6 \cdot 1^2 = 6$. The ratio of volume:surface area is then 1:6. Doubling the edge length from 1 to 2 results in a volume of $2^3 = 8$, a surface area of $6 \cdot 2^2 = 24$ and a ratio of volume:surface area of 1:3. When the edge length is tripled from 1 to 3, the volume is $3^3 = 27$, the surface area is $6 \cdot 3^2 = 54$ and the ratio of surface area to volume is 1:2. Transferred to animals of different sizes, this means that **small animals have a large relative body surface area**. For large animals, this is reversed.

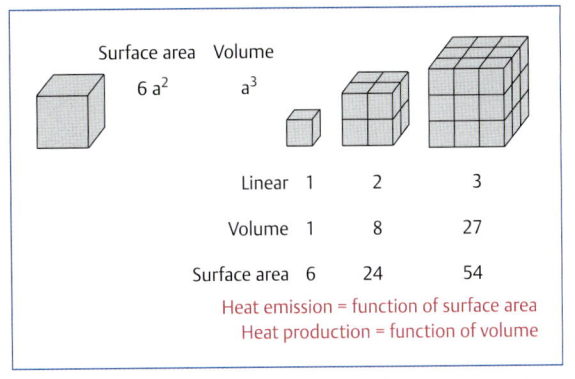

Fig. 19.6 The significance of the volume:surface area ratio using the example of a cube for the measured dependence of the energy turnover on the body size of the animals.

The **heat generation** of an animal takes place largely in the **body core** and depends on the **volume** or **body mass**. In most animals, however, **heat dissipation** or **heat loss** in most animals occurs predominantly via the **body surface** or the **respiratory tract**. **Small animals** have a **larger relative body surface per kg body mass** and thus also a **greater relative heat loss** to the environment per kg body mass, than large animals. Small animals can therefore cool down quickly. They can only maintain their core body temperature because of their high energy turnover. **Large animals**, on the other hand, would overheat with the high energy turnover of small animals, because their relative body surface area is too small to allow such high heat production.

The high relative energy turnover of small animals is possible because the proportion of **metabolically intensive internal organs** (heart, liver, kidneys) in the mass of the body is higher than that of the **supporting organs** (bones, connective tissue), which **have a low metabolic rate**. In large animals, this is reversed for mechanical reasons. This is another reason for the relatively higher metabolic rate of small animals compared to large animals (the so-called structural theory).

> **IN A NUTSHELL**   !
>
> The higher relative energy turnover in small animals compared to large animals is explained by their higher relative heat loss to the environment and their larger relative share of metabolically intensive organs in the total body mass.

In the basic turnover measurements carried out by Kleiber, the exponent of the exponential equation $MR = a \cdot M^n$ was approximately n = 0.75 (rounded up), **Fig. 19.7**). This means that when comparing species of different sizes, the resting energy turnover follows the ¾-potency rather than the ⅔-potency of the body mass. Despite some hypotheses to explain the allometric principle and the exponent determined (theory of external and internal surfaces, structural theory, transport theories), the physiological causes for the exponential relationship between body mass and energy turnover are not precisely known.

Nutrition, energy

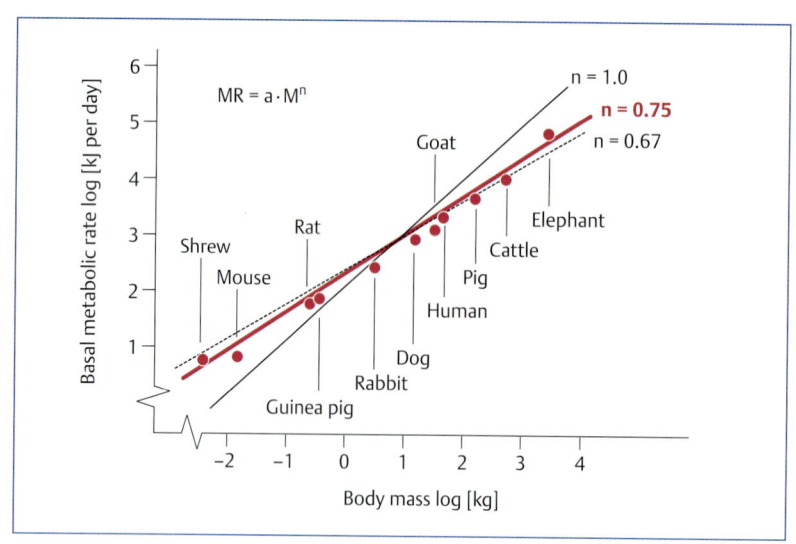

Fig. 19.7 Basal metabolic rate and body mass in mammals (basal metabolic rate = a · body mass^n = a · M^n. The following lines are plotted on a double logarithmic scale. **1.** if the values for basal metabolic rate were to increase proportionally to **body mass** (black line, n = 1); **2.** if the values for basal metabolic rate were to increase proportionally to **body surface area** (dashed line, n = 0.67); **3.** if the values for basal metabolic rate increase according to the dependence **described by Kleiber** (red, thickly highlighted line, n = 0.75). MR: metabolic rate; a: intersection with the y-axis; n: Slope of the respective straight line.

Kleiber carried out measurements with different animal species and with animals of different weights and thereby determined the following relationship between basal metabolic rate (BMR) and body weight:

$$BMR\ (kJ/day) = 283 \cdot M^{0.75} \qquad (19.4)$$

Subsequently, attempts were made to empirically determine the maintenance metabolic rate in the same way. Today the maintenance energy requirement is specified on the basis of the metabolizable energy ME. The maintenance requirement also correlates with the metabolic body weight, i.e. M$^{0.75}$, whereby, as expected, the factor a, i.e. the constant, takes on a greater value than with the basal metabolic rate. However, here too there is good agreement between animal species (with the exception of piglets), so that the following relationship can be given for the maintenance energy requirement.

$$MER\ (kJ/day) = (370 - 530) \cdot M^{0.75} \qquad (19.5)$$

However, the values for the constant are only valid for a thermoneutral environment. The values rise sharply when an animal is in an environment below its thermoneutral range.

MORE DETAILS The mass exponent of about 0.75 when determined for various animal species, indicates a uniform regularity for the **disproportionately small increase in basal metabolic rate** associated with **increasing body mass**. It should be noted, however, that when further measurements were made on numerous other species, the exponent 0.75, (which was rounded up anyway), seems to be somewhat too high and could possibly only be 0.71. This, however, is based on differences between animal species. Thus, there does not seem to be a uniform exponent valid for all animal species. A clear species-dependent variability can also be observed in the relationship between maximum oxygen uptake and body mass of animals of different weights **(Fig. 26.8)**.

19.7   Pathophysiological aspects

In a state of **starvation** (insufficient or no food intake), and also in a high-performance cow with a negative energy balance (p.601), the energy for all the vital processes (circulation, respiration, heat balance, muscle and nerve activity) must be obtained from the breakdown of the body's own molecules/tissues. Since glycogen stored in the body is rapidly depleted, depot fat is then used as the source of energy, by oxidation of fatty acids. In the longer term, the acetyl-CoA being produced from fatty acid oxidation is not able to enter the citric acid cycle because of a lack of oxaloacetate (which is needed for gluconeogenesis), and ketone bodies are formed These are also released into blood and can cause ketoacidosis. As the fat depots decrease, protein breakdown eventually also occurs, with released amino acids being either oxidised as an energy source or used for gluconeogenesis.

MORE DETAILS The **survival time** in a starvation state depends mainly on the **body fat reserve**. Young and small animals with low fat reserves thus survive starvation less well than adult, well-fed animals. Examples of genetically determined survival advantages in a starvation state are provided by fat-tailed sheep and camels with their extensive storage fat reserves in the tail and hump, respectively. Hibernators and ectothermic animals (p.494), on the other hand, can remain without food for a very long time. After losing 25–50% of their body mass, they often die of starvation. However, a weight loss of about 30% is not uncommon in winter in non-hibernating species. The weight loss of organs during starvation varies and vital organs are spared. While body fat can decrease by up to 97%, muscles by 30%, digestive tract by 28%, glands, such as the pancreas, by 17%, and the liver by up to 54%, the heart and central nervous system only lose 2–3% of their weight.

Various other pathophysiological conditions directly affect energy metabolism (basal metabolic rate). In a catabolic metabolic state from injuries, burns, fractures and febrile illnesses, there is an increase in energy metabolism. Conversely, in hypovolaemic shock (peripheral ischaemia), energy metabolism falls below the basal metabolic rate.

19.8 Regulation of energy metabolism

Some **hormones** or **neuronal components** (sympathetic or somatomotor nerves) have a direct effect on the level of energy turnover. Another factor that has a close causal relationship to the extent of energy turnover is the prevailing **temperature** in the organism. This is not only important in ectothermic animals, in which core body temperature can undergo strong fluctuations depending on the ambient temperature, and thus the intensity of metabolic processes also fluctuate. In endothermic animals, too, there can be temporary changes in core body temperature related to daily or seasonal environmental temperature changes, or by adapting to factors which influence energy metabolism. However, a lowering of the core body temperature is not a primary cause of lower energy metabolism. Rather, under certain conditions such as torpor and hibernation (p.509), energy consumption itself appears to be the primary regulated variable. In this case, reduced internal heat production is achieved by lowering the thermoregulatory set point (**Fig. 20.14**).

19.8.1 Hormonal influences on energy metabolism

The level of energy metabolism is influenced and regulated by a number of factors. The influence of the thyroid hormones (p.545) on basal metabolic rate is striking. Basal metabolic rate is significantly increased in hyperthyroidism and strongly depressed in hypothyroidism. Other hormones, with demonstrated enhancement of energy metabolism, are **adrenaline** and **progesterone**.

The hormone **leptin** produced by fat cells has an inhibitory effect on appetite, and hence on food intake (**Fig. 22.7**), and increases energy utilisation. Both effects are mediated centrally via leptin receptors in specific nuclear regions of the hypothalamus. The increase in energy turnover ultimately is mediated by central stimulation of the sympathetic nervous system.

19.8.2 Energy metabolism and temperature regulation

In ectothermic animals, metabolism is increased with an increase in environmental temperature. Hence, according to the van't Hoff rule (reaction rate of physiological processes as a function of temperature), O_2 consumption at least doubles with a temperature increase of 10 °C ($Q_{10} = 2$, **Fig. 20.1**). The metabolic rate of ectothermic species thus depends markedly on changes in ambient temperature. The van't Hoff rule also applies to endothermic animals. Thus, when there is a febrile increase in core body (p.508) temperature, there is a consequential increase in energy turnover of 12–22% per degree of temperature increase.

Regulated periodic changes in metabolic intensity are described in numerous endothermic animal species. During **sleep** and in circadian and seasonal **rest phases** in mammals, energy metabolism (10–20%) and core body temperature (0.5–2.0 °C) are reduced. In diurnal birds, the reduction in energy metabolism is as much as 30%, when core body temperature falls by up to 4 °C. Seasonal changes in metabolic intensity also serve to adapt energy consumption to external conditions, see ch. Rheostasis (p.509). One of the most effective physiological mechanisms for energy conservation is called **torpor**. This is a strictly regulated process in the course of which the animals are physically inactive. Their O_2 consumption (energy turnover) declines to very low levels, either briefly for a few hours in the course of the day, or for a longer period (**hibernation**), so that core body temperature is strongly reduced ("setpoint adjustment"). The reduction in metabolism in all these circumstances can be mediated by adaptative metabolic changes in cell metabolism (biochemical mechanisms). In the whole animal, complex neuronal and (neuro-)endocrine regulatory mechanisms modify energy metabolism in adaptation to the availability of nutrients, or unfavourable environmental conditions. Details of these regulatory mechanisms are not yet fully understood.

Suggested reading

Bergner H, Hoffmann L. Bioenergetics and substance production of farm animals. Amsterdam: Harwood Academic Publishers; 1996

Heldmaier G, Neuweiler G, Rössler W. Comparative animal physiology. Heidelberg: Springer; 2013

Heldmaier G, Werner D, eds. Environmental signal processing and adaptation. Heidelberg: Springer; 2003

Kleiber M. Der Energiehaushalt von Mensch und Haustier. Hamburg, Berlin: Parey; 1967

McMahon T. Size and shape in biology. Science 1973; 179: 1201–1204

Rolfe FS, Brown GC. Cellular energy utilization and molecular origin of metabolic rate in mammals. Physol Rev 1997; 77: 731–758

Sjaastad ØV, Hove K, Sand O. Physiology of Domestic Animals. Oslo:Scandinavian Veterinary Press; 2007

Wieser W. Bioenergetics. Stuttgart: Thieme; 1986

Nutrition, energy

20 Thermoregulation

Stephan Steinlechner, Walter Arnold

20.1 Heat production, heat emission, heat balance

ESSENTIALS ✖

- Mammals and birds maintain their body temperature at a high, relatively constant level, through internal heat production (endothermy). In most other animals, the body temperature is mainly determined by the ambient temperature (ectothermy). Endothermic animals have a much higher basal metabolic rate relative to body weight, than ectothermic animals.
- Heat is exchanged between the animal and its environment, but also within the animal via heat conduction at contact surfaces (conduction), heat transport through moving masses such as air and blood (convection), infrared radiation (radiation) and evaporation.
- The thermoneutral zone (TNZ) is the range of ambient temperature in which endothermic animals maintain their core body temperature within a normal range (physical thermoregulation) just by changing peripheral blood circulation or the body surface (body posture, plumage of fur or feathers). Below and above the TNZ, heat is produced or released by energy expenditure (critical thresholds, above which chemical thermoregulation sets in).
- Heat production below the TNZ occurs either by involuntary muscle tremor or, especially in small mammals, by short-circuiting the proton gradient at the inner mitochondrial membrane in brown fat, and/or in muscle cells, by uncoupling ATP hydrolysis from the transport of Ca^{2+} from the cytosol into the sarcoplasmic reticulum.
- Fur, feathers, subcutaneous fat deposits, changes in peripheral blood circulation, sweating and panting, countercurrent heat exchange and behavioural reactions (posture, choice of location, cuddling with conspecifics) protect against heat loss and overheating.
- Regulated increases in the normal temperature are defence reactions (fever, inflammation). Regulated decreases compensate for bottlenecks in daily energy supply. All animals are moderately hypothermic in their daily resting phase, and extremely so in "daily torpor". Over a year, many animals are moderately hypothermic in winter. Extreme examples of this are the hibernators.

20.2 Nomenclature

In most animals, body temperature and metabolic rate are mainly determined by the environmental temperature. They are therefore called **ectothermic animals** (Fig. 20.1 a). These include all the invertebrates and, among the vertebrates, fish, amphibians and reptiles. Mammals and birds, on the other hand, are **endothermic animals**. They have a high body temperature, usually well above the ambient temperature, which is kept within a narrow range that fluctuates only slightly, and is maintained by regulation of the body's own heat production. This allows them to live in a wide variety of habitats where marked changes in ambient temperature occur. They can also live in habitats with very low ambient temperatures, and can there develop ecological niches that are denied to ectothermic animals. The energetic cost for this is maintenance of a very high metabolic rate. The energy requirement of an endothermic animal is about 8–10 times higher than that of an ectothermic animal of the same size (Fig. 20.1 b).

The colloquial terms cold-blooded and warm-blooded should be avoided in the context of thermoregulation, as many ectothermic animals may well have higher body temperatures than endothermic animals at high ambient temperatures. The classical pair of terms (**poikilothermic animals** and **homeothermic animals**) should also be avoided, because they do not apply to ectothermic fish or invertebrates living at great depths in the ocean, These ectothermic animals have a much more constant body temperature throughout their lives than endothermic birds or mammals. Moreover, the body temperature of endothermic animals also fluctuates by up to several degrees Celsius during the course of the day. It also changes with the seasons and is influenced by physical activity and nutritional status. Losing weight in obesity, is also very difficult because the body's first reaction to hunger is to lower body temperature and thus the energy requirement.

The term **heterotherm** refers to animals that can switch between endothermic and ectothermic strategies. These include tunas, for example, which can reach a high temperature locally in their swimming musculature (**local heterothermy**), by means of a special countercurrent heat exchanger. Large insects, like grasshoppers or moths, can generate heat with their thoracic flight muscles to about 35 °C, before they become active. During resting phases such insects are ectothermic. However, mammals and birds can also exhibit quite high daily fluctuations in body temperature (e.g. daily or nocturnal **torpor**) or they can **hibernate** (temporary heterothermy (p. 509)).

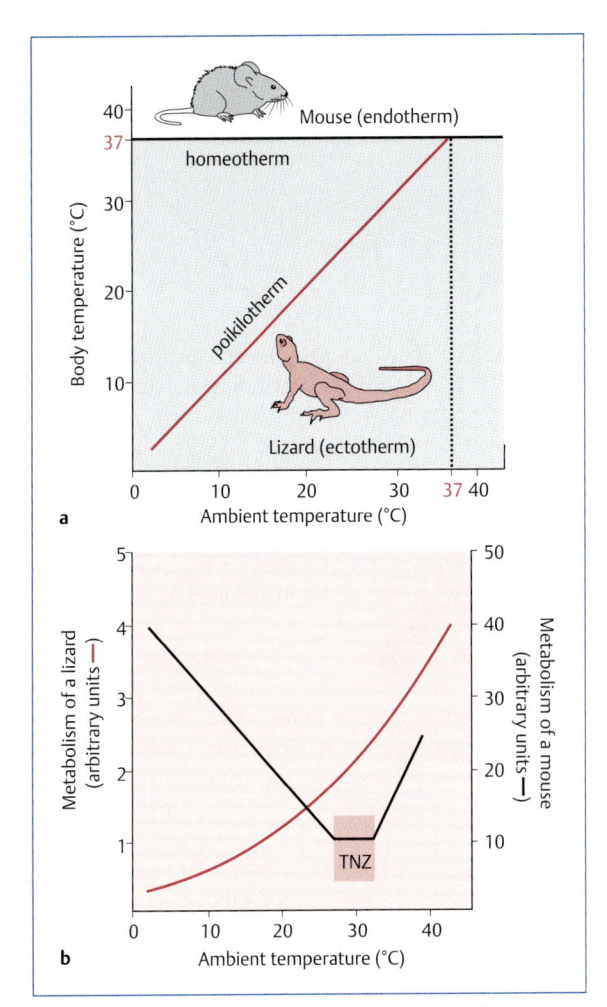

Fig. 20.1 Body temperature (**a**) and metabolism (**b**) of ectotherms (poikilotherms, red line) and endotherms (homeotherms, black line) as a function of ambient temperature. Note the different scales for mouse and lizard metabolism in **b**. TNZ = thermoneutral zone.

20.3 Heat balance

The body temperature of an animal depends on the amount of heat energy produced per unit of body weight. All living organisms produce heat in their cells from their metabolic reactions. The higher the metabolic rate, the greater the amount of heat produced. The rate of change of body heat thereby depends on

- the production of heat in the body,
- heat absorbed from the external environment
- heat emission to the environment.

In summary:

body heat =
heat generation + (heat absorption – heat emission)   (20.1)

Consequently, the heat content of a body and thus the body temperature of an animal, can be regulated both by changes in **heat production** (i.e. by changing metabolism) and by **heat exchange** with the environment. Or, to put it another way, any animal can only keep its body temperature constant if **heat production equals heat loss**. If more heat is lost than produced and absorbed, then the body

temperature falls. If more heat is produced and absorbed, than released to the environment, then body temperature rises.

In general, it can be said that in **small animals** (relatively large surface area in relation to volume) the risk of **cooling** predominates, but in **large animals** (relatively small surface area in relation to volume), especially during physical activity, there is more of a risk of **overheating** (see ch. Thermoregulation and sweat secretion (p. 627)).

> **IN A NUTSHELL**   !
>
> Only when heat production and heat emission are equal does the body temperature remain constant. If one of these two variables is changed, regulatory mechanisms are needed to restore the balance.

20.4 Heat exchange with the environment

Heat exchange between an animal and its environment is complex and can only be shown in a very simplified way (**Fig. 20.2**). In general, there are four possible ways for heat energy to be transferred between an animal's body and its environment: **conduction**), **convection**, **radiation** and **evaporation**.

20.4.1 Conduction

If two bodies with different temperatures are brought into contact, energy in the form of heat flows from the body with the higher temperature to the body with the lower temperature until the temperature of each is the same. Conduction can therefore also be understood as "heat diffusion", for which by analogy, Fick's law of diffusion (p. 32) applies. It follows that the higher the temperature difference, the larger the contact area, and the closer the contact between the bodies, the greater the conduction. A cat on a stone bench or a dog stretching out on cool tiles in a hot environment, make use of conduction. If the thermal conductivity of a stable floor is high (e.g. concrete floor), then the animal lying on it can loose too much heat. Bedding between the floor and the animal, counteracts this by reducing thermal conductivity.

20.4.2 Convection

Convection is heat transport by means of a moving medium (e.g. water, blood, air, etc.). The power of convection depends on the flow velocity and the heat capacity of the transporting medium: $air = 0.001 \ J \cdot ml^{-1} \cdot K^{-1}$, $water = 4.72 \ J \cdot ml^{-1} \cdot K^{-1}$. Water has an almost 5000 times better transport capacity for heat than air. Convection through the bloodstream is the physiologically most important way for heat distribution within the body and thus also for the exchange between the surface environment and the body core. For example, heat produced in muscles or in brown adipose tissue (**Fig. 20.6**) is distributed throughout the body via the blood circulation. In convective heat dissi-

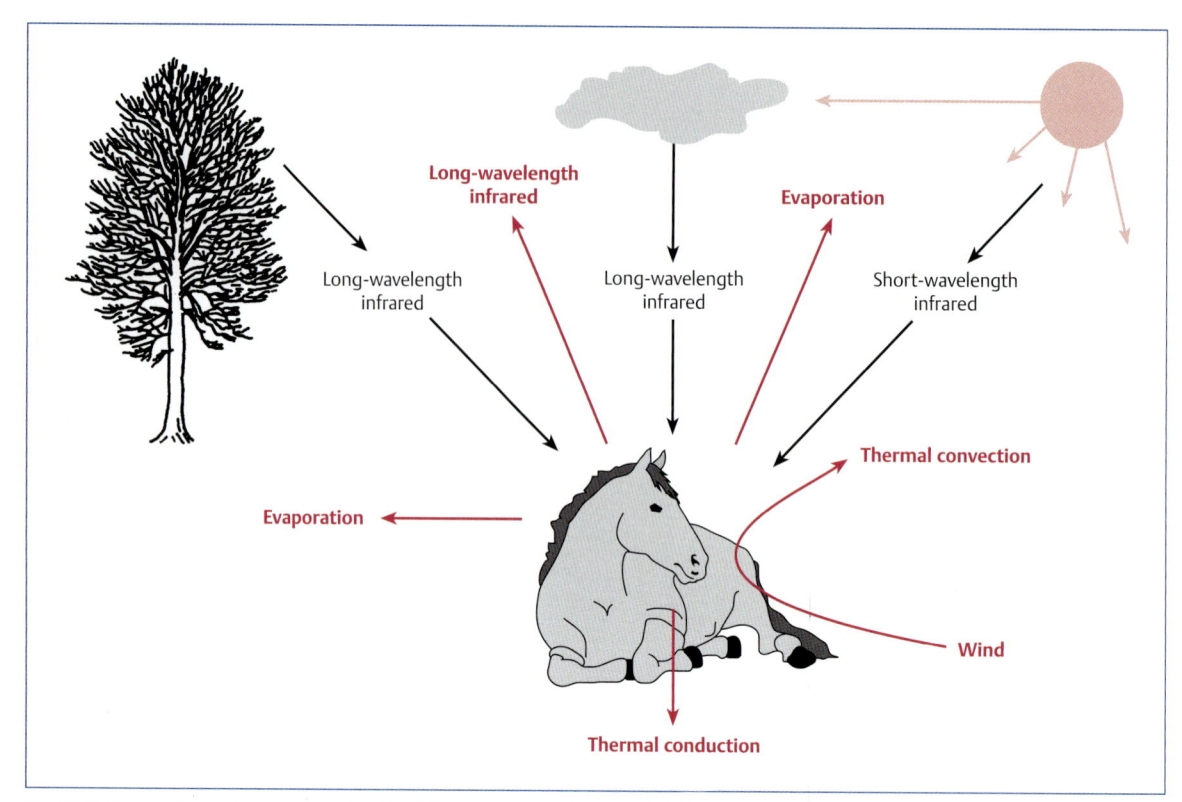

Fig. 20.2 Heat exchange between an animal and its environment. Outflow (red) by conduction (heat conduction through contact with the colder ground), convection (cool air passes over the fur and warms up in the process), radiation (from the warmer fur to colder objects in the environment) and cooling by evaporation of water (respiration and sweating). Inflow (black) through radiation from the sun and warmer objects in the environment.

pation over the surface of the body, the air adjacent to the coat first takes heat energy from the body by conduction. The resulting warmer air rises, so that colder air follows (**free convection**). Heat dissipation is proportional to the temperature difference between the air and the body surface. With increasing wind, convective heat emission increases (**forced convection; Fig. 20.10**). At low air temperatures, the cold load becomes considerably greater if it is also windy ("wind chill factor", "perceived temperature"). Air movement around a body is also achieved by an animal running. If a horse runs at a speed of $30\,km \cdot h^{-1}$ when there is no wind, this corresponds to a wind equivalent of about $8\,m \cdot s^{-1}$, which increases heat dissipation through convection and evaporation compared to a standing horse.

20.4.3   Radiation

Radiation is the transmission of heat in the form of electromagnetic waves in the infrared range. The warmer a body, the more and the shorter-wavelength is the infrared radiation it emits. The practical (and physiological) importance of radiation is often underestimated, because heat loss via radiation can be considerable. Especially at night, when there is no solar radiation on Earth, the cold universe is a heat drain ("heat sink") of infinite capacity (importance of shelters in open pasture!). Since water and clouds are almost impermeable to infrared radiation, it is much colder at night when the sky is clear than when it is cloudy. The sun's radiant energy influences an animal's heat balance either directly or indirectly by heating the environment.

Endothermic organisms use radiant heat to save energy for endogenous heat production. Ectothermic organisms use it to reach their preferred temperature.

MORE DETAILS   The importance of radiation also emerges from the **Stefan-Boltzmann law** which states that the flow of heat depends on the difference between the **fourth power of the temperature of the animal** and its environment. The heat radiation of an animal can be used to diagnose superficial tumours and inflammations with infrared cameras.

IN A NUTSHELL   !

Heat emission by conduction, convection and radiation, is proportional to the body surface area and the temperature difference between the body surface and the environment.

20.4.4   Evaporation

The "dry" heat released through conduction, convection and radiation is contrasted with the "moist" heat released through evaporation of water (**evaporation**) on the skin or in the respiratory tract. It is the only way animals can release heat against a temperature gradient, i.e. when the ambient temperature is higher than the body temperature. Evaporation of water from the body surface removes heat from the body (approx. **$2400\,J \cdot ml^{-1}\,H_2O$**). Animals that can sweat thus have a highly effective way of dissipating heat. For example, if a $600\,kg$ horse secretes only three litres of sweat (p. 627) per hour, its **evaporation** enables a

heat dissipation of 2000 watts. This is three times the heat production of a resting horse.

> MORE DETAILS   Cooling by evaporation depends on the **difference between the partial pressures of water vapour** on the skin and in the air (i.e. not on the temperature difference!). At a partial pressure difference of 1 kPa this leads to a heat emission of about $58\,W \cdot m^{-2}$. This value applies to still air and increases with increasing wind speed in a similar way to convective heat emission (**Fig. 20.10**). However, if the partial pressure difference is low because the humidity is very high, such as in the tropics, after rain on a hot day, or in a poorly ventilated stable with many animals, evaporation is greatly reduced and evaporative cooling approaches zero.
>
> An animal that neither sweats nor pants, still gives off heat through evaporation. The air breathed is heated in the lungs and thereby saturated with water vapour. When exhaling, a large part of this water is lost, which is particularly evident in winter, when the air is cold and dry, through the cloud of vapour that forms when exhaling. But water is also constantly diffusing through dry skin. This unregulated evaporation through the skin and the respiratory tract (**perspiratio insensibilis**) leads to a loss of heat, which usually amounts to about 20% of heat production at rest. In very dry, cold air (high mountains!), or in windy conditions, evaporation from the skin can reach much higher values. **Perspiratio sensibilis** is the visible release of water through the skin or mucous membranes, primarily through the activity of sweat glands or panting.

> **IN A NUTSHELL**   !
>
> Evaporative cooling is more effective, the higher the difference between the partial pressures of water vapour and of skin and air.

20.5   Temperature field of the body

20.5.1   Core and shell

Despite the accuracy with which endotherms can regulate their body temperature, it is not constant, but fluctuates both in spatial body regions and over time. The spatial fluctuations of body temperature can be seen particularly well in large mammals where the core body temperature is highest. The core consists of the brain and the metabolically active internal organs of the trunk, in which about 70% of the total heat is generated under resting conditions. At high ambient temperature, the thin outer parts of the body and parts of the extremities are at the temperature level of the core. In cold conditions, the body core is small, while the outer regions with a lower temperature is large (**Fig. 20.3**). In the outer body regions a temperature gradient develops, which reduces the heat loss from the body core. Regional changes in body temperature occur mainly through changes in the rate of blood flow (see ch. on heat transport (p.500).

> **IN A NUTSHELL**   !
>
> The temperature is highest in the core of the body. It is surrounded by the outer regions in which the temperature decreases towards the surface of the body – the colder it is, the more extensive are these outer regions. In a cold environment, the body core is small.

20.5.2   Countercurrent heat exchange

The heat exchange in the body via systemic circulation regulation is supported by anatomical structures. In particular, a **countercurrent heat exchange** can take place in the extremities. The blood cooled in the extremities flows back into the core in a thin-walled venous plexus that closely surrounds the large arteries carrying blood to the extremities (**Fig. 20.4**). As a result, the arterial blood transfers its heat to the returning venous blood. The large contact surfaces of the arterial and venous vessels (conduction) ensure that blood does not get too cold in the body core, and that much less heat is lost through the surface of the extremities. This mechanism is particularly important in birds with unfeathered legs and especially in waterfowl, such as ducks or gulls, when they swim in ice-cold water or stand on ice. Prolonged hypothermia of the extremities results in repeated, short-term vasodilations (Lewis-Hunting reaction) to protect the tissue from hypothermic damage (tissue necrosis).

In cloven-hoofed animals, the sinus cavernosus, where venous inflow brings cool blood from the nasopharynx, is a network of thin-walled arteries (**rete mirabile**). The sinus cavernosus is formed by hundreds of fine branches of the maxillary artery, which reunite before entering the cerebral arterial circulation (**Fig. 20.5 a**). This rete mirabile is a **heat exchanger** that cools the blood flowing to the brain. The cooling is regulated so that the cooler blood from the nasopharynx flows from the V. dorsalis nasi (VDN) either (1) via the V. angularis oculi (VAO) to the sinus cavernosus or (2) via the V. facialis (VF) directly to the V. jugularis. In the second case, the heat exchanger is bypassed so that no cooling takes place. Which path the blood takes is determined directly by the contraction state of the VAO or VF and indirectly by the brain temperature. At low brain temperature, cooling is switched off. When the temperature rises, more cool venous blood flows via the cavernous sinus, so that the brain temperature rises less than the temperature in the trunk (**Fig. 20.5 b**). In the control circuit, the regulator (hypothalamus) is not notified of a temporary hyperthermia of the trunk (e.g. in the case of escape-related hyperthermia) and an otherwise immediate temperature regulation is postponed. Limits of stress can thus be temporarily masked by brain cooling (see ch. Thermoregulation and sweat secretion (p.627)).

Countercurrent exchange also takes place during breathing. The exhaled air releases heat and water vapour in the nasal cavity to the mucous membrane. The inhaled air, which is much cooler and drier, partly takes up this heat and moisture, on its way into the lungs. In animals living in cold habitats (e.g. reindeer), deeply branched folds increase the mucosal surface of the nasal cavity, making this exchange more effective.

> **IN A NUTSHELL**   !
>
> During heat stress, the brain temperature can be kept at a lower level than the torso core temperature by countercurrent heat exchange.

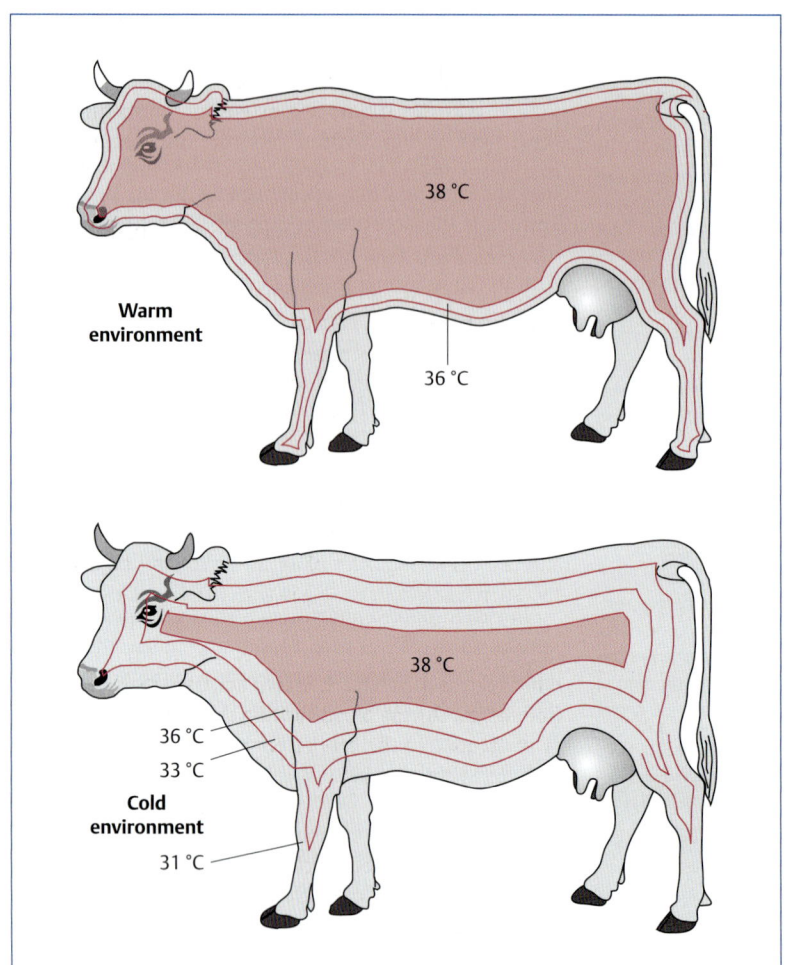

Fig. 20.3 Temperature distribution in the body of a cow in warm (top) and cold (bottom) environments. The lines of equal temperature (isotherms) indicate that the temperature in the body core remains high, but in cold conditions the core of equal temperatures is restricted to the interior of the trunk and the brain. The body outer regions, expand in cold conditions and form an insulating layer around the body core.

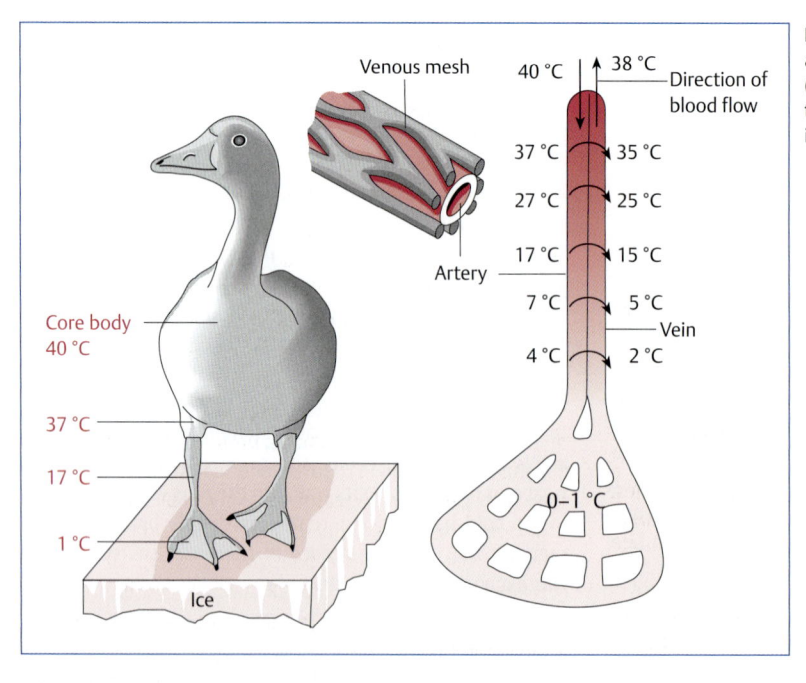

Fig. 20.4 Regional heterothermy (left), arrangement of blood vessels in the foot (centre) and schematic representation of the countercurrent heat exchanger (right) in the foot of a goose.

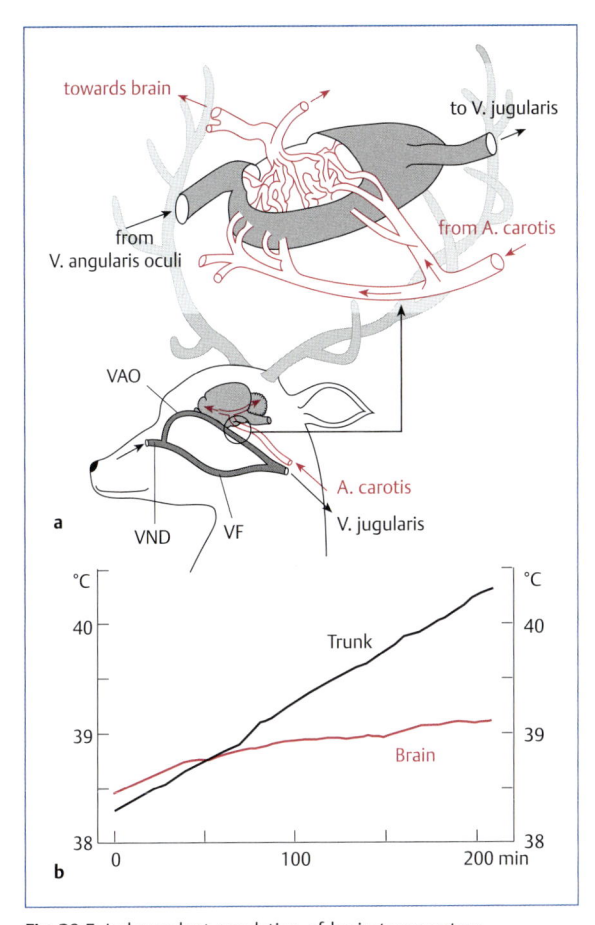

Fig. 20.5 Independent regulation of brain temperature.
a Heat exchange in a reindeer between the cool venous return flow from the nasopharynx in the rete mirabile sinus cavernosus and the warm arterial inflow to the brain. VND = Vena dorsalis nasi, VAO = Vena angularis oculi, VF = Vena facialis.
b As a goat's body temperature rises, the rate of increase in brain temperature declines; based on data from Kuhnen G, Jessen C. Threshold and slope of selective brain cooling. Pfl Arch Physiol 1991; 418: 176-183

20.6 Heat generation

The **resting heat production** in a thermoneutral environment (resulting from basal metabolic rate (p. 489). See also thermoneutral zone, **Fig. 20.1**) is an important parameter of heat balance. It is expressed in $J \cdot kg^{-1} \cdot d^{-1}$ or $W \cdot kg^{-1}$ $(1\,W = 1\ J \cdot s^{-1} = 3.6\,kJ \cdot h^{-1} = 86.4\,kJ \cdot d^{-1})$ and decreases with increasing body mass (p. 490). For most domestic animals, the resting heat production with normal feeding is between $2\,W \cdot kg^{-1}$ (dog) and $1\,W \cdot kg^{-1}$ (cattle). With increased feed intake (lactation, fattening, pregnancy), these values can increase considerably. In addition, hormonal (including thyroid hormones) and neuronal influences (sympathetic nervous system) play an essential role in energy metabolism and consequently in heat production (p. 493). The diurnal increase in glucocorticoids in diurnal mammals in the early morning is accompanied by an increase in resting metabolic rate, and thus in body temperature (see ch. 21 (p. 511)). In situations of increased cold stress, heat production (thermogenesis) must be increased above the resting value in order to maintain a steady core

temperature. One possibility, especially in larger animals with considerable muscle mass, is **cold shivering**. In mild cold stress, there is initially only an increase in tone in the muscle, with the flexors and extensors contracting at the same time. Stronger cold tremors are also perceptible as movement (**tremor**); however, the whole muscle does not shorten synchronously, but individual muscle fibres work in an uncoordinated way. Since no meaningful external work is done, the energy converted via ATP in the muscles, which corresponds to the normal efficiency of muscle contraction, is retained as heat. Thus, for a short time, heat production can be increased to 5 times the resting value. However, mammalian muscle tremor is not a very economical way of thermogenesis. Because it mainly takes place in the peripheral muscles, which have to be better supplied with blood for cold shivering, a lot of the generated heat is lost from the body surface. In addition, during violent shivering, fine motor skills are severely impaired and the insulating layer of air in the fur can be disturbed by the movement, resulting in additional heat loss.

Mammals especially that **weigh less than 10 kg**, including babies, also have a specialised tissue, the **brown fat**, which can generate **heat**. Brown adipose tissue acts like a flow heater for the blood flowing through it and, because of its location in the cervicothoracic region, it has a function like a heating jacket, which is worn under the skin (**Fig. 20.6**). The adipocytes of the brown adipose tissue are densely surrounded by fibres of the sympathetic nervous tissue and are densely packed with mitochondria (hence the colour!). During cold stress, noradrenaline is released, which binds to β_3-adrenergic receptors on blood vessels and adipocytes. This increases the blood supply to the brown adipose tissue and triglycerides are hydrolysed in the adipocytes. The released fatty acids activate a specific protein in the inner mitochondrial membrane (UCP1, uncoupling protein 1), which uncouples the respiratory chain from ATP synthesis. The activation of UCP1 collapses the proton gradient across the inner mitochondrial membrane, and with it ATP synthesis. This triggers maximum activity of the respiratory chain and almost all of the oxidation energy converted is released as heat instead of being stored as ATP. In contrast to white adipocytes, which have only one large lipid vacuole (unilocular), brown adipocytes have numerous small lipid vacuoles (multilocular), which provide a larger surface for lipolytic enzymes to attack. However, during prolonged active thermogenesis, most of the lipids metabolised in brown adipose tissue must be replenished from white fat. During prolonged "cold stress" in autumn/winter, chronic noradrenergic stimulation of the brown fat cells also increases the activity of type 2 deiodinase, which leads to an increased conversion of thyroxine (T4) into the bioactive triiodothyronine (T3). T3, in turn, activates the expression of UCP1, which results in an increase in the thermogenic capacity in brown fat and thus is an adaptation to cold.

When exposed to cold, small mammals mainly use shiver-free heat production. Only in extreme cold do they also use cold shivering in addition to metabolic heat generation. Shiver-free heat production is particularly important

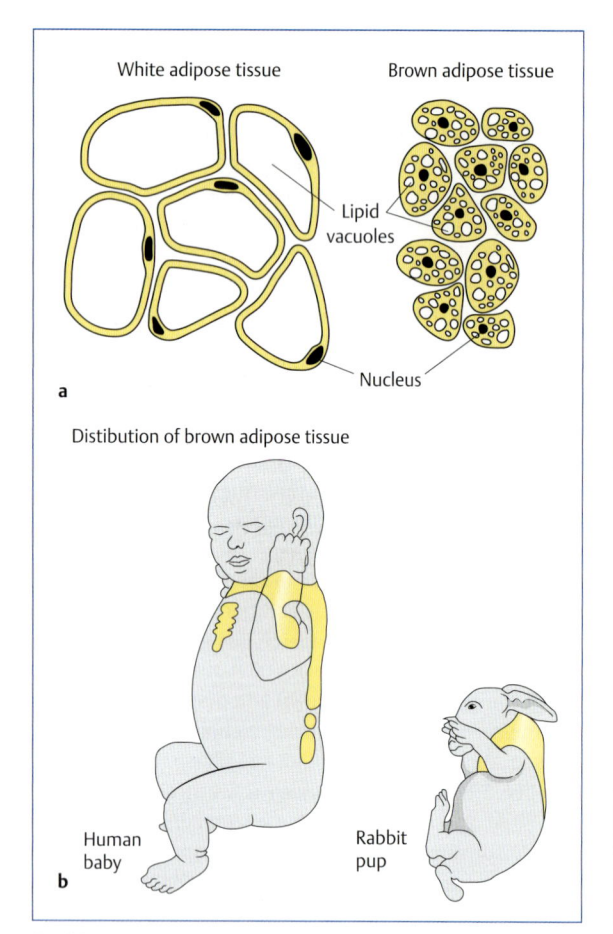

Fig. 20.6
a White (unilocular) and brown (multilocular) adipose tissue.
b Distribution of brown adipose tissue in the infant and the rabbit.

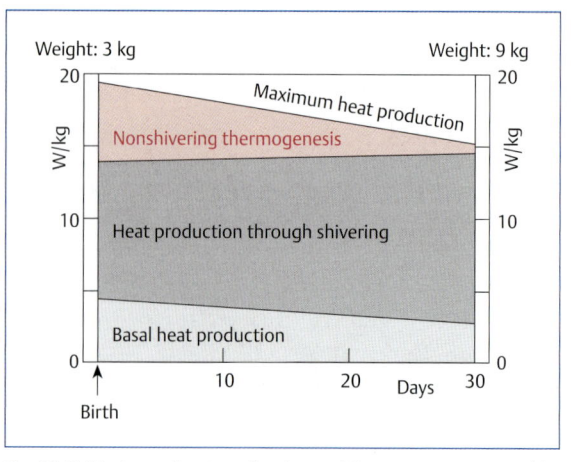

Fig. 20.7 Maximum heat production and its components in cold-stressed lambs. After birth, under severe cold stress (low temperature, wind, damp coat), the maximum heat production is almost $20\,W \cdot kg^{-1}$. Of this, about 30% is accounted for by shiver-free heat production in the brown adipose tissue. After 30 days and weight gain to 9 kg, the brown adipose tissue has almost completely regressed and the shiver-free heat production is replaced by cold shivering in the now increased muscle mass. [Source: Alexander G, Williams D. Shivering and non-shivering thermogenesis during summit metabolism in young lambs. J Physiol 1968; 198: 251–276]

for small mammals during hibernation, when their body temperature falls into the single-digit range. The first phase of the awakening (heating) process can only take place with shiver-free heat production, because heat production through muscle tremors is only possible from about 15 °C upwards. In larger species, shiver-free thermogenesis is particularly relevant in the postnatal phase, because the risk of severe cold stress is greatest in young small animals (**Fig. 20.7**). In the past it was believed that the ability to produce shiver-free heat was lost when a sufficiently large body size was reached. However, brown fat and active UCP1 are now thought to be retained to a small extent throughout life, even in larger animals, as recent findings in adult humans have demonstrated.

MORE DETAILS A most interesting exception is in pigs. Although pigs do not possess a functional UCP1 protein, newborn piglets develop the ability to produce shiver-free heat within a few days. They employ a different mechanism of shiver-free heat production. In skeletal muscle, the membrane-bound Ca^{2+}-ATPase of the sarcoplasmic reticulum (SERCA) transports Ca^{2+} ions from the cytosol back to the sarcoplasmic reticulum with ATP consumption – an essential part of muscle activity (p. 145). Depending on the isoform, SERCAs convert 42–125 kJ per mol ATP into heat during ATP hydrolysis. Heat generation by SERCAs can be further increased if the enzymatic activity is decoupled from Ca^{2+} transport by special proteins such as sarcolipin (SLN). The SERCA activity

then leads to the hydrolysis of ATP, but the binding of SLN to SERCA creates an idle cycle of the reaction ("futile cycle"). The Ca^{2+} ions are no longer transported from the cytosol into the sarcoplasmic reticulum, but are released back into the cytosol. The importance of shiver-free heat generation via this mechanism in the musculature has probably been greatly underestimated up to now. Tremor-free heat generation via the idling of SERCA could explain why a thermogenic UCP1 is absent in birds, monotremes and marsupials and, as is now known, also in other eutherian mammals in addition to pigs.

> **IN A NUTSHELL** !
>
> In acute cold stress, heat production is increased by cold shivering and/or by shiver-free heat production in the muscles and brown adipose tissue.

20.7 Heat transport

20.7.1 Internal heat transport

To dissipate heat produced in the body in various tissues and organs, it must first be transported to the cooler body surface. This heat transport from the body core to the outer regions is the **internal heat transport**, which is essentially by convection through blood, as thermal conductivity of the various tissues is relatively low. This internal heat transport is regulated by changing blood flow to the body periphery. **Vasoconstriction that occurs during exposure to cold is mediated by** activation of the sympathetic nervous system, as demonstrated in a simple experiment by Claude Bernard about 150 years ago (**Fig. 20.8**).

Peripheral blood circulation can also be partially regulated. This creates "thermal windows", i.e. regions of skin with a good blood supply, through which more heat can be released or radiant heat can be absorbed. Such thermal

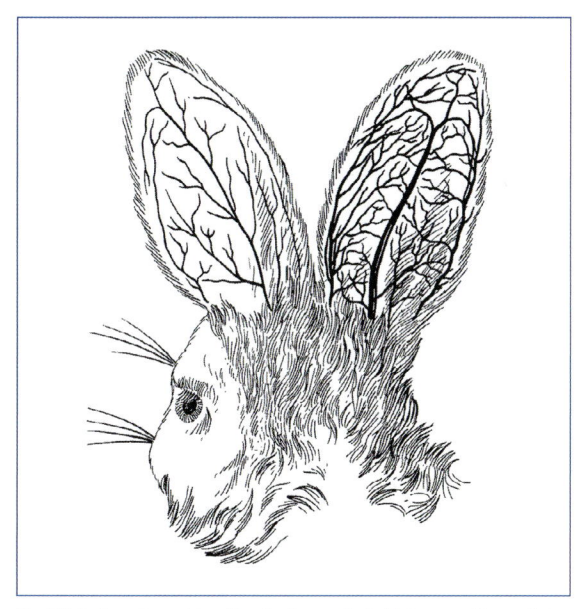

Fig. 20.8 Experiment by Claude Bernard: Rabbit ears after unilateral transection of the sympathetic innervation. The right ear is denervated and therefore shows no vasoconstriction during cold stress. [Source: Claude Bernard, from the 19th century]

windows can be found, for example, in the large ears of African elephants, or in the body of seals, which, when resting on ice, absorb radiant heat via thermal windows on their backs while at the same time, only releasing minimal amounts of heat into the ice below them. Another example of a thermal window is the breeding patch in birds (area incubationis), which increases the heat transfer to their clutch of eggs.

Increased internal heat production (e.g. due to physical work) or external heat stress, both lead to increased blood flow to large areas of the skin. The acra (hands, feet, ears) in particular have a large surface area in relation to their volume due to their structural geometry. This makes it easier for heat to be released into the environment. Conversely, heat dissipation and skin temperature both decrease when the skin is exposed to cold, as the skin vessels constrict and the blood flows into deeper layers via arteriovenous anastomoses (**Fig. 20.9**).

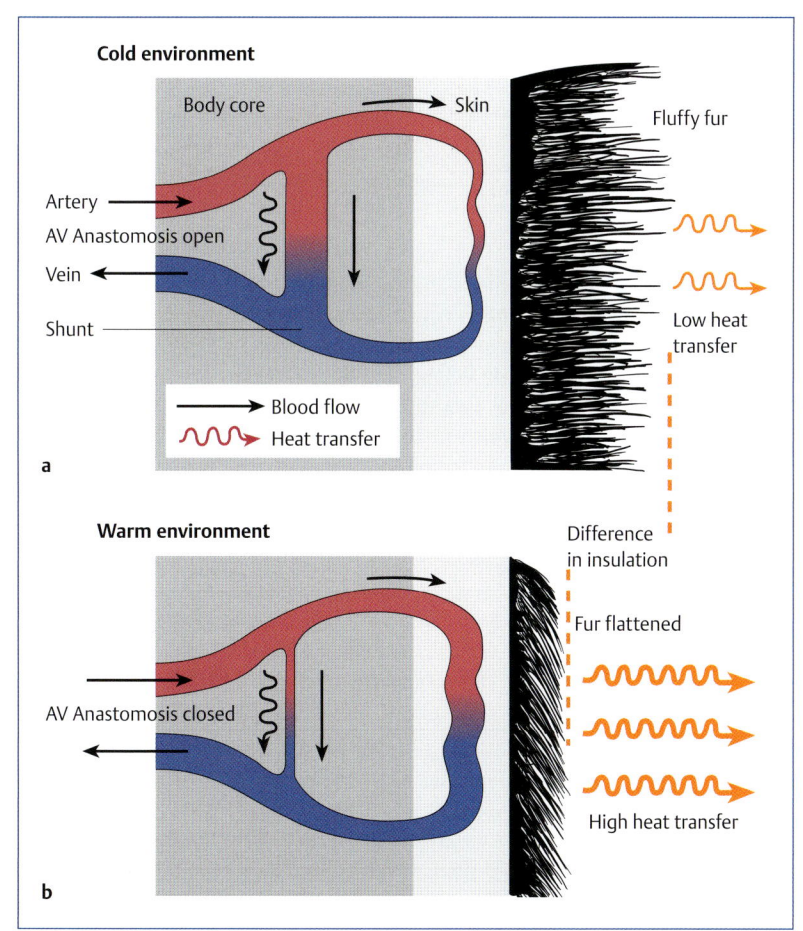

Fig. 20.9 Control of heat exchange at the body surface via regulation of blood flow and by fur insulation.
a At low ambient temperatures, the peripheral blood vessels are constricted so that warm blood does not reach the skin surface (pale skin), and passes via AV anastomoses to deeper layers. This insulation can be improved by fluffing up fur (or feathers in birds).
b At high ambient temperatures, the anastomoses are constricted so that more blood is conducted to the surface of the skin. By simultaneously fluffing the fur (or feathers in the case of birds), heat insulation is reduced and thus heat dissipation increases.

Nutrition, energy

20.7.2 External heat transport

■ Radiation

By lowering the skin temperature in a cold environment, long-wave infrared heat radiation is also reduced. When there is **internal heat stress (**e.g. during intense physical activity), the temperature of the surface should be higher than that of the air (vasodilation in the skin) to allow dry heat dissipation through radiation. When there is **external heat stress**, and the air is hotter than the core temperature, a high surface temperature is an advantage, because then less heat is absorbed via radiation. The **structure** and **colour of** the surfaces also play a major role in the amount of radiant energy absorbed. A shiny and light-coloured coat reflects more radiation, while a black and dull coat absorbs more radiation. Therefore, in a hot desert climate, animals need to be lighter in colour and shinier, than in polar regions, where darker coat colours would increase absorption of radiant heat.

> **MORE DETAILS**   However, there are many examples that do not meet this expectation: Polar bear or snow hare with their white fur, and the black Bedouin goat and the desert raven are dark in colour. In these examples, obviously other needs such as for camouflage are more important than that of thermal regulation. The Bedouin goat has been shown to be at a disadvantage in summer, but to benefit energetically from its dark coat in winter. In calm conditions, the desert raven absorbs more energy via radiation than a white bird, but even at wind speeds of $4\,\text{m}\cdot\text{s}^{-1}$ the black bird has an advantage because only the surface of its plumage is heated. Radiant heat can penetrate white plumage more deeply and is thus not so readily dissipated by the wind.

■ Subcutaneous fat tissue, hair and feathers

Hair and **feathers**, together with **subcutaneous fatty tissue**, provide resistance to heat dissipation. They thus increase the **insulation**. In aquatic mammals (seals, whales), a thick subcutaneous fat layer ("blubber") in particular serves as insulation from the cold water. Excellent insulation is indispensable for these animals, because **water has 25 times the thermal conductivity** and almost **5000 times the thermal capacity of air**. In large land-dwelling mammals, however, such a thick layer of fat would be a great hindrance to good heat flow through the skin. Large fat deposits are therefore often not spread evenly over the body, but are present as **ectopic fat pads** (camels, zebus, fat-tailed sheep).

> **MORE DETAILS**   **Heat conduction** through fur is a function of its thickness. At a thickness of 10 mm it is about $4\,\text{W}\cdot\text{m}^{-2}$ for a temperature difference of 1 °C between skin and air, but for a coat that is 40 mm thick, only $1\,\text{W}\cdot\text{m}^{-2}\cdot\text{°C}^{-1}$. This high degree of insulation is roughly equivalent to that of a still layer of air of the same thickness. **Air has very low thermal conductivity** and is therefore a very **good insulator**. The decisive factor, however, is the reduction of heat convection by fur or feathers, which place a layer of still air over the skin. A comparison shows the effectiveness of this. An unclothed person begins to shiver with cold after some time at an air temperature of 25 °C. In contrast, an ice fox or a husky, with enormous insulation from dense winter fur, can compensate for the slight heat loss with only resting heat production, even at temperatures far below freezing. With increasing wind strength, the layer of insulating, resting air is more and

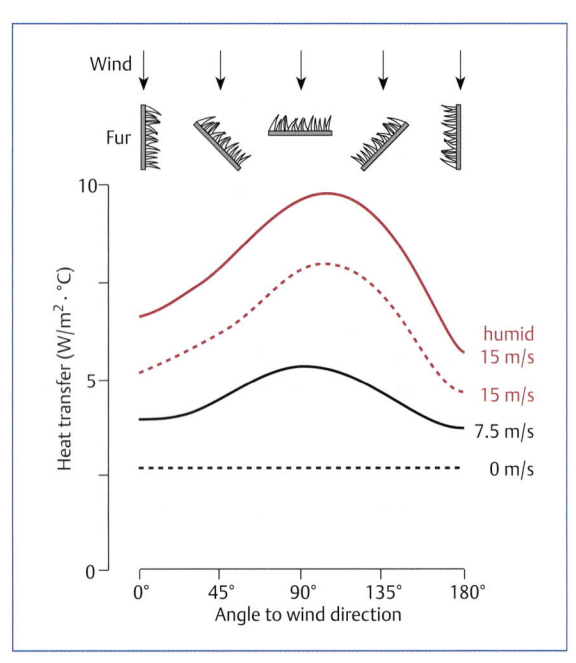

Fig. 20.10 Convective heat transfer through fur as a function of wind speed and wind direction. When the air is still (black dashed line), the heat transfer through the fur is approx. $2.5\,\text{W}\cdot\text{m}^{-2}\cdot\text{°C}^{-1}$. With increasing wind (black line and red dashed line) the heat loss increases sharply, especially when the wind hits the coat at right angles or when the coat is damp (red line); based on data from Lentz CP, Hart JS. The effect of wind on heat loss through the fur of newborn caribou. Can J Zool 1960; 38: 679–687

more disturbed (**Fig. 20.10**). Even a fresh breeze (wind speed $7.5\,\text{m}\cdot\text{s}^{-1}$) doubles the heat loss if the wind hits the coat at a right angle. If rain is added to the wind, the situation can quickly become critical.

In summer, a thick coat makes it more difficult to dissipate heat. This is why many mammals change from a winter to a summer coat. The summer coat is shorter-haired, often lighter in colour, and above all, has less undercoat. This seasonal change of coat is controlled by prolactin secretion, which in turn is controlled by the changes in day length, and thus by melatonin production in the pineal gland (**Fig. 21.8, Fig. 24.6**).

> **MORE DETAILS**   A well-insulating coat also protects against heat radiation because it reflects part of the short-wavelength radiation. In strong, direct sunlight, only a small part of the energy-rich radiation then reaches the body core. Camels therefore have a thick coat on their back that limits heat absorption, but a bare belly through which heat can be readily dissipated.

The insulation value of the coat can be additionally regulated by contraction of smooth muscles on hair shafts, especially the awn hairs. These hairs then become erect, followed passively by the downy hairs. The insulating layer of air thus becomes thicker (**Fig. 20.9**). Besides a change in blood circulation, this is the most important mechanism by which body temperature can be maintained, even when the ambient temperature drops.

In birds, the mechanism of "fluffing up" is of even greater importance, as the bird's plumage creates a more stable and thicker insulation layer relative to body size due to the stiffer feather shafts with down feathers in between.

IN A NUTSHELL !

Fur and feathers form an insulating layer of air around the body. As a result, fur and feathers not only protect against heat loss, but also against heat gain from intense radiation.

■ Evaporative cooling

As already mentioned in the chapter on evaporation, evaporative cooling is the only way to dissipate heat when the ambient temperature is higher than the body temperature. If the air above the skin is very dry, a lot of water evaporates, but if the humidity is high (close to 100%), very little water evaporates. In addition to perspiratio insensibilis, which can hardly be regulated, evaporative cooling can be achieved by sweating, panting, wallowing and salivation.

IN A NUTSHELL !

The higher the water vapour pressure in the ambient air (humid air, tropics), the more difficult it is to dissipate heat by evaporation.

Sweating

Sweat production consumes little energy. **Sweating** is very effective, especially in dry air. However, sweating can also lead to high water loss, because often only about ⅓ of the secreted sweat contributes to cooling by evaporation on the skin. The number and function of sweat glands vary greatly in different animal species. Many rodents (mouse, rat), the rabbit as well as birds lack sweat glands. Other species have very little sweat secretion (dog, sheep, pig) and this is usually restricted to small areas of skin. In animals with short or very thin fur, the skin provides a large evaporation surface. This therefore allows horses, for example, to use sweating for "whole-body cooling". However, the **loss of electrolytes** through sweating is high in horses because the electrolyte concentration in horse sweat is very high, compared to humans (**Table 26.6**).

MORE DETAILS   The loss of water and electrolytes has negative consequences for the circulation during prolonged exercise, as the plasma volume then decreases. Animals can therefore only afford to sweat if sufficient drinking water is available. A camel that has no drinking water available stops sweating and lets the body heat up passively (**Fig. 20.12**) (see ch. on heat storage (p.504)). For many animals, the danger of **dehydration** is so great that they almost completely forgo evaporative cooling.

IN A NUTSHELL !

Water and electrolytes are lost with sweat. If the fluid and electrolyte losses cannot be compensated immediately, there is a risk of dehydration and hyponatremia/hypochloridemia.

Panting

Panting allows regional evaporative cooling without salt loss, but has two potential disadvantages: Hyperventilation (p.270) which leads to respiratory alkalosis, and more muscle work from the increased ventilation, which in turn means an increased heat load. However, the muscle work required for panting is low because the elastic properties of the respiratory tract are utilised.

A dog exposed to only moderate heat stress pants at a high rate for a short time, interspersed with periods of normal respiratory rate. When a dog starts panting, it increases its respiratory rate quite suddenly from 30–40 breaths by about 10 times, i.e. to 300–400 breaths, which corresponds to the resonant frequency of its respiratory tract and thorax. To maintain this resonant frequency, only a very moderate muscular effort is required and this leads to only a small heat load. Panting without taking advantage of the elastic properties of the respiratory system would in fact generate more heat through muscular work than could be dissipated through increased evaporation.

A relatively large anatomical dead space (p.267) is important for avoiding respiratory alkalosis. Due to the shallow, high-frequency breaths during panting, only the dead space is ventilated and there is no ventilation of the alveoli. Only in severe heat stress does alveolar ventilation begin to increase.

IN A NUTSHELL !

In severe heat stress panting can lead to respiratory alkalosis.

MORE DETAILS   The dog can also control its heat output by exhaling either through the nose or the mouth. When exhaling through the nose, the exhaled air has a temperature of 29 °C. If the dog pants at the same frequency and switches to exhaling air through the mouth, the exhaled air will be close to body temperature, at about 38 °C. If 1 litre of air at 29 °C is exhaled fully saturated with water vapour, 62 J are released. However, if the air temperature is 38 °C when exhaled through the mouth, then almost twice as much heat (116 J) is given off. The dog can therefore vary its heat output at the same respiratory frequency and the same respiratory volume simply by discharging expiratory air via the nose or via the mouth (**Fig. 20.11**).

Wallow

By wallowing in mud or puddles, (usually larger) animals can also cool themselves. This is a mixture of direct cooling through mud/water and indirect cooling through evaporation of the water on the skin.

Salivation

Evaporative cooling by salivation is not a very efficient mechanism. It is most common in marsupials (kangaroos) and small mammals. The extremities and the pleura are licked and thus humidified with moisture. Since saliva contains electrolytes, salt loss also occurs.

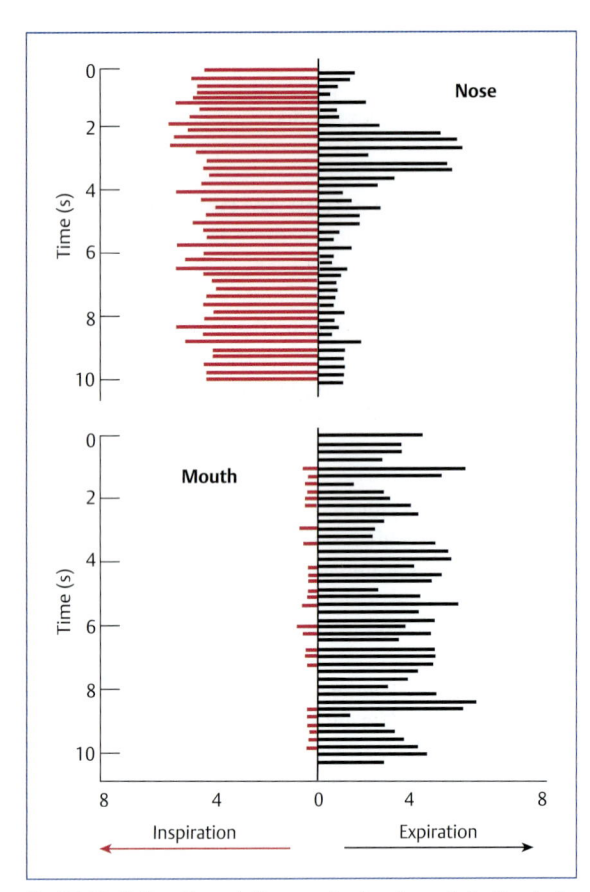

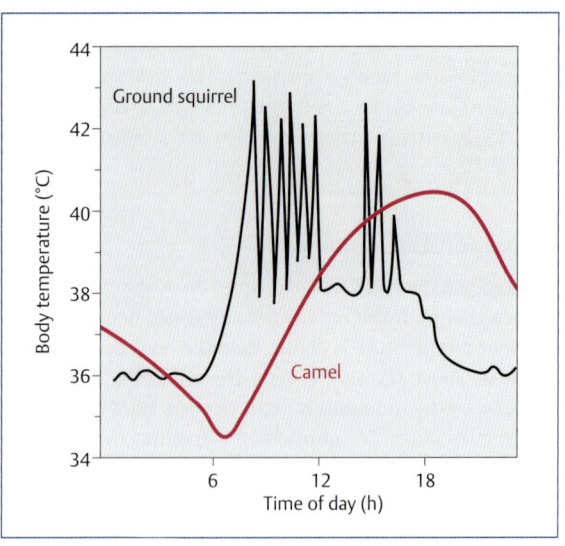

Fig. 20.12 Diurnal course of body temperatures of a ground squirrel and a camel under heat stress in the desert. The ground squirrel always returns to its burrow to cool down. The camel stores heat in its large body during the day and releases that heat again at night. [Source: Bartholomew GA. The roles of physiology and behaviour in the maintenance of homeostasis in the desert environment. Symp Soc Exp Biol 1964; 18: 7–29]

Fig. 20.11 Airflow through the nose (top) and mouth (bottom) of a panting dog. During inhalation, practically no air is taken in through the mouth, only exhaled air is released.
Red = volumes during inhalation; black = volumes during exhalation; based on data from Schmidt-Nielsen K. How Animals Work. Cambridge University Press; 1984

20.8   Heat storage

Some mammals, especially those living in arid regions, are surprisingly tolerant of transient hyperthermia due to hot ambient temperatures or high muscle activity. The larger the animal, the more heat it can store in its body under these conditions. A small rodent, such as the antelope ground squirrel (100–250 g), tolerates a rise in body temperature to almost 43 °C during short forays of about 30 min in the blazing sun. Then it returns to the burrow, allows itself to cool down to 38 °C and then resumes its outdoor activities. A camel (500 kg) can let its body temperature rise to 41 °C during a hot day and then reduce the excess heat to 34 °C during the cool night (**Fig. 20.12**). Hyperthermia has two advantages: (1) The higher body temperature reduces the temperature gradient to the hot ambient temperature and thus reduces the heat influx. (2) Above all, it conserves the water which would be used for evaporative cooling.

MORE DETAILS   The strategy of storing heat in the body instead of releasing it through evaporation saves the camel about 5 litres of water per day. This **adaptive hyperthermia** should not be confused with fever (p. 508). Local brain cooling via the mechanism described above (**Fig. 20.5**) is a prerequisite for keeping a "cool head".

20.9   Behaviour

Animals can greatly influence their heat exchange with the environment through **thermoregulatory behaviour**. They can modify their heat exchange by choosing their microclimate, by moving into the shade or by sunbathing. They can retreat into cool burrows. They can cool down in hot weather by bathing or rolling in mud. Birds and small mammals can protect themselves from the cold by building a well-insulated nest. The "cuddling" (**social thermoregulation**, is a strategy to reduce the ratio of surface area to volume. From the perspective of an individual animal, close contact with conspecifics reduces heat loss because the cold air of the environment is replaced by a warm neighbour. This behaviour is widespread among young animals in the nest. The effect of energy saving through group formation has been studied and quantified in newborn piglets (**Fig. 20.13**).

But even just by changing their **posture** and **orientation** relative to the sun, animals can influence the intensity of the incoming radiation and thus their body temperature.

MORE DETAILS   In the midday heat, most antelopes in shadeless savannah orient their longitudinal body axis towards the sun, whereas their orientation is purely random in cloudy conditions. By stretching out and lying flat on the ground or curling up, the exposed body surface can be maximised or minimised. When a python, which is approximately cylindrical in shape and thus has a large relative surface area, curls up, its exposed body surface area decreases by about 85%, which significantly reduces heat loss.

Social thermoregulation is regularly observed in animals in polar regions (e.g. penguins, musk oxen), which huddle closely together in circles during snowstorms (very high convective cooling!), but also in marmots, which defy the cold mountain winter by hibernating closely together.

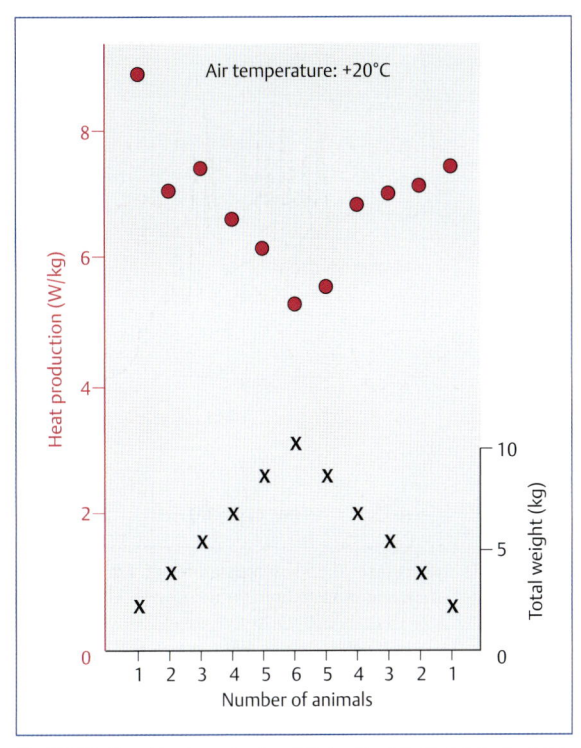

Fig. 20.13 Top: Heat production (W·kg⁻¹) of 1–6 piglets (individual weights 1.2–1.6 kg) during cold stress. The piglets were placed in a climate chamber at 30-minute intervals and their metabolism measured. After the metabolic rate was measured for the whole group in the chamber, the animals were removed from the chamber one by one at equal time intervals. Bottom: Total body weight of the piglets in the chamber. [Source: Mount LE. The influence of huddling and body size on the metabolic rate of young pigs. J Agric Sci 1960; 55: 101–105]

IN A NUTSHELL   !

Numerous behaviours support the physiological mechanisms of heat exchange with the environment.

20.10 Thermoregulatory control loop

The balance between heat production and heat release is subject to careful regulation by thermoregulatory centres (**regulators**) in the anterior **hypothalamus**. This requires **sensors** that measure the respective state in the periphery and in the body core (**actual value**) and pass it on to the regulatory centre. There, the actual value must be compared with a reference value, the **setpoint**, and any differences (control **deviations**) must be reported to the **effectors** (**actuators**) via control signals. This activates either mechanisms of heat emission or heat generation, which ultimately leads to a reduction or increase of the temperature in the **controlled system**: the **core temperature**. The term "setpoint" is used here to refer to the core temperature that occurs when heat emission and heat generation are in equilibrium (**Fig. 20.14**). However, the core temperature must first have fallen by a certain amount before the actuator "heat production" can be activated proportionally to this control deviation (**proportional control**).

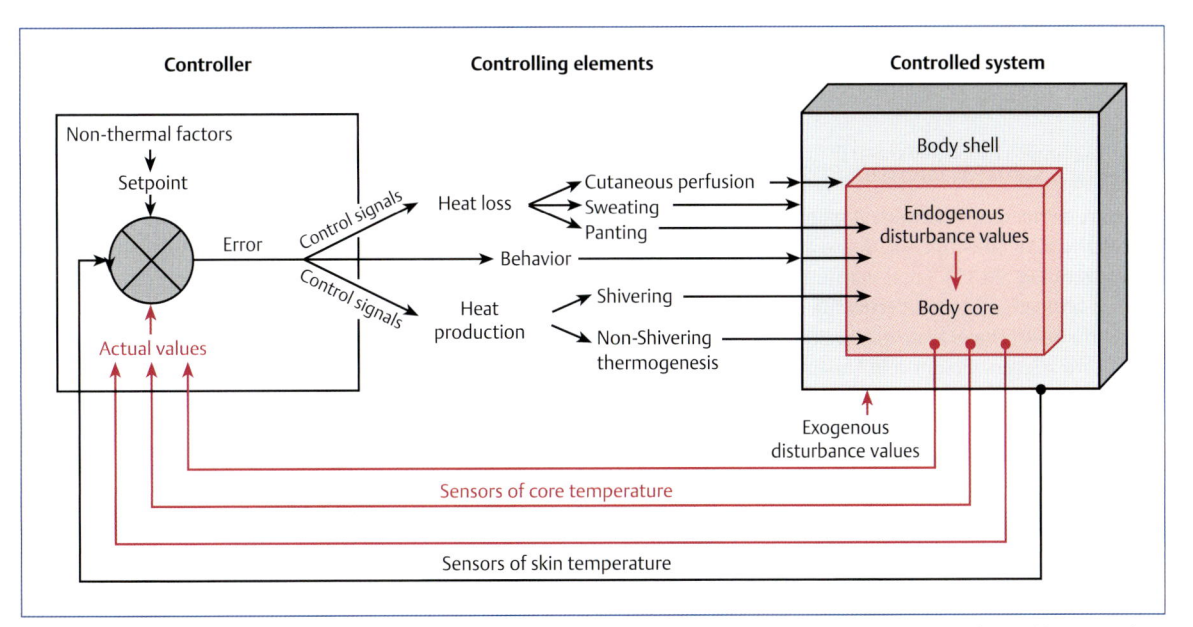

Fig. 20.14 Simplified illustration of the control circuit for temperature regulation. The body core temperature is changed by external disturbances on the skin and by internal disturbances. As a result, a difference between the actual and setpoint values occurs in the hypothalamus (regulator, controller) (control deviation). The control signals activate heat production when the core temperature is lower than the setpoint. If the actual value is higher than the setpoint, heat release is initiated. In both cases, the control deviation is limited (negative feedback).

Nutrition, energy

20.10.1   Peripheral thermosensitivity

Since all animals prefer certain temperatures and avoid others, they clearly have a **peripheral sense of temperature** on the surface of their skin. This temperature sensing is distributed over the body. However, in some places it is locally concentrated. On the face, especially around the nose and mouth, and on the extremities, the temperature points are located more closely together. These temperature sensors are free nerve endings. Their associated sensory neurons can be classified as either cold-sensitive or warm-sensitive neurons. In these thermo-sensitive neurons special ion channels have been identified that open in response to cold or heat and cause a Ca^{2+} and Na^+ influx into the dendrites. Each system thus becomes increasingly insensitive to one side of the detected gradient. The combination of the two receptor types compensates for this.

> **MORE DETAILS**   Both, the cold- and the warm-sensitive neurons are receptors from the large TRP (transient receptor potential) family. In the search for the receptors, it was found that menthol triggers a perception of cold. Analogously, capsaicin, the hot-tasting component of peppers and chillies, enabled the identification of the receptor of the warm-sensitive neurons. When capsaicin comes into contact with the sensory terminals of the sensory cells, a strong heat sensation (heat pain) is triggered.

20.10.2   Central thermosensitivity

There are temperature sensors at many places in the body core. Particularly sensitive and dense are the sensors in the spinal cord (**Fig. 20.15**). Local warming of the spinal cord leads to an increase in heat emission (panting, sweating), so that the core temperature drops. Conversely, cooling the spinal cord triggers violent cold shivering. Local cooling or heating of the **hypothalamus** can also trigger all thermoregulatory reactions of heat generation and heat release, depending on the temperature. Afferent signals from the thermosensors from all parts of the body converge, especially in the anterior hypothalamus (**area praeoptica**). Since the efferent signals to the thermoregulatory actuators also originate from the posterior hypothalamus, the hypothalamus plays a central role as integrator and processor of temperature information as well as a regulator and control unit.

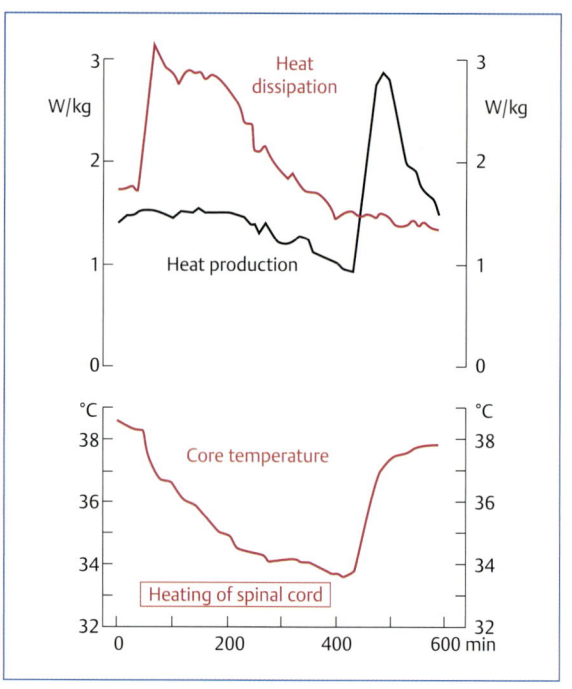

Fig. 20.15 Detection of temperature sensors in the spinal cord. When the spinal cord of a steer is heated locally, the steer begins to pant and sweat (increase in heat dissipation). This causes the core temperature to drop to 34 °C. After heating of the spinal cord has stopped, heat production increases sharply until the core temperature has returned to its initial value. Conversely, if the spinal cord were cooled, severe muscle tremors would occur and the core temperature would rise (not shown here). [Source: Jessen C. Temperature Regulation in Humans and Other Mammals. Berlin, Heidelberg: Springer; 2001]

Since it would not make much sense from an energy point of view to activate heat production and heat emission mechanisms simultaneously (this would be equivalent to heating with an open window), one must assume that there is a **reciprocal inhibition of signalling pathways**. Hypothalamic interneurons that activate the effector neurons of heat production simultaneously inhibit the effector neurons of heat release and vice versa.

> **MORE DETAILS**   Although the hypothalamus certainly plays an important role, no single central coordinator for all thermoregulatory actions has yet been found. Rather, it appears that core temperature is regulated by multiple, independently operating sensor-effector loops, each with its own afferents and efferents. It has been shown, for example, that for adequate thermoregulatory behaviour, an intact area praeoptica is not necessary. It has also been shown that the thresholds for individual effector mechanisms can be regulated independently of each other. In endotoxic shock, for example, the threshold at which cold-induced heat generation is triggered is lowered by 2 °C. At the same time, however, the threshold for cold-induced vasoconstriction hardly changes.

20.11 Normal range of body temperature

The core temperature of a mammal or bird at rest is called **normothermic** or **euthermic**. This normal range is typical for a species and lies between 37.5 and 40 °C in domestic and laboratory animals, and between 40 and 42 °C in birds (**Table 20.1**). Pathological deviations from this range are called either **hypothermia** or **hyperthermia**. These need to be distinguished from the adaptive changes in the **setpoint** of body temperature regulation described in ch. 20.13 (p. 508) and ch. 20.14 (p. 509).

Table 20.1 Normal core temperature ranges.

Animal species	Temperature range (°C)	Average temperature
Horse	37.5–38.5	37.8
Cattle	37.5–39.5	38.5
Sheep	38.0–39.5	39.3
Goat	38.0–39.5	39.5
Pig	38.0–40.0	39.0
Dog	37.5–39.0	38.4
Cat	38.0–39.0	38.8
Rabbit	38.5–39.5	39.0
Guinea pig	37.5–39.5	38.5
Goose	40.0–41.0	40.5
Chicken	40.0–42.0	41.0
Pigeon	41.0–43.0	42.0

Source: Kolb E (ed.). Lehrbuch der Physiologie der Haustiere. Stuttgart: Fischer; 1989 and Refinetti R. Circadian Physiology. 2nd ed., Boca Raton: Taylor & Francis; 2006

MORE DETAILS Despite the variability of core temperature, a representative value that can be measured in the rectum, vagina or cloaca is sufficient for clinical purposes. It should be determined after prolonged rest at neutral air temperature. These conditions often cannot be met in practice. In a racehorse, it may take more than an hour for work-induced hyperthermia to subside (see ch. Thermoregulation and sweat secretion (p. 627). In small animals, the stress of holding is enough to raise the temperature very rapidly and markedly. A value in the upper limit range can be regarded as an indication of fever (p. 508), the better the measuring conditions have been observed.

IN A NUTSHELL !

Temperature measurements to rule out fever should be taken at normal ambient temperature and after prolonged rest.

20.12 Hypothermia and hyperthermia

Heat production over a long term, cannot be increased by much more than 5 times the resting metabolic rate. If heat losses in a cold environment exceed this heat production, the core temperature drops continuously and a state of **hypothermia** then exists. Most adult farm animals in Central Europe are unlikely to experience problems, if they are adequately fed and their fur insulation is intact. However, the core temperature of newborn lambs or piglets, and also newly shorn sheep, can definitely reach these limits in a cold and especially damp environment and with strong wind at the same time. Mild hypothermia is when core body temperatures are 35–32 °C. This state is characterised by an increase in cold-shivering, hyperventilation and tachycardia. At temperatures below 32 °C, drowsiness, apathy and later unconsciousness occur. From about 28 °C, muscles and joints become rigid and cardiac arrhythmias are increasingly observed. At 25 °C, ventricular fibrillation may often occur. Even prolonged **deep anaesthesia** can lead to life-threatening hypothermia because of reduced metabolism and the simultaneous suppression of muscle tone.

IN A NUTSHELL !

With increasing hypothermia, the organism usually goes through a stage of excitation, exhaustion and paralysis before death occurs.

Hyperthermia is also characterised by disproportionate heat production and heat output, without the setpoint being adjusted. In this case, however, the heat output is always too low in relation to heat input and heat production. The upper limits of control are reached relatively quickly in the case of intense physical activity of larger animals with a high muscle content. Prolonged overheating at body temperatures above 42–43 °C leads to life-threatening **heat stroke** in mammals. This is characterised by pale, dry skin (vasoconstriction, no sweat production), which additionally hinders heat dissipation.

MORE DETAILS **Malignant hyperthermia**, which is not uncommon in **pigs**, is due to a genetic defect in the ryanodine receptor of the sarcoplasmic reticulum, which plays a key role in electromechanical coupling in muscle. Triggered by stress loads such as transport to the slaughterhouse and/or caging before slaughter, but also by fluorinated inhalation narcotics (halothane) or muscle relaxants (succinylcholine), there is an uncontrolled Ca^{2+} outflow into the cytosol, resulting in permanent contraction of the muscles, with consequent increased heat production. Since heat release is reduced at the same time, life-threatening hyperthermia can develop, which can lead to partial denaturation of the muscle proteins. After slaughter, the meat is often **p**ale (pale), **s**oft and watery (**e**xudative), which is why it is also called PSE meat.

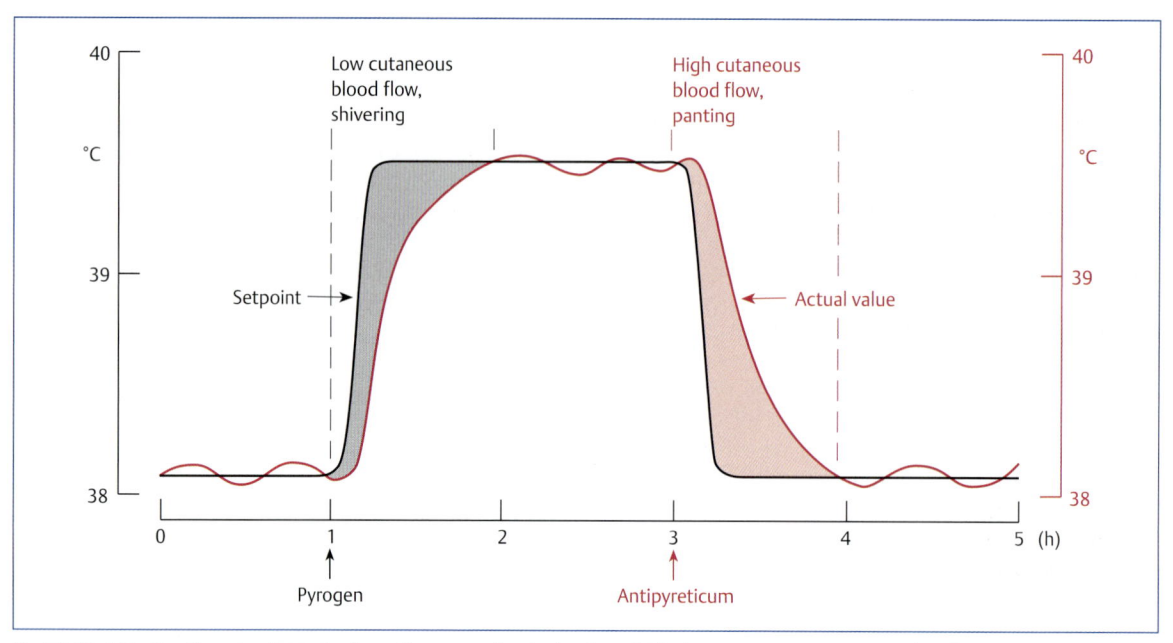

Low cutaneous blood flow, shivering

High cutaneous blood flow, panting

Setpoint →

← Actual value

Pyrogen

Antipyreticum

Fig. 20.16 Adjusting the set point in the fever. Pyrogens raise the level at which the core temperature is regulated. This results in a control deviation (grey area), which activates mechanisms of cold defence (heat production). Lowering the control level after the end of the fever or administration of fever-reducing medication again results in a control deviation (red area). Heat release is then activated until the normothermic core temperature is reached,.

20.13 Fever

Fever is associated with a variety of diseases and is accompanied by clearly visible symptoms of illness such as loss of appetite, listlessness and lack of energy, as well as increased need for sleep and hyperalgesia. An increase in body temperature above the normal range (animal species-specific, **Table 20.1**) is therefore considered a non-specific indicator of illness. Infections in particular, but also some tumours and non-infectious inflammations can be the cause of fever. Fever is an acute increase in core temperature, triggered by **pyrogens**. A distinction is made between exogenous and endogenous pyrogens. Exogenous pyrogens are viruses or bacteria or their components (e.g. lipopolysaccharides, LPS). They induce in granulocytes and macrophages the release of cytokines (including interleukin-1β, IL-6, TNF-α, and interferons) which are referred to as endogenous pyrogens. These cytokines reach the preoptic area of the hypothalamus via the fenestrated capillaries of the organum vasculosum laminae. There, prostaglandin E_2 is produced in endothelial and glial cells. The finding that cyclooxygenase inhibitors such as acetylsalicylic acid or indomethacin have a fever-reducing (**antipyretic**) effect, because they prevent the formation of prostaglandins, suggests that prostaglandin E_2 plays an important role in initiating fever.

The setpoint adjustment causes the core temperature to be below the new setpoint. The organism reacts to this as if it were exposed to a cold environment. Muscle tremors and vasoconstriction occur until the core temperature reaches the new, higher set point. This is followed by a plateau phase of varying length, depending on the disease. In contrast in hyperthermia, there is no increase in the activity of heat release mechanisms. It is only at the end of an episode of fever that the set point is again below the current core temperature., This becomes apparent through sweating or panting in this phase (**Fig. 20.16**).

MORE DETAILS Ectothermic animals can also react to pyrogens; however, since they do not have endogenous heat production, they achieve an increase in body temperature through their behaviour. When a lizard suffers from an infection, it seeks out a warmer environment ("behavioural fever"). It can therefore be assumed that fever is a phylogenetically ancient mechanism by means of which an organism fights infections. This also suggests that fever has an adaptive value, and several arguments suggest that the increased body temperature in fever has positive effects. Various components of the innate and acquired immune system are stimulated by fever, such as the mobility and activity of phagocytic cells, the production of antibodies and interferons, and the activation of T-helper cells. In addition, growth and multiplication of some (but not all!) pathogenic microorganisms may be inhibited by an increase in temperature. An elevated body temperature also leads to the synthesis of "heat shock" proteins, which repair any damage to the tertiary structure of proteins.

Excessive inflammatory reactions and high body temperatures are counteracted by endogenous **antipyretics in the periphery and central nervous system**. Peripherally acting antipyretics include glucocorticoids and anti-inflammatory cytokines (IL-4, IL-10). Centrally acting antipyretics include nitric oxide (NO) and eicosanoids. Fever and antipyretics are therefore subject to finely controlled regulation and are to be regarded as physiological reactions.

> **IN A NUTSHELL** !
>
> Fever is not uncontrolled hyperthermia, but a regulated thermoregulation at an elevated core temperature. Fever is therefore not pathological, but a physiological reaction of an organism to an infection.

20.14 Rheostasis

The concept of **homeostasis**, which can be traced back to Claude Bernard (1813–1878), assumes characteristic target values for all physiological processes. These are "defended" by their respective regulatory mechanisms and thus a constant internal milieu ("fixité du milieu intérieure") is maintained. However, the findings of chronobiology (p. 511) in particular, make it increasingly clear that there are endogenous, diurnal fluctuations of sometimes considerable proportions in practically all physiological parameters. Measurements in the field at different times of the year also show that many organisms regulate to very different levels, i.e. that the target values are variable depending on the season and the situation. To do justice to these findings, Nicholas Mrosovsky introduced the term **rheostasis**. This describes the regulation to a rhythmically changing setpoint, in contrast to the constant setpoint of a homeostatically regulated system. Rheostatic regulation has the great advantage of increased flexibility in the face of a variable environment. In addition, there can be anticipatory adaptation to periodically changing conditions rather than mere fixed reaction to the changes.

20.14.1 Daily periodicity and annual periodicity of body temperature

In all endothermic animals studied so far, the body temperature follows regular cycles during the course of a day and also during the course of a year. These cycles are endogenous in nature and also occur at very constant ambient temperatures and without physical exertion. They obviously follow a rhythmically changing set point, controlled by an endogenous, biological "clock" (p. 511). The amplitude of the daily fluctuations depends, among other things, on the body mass. In small mammals (mice, hamsters) the amplitude can be up to 4 °C, whereas in cattle and horses it is between 0.6 and 1.2 °C.

There are also hormonally determined rhythms (p. 511) of body temperature, such as during an oestrus cycle, see ch. 24.

20.14.2 Torpor and hibernation

In winter, endothermic organisms, especially small mammals and birds, need more energy to keep their body temperature constant. At the same time, however, their food supply may be limited, of poorer quality, and be less accessible because of ice and snow. Many species solve this problem by reducing their metabolic rate to a "low flame" of up to 0.02 ml $O_2 \cdot g^{-1} \cdot h^{-1}$ (approx. 100 mW$\cdot$kg^{-1}). As a result, the body temperature of smaller animals drops significantly (**hypothermia**). This lowering of the body temperature due to regulated reduced heat production is called **torpor**, as it is accompanied by an impairment or even loss of the ability to move. Torpor occurs either on a daily basis – see diurnal (p. 509) torpor – or persistently over many days in "true hibernation". Hibernation is a strategy of energy conservation for long periods of cold

and lack of food. Small mammals such as native bats, hedgehogs, dormice, field hamsters or marmots, before the onset of winter, seek out winter quarters that are protected as far as possible from frost., This is triggered by an endogenous annual periodicity. In deep hibernation, the core temperature of these hibernating animals drops to values close to the ambient temperature, the heart beats much slower, and in the case of marmots, beats only 4–6 times per minute (compared to 80–140 times in summer). The rate of breathing is also significantly reduced, often with very long pauses, followed by several deep breaths (**Cheyne-Stokes breathing**). The core body temperature of some gnats can even drop below freezing. The animals' body fluid does not freeze because there are no crystallisation nuclei to form ice ("supercooling"). If the core temperature in the torpor threatens to fall below a species- and situation-specific value, heat production starts again. This occurs through the cyclical activation of thermogenic mechanisms. In sum, heat production increases proportionally to the falling ambient temperature and thus prevents a further drop in body temperature. This shows that torpor is also a regulated state, but at a different temperature level.

MORE DETAILS The brown bear lowers its body temperature to values around 30–32 °C, for which the term "**hibernation**" has been used. Recent studies show that many animal species are able to maintain a **hypometabolic state** for some time. Przewalski's horses, deer, ibex and even prosimians (fat-tailed maki) are capable of lowering their energy metabolism. The core temperature drops only slowly and only by a few degrees Celsius in this process because of
their large body mass and/or very good thermal insulation (bear) or because the ambient temperature in the habitat is high (maki).

Hibernators can reduce their energy metabolism during the torpor phases, to one hundredth to one-twentieth of the normal resting value, depending on body size. However, hibernation is not continuous, but consists of individual episodes with regular awakenings (**Fig. 20.17**). If one accounts for the high energy costs during the waking and awake phases, there are still energy savings of 85–95% over the entire winter season. The question of why hibernating animals have to wake up regularly has not yet been definitively answered.

MORE DETAILS In a state of **daily torpor**, the core temperature only drops to values around 20 °C for a few hours during the daily resting phase. This form of torpor occurs in many small mammals and marsupials, but also in birds (humming birds, swifts). Not as much energy can be saved in this form of torpor (up to max. 67% per day) as in true hibernation. The advantage is probably that during the activity period with high body temperature, social and territorial needs can be maintained even during the food-poor period. In addition, the intensity and frequency of torpor can be varied from day to day and adapted to the current food supply.

> **IN A NUTSHELL** !
>
> Torpor and hibernation are not uncontrolled hypothermia, but regulated saving mechanisms at a lowered metabolic level.

Nutrition, energy

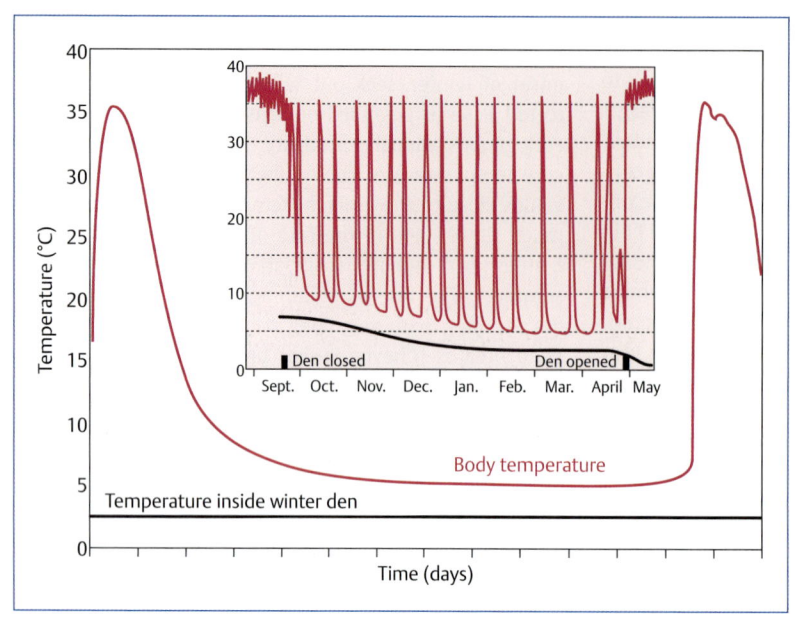

Fig. 20.17 Course of body temperature of a marmot during a single hibernation episode (large image) and during the entire hibernation season (top). In the course of winter, torpor phases of about twelve days' duration with a drop in body temperature to 2 °C regularly alternate with normothermic phases of 28 hours' duration on average. However, the core body temperature remains about 2–3 °C below the summer level even during these phases. [Source: Arnold W, Ruf T, Frey-Roos F et al. Diet-independent remodelling of cellular membranes precedes seasonally changing body temperature in a hibernator. PLoS One 2011; 6: e18641]

Suggested reading

Arnold W, Ruf T, Kuntz R. Seasonal adjustment of energy budget in a large mammal, the Przewalski horse (*Equus ferus przewalskii*) II. Energy expenditure. J Exp Biol 2006; 209: 4566–4573

Berg F, Gustafson U, Andersson L. The uncoupling protein 1 gene (UCP1) is disrupted in the pig lineage: a genetic explanation for poor thermoregulation in piglets. PLoS Genet 2006; 2: 1178–1181

Brinkmann L, Gerken M, Riek A. Adaptation strategies to seasonal changes in environmental conditions of a domesticated horse breed, the Shetland pony (*Equus ferus caballus*). Exp Biol 2012; 215: 1061–1068

Cunningham JG. Textbook of Veterinary Physiology. 2nd ed. Philadelphia: WB Saunders; 1997

Dausmann KH, Glos J, Ganzhorn JU et al. Physiology: Hibernation in a tropical primate. Nature 2004; 429: 825–826

Heldmaier G. Tremor-free heat production and body size in mammals. Z Vergl Phys 1971; 73: 222–248

Jessen C. Temperature regulation in humans and other mammals. Berlin, Heidelberg: Springer; 2001

Klingenberg M, Huang SG. Structure and function of the uncoupling protein from brown adipose tissue. Biochim Biophys Acta 1999; 1415: 271–296

McGaugh S, Schwartz TS. Here and there, but not everywhere: repeated loss of uncoupling protein 1 in amniotes. Biol Lett 2017; 13: 20160749

Mrosovsky N. Rheostasis. The Physiology of Change. New York: Oxford University Press; 1990

Nowack J, Giroud S, Arnold W et al. Muscle non-shivering thermogenesis and its role in the evolution of endothermy. Front Physiol 2017; 8: 889

Nowack J, Vetter S, Stalder G et al. Muscle non-shivering thermogenesis in a feral mammal. Sci Rep 2019; 9: 6378

Riek A, Brinkmann L, Gauly M et al. Seasonal changes in energy expenditure, body temperature and activity patterns in llamas (Lama glama). Sci Rep 2017; 7: 7600

Romanovsky AA. Thermoregulation: some concepts have changed. Functional architecture of the thermoregulatory system. Am J Physiol Regul Integr Comp Physiol 2007; 292: R37–46

Roth J, Blatteis CM. Mechanisms of fever production and lysis: Lessons from experimental LPS fever. Compr Physiol 2014; 4: 1563–1604

Signer C, Ruf T, Arnold W. Hypometabolism and basking: The strategies of Alpine ibex to endure harsh over-wintering conditions. Functional Ecology 2011; 25: 537–547

Turbill C, Ruf T, Mang T et al. Regulation of heart rate and rumen temperature in red deer: effects of season and food intake. J Exp Biol 2011; 214: 963–970

Wascher CA, Kotrschal K, Arnold W. Free-living greylag geese adjust their heart rates and body core temperatures to season and reproductive context. Sci Rep 2018; 8: 2142

21 Biological rhythms

Walter Arnold, Stephan Steinlechner

21.1 The "inner" clock

ESSENTIALS ✖

- All biological processes show periodic fluctuations of specific duration.
- Many are controlled by "internal clocks", i.e. by endogenous rhythms that are synchronised with exogenous factors.
- Internal clocks enable the organism to act with foresight and not just react to environmental stimuli.
- The most important events in time are the day/night change and the seasonal changes in day length (photoperiod).
- The length of time of endogenous rhythms coincides only approximately with the lengths of time of variable environmental factors. Hence the terms "circadian" or "circannual" rhythms, are used.
- The endogenous daily rhythm is created by complex molecular feedback loops. Proteins encoded by "clock genes" form heterodimers in the cytosol, which migrate back into the cell nucleus and inhibit further transcription of the clock genes. The subsequent decrease in the concentration of the heterodimers in turn releases the blockade of transcription and thus closes the feedback loop.
- The molecular mechanism of endogenous rhythms with period lengths other than about 24 hours is still unclear.
- Interference with the pattern of endogenous rhythms leads to disturbances of well-being or even illness.

21.2 Phenomenology

Animal physiology and behaviour, may have time-related programmes such as sleeping, feeding, reproductive readiness, or moulting. Precise temporal organisation of life functions and behaviour is necessary to meet the constantly changing needs of an organism (e.g. well fed or hungry; tired or awake) and changing environmental conditions (e.g. seasons, food availability). This applies also to unicellular organisms and plants. **Chronobiology** (from Greek Χρόνος – chrónos, "time") studies the temporal structure and organisation of physiological processes and has contributed significantly to the concept of rheostasis (p. 509).

Since most organ functions and metabolism exhibit rhythmicity, the effect or side effect of a drug is also dependent on the time of its administration. **Chronopharmacological** studies have shown, for example, that the side effects of a therapy with corticosteroids can be significantly reduced if the natural rhythm of the body's own corticoid secretion is taken into account. An animal's sensitivity to toxic substances also depends on the time of day. **Chronotoxicological** studies have shown that the same dose, administered at different times of the day, can either be lethal or tolerated by the organism. Anaesthetics and painkillers also have a diurnal effect, and possibly also a seasonal effect.

However, the application of chronobiological knowledge requires knowledge of the biological rhythms and the timing of phases of the individual to be treated. This is a topic where there is still a need for further studies in practical veterinary medicine, especially in relation to farm and laboratory animals.

21.2.1 Spectrum of biological rhythms

The frequency range of biological rhythms extends from milliseconds for molecular and neuronal rhythms (e.g. action potential) to decades for population cycles (**Table 21.1**).

Rhythms that are distinctly shorter than 24 hours are called **ultradian** (from Latin: dies=day), those that are significantly longer than 24 hours are called **infradian**.

Many biological rhythms are generated by **endogenous pacemakers** in an organism ("internal clock"), analogous to the pacemaker cells in the heart. They are self-excited and continue to operate even in the absence of an external stimulus. Four of these biological rhythms (diurnal, annual, lunar and tidal) have developed in the course of evolution as adaptations to cyclical environmental changes. Since lunar and tidal rhythms are mainly relevant for marine or intertidal organisms and do not play a role for domestic animals, they will not be discussed further in this chapter. It must also be emphasised that not all biological rhythms are of endogenous origin or have endogenous components, but are determined by exogenous factors.

21.2.2 Importance of biological rhythms

Internal clocks developed during evolution because they offer decisive advantages. For example, competition can be avoided or predators can be better evaded by appropriate timely interactions when searching for food. Furthermore, physiological or morphological adaptations that require a longer period to become established, can be started before the time of activation, and thus be completed when they are needed. If, for example, cold alone were to trigger the change from summer to winter coat, then high energy costs would be incurred for thermoregulation during the time needed for the growth of a dense undercoat. Internal clocks thus enable – in contrast to an acute reaction – timely preparation for something to come (**feed forward coupling**).

Table 21.1 Spectrum of biological rhythms[1].

Biological rhythm	Typical period lengths	Example
Neuronal rhythms	0.001 to 1 second	Spontaneous frequency of cold sensors in the cat lingual nerve
Heart rate	0.05 to 3 seconds	Depending on species and activity
Breathing rate	0.1 to 10 seconds	Depending on species and activity
Biochemical oscillations	30 seconds to 20 minutes	Glycolysis
Hormonal rhythms	10 minutes to 3–5 hours[2]	GnRH secretion
Tidal rhythms	12.4 hours	Activity of fiddler crabs; hatching of the sea midge (*Clunio marinus*)
Daily rhythms	24 hours	Body temperature, metabolic rate
Sexual cycles	1 day until 1 year[2]	**Table 24.2**
Lunar rhythms	29.5 days	Spawning in spurdogs and shore crabs
Annual rhythms	1 year	Coat change, hibernation
Population rhythms	1 to 20 years[2]	May beetles, cicadas, voles, lemmings, snowshoe hares, Canadian lynx

[1] based on data from Goldbeter A. Biological rhythms: Clocks for all times. Curr Biol 2008, 17: R751–R753
[2] possibly even longer

MORE DETAILS   A good example of anticipatory activity can be observed in the rabbit: The mother rabbit hides her young in a well-insulated nest after birth and returns to the nest only once a day for about five minutes to suckle the young. Presumably, this very short presence of the mother prevents the young from being discovered by predators through noises or smell. However, the young must take in enough milk for the next 24 hours in this short time. The infants anticipate the mother's arrival and free themselves from the dense nest material about five minutes beforehand in order to be able to start suckling immediately. The control of this anticipatory activity by an internal clock is evidenced by the fact that the young free themselves from the nest at the "right" time even if the mother repeatedly does not appear.

IN A NUTSHELL   **!**

Biological rhythms enable the organism to act "ahead" and not just react.

21.3   Daily periodic rhythms

21.3.1   Period lengths

The endogenous component of a biological rhythm becomes visible when organisms are deprived of time information from their environment. For example, if animals are kept in constant darkness, their daily sleep-wake cycle is maintained. However, the period length (symbolised by the Greek letter tau: τ) deviates somewhat from 24 hours (**Fig. 21.1**), which is why the endogenous daily rhythm is **circadian** (from Latin: circa = about and dies = day). Most of our farm animals are diurnal, whereas many mice, rats, hamsters, rabbits or domestic cats are predominantly nocturnal. The period length of a cycle under free-living conditions is also an individual characteristic, referred to as **chronotypes** (**Fig. 21.1**).

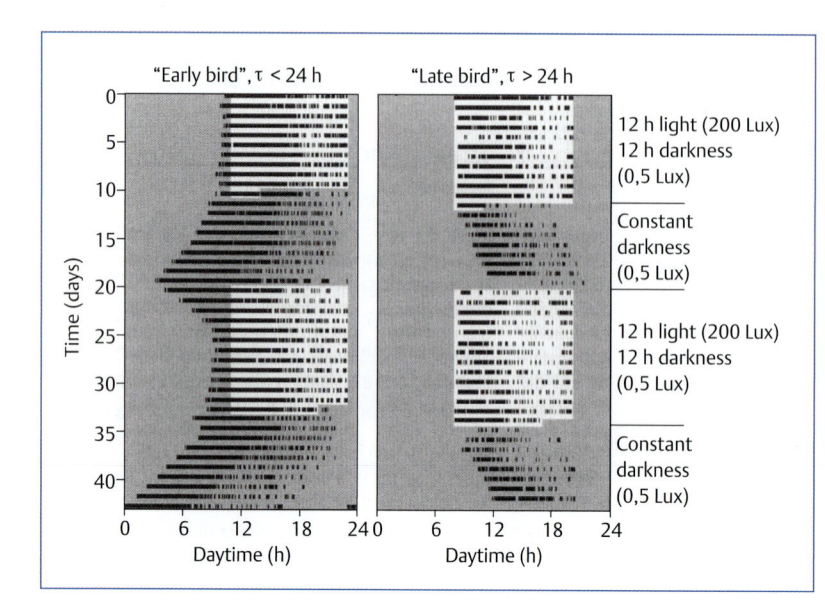

Fig. 21.1 The free-running circadian rhythms of two Chaffinches with period lengths smaller and larger than 24 hours. Along the x-axis, a bar indicates in dark when the animals were active in the 24 hours of a day. Consecutive days of the measurement are plotted on the y-axis. After switching off the external time information light/dark alternation, the endogenous rhythm emerges (i.e. during the "permanent darkness" (0.5 lux) of day 10–20 and day 33–43). The endogenous rhythm τ is somewhat shorter than 24 hours in the individual shown on the left, and somewhat longer in the individual on the right; based on data from Aschoff J (ed.). Biological Rhythms. Handbook of Behavioural Neurobiology. New York: Plenum Press; 1981

21.3.2 Genetic and molecular basis of the day clock

The discovery of mutations in a single gene of the fruit fly *Drosophila* that alter the circadian phenotype has provided the final proof that circadian rhythms have a genetic basis. The gene *Per* - for period – occurs in three different alleles besides the wild type: *Per*^{S} shows a shortened ($\tau = 19$ hours), *Per*^{L} a prolonged ($\tau = 28$ hours) period, while *Per*^{0} mutants showed no rhythm at all. This gene *Per*, which is localised on the X chromosome of *Drosophila*, must therefore be actively involved in the generation of the circadian rhythm and at the same time co-determine its period length.

In particular, the use of molecular biological methods and the generation of transgenic mice and knock-out mice have contributed to the elucidation of the mechanism of the internal daily clock in the last two decades. The functioning of the intracellular clock mechanism is based on repetitive positive and negative feedback loops that inter-act with each other both at the level of activation of specific clock genes and at the protein transcription level. The first "**clock gene**" in mammals was found using a mutagenicity screen performed on 10,000 mice and was named **Clock** (acronym for circadian locomotor output cycle kaput) because homozygous mutants lose their activity rhythm in continuous darkness. To date, at least eleven clock genes are known in mammals, and up to 18 are suspected (**Fig. 21.2**).

21.4 Annual periodic rhythms

A large number of biological processes are also subject to seasonal periodic changes. The endogenous component of year-periodic rhythms can be seen, as with diurnal periodicity, in the experimental elimination of the most important timer (**Fig. 21.3**). For annual periodicity, this is the length of day (**photoperiod**), which changes rhythmically over the course of a year, at latitudes away from the equator. In many vertebrates, the **pineal organ** plays an impor-

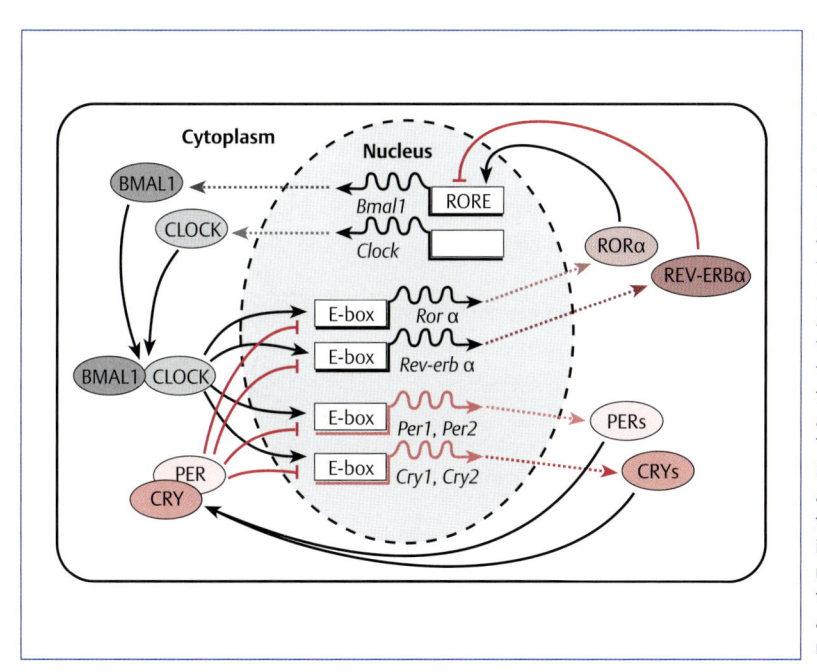

Fig. 21.2 Simplified model of the molecular mechanism of the circadian clock. The protein CLOCK and another protein BMAL1 form CLOCK-BMAL1 heterodimers in the cytoplasm and activate the transcription of *period genes* and *cryptochrome genes*. The PER and CRY proteins when produced, migrate into the nucleus as heterodimers, where they serve as a negative regulator. They block activation by CLOCK-BMAL1 and thus prevent transcription of their own *Per* and *Cry* genes, closing the negative feedback loop. The positive feedback loop that runs simultaneously begins with the transcription of *Rev-Erbα*, which is also activated by CLOCK-BMAL1 heterodimers. The Rev-Erbα protein formed represses BMAL1 transcription, so that overall the amount of BMAL1 RNA decreases, while at the same time the levels of *Per* and *Cry RNA* increase. When CRY and PER proteins migrate into the nucleus as heterodimers to repress *Per* and *Cry* transcription, they also inhibit Rev-Erbα protein transcription, resulting in BMAL1 activation.

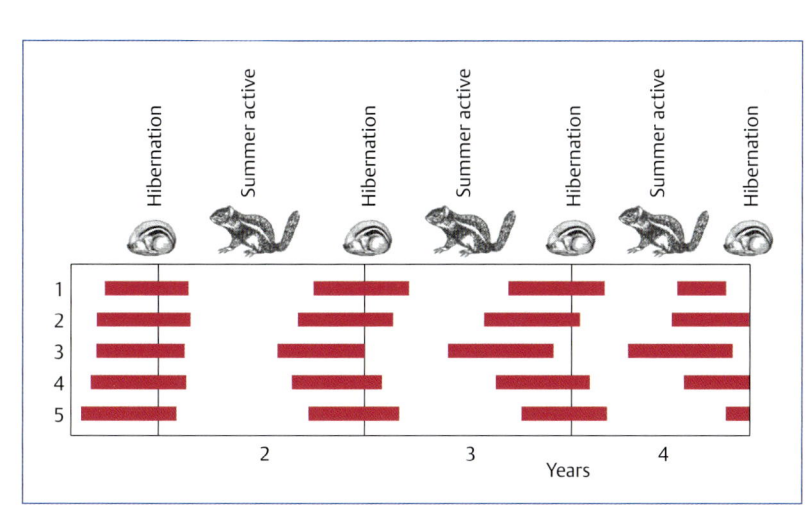

Fig. 21.3 Free-running "circannual" endogenous rhythm of hibernation and summer activity in the golden-mantled gopher (*Callospermophilus lateralis*). Five animals were kept in constant darkness and temperature for four years, yet they hibernated year after year (red bars).

tant role in detecting the photoperiod. Corpus pineale (as in **Fig. 5.22** to keep nomenclature consistent) plays a special role; syn. pineal gland, epiphysis cerebri, see ch. 5.2.2 (p. 122) and **Fig. 5.22**. The C. pineale is a dorsal protrusion of the diencephalon above the hypothalamus. It synthesises the hormone **melatonin** only during the time of darkness and thus reflects the duration of night. Melatonin (p. 556) is therefore a hormone that acts mainly during the time it is being secreted and not justthrough its concentration.

Endogenously controlled annual rhythms are called "circannual" in analogy to circadian rhythms. Here, too, the period lengths of the endogenous rhythm and the environmental timer do not coincide exactly. With circannual rhythms, the deviation is usually even more pronounced, as are the differences between individuals. In contrast to the endogenous daily clock, the mechanism of the circannual clock and its anatomical localisation are still unclear.

Circannual rhythms control a whole range of adaptations that enable animals to cope with seasonally changing living conditions (**Fig. 21.4**, **Table 21.2**). In northern or southern latitudes, winter in particular presents a challenge. Food shortages and cold weather can only be survived by those who evade them in time or who adapt physiological processes and organ systems accordingly (**acclimatisation**). In summer, however, these latitudes have a high productivity, which favour the opportunity to build up fat reserves and produce offspring.

Table 21.2 Examples of year-period adjustments with endogenous control.

Feature	Examples
Reproduction	Most animal species regulate reproductive readiness so that young are born in the season with the best food availability (**Fig. 21.4**). In many species, reproductive organs (testes) and secondary sexual characteristics (e.g. antlers) are only functional during the rut. A distinction is made between so-called "short day breeders" (e.g. sheep, goat), which become sexually active when day length decreases, and "long day breeders" (e.g. horse), which become sexually active in spring when day length increases (**Fig. 21.4**) (see ch. on the sexual cycle (p. 560).
Height	Because of their high metabolic rate (p. 490), small mammals cannot adjust to long periods with limited food supply by utilising fat reserves. Instead, they reduce their total energy requirements by becoming even smaller in winter (Dehnel effect). Even the skeleton and skull capsule can shrink (shrews).
Activity and food intake	Hibernators, winter resting animals and many species not previously so categorised (e.g. red deer, chamois, ibex, Przewalski's horses, Shetland ponies) reduce activity and foraging during the winter months.
Metabolism	In summer, these species consume a lot of food and build up fat deposits (high, anabolic metabolism), which they draw on in winter (low, catabolic metabolism), see ch. on energy (p. 483) metabolism and temperature regulation (p. 494). Subadult animals hardly grow at all in winter. The frugal winter state is not prevented even by ad libitum feeding.
Digestion	The organs that are less active in winter (rumen, intestine, liver, kidney) become considerably smaller in some cases (**Fig. 21.5**). This reduces their maintenance requirement.
Fur and feathers	Denser undercoat or down in the winter coat and increased vasoconstriction in the periphery improve insulation of the warm body core and reduce thermoregulatory costs in the cold (**Fig. 20.1 b**). White winter coat protects against detection (snow hare, Dzungarian dwarf hamster, stoat).
Thermoregulation	The lowering of the metabolic rate (p. 493) in winter means above all lower endogenous heat production, which is why the body temperature is lower in winter in all endothermic species studied so far. However, the extent of the lowering varies greatly from species to species (see ch. Rheostasis (p. 509).
Fatty acids	In preparation for the cold season, unsaturated fatty acids with a higher melting point are increasingly incorporated into cell membranes so that they remain functional in the cold and membrane-bound key enzymes of muscle activity and energy metabolism (p. 493) work faster, thus counteracting the temperature-related reduction of enzyme activities (Q_{10} effects).
Stockpiling	Crows, titmice, field hamsters, squirrels build up food stocks during summer which they then use over winter.
Hikes	Migratory birds migrate seasonally over long distances, to evade local unfavourable weather and feeding conditions. Red deer use the highly productive alpine meadows above the timberline in summer, but spend the winter at lower altitudes. Bats migrate to regions with caves that are suitable for hibernation.
Social behaviour	Many species show increased social thermoregulation ("cuddling", e.g. small mammals, horses, pigs) in winter. Increased tolerance leads to the formation of larger flocks (birds) or herds (e.g. deer) in winter. This reduces the individual risk of severe hypothermia ("selfish herd" effect).

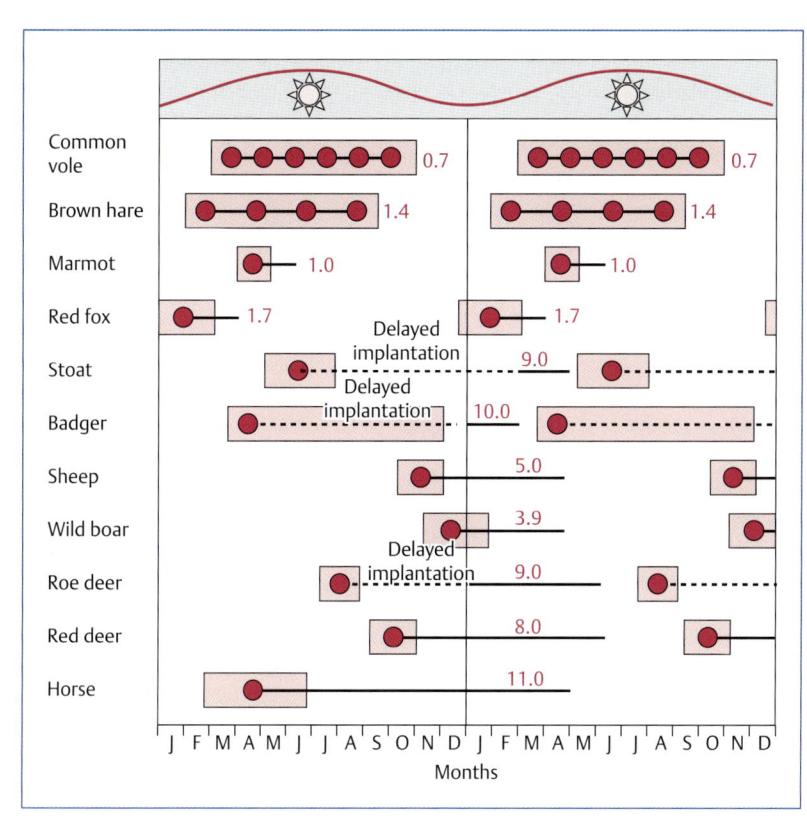

Fig. 21.4 Mammals coordinate their sexual cycles so that young are born during seasons when there is a good food supply. Some species have developed the phenomenon of dormancy. The zygote is dormant after fertilisation until an endocrine signal, controlled by the annual clock, triggers implantation and further development (see ch. 24 (p. 553)). The oestrous cycles and their duration of domestic animals are listed in **Table 24.2**.
Red dots: probable times of fertilisation; pink bars: range of variation; lines with red numbers: total gestation period (in months); dashed lines: dormancy; red wavy line at top: Day length.

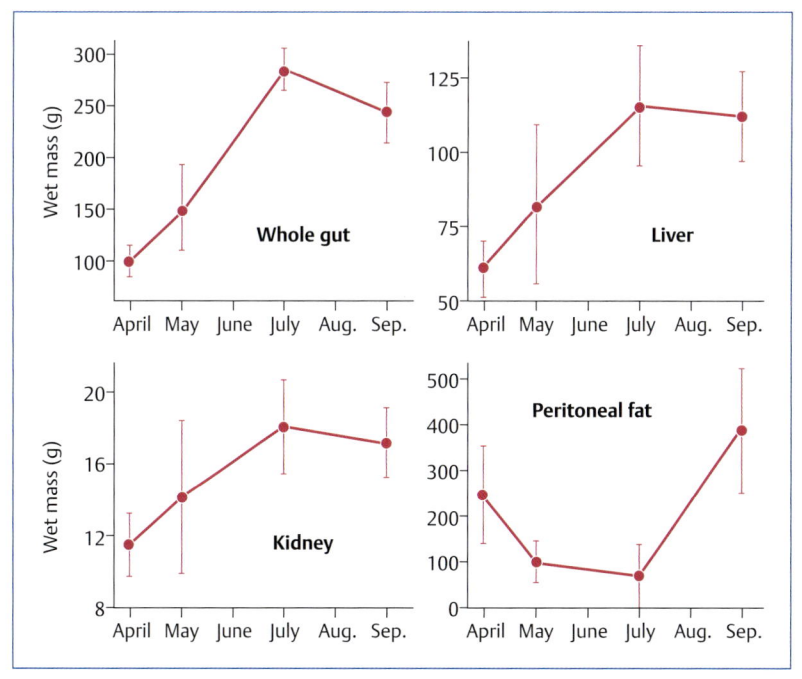

Fig. 21.5 The digestive organs are used less in winter due to reduced or no food intake. As seen here in the example of the Alpine marmot, the intestine and visceral organs enlarge during anabolic metabolism in summer and shrink in winter, when the animals cover their energy needs from fat reserves; Diagram above left is based on data from Hume ID et al. Seasonal changes in morphology and function of the gastrointestinal tract of free-living alpine marmots (Marmota marmota). J Comp Physiol B 2002; 172: 197–207

Special annual rhythms are seen in rather short-lived mammals (< 1–3 years life expectancy). Although their annual rhythm has an endogenous component, it does not persist for longer than one cycle without the influence of environmental signals. Such an "hourglass" timer regulates adaptation to winter of the Dzungarian dwarf hamster. If these animals are exposed to alternate light/dark periods with a short light phase (winter), they develop their white winter coat and often show "daily torpor" (p. 509). After about six months, the animals spontaneously return to their summer state, in which they then remain. The hourglass is only triggered again when the animals have been exposed to long-day conditions (summer) for sometime, and then followed by a period of short-day exposure.

21.5 Timer

Endogenous rhythms are synchronised with regularly recurring environmental stimuli, so-called **timers**. The most important of these is light, but the time of feeding, large changes in temperature (especially in ectothermic animals) or social interactions are also timing activators. Social interactions seem to be as important in humans or social animals as the change between light and dark.

Since the endogenous period length τ only corresponds approximately to the period length of a timing activator, internal clocks must be synchronised with the timer, a process called **entrainment**. Depending on the period length τ, the phase position of the inner clock is accelerated or slowed down. This succeeds without problems in the so-called **entrainment range**, in which the phase position of the two rhythms does not differ substantially. If the differences are too great, the endogenous rhythm **decouples from** the timer and runs independently. We humans experience a decoupling of our inner daily clock, for example, as „jet lag" when flying across several time zones. This can also lead to a desynchronisation of individual endogenous rhythms (body temperature, hormonal rhythms, activity rhythms, etc.), a phenomenon known as **internal desynchronisation** (Fig. 21.6). After such events, it takes some time for the endogenous rhythm to resynchronise with the exogenous timer. Since social stimuli also act as timing activators, the unpleasant side effects of "jet lag" can be shortened by forcing oneself to adapt to the rest and activity phases of the new local environment.

A rapid transport from the northern to the southern hemisphere produces a similar phase shift of the circannual clock with the photoperiod timer (**Fig. 21.7**). Again, resynchronisation may require several days to adapt to the new location.

MORE DETAILS Decoupling and the associated internal desynchronisation can be both the cause and the consequence of illnesses (**chronopathology**). Thus, the problems arising from alternating shift work are not only because the work has to be done partly at "biologically unfavourable" times (night and early morning hours), but also because of the lack of synchronicity with the social timers of the personal environment.

The great importance of light in controlling endogenous rhythms has also been used in animal husbandry (**light regime**). When **cattle** and **horses housed in stalls, were exposed to** lighting of 100–140 lux for 14 hours each day in the winter months, their reproductive performance improved. When **sows were housed in** this lighting regime, there was an increase in the number of piglets they produced. However, an exclusively artificial light regime is no longer permissible in farm animal husbandry in Germany. The Ordinance on Animal Welfare and Farm Animal Husbandry of October 2001 requires adaptation to a natural daily pattern of lighting according to season.

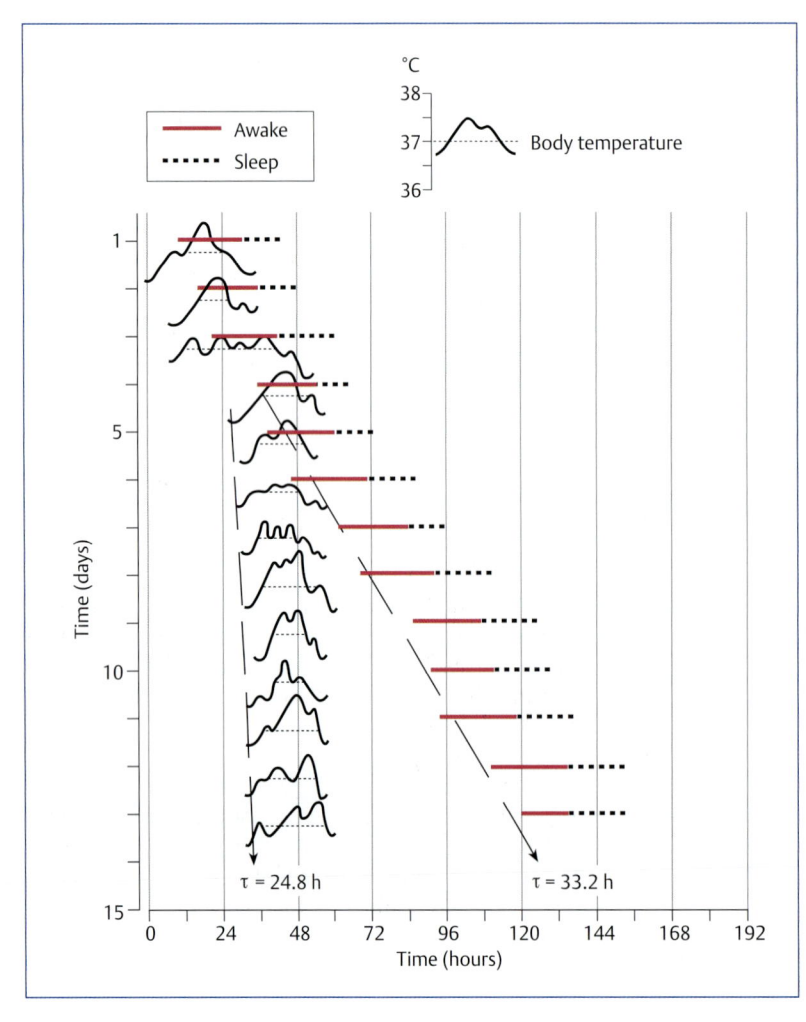

Fig. 21.6 Internal desynchronisation using the example of the diurnal rhythms of body temperature and the sleep-wake cycle of an experimental subject, in which both rhythms ran independently due to the withdrawal of external time information. Since τ was > 24 hours for both rhythms, the start of the period from the beginning of the experiment (day 1, y-axis) drifted further and further apart with each day to a later time than on the previous day, since the sleep-wake rhythm in this subject had a significantly longer τ than the daily rhythm of body temperature; based on data from Aschoff J, Gerecke U, Wever R. Desynchronization of human circadian rhythms. Japanese J Physiol 1967; 17: 450–457

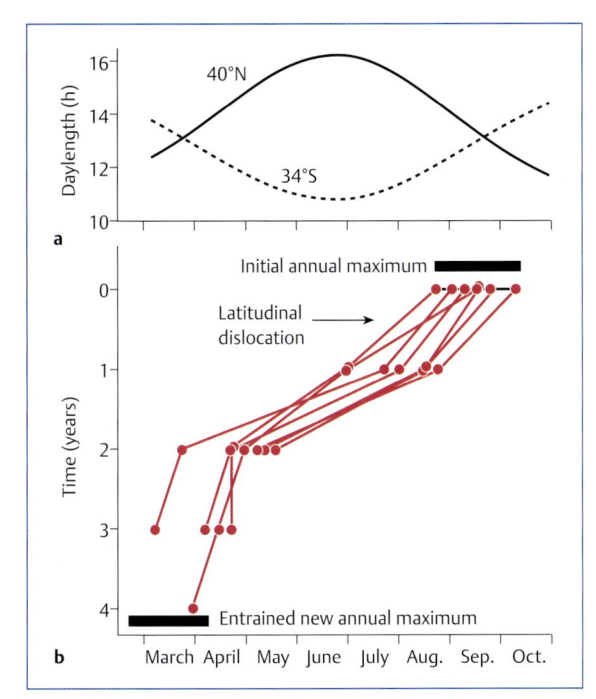

Fig. 21.7 Experimentally generated "jet lag" of the annual clock of American woodchucks shipped by plane from the northern to the southern hemisphere.
a Day length in the course of a year at the place of origin (40° N) and at the destination (34° S).
b The black bar at the top indicates the period during which the animals had maximum fat reserves at the place of origin in preparation for hibernation. The red dots (connected with red lines) indicate the individual maximum body weights of the original seven animals during the course of the experiment. The animals needed several years of resynchronisation until they were at maximum body fatness again at the appropriate time of the year in the southern hemisphere, namely in the autumn month of March (black bar below). [Source: Gwinner E. Circannual Rhythms. In: Aschoff J (ed.). Biological Rhythms. Handbook of Behavioural Neurobiology. New York: Plenum Press; 1981]

The influence of light regulation has been used particularly for intensive **poultry production**. Periods of light for one hour followed by periods of darkness (less movement = better fattening performance) are sufficient to control the circadian rhythm in growing birds. A different lighting regime has been applied to laying hens. Since they only lay eggs during a period of exposure to light, an artificial light/dark alternation, with 16–18 hours of light, creates a long "day phase".

The influence of an external timer on the internal clock can be used to alter patterns of behaviour. If, for example, nocturnal animals such as laboratory rats need to be observed during their activity phase, this would result in unfavourable working times for the observer. The solution to this problem is to swap the light-dark phases with the actual day-night rhythm. After resynchronisation, the animals continue to be active in the dark but during the hours of daylight for the observer. The same manipulation is used in the so-called night animal houses of zoological gardens to be able to present the animals to the public during their activity phase.

IN A NUTSHELL   !

Biological rhythms are adapted (synchronised) to environmental conditions by external timers. Light plays the most important role in this.

21.6 Central and peripheral clocks, transduction of the light signal

In mammals, the coordination of the temporal patterns of physiological processes is under the control of a paired nucleus of the ventral hypothalamus, above the junction of the optic nerves (nucleus suprachiasmaticus, **SCN**). The SCN is part of the so-called "**photoneuroendocrine system**". The pattern of light as an external timer of circadian rhythms is detected, by the visual pigment **melanopsin**, in special light-sensitive ganglion cells in the retina. The neural signal is transmitted via the retinohypothalamic tract to the SCN. From there, polysynaptic efferents lead via pre- and postganglionic sympathetic fibres to the **pineal gland**, where melatonin is produced, but only during the night (**Fig. 21.8**). In reptiles and birds, the pineal gland itself is directly sensitive to light and thus also assumes the function of an internal central clock.

Mammals perceive the photoperiod exclusively from the duration of melatonin secretion. For the annual clock of birds, however, melatonin plays a subordinate role. They perceive the length of day directly with light-sensitive photoreceptors located deep in the brain. However, the subsequent conversion of the photoperiodic signal is the same in both, birds and mammals. A change in day length causes a reciprocal change of either activation or inhibition of the enzymes that convert thyroxine into the bioactive form triiodothyronine. This fine-tuning of the concentration of thyroid hormones in the mediobasal hypothalamus triggers the further cascade of short-day and long-day reactions (**Fig. 21.9**). Whether this triggers activation or deactivation, of reproduction or moulting, depends on the species of animal. In sheep, for example, a sequence of short days stimulates gonadal activity (p. 542) and mating then occurs around the winter solstice, whereas in small mammals the exact opposite happens. They are only reproductively active under long-day conditions.

As well as the central pacemakers – SCN in mammals and pineal organ in birds – other clocks have now been detected in practically all organs of the body. These peripheral "slave clocks" can generate their own rhythm. Rhythmic expression of genes in the liver particularly affects key enzymes of energy metabolism, the redox status of cells, and digestive and detoxification reactions of xenobiotics. Therefore, it is now assumed that peripheral clocks fulfil three essential tasks: 1. anticipatory activation of metabolic pathways to optimise food utilisation; 2. temporal limitation of metabolic processes with harmful side effects (e.g. formation of reactive radicals); and 3. separation of chemically incompatible reactions into different time windows.

Nutrition, energy

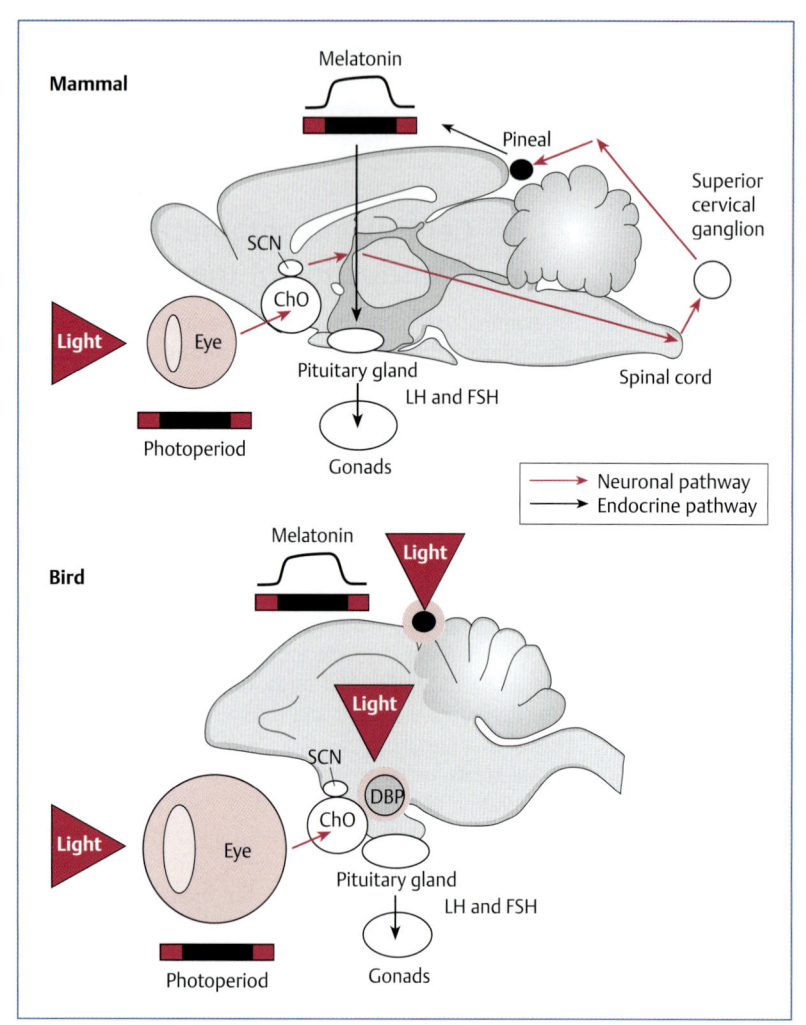

Fig. 21.8 Physiological measurement of day length in the photoneuroendocrine system: mammals perceive the length of the night exclusively via the duration of melatonin secretion; birds, on the other hand, additionally measure day length with light-sensitive regions in the brain. DBP = deep brain photoreceptors; ChO = Chiasma opticum; SCN = paired suprachiasmatic nucleus; LH = luteinising hormone; FSH = follicle-stimulating hormone.

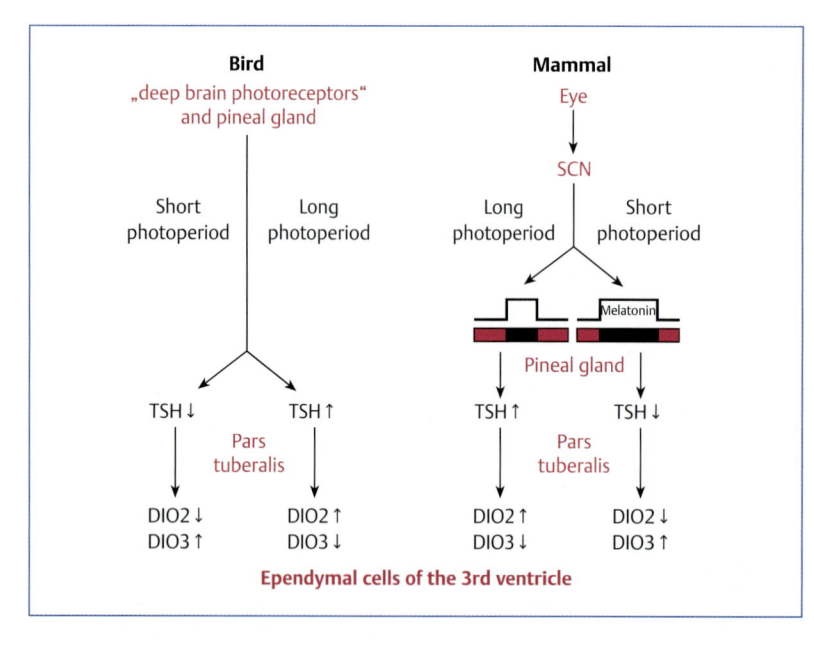

Fig. 21.9 Physiological conversion of day-length information in the brain of birds and mammals. Long photoperiod leads to increased expression of TSH, the thyroid-stimulating hormone in the pars tuberalis. This causes a local increase in the expression of type 2 iodothyronine deiodinase (DIO2), in the ependymal cells along the ventrolateral wall of the 3rd ventricle in the mediobasal hypothalamus. DIO2 is the enzyme that converts the prohormone thyroxine (T4) into the bioactive form triiodothyronine (T3) (see ch. Endocrinology (p.531). At the same time, under these long-day conditions, the thyroid hormone-deactivating enzyme type 3 deodinase (DIO3) is suppressed. Short photoperiods have the opposite effect.

Suggested reading

Arnold W. Review: Seasonal differences in the physiology of wild northern ruminants. Animal 2020; 14 (S1): s124-s132

Arnold W, Ruf T, Loe LE et al. Circadian rhythmicity persists through the polar night and midnight sun in Svalbard reindeer. Sci Rep 2018; 8: 14466

Aschoff J. Free running and entrained circadian rhythms. In: Aschoff J, ed. Biological rhythms. Handbook of Behavioral Neurobiology. New York: Plenum Press; 1981

Barnard Alun R, Nolan PM. When Clocks Go Bad: Neuro-behavioural Consequences of Disrupted Circadian Timing. PLoS
Genet 2008; 4:e1000040

Davis DE, Finnie EP. Entrainment of circannual rhythm in weight of woodchucks. Journal of Mammalogy 1975; 56: 199–203

Goldbeter A. Biological rhythms: clocks for all times. Curr Biol 2008; 18: 751–753

Gwinner E. Circannual Rhythms. Endogenous Annual Clocks in the Organization of Seasonal Processes. Berlin, Heidelberg, New York, London, Paris, Tokyo: Springer; 1986

Lemmer B. Chronopharmacology: cellular and biochemical interactions. New York: Dekker; 1989

Lincoln, G. A brief history of circannual time. J Neuroendocrinol 2019; 31

Pengelley ET, Asmundson SJ. Circannual clocks. New York: Academic Press; 1974

Steinlechner S. Biological rhythms of the mouse. In: Hedrich HJ, ed. The Laboratory Mouse. Oxford: Elsevier; 2012

Stevenson TJ, Visser ME, Arnold W et al. Disrupted seasonal biology impacts health, food security and ecosystems. Proc R Soc B 2015; 282: 20151453

22   Control of food intake

Wolfgang Langhans, Thomas A. Lutz

22.1   Food intake and homeostasis

> **ESSENTIALS**   ✘
>
> The control of food intake is integrated with other vital homeostatic control circuits (energy stores, metabolites and essential nutrients). Feedback signals from the digestive tract and general metabolism determine the start and end of individual meals. Endocrine adiposity signals from adipose tissue modulate meal-related signals. Control of choice is from learned preferences and aversion to some taste stimuli. A complex neural network with centres in the caudal brainstem, diencephalon and telencephalon, processes the peripheral signals and adapts to different physiological states and environmental conditions.

The intake of food provides energy-supplying substrates and essential nutrients for general metabolism and is thus part of the vital **homeostatic control circuits** of **an animal**, that maintain a constant internal milieu.

Complex central nervous networks control how much and what food is consumed. **Fig. 22.1** shows this control as part of the regulation of **energy homeostasis**. Its most reliable long-term indicator is body mass (fat mass and fat-free mass), which, over the long term, remains remarkably constant in healthy adult individuals, despite sometimes considerable fluctuations in food intake and energy expenditure. Energy homeostasis (E stored = E absorbed – E released) is thus relatively well regulated. The brain integrates (Σ) **peripheral feedback signals** (1) and controls **consumption and metabolism** (2) in such a way that the

body mass remains within a **certain range** (3). Food intake and energy expenditure are the controlled variables. The brain also processes feedback from the amount and composition of food consumed (4) as well as a variety of other external and internal factors that are independent of **body mass** or the **controlled variables** (5).

> **IN A NUTSHELL**   !
>
> The control of food intake is part of the regulation of various systems (energy homeostasis, nutrient homeostasis, etc.).

22.2   Control of frequency and size of meals

22.2.1   General

The frequency and circadian distribution of meals (= **meal patterns**) are species-specific. With free access to food, humans and pigs consume about 3–5 meals per 24 hours, while most other domestic animals and rats consume 6–12 meals over that time. Meal frequency is significantly higher (about 30 meals per 24 hours) in mice, rabbits, guinea pigs and chickens. In growing animals, the meal frequency is higher than in adults.

Feedback signals from the digestive tract and general metabolism control the beginning and end of each meal (**Fig. 22.2**). These include orosensory and pre-absorptive gastrointestinal signals, directly related to food intake, and also postabsorptive signals from metabolism of the absorbed nutrients.

Nutrition, energy

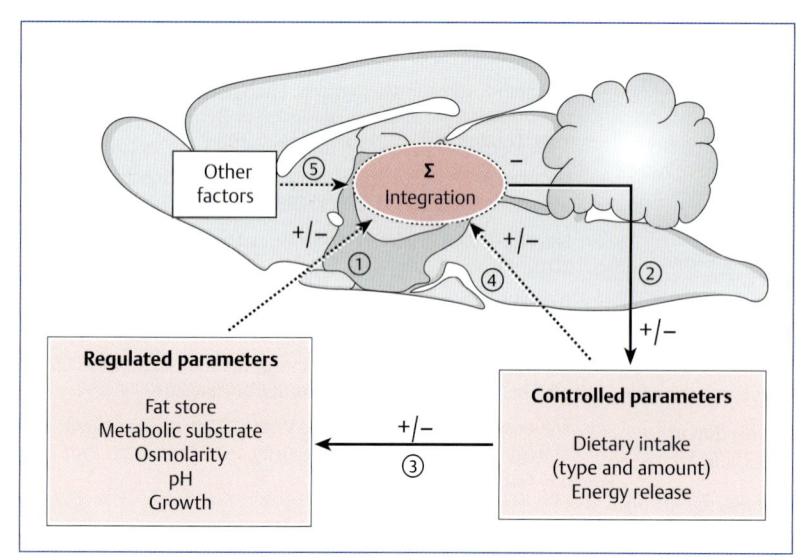

Fig. 22.1 The control of food intake as an essential part of the regulation of energy homeostasis. Peripheral feedback signals are registered in the brain (1) and cause (2) compensatory changes in food intake and energy output. (3). The intake of food itself also generates **feedback signals** (4), which control the beginning and end of meals. Other endogenous and exogenous factors can influence this control system (5). The drawing shows the sagittal section through a rat brain.

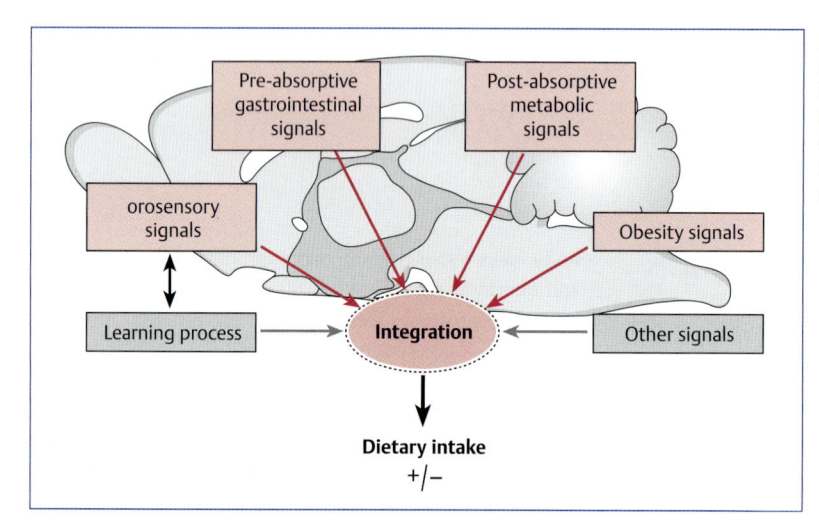

Fig. 22.2 Signals in the control of the start and end of individual meals. The arrow between orosensory signals and learning processes indicates that the orosensory signals described are the most important stimuli for the learning processes in food selection and acceptance.

> **IN A NUTSHELL**   !
>
> The interaction of these signals generates the meal pattern characteristic of each species.

22.2.2 Chemosensory signals

The combination of gustatory, olfactory, tactile and thermal stimuli in the mouth and nasal cavity results in the **taste** of the food. Taste and smell are important for locating and recognising food, for food selection (p. 526) and for the **hedonic response** to the food (**palatability, reward effects**), which can lead to increased or decreased consumption. In the longer term, the availability of preferred food may also result in an increase in body mass. The direct effect of palatability on food intake is shown in the so-called "sham feeding preparation" in rats. An artificial gastric fistula drains the ingested food directly to the outside and prevents food from accumulating in the stomach or entering the small intestine. Rats prepared in this way consume food for several hours without significant interruption,

with the increase in consumption being directly proportional to the intensity of taste (e.g. sugar concentration).

Taste receptors (e.g. sweet receptors) have also been found on enteroendocrine cells in the mucosa of the small intestine, where their activation contributes to the control of the secretion of gastrointestinal hormones such as glucagon-like peptide-1 (GLP-1) (p. 522).

> **IN A NUTSHELL**   !
>
> Orosensory signals can influence consumption positively or negatively in the short term (meal size) and longer term (amount of food).

22.2.3 Gastrointestinal signals

The presence of food in the digestive tract as well as its digestion and the absorption of nutrients trigger signals that are transmitted to the brain via vagal and spinal visceral afferents and also via circulating blood. Gastrointestinal peptides have a paracrine effect on afferent nerves or an endocrine effect via the blood.

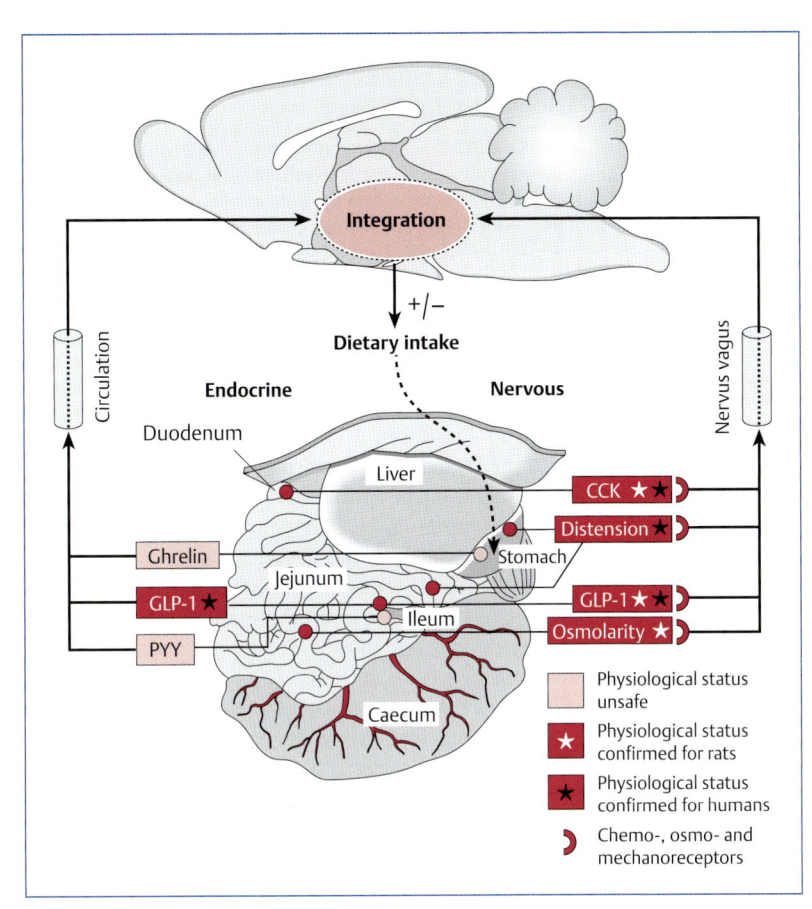

Fig. 22.3 Gastrointestinal signals in the control of food intake. The origin and nature of the signals, the mode of transmission to the brain (nervous or endocrine) and the physiological status based on current research are shown. The drawing below shows the ventral view of the digestive tract of a rat.
CCK = cholecystokinin; GLP-1 = glucagon-like peptide-1; PYY = peptide YY.

■ Stomach distension

The increase in volume of the stomach during food intake stimulates an **inhibitory signal** via **gastral stretch sensors**, which is transmitted via afferent **vagus fibres** to the **nucleus tractus solitarii (NTS)** in the caudal brainstem (**Fig. 22.3**). These same fibres also have receptors for cholecystokinin (CCK) (p.522) and GLP-1. At usual meal sizes, interaction with these hormonal signals from the small intestine causes satiety. The purely mechanical satiety effect of gastric distension is only significant when oversized meals are consumed, such as when eating bulky foods with low energy density. This also applies to satiety during milk intake in newborns, when other signals that would indicate the composition or energy density of food are not yet effective. The rapid emptying of energy-rich food of low viscosity can weaken the satiety signal from the stomach and can thus lead to an increase in food intake.

■ Ghrelin

Endocrine cells of the fundus glands synthesise the hormone **ghrelin**, which is often mistakenly called the "hunger hormone". In fact, in the rat, ghrelin increases food intake after peripheral injection. When it is neutralised by ghrelin antibodies, consumption is decreased. Therefore, it is not a hunger hormone. There is a conditioned increase in ghrelin secretion before meals. However, in food deprivation, there is an increased concentration in blood of an inactive, non-acylated form of ghrelin, rather than the ac-

tive, acylated form. The main action of ghrelin is directly on neurons in the hypothalamic nucleus arcuatus (p.528) (Arc). There it acts both, indirectly and directly on the reward system to make the available food more attractive. Ghrelin agonists are being tested for the treatment of tumour anorexia and cachexia. They are already in clinical use for the treatment of general anorexia in dogs.

> **IN A NUTSHELL** **!**
>
> The hormone ghrelin, which is secreted by the stomach, makes the available food attractive and thus stimulates food intake.

■ Intestinal chemo- and mechanosensitivity

Nutrients, osmotic and mechanical stimuli all trigger satiety signals in the small intestine. Intraduodenal nutrient infusions reduce food intake more than comparable intravenous infusions. An increase in osmolarity, as occurs in the course of a meal (approx. 700 mosmol·l^{-1}), also inhibits consumption. These signals reach the brain via vagal afferents. The reduction in food intake that occurs after intraduodenal lipid infusions disappears if pancreatic lipase is inhibited. Food intake suppression is therefore based (directly or indirectly) on the detection of fatty acids and monoacylglycerol from cleavage of triacylglycerol. Glucose, compared to other carbohydrates, has a particular intestinal effect that induces satiety. This is an effect that is independent of luminal glucose uptake into the enterocytes.

Various amino acids in the intestinal lumen also inhibit food consumption, partly via vagal afferents, but the underlying mechanisms are unknown.

The importance for satiety of mechanical stimuli in the small intestine has only become clear in recent years, especially through the molecular genetic characterisation of vagal afferents that transmit mechanical satiety signals to the brain. There are also receptors for gastrointestinal hormones on the mechanosensitive vagal afferents from the small intestine, thus providing the basis for these interactions.

■ Cholecystokinin (CCK)

CCK, which exists in several forms (e.g. CCK-8, CCK-33 and CCK-58), is secreted by I-cells in the proximal small intestine in response to intraluminal stimuli (primarily fatty acids and some amino acids). It activates vagal afferents in the intestinal wall even before it is absorbed into the intestinal capillaries (paracrine effect). In addition, CCK has an endocrine effect on vagal afferents in the portal vein at the entrance to the liver (**Fig. 22.3**) and also directly in the brain. CCK-58 is the most abundant form circulating in blood, and thus is responsible for the endocrine action of CCK. A specific effect of CCK, when parenterally administered, is to limit the amount of food being consumed. This effect is physiologically relevant because administration of CCK receptor antagonists leads to larger amounts of food being consumed, and blocking of the satiety response to intraduodenal fat infusions.

■ Glucagon-like peptide-1 (GLP-1)

GLP-1 is a product of the prepro-glucagon gene, which is expressed predominantly in L-cells in the small and large intestine and in a group of neurons in the NTS. Peripheral administration of GLP-1, and also when directly applied to the brain of laboratory animals, reduces the amount of food consumed. The main effect of GLP-1 in reducing meal size, is by a paracrine, vagally mediated action. Very high GLP-1 concentrations in blood (e.g. after bariatric surgery), are normally very unusual because it is rapidly broken down in the circulation. Its concentration can also be reduced by a direct endocrine effect on the area postrema (AP) (**Fig. 22.3**) to induce satiety. The primary action, with regard to food intake, of GLP-1 receptor agonists, used in the therapy of type 2 diabetes and obesity, is on more rostral brain regions, and they thus tend to copy the effect of the central GLP-1 system. The GLP-1-expressing neurons of this central GLP-1 system are located in the NTS and send axons to the hypothalamus and regions of the telencephalon. These GLP-1 expressing neurons may contribute to the inhibition of feed intake when there is taste aversion or disease, see ch. 22.5 (p.526) and ch. 22.7.

■ Peptide YY (PYY)

PYY is also secreted by intestinal L-cells. Two forms of PYY circulate in the blood, the full-length peptide (PYY1–36) and its biologically more active cleavage product PYY3–36. Peripheral administration of PYY3–36 reduces food intake, apparently by activating Y2 receptors. The exact site of action and the physiological relevance of the PYY effect are still not clear (**Fig. 22.3**).

MORE DETAILS Other gastrointestinal hormones and endogenous substances are also involved in the regulation of food intake (**Fig. 22.3**). These include the enterostatin pentapeptide cleaved from pancreatic pro-co-lipase, apolipoprotein-AIV (APO-A IV) and ethanolamides of fatty acids formed in the intestine from dietary fats. All these substances are thought to have a satiety effect, but their physiological relevance is still largely uncertain.

■ Special features of ruminants

Analogous to the gastric satiety signals in monogastric animals, the stimulation of reticuloruminal mechanosensors inhibits food intake in ruminants, especially in feeds rich in crude fibre (= low energy density). Of the short-chain fatty acids produced during rumen fermentation, acetic acid in particular reduces food intake when infused into the rumen. In contrast, infusing acetic acid into the abomasum, or directly into blood, has little influence on food intake. This suggests that chemosensors in the rumen, are directly involved in the control of food intake. However, the feedback signal is probably also based on activation of ruminal osmosensors, because an increase in the osmolarity of the rumen contents also promotes satiety. Under physiological conditions the pH sensors in the forestomach wall are probably insignificant in the control of food intake. However, in rumen acidosis, they could contribute to the suppression of food intake, because when the pH value in the rumen drops sharply, the rumen motor system is inhibited by activation of the pH sensors.

> **IN A NUTSHELL** !
>
> Different nutrient-dependent and nutrient-independent stimuli generate neural signals, especially transmitted via the vagus nerve, and also endocrine negative feedback signals that inhibit feed intake.

22.2.4 Pancreatic hormones

■ Glucagon

Glucagon is secreted by the α-cells of the endocrine pancreas, and stimulates hepatic glucose production when blood glucose concentration falls (see ch. growth (p.544)). However, it is also released during food intake, especially in response to protein intake. This seems to be particularly important in obligate carnivores (e.g. cats), as their physiological diet contains very few carbohydrates and the ingested amino acids are also used for gluconeogenesis. Glucagon also specifically reduces meal size after it is administered parenterally, whereas blocking the effect of endogenous glucagon by specific glucagon antibodies has the opposite effect. This indicates that the glucagon effect on limiting feed intake is of physiological significance. The satiety signal is transmitted to the brain via vagal afferents.

■ Insulin

Insulin is released from the β-cells of the endocrine pancreas in response to cephalic and intestinal signals during the course of a meal. Insulin also causes a reduction in meal size when it is administered parenterally, but only in non-hypoglycaemic doses, as hypoglycaemia itself induces hunger. The increase in meal size after infusion of specific insulin antibodies into the portal vein of rats indicates the physiological significance of the satiety effect of insulin. Furthermore, insulin is considered an endocrine signal that could contribute to the development of obesity (p. 524).

■ Amylin

Amylin is secreted together with insulin by the β-cells. Amylin and amylin agonists reduce meal size and meal frequency when given parenterally. Antagonising the action of endogenous amylin has the opposite effects in the rat. Amylin inhibits consumption via a direct effect on neurons of the AP in the medulla oblongata and possibly other brain regions (p. 527).

> **IN A NUTSHELL** !
>
> The pancreatic hormones glucagon, insulin and amylin reduce food intake mainly by reducing meal size. The glucagon effect is vagally mediated, while amylin and probably also insulin, act directly on the brain.

22.3 Metabolic signals

Food intake is also controlled by metabolic feedback signals (**Fig. 22.4**). Parenteral administration of various energy-providing substrates, and long-term parenteral nutrition both inhibit food intake whereas antimetabolites of glucose and fat metabolism stimulate it. Amino acids derived from the digestion of food protein are metabolised rapidly. However, the rapid pronounced satiety effect associated with the influx of amino acids, seems to be mediated by gastrointestinal hormones (p. 520) rather than directly by the metabolism of the absorbed amino acids. Carbohydrates and fats are more important as energy carriers in most species, with glucose in particular being the most important energy-providing substrate for the brain and other organs.

22.3.1 Glucose

The increase in food consumption that occurs after parenteral administration of **glucose antimetabolites** is likely to be a pharmacological effect. However, since in rats and humans the blood glucose level drops transiently, immediately before spontaneous meals, and the onset of meals is delayed if the drop in blood glucose is prevented by a glucose infusion, then blood glucose concentration sensors may be involved in initiating spontaneous meals. Importantly, this is an anticipatory signal that occurs long before hypoglycaemia develops and can also be a learned response.

Nutrition, energy

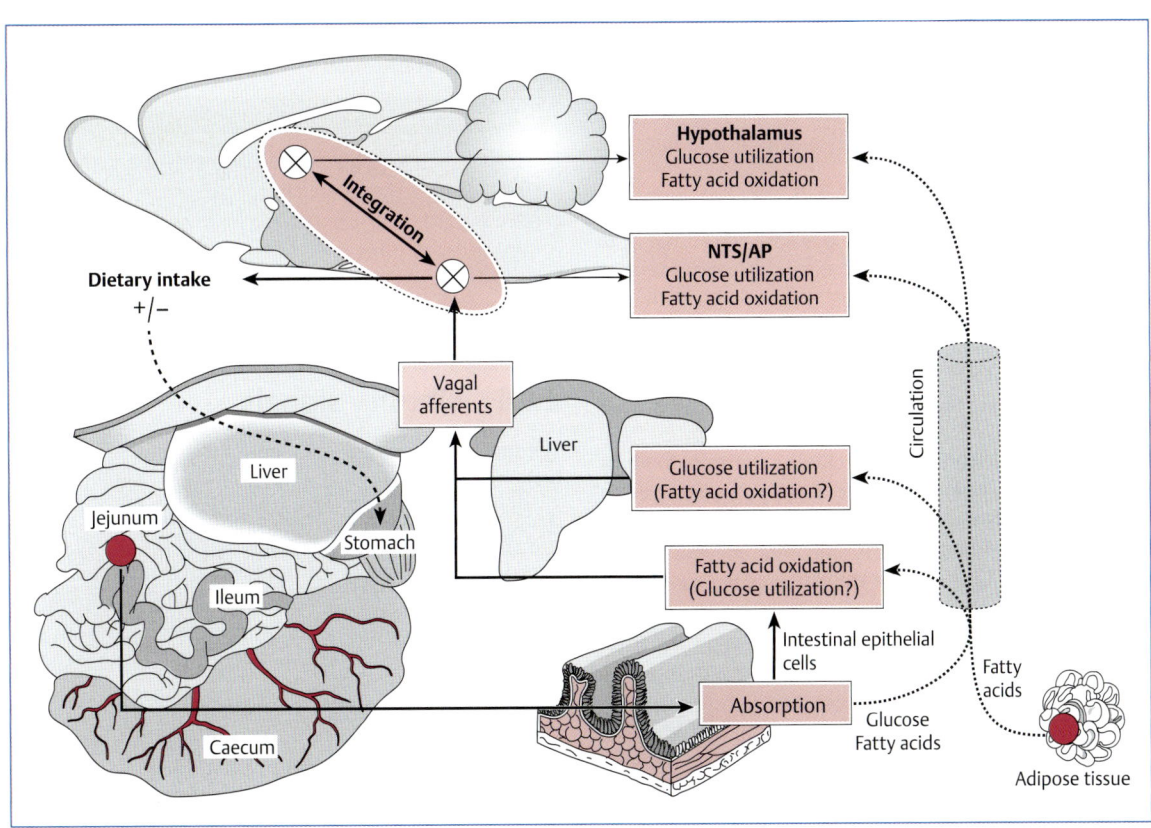

Fig. 22.4 Metabolic signals in the control of food intake. The metabolism of glucose and fatty acids is detected at different levels in the periphery and in the brain and can thus influence food intake. Detection in the periphery of glucose and fatty acids derived from food, modulates action potential frequency in afferent fibres of the vagus nerve.
(?) = not definitely proven assumption.

The storage capacity of an animal for carbohydrates is limited, because only the liver and muscle store glycogen to any significant extent. The conversion of carbohydrates into fat is energetically costly. Under normal nutritional conditions, ingested carbohydrates are therefore mostly rapidly catabolised. Accordingly, glucose catabolism increases during a meal. Parenteral administration of glucose antimetabolites (e.g. 2-deoxy-D-glucose) leads to an increase in food consumption in monogastric animals, whereas parenteral administration of glucose often leads to a reduction in consumption. Neurons in the medulla oblongata and vagal afferents in the wall of the portal vein function as glucose sensors and contribute to the control of food intake. Thus, infusions of glucose solution into the portal vein reduce consumption more than corresponding infusions into the jugular vein. This is important because the portal blood glucose concentration rises more rapidly during a meal and remains higher than in other blood vessels during the time glucose is being absorbed.

22.3.2   Fatty acids

As carbohydrate oxidation increases during and immediately after a meal, less of the fat ingested at the same time is oxidised and more is stored. This is thought to be partly responsible for the so-called obesogenic effect of high-fat overeating in humans. Nevertheless, the oxidation of fatty acids influences food intake. Thus, inhibitors of mitochondrial fatty acid oxidation stimulate food consumption, except in low-fat diets. Conversely, stimulation of fatty acid oxidation is accompanied by a limitation in food consumption. The sensors involved are partly located directly in the brain (**Fig. 22.4**), probably in glial cells, which in turn transmit the signal to neurons. Peripheral sensors for fatty acid oxidation could be localised mainly in the intestine (enterocytes) (**Fig. 22.4**).

> **MORE DETAILS**   The increased mobilisation of fat, and increased fatty acid oxidation, in a state of hunger is an attempt to compensate for a deficiency of food energy, by mobilising energy reserves. In fact, inhibition of fat mobilisation during food deprivation leads to increased hunger.

22.3.3   Energy flow

The ultimate mechanism for metabolic control of food intake is likely to be some indicator of energy turnover, common to all substrates. This could be the intracellular ATP concentration or the ATP/ADP ratio. The enzyme adenosine monophosphate kinase (AMPK), probably has an important role, as it is an ubiquitous sensor of cellular energy flow. In particular, changes in AMPK activity in hypothalamic neurons, affect food consumption. AMPK interacts with another kinase, the mammalian target of rapamycin (mTOR). The level of activity of AMPK and of mTOR are inversely proportional, and have opposite effects on food consumption. AMPK and mTOR also partially mediate the effect of hormones such as leptin and ghrelin on consumption. Thus, they integrate information about the cellular availability of energy and relevant endocrine status, con-

trolling the activity of the hypothalamic neurons involved in regulating food consumption (p. 528).

22.3.4   Special features of ruminants

Despite their central role in ruminant energy metabolism, the short-chain fatty acids absorbed from the rumen, do not have a significant effect on determining satiety. In ad libitum feeding, there is no significant meal-induced increase in the concentration of short-chain fatty acids in plasma, and their intravenous infusion does not generally inhibit food intake. Only the infusion of propionate into the portal vein reduces consumption. This effect does not occur after denervation of the liver and is therefore likely to be mediated by hepatic sensors. This is compatible with the fact that propionate, as an important gluconeogenic substrate in ruminants, is predominantly metabolised in the liver.

Because ruminant food has a low fat content, the physiological importance of long-chain fatty acids as a metabolic signal in ruminants is low. However, in dairy cows in the first third of lactation, any effect of fatty acid oxidation on restricting food consumption, could limit the increase in supply of energy from food, that is needed to compensate for the greatly increased energy requirement at that stage of lactation. Ultimately this would lead to a negative energy balance. The greatly increased mobilisation of body fat often leads to clinically manifest ketosis, in which food intake is reduced. Ketone bodies also seem to inhibit food consumption in ruminants. In contrast, even unphysiologically high or low blood glucose levels do not have any effect on food intake in ruminants.

> **IN A NUTSHELL** !
>
> Metabolic signals are generated by energy-providing substrates. They are registered by special sensors in the brain (glucose, fatty acids), portal vein (glucose, perhaps also fatty acids and other metabolites) and perhaps also in the small intestine. In hypothalamic neurons, AMPK and mTOR function as intracellular sensors of energy flow.

22.4   Obesity signals

The most reliable long-term indicator of energy balance is body mass. Changes in adult body weight are mainly based on changes in the size of fat depots. Energy homeostasis is also regulated by food intake, and indeed the size of fat depots directly influences consumption. In experimental animals, where the size of fat depots has been altered by some treatment, the amount of food consumed is also altered. The **adiposity signals** underlying this effect could also contribute to the negative energy balance occurring in the first third of lactation in high-yielding dairy cows, as more fat is stored towards the end of gestation.

IN A NUTSHELL !

Food intake and energy expenditure are also modulated by endocrine adiposity signals that reflect the size of fat depots.

Three hormones in particular are considered as obesity signals. These are **leptin**, the only one of the three that is synthesised in the adipose tissue itself, and the pancreatic hormones **insulin** and **amylin** (Fig. 22.5). The basal plasma levels of all three hormones are correlated with the size of the fat depots, at least under static equilibrium conditions. Injection of any of these into the brain ventricles, reduces food consumption in doses that if injected peripherally would have no effect on food consumption.

MORE DETAILS The absence of leptin or the leptin receptor (LRb) as a result of monogenetic mutations was identified in 1993–1994 as the cause of obesity and diabetes in the so-called ob/ob and db/db mice. Leptin is rapidly transported across the blood-brain barrier and binds to the LRb in the hypothalamic arc, to other hypothalamic nuclei and to the NTS of the medulla oblongata.

Leptin reduces meal size by enhancing the satiety effect of intestinal peptides such as CCK, GLP-1 and also amylin. Antagonising the action of leptin with an LRb blocker increases feed intake, suggesting a physiological role for the hormone. More important than this permissive consump-

tion-inhibiting effect of leptin, however, is that the decrease in leptin blood concentration that occurs during prolonged abstinence of food intake, acts as a strong hunger signal. In addition, other energy-consuming processes (metabolism, reproduction, etc.) are shut down as a result of lower blood concentrations of leptin.

With the exception of the very few people with a defect in the leptin gene, overweight people do not have reduced leptin production, but usually have elevated levels of leptin in their blood. The same is true for most domestic animal species. Obesity thus leads to a pronounced leptin resistance, i.e. leptin no longer reduces food consumption. Put simply, (low) leptin protects against starvation, but (high leptin) does not protect against getting fat. The leptin system thus works asymmetrically, probably because a protective mechanism against too high food intake is not relevant in animals in the wild and therefore has not been an evolutionary development.

MORE DETAILS The brain's information about the size of available body fat reserves is important for the overriding influence of numerous bodily functions. It is worth noting that reproduction is affected by both, leptin and insulin. If energy reserves are too low, i.e. low basal leptin and insulin levels in very lean animals (or in the pathological state of anorexia nervosa in humans) hormonal control of reproduction in the hypothalamus and anterior pituitary (GnRH or LH and FSH secretion) is suppressed. Puberty may also be delayed, and in adults, the sexual cycle may cease.

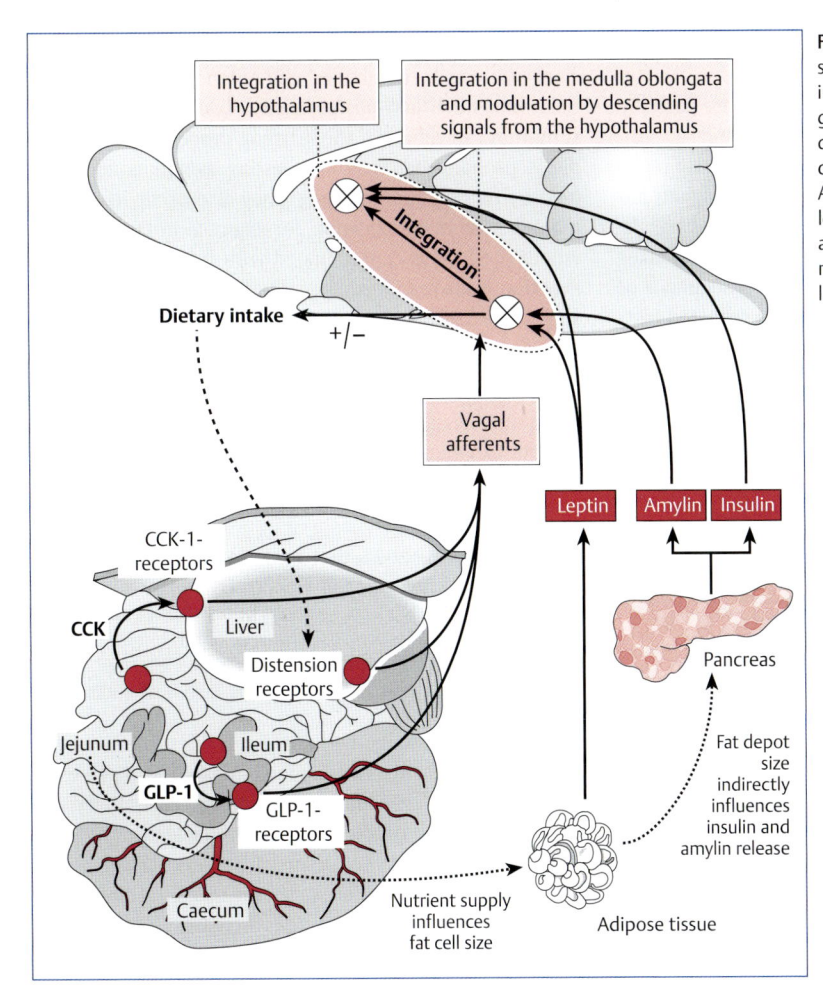

Fig. 22.5 Mode of action of the obesity signals leptin, insulin and amylin. They inhibit food intake primarily by enhancing gastrointestinal signals such as gastric distension, cholecystokinin (CCK) and glucagon-like peptide-1 (GLP-1) in the brain. At least for leptin, a decrease in blood leptin levels during food abstinence is an alarm signal for the brain and thus much more important than an increase in leptin levels.

Figure labels: Integration in the hypothalamus; Integration in the medulla oblongata and modulation by descending signals from the hypothalamus; Integration; Dietary intake; +/−; Vagal afferents; Leptin; Amylin; Insulin; CCK-1-receptors; CCK; Liver; Distension receptors; Pancreas; Jejunum; Ileum; GLP-1; GLP-1-receptors; Caecum; Nutrient supply influences fat cell size; Adipose tissue; Fat depot size indirectly influences insulin and amylin release

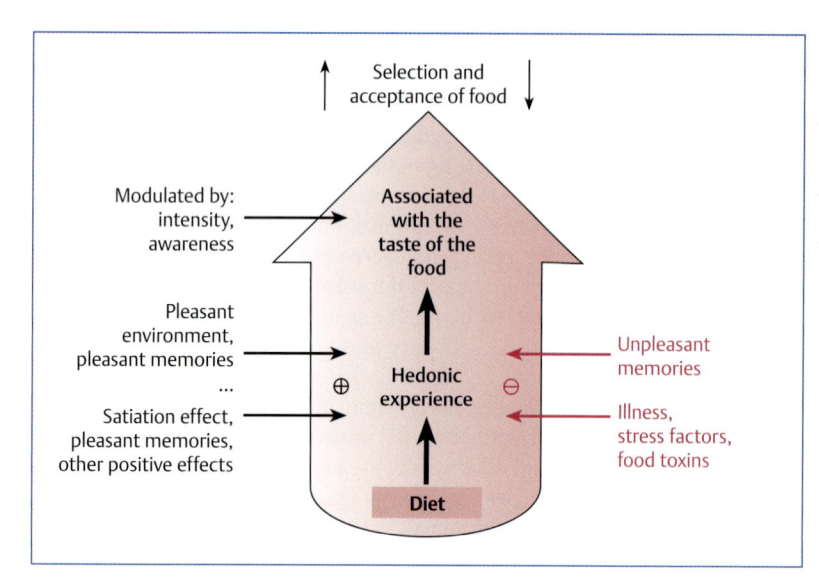

Fig. 22.6 Schematic of the learning processes that control the selection and acceptance of food. Positive and negative experiences with a particular food are associated with the taste and subsequently lead to preference or aversion to food with that taste. The learning processes are particularly efficient when the taste is intense and previously unknown.

Similar experimental findings to those for leptin, suggest that insulin and amylin also function as adiposity signals in the control of food intake. In principle, however, the function of adiposity signals in the regulation of energy homeostasis seems to be more dynamic than generally assumed. For example, the release of leptin from adipose tissue, not only varies with the size of fat cells, but also reflects changes in the cellular uptake or release of energy-providing substrates.

An interesting therapy option for the treatment of obesity could be the combination of amylin and leptin. Amylin in fact enhances the effect of leptin by at least partially overcoming leptin resistance in overweight people.

Several findings show that lean body mass is also regulated independently of body fat. The underlying signals are largely unknown. However, it is clear that the establishment of lean body mass after body weight changes, takes longer than the recovery of fat mass. One consequence of this is the relative increase in fat mass with repeated fasting cycles (yo-yo effect).

> **IN A NUTSHELL** !
>
> The blood concentration of adiposity signals reflects the size of the body fat depots. Leptin, insulin and amylin each function as signals for controlling food intake. Lean body mass is also regulated, but independent of the regulation of fat mass.

22.5 Food choice control

Mammals can feed on a diverse range of foods, according to their specific needs, i.e. they recognise and select food based on its sensory qualities. Taste (p. 520) and palatability are of particular importance. Some **preferences** (sweet, salty in the case of salt deficiency) and **aversions** (bitter, less pronounced also sour) for gustatory stimuli are **innate**. However, the cat, as a true carnivore, has no sweet receptors and accordingly shows no innate sweet preference.

In general, the acceptance of taste stimuli and thus the **choice of food** is primarily by **learned preferences** and **aversions**. In this process, positive or negative consequences of ingesting a food are associated with its sensory properties and henceforth lead to its preference or rejection (**Fig. 22.6**). Such associations take place each time food is consumed, i.e. the current sensory impression retrieves the stored information that decides on acceptance or rejection of the food; so that this information is continuously "updated". These learning processes are particularly efficient with new, unfamiliar and intensely tasting foods. Gastrointestinal and postabsorptive consequences of consumption can reinforce the learning processes. One example is pronounced, very long-lasting aversions accompanied by nausea and vomiting. They also occur in cases of malnutrition or intoxication, for example in farm animals where the food is contaminated with fungal toxins. **Taste aversion** leads to inappetence when no other food is available. Conversely, learned **taste preferences** can cause animals with nutrient deficiencies (e.g. also individual amino acids) to prefer a food that contains the nutrients in question.

MORE DETAILS Also food-independent disturbances of well-being can lead to taste aversion, for example through injection of toxins and through many other manipulations that cause discomfort. This is true even if the food is familiar and where positive experiences have previously been associated with the taste of that food. Therefore, learned taste aversions are also likely to contribute to decreased food consumption in some diseases. Furthermore, taste aversions are clinically important in tumour anorexia and in the inappetence that occurs as a side effect of various treatments (e.g. cytostatics, radiotherapy, high-dose antibiotics).

In addition to these learned processes, the subjective evaluation of taste changes during food intake. These processes are particularly relevant in omnivores. Palatability decreases during the course of a meal, which leads to the cessation of consumption of a particular food (**taste-specific satiety**). Food with a different taste is usually still willingly consumed. Therefore, meal size increases when several foods are offered in one meal. This effect is not limited to just one meal. Rats inevitably become fat if they are continuously offered a choice of different tasty foods (cafeteria diet). Similar factors could also be causal of obesity in both humans and their pets. From a teleological point of view, taste-specific satiety favours switching from one nutrient source to another and thus increases the likelihood of a balanced diet, especially in omnivores.

> **IN A NUTSHELL** !
>
> Food choice control is mainly based on learned preferences and aversions to taste stimuli. Greater food choice leads to increased food intake.

22.6 Brain areas involved

Food intake is controlled by a widely ramified neuronal network. Three important centres in this network are (1) **the caudal brainstem**, (2) a very closely linked group of **hypothalamic nuclei**, and (3) an equally closely linked regional group in the **telencephalon**.

> **IN A NUTSHELL** !
>
> Central nervous integration of peripheral satiety signals occurs via a complex network of neurons, with centres in the caudal brainstem, hypothalamus and telencephalon.

22.6.1 Caudal brainstem

Sensory, integrative and motor functions are located in the caudal brainstem and the medulla oblongata (mainly NTS and AP) and the parabrachial nucleus (PBN) (Fig. 22.7). These are all essential for the control of food intake. The information coming from the digestive tract about the size and nutritional composition of a meal is mainly via **vagal** and **spinal visceral afferents**, which are first switched in the **NTS**. Taste afferents are also switched in the NTS. Signalling molecules circulating in the blood, such as amylin and GLP-1, can be detected via the **AP**. The AP, located in the roof of the 4th cerebral ventricle, is in close contact with the NTS and as a **circumventricular organ** has a **permeable blood-brain barrier**. The convergence of gastrointestinal signals and taste information, and also of descend-

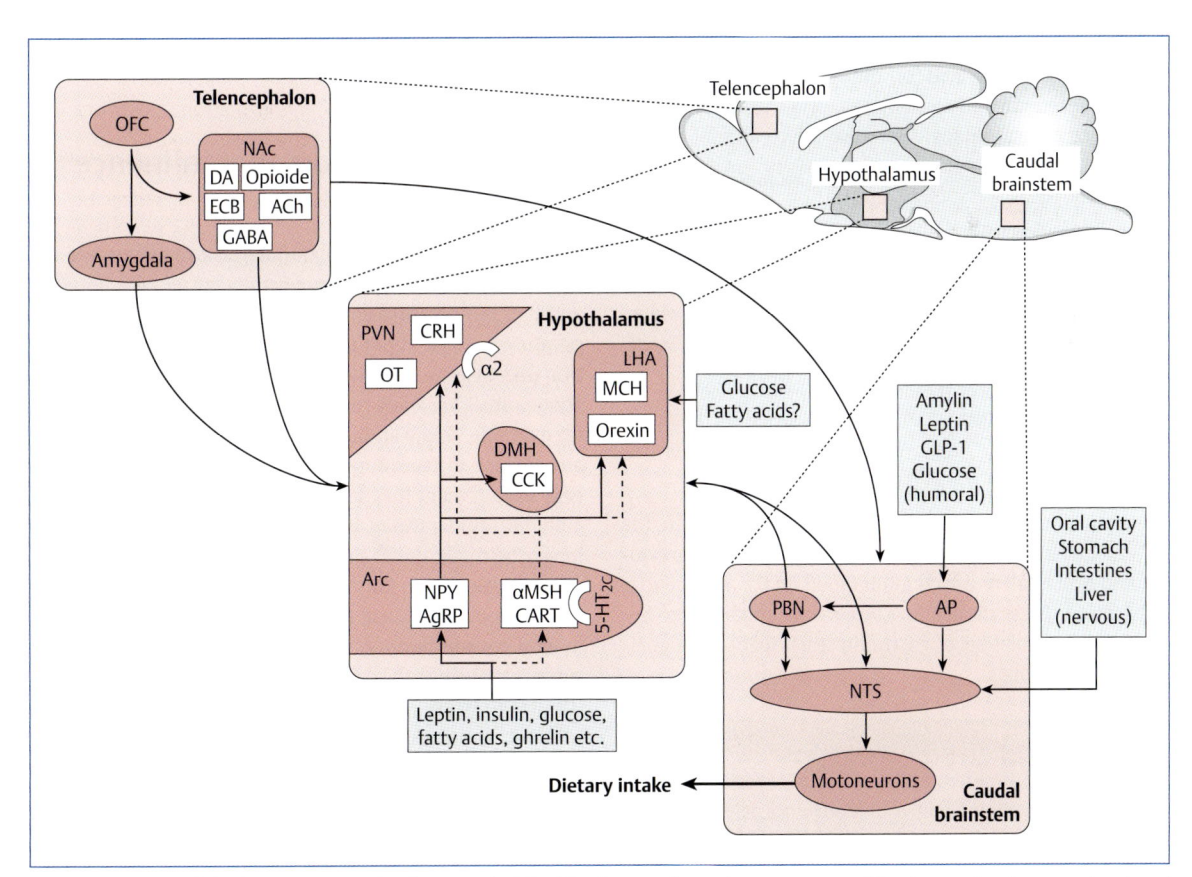

Fig. 22.7 Regions of the brain important for the control of food intake as well as relevant neuropeptides, humoral and nervous input and important ascending and descending connections.
ACh: acetylcholine; AgRP: Agouti-related peptide; αMSH: α-melanocyte-stimulating hormone; AP: area postrema; Arc: nucleus arcuatus.
CART: cocaine-/amphetamine-regulated transcript; CCK: cholecystokinin; CRH: corticotropin-releasing hormone; DA: dopamine;
DMH: dorsomedial hypothalamus; ECB: endocannabinoids; GABA: γ-aminobutyric acid; GLP-1: glucagon-like peptide-1; LHA: lateral hypothalamus; MCH: melanin-concentrating hormone; NAc: nucleus accumbens; NPY: neuropeptide Y; NTS: nucleus tractus solitarii; OFC: orbifrontal cortex; OT: oxytocin; PBN: nucleus parabrachialis; PVN: nucleus paraventricularis; PYY: peptide YY; α_2: α_2-noradrenergic receptors; 5HT$_{2C}$: serotonin-2c receptors.

ing projections from the hypothalamus in the NTS and PBN, are all important for the control of food intake. In addition, motoneurones of the medulla oblongata function as "**final common pathways**" for regulating **chewing** and **swallowing**. These common pathways require connections to rostral parts of the brain.

22.6.2 Hypothalamus

The hypothalamus processes adiposity signals, and also orosensory and gastrointestinal signals. The most important nuclei in this context are shown in **Fig. 22.7**. Receptors for leptin, insulin, amylin and ghrelin are mainly located in the Arc. Metabolic sensors are also present in other nuclei. Two groups of neurons are especially involved in regulating food intake. These are connected from the Arc to the nucleus paraventricularis (PVN) and to the lateral hypothalamus (LHA). One group expresses the consumption-enhancing neuropeptides neuropeptide **Y (NPY)** and **Agouti-related peptide (AgRP)**. The other group expresses the consumption-inhibiting neuropeptides α-melanocyte-stimulating hormone **(αMSH)** and **cocaine/amphetamine-regulated transcript (CART)**. The inhibition of consumption caused by αMSH is mediated by MC-4 receptors on target cells. Serotonin (5-hydroxytryptamine, 5-HT) inhibits consumption primarily by activation of the $5HT_{2C}$ receptors which are located, on the αMSH/CART neurons of the Arc. Serotonin and serotonergic drugs lead to a reduction in body mass when given repeatedly.

> **MORE DETAILS**   Downstream of these neurons, other neurotransmitters act, such as melanin-concentrating hormone (MCH, anabolic), endogenous opioids (essentially anabolic) or corticotropin-releasing hormone (CRH, catabolic). Furthermore, noradrenaline stimulates consumption via $α_2$ -adrenergic receptors in the PVN, an effect specific to carbohydrates when multiple nutrients are offered. This noradrenergic system is inhibited by high blood glucose levels and activated by low blood glucose levels. Glucocorticoids enhance the effect of noradrenaline, which, in addition to the reduction in CRH release triggered by glucocorticoids, could partly explain the often observed consumption-increasing effect of glucocorticoid treatments.

Descending connections from the hypothalamus to the NTS include, in particular, the neuropeptides CRH, oxytocin and αMSH, all of which inhibit food intake after central application. These descending projections mediate the homeostatic modulation of gastrointestinal feedback signals by adiposity signals.

> **IN A NUTSHELL**   !
>
> Many neurotransmitters and neuropeptides are involved in the central nervous control of food intake. NPY, AgRP, MCH, orexin and some endogenous opiates stimulate food intake; αMSH, CART, CRH, OT and 5-HT inhibit food intake.

22.6.3 Telencephalon

The regions of the telencephalon (e.g. nucleus accumbens, amygdala, orbitofrontal cortex) and the projections of dopaminergic, noradrenergic and serotonergic neurons from cell groups in the caudal brainstem and diencephalon leading to them, are all particularly important for various **hedonic aspects of** food intake (reward effect or aversion), and thus also for the influence of taste on the amount of food consumed.

Two other aspects are worth mentioning. (1) The circuits that mediate the reward effect of food and those mediating the reward effect of other natural (e.g. water for thirst, sex) or unnatural (e.g. drugs) stimuli are almost congruent and are also involved in the development of addiction. (2) With regard to the reward effect of food, a distinction is made between the impulse to eat food based on the affective evaluation of its taste (referred to in the literature as "liking") and the motivation to seek food (the desire or "wanting"). For both components, partially different neural substrates and neurochemical mediators can be identified.

> **MORE DETAILS**   Within the NAc, in particular dopamine (DA), opioids endocannabinoids (ECB), acetylcholine (ACh) and GABA, determine the reward effect of food. It is likely that the same mechanisms contribute to food preferences in other species, with the orbitofrontal cortex and parts of the insula in particular playing these roles.

22.7 Other factors that influence food intake

Food intake is modulated by numerous exogenous and endogenous factors. One example is the correlation between ambient temperature and food intake. If the ambient temperature rises far above the thermoneutral zone, consumption decreases, sometimes despite an increased basal metabolic rate. This leads to reduced milk yield in dairy cows, for example. A low ambient temperature probably leads to an increase in consumption because of the increased energy requirement for thermogenesis. However, at very low ambient temperatures, when the core temperature can no longer be maintained, animals often stop eating, with negative consequences for their energy balance.

Stressors can cause both, an increase and a reduction in food consumption. Activation of the endogenous opiate system as well as the dopaminergic system, probably contributes to stress-induced increase in food consumption. In contrast, the stress-induced suppression of food intake, is probably mainly due to the activation of the sympathetic nervous system and the increased production of CRH and urocortin. Whether the anorexia that occurs in many pain conditions is also due to a stress response is unclear.

Close interactions exist between food and water intake. Typically, a good 80% of the daily water intake of animals takes place in relation to meals. The amount and composition of the food consumed are important determinants of water intake. This is particularly evident in dry-fed pets. Cats naturally take up most of their water requirements with food (mice, birds). When feeding dry food, the "water deficit" is often not fully compensated by drinking. Food intake is significantly reduced when there is a lack of water. The mechanisms of this phenomenon are largely unknown; however, it is of practical importance especially for ruminants, which are regularly exposed to periods of dehydration in many parts of the world. Lack of water also inhibits rumination, which per se also inhibits food intake. Lactating ruminants also react to a lack of water with significantly reduced milk production. The water requirement of lactating animals is particularly high not only because of the quantity required for milk secretion, but also because of the increased energy metabolism during lactation.

In females, food intake fluctuates during the sexual cycle. Consumption decreases during proestrus and reaches a minimum in oestrus because of the food intake suppressive effect of oestrogens. Oestrogens enhance the effect of peripheral satiety signals such as CCK and GLP-1, via oestrogen receptors in the NTS. The tendency to weight gain after ovariectomy, seen in many species, is due to the discontinuation of this oestrogen effect.

For some species during gestation, the energy requirement increases by approx. 50% compared to the maintenance level in adult animals. In some cases, energy requirement may increase 2 to 3 times more than the maintenance requirement and food intake normally increases, but the underlying mechanisms are only partially known. For example, pregnant animals are often hyperleptinaemic, but develop leptin resistance due to reduced expression of the leptin receptor in the hypothalamus and reduced signalling at the MC receptor level. Such leptin resistance does not occur in pseudopregnancy, which is often accompanied by hyperphagia. Thus, foetal or placental factors seem to be involved in the development of leptin resistance. Finally, the decrease in food intake, often observed in cows towards the end of pregnancy, could also be related to the marked increase in plasma levels of oestrogen at that time.

In lactating animals, prolactin could be involved in the increase in food consumption. However, despite this increased food intake, most species are in negative energy balance during the first phase of lactation. Especially in the high yielding cow, this often develops into ketosis. Why the dairy cow does not eat according to her energy needs during this phase is unknown.

During growth, food intake is increased as a result of the increased demand for energy. Ghrelin also increases the secretion of growth hormone and may therefore be involved in the coordination of these processes. The choice of food also reflects the altered nutrient requirements for protein and fat synthesis in growing animals.

The depression of food intake in the course of a disease is of great clinical importance. It is part of the generalised defence reaction of an animal to infections and other noxious agents. Short term inappetence is interpreted as contributing to the defence against a noxious agent, because forced feeding is initially associated with increased mortality in experimentally induced infections. The positive effect of inappetence is associated with 1) saving energy available for defence mechanisms in the short term by avoiding foraging, 2) depriving microorganisms of essential nutrients and 3) promoting apoptosis of infected cells. In the longer term, however, depression of food consumption harms an animal by depleting protein and energy reserves, which delays recovery. The central event in the development of the acute-phase response is the production of proinflammatory cytokines which are released by monocytes, macrophages, epithelial and other cells when they come into contact with antigens. Basically similar processes take place in tumour anorexia and cachexia, which is very often observed in the final stage of tumour diseases. Here, too, there is a massive release of cytokines.

Many cytokines (especially interleukin-1, interleukin-6, tumour necrosis factor-α, interferon-γ and growth differentiation factor-15) have a pronounced consumption-reducing effect. Of particular importance is signal transmission at the blood-brain barrier, where the release of certain neuroactive mediators such as prostaglandins and nitric oxide (NO) is triggered. Ultimately, cytokines inhibit food consumption by modulation of the aforementioned neurotransmitter and neuropeptide systems.

MORE DETAILS   Cytokines and other immune stimuli activate the enzyme cyclooxygenase-2 (COX-2) in the capillary endothelial cells of the blood-brain barrier. This results in the production of eicosanoids (arachidonic acid derivatives, e.g. prostaglandin E_2), which are linked via 5-HT, GLP-1 and the hypothalamic circuits mentioned above. The involvement of eicosanoids in this signalling is of practical importance because inhibitors of eicosanoid synthesis (e.g. COX-2 inhibitors) are commonly used in the clinic for their analgesic, antiphlogistic and antipyretic effects. Similarly, learned aversions are likely to play a role in some forms of disease-related inappetence. This is consistent with the observation that eating can often be stimulated, at least temporarily, in patients by offering them new, good-tasting food.

IN A NUTSHELL !

Food intake is influenced by many external and internal factors that a priori have nothing to do with the physiological control mechanisms. Most such effects are based on a modulation of the hunger or satiety mechanisms.

Nutrition, energy

Suggested reading

Bai L, Mesgarzadeh S, Ramesh KS et al. Genetic identification of vagal sensory neurons that control feeding. Cell 2019; 179: 1129–1143

Berridge KC, Kringelbach ML. Affective neuroscience of pleasure: reward in humans and animals. Psychopharmacol 2008; 199: 457–480

Carter ME, Soden ME, Zweifel LS et al. Genetic identification of a neural circuit that suppresses appetite. Nature 2013; 503 (7474): 111–114

Langhans W, Harrold J, Williams G et al. Control of eating. In: Williams G, Fruehbeck G, eds. Obesity: Science to Practice. Chichester: Wiley-Blackwell; 2009: 127–166

Langhans W, Leitner C, Arnold M. Dietary fat sensing via fatty acid oxidation in enterocytes – possible role in the control of eating. Am J Physiol 2011; 300: R554-R565

Robertson SA, Leinninger GM, Myers MG Jr. Molecular and neural mediators of leptin action. Physiol Behav 2008; 94: 637–642

Schwartz MW, Porte D Jr. Diabetes, obesity, and the brain. Science 2005; 307: 375–379

Steinert RE, Feinle-Bisset C, Asarian L et al. Ghrelin, CCK, GLP-1, and PYY(3–36): secretory controls and physiological roles in eating and glycemia in health, obesity and after RYGB. Physiol Rev 2017; 97: 411–463

Woods SC, Lutz TA, Geary N et al. Pancreatic signals controlling food intake – insulin, glucagon and amylin. Phil Trans R Soc B 2006; 361: 1219–1235

Zakariassen HL, John LM, Lutz TA. Central control of energy balance by amylin and calcitonin receptor agonists and their potential for treatment of metabolic diseases. Basic Clin Pharmacol Toxicol 2020; 127: 163–177

Endocrinology and reproduction

23 Endocrinology

Mirja Wilkens, Alexandra Muscher-Banse

23.1 General endocrinology

Mirja Wilkens

ESSENTIALS ✘

Endocrinology is the study of **humoral signal transmission** mediated by **extracellular messenger molecules**, i.e. hormones, tissue hormones and cytokines. Together with the signal transmission of the nervous system, the endocrine system is responsible for the regulation and coordination of all physiological processes in an animal. Endocrine malfunction can result in severe disease and functional disorders at all stages of an animal's life. To limit the amount of a hormone being secreted and to adjust the secretion rate to the demand, there are complex **control circuit systems**.

The term "extracellular messenger molecules" is used because in endocrinology there are not only **hormones** secreted by endocrine glands, but there are also **non-glandular hormones** secreted by other tissues, such as bone, adipose tissue, heart, kidneys or intestinal epithelium. Furthermore, there are not only endocrine-acting molecules that reach their distant target cells and tissues via the blood circulation, but there are also tissue hormones and cytokines, transported via the extracellular fluid, acting as **auto- and paracrine agents** on cells in the immediate vicinity of the sites of secretion. All these messenger molecules must bind to **specific receptors**, and can therefore only elicit responses in target cells and tissues equipped with these receptors. The type and speed of this cellular response depends on the chemical properties of a hormone. Lipophilic **steroid hormones**, such as the oestrogens or cortisol, bind to **intracellular receptors** and influence gene expression as a hormone-receptor complex, resulting in medium- to long-term changes in cell function. In contrast, **peptide hormones** such as insulin or luteinising hormone bind to **membrane receptors** that transmit the signal into the cell **by coupling to an enzyme or by activating** a second-messenger system. These messenger peptides act by stimulating or inhibiting the activity of proteins such as enzymes.

In contrast to the action of steroid hormones, the effect of peptide hormones is much faster and is primarily directed at changing the **activity of already existing transport systems and enzymes**.

23.1.1 Introduction

In multicellular organisms, where the different cells and organs have a high degree of specialisation, there is a need for regulatory signals to mediate the complex coordination and control of physiological processes such as digestion, the metabolic utilisation of nutrients, reproduction, maintenance of electrolyte and water balance, and for growth and development. These signals are both **neurogenic**, from the somatic or autonomic nervous system, and **humoral**, as **extracellular messenger molecules**, i.e. glandular hormones from endocrine glands, as well as non-glandular hormones and cytokines from other tissues.

Neurogenic control signals are transmitted rapidly along nerve pathways, while humoral signals are transmitted more slowly via the bloodstream or the extracellular fluid. Nevertheless, there are many examples of a close link between the two systems (p.119) such as the release of adrenaline from the adrenal medulla in response to neural stimulation via preganglionic sympathetic fibres.

Depending on the spatial relationship of the messenger secreting cell and the target cell, the effect is described as autocrine, paracrine or endocrine. **Autocrine** means that the messenger molecule acts on the cell secreting it, or on cells of the same type in the immediate vicinity. Interleukin-2 released by T cells is an autocrine signal that serves to amplify its action by a positive feedback loop. However, autocrine hormones may also provide a mechanism to limit their own release by negative feedback, or to coordinate the function of cells of the same type, such as in the processes of growth. If the signal is transmitted via the interstitial fluid to cells of other types in the immediate vicinity, this is a **paracrine effect**. In this way, D-cells in the gastric mucosa secrete somatostatin to inhibit nearby G-cells, which consequently release less gastrin, and then acid secretion by the parietal cells is decreased. During **endocrine** transmission, the messenger substance is transported from the endocrine gland via the bloodstream to influence the function of organs and tissues further away. In principle, hormones influence enzyme activities, transport processes, cell proliferation and apoptosis as well as the secretion of other messenger substances.

The mediation of the effect always takes place via **specific receptors**. Only a cell with a receptor that has an affinity for the specific messenger molecule can respond to that messenger. The effect is not only dependent on the concentration of the messenger molecule, but also on the number and affinity of the receptors. For example, ovulation of a follicle can only occur through a big increase in the secretion of luteinising hormone (LH) from the pituitary gland, and only if the granulosa cells of the follicle have developed a sufficient number of LH receptors during its maturation.

Depending on the type of hormone and receptor, there is either a very rapid (milliseconds to seconds) influence on metabolic processes via an intracellular signalling cascade, or a change in gene expression where the functional manifestation takes a longer time to develop (hours to days).

> ### IN A NUTSHELL   !
>
> Extracellular messenger molecules bind to specific receptors and thus only influence cells that are equipped with those receptors. They exert their effect via a change in gene expression or via the formation of intracellular signal molecules (second messengers), by changing the conductivity of the cell membrane or by direct coupling of the receptor to an enzyme. Depending on the spatial relationship between the secreting cell and the target cell, the hormonal action is either autocrine, paracrine or endocrine.

23.1.2 Synthesis and chemical properties of extracellular messenger molecules

Four groups of messenger molecules can be defined on the basis of their chemical structure. Most hormones are **proteins or peptides**. The biogenic amines, such as the tissue hormone histamine from histidine, and the tyrosine derivatives, which include the catecholamines, i.e. adrenaline, noradrenaline and dopamine, as well as the **thyroid hormones**, are produced from individual amino acids. The **steroid hormones**, which include the hormones of the adrenal cortex and the vitamin D hormone in addition to those involved in the reproductive process, are derived from the structure of cholesterol. The **eicosanoids**, with the prostaglandins as the best-known representatives, are derivatives of arachidonic acid. The basic properties of these hormones, determined by their chemical structure, are described below, with the exception of the catecholamines (p. 116).

■ Peptide hormones

Although their size can vary from three to 200–400 amino acids, the hormones belonging to this group are called peptide hormones. First, so-called preprohormones are synthesised, which have no endocrine activity. These long polypeptide chains enter the interior of the endoplasmic reticulum, where a prohormone is formed in the Golgi apparatus, by cleavage of a signal sequence. Further post-translational modification leads to the formation of the actual hormone (**Fig. 23.1**), which is stored in vesicles near the cell membrane and released by **exocytosis**, in response to an adequate stimulus. Exocytosis requires adenosine triphosphate and calcium. In most cases, the secretion of peptide hormones is always accompanied by their continuous formation, so that the **intracellular stores** are usually always sufficiently filled to allow for their future secretion and function. Their **plasma half-life** is a **few minutes to hours**. Inactivation takes place through proteolysis, especially in the liver and kidney.

MORE DETAILS   Different hormones can also be formed from a single preprohormone. During physical or mental stress, adrenocorticotropic hormone (ACTH) is secreted from the pituitary gland, and acts on the adrenal cortex to cause the secretion of glucocorticoids. The precursor protein of ACTH is proopiomelanocortin (POMC). In addition to ACTH, POMC also produces β-endorphin, which has an analgesic effect, and α-melanocyte-stimu-

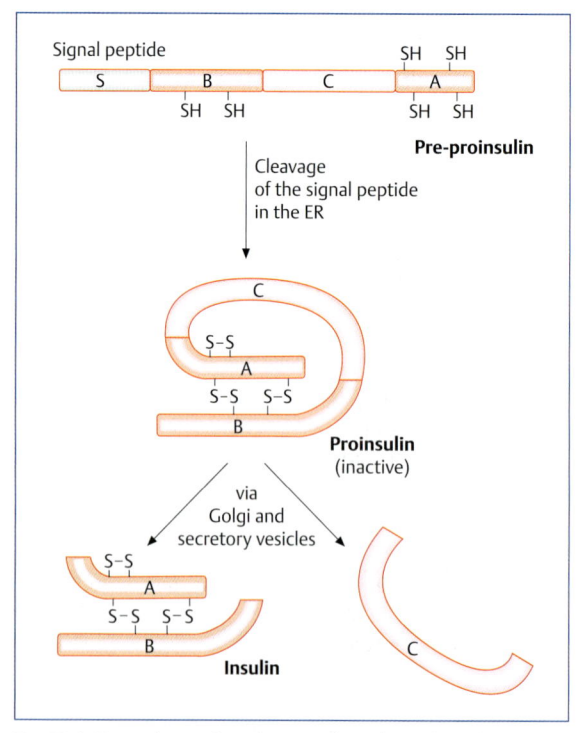

Fig. 23.1 Biosynthesis of insulin. Based on the coding mRNA, the preproinsulin is synthesised first. The signal peptide is cleaved off after transport into the endoplasmic reticulum. In the course of posttranslational modification, the C-peptide is cleaved off and the A- and B-chain are connected via disulphide bridges, so that biologically active insulin is finally produced, and is stored in secretory vesicles of the cell. [Source: Königshoff M, Brandenburger T, eds. Kurzlehrbuch Biochemie. 4th, completely revised edition. Stuttgart: Thieme; 2018]

lating hormone (α-MSH), which limits fever reactions, influences food intake behaviour, and promotes the production of pigments in melanocytes. For this reason, brown colouration of the skin occurs in humans in Addison's disease, where there is adrenal cortex insufficiency. This results in a greatly increased production of ACTH, and consequently, also of α-MSH, as an attempt to compensate for inadequate glucocorticoid hormone release from the adrenal gland.

■ Steroid hormones

In contrast to peptide hormones, steroid hormones are **not stored** but, due to their lipophilic properties, are released by simple diffusion as soon as they are synthesised. The first step in their synthesis is the oxidative shortening of the side chain of **cholesterol**. Thus, pregnenolone with 21 C-atoms is formed from the molecule originally having 27 C-atoms. Further modifications take place depending on the cellular enzymes for oxidation and reduction of hydroxy and keto groups, introduction, rearrangement and hydrogenation of double bonds, hydroxylation, etc. In the adrenal cortex, **mineralo- and glucocorticoids** are formed by hydroxylations at C21 and C11, while in the organs involved in the reproductive process, **gestagens** (21 C-atoms), **androgens** (19 C-atoms) and **oestrogens** (18 C-atoms) are synthesised (**Fig. 23.2**). These individual reactions can also serve as important points for endocrine regulation of steroid hormone production. This type of control is seen in the endocrine changes that precede birth. Even before there is a reduction in the production of progesterone, the hormone that plays a key role in the maintenance of pregnancy, an increased conversion to oestrogen is induced in the placenta. This results in a significant change in the progesterone/oestrogen ratio in plasma, in favour of oestrogen. **Fig. 23.3** shows the increase in mRNA expression of steroid 17α-hydroxylase (CYP17A1) at the end of gestation in the placenta of a cat. CYP17A1 is an enzyme of the cytochrome P450 superfamily that initiates the transformation of progesterone into oestrogen by hydroxylation at position 17 and subsequent deacetylation.

Calcitriol, the so-called vitamin D hormone, is also a steroid hormone. **Vitamin D** is formed in the skin from 7-dehydrocholesterol under the influence of UV light and/or is ingested with food. After its 25-hydroxylation in the liver and 1-hydroxylation in the kidney, 1,25-dihydroxycholecalciferol (calcitriol), is formed.

Because of their low water solubility, the transport of lipophilic steroids and also thyroid hormones in blood is mainly by binding to plasma proteins such as **albumin** and **special binding proteins**, synthesised in the liver. Some of the binding proteins have a high affinity for a specific hormone, but in principle they also bind all other, chemically closely related molecules. Transcortin, for example, shows the highest affinity for cortisol and corticosterone, but also binds progesterone. Since the duration and extent of binding is determined by classical binding kinetics, an **equilibrium is established between free and bound hormone in plasma**, whereby the proportion of free, and thus effective hormone, is relatively low (1–10%). Since only the free hormone is taken up into cells, its binding to a protein in

blood prevents an excessive increased effect of these hormones, including feedback mechanisms inducing their metabolism and inactivation, thus ensuring that a reservoir of the hormone in plasma continues to be available. Protein binding is the reason why the plasma half-lives of steroid hormones are significantly longer than those of peptide hormones, and range from several hours to days. The binding to protein also provides a mechanism for fine-tuning the functional hormone concentration and its effect.

■ Thyroid hormones

In the follicle cells of the thyroid gland, thyroid hormones are produced by the formation of an ether linkage between two iodinated **tyrosine molecules**. Depending on the number of iodine substituents, the thyroid hormones are either **triiodothyronine (T3)** or **tetraiodothyronine (T4)** which is also called **thyroxine**. The incorporation of iodine into thyroid hormones is the only known physiological function of iodine. Iodide is actively co-transported with sodium from blood into the **thyrocytes**, and transported via a channel into the lumen of the follicle. Thyrocytes are also referred to as follicular epithelial cells, because the thyroid gland is organised into follicles. In the Golgi apparatus of thyrocytes, the glycoprotein **thyroglobulin** is formed. This glycoprotein contains over 100 tyrosine residues and is released into the follicular lumen by exocytosis. There, iodination of about 20 of these tyrosine residues takes place, for which iodide must first be converted into iodine by **thyroperoxidase** with the aid of hydrogen peroxide. This leads to the combination of two tyrosine molecules into T3 and T4, usually in a ratio of 1:9, which initially remain part of thyroglobulin, which is stored in this form in the colloid inside the thyroid follicle. The oxidation of iodide to iodine is of central importance and therefore also the starting point for one of the standard therapies of hyperthyroidism, the most common endocrine dysfunction in older cats. By administering a competitive inhibitor of thyroperoxidase, this step is prevented and thus thyroid hormone synthesis is reduced.

In order to secrete thyroid hormones, thyroglobulin must first be reabsorbed from the colloid into the thyrocytes by endocytosis. After fusion of these vesicles with lysosomes, triiodothyronine and thyroxine are enzymatically cleaved from thyroglobulin. The processes described are summarised in **Fig. 23.4**.

Due to their lipophilic nature, the two hormones can cross the basolateral plasma membrane by diffusion. In blood, the thyroid hormones, except for a **free fraction of approx. 0.3%**, are bound to a high-affinity thyroxine-binding globulin, the thyroxine-binding prealbumin transthyretin) and albumin. It is assumed that there are species-specific differences with regard to the relative amounts of each protein involved in binding the thyroid hormones. Since there is always a balance between the bound and the free form, there is always a sufficient amount of thyroid hormones in blood for several days because of this protein binding. Thyroxine, which is the main hormone released from the thyroid gland is biologically less effective than triiodothyronine, but it has a significantly longer plasma

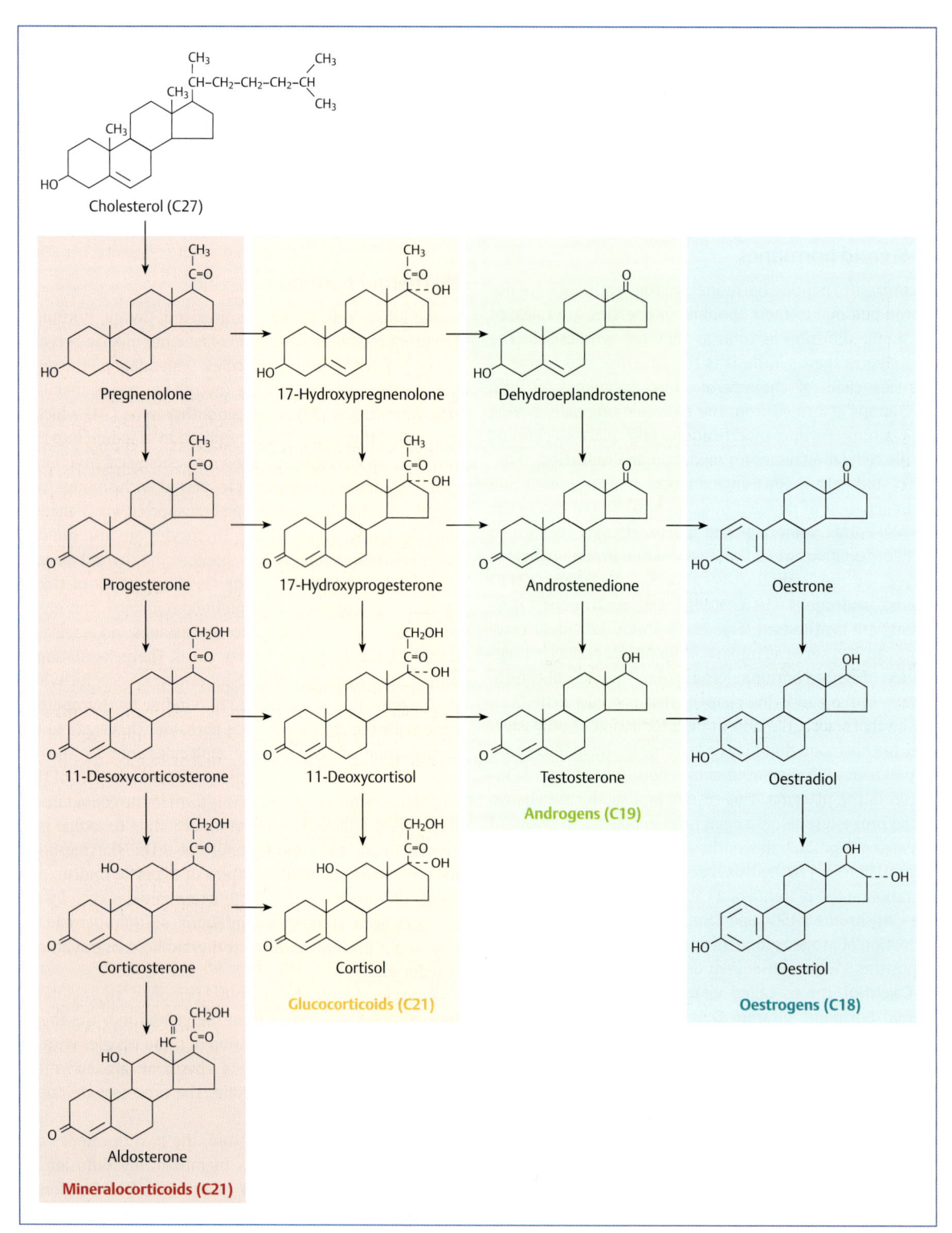

Fig. 23.2 Mineralo- and glucocorticoids, gestagens, androgens and oestrogens are synthesised from cholesterol by specific enzymes. Many of the individual metabolites are precursors for other hormones. It should be noted that in these transformations the number of C-atoms can be reduced, but not increased. This means that oestrogens can be produced from androgens, but the reverse is not possible.

half-life of about one week compared to triiodothyronine, which has a half-life of only about one day. The thyroid hormones undergo hepatic biotransformation to hydrophilic metabolites which are excreted via bile and in urine.

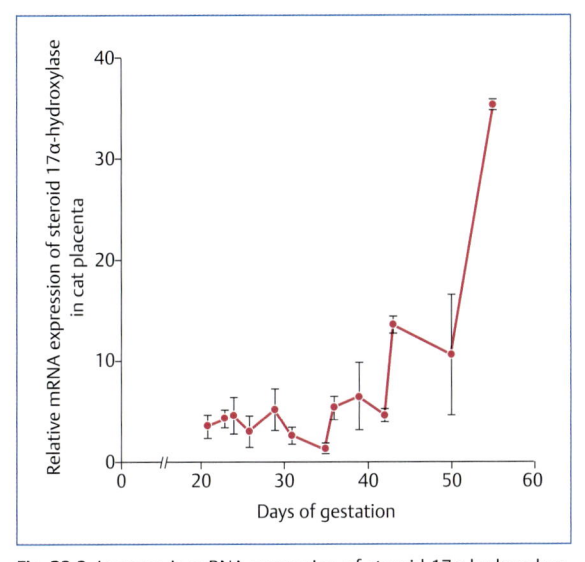

Fig. 23.3 Increase in mRNA expression of steroid 17α-hydroxylase, which initiates the conversion of progesterone to oestrogen, in the placenta of a cat at the end of gestation. [Source: Braun et al. Progesterone and oestradiol in cat placenta – biosynthesis and tissue concentration. J Steroid Biochem Mol Biol 2012; 132: 295–302]

■ Eicosanoids

The eicosanoids, which can be formed in various tissues, and also in thrombocytes, are **prostaglandins**, **thromboxanes** and **leukotrienes**. Their physiological roles include the local regulation of blood flow, vascular permeability and haemostasis, influencing the secretion activity of certain cells, and induction of pain and fever. Specific effects of eicosanoids can be found, among others, in ch. 3.3 (p. 76), ch. 8.5.1 (p. 208), ch. 9.4 (p. 234), ch. 10.3.7 (p. 250), ch. 20.13 (p. 508), ch. 24.2.1 and ch. 24.2.2.

For biosynthesis, the quadruply unsaturated **arachidonic acid** is first cleaved from membrane phospholipids by the specific, regulable phospholipase A_2. This process is stimulated by inflammatory mediators such as histamine and bradykinin and inhibited by glucocorticoids. The formation of leukotrienes is subsequently initiated by the action of **lipoxygenase**. A **peroxidase** and a **cyclooxygenase** (COX) mediate the formation of prostaglandin H_2 from arachidonic acid, from which the prostaglandins I_2, E_2 and F_2 as well as thromboxane A_2 can subsequently be formed. The cyclooxygenase COX-1 is expressed ubiquitously, for example in the stomach and kidney, whereas the activity of COX-2 is inducible and plays a role above all in inflammatory processes. Drugs with an inhibitory effect on these enzymes, the so-called non-steroidal anti-inflammatory drugs, are often used to treat pain and reduce fever due to their anti-inflammatory properties. It should be noted that side effects such as damage to the gastric mucosa may occur with treatment by non-specific COX inhibitors, as the secretion of protective gastric mucus is mediated by the

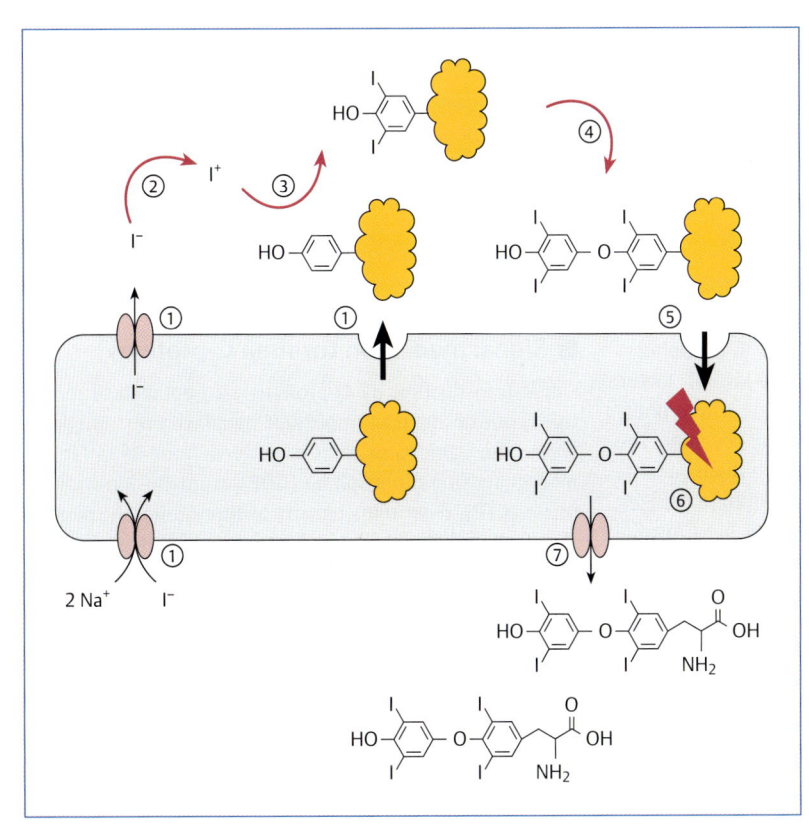

Fig. 23.4 After the transport of iodide and thyroglobulin into the follicular lumen (**1**), oxidation to iodine (**2**) and iodination of the tyrosine residues of thyroglobulin (**3**) takes place there. After two tyrosine residues have been linked together by an ether bond (**4**), thyroglobulin is resorbed into the thyrocytes by endocytosis (**5**). There, thyroxine and triiodothyronine are cleaved from thyroglobulin (**6**) and, after partial deiodination of thyroxine, triiodothyronine is released into blood via a transporter (**7**).

Endocrinology, reproduction

paracrine action of prostaglandin E_2, the synthesis of which may be suppressed by therapy with COX inhibitors.

Eicosanoids are eliminated from tissues quite quickly (within two minutes). Some of their metabolites are associated with pathophysiological processes and have proinflammatory and possibly carcinogenic effects. It is possible that the concentration of eicosanoids with adverse effects can be influenced by the ratio of omega-3/omega-6 fatty acids in the diet.

> ### IN A NUTSHELL !
>
> Peptide hormones are present, preformed in a cell, and are secreted within seconds to minutes in response to a stimulus. After secretion, they have a short half-life in blood plasma. Steroid hormones are synthesised from cholesterol and are then released continuously. Thyroid hormones are tyrosine derivatives, stored in the follicles of the thyroid gland, and are released when needed. Because of their lipophilic nature, steroid and thyroid hormones in blood are mainly bound to specific proteins, which also give them a relatively long plasma half-life. Eicosanoids are synthesised from arachidonic acid.

23.1.3   Membrane receptors

The hydrophilic peptide hormones, as well as the eicosanoids, are not able to pass through the cell membrane and therefore bind to **membrane receptors**. Some lipophilic messengers also bind to membrane receptors. Hormone binding leads to a conformational change of the receptor, which activates a complex **signalling cascade** in the cell, mediated by so-called second messengers. These signalling molecules are **not specific**, so that the effects of different hormones can be mediated by the same pathway. However, the targeted effect of a hormone is ensured by its specific receptor on the cell. Receptors are classified according to their structure. A classification of the signal transmission pathways according to the second messengers involved, can be found in ch. Second messenger (p.39).

■ Signal mediation via tyrosine kinases

Almost all **growth factors** and **insulin** act via tyrosine kinases. Binding of the hormone leads either to phosphorylation of the receptor itself (e.g. epithelial growth factor, EGF, and insulin-like growth factor, IGF-1) or also to phosphorylation of proteins associated with the receptor. The latter is the case with the **insulin receptor** which consists of **two polypeptide chains linked by** disulphide bridges. The two **extracellularly localised α-subunits** bind insulin, triggering a conformational change through the transmembrane domain of the two β-subunits. These have an **extracellular** and an **intracellular component** with **tyrosine kinase-activity** (Fig. 23.5). After **autophosphorylation** at several sites, binding and phosphorylation of various adapter proteins, the so-called insulin receptor substrates (**IRS**), occurs. These subsequently modify various metabolic pathways by activation of phosphoinositide 3-kinase (**PI3K**), which is associated with an increase in the concen-

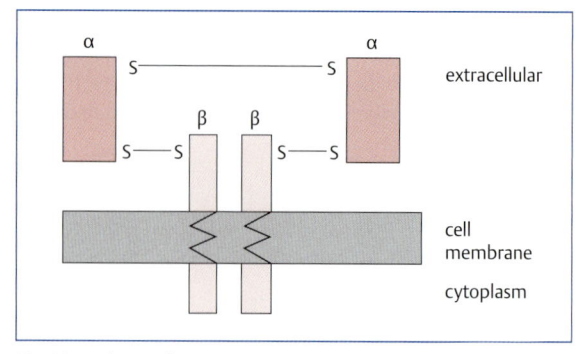

Fig. 23.5 The insulin receptor consists of two polypeptide chains connected by disulphide bridges. After binding of insulin to the two extracellularly localised α-subunits, a conformational change occurs, which results in activation of the tyrosine kinase activity of the intracellular portions of the β-subunits. S-S = disulphide bridge

tration of **phosphatidylinositol-3,4,5-trisphosphate (PIP₃)** and activation of **protein kinase B (PKB)**. Phosphorylation by PKB, inactivates glycogen synthase kinase. This inactivation then prevents the phosphorylation of glycogen synthase. Since glycogen synthase is also active in the dephosphorylated state, an increased synthesis of glycogen from glucose will still occur. Activation of phosphodiesterase (**PDE**) depresses the intracellular concentration of cyclic adenosine monophosphate (**cAMP**). This inhibits various processes that are stimulated by high cAMP levels, such as lipolysis by hormone-sensitive lipase (HSL). The stimulation of glucose uptake into muscle and adipose tissue by incorporation of the glucose transporter GLUT4 into the plasma membrane is mainly triggered by the **SH2 adapter protein cascade**. The **MAP kinase pathway** (mitogen activated protein) is also induced by receptors with tyrosine kinase activity. Hence, any disturbance of these regulatory mechanisms can favour the development of tumours by modifying differentiation and growth.

The **internalisation** of the phosphorylated receptor serves to limit the insulin effect. Proton pumps in the vesicle membrane cause acidification and thus dissociation of insulin from its receptor. After its subsequent dephosphorylation, the receptor is then translocated back into the membrane.

■ Signal mediation through G-proteins

Signal transduction by G-proteins via heptahelical receptors is one of the most important signal transduction pathways. The name **G-protein** is derived from its ability to bind guanosine diphosphate (**GDP**) or guanosine triphosphate (**GTP**). G-proteins consist of three different peptide chains (heterotrimers), which are called **α-, β- and γ-subunits** depending on their size. When a hormone binds to its receptor, the hormone-receptor complex associates with the G-protein, which then releases **GDP** from the α-subunit and binds **GTP** instead. The formation of this **GTP-protein complex** dissociates the β- and γ-subunits from the receptor, enabling the α-subunit to interact with the **adenylate cyclase** located on the inside of the cell membrane. Depending on whether it is a **stimulating G_s-** or an **inhibiting G_i-protein**, the activity of the adenylate cy-

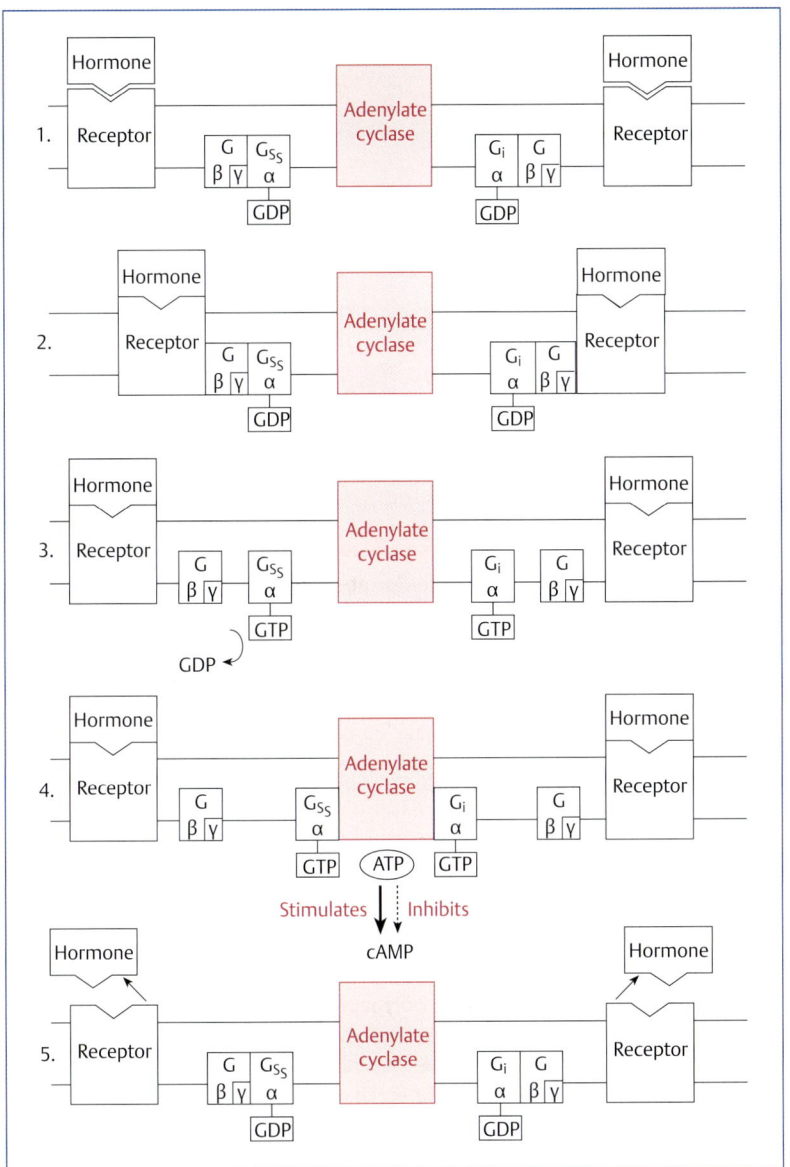

Fig. 23.6 Activation of adenylate cyclase by G-protein-mediated signal transduction.
1. Initial situation: the hormone in the extracellular fluid diffuses to the receptor.
2. The hormone is bound by the receptor, and the hormone-receptor complex in the cell membrane is transported to the α-β-γ-GDP molecule.
3. The GDP bound to Gα is exchanged for GTP. The Gα-subunit "migrates" to the adenylate cyclase.
4. The Gα-subunit binds to adenylate cyclase. Depending on whether it is a stimulatory (4a) or an inhibitory (4b) G-protein, the Gα-subunit exerts a stimulatory (G_s α) or an inhibitory influence (G_i α) on the adenylate cyclase, so that more or less cAMP is produced.
The GTP is then hydrolysed and the Gα-subunit binds to the Gβ-γ molecule again. Finally, the hormone dissociates from the receptor.

clase is increased or decreased (**Fig. 23.6**). As a result, the intracellular concentration of **cAMP** changes. Cyclic AMP, one of the most important second messengers, activates **protein kinase A (PKA)**, which is then able to phosphorylate other proteins and thus change their activity.

This process is limited by the fact that the α-subunit also has **GTPase activity**, so that the bound GTP is promptly hydrolysed to GDP. The resulting GDP-α subunit dissociates from the adenylate cyclase, terminating its stimulation, and associates again with the β- and γ-subunits to form the original α-β-γ-GDP molecule. The physiological effect of the hormone is thus rapidly terminated, if is not continuously being supplied.

Just as important as the **tight control of hormone action** provided by this signalling pathway, is the **amplifier function**. The receptor and G-protein are mobile within the membrane, so that a single receptor, activated by a hormone molecule, can produce many Gα-GTP complexes. Each of these Gα-GTP complexes stimulates or inhibits an

adenylate cyclase. The activated enzyme and a G_s-protein-coupled receptor can then produce numerous cAMP molecules.

The messenger molecules that mediate their effect via G_i-protein-coupled receptors include melatonin and somatostatin. An increase in the concentration of cAMP and thus the activity of protein kinase A via G_s-protein-coupled receptors is triggered, for example, by ACTH, FSH and glucagon. It should be noted that some messenger molecules, such as adrenaline, noradrenaline, dopamine and adenosine, can act on various target tissues via different receptors (**Table 4.1**). In addition, the receptors specific to the messenger molecule can also differ in their affinities. In this way, the catecholamines cause both vascular dilatation and vasoconstriction, depending on their localisation and concentration.

In addition to the G_s- and G_i-proteins described so far, there are also other types of G-proteins. In the case of **G_q-protein-coupled receptors**, signal transmission takes place through activation of **phospholipase C (PLC)** via an increase in the concentration of **DAG** and **IP$_3$** and thus a **release of Ca^{2+}** takes place. Adrenaline, noradrenaline and oxytocin, for example, act on smooth muscle cells via this pathway. In the case of signal transduction in the retina, photons impacting a G-protein called **transducin (G$_t$)**, leads to an increase in the activity of **phosphodiesterase** and thus to a reduction in the intracellular concentration of **cGMP** and the closure of cGMP-controlled cation channels. The receptors of the olfactory mucosa also mediate their signal via G proteins (**G$_{olf}$**), which activate adenylate cyclase.

■ Signal mediation through direct binding to a guanylate cyclase

The right atrial natriuretic peptide (**ANP**) receptor is a **membrane-bound guanylate cyclase**. After binding of the ligand to the extracellular domain, a conformational change occurs that removes the inhibition of the enzymatic activity, so that the second messenger cyclic guanosine monophosphate (**cGMP**) is increasingly formed. Nitric oxide (**NO**) acts via a soluble guanylate cyclase. Since it is a gas, it can diffuse through the cell membrane and thus does not require a membrane receptor. Nitric oxide, which plays (p. 362) an important role in the regulation of vascular tone and intestinal motor (p. 362) function (**Table 16.4**), functions as a neurotransmitter. Details are described in ch. 4.4.5.

The increase in cGMP concentration leads to an activation of **phosphodiesterase** and thus to a decrease in cAMP concentration, an activation of **protein kinase G (PKG)** and a **modification of transmembrane ion transport**. This mechanism modifies ion transport in the kidney, and also mediates vasodilatative effects and dilation of the bronchial tubes. For the role of cGMP in signal transduction in the retina, see ch. Photoreception and transduction (p. 94).

IN A NUTSHELL   !

After hormone binding, the insulin receptor initiates tyrosine kinase activity and phosphorylates cellular proteins, which are thereby activated or deactivated. Eicosanoids and most peptide hormones bind to membrane receptors and mediate their effect via second-messenger systems, especially via adenylate cyclase, where cAMP production is activated or inhibited depending on the receptor type.

23.1.4   Nuclear receptors

Even though membrane receptors are now known for some of the steroid and thyroid hormones, the main receptors mediating their effects are in the cytosol, in cell organelles or in the cell nucleus. The cell membrane is quite permeable to these lipophilic messengers. Since steroid and thyroid hormones are **ligands and activators of transcription factors** that induce an increase or a decrease in the expression of certain genes, this is also called a genomic action.

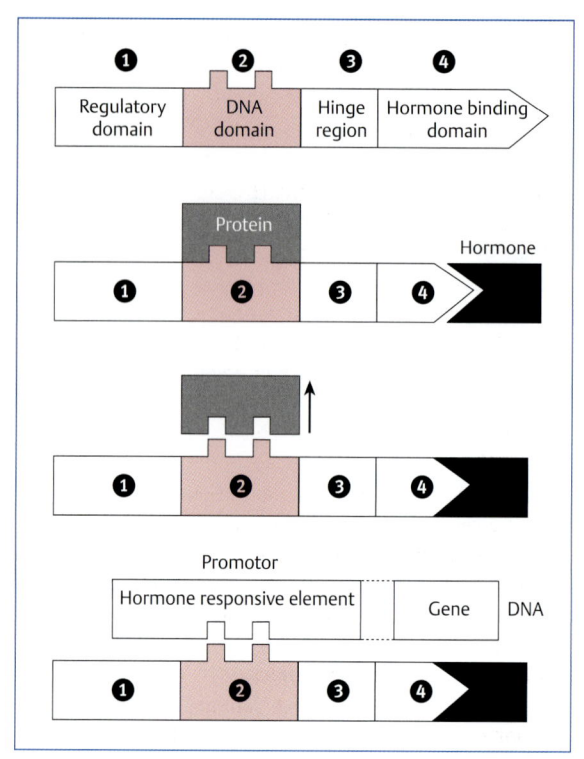

Fig. 23.7 Domain structure and function of a steroid hormone receptor. The DNA domain carries a zinc finger-like structure protected by a protein. With the binding of the steroid hormone to the receptor, the protein dissociates and the DNA domain of the hormone-receptor complex can bind to the DNA (promoter) and activate the associated gene. Hinge region: Connecting region.

The structure of these intracellular receptors is invariably only one **polypeptide chain** (**Fig. 23.7**). It is therefore not surprising that different hormones can react with more than one receptor within this receptor family. The **DNA domain** of the steroid hormone receptors has a characteristic amino acid sequence. In this section of the receptor there are two structures characterised by accumulations of the amino acid cysteine, where four cysteine molecules, fixed by a zinc atom, form the basis for a finger-like amino acid loop. These **zinc fingers** differ in each of the various steroid hormone receptors. Nutritional zinc deficiency can cause, among other things, delayed sexual development. This symptom can be attributed to the inability of oestrogen and androgen receptors to form the appropriate link to their DNA domain in the absence of zinc.

Glucocorticoids such as cortisol bind, in the cytoplasm to a glucocorticoid receptor which is complexed with the heat shock protein, Hsp 90 and p59. This leads to the dissolution of the complex and the dimerisation of the receptor. The receptor dimer is translocated into the cell nucleus together with the bound glucocorticoid. There, as a ligand-activated transcription factor, it binds to so-called glucocorticoid responsive elements and thus influences the transcription of downstream genes.

Such **hormone responsive elements** in the promoter regions of the target genes, to which the DNA domain of the respective receptors binds hormone-specifically with their zinc fingers, consist of about 70 base pairs and improve the recognition of the promoter by the RNA polymerases that translate the gene into mRNA. **Promoters** are DNA sequence regions about 100 base pairs long that control the transcription of a gene. They are located in front of the gene that is to be transcribed.

To mediate the effect of the **thyroid hormones** the iodine on the 5'-C atom of the outer ring is cleaved from thyroxine (T4) to form triiodothyronine (T3). The exact localisation is important because cleavage of the iodine on the inner ring produces biologically inactive, so-called reverse triiodothyronine. The formation of this type of T3 probably plays a role in prolonged fasting and severe general diseases.

In the cell nucleus, T3 activates the **T3 receptor** which bears a close resemblance to the steroid hormone receptors. After the formation of homodimers and heterodimers with the **retinoid X receptor**, the complex functions as a **ligand-activated transcription factor** which influences the expression of specific genes. The increased expression of receptors and parts of intracellular signalling cascades also have a role in altering sensitivity to other hormones. An example of this **permissive effect** is the increased responsiveness of the heart to catecholamines by increased expression of β-receptors in hyperthyroidism.

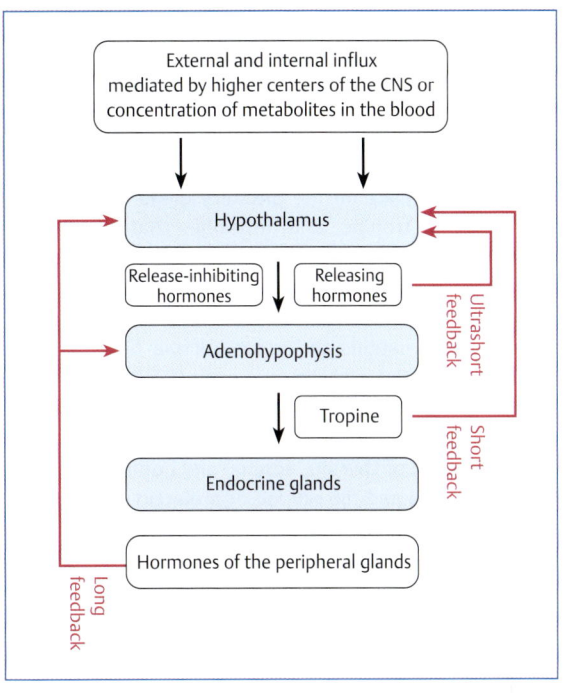

Fig. 23.8 Basic principles of the endocrine axes controlled by the hypothalamus and pituitary gland. The hierarchy of hormone secretion is controlled by the respective downstream levels via feedback loops (cf. **Fig. 24.11**). As a rule, there is a negative feedback loop, but in some cases a high concentration of a subordinate hormone also causes a stimulation of the secretion of the corresponding tropin (positive feedback loop, see ovulation (p. 561)).

> **IN A NUTSHELL** !
>
> Steroid and thyroid hormone receptors consist of a single polypeptide chain with four characteristic domains. After binding of the ligand to its receptor, the hormone-receptor complex migrates into the cell nucleus, binds to DNA and activates transcription of specific genes. This changes the expression of proteins in the cell, so that there are usually medium- to long-term changes in the functionality of the affected tissues. Thyroid hormones primarily have a permissive effect, i.e. the responsiveness of the stimulated cells to other messenger molecules is modulated.

23.1.5 Principles of hormone secretion

Extracellular messenger molecules allow an animal to adapt to physiological changes. This adaptation is only necessary until a certain state is reached, such as a particular reproductive status, a change in energy metabolism, the physiological plasma concentration of sodium, etc. Therefore, these messenger molecules are components of a **regulatory circuit** (**Fig. 23.8**), which in most cases, with the help of feedback loops, the controlled variable or a hormone concentration regulating it – in turn influence the secretion and the action of the hormone.

■ Neuroendocrine control

The endocrine systems controlling reproduction, growth and adaptation to challenging environmental conditions (stress) are under neuroendocrine control. Each is a cascade of hormones from different, hierarchically arranged endocrine glands: **axes from the hypothalamus, the pituitary gland and downstream endocrine glands**.

The **hypothalamus**, a component of the diencephalon, situated ventral to the thalamus, is the crucial **link between the central nervous system and the endocrine system** for maintaining **homeostasis**, i.e. keeping the internal environment constant, and **homeorhesis**, i.e. the long-term adaptation to various physiological conditions such as growth, pregnancy and lactation. The neurons of the hypothalamus represent the link between the central nervous system and the endocrine system for the maintenance of homeostasis, and homeorhesis. Certain neurons of the hypothalamus are able to synthesise hormones, package them into vesicles and release them at the end of neurites, a process called **neurosecretion**.

The **lateral zone of** the hypothalamus is connected by fibrous cords to the limbic system, the thalamus and the midbrain (mesencephalon). With its **periventricular zone**, it borders on the humoral compartment via the 3rd ventricle (**Fig. 5.22**). In this way, information from the **non-hypothalamic brain regions**, about **core body temperature** and important **parameters of blood and cerebrospinal fluid**, i.e. the concentrations of hormones, nutrients, ions etc., are collected and integrated. The pituitary stalk originates in the **medial zone**. (**Fig. 5.21**). The hypothalamus is in neuronal contact with the **neurohypophysis** (posterior lobe of the pituitary gland). Antidiuretic hormone (ADH) and oxytocin are directed via **axoplasmic transport** to the pituitary gland and secreted from there into the bloodstream. All other hypothalamic hormones are secreted into

Endocrinology, reproduction

a **portal vein system** and thus reach the **adenohypophysis** (anterior pituitary). The secretion is not continuous, but pulsatile. As a rule, 12–14 peaks are observed over 24 hours. A tuning of the effect is possible via the frequency as well as the amplitude.

These hormones are releasing and release-inhibiting hormones. They act on the **pituitary gland** and regulate the release of **tropine, and hormones that stimulate** a downstream endocrine gland (stimulating hormones), **prolactin** and **growth hormone** (somatotropin). Negative feedback occurs at each level, i.e. the messenger substance released, then inhibits the release of the hormone that stimulates the release of the messenger (**Fig. 23.8**).

Pulsatile secretion also occurs at the adenohypophysis. An overview of the hormones of the **axes** for the **neuroendocrine control of thyroid, adrenal and gonads** as well as the **growth axis** and the **release of prolactin** can be found in **Table 23.1**. Not all axes contain statins and, according to current scientific knowledge, there is no liberin for prolactin. The release of prolactin is inhibited by dopamine. Corresponding agonists, i.e. substances that bind to the dopamine receptor type 2 (G_i-protein-coupled, **Fig. 23.6**) and can trigger a signal transduction, are used in both, human and veterinary medicine to reduce or stop milk production, for example in the treatment of bitches in false pregnancy.

MORE DETAILS

Reversible suppression of reproduction with the aid of GnRH implants

Endogenous GnRH from the hypothalamus, which induces the secretion of the gonadotropins, FSH and LH, by the pituitary gland, is not released continuously but has a pulsatile secretion. In the male beagle, for example, 4.5 peaks were detected within six hours. Implants that continuously release a synthetic GnRH analogue (deslorelin acetate) are often used to temporarily and reversibly suppress reproductive ability and sex-specific behaviour. While a single administration of a GnRH analogue would result in stimulation of the release of FSH and LH, the persistently increased GnRH concentration at the pituitary gland results in a compensatory reduction of the GnRH receptors ("down-regulation") after a period of 7–27 days, resulting in their loss of responsiveness. In contrast to the endogenous, pulsatile GnRH, the exogenously supplied GnRH analogue, which is constantly released from the implant, does not cause the secretion of FSH and LH. This also means that the gonads are not stimulated. In the male dog, in addition to the loss of reproductive capacity, a reduction in the size of the testicles and, as a rule, behavioural changes can be observed. In contrast to surgical castration, these processes are reversible. If the implant is removed, or if there is no longer sufficient active substance in the implant after about eight months, GnRH receptors are again expressed on the pituitary gland and responsiveness to endogenous GnRH is restored. Of course, GnRH analogues can also be used in female animals to suppress the sexual cycle. Such preparations are used, for example, in zoo animals.

Table 23.1 Overview of the endocrine axes controlled by the hypothalamus and pituitary gland.

Axis	Hormones from the hypothalamus	Hormones from the pituitary gland	Effects
Stress	**CRH:** Corticoliberin	**ACTH:** Adrenocorticotropic hormone	Production of **glucocorticoids** in the adrenal cortex
Growth	**GH-RH:** Somatoliberin **GH-IH:** Somatostatin	**GH:** Somatotropin, growth hormone	Release of **IGF-1** (insulin-like growth factor 1, somatomedin C) from the liver Stimulation of lipolysis in the adipose tissue, bone growth, stimulation of the alveolar cells in the mammary gland
Thyroid gland	**TRH:** Thyrooliberin	**TSH:** Thyroid-stimulating hormone	Release of **T3/T4** (triiodothyronine, thyroxine) from the thyroid gland
Reproduction	**GnRH:** Gonadoliberin	**Gonadotropins: FSH:** Follicle-stimulating hormone **LH:** luteinising hormone	Production of **oestrogens, gestagens** and **androgens** Effect on the gonads of both sexes, see ch. 24.1.1)
Milk production	**Dopamine**	**Prolactin**	Regulation of mammary gland function: initiation and maintenance of milk production (species differences).

■ Humoral control

Control through the composition of the blood

The secretion of messenger substances can be controlled by the **concentration of a particular substance in a body fluid**. A simple example of this is the secretion of parathyroid hormone (PTH). On the parathyroid gland there is a so-called **Ca sensing receptor (CaSR)**. As long as this G_q protein-coupled receptor (effect mediated via phospholipase C, IP_3 and DAG, intracellular Ca^{2+} (p. 536)) is occupied by Ca^{2+}, **the release of PTH is** inhibited. However, if the blood concentration of Ca^{2+} decreases, the proportion of ligand-occupied receptor decreases, which leads to the inhibition of PTH release being lifted. Exocytosis of PTH then occurs. It is remarkable in this context, that the parathyroid gland is the only known organ in which it is not an increase but rather a decrease in the intracellular Ca^{2+} concentration that leads to the fusion of messenger-filled vesicles with the cell membrane. Various physiological processes are triggered by PTH, all of which lead to an increase in the **blood concentration of Ca^{2+}**. When the CaSR is reoccupied as a result of PTH actions, the secretion of PTH is instantly reduced.

This example shows that not only **regulation of the release of a hormone**, but also sensitive **detection of the controlled variable** are important prerequisites for this feedback mechanism. In human medicine, both, gain-of-function and loss-of-function mutations of the CaSR are known to lead to severe disturbances of mineral balance.

Another example of humoral control of hormone release is the **secretion of insulin** from the β-cells of the **endocrine pancreas**. Glucose enters the pancreatic β-cells via **insulin-independent glucose uniporters**, so the amount taken up correlates directly with the current blood glucose concentration. In the cell, metabolism of glucose leads to the **formation of ATP**, the concentration of which also correlates directly with the blood glucose concentration. ATP then inhibits **ATP-sensitive K^+ channels**, which are responsible for maintaining the resting membrane potential. Thus, at high blood glucose concentrations, **depolarisation of the cell** occurs, causing **voltage-dependent Ca^{2+} channels to** open. The resulting increase in the intracellular Ca^{2+} concentration causes the **insulin-filled vesicles to fuse with the cell membrane**, leading to insulin secretion. Insulin then has the effect of lowering glucose concentration, by influencing gluconeogenesis, glycogen synthesis and glucose uptake in insulin-dependent tissues such as muscle, fat and liver, and ultimately its own secretion. (**Fig. 23.9**). These processes of the β-cell can also be **modulated by other stimuli**. For example, increased parasympathetic tone, gastric inhibitory polypeptide (GIP) and glucagon-like peptide (GLP) from the small intestine, have a stimulating effect on insulin release, while somatostatin and increased sympathetic tone inhibit insulin release.

The release of **ADH** (antidiuretic hormone) from the neurohypophysis, i.e. the **posterior pituitary lobe**, is primarily dependent on the **osmolarity** of **plasma**. In this case, the controlled variable is not the concentration of a specific metabolite, but the total sum of all the osmotically active substances. This is detected by **osmosensors** of the **medial hypothalamus**, which is connected to the 3rd ventricle and thus to both, the blood and the cerebrospinal fluid. An increase in osmolarity by only 1–2%, is already enough to induce the release of ADH from the posterior pituitary lobe via neuronal efferents, which causes the osmolarity to decrease again through increased reabsorption of water in the kidney. The exact identity of the central osmosensors is still unknown.

Control through the composition of ingested food

Humoral control also includes regulation of the release of messengers through the **concentration of substances in ingested feed**, which has an important role in regulating secretion of gastrointestinal hormones. This is also known as **intestinal chemosensitivity**.

Ghrelin can be secreted along the entire gastrointestinal tract, but the main site of production is the **gastric mucosa**. In addition, ghrelin synthesis also occurs in the pan-

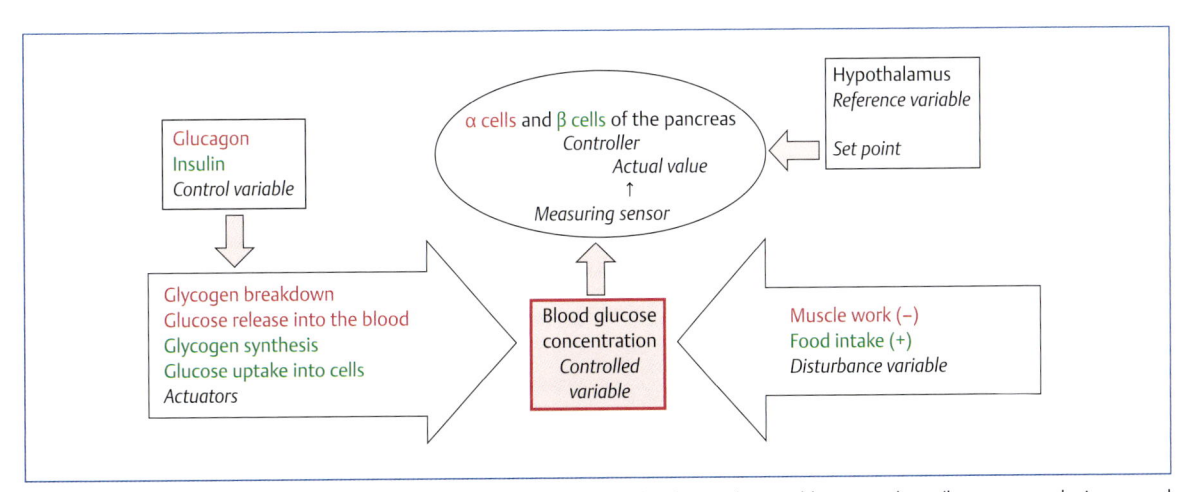

Fig. 23.9 Regulation of blood glucose concentration, as an example of a biochemical control loop: regulator (hormone-producing α- and β-cells of the pancreas), manipulated variable (e.g. insulin and glucagon), actuators (e.g. activity of enzymes and transport systems), controlled variable (extracellular glucose concentration), sensor (K^+_{ATP} channel), disturbance variable (e.g. muscle work or food intake), reference variable (hypothalamus).

Endocrinology, reproduction

creas, lungs, gonads, adrenal cortex, placenta and kidney. It is a hormone involved in (p.521) the regulation of food intake. The name is derived from the term "GH-releasing hormone" and thus describes another important function of ghrelin: it stimulates the secretion of growth hormone (GH (p.544)) during periods of fasting or food restriction. The gastric content also controls secretion of **somatostatin** from the D-cells of the gastric mucosa. The stimulus for this is a **drop in the pH** of the stomach contents. Somatostatin counteracts this drop by inhibiting the release of **gastrin** from the G-cells of the stomach. Gastrin stimulates the parietal cells of the gastric mucosa to secrete hydrochloric acid. The G-cells, in turn, are controlled (p.413) not only neurogenically via the gastrin-releasing peptide produced by parasympathetic neurons, but also by **amino acids** and **peptides** in the stomach contents (p.413).

This principle of chemosensitivity continues in the proximal small intestine. Here, a low **pH** leads to the release of **secretin** from the S-cells, which induces enrichment of pancreatic juice and bile with bicarbonate, and also has an inhibitory effect on the G-cells, similar to that of somatostatin. Secretin also delays gastric emptying. In contrast, the onward transport of ingesta into the intestine is promoted by **motilin** from the duodenal M cells, released in response to high concentrations of **free fatty acids** and **bile acids** along with **low concentrations** of **amino acids** and **glucose**. An increase in the concentration of long-chain **fatty acids** and some **amino acids** alone, leads to the secretion of **cholecystokinin** (CCK) from the I cells. CCK stimulates pancreatic secretion and gallbladder contraction, delays gastric emptying and stimulates vagal afferents in the intestinal wall and portal vein. CCK is also found in the central nervous system and plays a role in the regulation of food intake.

Carbohydrate- and fat-rich meals lead to the release of **GIP** (glucose-dependent insulinotropic polypeptide, also called gastric inhibitory polypeptide), **GLP-1** and **GLP-2** (glucagon-like peptide), **oxyntomodulin** and **peptide YY** from the L-cells of the distal small intestine. The incretins GIP and GLP-1 mainly increase glucose-dependent insulin secretion from pancreatic β-cells, while GLP-2 is a growth factor. Oxyntomodulin and peptide YY produce a feeling of satiety. Peptide YY also inhibits gastric emptying ("ileum brake" (p.385)).

MORE DETAILS

Incretin therapy of diabetes mellitus type 2

In human medicine, a long-acting GLP-1 analogue has been used since 2005 in the treatment of type 2 diabetes mellitus, i.e. so-called insulin-independent diabetes, which is associated with disorders of insulin secretion and sensitivity. It has also been used, in combination with insulin preparations, in treatment of cats. Since GLP-1 does not increase insulin secretion per se, but rather, depending on blood glucose concentration, it facilitates the appropriate response to insulin, so that the risk of a dangerous drop in blood glucose concentration from insulin therapy is avoided.

■ Control through mechanical stimuli

Mechanical stimuli can also lead to the release of hormones. This applies to myocytes of the right atrium, where increased **stretch** most likely leads to activation of **cation channels**, which in turn results in depletion of **ANP** (atrial natriuretic peptide)-filled vesicles. The main function of ANP is long-term regulation of blood pressure by inhibiting renal reabsorption of Na and thus also of water from the glomerular filtrate. In contrast to the regulators of mean arterial blood pressure, the action of ANP is a regulator of variable intravascular volume, see ch. 8. The strain-sensitive cells in the right atrium thus serve as sensors for **central venous pressure**.

ADH (antidiuretic hormone) is also controlled by stretching in the right atrium. However here, the site of stimulation and the site of release are not identical. Distension of the right atrium is detected by **B receptors** during the filling phase, and the signal is then transmitted by **vagal afferents** to the **hypothalamus**, which controls the release of ADH from the posterior pituitary. Reduced distension leads to stimulation of ADH secretion and thus to an increase in renal water reabsorption (Gauer-Henry reflex (p.191)).

Induction of the secretion of **oxytocin** from the posterior pituitary lobe is similar. Mechanical stimulation of the vagina or the mammary teats is transmitted via sensory afferents and the spinal cord. The secretion of oxytocin causes contraction of the uterus and thus expulsion of the foetus (p.571), or contraction of the myoepithelial (basket) cells in the mammary gland, and thus the ejection of milk (p.613).

■ Endocrine rhythms

Many physiological functions of an animal are subject to **periodic changes**. This applies, for example, not only to the core body temperature, which is lower at night than during the day in diurnal animals, but also to the release of various hormones. The mechanisms already mentioned, which control plasma concentrations by feedback regulation, maintain an equilibrium by modifying internal variables. In contrast, **endocrine rhythms** serve to **release hormones without preceding changes in the internal milieu**, to enable an animal to make longer term adaptations to the changing seasons or to its activity associated with the time of day. This applies to control of both, reproduction and metabolism, and as a protective mechanism to prevent wide fluctuations in homeostasis caused by varying external and internal factors over the course of a day.

Circadian secretion rhythms have a **periodicity of about 24 hours**. Such regular fluctuations apply to cortisol concentration in plasma of various species and to aldosterone-dependent excretion of soft faeces in animals which demonstrate caecotrophy.

Rhythms that depend on the light/dark phase or on the seasonal increase or decrease in the length of daylight are controlled by complex interactions of various neurogenic signals and hormones, and periodic changes in the responsiveness of their target cells in the central nervous system, some of which are still poorly understood. The **pineal** (pineal gland; pineal organ) plays a decisive role in this process. In dark phases, the **suprachiasmatic nucleus of** the hypothalamus stimulates the pineal gland to release **melatonin,** which is synthesised from tryptophan via serotonin. This secretion is inhibited during exposure to light. Melatonin is also used in human medicine to support the synchronisation of circadian rhythms that are disturbed by shift work, movement between geographical time zones, or complete blindness.

Melatonin also influences seasonal endocrine rhythms. Sheep, with an average mammalian gestation length, typically mate in autumn (**"short day breeders"**), and their fertility can be improved by administering melatonin. Smaller mammals with very short gestations, and species with very long gestations, mate in spring (**"long day breeders"** e.g. rabbits, horses), so that the production of offspring coincides with the time of optimum feed availability. This **seasonality** of reproduction is controlled by secretion of gonadotrophin-releasing hormone from the hypothalamus. The subsequent secretion of gonadotrophins increases or decreases the response of the gonads. Outside the mating season, females stop cycling (seasonal anoestrus). In male deer, for example, the size of the testicles decreases significantly due to reduced endocrine stimulation. More details can be found in ch. 21 (p. 511).

> ### IN A NUTSHELL !
>
> The secretion of hormones from the thyroid gland, the adrenal cortex and the gonads is controlled by neuro-endocrine axes, i.e. by the influence of higher-level hormones from the hypothalamus and the pituitary gland. Humoral control is when changes in the composition of body fluids stimulate or inhibit the secretion of a hormone. Mechanical stimuli, such as dilation of the right atrium, can also control the secretion of hormones. Feedback mechanisms always apply. The changes in a hormone-controlled variable, such as the blood concentration of a downstream hormone, can have a direct or indirect effect on the secretion of the hormone which regulates it. There are also so-called endocrine rhythms that independently modulate the secretion of hormones, according to the time of day or the season.

23.1.6 Diagnostics and therapy

Some hormones (e.g. FSH, LH, GH) are not released (p. 539) continuously but have a pulsatile pattern of secretion (p. 539) (ch. 24 (p. 553)). For others, (e.g. cortisol) the release is subject to a circadian rhythm (p. 542) (ch. 21 (p. 511)). Because of these **dynamic variations,** the significance of a hormone concentration at any single point in time is often limited. In addition, endocrine disorders often involve a **decoupling or insufficiency of the regulatory circuits,** so that diagnosis of such diseases requires more than a single measurement of hormone concentration.

For example, in suspected **hypofunction of the adrenal cortex** (Addison's disease), a diagnosis cannot be made just on the current concentrations of gluco- and mineralocorticoids in blood. When an animal shows clinical signs of adrenal insufficiency, which may be quite variable and relatively non specific, an **ACTH-stimulation test** could be performed. This would involve first taking a basal blood sample, and then another sample one hour after administering a synthetic analogue of pituitary tropin. The cortisol value should not only be in the standard reference range, but should also have increased significantly after ACTH stimulation of the adrenal cortex. It may also be necessary to determine other messengers involved in regulation (e.g. Cushing's syndrome, see below) in order to clarify clinical pictures that can be traced back to a chronic increase in a particular hormone.

> **MORE DETAILS**
>
> ### Cushing's syndrome in dogs
>
> Cushing's syndrome, one of the most common endocrinological disorders of dogs, is a summation of all the clinical signs associated with a chronically increased concentration of glucocorticoids in blood, regardless of whether the glucocorticoids are endogenous or exogenously supplied. Because of the role of glucocorticoids on intermediary metabolism (p. 547), an increase in blood glucose concentration leads to polyuria and polydipsia, i.e. increased urination and fluid intake, muscle breakdown, truncal obesity and hair coat and skin changes. In the majority of clinical cases, an ACTH-producing tumour of the adenohypophysis is the cause of the persistent activation of this stress axis. When there is ACTH-dependent hypercortisolism, increased plasma concentrations of ACTH are detectable, in addition to increased cortisol levels, which cannot be lowered by administration of synthetic glucocorticoids (dexamethasone suppression test). However, the cause of Cushing's syndrome can also be an ACTH-independent increase in the production of cortisol by a tumour of the adrenal cortex. In this case, elevated cortisol, but low ACTH plasma concentrations would typically be found. Differentiation of these two types of hypercortisolism is necessary in determining treatment. Iatrogenic Cushing's syndrome can develop as a side effect of exogenously supplied glucocorticoids, such as in treatment of allergic diseases.

Because exogenously supplied hormones, or their analogues, influence the endocrine regulatory circuits, in any **therapy with endocrine messengers,** the effect of such interactions must be considered. For example, the use of glucocorticoids in high doses over a long period of time, inhibits the secretion of CRH, ACTH and endogenously produced cortisol via **Fig. 23.8.** If such drugs are suddenly discontinued, there is a temporary insufficiency of the stress axis, as the body's own production must first re-adapt to the changed endocrine state.

Hormone concentrations are usually determined in **peripheral blood plasma.** However, in some clinical conditions, or for special reasons, hormones and their degradation products can also be quantified in **cerebrospinal fluid, urine, milk** or **eggs.** For example, the progesterone content in milk is measured to monitor fertility in dairy cows. Endocrinological techniques can also be used to determine the sex of hatching eggs, to eliminate male chicks before they hatch, thus avoiding the need to kill day-old male chicks. In zoo and wild animals, hormone concentrations, such as those of glucocorticoids can be determined in faeces, to detect stress.

Knowledge of the specific physiology of each species is needed for accurate diagnosis: The plasma concentration of progesterone in the bitch cannot be used for pregnancy diagnosis, because in pseudo-pregnancy, progesterone is still secreted by the corpus luteum, independent of fertilisation. There are considerable differences in endocrine regulation of reproduction, between various species of domestic mammals (ch. 24 (p. 553)).

> **IN A NUTSHELL** !
>
> For diagnosis and therapy, it is important to know the species differences in physiological feedback loops, and in the chemical properties of the hormones being used or analysed, their secretion patterns, which can be continuous, pulsatile or characterised by an endocrine rhythm.

Suggested reading

Bertin F-R, Fraser NS. Equine Endocrinology. CABI 2020

Feldman EC, Nelson RW, Reusch C et al. Canine and Feline Endocrinology. Elsevier Saunders 2015

Squires EJ. Applied Animal Endocrinology. 2nd ed., CABI 2010

23.2 Special endocrinology

Alexandra Muscher-Banse, Mirja Wilkens

> **ESSENTIALS** ✖
>
> Hormones are involved in homeostasis, i.e. the regulatory mechanisms for maintaining internal equilibrium, in which the short-term control of vital functions (e.g. constant blood glucose concentration) is by a control loop with regulators, sensors, actuators and manipulated variables. Hormones are also important in homeorhesis, the coordinated control of metabolism required for medium- to long-term adaptation to changes in physiological status (pregnancy, lactation, growth).

23.2.1 Introduction

The functional role of endocrine regulatory mechanisms of an animal will now be considered. Control of physiological processes, explained in individual chapters, often cannot be completely separated from one another. This is seen particularly, in the interaction between growth, lactation and intermediary metabolism. The endocrine control of reproductive processes is described in the chapters on Reproduction (ch. 24 (p. 553)) and Lactation (ch. 25 (p. 601)). The regulation of water and electrolyte balance is dealt within the chapters on water and sodium balance (ch. 13.8 (p. 334)) and regulation of blood circulation (ch. 8.5 (p. 208)).

23.2.2 Growth

Growth is defined as the accumulation of body substance that results in an increase in body size and weight. It is an anabolic process that is not limited to the skeleton and musculature, but also includes the development of the various organs. **Anabolic processes** also play an important role in the adult body in **building up, replacing and maintaining functional body substance**. Changing the physical loads of the whole animal or of individual organs, such as by physical training, or in diseases of the respiratory tract, or the pathophysiological load on the heart, can result in pathophysiological growth processes. In addition, **catabolic processes** can predominate in various illnesses, food restriction (particularly pronounced in hibernators), and in reproduction This physiological or pathophysiological mobilisation of existing body substance is usually compensated for by anabolic processes.

Because these are very **complex, dynamic processes**, sufficient energy must be available to **build up body substance**, i.e. for the anabolic metabolic processes. There is also an increased demand for the chemical building blocks of growth such as amino acids, certain fatty acids and minerals. In addition, the different organs and tissues vary in composition and growth rate. The development of bones, for example, has different requirements than the development of muscles. In order to ensure the necessary **flow of nutrients**, there are therefore interactions between the superordinate regulation by the so-called **growth axis** and the systems for **regulating intermediary metabolism, mineral balance and the regulation at the level of individual tissues and cells**. This is partly by specific growth factors, which control an increase in the size of cells (hypertrophy) and a proliferation of cells (hyperplasia). This also enables organ-specific regulation of **nutrient distribution** for simultaneous anabolic processes. This is particularly apparent at the end of pregnancy and during lactation, when the flow of nutrients is first diverted from the uterus to the mammary gland, and then fat and protein are mobilised (p. 545) from the existing body substance (ch. 25.10 (p. 615)).

Growth axis

The increase in body mass and the growth in bone length, and also the redistribution of nutrients during feed restriction and lactation, are regulated by **growth hormone** (GH, growth hormone, somatotropin). The release of GH from the adenohypophysis is in turn under the control of GH-releasing hormone (GH-RH, **somatoliberin)** and **somatostatin** (growth hormone-inhibiting hormone, GH-IH) from the hypothalamus (p. 539). Since growth is optimally adapted to environmental conditions, and depends on the availability of nutrients, the activity of the hypothalamus is under complex control. **Physical activity, sleep** (there is a distinct circadian rhythm), **food restriction, lactation** and **stress**, partly mediated and modified by **thyroid hormones, oestrogen** and **testosterone, glucagon and ghrelin**, as well as a high availability of **amino acids in the plasma** and **low blood glucose levels**, increase the release of

GH-RH, and thus secretion of growth hormone. This in turn leads to increased production of the **somatomedins** IGF-1 and IGF-2 (insulin-like growth factor) in the liver. IGF-1 is of importance for growth, while IGF-2 mainly has a role in embryonic development. The somatomedins not only have specific actions in the peripheral tissues, they also have an inhibitory effect on the release of GH-RH and GH by negative feedback. Other factors that shift the ratio of GR-RH and GH-IH, and **reduce the growth rate**, are a high percentage of body fat and thus a high leptin level, as well as high blood concentrations of glucose and fatty acids. There is hence a close link between growth and intermediary metabolism.

Development of the growing body

Growth in body length takes place in the **growth plates** of the long bones, where ossifying cartilage tissue is being layed down. As soon as the cartilage tissue is completely ossified, the bone loses its ability to increase in length (closure of the growth plates). Under the influence of **GH**, the immature cells in the growth plate produce **IGF-1** which in turn increases the **mitotic rate** of the **chondrocytes** and thus contributes substantially to the increase in bone length. **Protein biosynthesis** is also increased in various tissues – an **anabolic effect** in the muscles, heart, liver, spleen, etc. The half-life of IGF-1 is significantly longer than that of GH, being protected from inactivation by linkage to its specific binding proteins, **IGFBP 1–6** (IGF binding proteins).

Body composition is modified by the simultaneously increasing concentrations of sex-specific steroid hormones during growth. **Testosterone** promotes the development of **muscles**. Thus, by rearing intact boars, higher lean meat percentages can be achieved than by fattening castrates. At the same time, increasing concentrations of testosterone and oestrogen lead to the closure of the growth plates and thus to the termination of growth in body length. Animals castrated before the onset of puberty can therefore reach a greater body height than those that remain intact. The increase in **body fat content** with age and maturity is accompanied by increasing secretion of **leptin**. Leptin leads to a **reduction in food intake**, so that energy intake is adjusted to the adult animal's lower requirements as the rate of body weight increase slows approaching maturity. More details can be found in ch. 19 (p.483) and ch. 22 (p.519).

MORE DETAILS

Use of hormones in fattening

In order to optimise fattening, numerous experiments on the effect of GH in pigs have been carried out since the 1950s, especially in the USA. These studies show that daily weight gain and feed efficiency, (i.e. the food input in relation to weight gain), increase significantly as a result of treatment. At the same time, there is an increase in lean meat content compared to untreated animals due to a reduction in fat and an increase in muscle mass. However, since the meat quality is slightly lower than in untreated pigs, and the peptide hormone cannot be administered orally, it was assumed that this method would not meet with consumer acceptance. Its use in pig fattening has therefore not become established practice.

GH is also not used in cattle fattening. However, to improve feed efficiency and to influence carcass composition, a number of steroid hormones have been approved by the US Food and Drug Administration for use in beef cattle and sheep. Typically, these are depot preparations that are implanted subcutaneously behind the ear, and release the active hormone over a longer period of time than would occur with rapid absorption injection preparations. In the EU, the use of substances with hormonal effects as performance enhancers is prohibited for fattening.

Thyroid axis

The hormones of the thyroid axis are also of great importance for growth and development. During **embryonic development**, especially in the intrauterine development of the nervous system, and also at later stages of foetal growth, the thyroid hormones affect numerous **differentiation processes** in ways that are still not fully understood. They stimulate **protein biosynthesis** and thus anabolic processes, but are also involved in the **maturation** of the intestinal epithelium, lymphocytes, skin, sexual and sensory organs. **Regulation of energy turnover** creates the conditions for the cellular functions that determine growth. An essential mechanism here is the increase in the responsiveness of certain organs to other hormones (permissive effect (p.539)), so that synergistic effects occur. There are also **direct effects** on the activity of the **growth axis**, through stimulation of GH secretion and increased expression of IGF-1 (p.544).

MORE DETAILS

Case report: Congenital hypothyroidism in dogs in the dog

In several litters from a mating with a male of the American Toy Terrier breed, the following were found in some puppies: inactivity, stenosis of the auditory canal, delayed opening of the eyes, hair coat changes, and a developing goitre. The concentrations of T4 in blood were strikingly low, while those of TSH were markedly elevated. Treatment with L-thyroxine led to a clear improvement in the developmental disorders. At the age of eight weeks, imaging the thyroid gland of the affected puppies after administration of radioactive iodine showed that the uptake of iodine was initially greatly increased compared to that in the unaffected animals, but after 24 hours detectable radioactivity had dropped significantly more in the affected pups. Iodine can therefore apparently be absorbed into the thyroid gland but not retained there. After an additional genome analysis, it becomes clear that there was a mutation that disturbed the oxidation of iodide by thyroperoxidase. The resulting insufficient formation of T3 and T4 led to increased TSH levels, and a consequent stimulated uptake of iodine by the thyroid, because the physiological control loop had been interrupted by this malfunction.

Nutrient distribution

Independent of its affect on IGF-1, GH also stimulates **lipolysis** via a tyrosine kinase-associated receptor (p.536), and reduces **glucose utilisation in the periphery**, especially in muscles, by decreasing **sensitivity to insulin**. At the same time, **gluconeogenesis** is also promoted. This increases blood concentrations of free fatty acids, glycerol and glucose, known as a **diabetogenic effect** as these responses are opposite to those of insulin. These functions of GH play a special role during prolonged **fasting**, especially when there is an undersupply of protein, and during **lactation**. In these situations, the **somatotropic axis is uncoupled**, which is associated with high GH levels in the absence of IGF-1 synthesis. Thus, the effects of GH, independent of IGF-1, become predominant. Through this mechanism, the **anabolic and catabolic effects of GH** can be mediated independently, in appropriate adaptation to any particular physiological state.

■ Mammary gland

In the mammary gland, the mammary duct system develops under the influence of **oestrogen**, while the alveolar epithelium, which is capable of secretion, is formed under the influence of **progesterone**. The role of **prolactin** in the onset and maintenance of lactation through differentiation of mammary gland tissue, varies from species to species. In rabbits, the administration of prolactin alone can induce lactation. In ruminants, prolactin is involved in the regulation of **lactation**, in association with **placental lactogen**, **GH**, **insulin**, **thyroid hormones**, and **steroid hormones** (ch. 25 (p. 601)).

> MORE DETAILS
>
> **Use of GH to enhance performance**
> Recombinant bovine somatotropin (bST), i.e. growth hormone produced in bacteria using genetic engineering techniques, is used in the USA to increase performance in dairy farming. Its effect, especially in late lactation, is based on two mechanisms. One is modification of nutrient distribution so that there is less adipose tissue development, and increased mobilisation of fatty acids, to ensure that more nutrients are available for milk production. For the second mechanism, apoptosis of the milk-producing alveolar cells, which occurs naturally in the course of lactation, is counteracted and thus there is less of a decline in milk yield over time. Depending on how this is managed, the milk yield can be increased by 10–25%. This method is not approved in Europe.

23.2.3 Intermediary metabolism

> **IN A NUTSHELL** !
>
> Insulin (from β-cells) and glucagon (from α-cells) are produced in the pancreas. Insulin lowers the blood glucose level by facilitating the uptake of glucose from blood into cells. Glucagon has the opposite effect and increases glucose concentration in blood. Adrenaline, growth hormones, thyroid hormones and cortisol also have blood glucose-increasing effects.

Intermediary metabolism describes the utilisation of substrates in different organs. Catabolic and anabolic metabolic pathways, required for growth, development and reproduction are integrated. Intermediary metabolism provides the chemical energy as **ATP**, needed for biosyntheses as well as for mechanical and osmotic work.

■ Insulin, the blood glucose-lowering hormone

The maintenance of an almost constant blood glucose concentration, and the regulatory mechanisms for this in the various organ systems is a central role of intermediary metabolism. The transporter-mediated uptake of glucose into cells is insulin-dependent in most organs, but not in the brain, intestine, kidney, mammary gland and erythrocytes (**Fig. 23.9**). The secretion of **insulin** from the β-cells of the **pancreas** is determined primarily by the level of blood glucose concentration. The set point can be changed by external factors (**Fig. 23.9**). However, insulin secretion can also be (p. 541) mediated by increased amino acid concentrations in blood, signals from the parasympathetic nervous system, or by intestinal hormones (**incretins**: glucagon-like peptide 1, **GLP-1**) in response to food intake. Thus, the endocrine cells of the pancreas must evaluate and assess input signals from different sources.

The primary target tissues for insulin are the liver, adipose tissue and skeletal muscle, where it stimulates glucose metabolism. In the brain, insulin acts as a satiety signal and thus influences eating behaviour and body weight, in addition to its roles in regulating blood glucose concentration and energy balance.

In some target cells, such as adipose tissue and resting skeletal muscle, insulin enables the vesicles incorporating GLUT4 uniporter to fuse with the cell membrane, thus stimulating the uptake of glucose into cells and lowering the concentrations of glucose in blood. Insulin is the only hormone capable of doing this. Incorporation of GLUT4 uniporters into the cell membranes of contracting skeletal muscle cells also occurs by an insulin-independent mechanism. Hence increased physical exercise can be used as an important non-pharmacological intervention to improve glycaemic control in obese and diabetic patients. Both Ca^{2+} and P_i are considered here as intracellular control signals.

In liver cells, insulin does not directly regulate the uptake of glucose from blood (ch. 17 (p. 463)), but it does influence it by ensuring that the concentration of free intracellular glucose is low. Insulin activates hepatic hexokinase, the enzyme that phosphorylates glucose to glucose-6-phosphate, so that glucose continuously diffuses into cells via GLUT2 uniporters. When the blood glucose concentration decreases, insulin secretion (**negative feedback signal**) from the pancreas ceases. Insulin-dependent glucose uptake into fat cells and striated muscle cells via GLUT4 uniporters is thus inhibited, to ensure the availability of blood glucose for obligate glucose-dependent tissues such as the brain, renal medulla or erythrocytes. In these tissues, metabolic energy cannot be obtained from the oxidative breakdown of fats. To increase glucose concentrations in blood, glucose from the breakdown of glycogen and from amino acids (gluconeogenesis), can diffuse out of hepatocytes via insulin-independent GLUT2 uniporters in the liver when insulin levels are low. If blood glucose concentrations drop further (severe hypoglycaemia), there is no longer enough glucose available to the brain. This leads to seizures, coma or death.

In addition to stimulating glycolysis, insulin activates enzymes of glycogenesis and, in the liver (p. 463), it inhibits glycogenolysis as well as gluconeogenesis. In adipose tissue, insulin inhibits lipolysis (p. 478) and promotes the formation of triacylglycerol (p. 479). In addition to the increased uptake of glucose into skeletal muscle, insulin promotes protein synthesis (p. 145). Under the influence of insulin, glucose, fatty acids and amino acids are taken up by muscle, fat, and liver cells to stimulate anabolic metabolic pathways. If there is a lack of insulin, these cells switch to catabolic metabolism.

■ Glucagon, a blood glucose-increasing hormone

The counter-regulatory hormone systems react in proportion to the degree of any decline in blood glucose concentration. In the postabsorptive state, when the concentration of glucose in blood begins to decrease, insulin secretion slows down, and the secretion of the peptide hormone **glucagon** from the **pancreatic α-cells** is stimulated to counteract hypoglycaemia. Glucagon is the most important antagonist of insulin, so that the ratio of insulin to glucagon determines the direction of metabolism (anabolic versus catabolic).

In the liver, glucagon activates the phosphorylation of glycogen phosphorylase via **cAMP** which is responsible for the breakdown of glycogen, whereas glycolysis is inhibited. At the same time, glucagon stimulates the de novo synthesis of glucose from amino acids, to increase blood glucose concentration (ch. 17 (p. 463)), (**Fig. 23.9**). This provides a **negative feedback signal** to the pancreas and thus inhibits glucagon secretion. In adipose tissue, glucagon promotes lipolysis, β-oxidation of fatty acids, and the formation of ketone bodies, while inhibiting lipogenesis (ch. 18.2.1 (p. 478)). In skeletal muscle, glucagon stimulates proteolysis to provide required free amino acids. However, in contrast to the liver, glucagon has no influence on the breakdown of muscle glycogen, and glycolysis is not stimulated in muscle.

The release of glucagon is also stimulated by amino acids in the plasma. A protein-containing, low-carbohydrate diet (e.g. in cats) leads to a secretion of insulin under the influence of the amino acids absorbed from protein digestion, and thus to a drop in glucose concentration in blood. Theoretically, the brain and the erythrocytes would be threatened with an undersupply of glucose, as no energy reserves can be stored here. However, the simultaneous release of glucagon, stimulated by the increasing concentration of amino acids in blood, prevents this hypoglycaemia by promoting the glucose release mechanisms (glycogenolysis and gluconeogenesis) in the liver.

■ Adrenaline, growth hormone and cortisol – other blood glucose-increasing hormones

Normally, the function of insulin and glucagon maintains a constant glucose concentration in blood. When there is an increased energy demand, such as in hard work, stress, or hunger, other hormones come into play as counterparts of insulin. In addition to the secretion of glucagon, **adrenaline** is also secreted from the **adrenal medulla** through the activation of sympathetic nerve fibres. Adrenaline acts on the liver, adipose tissue and muscles to mobilise energy reserves to raise the lowered blood glucose concentrations again. In the liver, adrenaline stimulates glycogen breakdown and gluconeogenesis (p. 470), and in adipose tissue, lipolysis (ch. 18.2.1 (p. 478)). In muscle, adrenaline increases glycogen breakdown to generate ATP for muscle contraction, while simultaneously inhibiting proteolysis.

Stimulation of the secretion of **growth hormone** from the pituitary gland occurs when the concentration of blood glucose falls below a certain threshold. Growth hormone is anabolically active. It stimulates gluconeogenesis as well as protein synthesis in the liver, and it inhibits glucose utilisation so that blood glucose concentration increases again (ch. 17 (p. 463)). In adipose tissue, growth hormone causes the release of fatty acids into blood (ch. 18.2.1 (p. 478)). In muscle, growth hormone facilitates the uptake of amino acids and stimulates protein synthesis.

If the glycogen stores are low for a prolonged period of time, and blood glucose concentrations continue to fall, there is activation of the **stress axis** through **ACTH**, and thus the release of **cortisol** from the adrenal cortex. Cortisol stimulates the breakdown of proteins in muscles and thus provides amino acids for gluconeogenesis in the liver (ch. 17 (p. 463)). At the same time, cortisol inhibits the uptake of glucose into cells and increases the cleavage of triacylglycerols in adipose tissue (lipolysis, ch. 18.2.1 (p. 478)) to increase the level of fatty acids in blood. All insulin antagonists (glucagon, adrenaline, growth hormone and cortisol) have the function of bringing the reduced blood glucose concentrations back into the physiological range.

■ Insulin secretion in ruminants

In ruminants, the secretion of insulin is primarily controlled by the concentrations of short-chain fatty acids, especially propionate, and less by the blood glucose concentration, which is quite low in ruminants, even after feed intake (approx. $3.3 \, \mathrm{mmol \cdot l^{-1}}$ in cattle and approx. $2.8 \, \mathrm{mmol \cdot l^{-1}}$ in sheep). In regulating intermediary metabolism, insulin is only of minor importance in ruminants compared to monogastric animals.

■ Biological half-lives

The approximate half-life of insulin in humans is five minutes, in dogs three minutes, in horses five minutes and in sheep 14 minutes. Insulin is inactivated and degraded in the liver and kidney by glutathione-insulin transhydrogenase. Glucagon is degraded in the liver after a biological half-life of about 4–6 minutes. Adrenaline has a plasma half-life of 1–3 minutes. The enzymes catechol-O-methyltransferase (COMT) and monoamine oxidase (MAO) are involved in the breakdown of adrenaline. Growth hormones have a biological half-life of 10–60 minutes and are broken down in the kidney by hepatic peptidases. The half-life of the steroid hormone cortisol is about 90 minutes. Inactivation takes place in the liver.

The effects of hormones with short half-lives are more readily apparent, than those of hormones with long half-lives. Hormones with long half-lives are less subject to fluctuations in their blood concentrations than those with short half-lives.

MORE DETAILS

Diabetes mellitus

Diabetes mellitus is a group of metabolic defects in the pancreatic endocrine system. Typical findings are enormously high blood glucose levels (hyperglycaemia), which are a result of an absolute or relative lack of insulin, or an insulin insensitivity of the insulin receptors.

In type 1 diabetes, there is an absolute lack of insulin, caused by the destruction of the pancreatic β-cells. In most cases, type 1 diabetes is an autoimmune disease in which the the β-cells are mistakenly classified as "foreign to the body" and the response is to destroy them with antibodies and white blood cells.

A functional insulin deficiency is present in type 2 diabetes, which is also called insulin-resistant diabetes. In this case, sufficient insulin is available, sometimes even at an elevated level. Often the sensitivity of the receptors for insulin is reduced. A so-called receptor desensitisation occurs, or else there are defects in the receptor or in the cellular signal transmission from the receptor.

Despite hyperglycaemia, the cells in diabetes mellitus are deficient in glucose. For energy production, there is now increased β-oxidation of fatty acids and formation of ketone bodies, which are metabolised by extrahepatic tissues (cardiac and skeletal muscle, renal cortex and brain) as alternative energy sources. In addition, glycogen breakdown in the liver is stimulated, as is gluconeogenesis, and even more glucose is released into the blood. The concentration of glucose in blood continues to rise, resulting in the typical symptoms of type 1 or type 2 diabetes: glucosuria, polyuria and polydipsia. Excretion of glucose (glucosuria) in the urine occurs because the tubular maximum for transporter-mediated reabsorption of glucose (p. 323) is exceeded. Because of the high concentration of glucose in the ultrafiltrate, polyuria (osmotic diuresis) occurs because osmotically active glucose in the tubule prevents water reabsorption. This leads to the expression of a massive feeling of thirst in the nucleus supraopticus of the hypothalamus.

Type 1 diabetes is very rare in cats, but the most common form of diabetes in dogs. Cats often suffer from type 2 diabetes. Diabetes mellitus that is not treated or is inadequately treated, leads to kidney failure, neuropathies, infarctions and also blindness.

23.2.4 Calcium and phosphate balance

The regulation of calcium and phosphate balance is mainly under the control of parathyroid hormone (PTH), calcitriol, (the biologically active form of vitamin D hydroxylated at positions 1 and 25), calcitonin from the C-cells of the thyroid gland, and fibroblast growth factor 23 (FGF23) from bone (**Fig. 23.10**).

Calcium and phosphate are the main components of bone mineral as hydroxyapatite and bruschite. Because calcium functions in cells as a second messenger, and is important for muscle contraction, and for blood clotting, a constant calcium concentration in the blood is of considerable importance for many physiological processes and is therefore subject to strict control. Phosphate is involved in chemical energy transfer (e.g. ATP) and in information-bearing molecules (nucleotides), as well as being a significant factor in the regulation of intracellular pH (p. 351). The concentrations of phosphate in blood fluctuate within a wider physiological range than those of calcium.

■ Parathyroid hormone

Depending on blood pH and blood protein concentration, about 55% of calcium in the blood is in the free, i.e. non-protein-bound, ionised form (Ca^{2+}). A decrease in the concentration of Ca^{2+} leads to the release of the peptide hormone PTH (p. 541) in the parathyroid gland. In monogas-

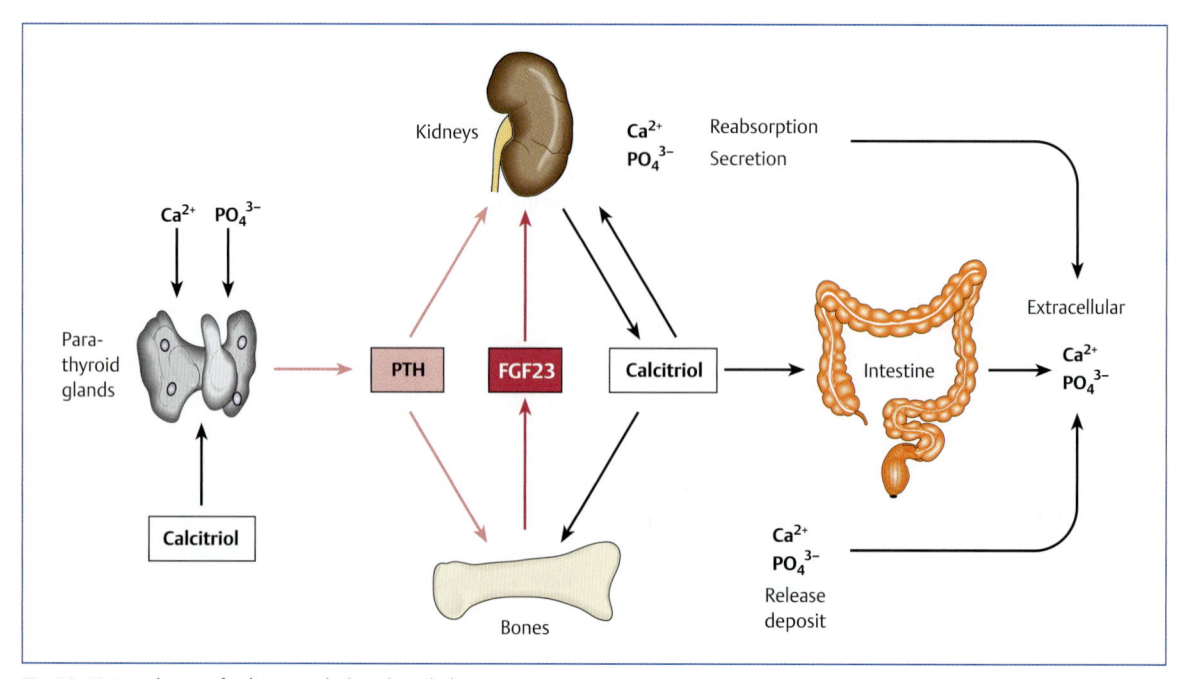

Fig. 23.10 Regulation of calcium and phosphate balance.

tric animals, PTH leads to an increase in the renal resorption of calcium and excretion of phosphate. In ruminants, these effects are quantitatively of secondary importance.

In all animals, however, PTH leads to the mobilisation of calcium and phosphate from bone through the activation of osteoclasts. RANK (receptor activator of NFκB) is expressed on the surface of immature osteoclasts. When RANK and RANKL (receptor activator of NFκB ligand) interact, a signalling cascade is induced that leads to the differentiation and maturation of osteoclasts, and thus to bone resorption. This process is limited by OPG (osteoblast-derived soluble decoy receptor). Just like RANK, OPG can also bind RANKL, but the interaction does not lead to increased stimulation of bone resorption. Rather, OPG serves as a kind of bait trap to keep the concentration of RANKL low in the vicinity of RANK-expressing osteoclasts. The resorption and formation processes on the skeleton are thus ultimately dependent on the balance of RANK, RANKL and OPG. That PTH decreases the secretion of OPG and increases that of RANKL has been shown both in vitro and in vivo.

Another important function of PTH is the stimulation of calcitriol (1,25-(OH)2D3, 1α,25-dihydroxyvitamin D3) formation (p. 322) from calcidiol through activation of 1α-hydroxylase in the kidney **Fig. 23.11**).

■ Calcitriol

Vitamin D_3 as well as the fungus-derived form, vitamin D_2, found on plants (e.g. hay) can be obtained from food, but mainly vitamin D_3 is obtained from synthesis in skin from exposure to UV radiation. This process differs in various animal species. In carnivores, especially the cat, cutaneous production is very low, presumably an evolutionary adaptation to a carnivorous diet which supplies vitamin D, calcium and phosphorus. The comparatively low vitamin D synthesis in the skin of New World camelids also represents an adaptation to their natural habitat in the high altitudes of South America, where intensive UV radiation ensures that the synthesis in skin is still sufficient to meet requirements. In Europe these animals often suffer from vitamin D deficiency during the winter months.

The action of the biologically active form, the steroid hormone calcitriol (1,25-dihydroxycholecalciferol, 1,25-(OH)₂D), is implemented after binding to the intracellular vitamin D receptor (VDR). Calcitriol is the doubly hydroxylated form of vitamin D. The first hydroxylation at position 25 takes place by various enzymes in the liver, and is almost unregulated. The concentration of the resulting calcidiol (25-hydroxycholecalciferol, 25-OHD) in blood, thus depends on the supply of vitamin D so that its blood concentration can be used as an indicator for the vitamin D status of an individual. The second hydroxylation at position 1, takes place in the kidney by the 1α-hydroxylase, which is stimulated by PTH. A connection to the growth axis arises via the likewise stimulating effect of IGF-1 (p. 544). 1α-Hydroxylase is inhibited by Ca^{2+}, FGF23 and calcitriol itself, in the sense of a negative feedback. These factors also initiate the inactivation of vitamin D metabolites by hydroxylation at position 24 to 1,24,25-(OH)₃ D and 24,25-(OH)₂ D. All vitamin D metabolites are mainly bound (p. 533) to plasma proteins, particularly to the vitamin D-binding protein, and with lower affinity to albumin.

Calcitriol induces the expression of calcium transport proteins in the intestinal tract and distal tubule, so that the absorption of calcium from the ingesta and reabsorption from the ultrafiltrate are increased, with a resultant rise in blood calcium concentration (p. 435). The regulatory mechanism for the active absorption of calcium from the rumen in ruminants has not yet been identified, but it is most likely not controlled (p. 407) by calcitriol.

In addition, calcitriol is involved in bone metabolism. While the observed anabolic effect of calcitriol on bone seems to depend on an adequate supply of calcium from the diet, and is thus probably due to increased intestinal absorption of calcium, and mobilisation of bone mineral

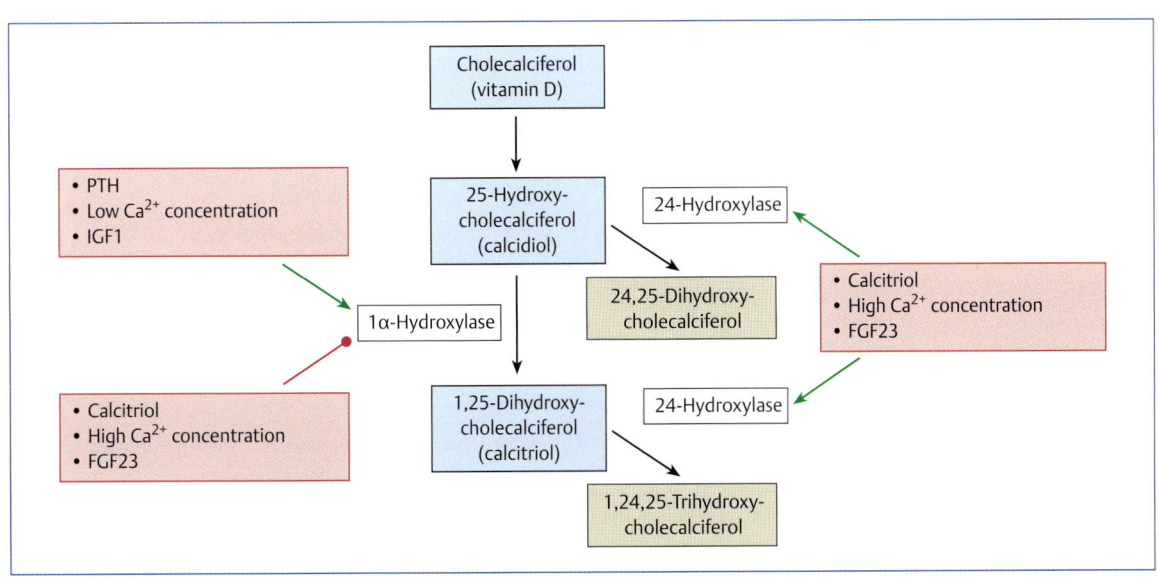

Fig. 23.11 Vitamin D metabolism. Explanations in the text.

when calcium supply is limited. Calcitriol, like PTH, promotes the differentiation and maturation of osteoclasts and can thus cause mobilisation of calcium from the skeleton. This process is also mediated by an increased expression of RANKL and a reduced secretion of OPG (p. 549). In the parathyroid gland, calcitriol inhibits the transcription of PTH.

■ Calcitonin

The secretion of the peptide hormone calcitonin (32 amino acids) from the parafollicular C cells of the thyroid gland is stimulated by increased calcium concentrations in blood and is inhibited by falling calcium levels. Calcitonin is considered an antagonist of PTH because it has a calcium-lowering effect. In bone, calcitonin has an inhibitory effect on the activity of osteoclasts after binding to calcitonin receptors, so that calcium release is inhibited and less bone mineral is mobilised.

■ Fibroblast growth factor 23

Fibroblast growth factor 23 (FGF23) is mainly produced by osteocytes in bone tissue. The synthesis of FGF23 is stimulated by increased phosphate concentrations in blood and also by calcitriol. FGF23 acts as a phosphatonin in the kidney by stimulating renal excretion of phosphate after binding to FGF receptors, which form receptor complexes together with Klotho co-receptors. At the same time, FGF23 stimulates the reabsorption of calcium in the distal tubule

of the kidney and inhibits the synthesis of renal 1α-hydroxylase and thus the production of calcitriol.

MORE DETAILS

Hyperparathyroidism

In hyperparathyroidism, the secretion of PTH from the parathyroid glands is persistently increased. A distinction is made between primary and secondary hyperparathyroidism.

In primary hyperparathyroidism, the increased uncontrolled PTH secretion is usually caused by an adenoma in the parathyroid gland. Inhibition of PTH secretion by rising blood calcium concentrations is absent. This type of disease occurs very rarely and mostly affects older animals.

Secondary hyperparathyroidism results from persistently low blood calcium concentrations. In most cases, the cause of the low calcium level is chronic kidney disease, and thus reduced hydroxylation of calcidiol to calcitriol, or malnutrition during growth. Incorrectly composed BARF rations ("biologically species-appropriate raw feeding") with a high meat content without appropriate additions of mineral feeds or bone meal lead to secondary hyperparathyroidism and corresponding abnormalities in the skeleton, with reduced bone mineralisation, especially in puppies.

23.2.5 Summary of the primary sites of origin and major effects of various hormones

Table 23.2 gives an overview of different hormones, their sites of origin and main effects.

Table 23.2 Overview of the different hormones according to place of origin and effects.

Place of origin	Hormone	Major effects	Regulated physiological processes
Epiphysis	Melatonin	Influencing the hypothalamus	Endocrine rhythms, sleep
Hypothalamus	CRH	Release of ACTH, β-endorphins and α-MSH from the pituitary gland.	Adaptation to stress, water balance, regulation of intermediary metabolism
	GH-RH, GH-IH	Stimulation or inhibition of the release of GH from the pituitary gland.	Growth, lactation, regulation of intermediary metabolism
	TRH	Release of TSH from the pituitary gland	Regulation of energy turnover, growth and development
	GnRH	Release of FSH and LH from the pituitary gland	Development, reproduction
Adenohypophysis	ACTH	Release of glucocorticoids from the adrenal cortex	Adaptation to stress, regulation of intermediary metabolism, water balance
	β-Endorphins	Modulation of the sensation of pain	Adaptation to loads
	α-MSH	Reduction of feed intake, stimulation of melanocytes	Regulation of feed intake, pigmentation of the skin
	GH	Formation of IGF-1 in the liver, stimulation of protein biosynthesis, lipolysis, increase in blood glucose concentration.	Growth, lactation, regulation of intermediary metabolism
	TSH	Release of T3 and T4 from the thyroid gland	Regulation of energy turnover, growth and development
	FSH	Ovary: follicle maturation, oestrogen synthesis Testis: sperm maturation	Development, reproduction

Table 23.2 continued

Place of origin	Hormone	Major effects	Regulated physiological processes
	LH	Ovary: Ovulation, development of the corpus luteum, oestrogen and progestogen synthesis (progesterone) Testis: Androgen synthesis (testosterone)	Development, reproduction
	Prolactin	Development of the mammary gland, influence on the reproductive process	Reproduction, lactation
Neurohypophysis	ADH	Increase in renal water reabsorption, vasoconstriction in high concentrations.	Water balance and osmoregulation, circulatory regulation
	Oxytocin	Contractions of the myometrium and myoepithelia on the alveolar cells, brood care behaviour	Reproduction, lactation
Adrenal cortex	Glucocorticoids (cortisol)	Increase of blood glucose concentration, inhibition of protein biosynthesis, immunomodulation	Adaptation to stress, regulation of intermediary metabolism
	Mineralocorticoids (aldosterone)	Increase of renal and intestinal Na and water reabsorption, decrease of K reabsorption	Water balance, circulation regulation
Adrenal medulla	Catecholamines (adrenaline and noradrenaline)	Alertness and performance through effects on heart and respiratory rate, changes in blood flow, increase in blood glucose concentration, etc.	Adaptation to stress, regulation of intermediary metabolism, circulatory regulation
Liver	IGF-1	Stimulation of protein biosynthesis, longitudinal growth of the bone, growth factor, e.g. in the mammary gland.	Growth, lactation, regulation of intermediary metabolism
	Angiotensin (activation in the lungs)	Vasoconstriction, stimulation of the release of aldosterone	Water balance, circulation regulation
	Thrombopoietin	Stimulation of thrombocyte production	Blood clotting
Thyroid gland	T3, T4	Increase in the responsiveness of tissues to other hormones (permissive effect), uncoupling of the respiratory chain in adipose tissue.	Regulation of energy metabolism, thermoregulation, growth and development
C cells of the thyroid gland	Calcitonin	Inhibition of osteoclasts	Bone metabolism, Ca and P_i balance
Ovary (follicle)	Oestrogen	Growth and differentiation of the female reproductive organs including the mammary gland, control of the sexual cycle	Development, reproduction, lactation
	Inhibin	Inhibition of FSH secretion	Reproduction, control of the sexual cycle
Ovary (corpus luteum) and placenta	Progestogens (progesterone)	Growth and differentiation of the female reproductive organs including the mammary gland, control of the sexual cycle, "pregnancy-protective hormone	Development, reproduction, lactation
Ovary (corpus luteum)	Oxytocin	Stimulation of the synthesis of $PGF_{2\alpha}$ in the endometrium	Reproduction, control of the sexual cycle
Endometrium	$PGF_{2\alpha}$	Luteolysis	Reproduction, control of the sexual cycle
Placenta	Relaxin	Slackening of the pelvic ligaments, opening of the cervix	Reproduction, birth
Mammary gland	PTHrP	Stimulation of the osteoclasts	Lactation, bone metabolism, Ca and P_i balance

Endocrinology, reproduction

Table 23.2 continued

Place of origin	Hormone	Major effects	Regulated physiological processes
Testis (Sertoli cells)	Inhibin	Inhibition of FSH secretion, paracrine influence on spermatogenesis.	Reproduction, sperm maturation
Testis (Leydig cells)	Androgens (testosterone)	Growth and differentiation of the male sex organs, muscle development, sex-specific behaviour, stimulation of Sertoli cells	Development, reproduction, sperm maturation
Parathyroid gland	PTH	Reduction of renal Ca and increase of renal P_i excretion, stimulation of osteoclasts, production of calcitriol	Bone metabolism, Ca and P_i balance
Endocrine pancreas	Insulin	Inhibition of glycogenolysis and gluconeogenesis, stimulation of glucose uptake into insulin-dependent tissues, stimulation of lipogenesis.	Regulation of the intermediary metabolism
	Glucagon	Stimulation of glycogenolysis and gluconeogenesis, inhibition of lipogenesis	Regulation of the intermediary metabolism
	Amylin	Reduction of meal size and frequency	Regulation of feed intake
Heart	ANP, BNP	Increase in Na and water excretion	Water balance, circulation regulation
Kidney	Erythropoietin	Stimulation of erythrocyte production	Adjustment of the oxygen transport capacity of the blood
	Calcitriol	Reduction of renal Ca excretion, increase of intestinal Ca and P_i absorption, stimulation of osteoclasts	Bone metabolism, Ca and P_i balance
Gastrointestinal tract (stomach)	Ghrelin	Stimulation of GH secretion and feed intake	Growth, regulation of feed intake
	Somatostatin	Inhibition of G cells	Regulation of gastric secretion
	Gastrin	Stimulation of the follicular cells	Regulation of gastric secretion
Gastrointestinal tract (proximal small intestine)	Secretin	Stimulation of bicarbonate secretion in pancreas and bile, inhibition of G-cells, delay of gastric emptying	Regulation of gastric secretion and pH in the gastrointestinal tract
	Motilin	Promote gastric emptying	Digestion
	CCK	Stimulation of pancreatic and bile secretion, delay of gastric emptying, reduction of feed intake	Digestion, regulation of feed intake
Gastrointestinal tract (distal small intestine)	GIP, GLP-1	Stimulation of insulin secretion in the endocrine pancreas	Regulation of the intermediary metabolism
	GLP-2	Growth factor with local effect	Development, digestion
	Oxyntomodulin	Reduction of feed intake	Regulation of feed intake
	Peptide YY	Delay of gastric emptying, reduction of feed intake	Digestion, regulation of feed intake
Bones	FGF23	Increase of renal P_i-excretion, inhibition of calcitriol synthesis	Bone metabolism, Ca and P_i balance
Fatty tissue	Leptin	Reduction of feed intake, increase of basal metabolic rate	Regulation of feed intake, regulation of intermediary metabolism
	Adiponectin	Increase insulin sensitivity	Regulation of the intermediary metabolism

Suggested reading

Hewison M, Bouillon R, Giovannucci E et al. Vitamin D. 2017

Judge A, Dodd MS. Metabolism. Understanding Biochemistry 2020; 64(4): 607–647

Kuhn M. Molecular physiology of membrane guanylyl cyclase receptors. Physiol Rev 2016; 96: 751–804

Levin ER, Gardner DG, Samson WK. Natriuretic peptides. New England Journal of Medicine 1998; 339: 321–328

24 Reproduction

Christine Aurich, Jörg Aurich, Almuth Einspanier, Susanne Reitemeier

24.1 Basics of reproduction in domestic mammals

Christine Aurich, Jörg Aurich

ESSENTIALS ✖

- Knowledge of the physiology of the reproductive system is needed to understand malfunctions and diseases of that system. During sex differentiation of an embryo or foetus, defects can develop that affect later health or fertility. Furthermore, comprehensive knowledge of the physiology of mating behaviour, spermatogenesis and fertilisation is required to perform various practical reproductive biotechnologies. This applies in many animal species particularly to artificial insemination, and also increasingly to embryo transfer and associated reproductive techniques, which are now important in the breeding of all domestic animal species.
- Hormones are among the most important signalling molecules in the reproductive process. Knowledge of their physicochemical properties and secretion profiles can be used to modify their specific functions. During the transition from juvenile to adult animals, changes especially in the hypothalamus, lead to puberty. As a result, an animal acquires the ability to reproduce. In the female this is demonstrated by the development of regular oestrous cycles, and in the male by the production of sperm.
- The frequency per year and the duration of oestrous cycles are species-specific. Only during oestrus do females show a readiness to mate, which, like ovulation, is influenced by sex hormones from the maturing follicle, and thus makes mating close to ovulation more likely.
- The control systems of the **oestrous cycle** develop during puberty, and characterise female reproduction. At regular intervals, depending on the species, one or more **endocrine active follicles** mature and provoke a **readiness to mate**. After **ovulation, the granulosa** and **theca cells** differentiate into **lutein cells**, which secrete **progesterone**, the **pregnancy-maintaining hormone**. The life span of the corpus luteum is prolonged during pregnancy by the embryo itself, which as a differentiated foetus, finally also induces its own birth. The physiological regulation of these processes is mediated by finely tuned communication between the **hypothalamus**, **pituitary gland** and **ovary**.
- During pregnancy, the conceptus develops all organs and grows to a size and maturity, typical for each species. The foetus or foetuses, with the help of hormones, signal the mother that they are ready for birth, and thus play a major role in determining the time of parturition. The opening of the reproductive tract, the expulsion of the foetus, and the postpartum changes, all characterise the birth process and are species-specific.

24.1.1 Reproductive hormones, and regulation of their synthesis and secretion

The gonads are under the control of the hypothalamus and pituitary gland. These organs work closely together in the regulation of reproduction in both, male and female animals via neuronal and endocrine mechanisms. The frequently used term **hypothalamus-pituitary-gonadal axis** implies a predominantly hierarchical structure, but in fact regulation of reproduction is based on different, but interconnected regulatory circuits. The most important reproductive signals within these regulatory circuits are either **peptide** or **steroid hormones**.

> **IN A NUTSHELL** !
>
> The central nervous system, pituitary gland and gonads interact through various endocrine regulatory circuits and form a functional unit.

The hypothalamus, in the central nervous system is an important integration centre in reproduction. It processes incoming external and internal information and converts this into either neuronal or endocrine signals. Hypothalamic nuclei, which pass on their "orders" by secreting hormones, consist of highly specialised cells. Because they integrate the properties of neurons and endocrine gland cells, they are called neurosecretory cells. Short-chain peptide hormones (neuropeptides) are synthesised in the region close to the nucleus, and are transported along the axons, stored in the nerve cell terminals and secreted from there into blood. The neurocrine cells of the ganglia in the preoptic region and the mediobasal hypothalamus produce a peptide hormone, **gonadotropin-releasing hormone (GnRH)** which travels via a hypothalamo-pituitary venous portal vein directly to the anterior pituitary (adenohypophysis), where it stimulates the synthesis and release of the gonadotropins: **luteinising hormone (LH)** and **follicle-stimulating hormone (FSH)**.

The secretion of GnRH is pulsatile. The pulse frequency is determined by an anatomically not yet localised timer (pulse generator). Centres in the brain are superordinate to the pulse generator, i.e. they modulate the pulse frequency,

Endocrinology, reproduction

and they register and process stimuli and signals that influence the reproductive process. This information can come from the animal itself (e.g. concentrations of sex steroid hormones during the oestrous cycle or pregnancy in female animals) or it can come from the environment. Environmental factors that influence sexual function via GnRH release can be the season (length of daylight), climate (temperature, humidity), food supply or social status of an animal. In addition, stress factors, such as excessive psychological or physical stress, can also have an effect on GnRH secretion. Since the approximately 1000 GnRH neurons have no receptors for steroid hormones, a steroid hormone signal is first transcribed into a dopamine, adrenaline, or endorphin message before being passed on to the GnRH neurons. The peptide hormone **kisspeptin** belongs to a family of peptide hormones that are all products of the Kiss1 gene. Kisspeptin binds to the G-protein-coupled Kiss1 receptor, also known as GPR54. Among other functions, kisspeptin has been shown to play a role in the regulation of GnRH release at puberty, and also as a mediator of the feedback of sex steroid hormones on GnRH secretion.

> **MORE DETAILS**   Only in the portal system of the pituitary gland does endogenously released GnRH occur in such high concentrations that it can stimulate pituitary gonadotropin release. In the peripheral blood circulation, the concentrations of GnRH are very low due to its short biological half-life of 2–4 minutes, and from its dilution in total blood volume. It is therefore not possible to quantify GnRH in blood samples from the peripheral circulation, for diagnostic purposes in animals with fertility disorders.

The ganglion cells of the hypothalamic nucleus supraopticus and nucleus paraventricularis synthesise two further peptide hormones, oxytocin and antidiuretic hormone (ADH), of which oxytocin has particular relevance for various reproductive functions. The nerve axons of these nuclear regions end in the posterior lobe of the **pituitary gland (neurohypophysis)**, so that the hormones are transported directly via the axons, and stored there. Thus, although oxytocin and ADH are released from the posterior pituitary, they are hormones of hypothalamic origin.

The most important subordinate organ of the hypothalamus is the **pituitary gland**. This is identical in both male and female animals and consists of an anterior lobe **(adenohypophysis)** and a **posterior lobe (neurohypophysis)**. The anterior pituitary lobe consists of various glandular epithelial cells where pituitary hormones are synthesised and stored. The gonadotropins, LH and FSH, are synthesised in the basophilic cells of the anterior pituitary, which are therefore also called gonadotropic cells. Structurally, the gonadotropins are **glycoproteins** LH and FSH, each having two peptide chains, an α- and a β-chain. The α-chains of LH and FSH are identical. The specificity of these two hormones is determined by their β-chains as well as by numerous carbohydrate side chains. FSH and LH are essential for the regulation of gonadal function. Their synthesis and secretion occur identically in male and female animals. However, LH and FSH secretion are subject to quite different control mechanisms.

> **MORE DETAILS**   Only a small percentage of gonadotropic cells synthesise LH or FSH exclusively, and synthesis often occurs side by side in the same cell. Both gonadotropins have a common **basal** (tonic) pattern of secretion, which is **independent** of the GnRH pulses. **LH** is stored in granules in the gonadotropic cells of the pituitary gland, and is released in a pulsatile manner under the influence of GnRH (**Fig. 24.7**, **Fig. 24.11**). Thus, the GnRH pulse frequency directly controls the LH pulse frequency. **FSH**, on the other hand, is not stored in the gonadotropic cells, but is usually secreted continuously into blood as it is being synthesised. FSH synthesis is activated by GnRH pulses, but these have no influence on the pattern of secretion of FSH. Consequently, LH secretion is much more closely coupled to the GnRH pulse frequency than FSH release.
>
> The gonadotropins FSH and LH inhibit their own synthesis and release via a short **feedback loop** which suppresses GnRH secretion. Finally, secreted GnRH also reduces its own synthesis by feedback to its own neurons (**ultra short feedback; Fig. 24.9**).

Gonadotropin. In a female animal, FSH stimulates **follicle growth** and is responsible for the synthesis of **oestrogens** in the **granulosa** cells of the follicle. LH stimulates the maturation of the preovulatory follicle and the oocyte it contains. **Ovulation is** also triggered by LH. After ovulation, LH is responsible for the remodelling of the follicular wall into a corpus luteum and for its maintenance.

In a male animal, LH stimulates the synthesis and secretion of androgens from the steroid hormone-producing Leydig cells of the testis. FSH, on the other hand, controls the function of the Sertoli cells and is essential for the stimulation and maintenance of **spermatogenesis**. FSH has some direct effects on the development of sperm cells. It also stimulates the Sertoli cells to synthesise and secrete other factors that have paracrine and autocrine effects in the regulation of spermatogenesis. These include prolactin, growth hormone and insulin-like growth factor-1 (IGF-1).

Prolactin. Prolactin is a single-chain proteohormone. It is synthesised in the **lactotropic cells of the adenohypophysis**. As with the gonadotropins, different isohormones are produced along with prolactin. These are isohormones with different glycosylation, and others with different lengths of the peptide chain. The synthesis and secretion of prolactin is influenced by sex steroid hormones and the length of daylight, among other factors. In female animals, prolactin is involved in the regulation of growth of the mammary gland during pregnancy and in the induction and maintenance of lactation. In addition, prolactin influences the function of the ovaries, where it can be either inhibitory or stimulatory, depending on the species.

Little is known about the function and importance of prolactin in the reproductive physiology of the male animal. There is evidence that prolactin has a role in the control of testicular and epididymal function, and is involved in the regulation of seasonal changes in gonadal activity in sheep and horses.

> **MORE DETAILS**   The release of prolactin from the pituitary gland is controlled by dopamine which has an inhibitory effect on prolactin secretion and is therefore also called prolactin-inhibiting hormone. A separate hypothalamic releasing hormone for prolactin has not yet been reliably demonstrated, but the application of thyreotropin-releasing hormone (TRH) can experimentally stimulate prolactin secretion.

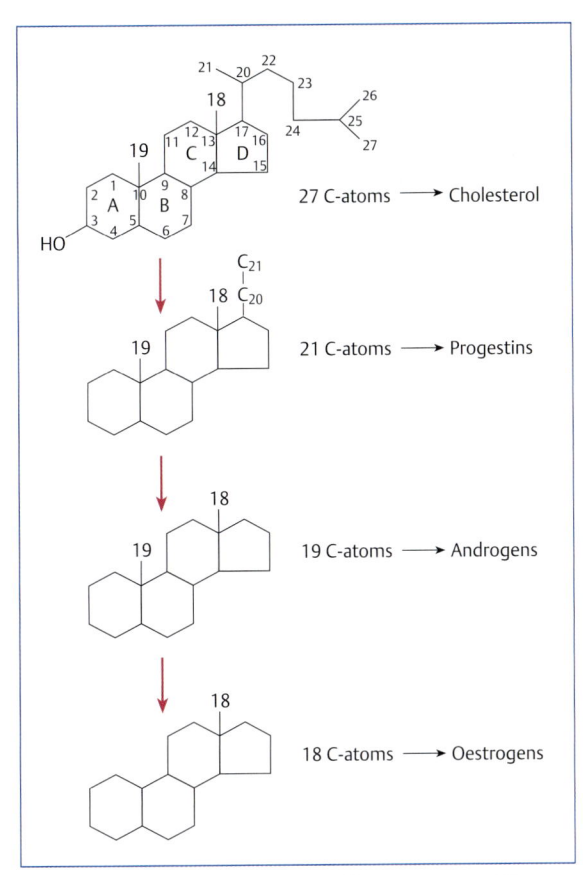

Fig. 24.1 Classification of the sex steroid hormones. Steroid hormones are synthesised from cholesterol. During enzymatic conversion, the number of C atoms can only be reduced, never increased.

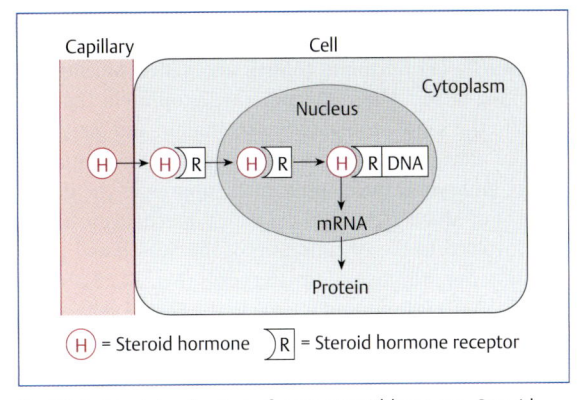

Fig. 24.2 Principle of action of a sex steroid hormone. Steroid hormones enter cells from the blood by diffusion. After binding to a receptor in the cell, the receptor-hormone complex then links to DNA. Steroid hormones activate the transcription of specific genes.

■ Steroid hormones

The **sex steroid hormones** are divided into **three groups** according to the **number of carbon atoms** (**Fig. 24.1**). Their mode of action at the cellular level is shown in **Fig. 24.2**.

In the female animal, reproductively relevant steroid hormones are synthesised in the ovary – the follicles and corpus luteum – and during pregnancy, depending on the species, also in the placenta. In the process, follicles produce various **oestrogens** of which **oestradiol-17β** has the greatest biological potency and significance. It is usually referred to as oestradiol. Of the **progestogens**, progesterone is the most important. The corpus luteum of the various domestic animal species produces **progesterone** exclusively, and only in the horse does the corpus luteum produce other gestagens. In those species in which the maintenance of pregnancy is not only achieved by progesterone of luteal origin, but also by progestogens synthesised in the placenta, progesterone is still the most important progestogen, although other gestagens are also detectable in blood during pregnancy.

In the male animal, androgens and, in some species, oestrogens (in varying concentrations), are **synthesised** and secreted by the testis. In the Leydig cells, **steroid hormones are synthesised** from cholesterol, in a similar manner to the steroid hormones synthesised in the adrenal cortex. The most important product is the C-19 steroid, **testosterone**.

■ Endogenous opioids

In addition to the classical peptide hormones, there are other **peptides** involved in the neurocrine regulation of synthesis and release of reproduction-relevant hormones in the **CNS**. Among these is the group of endogenous opioids, which are subdivided into endorphins, enkephalins and dynorphins. Endogenous opioids modulate the secretion of gonadotropins and, in seasonally cyclic animal species, are mainly inhibitory on the secretion of GnRH, in the corpus luteum phase of the sexual cycle, and during anoestrus.

■ Inhibin and Activin

Inhibin and activin are peptides that belong to the TGF-β (transforming growth factor-β) family. **Inhibin** consists of two subunits connected by disulphide bridges. It exists in two forms: Inhibin A and Inhibin B. In both forms, the α-subunit is identical, while the β-subunit differs.

In the female animal, inhibin is synthesised by the **granulosa cells** of the ovarian follicle, and reaches the anterior pituitary via the bloodstream. There it selectively **inhibits** FSH secretion. In male animals, inhibin is synthesised and secreted by the **Sertoli cells**, under the control of FSH. Inhibin exerts paracrine effects on various stages of spermatogenesis and also regulates the synthesis and secretion of FSH (**Fig. 24.22**).

Activin is also synthesised and secreted by the **granulosa or Sertoli cells**, and also in the gonadotropic cells of the **pituitary gland**. Activin has exclusively paracrine effects and does not leave the ovarian follicle or the pituitary gland. In contrast to inhibin, activin stimulates FSH secretion.

Follistatin is an activin-binding protein that is secreted by the gonadotropic cells of the **pituitary gland**, but is also found in the **follicular fluid**. It **inhibits** FSH synthesis and secretion in the pituitary gland, and reduces the FSH response to GnRH pulses. Follistatin binds to activin and thus reduces the increase in FSH secretion caused by this peptide. The common feature of the peptides inhibin, activin and follistatin in reproductive biology, lies in their effect of inhibiting or promoting FSH secretion.

■ Anti-Muellerian hormone

Anti-Muellerian hormone (AMH), also called Muellerian-inhibiting factor (**MIF**), is a dimeric glycoprotein that belongs to the same protein family as inhibin and activin. It initially plays an important role in sexual differentiation during **embryonic development**. It suppresses the development of Muellerian ducts via a local mechanism, and is also involved in the organisation of the Sertoli and germ cells into the primitive spermatic cords (**Fig. 24.28**). In the embryo, AMH is produced mainly in the Sertoli cells of the embryonic testis. Postnatally, AMH is produced in female animals in the granulosa cells of preantral and early antral follicles, and in male animals in the Sertoli cells. The hormone is of particular interest as a biomarker for assessing gonadal activity. In female ruminants and mares, there are correlations between ovarian follicular reserve and blood AMH concentration. The determination of the AMH concentration is also used for the diagnosis of granulosa cell tumours in various animal species. In addition, AMH blood concentration can be used to determine whether gonads are present in animals of uncertain reproductive status, such as cryptorchids, i.e. male animals with testes that have not descended from the abdominal cavity into the scrotum.

■ Oxytocin

Oxytocin is a peptide consisting of nine amino acids. It is synthesised by **neurosecretory cells** of the **nucleus supraopticus** and **nucleus paraventricularis** in the hypothalamus. It travels via axons of the neurosecretory cells to the posterior hypophysial lobe and is there **released** into blood. In some species, **oxytocin** is also synthesised in the **ovary**, so that it may have two sites of origin (**Fig. 24.3**).

Oxytocin induces the **contraction** of the muscular wall layers of the **uterus** and the **fallopian tube** and the **myoepithelial cells** of the **mammary gland**. It is therefore of great importance for the transport of sperm in the female genitals, the emptying of uterine contents at parturition, and for milk secretion.

In some animal species (e.g. cattle and pigs), oxytocin is also produced in the corpus luteum and is involved in regulating the life span of the corpus luteum. In the absence of pregnancy, it stimulates the release of prostaglandin $F_{2\alpha}$ from the endometrial cells, which then initiates luteolysis.

In addition to its primary contractile effect on the smooth musculature of the sexual organs, oxytocin is also important in the expression of emotionally controlled behaviour. These are, in particular, mother-child bonding, partner bonding, and sexually stimulating effects in both, males and females.

■ Melatonin

Melatonin (chemically N-acetyl-5-methoxy-tryptamine) is the main product of the **pineal gland**. This gland develops during embryogenesis as an extension of the third ventricle of the brain. After birth, the pineal gland loses all afferent and efferent neuronal connections with the brain. The parenchymal cells then acquire new sympathetic innervation, allowing this gland to actively neurosecrete and respond to hormonal and environmental stimuli.

Melatonin secretion is inhibited by an animal being exposed to light. Light is detected by the retina of the eye and this signal is neuronally transmitted to the pineal gland. As a result, melatonin secretion is subject to a clear **circadian rhythm** (low release during the day, increased release at night in darkness). In the context of reproduction, melatonin mediates the influence of increasing or decreasing daylight length on gonadal function in seasonally reproducing species.

■ Relaxin

Relaxin is a polypeptide hormone consisting of an α- and a β-subunit, which is synthesised in the corpus luteum, and in the placenta during pregnancy. In the preparatory stage for birth, relaxin influences the properties of the connective tissue, and thus enables the widening and stretching of the birth canal.

■ Prostaglandins

Prostaglandins can be synthesised in most tissues of the body and have autocrine, paracrine and endocrine effects. Chemically, prostaglandins are unsaturated hydroxy fatty acids. They are synthesised from membrane phospholipids

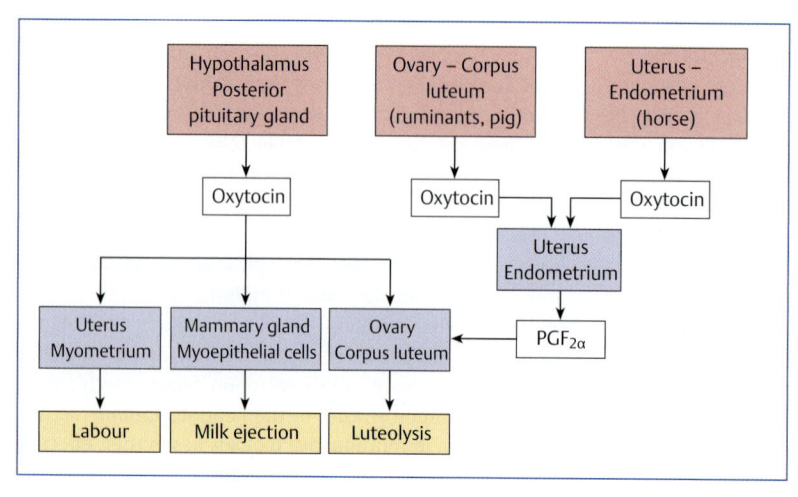

Fig. 24.3 Sites of synthesis and target organs of oxytocin. Oxytocin is a nonapeptide (nine amino acids) synthesised in the hypothalamus and secreted via the posterior pituitary. It causes the milk ejection reflex in the udder, the contraction of the myometrium during birth, and, together with the oxytocin produced by the corpus luteum, it is involved in the release of $PGF_{2\alpha}$ from the endometrium (luteolysis).

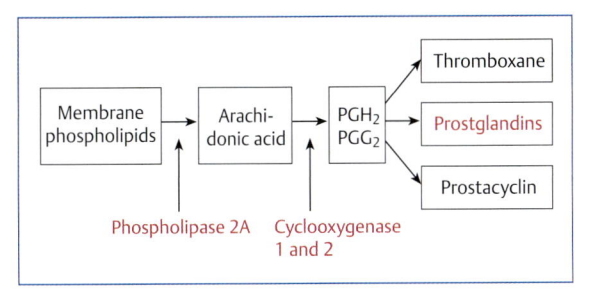

Fig. 24.4 Schematic representation of the synthesis pathway of prostaglandins.
Membrane phospholipids are hydrolysed by a phospholipase (2A) to release arachidonic acid. From arachidonic acid, cyclooxygenase-1 (constitutive) and cyclooxygenase-2 (hormone-induced) produce prostaglandin H_2 (PGH$_2$) and PGG$_2$ from which a terminal synthase generates the prostaglandins.

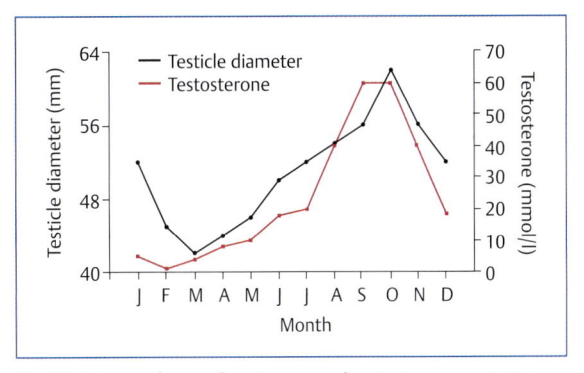

Fig. 24.5 Dependence of testis size and testosterone secretion on daylight length in seasonally reproductively active Soay rams. In the months with short nights (= long phase of melatonin release), testis size and testosterone synthesis and secretion are increased.
[Source: Ebling FJP, Lincoln GA. Endogenous opioids and the control of seasonal LH secretion in Soay rams. J Endocrinol 1985; 107: 341–353]

and, after their secretion, are completely degraded within seconds or minutes (**Fig. 24.4**).

Prostaglandin F$_{2\alpha}$ (PGF$_{2\alpha}$) causes regression of the corpus luteum (luteolysis) when there is no pregnancy, and thereby this triggers the start of a **new cycle**. In species in which progesterone is necessary for maintaining pregnancy, its secretion by one or more corpora lutea is maintained throughout the entire gestation period. Luteolysis must then take place to induce birth.

Clinically, PGF$_{2\alpha}$ can be used to terminate an unwanted pregnancy in many animal species. However, this is only possible if pregnancy is maintained exclusively via one or more corpora lutea. Prostaglandin F$_{2\alpha}$ and PGE$_2$ also play a role in ovulation, leading to changes in the follicle wall that allow the release of the egg. Therefore, in most species, ovulation can be inhibited by drugs that suppress PGF$_{2\alpha}$ synthesis (treatment with cyclooxygenase inhibitors). During parturition, prostaglandins, together with oxytocin, stimulate contraction of the uterine muscles by increasing intracellular Ca^{2+} in the myometrium, which activates myosin light chain kinase, which phosphorylates the myosin light chain, and thus initiates contraction.

24.1.2 Seasonality

Numerous animal species living in temperate climates reproduce according to season. Seasonal reproductive activity is mainly controlled by changes in the length of daylight. Among domestic animals, **goats, sheep, horses**, but also **cats**, show a clear seasonal influence on reproductive activity. Due to the seasonal **sexual rhythm**, the females of these species are called seasonally polyoestrous. In **cattle** and **domestic pigs**, seasonal influences have almost completely **disappeared** through domestication, and their oestrous cycles are regular and unaffected over the course of a year (polyoestrous animals). In contrast, wild boars have seasonal reproductive activity.

The seasonality of reproduction is genetically fixed and is synchronised to a rhythm over twelve months, by the change in seasons. In some species, reproductive activity begins with decreasing daylight length ("short-day breeding-active" species such as sheep and goats) or with increasing daylight length ("long-day breeding-active" spe-

cies such as horses, hamsters). Whether the reproductive season is in autumn and winter or in spring and summer, is essentially determined by the length of gestation. For example, the mating season for mares with a gestation period of about 340 days is in spring and summer, while goats and sheep with a gestation length of about 150 days, initiate reproduction in autumn and winter. In both cases, the young are born in spring and summer when, for free-ranging animals, sufficient green fodder growth ensures lactation of the dam and adequate nutrition for the young offspring. Seasonality in reproductive behaviour thus represents an evolutionarily acquired selection advantage.

> **MORE DETAILS** Seasonal changes in reproductive activity are regulated by fluctuations in GnRH synthesis and secretion in the hypothalamus, which in turn are determined by **photoperiodicity**. Light impulses are received by the retina, conducted to the pineal gland in the form of afferent nerve signals, and converted there into an endocrine signal. This endocrine signal consists of the secretion of the hormone **melatonin**. Exposure to light inhibits melatonin secretion, while darkness stimulates its release. Alternation between day and night causes fluctuations in the melatonin concentrations in blood, so that a circadian rhythm is established. Melatonin influences the **release of GnRH** in the CNS via neuromodulators. Depending on whether it is a long-day or short-day active species, melatonin has an inhibiting or stimulating effect on reproductive functions. Inhibition of GnRH release outside the respective mating season leads to reduced gonadotropin synthesis and secretion, and thus to reduced gonadal function (**Fig. 24.6**).
>
> Melatonin also directly inhibits the release of **prolactin** from the **pituitary gland**. Prolactin may be involved in the control of seasonal reproductive activity via effects on the gonads. Independent of its possible role in controlling reproductive activity, prolactin is also involved in seasonal adaptation and regulates, for example, the change in hair coats between summer and winter.

Gradual differences have developed between species, and between breeds within a species, in the seasonal changes in reproductive functions. In less domesticated species and breeds, the effects of **photoperiodicity** are often more pronounced than in **highly domesticated species**. In males, with strictly seasonal reproductive behaviour, there may be pronounced **testicular regression** outside of the mating season (**Fig. 24.5**). In some sheep breeds, testicular mass is

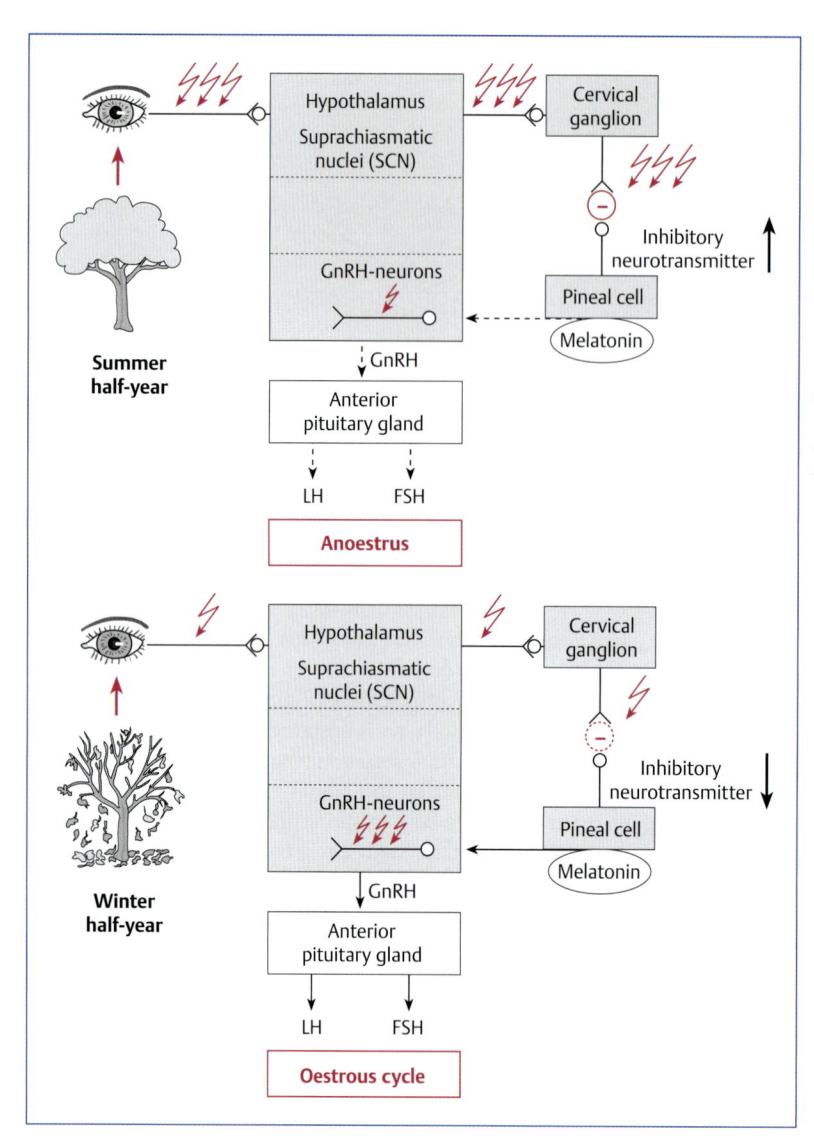

Fig. 24.6 Scheme of the inhibitory effect of light in sheep and goats. Melatonin is secreted during the night and stimulates GnRH secretion leading to increased LH and FSH release. In the summer half-year, light excites downstream inhibitory neurons via the retina. Thus, during the already short-night phase, little melatonin is released and GnRH secretion is reduced. In the winter half-year, the inhibitory neurons are only slightly excited. The pineal cell receives hardly any inhibitory signals during the long winter nights and secretes melatonin, which excites the GnRH neurons. The increased GnRH secretion causes the anterior pituitary to release more LH and FSH, thus controlling the oestrous cycle.

reduced to about 10% of that in the mating season. **Spermatogenesis** and **androgen synthesis** almost completely cease, the accessory sex glands atrophy, and the animals become infertile. In contrast, in species and breeds with less pronounced seasonal reproductive behaviour, such as male horses, the fluctuations in reproductive activity caused by daylight length are not so marked. Outside the breeding season, there is some decline in androgen synthesis and spermatogenesis, but the males still remain fertile throughout the year.

Through domestication, selection, and changes in environmental conditions such as stabling, and needs-based feeding, the seasonal character of the breeding season has been increasingly lost in some breeds that originally were seasonal breeders. While mares of less domesticated pony breeds do not show any oestrous cycles in the autumn and winter months, up to 70% of warm-blooded mares in temperate climates show regular oestrous cycles throughout the year. Similarly, in sheep, there are original breeds with strong seasonality, and highly domesticated breeds (e.g.

Merino sheep) that are reproductively active almost all year round. The degree of seasonal reproductive behaviour controlled by daylight length is also influenced by environmental factors such as climate (temperature and humidity) and food supply.

If breeding is required before the mating season, for species with seasonal reproduction, their reproductive activity can be brought forward by the use of controlled lighting programmes. In sheep, a lighting programme with long nights and short days could be applied during summer. However, this requires the animals to be kept indoors. More practical is the possibility of increasing the endogenous melatonin concentration of the sheep in summer, by administering melatonin in the form of implants, thus bringing forward the start of the reproductive season by a few weeks. In mares, the onset of fertile reproductive cycles in the Northern hemisphere spring, can be brought forward by about two months, by implementing a lighting programme that mimics long days (16 h) with short nights (8 h) from the beginning of December.

24.1.3   Puberty

Puberty is a process that enables an animal to reproduce. However, puberty is not a sudden change, but a **slowly progressing process of maturation**.

The time of onset of puberty in the female is defined by the **first ovulation**, which gives rise to measurable concentrations of the steroid hormone progesterone, through the development of one or more corpora lutea. In many species, the first ovulation is not marked by any preceding oestrous behaviour. Typical oestrous behaviour is often only apparent after completion of the first corpus luteum phase. In males, the onset of puberty is defined as the time when there is a noticeably increased concentration of testosterone in blood. The prerequisite for both males and females, is sufficient secretion of GnRH from the hypothalamus, to stimulate the synthesis and secretion of FSH and LH in the anterior pituitary. Before puberty, GnRH secretion is suppressed by a centrally acting mechanism that has not yet been conclusively identified. Of central importance for the onset and course of puberty are the genes KiSS1 and KiSS1 R, also known as the "puberty genes", the products of which, **kisspeptin** and its receptor, form a part of the GnRH pulse generators, and are crucial for the onset of GnRH secretion at the onset of puberty.

The **GnRH pulse**s initially lead to increased secretion of FSH, while LH release is still low. This activates follicle growth, but does not yet trigger ovulation. GnRH also leads to an induction of its own receptors on the cells of the AP in this early phase, so that there is increased response of the gonadotropic cells to GnRH. **Oestradiol** secreted by the maturing follicles progressively increases the secretory LH response (**Fig. 24.7**) to GnRH pulses (positive feedback), while inhibin (secreted by maturing follicles) progressively reduces the FSH response to GnRH pulses (negative feedback).

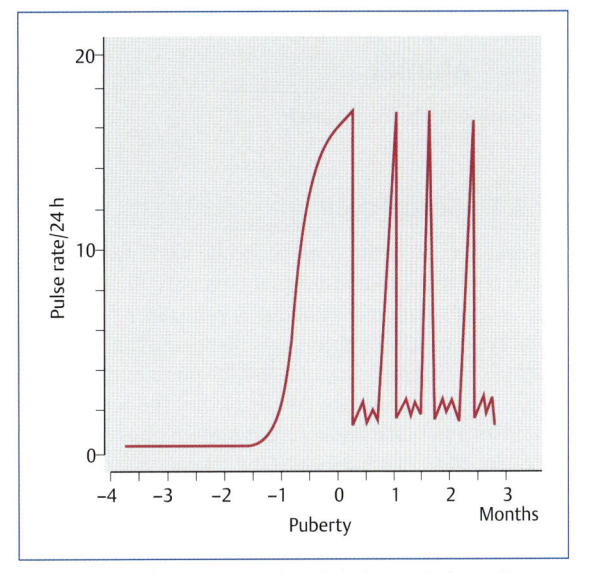

Fig. 24.7 LH pulse frequency of cattle before and after puberty. The LH pulses reflect the GnRH pulses. In cattle, about two months of GnRH secretion is needed before its pulse frequency is sufficient to trigger the first preovulatory LH peak. [Source: Senger PL. Pathways to Pregnancy and Parturition. REV. 2011. New York: McGraw-Hill; 2011]

The age at which sexual maturity occurs varies significantly between, but also within, species (**Table 24.1**). In cattle, significant differences in the age at which animals enter puberty have been reported. Dairy cattle breeds become sexually mature at 7–9 months of age, whereas beef cattle breeds do not enter puberty until they are 12–13 months old. The season also influences the time of puberty in seasonally reproducing animals (sheep, goats, horses). Lambs born in spring start their sexual cycle at 4–8 months of age, in the autumn of the year they were born. If lambs are born in autumn (October in the Northern hemisphere), they do not enter puberty (at 10–12 months of age) until autumn of the following year.

Table 24.1 Average age (range of variation of onset) of sexual maturity in different domestic animals.

Animal species	Age (months)	
	male	**female**
Horse	13 (12–19)	14 (10–14)
Cattle	11 (9–24)	11 (7–18)
Pig	6 (5–7)	7 (5–8)
Sheep	7 (4–14)	7 (6–9)

Endocrinology. reproduction

24.2   Reproduction in the female animal

Christine Aurich, Jörg Aurich

24.2.1   Sexual cycle

The **sexual cycle** is the **time** period between two physiological ovulations in non-pregnant animals. In contrast to other mammals, humans and many primates have a **menstrual cycle** which comprises the time period between the onset of the first menstruation and the onset of the following one (**Fig. 24.8**). Independently of this, the sexual cycle comprises a **follicular** and a **corpus luteum phase** (biphasic cycle, **Fig. 24.8**). Physiologically, the sexual cycle can be interrupted by pregnancy, and in some species also by the duration of lactation or by the season (seasonal anoestrus). As these animals then do not show oestrous behaviour, these phases are called **anoestrus**. In the bitch, oestrus (heat), and the subsequent luteal phase, are physiologically followed by several months of anoestrus, with only minimal, or dormant, ovarian function. In addition to the physiological suspension of the sexual cycle, a number of pathological processes can cause anoestrus, such as chronic endometrial infection, dead and mummified foetuses, malnutrition, and continuous milk production in dairy cows.

The females of domestic mammal species usually show **readiness to mate** only during **oestrus** (Mare: heat, the mare is in heat; cattle: oestrus, the cow is in heat; sheep/goat: oestrus, the sheep, the goat is in heat; dog: heat, the bitch is in heat; cat: rutting, the queen is in heat). An exception here are mares, which sometimes also mate during the luteal phase in pregnancy, or during the winter anoestrus. The mating act by a stallion strengthens the bond between him and the mares in the so-called harems, typical for horses in the wild.

The **behavioural patterns** displayed by females during oestrus are species-specific and are necessary signals to the males that they are ready to mate. Often oestrus is also associated with the secretion of pheromones (olfactory perceptible hormones) in urine or vaginal secretions, which can be perceived by the male. Most species in oestrus show an increase in typical locomotor activity and seeking contact with others. In some species such as cattle, the females may also jump on other cows, and become increasingly tolerant of approaches by a male. At the peak of oestrus, the duration and expression of which vary according to species and between individuals, the male courtship signals are answered by remaining in one place ("standing") and bending the spine (lordosis) with the pelvis raised (mating posture, often sawhorse-like with hind legs out and exposing the vulva by holding the tail/tail to the side). The presentation of this mating posture is a specifically female stimulus response (receptivity: acquiescence and invitation to mate), which additionally stimulates the male sex partner so that mounting and copulation follow. Disturbances of these behavioural patterns due to incorrect mating management, faulty interpretation of oestrous expressions, or too vigorous regimentation of the animals, not infrequently lead to an interruption of the finely tuned reflex chain.

The frequency of the sexual cycle over the course of a year has species-specific characteristics. In cattle, pigs, mice and rats, the oestrous cycles are regularly distributed throughout the **year**. These animals are therefore called **polyoestrous**.

Seasonally polyoestrous animals (horse, sheep, goat, cat) show regularly recurring oestrous cycles only during a certain phase of the year. For example, sheep and goats are short-day breeding animals, whereas cats and horses are long-day breeding animals.

Monoestrous animals (dogs) are cyclic only **once** a **year**. In many dog breeds, two or even three heat cycles per year are observed, but dogs are still formally regarded as a monoestrous species.

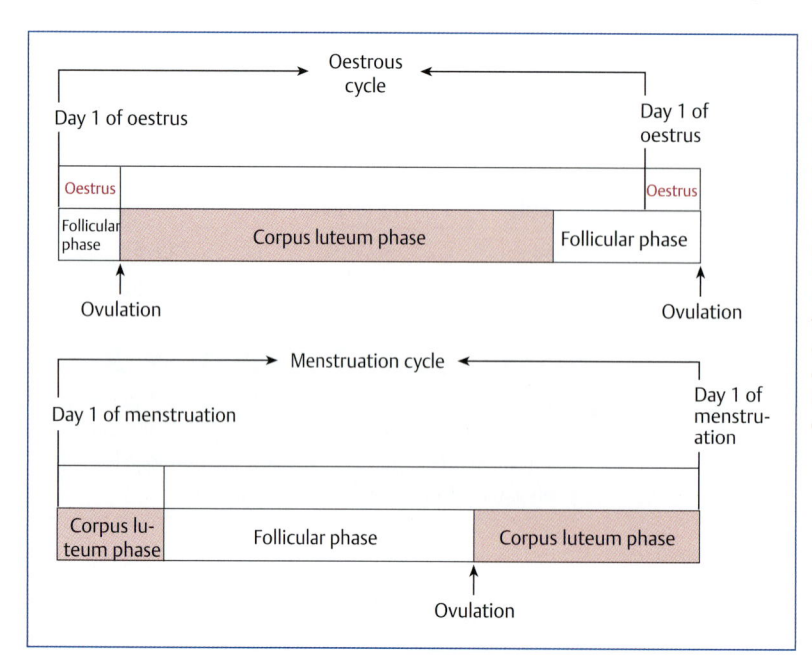

Fig. 24.8 Comparative representation of the oestrous and menstrual cycle. The oestrous cycle of animals begins with the first day of oestrus and ends with the start of the next oestrus. Animals usually ovulate towards the end of oestrus or shortly after. Depending on the species, the oestrous cycle is characterised by a short follicular phase and a long luteal phase (1:4). The menstrual cycle begins with the first day of menstruation and ends with the start of the next menstruation. Ovulation usually occurs in the middle of the menstrual cycle. The menstrual cycle is characterised by an equal length of the follicular and corpus luteum phases (1:1).

Table 24.2 Duration of the sexual cycle and oestrus in different domestic animal species.

Species	Ovulation type	Cycle duration (days)		Oestrus duration	Timing of ovulation	
		total	Follicular phase		Hours after the LH peak	in relation to the cycle
Horse	spontaneous	19–25	4–8	5–8 d	–	1–2 d before end of heat
Cattle	spontaneous	21–22	3–5	18–19 h	24–30 h	25–30 h after onset of oestrus
Sheep	spontaneous	17	2–3	24–36 h	21–23 h	24–27 h after onset of oestrus
Goat	spontaneous	20–21	2–3	32–40 h	–	30–36 h after onset of oestrus
Pig	spontaneous	20–21	3–5	40–60 h	40 h	38–42 h after onset of oestrus
Dog	spontaneous	203–224	13–14	7–9 d	38–44 h	1–3 d after onset of oestrus
Cat	spontaneous or induced	14–21	5–6	4–6 d	25–26 h	24–36 h after coitus

The duration of the oestrous cycle and the mean length of time during which females show signs of oestrus, varies with species. Even within a species, there can be considerable physiological variation between individuals, or variation related to environmental factors. **Table 24.2** provides information on the duration of the sexual cycle and oestrus in different domestic animals.

■ Endocrine control of the sexual cycle and ovulation

The secretion pattern of GnRH is subject to large individual variations in pulse amplitude and frequency. As a general rule, the pulse frequency is higher during the follicular phase, and the amplitude is smaller than during the corpus luteum phase (**Fig. 24.9, Fig. 24.10**).

In the early follicular phase, i.e. immediately after luteolysis, the anterior pituitary secretes sufficient FSH to support the growth of multiple tertiary follicles. Depending on whether the species is monoovulatory or polyovulatory, one or more follicles are selected and become dominant follicles that develop to the preovulatory stage. These follicles produce the oestradiol necessary for the signs of

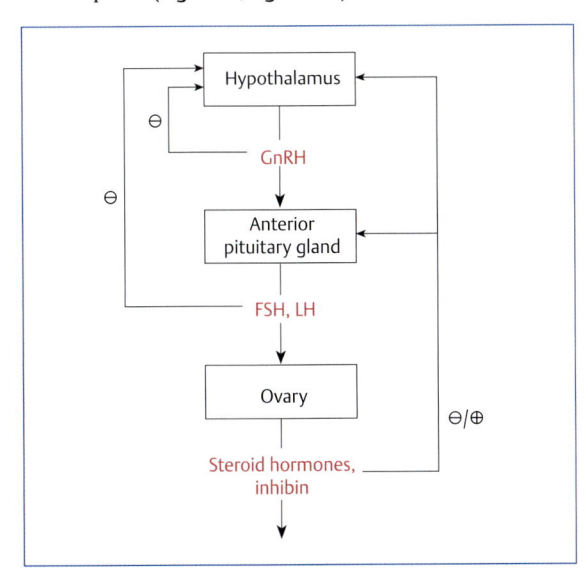

Fig. 24.9 Diagram of important feedback loops in endocrine control of the sexual cycle. The steroid hormones inhibit (although oestrogens can also promote) the secretion of GnRH, and partly also directly that of FSH and LH. FSH and LH inhibit the secretion of GnRH. GnRH inhibits its own secretion.

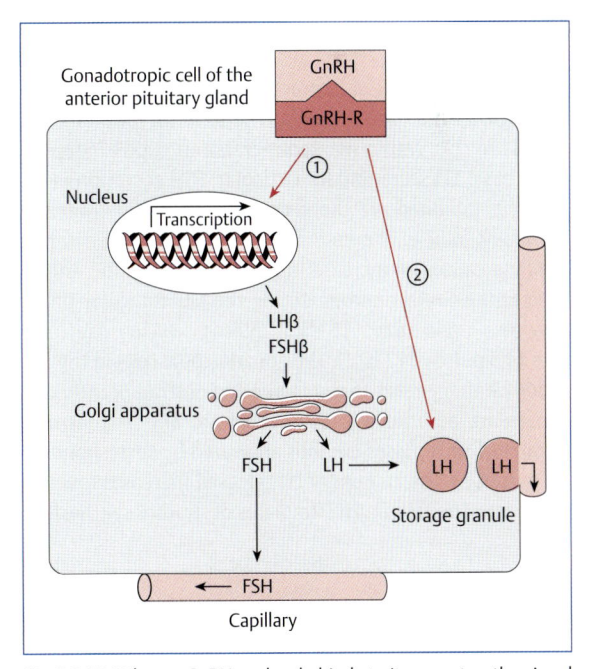

Fig. 24.10 When a GnRH molecule binds to its receptor, the signal can activate different signalling pathways in the cell.
1: GnRH causes the transcription of the β-subunits of LH and FSH, which are processed in the Golgi apparatus to form biologically active LH and FSH molecules. The FSH molecules are usually secreted immediately, while the LH molecules are usually stored.
2: During the preovulatory LH release, GnRH receptor binding causes a rapid depletion of the stored LH. In the process, any stored FSH is also secreted, so that the LH peak is accompanied by an FSH peak.

Endocrinology, reproduction

oestrus, and for preparing the reproductive organs for mating and conception. At the same time, the follicles also secrete inhibin which inhibits pituitary FSH secretion. During oestrus, when oestrogen synthesis of the preovulatory follicle reaches its maximum, the blood concentration of FSH decreases (**Fig. 24.11**). Preovulatory follicles are FSH-independent and also have a high number of LH receptors, which enables them to mature and ultimately to ovulate under the influence of LH released by the anterior pituitary.

> **IN A NUTSHELL**   !
>
> The increasing oestradiol secretion of the maturing follicles exerts a negative feedback on the FSH secretion of the anterior pituitary. Only the preovulatory follicle(s) that come to ovulation later, continue to develop independently of FSH, because they express enough LH receptors in time to ensure adequate oestradiol synthesis.

Oestradiol exerts either negative or positive feedback on GnRH and LH secretion, depending on its blood concentration. Thus a low oestradiol concentration, together with progesterone, has an inhibitory effect, but a high oestradiol concentration in the absence of progesterone, has a stimulating effect on GnRH secretion. The most significant of these oestradiol effects is the stimulation of GnRH neurons in the hypothalamus and the gonadotropic cells of the anterior pituitary, which is effective for a minimum time after exceeding the minimum concentration required for each species. This **positive oestradiol feedback** is the main ovulation-triggering mechanism. In the early follicular phase, and the onset of luteolysis, the blood concentration of progesterone drops rapidly. The anterior pituitary responds to this with a marked increase in GnRH-independent, basal LH secretion. In particular, FSH secretion is selectively inhibited via the secretion of inhibin from the dominant follicle. The increasing oestradiol concentration in blood causes an increase in pulse frequency and amplitude at the GnRH neurons during the late follicular phase (bovine: cycle day $15 = 3.5$ pulses, cycle day $17–19 = 14.5$ pulses $\cdot [12\ \mathrm{h}]^{-1}$). The gonadotropic cells in the anterior pituitary react to the increasing oestradiol influx by expressing additional GnRH receptors. The increasingly frequent GnRH pulses are thus answered by corresponding LH pulses, i.e. the amount of LH released increases towards ovulation. The LH in turn stimulates oestradiol synthesis in

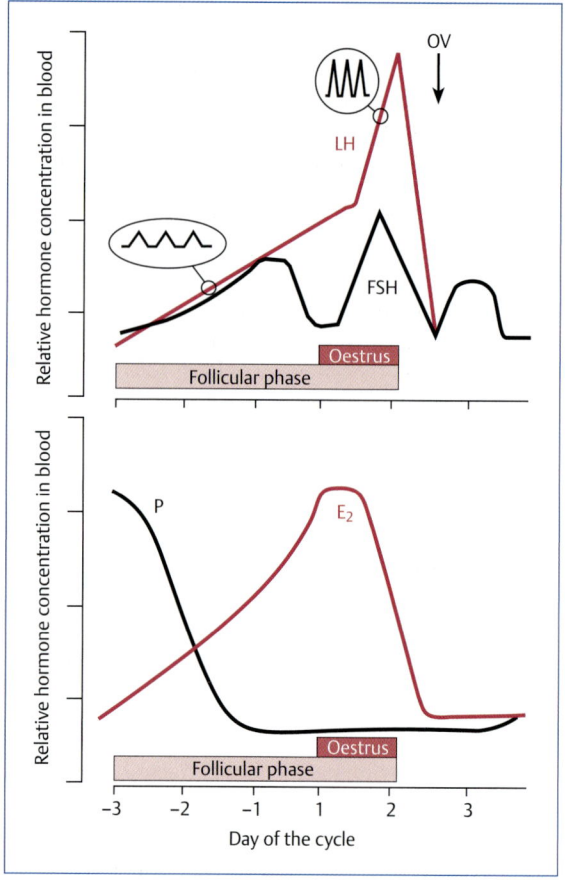

Fig. 24.11 Schematic representation of the blood concentrations of the gonadotropins LH and FSH, and the steroid hormones oestradiol (E_2) and progesterone (P), during the follicular phase of the oestrous cycle. As E_2 (and inhibin) concentrations increase, FSH secretion decreases. During oestrus, E_2 stimulates increased release of LH from the AP (LH peak). The LH release is also accompanied by more FSH release. This postovulatory FSH surge then initiates the development of a subsequent set of follicles for the next cycle. [Source: Senger PL. Pathways to Pregnancy and Parturition. REV. 2011. New York: McGraw-Hill; 2011]

the preovulatory follicles. The gonadotropic cells of the AP respond by rapidly (cattle and sheep: 10–12 h) emptying the LH stores. Until the onset of oestrus, only about 20% of the gonadotropic cells of the anterior pituitary release LH. During oestrus, not only does the responsiveness of LH-synthesising cells to GnRH increase, but they also increase in number.

Table 24.3 Characteristics of the follicular phase of the oestrous cycle in different domestic animals.

Feature	Horse	Cattle	Sheep	Pig
Number of ovulations per heat	1	1	1–3	12–20
Duration of the follicular phase of the oestrous cycle (days)	6–8	3–4	3–4	5–7
preovulatory follicle diameter (mm)	35–45	16–22	5–7	8–10
Diameter (mm) from which the follicles are FSH-dependent	6	3–4	2–3	4–5
Diameter (mm) from which the granulosa cells express LH receptors	10	9–10	3.5	5

During preovulatory LH release, which in most species lasts only a few hours and is characterised by a very rapid rise and fall that is graphically represented as a peak in the LH concentration curve (LH peak), 80% of the total LH in the anterior pituitary enters the bloodstream. This ensures that a sufficient amount of LH reaches the follicle, so that ovulation is triggered. The time that elapses between the LH peak and ovulation is species-specific (**Table 24.2**). In the female horse, the increase in LH concentration in oestrus, occurs gradually over several days and only reaches its maximum shortly after ovulation.

Considering the manifold interdependencies of the cellular responses in this interplay of hypothalamus (GnRH), pituitary (FSH, LH) and ovary (oestrogen, inhibin), **oestradiol** plays a central role in the endocrine regulation of ovulation.

> **IN A NUTSHELL** !
>
> The oestradiol synthesised and secreted by the preovulatory follicle is of central importance in the regulation of ovulation, i.e. the preovulatory follicle determines whether and when it ovulates, from the concentration of the oestrogen it is secreting.

Ovulation characteristics of different animal species

Some species such as rabbits or camelids (camel, llama, alpaca) only ovulate when they have been mated. This type of ovulation is called **induced ovulation**, whereas ovulation occurs **spontaneously** in the vast majority of species. Ovulation can be induced by various mechanisms. In rabbits, the mechanism is the mechanical stimulus of the mating act, which is perceived in the region of the vagina and/or cervix, and leads ultimately to increased release of GnRH, and subsequently of LH. In camelids, the **seminal plasma** contains **NGFβ** (**nerve growth factor β**) which has been identified as the factor that induces the release of LH at the anterior pituitary, and thus triggers ovulation. NGFβ also stimulates ovulation and corpus luteum function in rabbits and cattle. In spontaneously ovulating animals, ovulation can be accelerated by mechanisms related to mating, but usually ovulation is not induced by the act of mating.

■ Growth dynamics of the ovarian follicle during the sexual cycle

In the ovary, follicle growth is continuous, i.e. it already has begun during foetal development and only ends when all the eggs have been used up by cell death (atresia) or ovulation. Neither pregnancy, nor age, nor the phases of oestrus, interrupt this process. Before puberty, the follicles go through only a few developmental steps before they undergo atresia. Only when sexual maturity is reached and the feedback mechanisms are sufficiently synchronised does the **biphasic cycle** establish itself with its regular alternation between follicular and luteal phases. While in women the so-called menopause occurs around the age of 50 due to

the loss of most or all eggs, (i.e. there is no longer an ovarian cycle), such cessation of ovarian activity is only observed in exceptional cases in female domestic animals, i.e. they usually maintain sexual cycles throughout their lives.

The **initial growth** of a **primordial follicle**, which is **irreversible**, involves an increase in size of the oocyte and a change in shape and proliferation of the granulosa cells. Once a primordial follicle begins to grow, it continues its development until either **ovulation** or **atresia**. The number of ovulating follicles, recruited and selected from the total ovarian pool of follicles, is specific for each animal species and breeds. Recruitment initially leads to the growth of a so-called **follicular wave**, from which one or more follicles, growing to preovulatory size, are ultimately selected. The follicle group, which initially begins to grow independently of gonadotropin, comprises 100–300 primordial follicles, depending on the species, while the majority of primordial follicles remain in a resting state. Dependence of the follicles on FSH only begins after a certain diameter is reached, specific for each species (**Table 24.3**). One or more follicles, selected from the growing follicle wave, become **dominant** over the other follicles and develop to ovulation, while the subordinate follicles **undergo atresia**. **Follicle recruitment** and **selection** are subject to precise endocrine and paracrine regulation involving gonadotropins released by the anterior pituitary, and steroid hormones of follicular origin, as well as numerous growth factors and other locally produced factors.

The number of follicles progressing to ovulation can be modified by mutations in the genes coding for growth factors. Such mutations can lead to above-average ovulation rates in some breeds or in subpopulations of a species. Furthermore, the expression of angiogenic factors and their receptors in the wall of the growing follicle plays an important role, also for the blood supply of the corpus luteum after ovulation (**Fig. 24.12**).

Since the transition from dormant to growing follicle population is continuous, there are always growing follicles originating from different **follicle growth waves** in

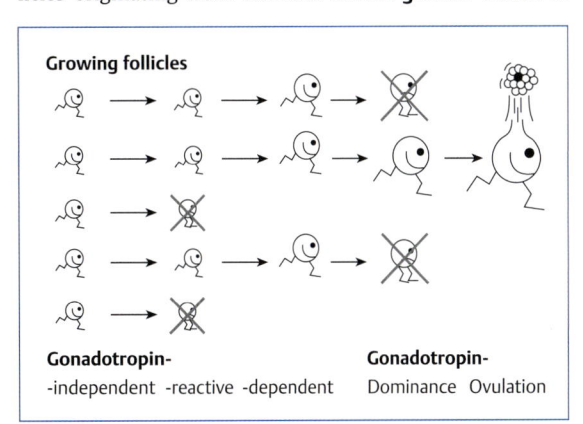

Fig. 24.12 Functional processes in folliculogenesis. The gonadotropin-independent pre-antral follicle begins to grow in response to an unknown earlier signal. It develops an antrum and receptors on its granulosa and theca cells that make it reactive to FSH and LH. The progression of maturation subsequently becomes dependent on FSH and LH supply. On the way to ovulation, one follicle or, in multiparous species, several follicles, become dominant and inhibit the development of the other follicles.

Endocrinology, reproduction

the ovaries. Some species (**horse, cow, sheep, goat**) have progressive follicle maturation, independent of oestrous cycle status, so that individual follicles can develop to pre-ovulatory diameters. Therefore, in addition to an endocrine-active **corpus luteum**, there is often also a **large**, maturing **follicle** which only fails to ovulate because the progesterone secreted by the corpus luteum suppresses it by inhibiting LH secretion. In other species (**pigs, rats, primates**), **follicular growth** is terminated early during the **corpus luteum phase**, so that only small, antral follicles can be seen in the ovary, in addition to the functioning corpus **luteum**. Here, further growth and maturation of follicles only takes place after luteolysis (**Fig. 24.13**).

MORE DETAILS   Stimulation of several follicles that grow to preovulatory sizes and ultimately ovulate, can also be achieved by exogenous treatment with FSH-acting hormones. This is known as **superovulation** and is used, for **embryo transfer** in various species, to produce more than the typical number of embryos for those species. These are then collected from the uterus of a donor animal and transferred to recipient animals ("surrogate mothers").

IN A NUTSHELL   !

Follicle growth is a continuum that initially occurs independently of gonadotropins. Only when follicles reach a particular size, specific for each species, do gonadotropic hormones stimulate further follicle growth and final maturation. The functional development of a follicle includes: recruitment, selection, dominance, and ovulation or atresia.

■ Endocrine control of follicle maturation

The endocrine control of follicle maturation is through receptors on the **granulosa** and **theca cells**. When a follicle has reached its gonadotropin-dependent stage of development, its **granulosa cells** express **FSH receptors** and its **theca-interna cells** express **LH receptors**. LH released from the anterior pituitary in basal amounts, binds to specific receptors on theca cells and through the second messenger

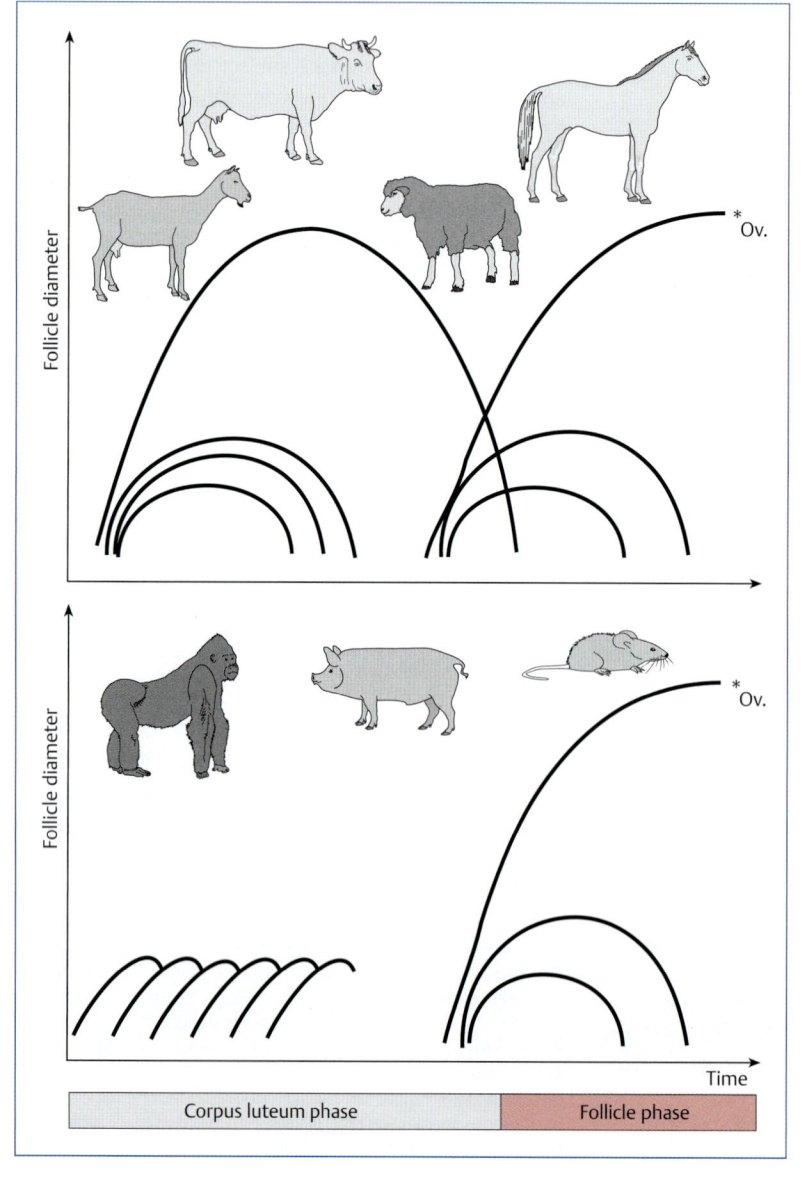

Fig. 24.13 Follicle development in different mammals. In cattle, sheep, goats and horses, follicles grow in several waves (1–3) during an oestrous cycle, reaching preovulatory diameters. In primates, pigs and rats, many waves of follicle formation are found during the corpus luteum phase, but the follicles remain small and soon undergo atresia.

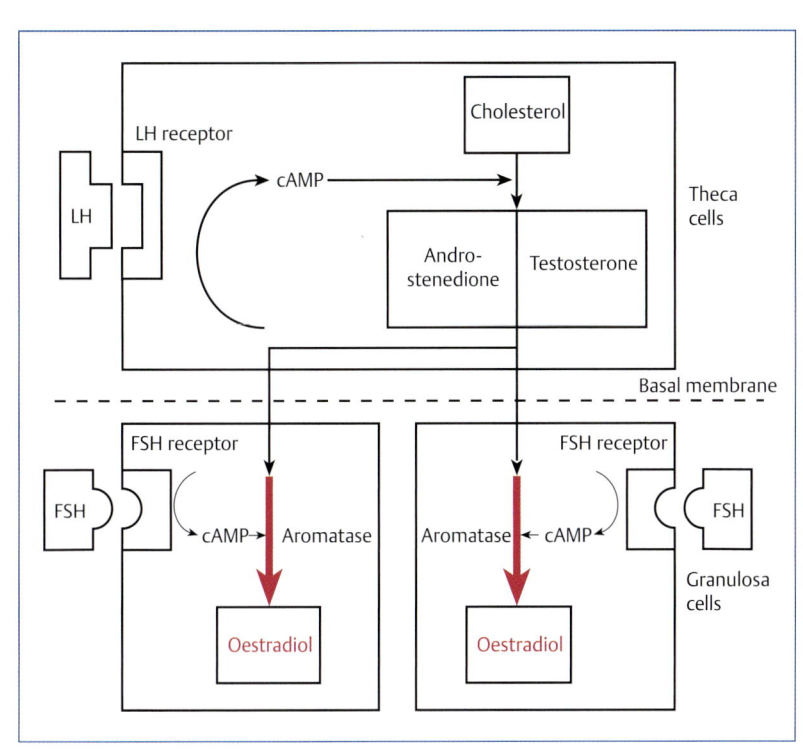

Fig. 24.14 Oestradiol synthesis in the follicle occurs under the influence of two gonadotropins (FSH and LH) in two cell types (granulosa and theca cells). LH stimulates the synthesis of androgens in the theca cells. These androgens are transported into the granulosa cells where they are converted into oestradiol by the FSH-dependent enzyme, aromatase.

cAMP, stimulates synthesis of androgens (androstenedione, testosterone) from steroid hormone precursors. These androgens are transported into the granulosa cells. Granulosa cells have specific receptors for FSH, which promotes expression of the enzyme **aromatase**, which then catalyses the synthesis of oestradiol from testosterone. For all species, mature preovulatory follicles are characterised by the enzyme aromatase, a high concentration of oestradiol in the follicular fluid, and the presence of numerous LH receptors on the granulosa cells (**Fig. 24.14**).

The number of FSH receptors on a granulosa cell is initially limited, i.e. there is only a limited increase in the number of FSH receptors on a granulosa cell in a growing follicle. Oestradiol has a **mitogenic** (mitosis-stimulating) effect on the granulosa cells. So, by increasing the number of granulosa cells, the total number of FSH receptors can increase rapidly. The proliferation of FSH receptors therefore takes place in an oestradiol-dependent manner via increased division of granulosa cells. Only if the androgens originating from the theca interna are converted to oestradiol does the microenvironment of the follicle remain characterised by oestrogens. If this does not happen, the follicle is under androgen control and undergoes atresia.

The **increasing number of granulosa cells** leads to a steady **increase in oestradiol synthesis** and **secretion** in a maturing follicle. Oestradiol has actions both at the follicular and pituitary level. At the follicle, it induces the spread of blood vessels into the theca interna. This enables better follicular development than in those follicles exposed to lower levels of oestradiol. In the pituitary, the increasing concentration of oestradiol reduces FSH release. However, since the oestradiol-rich, and thus also capillary-rich follicle, receives more blood, more FSH molecules reach it, and bind to the numerous FSH receptors. Thus more synthesis of oestradiol is again stimulated. In this way, the development of the follicle is enhanced, compared to other follicles in the cohort, and so it exerts **dominance** over them. In the advanced follicular phase, the dominant follicle becomes LH-dependent and FSH-independent. This is made possible by an increased formation of LH receptors on the granulosa cells, which is also stimulated by LH and oestradiol.

In the **final phase** of **maturation** (preovulatory development), LH induces **ovulation** by the effect of its peak concentration.

> **IN A NUTSHELL**   !
>
> Oestradiol synthesis in the maturing follicle follows the 2-gonadotropin, 2-cell model. LH stimulates androgen synthesis in the theca cells, while FSH enables the aromatisation of androgens to oestradiol in the granulosa cells.

■ Ovulation and formation of the corpus luteum

The preovulatory secreted LH binds to granulosa and theca cells of the preovulatory follicle(s) and stimulates enzyme systems that induce ovulation and luteinisation. During ovulation, the **increasing PGF$_{2\alpha}$ and PGE$_2$ concentrations** in the follicular fluid degrade a small region of the follicle wall so that it ruptures (stigma formation). The oocyte is flushed out together with the cumulus oophorus and the follicular fluid and can be taken up by the fimbrial funnel of the fallopian tube. The internal pressure of the follicle remains constant towards ovulation, or even decreases in many species.

Endocrinology, reproduction

The **lutein cells** of the corpus luteum are formed from the **granulosa** and **theca cells** of the ovulated follicle. First, the basement membrane, which separates the vascularised theca cell layer from the vascularised granulosa cell layer before ovulation, is dissolved. Vascular cells, along with blood, migrate through the resulting gaps, accompanied by fibroblasts. **Large** and **small luteal cells** settle in the resulting network, both of which synthesise **progesterone**. In most species the lutein cells are formed by both, granulosa and theca cells, but in the horse they are derived exclusively from granulosa cells and only large luteal cells are capable of progesterone synthesis. Irrespective of species, the endothelial cells of the numerous capillaries arise from the vascular endothelium of the preovulatory follicle. In addition, a corpus luteum also contains smooth muscle cells, fibroblasts and macrophages.

In the first days after ovulation, the lutein cells are autonomous with regard to progesterone production. Progesterone synthesis occurs independently of pituitary signals because the preovulatory LH release was sufficient to maintain the initial production of progesterone. This phase comprises about one third of the entire life span of the cyclic corpus luteum. In addition to **progesterone**, other gestagens can also be produced, depending on the species, such as the horse. The progesterone concentration increases in some animal species, for example in dogs, shortly before ovulation. It increases considerably in the first few days of the **luteal phase** and then reaches a plateau, i.e. a constant concentration, in the productive phase of the corpus luteum. At high progesterone concentrations, **negative feedback** at the hypothalamus leads to an inhibition of **GnRH secretion**, whereby both the frequency of GnRH pulses and basal GnRH secretion are reduced. This suppression of GnRH secretion stimulates FSH secretion from the AP, thus allowing follicle development in the corpus luteum phase, but does not allow ovulation. In addition to progestins, the corpus luteum also produces **oxytocin** in various domestic animal species, studied in particular detail in ruminants. Expression of the oxytocin gene can already be detected in the preovulatory follicle and is stimulated by LH. Maximum luteal oxytocin concentrations are detectable during the productive phase of the corpus luteum, after which its concentration falls away.

Hormones that stimulate the growth of lutein cells and their progesterone synthesis are called **luteotropic hormones**. The most important luteotropic hormone in domestic animals is **LH**, the basal secretion of which from the anterior pituitary, ensures adequate progesterone secretion from the lutein cells. In some animal species (rat, pig, dog), **prolactin** also exerts a luteotropic effect on the corpus luteum. In addition to these two pituitary luteotropic hormones, progesterone synthesis in the corpus luteum is subject to numerous paracrine influences, with growth factors playing a particularly important role. Thus, intensive angiogenesis is stimulated by VEGF (vascular endothelial growth factor).

> ### IN A NUTSHELL   !
>
> In the corpus luteum, large and small lutein cells develop from the granulosa and partly also from theca cells, during or after ovulation. These produce progesterone, which, by negative feedback, reduces the frequency and amplitude of GnRH secretion during the luteal phase.

If a female animal is not mated or does not conceive, the breakdown of the corpus luteum is actively promoted at a time after ovulation characteristic for each species, (bovine: 16–17 days, mare: 13 days), so that a new follicular phase can begin. In most domestic species, the breakdown of the corpus luteum is induced by the release of **$PGF_{2\alpha}$**, which originates from the **endometrial cells**. This process is called luteolysis and only occurs when the endometrium has not received an embryonic signal that prevents this process. In ruminants and pigs, $PGF_{2\alpha}$ enters the **ovarian artery** directly from the venous blood outflow of the uterus, via a countercurrent system, thus bypassing the peripheral circulation to reach the corpus luteum. Since $PGF_{2\alpha}$ is inactivated very quickly (in one lung passage its efficacy is reduced by > 90%), this transport route ensures the **luteolytic** effect (**Fig. 24.15**). In the **horse**, this countercurrent system does not exist, and therefore much higher concentrations of $PGF_{2\alpha}$ are secreted into the peripheral circulation so that sufficient quantities still arrive at the corpus luteum. **Oxytocin** which is of luteal origin in ruminants and pigs, and of endometrial origin in horses, further stimulates the secretion of $PGF_{2\alpha}$, and the release of oxytocin is in turn sustained by $PGF_{2\alpha}$, so that a **positive feedback** develops. Although $PGF_{2\alpha}$ is known as the initial **luteolytic factor**, its effect on the corpus luteum is achieved by intraovarian factors. Among these, **tumour necrosis factor-α** (TNF-α) and **nitric oxide** (NO) in particular lead to the induction of **apoptosis** (programmed cell death) of the luteal cells. This is achieved at least in part by reduced

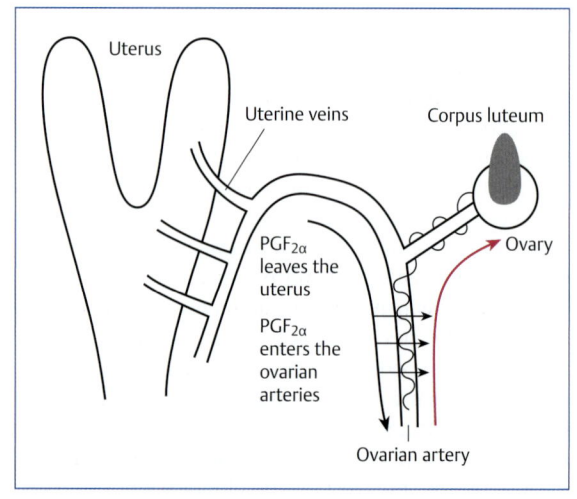

Fig. 24.15 Secretion pathway of uterine $PGF_{2\alpha}$ into the ovarian artery. $PGF_{2\alpha}$ is synthesised in the endometrial cells and released into the uterine veins in the absence of pregnancy. In cattle, pigs and sheep, $PGF_{2\alpha}$ passes through the vascular walls into the ovarian artery, which then flows to the ovarian vein.

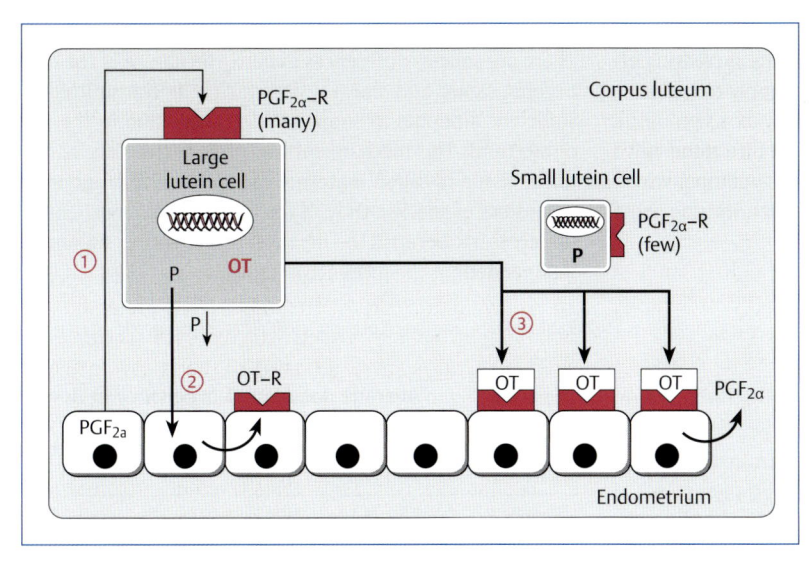

Fig. 24.16 Process of luteolysis at the cellular level in ruminants (model).
1: $PGF_{2\alpha}$ from the endometrium binds to its receptor on the large lutein cells.
2: Progesterone secretion by the large lutein cells decreases. More oxytocin receptors (OT-R) are then expressed on the endometrial cells.
3: OT secretion increases and OT binds to the increasingly expressed OT-R, resulting in increased $PGF_{2\alpha}$ secretion from the endometrial cells (positive feedback!).
P: Progesterone, OT: OxytocinOT-R: oxytocin receptorPGF$_{2\alpha}$: Prostaglandin F$_{2\alpha}$.

blood flow to the corpus luteum due to vascular constriction. The consequence of luteolysis is a rapid drop in the concentration of progesterone in the peripheral blood, so that the inhibitory effects of this hormone on gonadotropin release from the AP cease, and a new follicular phase with development of preovulatory follicles can then occur.

In **dogs**, the duration of the luteal phase is largely independent of whether the bitch is pregnant or not. The corpus luteum breaks down in non-pregnant bitches after a life span of about 63 days, without any active luteolytic mechanism being detectable. In contrast, in pregnant bitches, active luteolysis occurs after a mean gestation period of 60–66 days and thus at the time of onset of parturition, induced by a foetal signal. After the breakdown of the corpora lutea, the non-gravid bitch becomes **anoestric**, which lasts for several months before the next follicular phase begins (**Fig. 24.16**).

■ Cycle-related changes in the uterus, cervix and vagina

Due to the cycle-related changes in the steroid hormone milieu, with **oestradiol dominance** during the follicular phase and **progesterone dominance** during the luteal phase, there are striking changes in the uterus, cervix and vagina which can be detected by **clinical examination** and therefore provide valuable veterinary information on the stage of the oestrous **cycle**. During the follicular phase there is increased blood flow and accumulation of water, so that the walls of the hollow organs of the female reproductive tract become more elastic and softer. The **cervix** in particular becomes increasingly open. Histologically, the development of **oedema** is particularly evident in the stratum compactum of the endometrium. In contrast, during the luteal phase, the walls of the hollow organs are firmer in consistency and the cervix closes. In addition, **glands** in the mucous membrane of the endometrium, cervix and vagina produce larger amounts of a more fluid mucus during the follicular phase, and smaller amounts of a viscous mucus during the luteal phase. Taken together, the changes in **oestrus** serve to facilitate the mating act and,

depending on the species, allows the direct introduction of ejaculate into the uterus, or the active migration of sperm from the the external cervix into the uterus. During the **luteal phase**, these changes serve to protect the uterus against the invasion of pathogens via the vagina and the cervix.

In connection with the cycle-related changes in the uterus, there is also a modification of the cell types in the endometrium. The epithelial cells of the endometrium are characterised by predominantly **proliferative** activity during the follicular phase, and then by **secretory** activity in the luteal phase. The secretion produced by the endometrium in the luteal phase serves to nourish the embryos during pregnancy until the onset of placentation. It is therefore also called **uterine milk** or **histotrophs**. This secretion in the uteri of all mammalian species is a complex mixture of proteins, amino acids, carbohydrates and other molecules. In the sheep endometrial fluid, between day 10 and 15 after ovulation, the concentrations of glucose as well as the amino acids arginine, leucine, and glutamine, increase greatly, because of increasing expression of relevant **transport molecules**. The secretory activity of the endometrium is induced by progesterone, acting through **progesterone receptors**. It seems paradoxical, but it has been demonstrated for several domestic animal species that after ovulation, progesterone concentrations increase and then having reached a high level plateau, there is **downregulation of endometrial progesterone receptors** that had stimulated these changes. Therefore, the number of endometrial progesterone receptors is maximal in oestrus and minimal at the peak of the luteal phase. In sheep, embryonic interferon τ has an additional stimulatory effect on histotroph formation, i.e. more histotrophs are formed in this species in the presence of intact embryos than in the non-pregnant luteal phase.

In domestic mammals, the histological changes of the endometrium are comparatively subtle and there is no active shedding of the upper layers of the endometrium at the end of the luteal phase, accompanied by bleeding, as is observed in women with **menstruation**. In the bitch, how-

Endocrinology, reproduction

ever, bleeding from the endometrium occurs during the early follicular phase in connection with the increasing effect of oestradiol and the massive blood supply to the genital tract, which can be observed externally as a sign of the **onset of heat**. In cattle, light haemorrhages from the vulva are occasionally seen in connection with ovulation, which are called "bleeding off" and indicate the end of the short oestrus in this species.

24.2.2   Gestation

■ Establishment of pregnancy

Pregnancy covers the period from conception to birth, with a length that is specific for each species (**Table 24.4**).

After fusion of the male pronucleus from the sperm, and the female pronucleus within the egg (**syngamy**), a diploid zygote is formed. This is now equipped with a diploid set of chromosomes and thus is capable of **mitosis**. At different intervals, depending on the species, the zygote first divides into a two-cell structure, which is then called a **conceptus** (embryo). Continued mitotic divisions lead to 4-cell, 8-cell and finally 16-cell stages. From then onwards, the conceptus is called a **morula** (mulberry) because of the cluster-like arrangement of its cells. Further divisions and the formation of a fluid-filled cavity (**blastocoel**) give rise to the **blastocyst**, the cells of which are called blastomeres. Through expansion of the blastocoel and initial differentiation of the cells, an **inner cell mass develops**, which becomes the **actual embryo**, along with the **trophoblast**, from which the egg membranes (**placenta**) develop. Regardless of species, the conceptus continues to be held in its spherical form by the **zona pellucida**, which surrounds the ovum. As the number of cells and fluid in the blastocoel increase, the blastocyst increases in size and the zona pellucida becomes thinner. This developmental step is called expansion. Thereafter, the blastocyst actively breaks through the zona pellucida in ruminants, pigs, and carnivores. The conceptus thus loses its spherical shape and acquires a spindle-shaped appearance through differentiation and growth of the trophoblast. This is also called **elongation**. In pigs, each conceptus reaches a length of about 8–10 mm on day 10 after ovulation. In the horse, however, an acellular capsule develops between the zona pellucida and the trophoblast during the development of the blastocyst. As the blastocyst expands, this capsule maintains the spherical shape of the conceptus and massive influx of fluid into the blastocoel causes this spherical tissue to increase in size rapidly. The zona pellucida gradually sloughs off from the capsule, but there is no slippage from the zona.

Pregnancy requires continuous synthesis and secretion of the steroid hormone progesterone. To ensure that this occurs, the luteal phase must be prolonged by omitting luteolysis of the corpus luteum(s), i.e. the cycle corpora lutea are converted into pregnancy corpora lutea. In most domestic mammals (pigs, sheep, goats, cattle) this occurs through an **embryonic signal** which suppresses endometrial synthesis and secretion of $PGF_{2\alpha}$ shortly before the time of luteolysis. This requires that the embryo has devel-

oped to the stage where it is able to produce this signal. There are species differences in both, the nature of the embryonic signal and the way in which it is transmitted in sufficient amounts to suppress $PGF_{2\alpha}$ secretion in the endometrium. The mechanism that prolongs the life of the luteal tissue is called **maternal recognition of pregnancy**, regardless of species. Only in the dog is such a mechanism unnecessary, because the life span of the corpus luteum is independent of the presence of embryos.

Table 24.4 Duration of pregnancy in different domestic animal species.

Species	Average duration of pregnancy in days
Horse	336 (320–360)
Cattle	280 (270–295)
Sheep	150 (144–157)
Goat	150 (144–157)
Pig	114 (110–118)
Dog	63 (60–66)
Cat	63 (56–71)

■ Signals from the embryo

In **ruminants**, from the beginning of its elongation, the conceptus secretes a protein that belongs to the interferon family and is called interferon tau (τ) (**Fig. 24.17**). The homogeneity between ovine and bovine **interferon τ is** very close. In sheep it is produced by the conceptus from day 10 and in cattle from day 14. This embryonic protein has pronounced **antiluteolytic properties** that can be attributed to inhibition or modification of the oxytocin receptors in the endometrium. This prevents the binding of oxytocin, whether of endometrial or luteal origin, to oxytocin receptors in the endometrium and suppresses the pulsatile secretion of $PGF_{2\alpha}$ so that luteolysis cannot occur. In **pigs**, maternal recognition of pregnancy requires the presence of multiple concepti, which, after entry from the oviduct into the uterus around day 4, become evenly distributed in the two uterine horns until day 12. This process is also

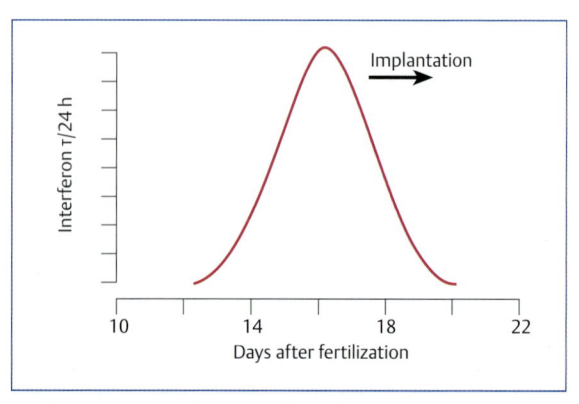

Fig. 24.17 Secretion dynamics of interferon τ in vitro. If sheep embryos are removed from the uterus at different times after fertilisation and cultivated in vitro, they secrete increasing and then decreasing amounts of interferon τ into the medium, according to the stage of development.

known as **"spacing"**. Porcine conceptuses synthesise various oestrogens, including **oestradiol-17β**. As elongation increases, oestradiol synthesis increases and the even distribution of embryos in the uterus ensures that the steroid hormones are delivered to the endometrium over a large area. They act luteotropically and maintain corpus luteum function by changing the transport pathway of $PGF_{2\alpha}$ from endocrine, (i.e. into the maternal blood circulation), to exocrine, (i.e. into the uterine lumen), thus preventing endometrial $PGF_{2\alpha}$ from reaching the corpora lutea. In addition, porcine conceptuses also synthesise interferons, but their importance in the context of maternal recognition of pregnancy is not yet clear.

In **horses**, there is a different strategy for maternal recognition of pregnancy. The spherical rapidly growing conceptus develops a distinct **intrinsic motility** in utero, made possible by embryonic prostaglandin synthesis. Prostaglandins of embryonic origin are secreted by the conceptus into the uterine lumen of the mare and cause local contractions of uterine smooth muscle. These propel the conceptus through the uterine lumen. The constantly changing position of the conceptus in the uterus can be easily detected by ultrasound examination. The smooth surface of the conceptus, which is caused by the **acellular capsule**, facilitates this movement. It is assumed that this mechanism enables the conceptus to synthesise and spread a substance over a large area, which prevents the synthesis and secretion of $PGF_{2\alpha}$ by the endometrium, and thus preventing luteolysis. Maternal recognition of pregnancy takes place in the mare between days 11 and 13. However, the substance derived from the embryo, that is involved in this process has not yet been identified. Neither oestrogens, which are also synthesised in large quantities by the equine conceptus, nor interferon τ perform this task in the horse. After completion of the maternal recognition of pregnancy, **fixation** occurs on day 16. of the still spherical equine conceptus at the base of one of the two uterine horns. This fixation is achieved by a pronounced contraction of the uterine smooth muscles with a simultaneous change in the surface of the capsule from smooth to "sticky".

For a carnivore, the **cat's** corpus luteum is a special case. It remains functionally intact for only about 40–45 days after ovulation in pseudopregnancy, but in pregnancy it remains intact for about 20 days longer, i.e. until parturition. Obviously, there is maternal recognition of pregnancy here, but the mechanism is unknown. While corpus luteum function in the cat is maintained by LH until day 45, prolactin increasingly takes over this role in the second half of pregnancy. If pregnant cats are treated with the dopamine agonist cabergoline in the second half of pregnancy, the prolactin concentration in blood decreases and abortion then follows.

■ Signals of the dam

Maintenance of early pregnancy is achieved by the corpora lutea of the dam providing the progestogens required to maintain pregnancy (**progesterone**, and in some species, in association with oestrogens; **Table 24.5**). In sheep and horses, pregnancy is subsequently maintained by placental synthesis of gestagens. The gestational corpus luteum then gradually relinquishes this task. In some species, the placenta produces progesterone as well as other gestagens, which enter the mother's blood circulation. Depending on the species, the precursor substrates for placental gestagen synthesis come partly from the foetal circulation. This functional combination of foetus and placenta is also called the **fetoplacental unit**. Progesterone causes the uterine muscles to become inactive (progesterone block) during pregnancy so that the growing foetus can develop undisturbed in an expandable uterus. The electrical conductivity of the myometrial cell membrane is reduced, so that its excitability and the transmission of an excitation is largely blocked.

Table 24.5 Progestogen synthesis during pregnancy in domestic mammals (day of gestation).

Species	Gestation period (days)	Corpus luteum	Placenta	Comments
Cattle	280	+	+ (>160–<240)	–
Horse	340	+ (<150)	+ (>60)	+ Accessory corpus luteum (>37–<120)
Goat	150	+	–	–
Sheep	150	+ (activity ↓)	+ (>70)	–
Pig	114	+	–	–
Dog	63	+	–	–
Cat	63	+	–	Prolactin as a luteotropic hormone in the second half of gestation

MORE DETAILS The importance of luteal progestin synthesis in the maintenance of pregnancy can be demonstrated by the removal of the ovaries during pregnancy. If cattle, goats, pigs and dogs are ovariectomised during pregnancy, they will abort, regardless of the time of that surgery. If sufficient progesterone is administered to such ovariectomised animals as a substitute for its endogenous synthesis, pregnancy can continue. In these species, therefore, progesterone production is carried out by the gestational corpus luteum until birth. Horses and sheep, on the other hand, are able to maintain pregnancy after ovariectomy at particular times in gestation (horse: day 70, sheep: day 55), because the placenta produces sufficient progesterone from that point on.

Among domestic animals, the **horse** exhibits compartmentalisation of steroid hormone synthesis during pregnancy. The mare's placenta increasingly synthesises progestins from about day 50 of gestation, with precursors being provided from the maternal circulation. The progestin concentration in the maternal blood plasma initially remains relatively low until the last 4–6 weeks of gestation, when additional pregnenolone is synthesised by the foetal adrenal gland which is then converted in the placenta to progestin, which enter the maternal circulation. As a result, the total progestin concentration in the blood of the mare increases considerably in the last weeks of gestation. In the second half of pregnancy, the foetal gonads, in both sexes, hypertrophy and the interstitial cells produce C19-steroid hormones. In the placenta, these steroids are further metabolised to oestrogens, which can then be detected in high concentrations in both, blood and urine of the mare. Their concentration then decreases in the final stage of pregnancy.

Chorionic gonadotropins

Cells of the equine trophoblast migrate from the so-called chorionic girdle into the maternal endometrium around gestation day 35 and form anatomical structures called "endometrial cups". From the 37th to the 120th-150th day of pregnancy, these structures synthesise a gonadotropin called **equine chorionic gonadotropin (eCG)**. Unlike human chorionic gonadotropin (hCG), eCG does not serve to maintain the corpus luteum during early pregnancy, because its secretion does not begin (day 38) until after regression of the corpus luteum has been prevented (day 16). In the mare, eCG has predominantly an effect like LH and leads to the formation of accessory corpora lutea in the ovaries, which produce progesterone in addition to the primary corpora lutea. In other species, administration of eCG has an effect comparable to FSH. Therefore, for assisted reproduction, it can be used to stimulate follicle growth and lead to so-called superovulation, i.e. the ovulation of a greater number of follicles than is usual for that species.

Maternal tolerance of pregnancy

Since the conceptus also expresses antigens in its tissues that are determined by the paternal genetic make-up, both, the embryo or foetus and the placenta, would be recognised and treated by the maternal immune system as an organ transplanted from a foreign individual, as an **allograft**. In order to prevent such recognition and consequent destruction of the conceptus, there must be changes in the **maternal** immune system during pregnancy. This process begins at coitus in a species-specific manner, through contact of maternal tissues with the paternal antigens in seminal plasma. Various regulatory mechanisms ensure that fertilisation, placentation, and development of the conceptus, can proceed unhindered and that neither the mother nor the offspring are endangered. In addition to mechanisms at the uterine level, massive systemic changes also occur on the maternal side, in which the endocrine dominance of progesterone plays an important role. Lymphocytes are mainly involved here, with the subpopulation of **regulatory T cells** being of particular importance. These cells check and balance the different possibilities of the immune response on the maternal side. Insufficient maternal tolerance of pregnancy can contribute to abortions, but also to maternal diseases.

Placental metabolism

The placenta ensures the development of the embryo and foetus during pregnancy. It **transports** nutrients as well as oxygen (O_2) from the maternal to the foetal bloodstream, absorbs **excretory substances** including carbon dioxide (CO_2) from the foetus (exchange function), **synthesises** and **secretes enzymes** and **hormones**, and ensures **thermoregulation**. The mechanisms for these exchange functions are: simple diffusion, facilitated diffusion and active transport. Depending on the type of placenta, there can be a range of tissue layers between the maternal and the foetal circulation. The number of these tissue layers determines which molecules can be exchanged between the two circulations, and in what quantity.

Gases and H_2O pass through the placenta by simple diffusion down a concentration gradient. The transport of glucose as the most important energy supplier, and the transport of amino acids take place with the help of special carrier molecules, while sodium, potassium and calcium ions pass through the placenta via specific ion pumps (active transport). The high glucose requirement of the foetus in the final stage of pregnancy, especially in horses or in the case of multiple pregnancies in sheep, can lead to glucose depletion (hypoglycaemia) and ketone body formation (ketosis) in the dam.

Proteins and lipids cannot pass through the placenta. The placentas of the **haemochorial** type (e.g. human, mouse) and the **endotheliochorial** type (e.g. dog, cat) are exceptions, because immunoglobulins pass from the maternal circulation to the foetal side, thus providing the growing foetus with important antibodies. In those **species** where the placenta does **not allow immunoglobulin passage**, these protective proteins from maternal blood are delivered postnatally to the newborn, in **colostrum**.

MORE DETAILS An adequate supply of **immunoglobulins** to the newborn is possible, especially in ruminants, pigs and horses, and also in carnivores, exclusively through the timely intake of colostrum. A lack of uptake of maternal antibodies via the colostrum is referred to as **"failure of passive transfer"**. This is one of the most frequent causes of neonatal death, because the lack of colostral antibodies usually leads to a life-threatening bacterial infection (sepsis) in the first hours or days of life.

Lipids and phospholipids are enzymatically cleaved by the placenta and the low-molecular products are made available to the foetus for further metabolism.

Trace elements and water-soluble vitamins cross the placenta and thus easily pass from the mother to the foetus. Larger peptide hormones (e.g. TSH, ACTH, insulin) cannot pass through the placenta, whereas lipophilic hormones with a small molecular size (e.g. steroid hormones, catecholamines) pass through the placenta unhindered.

Of clinical significance is the possible passage from the dam to the foetus, of drugs such as narcotics and some antibiotics, which, depending on their solubility and the administered dose, could be harmful to the foetus.

■ Parturition

Preparation of the myometrium for birth

A change in the progesterone-oestrogen concentration ratio is the most significant hormonal change in the maternal blood circulation at the stage of imminent parturition. While there is always a **progesterone** or **progestogen dominance during pregnancy**, **progesterone concentration** in blood decreases in most species, towards the **end of gestation**. In species where there are one or more corpora lutea, this fall in progesterone occurs through luteolysis. In horses and sheep there are changes in **fetoplacental progestogen synthesis** induced by foetal maturation. One of the most important consequences of the cessation of progesterone action, and the decrease in the progesterone-oestrogen ratio, is the restoration of myometrial responsiveness to contractile stimulation by oxytocin. At the end of gestation, until the onset of labour, there is a marked increase in oxytocin receptors in the myometrium, placenta and also in the smooth muscle cells of the mammary gland. The number of **calcium channels** in the membrane of the uterine muscle cells also increases by more than 60%. This significantly increases the responsiveness of these tissues to oxytocin. After expulsion of the foetus(es), there is a very rapid decrease in the number of oxytocin receptors in the myometrium, although these remain in the smooth muscle cells of the mammary gland.

The electrical and metabolic coupling of the myometrial cells is mediated by intercellular gap junctions. These ensure the transmission and synchronisation of the contraction waves in the uterus. During pregnancy, the number of **gap junctions** in the myometrium is low. However, under the influence of increasing oestrogen concentration, the number of gap junctions in the myometrium increases sharply, and prepares the uterus for labour.

> **IN A NUTSHELL** !
>
> The decrease in the progesterone-oestrogen ratio towards the end of gestation favours, at the cellular level, all those processes that allow contraction of the myometrium.

Endocrine control of parturition

The **maturation** of the **foetal adrenal cortex** is an essential prerequisite for the birth of viable young animals at term. The weight of the foetal adrenal glands increases significantly in the last phase of gestation, both in absolute and relative terms. For example, the weight of the adrenal glands of an equine foetus is 60 mg/kg of foetal body weight on day 300 of gestation, but 100 mg/kg of foetal body weight on day 335, i.e. at term. In the ovine foetus, corresponding endocrine changes are detectable about three weeks before the end of gestation. Initially, there is an increase in ACTH concentration in foetal blood, which is followed about a week later by an increase in the **secretion of cortisol** from the adrenal cortex. In the equine foetus, increases in ACTH and cortisol concentrations in the circulation do not occur until much later, in the last five days of

gestation. These concentration changes last more than twice as long in horses than in sheep. Hence, premature birth is much more frequently associated with foetal immaturity in horses, than in sheep or cattle. The increased glucocorticoid concentration in the foetal blood is not only the signal to induce birth, but also an important prerequisite for the **final maturation of foetal organ systems**, and thus for preparation for extrauterine life. A prerequisite for this effect of glucocorticoids is the expression of glucocorticoid receptors in the various foetal organs.

Removal of the foetal adrenal cortex or foetal pituitary gland prolongs gestation, while infusion of ACTH or glucocorticoids into the foetal circulation induces premature parturition. The mechanisms by which increases in foetal pulsatile ACTH and cortisol concentrations are stimulated at the end of gestation, are not fully understood. They can be triggered experimentally towards the end of gestation, by inducing foetal hypoglycaemia. It is therefore assumed that an increasingly inadequate nutrient supply across the placenta to the foetus, towards the end of pregnancy, ultimately triggers parturition.

The increase in foetal glucocorticoid secretion is followed by a decrease in maternal progesterone concentration in blood. This decrease is caused in sheep by the induction of the enzyme 17_α-hydroxylase in the placenta. This increase in enzyme activity leads to an increase of a dihydroxyprogesterone metabolite ($17_\alpha,20_\alpha$-dihydroxypregn-4-en-3-one), which can be converted to oestrogens. In sheep, although there is no direct decrease in progesterone production towards the end of gestation, the increasing conversion of progesterone to a 17_α-hydroxylated product, consequently results in decreased availability of **progesterone**. In horses, on the other hand, the enzymes of the foetal adrenal gland change during the final phase of pregnancy due to tissue maturation, so that synthesis of the progestogen precursor molecule, pregnenolone, decreases and that of cortisol increases.

The final endocrine change in the induction of parturition is the increase in $PGF_{2\alpha}$ production a few hours before the onset of labour. The **increase in $PGF_{2\alpha}$ secretion** is triggered by stimulatory effects of placental oestrogens on the activity of the enzyme phospholipase-A_2. This leads to arachidonic acid, the precursor of all prostaglandins, to be released from phospholipids in cell membranes. In those species where pregnancy is maintained until birth, by one or more **corpora lutea**, the increase in $PGF_{2\alpha}$ concentration leads to their **luteolysis**, so that progesterone synthesis ceases and the influence of progesterone on the myometrium rapidly diminishes. In addition, prostaglandins **sensitise** the myometrium to **oxytocin** (Fig. 24.18 and Fig. 24.19).

The process of parturition

There are marked differences between species in the length and development of the **preparatory, opening, expulsion** and **postnatal stages of parturition** (Table 24.6). Under the increasing influence of oestrogen, and the increasing concentration of the hormone **relaxin** (synthesised in the ovary in cattle and pigs, and in the placenta of

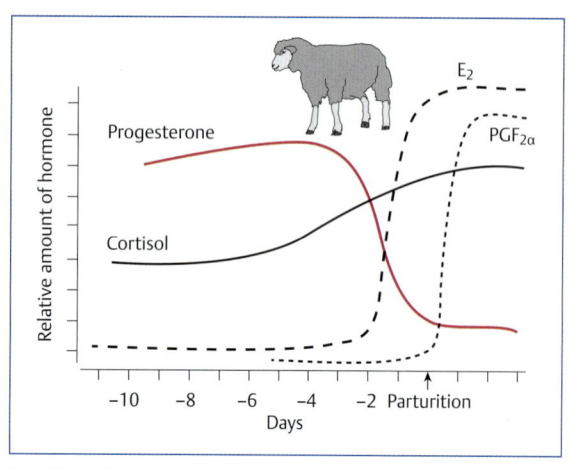

Fig. 24.18 Endocrine changes in the peripartum period of sheep. Foetal cortisol induces placental enzymes that convert progesterone to oestrogens. Oestrogens promote PGF$_{2\alpha}$ secretion by the placenta.

horses, sheep, and cats), there is a loosening of the tissue structure in the female genital tract and an increasing accumulation of water, so that the cervix and vagina dilate, the pelvic ligaments slacken, and the birth canal is prepared for the passage of the foetus. The change in dominance from progesterone to oestrogen in the mucous membrane, modifies the characteristics of mucus from the glandular cells from viscous to watery, in a similar manner to that in oestrus. The tough, sticky mucus plug that closes the cervix during gestation then dissolves, and the watery

mucus provides a slippery mucosal surface. In the mother animal, preparation for birth is usually characterised by increasing oedema in the lower abdomen, udder, and vulva, and the slackening of the maternal ligaments in the pelvis.

If the normal duration of parturition is exceeded, this is known as a birth disorder (**dystocia**).

The **preparatory stage** of parturition is characterised by more or less pronounced behavioural changes that are typical for each species. In many species, the hormonal changes in the dam are responsible for behavioural changes such as increasing restlessness. These are triggered, at least in part, by the repeated onset of myometrial contractions ("contractures") and can even lead to colic-like episodes of pain, especially in the mare. These contractures occur approximately during the last 24–48 hours before birth. Coordinated contractions of the myometrium do not occur until the final 12 hours before birth, depending on the species. Sometimes other behavioural changes can be observed, such as nest-building behaviour in pigs and dogs. Also, milk filling the udder as well as specific changes in the udder secretion (e.g. in horses a drop in the pH value to below 6.4 in the last hours before birth) can be perceived as signs of approaching parturition. In some species, like dogs, there is a drop in core body temperature of about 1 °C in conjunction with decreasing progesterone concentration in blood, which can be used clinically as an indication of approaching parturition. Particularly important in this phase is the gradual preparation of the birth canal for parturition.

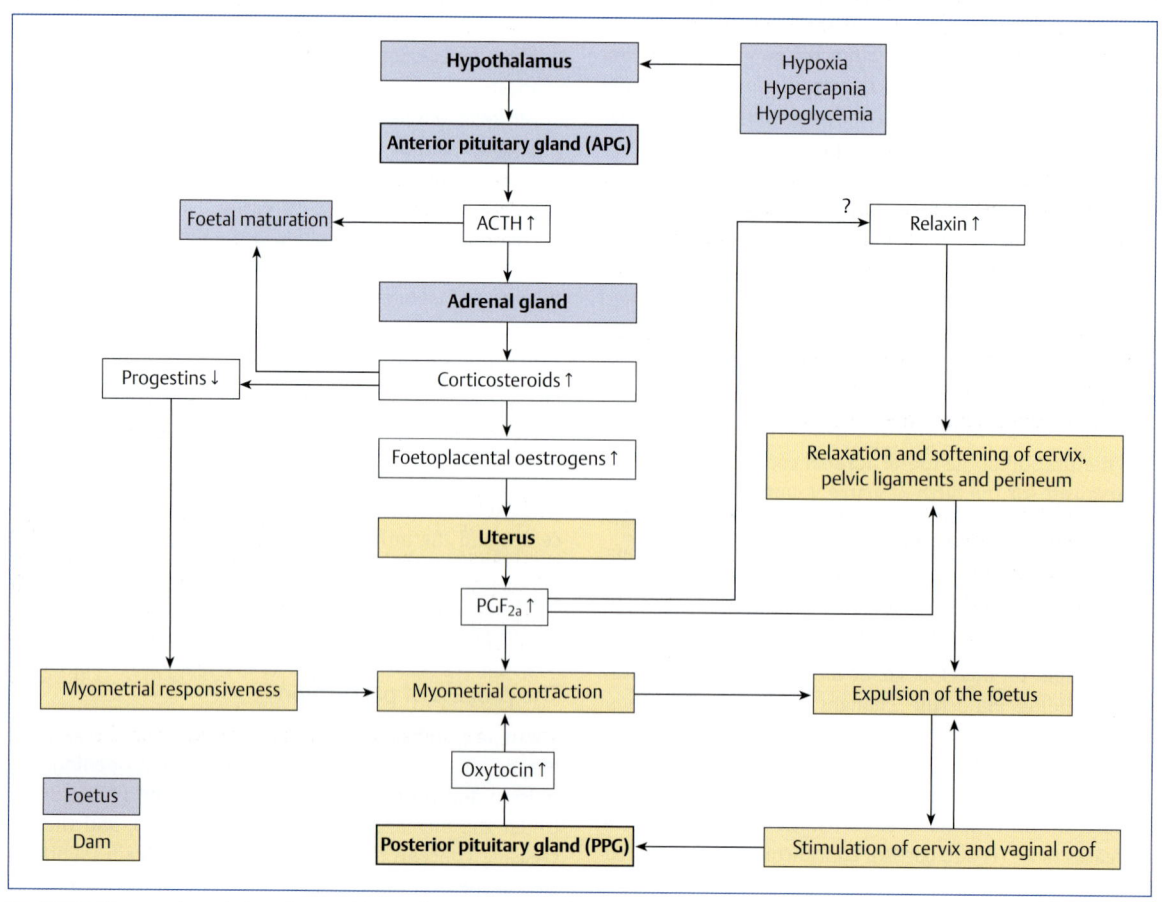

Fig. 24.19 Hormonal regulation of parturition in domestic mammal species.

Table 24.6 Duration of birth stages.

Animal species	Opening phase (hours)	Birth stage Expulsion stage (minutes)	Postpartum phase (hours)
Horse	1–4	10–15	1
Cattle	2–6	10–15	6–12
Sheep	2–6	30–120	5–8
Pig	2–12	150–180	1–4

The actual birth begins with the **opening phase** of the birth canal. During this phase, the foetus or, in animals with several foetuses, the first foetus enters the birth canal. In cattle and horses, the foetus rotates from a **lower position** (i.e. the foetal spine points ventrally) with the head and limbs tucked in, to an **upper position** (foetal spine points dorsally) with the head and forelimbs extended. At this stage, the **amniotic sacs** are still closed so that the amniotic fluid within them provides a cushion for the foetus and also helps to dilate the birth canal.

The first **spontaneous contractions** propel the foetus in its amniotic sacs into the opening inner cervix, exciting localised receptors there and leading to the release of **oxytocin** from the posterior pituitary via a **neurohormonal reflex arc** (**Ferguson reflex**). The duration and frequency of contractions are approximately the same in all domestic animals (6 contractions/15 min; duration of each contraction: 1–2 min). With entry of the foetus into the vagina, rupture of the allantochorion occurs, i.e. rupture of the **membranes**. This marks the beginning of the **expulsion** phase. Shortly afterwards, the allantoic membrane which directly surrounds the foetus, also ruptures, and the slightly viscous contents help to increase lubrication of the birth canal. In domestic mammals, the mother usually lies in a lateral position during the expulsion phase, which improves the mobility of the pelvis and thus enables further opening of the birth canal. Only in cattle does the expulsion of the calf not immediately follow rupture of the membranes, because the birth canal must first dilate. The duration of this **widening phase** is 1–3 hours, but in heifers (first-time mothers) it can be up to 6 hours. The **physiological expulsion** stage, when the calf's forehead passes through the cow's vulva, lasts about ten minute.

With advancement of the foetus into the vagina, **mechanosensors** in the dorsal **vaginal roof** are stretched, which reflexively trigger the **abdominal press** (contraction of the abdominal muscles) and thus supports **expulsion of the foetus (voiding reflex)**. With completion of foetal expulsion, the **postpartum phase** begins, in which the placenta detaches and is expelled (**Table 24.6**). In ruminants and horses, the hind legs of the foetus usually remain in the vagina for some time until the dam stands up, whereupon the umbilical cord breaks spontaneously.

24.3 Reproduction in male domestic mammals

Christine Aurich

> **ESSENTIALS**
>
> – Control of reproduction in the male takes place through complex interconnected hormonal regulatory circuits that link the organs involved (hypothalamus, pituitary gland, testis, epididymis, accessory sex glands and penis), into a functional unit.
> – The testicles produce male hormones (androgens), essential for all reproductive functions, and sperm, which pass genetic material to the next generation when mating with a female animal in heat.
> – The sperm develop in the testicular parenchyma. A characteristic morphology develops and the male's genes are redistributed.
> – After leaving the testes, sperm acquire the ability to fertilise through maturation processes in the epididymis, contact with the secretions of the accessory sex glands, and specific processes in the female genital tract.
> – The sex of a mammal is determined at fertilisation and depends on the combination of its sex chromosomes. The Y chromosome leads to male development, which depends on the function of the early developing Sertoli cells and the presence of male hormones.

24.3.1 Testicular function

The parenchyma of the male gonads, the **testis**, consists of a network of seminiferous **tubules**, the **tubules seminiferi**, and interposed collections of interstitial cells, the **Leydig cells** (Fig. 24.20). The epithelium of the seminiferous tubules is formed jointly by **Sertoli cells**, spermatogonia, spermatocytes and spermatids. The different developmental stages of spermatogenesis are closely associated with Sertoli cells, which have nutrient and support functions in the development of the male gametes. Leydig cells synthesise the steroid sex hormones (**Table 24.7**), (**Fig. 24.1**, **Fig. 24.2**). In males, the sex hormones of importance are androgens, and also oestrogens, depending on the species.

Table 24.7 Important hormones involved in the regulation of reproductive functions and their effects in the male animal.

Hormone	Origin	Structure	Effect
GnRH	Hypothalamus	Decapeptide	Synthesis and secretion of LH and FSH
endogenous opioids	CNS	Peptides	Inhibition of GnRH release
LH	Adenohypophysis	Glycoprotein	Synthesis and secretion of androgens and oestrogens from Leydig cells
FSH	Adenohypophysis	Glycoprotein	• Stimulation of spermatogenesis • Synthesis and secretion of factors involved in the control of spermatogenesis from Sertoli cells.
Prolactin	Adenohypophysis	Protein	• Testicular function (?) • seasonal coat change
Melatonin	Epiphysis	Indolamine	seasonal inhibition of hypothalamic-pituitary function
Inhibin	Sertoli cells	Glycoprotein	Inhibition of FSH release
Androgens	Leydig cells	Steroids	male genitalia: • Stimulation of spermatogenesis • Influencing the formation and function of the male sex organs Skin, hair and skin appendages: • Development of the secondary sexual characteristics Kidney and haematopoietic organs: • Stimulation of haematopoiesis Skeleton: • in low concentration: promotion of length growth • in high concentration: closure of epiphyseal joints, calcification Metabolism: • anabolic effect through increased nucleic acid and protein synthesis • Influencing the fat metabolism CNS: • Stimulation of male reproductive behaviour

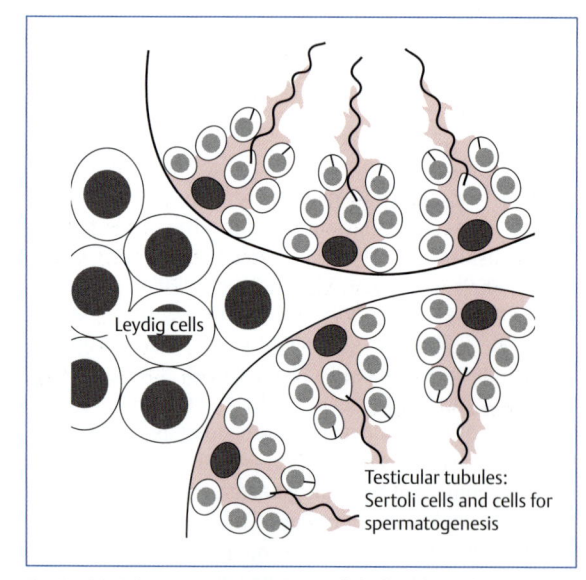

Fig. 24.20 Schematic representation of the histological structure of the testis. The testicular tubules are formed by the Sertoli cells arranged on a basal membrane, with the germ cells embedded between them at different stages of spermatogenesis. Between the testicular tubules are Leydig cells, in groups of different sizes.

Labels in figure: Leydig cells; Testicular tubules: Sertoli cells and cells for spermatogenesis

■ Steroid hormones and Leydig cell function

The cholesterol required for androgen synthesis comes partly from blood, and partly by synthesis from acetate in the Leydig cells. Intracellular cholesterol is stored in cytoplasmic fat depots, and from there, it enters the mitochondria where it is converted to pregnenolone in the inner mitochondrial membrane. This steroid is then metabolised in the endoplasmic reticulum of Leydig cells by various enzymes. These enzymes are not able to convert all the pregnenolone to testosterone, so other androgens are also produced. Pregnenolone can be oxidised to Δ16-androgens, which in various species are metabolised in the sweat glands to **pheromones** (sexual scents) (p. 104). Other metabolites of pregnenolone influence FSH secretion and spermatogenesis.

The pheromones produced by the boar give an unpleasant smell to the meat. Therefore, to prevent this, male fattening pigs are castrated as piglets. Immunological castration is also possible, where the GnRH effect is switched off by immunising against GnRH. This suppresses LH and subsequent androgen synthesis, so that no pheromones can be produced. However, castration – regardless of the method – is always associated with poorer fattening performance, as the anabolic effect of the androgens is also missing.

LH plays a central role in the regulation of steroid biosynthesis in the **Leydig cells** and affects testosterone synthesis (p.585) at several sites. The LH receptors are membrane-bound, so that LH does not act intracellularly in Leydig cells, but its effect is mediated by the release of second-messengers, especially cAMP. The second messengers stimulate the intracellular transport of cholesterol into mitochondria, as well as gene expression and activity of particular enzymes. This process of activation by LH is very short-term, but by stimulating enzyme synthesis, LH also has long-term effects on testosterone production in Leydig cells. If there are male fertility problems, the function of Leydig cells can be checked diagnostically by measuring short-term and long-term changes in testosterone concentration in blood after administration of LH or an LH-agonist. If there are no increases in testosterone concentration, impaired Leydig cell function is indicated.

Androgens leave the Leydig cells by diffusion and are rapidly distributed to all organ systems via the bloodstream. Testosterone is the most common androgen in both blood and testis. In blood, 98% of testosterone is bound to proteins (albumins, sex hormone-binding globulin). Since only the free, i.e. non-protein-bound **testosterone** is biologically active, the bioactivity of circulating testosterone is low. Free androgens enter the target cells mainly by diffusion, and partly by specific transport systems. In many target organs, it is not testosterone itself that is active, but rather its metabolites, either dihydrotestosterone or oestradiol-17β (p.533).

> **MORE DETAILS** Testosterone and **dihydrotestosterone** bind to the same steroid receptor (androgen receptor; (p.555) **Fig. 24.2**) in the cell nucleus. Dihydrotestosterone has a greater biological effect than testosterone because of its higher receptor affinity. **Oestradiol** has its own nuclear receptors in target cells. Testosterone can also be converted by various enzymes to metabolites for which no receptors exist, and which are therefore not biologically active. The actual metabolites produced depend on the enzyme profile of cells. Mutations of the androgen receptor can negatively influence fertility by inhibiting the effect of androgens on their target cells in the genitals, because of reduced androgen receptor affinity. In domestic mammals, very little is known about mutations of the androgen receptor, but in humans, more than 200 androgen receptor mutations have been documented, some of which can be linked to certain diseases. Genetic alterations of the oestradiol receptor, on the other hand, are much less common.

Androgens influence their own synthesis through inhibitory effects on hypothalamic **GnRH** and thus indirectly inhibit pituitary LH release (feedback mechanism). A high testosterone concentration in peripheral blood leads to an inhibition of GnRH release (negative feedback). The inhibitory effect of testosterone on GnRH-releasing neurons is mediated in the CNS by neuromodulators (**Fig. 24.21**). This reduces LH secretion so that there is no further stimulation of Leydig cell function, and androgen synthesis decreases.

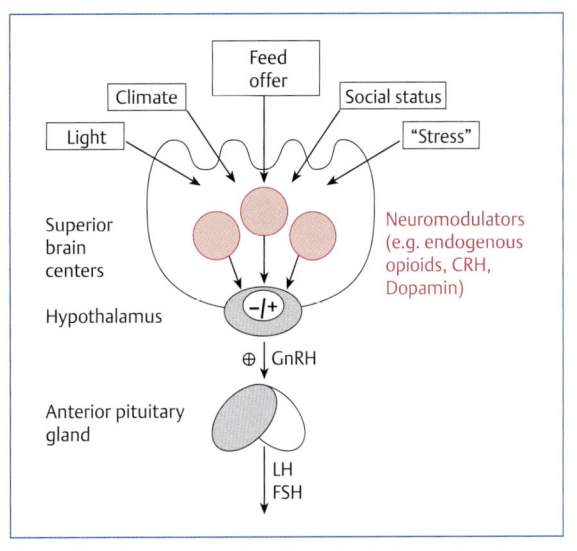

Fig. 24.21 Influence of the hypothalamic-pituitary system by exogenous factors, mediated via neuromodulators.

In the male, androgens have a variety of effects both on sexual organs and other organ systems. Testosterone is essential for the continuous process of **spermatogenesis**. Spermatogenesis is influenced indirectly by the **Sertoli cells**. Maturation of sperm cells in the **epididymis** is under the influence of **dihydrotestosterone** which is produced from testosterone in the Sertoli cells and secreted into the testicular tubules. Testosterone reaches numerous other target organs via the peripheral blood circulation.

During **puberty**, androgens stimulate the complete development of the male **sexual organs** (penis, accessory sex glands), the function and morphology of which are only appropriate for adult function when there is adequate androgen influence. Androgens are also responsible for the species-specific **masculine appearance** (physique, secondary sex characteristics) by effects on bone, muscle and skin function. By acting in the CNS, androgens promote male behavioural patterns. Androgens synthesised and secreted in the CNS are also important. Male behavioural patterns are mainly related to reproductive behaviour, such as aggressive behaviour towards other males, fighting to establish rank, or the entire sequence of mating behaviour. Sufficient testosterone production is necessary for the development of the reproductive instinct (libido sexualis) in males, but there is no direct correlation between the expression of the **libido sexualis** and the **level of endogenous androgens**.

> **IN A NUTSHELL** !
>
> Most reproductive-related functions in males depend on the presence of androgens.

Endocrinology, reproduction

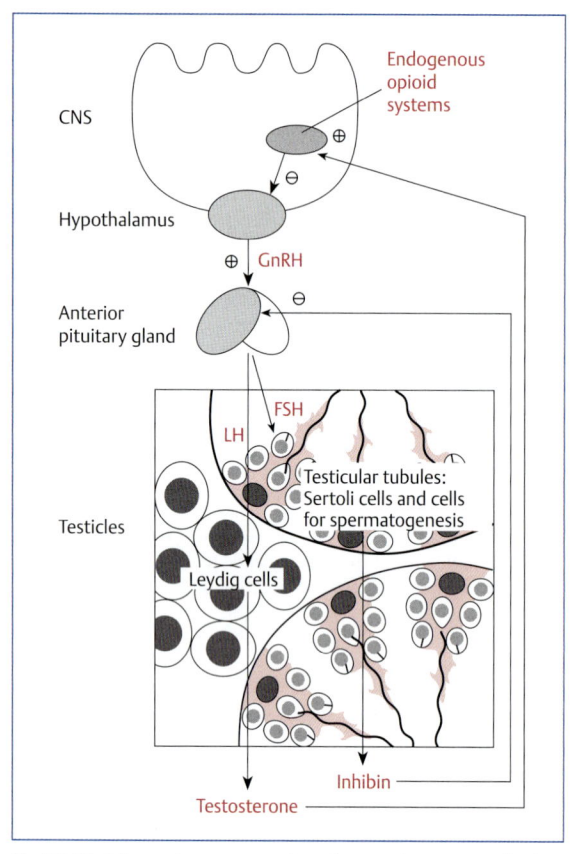

Fig. 24.22 Schematic representation of testicular negative feedback mechanisms: testosterone (synthesis site: Leydig cells) inhibits hypothalamic GnRH secretion, thus indirectly inhibiting pituitary LH release and its own synthesis and secretion. Inhibin (synthesis site: Sertoli cells) selectively inhibits FSH secretion by the pituitary gland, and thus spermatogenesis.

24.3.2 Spermatogenesis and Sertoli cell function

■ Spermatogenesis

Early germ cells, like all other cells, are diploid and have one paternal and one maternal **set of chromosomes**. In order to maintain diploidy in the next generation, the gametes, spermatozoon and egg, must each have only one set of haploid chromosomes. Only germ cells have the specialised ability to carry out the necessary maturation division or **meiosis**. During meiosis, not only the set of chromosomes is halved, but there is also random distribution of different maternal and paternal homologous chromosomes, by so-called **crossing over**, in which chromosome segments are exchanged between homologous chromosomes, so that there is a complete redistribution of maternal and paternal genetic material. The gametes of the offspring thus carry a different, new combination of genetic material. A haploid set of chromosomes is sufficient for the function and preservation of an organism. Diploid organisms are superior, however, because they have a reserve copy that increases the chances of survival in cases of lethal or harmful mutations. This also applies to mutations and gene duplications that introduce a new valuable function. Diploidy allows the organism to use both new and old

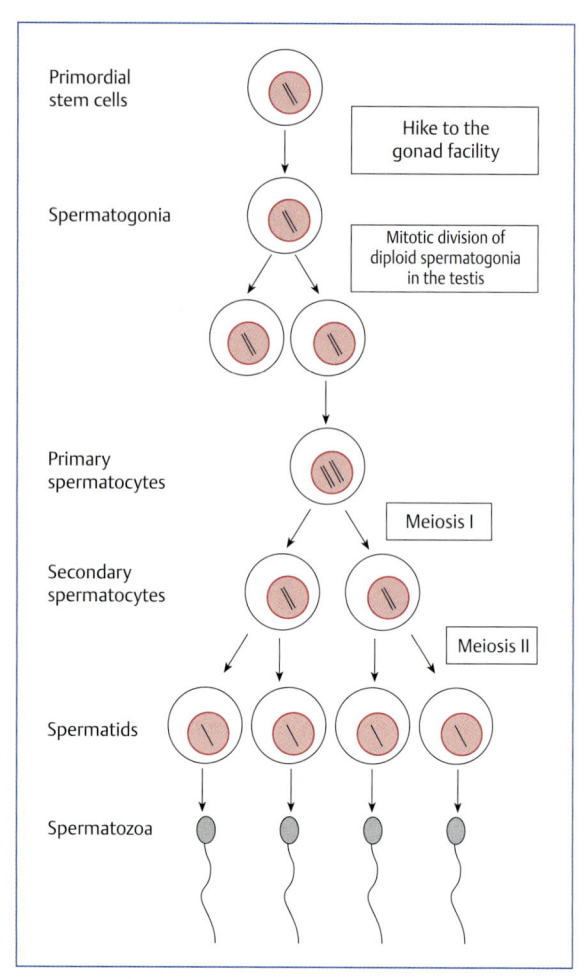

Fig. 24.23 Schematic representation of spermatogenesis in the mammal. The primordial germ cells migrate into the **gonadal system** and are then called spermatogonia. They initially reproduce mitotically. While a part of the spermatogonia remains as a stem cell population, the other part enters meiosis-I after duplication of the chromosome set (primary spermatocytes) enters meiosis-I and forms the already haploid secondary spermatocyte population, which immediately distributes its chromosomes to the developing spermatids by meiosis-II. Through spermatogenesis these differentiate into the morphologically characteristic spermatozoa.

functions. Through the redistribution of genes associated with sexual reproduction, such new hereditary traits can assert themselves better and faster.

Spermatogenesis is the process by which diploid male germ cells form haploid spermatozoa by meiosis (**Fig. 24.23**). During embryonic development, the primordial germ cells undergo several stages of multiplication and differentiate into **spermatogonia**. These are initially subject to a **meiosis block**, which prevents spermatogonia from entering meiosis. It is not until the onset of puberty that the hypothalamic-pituitary-gonadal axis is activated and, under the influence of FSH and testosterone, spermatogenesis is induced, i.e. the meiosis block is lifted.

The **spermatogonia** first divide mitotically. Some of these new spermatogonia remain as a stem cell population, while others differentiate further and enter meiosis. The first step of meiosis is the duplication of the diploid chromosome set. These **primary spermatocytes** are the largest germ cells of the germinal epithelium. They are still diploid, and each chromosome consists of two identical DNA strands, the chromatids. They therefore contain a total of four sets of DNA (4 n DNA). During division-I of meiosis, the haploid **secondary spermatocytes** are formed. They each contain only one homologous chromosome consisting of two chromatids (2 n DNA). In the **secondary spermatocytes**, there is no reduplication of the DNA. These spermatocytes immediately enter division-II of meiosis, in which the two chromatids of each chromosome are distributed to the daughter cells, so that the now newly formed spermatids each have a single copy of the entire set of chromosomes. Four haploid spermatids have thus arisen from one diploid primary **spermatocyte**. In the subsequent process of spermiogenesis, the spermatids differentiate into highly specialised **spermatozoa**.

> **IN A NUTSHELL** !
>
> Spermatozoa are only formed at the onset of sexual maturity, before which the male germ cells are subject to meiosis block.

Spermiogenesis can be divided into four phases, in the course of which a compact, streamlined spermatozoon with a locomotor system is formed from the round spermatid, with the loss of superfluous cytoplasm and cytoplasmic organelles.

MORE DETAILS

The spermiogenesis process

– In the **Golgi phase**, the acrosomal vacuole is formed by fusion of small vesicles from the Golgi apparatus, which attaches to the nuclear membrane. At the same time, two centrioles migrate to the opposite nuclear pole. While the proximal centriol attaches to the basal plate of the nucleus, the axonema grows from the distal centriol, which later forms the spermatozoa tail.
– In the **cap phase** the acrosomal vacuole flattens and spreads over the upper part of the nucleus.
– During the **acrosome phase** the cell elongates with increasing compaction of the nucleus. During this process, nuclear proteins typical of somatic cells, the histones, are exchanged for the sperm-specific protamines, which are responsible for the particularly compact packing of chromatin. In this phase, the spermatid rotates so that its tail points towards the tubule lumen. The mitochondria arrange themselves around the upper region of the flagellum and form the middle piece. The cytoplasm increasingly shifts and now surrounds the proximal region of the flagellum.
– In the subsequent **maturation phase** the transformation to the typically shaped spermatozoon is completed. The superfluous cytoplasm is detached in the form of a residual body and, after release of the complete spermatozoon into the tubular space, this residual body is degraded in the Sertoli cell.

Disorders of spermiogenesis

These are either permanent, such as from hormonal imbalances, or temporary, when there is a rise in temperature from some disease process, and the sperm released have some change in shape (pathological sperm forms). Such shape changes are tails that are too short, shape-changed acrosomes or plasma droplets containing superfluous cytoplasm that has not separated from the sperm. Depending on the extent of the shape deviation, sperm function and thus fertilisation ability may also be impaired.

The release of the spermatozoon from the germinal epithelium is called **spermiation**. The duration of a spermatogenesis cycle varies in domestic animals at, for example, 34 days in pigs, 43 days in cattle and 57 days in horses.

MORE DETAILS Throughout spermatogenesis, the germ cells resulting from a spermatogony remain connected to each other via cytoplasmic bridges. This ensures that the haploid germ cells are also supplied with all the products of the complete diploid genome. Thus, spermatids with a **Y chromosome**, which has only a relatively small number of genes, and those carrying a gene with a recessive deleterious mutation, are able to survive.

In most mammals, spermatogenesis only occurs at a temperature lower than body temperature. This is achieved by "externalisation" of the testes from the abdominal cavity into the scrotum. If there are "inhibition malformations", and one or both testicles do not descend into the scrotum, but remain in the abdominal cavity, or in the inguinal cleft ("**cryptorchidism**"), the affected testis does not produce sperm. However, Leydig cell functions including androgen synthesis, still occur at core body temperature, so that bilateral or unilaterally castrated cryptorchids are infertile, but show typical male behavioural patterns. In a few species, such as elephants, klipsliders and whales, the normal location of the testes is within the abdomen, but nevertheless, Sertoli cell function and spermatogenesis are maintained.

■ Function of the Sertoli cells

The **Sertoli cell** is the somatic cell of the germinal epithelium. Sertolic cells are essential for the germ cells to develop and are associated with germ cells during the entire process of **spermatogenesis**. Germ cells that lose contact with Sertoli cells cannot undergo spermatogenesis.
Sertoli cells have the following important functions:

- They transmit hormonal stimuli to the germ cells.
- They provide an optimal environment for the developing germ cells.
- They organise the germ cell population, and their transfer towards the tubule lumen.
- They establish a **blood-testicle barrier** which protects the germ cells from negative external influences and harmful effects by the body's own immune system.
- They also regulate FSH secretion from the pituitary gland through negative feedback.

MORE DETAILS Germ cells have no androgen receptors and, with the exception of the spermatogonia, also no receptors for FSH. The germ cell population is therefore dependent on the intervention of Sertoli cells for hormonal control. FSH and testosterone stimulate Sertoli cells to produce various factors that are essential for germ cell development. The influence is interactive because each germ cell stage produces factors that in turn stimulate the Sertoli cells to produce the necessary substances and factors. There is communication between germ cells and Sertoli cells that optimises the conditions for the different germ cell stages and coordinates the various functions. This paracrine and autocrine regulation is not limited to the germinal epithelium, but includes the neighbouring **Leydig cells** and peritubular cells. Thus, an information network exists between the different compartments and individual cells of the testis that is responsible for the fine regulation of spermatogenesis. Only some of these regulating factors have so far been identified. These include the **androgen-binding protein** (ABP) from Sertoli cells. It binds testosterone and ensures adequate steroid hormone concentration in Sertoli cells, and also testosterone transport into the epididymis.

Table 24.8 Animal species differences and peculiarities with regard to penis type and ejaculation.

	Ruminants	Pig	Horse	Dog
Penis type	fibroelastic	fibroelastic	musculocavernous	musculocavernous
Ejaculation duration	1–2 s (during the "after-push")	2–10 min	15–30 s	5–40 min
Semen depot in the female genital tract	Vagina, immediately before the cervix	Cervix/Uterus	Uterus (Cervix)	Vagina (and uterus)
Special features	in sheep and goats: urethral process over-hangs the glans penis by several centimetres, contains erectile tissue itself	Penis tip turned cork-screw-like, is fixed in the cervical rings during mating and prevents backflow of semen	greatly enlarged glans penis dilates the cervix so much that ejaculate is partially deposited directly into the uterus	greatly enlarged bulbus glandis anchors the penis in the vagina for minutes ("hanging"), male animal descends during ejaculation ("changing")

Another important function of the Sertoli cell is the formation of the **blood-testis barrier**. When the first germ cell enters meiosis at the onset of puberty, the zonulae occludentes or tight junctions form between neighbouring Sertoli cells, dividing the germinal epithelium into a basal and luminal part and allowing only a selective exchange of substances between the two compartments. This ensures that the very sensitive haploid germ cell stages are protected from toxic and harmful influences. During spermatogenesis, a number of proteins and antigens are expressed on the surface of the germ cells that are recognised as not being endogenous. Without this protective measure of the blood-testis barrier, the germ cells would therefore be damaged and degraded by the cells of the body's own immune system. A disturbance of the blood-testicle barrier can occur as a result of testicular inflammation or traumatic damage to the testicular tissue which results in **fertility disorders**.

> **IN A NUTSHELL**   !
>
> The Sertoli cell is the most important partner of the male germ cells.

24.3.3   Sexual behaviour

Sexual behaviour is controlled by a centre in the **central nervous system** that is responsible for behaviour. During foetal development, androgens promote the masculinisation of this centre. In the growing and adult animal, increasing production of **androgens** in the testes activates male sexual behaviour and sexual desire (libido sexualis). The climax of male sexual behaviour is mating with a female in heat. This requires that the male is able to be aroused in the presence of a female in heat, and to react appropriately, i.e. approaching and making direct contact with the female. This is followed by the mating act: a chain of interdependent innate reflex actions, with only limited self determination. The mating reflex chain is controlled by a nerve centre in the lumbar and sacral medulla (erectile centre). Unpleasant or painful experiences during the mating act can reduce or even completely switch off libido sexualis.

The **mating reflex chain** begins with a **prelude** characteristic for each species. The male makes visual, olfactory and tactile contact with the female. This is followed by the advancement (**excavation)** and **erection of** the penis. These are made possible by an increased blood inflow with reduced blood outflow, which is caused by vasodilation of the arteries with simultaneous vasoconstriction of the veins in the region of the penile corpus cavernosum. The penis differs in anatomical structure in different species, with two basic types of a fibroelastic and a musculocavernous **penis** (Table 24.8). Excavation and erection are under the influence of the parasympathetic nervous system. In cattle, this is triggered by the "archway reflex" (outline of the hindquarters of the mating partner). The female jumps up and clutches, followed by searching movements of the male and insertion of the penis into the vagina. Tactile stimuli, especially the temperature of the vulval mucosa, are essential for the male to locate the female vulva.

Ejaculation is preceded by frictional movements (horse, dog, pig), depending on the animal species, or it takes place during the after thrust (ruminant). The actual ejaculation (expulsion of sperm) is from waves of contractions of the smooth muscles of the epididymis, ductus deferens (vas deferens), and urethra (urethra). The sperm-rich contents of the **epididymis** are **first** expelled, accompanied by secretions of the **accessory sex glands**, and then followed by secretions of the urethra and the accessory sex glands. The volume and composition of the secretions of the accessory sex glands vary according to species. There are also individual differences in the volumes of these secretions, influenced, for example, by the length of foreplay. The expulsion of sperm from the urethra is assisted by contractions of the ischiocavernosus and bulbocavernosus muscles. After ejaculation, the male descends from the mating partner. The penis gradually becomes flaccid as the blood volume subsides. Depending on the species, a more or less pronounced after-play takes place. In the dog, a so-called transfer occurs at the beginning of ejaculation, i.e. the male rises from the bitch and turns his back to her. This species-specific position during the mating act is made possible by rotation in the proximal area of the penis. The penis is thereby fixed by a very strong swelling of the glans in the vagina of the bitch ("hanging"). In stallions used in riding or racing, sexual behaviour is often suppressed by the rider or trainer through punishment. This leads to conditioning, i.e. the stallion associates the sight of a mare with a negative, often painful experience, and shows no or at least a reduced libido sexualis. When such stallions are later used for breeding, it often takes some time until they overcome this negative experience and the mating reflex chain up to ejaculation, can then operate successfully.

If semen is to be obtained from a male animal, an artificial vagina similar in size and shape to the anatomical structure of the vagina is offered, using the **reflex chain**, after complete excavation and erection of the penis and jumping onto a female animal. To trigger ejaculation, a disproportionate stimulus is usually required in terms of temperature, i.e. the internal temperature of the **artificial vagina** must be approx. 4–8 °C above the internal body temperature (38 °C). In dogs and pigs, as well as in some stallions, ejaculation can also be achieved by a hand massage technique, if necessary after jumping on a female surrogate. In cattle, pigs and horses, the female is often replaced by a dummy, a jumping phantom. This must imitate in form the "archway stimulus" of the real female. For stimulation, the presence of a female in heat is helpful at first, but this can often be omitted after appropriate conditioning with semen collection using the phantom. Semen collection without using the reflex chain is possible with the help of an **electroejaculator**. Here, excavation, erection and ejaculation are triggered by electrical stimulation of the spinal cord and the male sexual apparatus. This is mainly used in wild animals to **obtain semen** under general anaesthesia, but is also possible on conscious tolerant animals such as cattle or sheep. For reasons of animal welfare, electroejaculation on non-anaesthetised ruminants should be limited for specific individual veterinary diagnosis, and not for regular semen collection. The composition of ejaculates obtained by electroejaculation often differs from ejaculates obtained with an artificial vagina, as increased secretion of the accessory sex glands may occur.

> **IN A NUTSHELL** !
>
> The mating act is a chain of interdependent innate reflexes that have only limited self control.

24.4 Fertilisation, sex determination and assisted reproduction

Christine Aurich

24.4.1 Fertilisation

In order for a new individual to develop from a spermatozoon and an egg cell, both gametes must meet during the fertilisation process, recognise each other, and the spermatozoon must penetrate the egg cell. Only then can the haploid genome of the spermatozoon unite with the haploid genome of the egg cell, and form the diploid zygote.

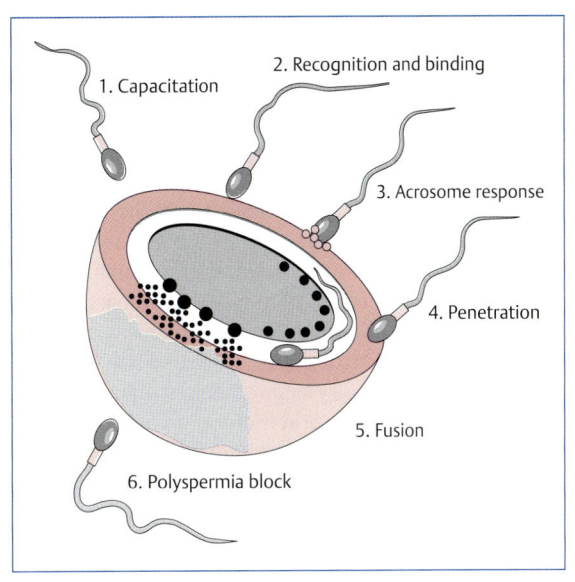

Fig. 24.24 Fertilisation sequence: 1./2. Capacitated spermatozoa bind to the zona pellucida. 3. The binding induces the acrosome reaction. 4. the spermatozoon can penetrate the zona pellucida with the help of released enzymes and hyperactivated movement. 5. fusion of the acrosome-reacted spermatozoon with the vitelline membrane (oolemn) of the oocyte results in oocyte activation, i.e. the oocyte completes meiosis and starts the embryonic developmental programme. 6. exocytosis of the cortical granules (black spots) triggers the polyspermy block (cortical reaction, zona hardening).

The fertilisation process is a complex sequence of events in the female genital tract. Prior to **fertilisation**, spermatozoa must undergo a subtle functional change known as **capacitation**. Only capacitated spermatozoa can recognise an egg and, when bound to the egg zona pellucida, can carry out the **acrosome reaction**. The acrosome reaction is the exocytosis of the acrosome, through which acrosomal enzymes are activated and released. With their help, a **hyperactivated spermatozoon** can penetrate the **zona pellucida** and finally fuse with the oocyte. The oocyte has developed a mechanism of **polyspermy block** that prevents more than one spermatozoon from penetrating the oocyte (**Fig. 24.24**).

■ Sperm maturation in the epididymis

Despite being morphologically complete, spermatozoa from the testis are not yet capable of fertilisation. They are not able to move independently, recognise the ovum and penetrate the zona pellucida. They only acquire these abilities during their transport through the **epididymis** – a process called **sperm maturation**.

Spermatozoa leave the germinal epithelium in a highly differentiated state, and are transported into the epididymis by the secretory flow and peristalsis of the tubules of the testis via rete testes and ductuli efferentes. To transport paternal DNA to the ovum and link it with maternal DNA, spermatozoa differentiate into various functional structures called domains. The head, which is almost completely occupied by the nucleus, is enclosed by the **acrosome** in the upper third to half, depending on species. The acrosome contains a number of proteolytic enzymes (e.g. the serine proteinase, acrosin), which faciliate spermatozoon penetratation of the outer egg membrane, especially the zona pellucida, to finally reach the egg cell (**Fig. 24.25**). The following **equatorial segment** and the **postacrosomal region** are specialised to fuse with the cell membrane of the oocyte (**oolemma**). The **midpiece** with its mitochondria maintains energy supply of the sperm, and the tail provides independent locomotion. Corresponding to the different functional regions of the spermatozoon, the plasma membrane is also organised into domains with different properties and functions. The shape and size of a spermatozoon can vary greatly among different animal species.

The mechanisms of **sperm maturation** and the resulting protective measures for the spermatozoa are extremely complicated and not yet fully elucidated. In the course of epididymal passage, stabilisation of tail and nucleus structures occurs through the formation of disulphide bridges and metabolic changes. A main feature of **maturation** is the functional change of the **plasma membrane** of the spermatozoon. Through interactions with the secretion products in the various sections of the epididymis, there is a gradual change in the exposed spermatozoon surface. The lipid bilayer itself also changes in composition and distribution of individual components. Some membrane proteins redistribute completely within the plasma membrane. This redistribution of proteins and the changes in the lipid bilayer contribute to the formation of the domain structure typical of the plasma membrane of a mature spermatozoon.

While the maturation processes occur mainly in the **head** and **body of the epididymis**, depending on species, the **tail of the epididymis** serves as a storage organ for mature spermatozoa. The differentiation of the epididymis as a storage organ is particularly well developed in placental mammals. It is probably linked to the principle of internal fertilisation and the need to store the spermatozoa population until ejaculation. The entire passage of a sperm through the epididymis takes 10–14 days. During that time, in addition to maturation, the spermatozoa must survive while stored in the epididymis, Thus, the processes of functional maturation are also associated with those that protect the spermatozoa. The **blood epididymis barrier** protects the spermatozoa from the immune system in a similar way to the blood-testicle barrier. However, there are also other protective measures. Incorporation of cholesterol into the spermatozoa plasma membrane helps to stabilise it. This is reinforced by a protective layer of proteins that masks functional proteins on the spermatozoa surface, such as receptors for the oocyte, or ion channels, or prevents their degradation by proteolysis. The epididymis has also developed several mechanisms that protect spermatozoa from oxidative stress from lipid peroxidation, which could severely restrict the ability to fertilise.

In males with low sexual activity, i.e. when ejaculation does not happen about once a day, a large reservoir of sperm produced over several days builds up in the epididymis. When an ejaculate is collected after several days or weeks of sexual rest, it is therefore not uncommon to find a disproportionately large number of dead and overaged sperm. The overaging of the sperm is indicated by pathological sperm shapes such as broken necks or kinked sperm tails. Only after repeated ejaculation, i.e. when the sperm reservoir has been drained, does sperm quality return to normal. However, special emptying mechanisms of the epididymal tails ensure that an excessive number of sperm do not accumulate, and sperm from the epididymal tails are regularly released during urination.

The **epididymal fluid** partly consists of secretions of the Sertoli cells, which leave the testicular tubules together with the spermatozoa. These secretions also nourish the spermatozoa. Their synthesis and secretion are stimulated by FSH in the presence of testosterone. Fluid production is continuous and the resulting fluid flow causes spermatozoa to be flushed out of the testicular tubules towards the epididymis. In the epididymis, the Sertoli cell secretions are modified by the resorptive and secretory activity of the epididymal epithelium, so that the composition of the fluid is constantly changing in the different sections. The possible effect of changes in blood plasma composition is prevented by the **blood-epididymal barrier**. Besides proteins and lipids, the epididymal fluid contains high concentrations of androgens, especially dihydrotestosterone. The resorptive and secretory activity of the epididymal epithelium as well as the maturation of the spermatozoa can only take place in the presence of androgens.

> ### IN A NUTSHELL   !
>
> Testicular spermatozoa are not yet capable of fertilisation and must first undergo a maturation phase in the epididymis, during which they acquire fertilisation competence.

■ Seminal plasma and ejaculation

The liquid part of the ejaculate is called seminal plasma. It consists of the secretions of the **accessory sex glands** (**seminal vesicle** (vas deferens, seminal vesicle glands, prostate and bulbourethral glands) and a small amount of the epididymal secretion.

There are differences in the development of the accessory sex glands and in the composition of **seminal plasma** in different species. Both, development and function of the accessory sex glands are androgen-dependent. Gonadectomy (castration) of a male animal stops the supply of testosterone and thus causes the accessory sex glands to become inactive. If castration takes place before sexual maturity, the accessory sex glands remain underdeveloped, and if castrated later, these glands atrophy and cease secretory activity. The secretions of the accessory sex glands are essentially protective and nutritive for spermatozoa. During ejaculation, proteinase inhibitors and other proteins of the seminal plasma associate with the surface of spermatozoa and enlarge the enveloping protein layer. They thus protect the sensitive membranes during migration through the female genital tract, where spermatozoa may encounter unfavourable conditions. Seminal proteins thus prevent phagocytosis of spermatozoa by polymorphonuclear neutrophil granulocytes. These proteins are known as **decapacitation factors** or negative regulatory factors. However, they can also have a positive influence on sperm functions and are then called positive regulatory factors.

In addition to protective and transport functions for sperm, seminal plasma also has direct effects on the female genital tract. In addition to the supportive effect on ovulation of the dominant follicle (p.565), seminal plasma factors are also involved in preparing the female genital tract for possible conception and pregnancy. Studies in mice, humans and horses show that contact with male antigens expressed in seminal plasma, induces primary immune tolerance of the female during coitus. This contributes to the conceptus not being recognised as "foreign tissue" and then being rejected (maternal tolerance of pregnancy). At the cellular level, regulatory T lymphocytes play a particularly important role in this process. They suppress any inflammatory reaction induced by antigens of the conceptus, and support important vascular changes in development of the placenta. In humans, exposure of the female to seminal plasma during coitus, considerably increases the chance of pregnancy. In horses and cattle, successful embryo transfer from a donor animal, is possible without the genitals of the recipient animal ever having had contact with seminal plasma.

In horses in particular, but to a lesser extent in other species, the introduction of seminal plasma into the uterus during oestrus, whether by natural mating or artificial insemination, causes an immediate inflammatory reaction of the endometrium. This self-cleaning mechanism quickly removes surplus sperm, other cells and especially bacteria, thus preventing infection of the uterine mucosa.

If an ejaculate is processed for artificial insemination, the at least partial removal of seminal plasma is advantageous for the preservation of semen in some species, such as horses and pigs. The seminal plasma is replaced by a preservation medium (semen diluent) that contains sugar, a pH buffer, plasma membrane stabilising factors, and other protective agents. In species with a high sperm concentration, removal of the seminal plasma is not necessary, but nevertheless, without the addition of seminal diluents, sperm viability cannot be maintained.

■ Sperm transport and storage in the female genital tract

Depending on species, the ejaculate is deposited either in the vagina (**vaginal inseminator**) or in the uterus (**uterine inseminator**) (Table 24.8). In vaginal inseminators, the cervix uteri and cervical mucus are the first barrier for the spermatozoa. In the strongly folded and mucus-filled **cervix**, immobile or malformed spermatozoa are retained, while fully functional spermatozoa accumulate in the folds and crypts of the cervix, or migrate by their own motility into the uterus. The cervix has some storage capacity for spermatozoa, so that passage of spermatozoa into the uterus can occur over several days. The viscosity of cervical mucus is under hormonal control and is therefore related to the oestrous cycle, so that spermatozoa are only able to pass through cervical mucus around the time of ovulation.

Transport of spermatozoa in the **uterus** itself is predominantly passive and is supported by antiperistaltic/retrograde contractions of the uterine musculature. For spermatozoa deposited directly into the uterus, the first barrier is the uterotubal junction, where like the cervix, sperm selection occurs. Only some of the spermatozoa in an ejaculate pass through this junction and reach the **fallopian tube**. The caudal segment of the **tubal isthmus** also acts as a **sperm reservoir** in where spermatozoa are retained until ovulation. Motile and fertilisation-capable spermatozoa make close contact with the epithelial cells of the isthmus, while dying or degenerating spermatozoa float in the lumen and eventually are removed by phagocytosis.

There are therefore three phases in sperm transport:
- the predominantly passive fast transport
- the accumulation in sperm reservoirs, a predominantly active process
- the slow detachment and directed transport of sperm

MORE DETAILS Some sperm reach the site of fertilisation in only a few minutes. However, these are not capable of fertilisation. Only after several hours does a largely fertilisation-competent sperm population establish itself in the fallopian tube. This leads to an extraordinary reduction in the number of sperm. For example in cattle, about 10^{10} sperm enter the uterus, and this number declines to about 10^6 in the uterus and in the caudal isthmus there are only about 10^4 sperm. At the site of fertilisation, only 10^2 or fewer spermatozoa actually meet the egg.

The **sperm reservoir** in the fallopian tube is of particular importance for both, vaginal and uterine inseminators. After actively overcoming the uterotubal junction, the spermatozoa enter the caudal **isthmus** of the **fallopian tube**. Here they reside in close contact with the ciliated fallopian tube epithelium. This so-called functional sperm reservoir in the fallopian tube is essential for successful fertilisation by:
- Selection of an intact sperm population
- Ensuring survival of spermatozoa for some time
- Enabling the capacitation process
- Reduction of sperm count by regulating their migration to the site of fertilisation as part of the process of polyspermy block

Binding to the oviduct epithelium is mediated by carbohydrate-protein interactions. For bound spermatozoa, the initial processes of capacitation are inhibited. This prolongs sperm life, since capacitation always destabilises spermatozoa. Around the time of ovulation, as yet unknown signals initiate capacitation and detachment of the spermatozoa from the fallopian tube epithelium. The spermatozoa begin to migrate into the tubal ampulla, the site of fertilisation, supported by a flow of fluid and movement of cilia of the fallopian tube.

> **IN A NUTSHELL**
>
> The fallopian tube synchronises sperm functions (capacitation) with ovulation so that fertilisation-competent gametes meet simultaneously at the right time at the site of fertilisation.

■ Interactions of sperm and seminal plasma with the female genital tract

Sperm capacitation

Capacitation refers to all the physiological changes in a spermatozoon that enable acrosome reaction and hyperactivated movement. Although the mechanisms are not yet fully understood, the **capacitation process** can be characterised by a sequence of intracellular changes in metabolism, ion concentration, membrane properties and protein phosphorylation. Only capacitated spermatozoa can enter the acrosome reaction, In which the outer acrosomal membrane fuses at many points with the overlying spermatozoon plasma membrane, creating openings and channels in the acrosome through which acrosomal enzymes pass (**Fig. 24.25**). As capacitation progresses, spermatozoa also change their pattern of movement. They develop a strong zigzag movement. This hyperactive motility is extremely energy-demanding and requires intense metabolic activity. The acrosome reaction and hyperactivated motility are both essential for **penetration** of the **zona pellucida** of the oocyte. Hyperactive motility also allows spermatozoa to separate from the epithelial cells of the oviduct isthmus, and subsequently to actively travel to the site of fertilisation.

MORE DETAILS   The first steps of **capacitation** are the removal of the protective protein envelope and the efflux of cholesterol from the sperm membrane. **Cholesterol efflux** is presumably mediated by lipid-binding proteins of the female genital tract. This reverses the protective measures taken during sperm maturation and ejaculation to allow sperm to survive during residence in the epididymis and passage through the female genital tract. The loss of cholesterol increases the fluidity of the plasma membrane and affects the membrane potential. This affects in particular the plasma membrane of the acrosome in the region of the spermatozoa head, which is involved in the **acrosome reaction**. In the fluid periacrosomal membrane, the membrane proteins are relocated and form aggregates. In this way, low-protein microdomains are formed, with particularly fluid and fusiogenic properties, thus enabling, the many point fusions with the outer acrosomal membrane during the subsequent acrosomal reaction. As a result of all these processes, as well as an initial influx of calcium, and phosphorylation reactions in the head and tail compartments, the spermatozoon is now ready for interaction with the egg.

Improper preparation or storage of semen to be used in artificial insemination, can initiate sperm capacitation even before transferrance into the female genital tract. This causes a significant reduction in the fertility of such semen preparations.

> **IN A NUTSHELL**   !
>
> Spermatozoa must undergo capacitation in order to fertilise an egg.

Spermatozoon oocyte interaction and acrosome reaction

The first contact point between a spermatozoon and an ovum is at the zona pellucida of the ovum. This is an extracellular matrix that surrounds the oocyte and protects it, and later the developing embryo, from mechanical damage. The zona pellucida (ZP) consists of three glycoproteins, produced by the egg itself, called ZPA, ZPB and ZPC according to the size of their coding genes. In some species, it is possible that the surrounding granulosa cells are also involved in the production of the zona pellucida. All three proteins are highly glycosylated. As long filaments they form an elastic network around the oocyte. In pigs, the zona pellucida has a thickness of about 20 μm.

The **zona pellucida** regulates the function of a capacitated spermatozoon and ensures the correct timing of acrosome reaction and penetration (**Fig. 24.26**). After fertilisation, the zona pellucida prevents the penetration of any other spermatozoa into the ovum (**Fig. 24.25**). The specific recognition in the interaction of both gametes is also a function of the zona pellucida. Proteins and carbohydrates are involved in this primary binding, in which defined carbohydrate side chains of the zona pellucida glycoproteins bind to complementary proteins or receptors on the spermatozoan surface. A number of such carbohydrate- and zona pellucida-binding proteins have been identified in spermatozoa.

After binding to the zona pellucida, the **acrosome reaction of** the spermatozoa is triggered (**Fig. 24.25**).

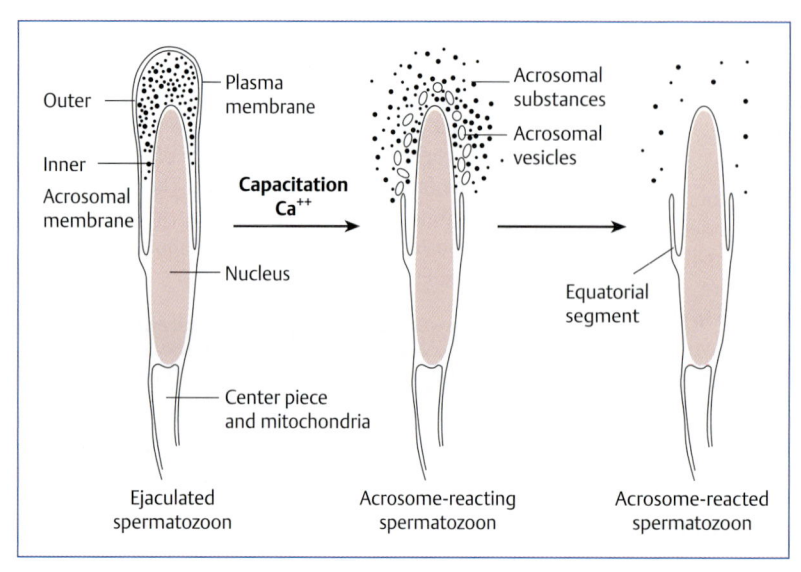

Fig. 24.25 Schematic representation of the acrosome reaction. The capacitation process results in reorganisation and alteration of the fluidity of the spermatozoon's plasma membrane. This enables the spermatozoon to trigger the acrosome reaction in response to binding to the zona pellucida. In this process, the plasma membrane fuses at many points with the overlying outer acrosomal membrane. The acrosomal enzymes can then be released through the resulting openings and channels.

Outer / Inner — Acrosomal membrane

Plasma membrane

Nucleus

Capacitation Ca++

Center piece and mitochondria

Acrosomal substances

Acrosomal vesicles

Equatorial segment

Ejaculated spermatozoon   Acrosome-reacting spermatozoon   Acrosome-reacted spermatozoon

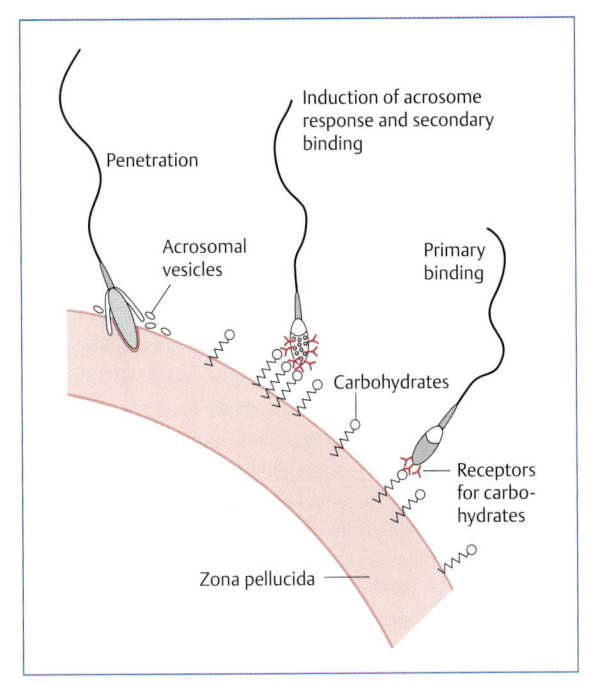

Fig. 24.26 Spermatozoa-zona pellucida interaction. Primary binding: The spermatozoon binds to defined carbohydrates of the zona pellucida via carbohydrate-binding proteins on the spermatozoon surface. Secondary binding: The acrosome-reacted spermatozoon is temporarily bound to the zona pellucida via acrosomal proteins such as acrosin.

MORE DETAILS The capacitation process has prepared the spermatozoa for several fusion processes at the acrosome. The acrosome reaction is finally induced by receptor-mediated signal transduction of the zona pellucida glycoproteins. The mechanism has not yet been fully elucidated. A voltage-dependent calcium channel is opened, involving G-proteins, a receptor tyrosine kinase, and possibly other signal transduction pathways. This allows a considerable influx of calcium which is ultimately responsible for the morphologically recognisable exocytosis (acrosome reaction). However, induction of the acrosome reaction is not always by this particular mechanism. It can also occur spontaneously, or be triggered by a number of other substances.

Triggering of the acrosome reaction at the zona pellucida ensures that enzymes such as acrosine, are released and can act directly on their target substrates. Spermatozoa that have already undergone the acrosome reaction before reaching the egg in the female genital tract fail to fertilise. From controlled proteolysis, the structure of the zona pellucida in the binding region is altered so that a hyperactivated spermatozoon is able to penetrate. The hybrid vesicles of plasma membrane and outer acrosomal membrane that form during the acrosomal reaction remain as so-called "ghosts" on the outside of the zona pellucida. By the action of enzymes (e.g. **acrosin**) associated with the acrosome-reacted spermatozoon, an opening is created in the zona pellucida through which the spermatozoon enters into the perivitelline space of the oocyte. Once in the perivitelline space, an acrosome-reacted spermatozoon can finally fuse with the oocyte.

■ Spermatozoon oocyte fusion and polyspermy block

During the acrosome reaction, the equatorial segment and the postacrosomal region of a spermatozoon also change and become conditioned for fusion with the oocyte oolemma. Fusion-enabling proteins concentrate in this region. The spermatozoon attaches to the side of the oocyte, the microvilli of the oocyte surface make contact with the fusiogenic region of the spermatozoon and envelop the spermatozoon until it is finally absorbed into the cytoplasm of the oocyte. During this process, the spermatozoon loses structures such as the tail and the midpiece. The nucleus begins to decondense and the male pronucleus is formed.

> **IN A NUTSHELL**   !
>
> Only acrosome-reacted spermatozoa can fuse with the egg.

The fusion of the two membranes of oocyte and sperm leads to a very rapid intermittent depolarisation of the oocyte plasma membrane and, by activation of various signal transduction pathways, to the intermittent release of Ca^{2+} from internal stores. These processes are essential for the further development of the fertilised oocyte. Usually, several spermatozoa can pass through the zona pellucida, but only one spermatozoon (with a few exceptions) actually penetrates the oocyte. The immediate depolarisation of the oocyte membrane prevents the fusion of further spermatozoa. This process is extraordinarily rapid. It is therefore referred to as **rapid polyspermy block**. The intracellular release of Ca^{2+}, then causes exocytosis of the cortical granules located below the plasma membrane of the oocyte (**Fig. 24.24**). This cortex-granule reaction is also called a **slow polyspermy block** because it takes a few seconds to develop. As a result of the release of enzymes from the cortical granules, the **zona pellucida** is structurally altered so that spermatozoa can no longer recognise and bind to it. The zona pellucida is also no longer penetrable by those spermatozoa already bound to it.

The developing oocyte is arrested in the prophase of the stage I maturation division. Only at ovulation does it resume meiosis and it then remains in the metaphase of the stage II maturation division until fertilisation. Upon fusion with the spermatozoon, the oocyte is activated and then completes stage **II maturation** with the **constriction** of a polar body. When the female and male pronuclei have reached their maximum size, the nuclear membranes dissolve and the two nuclei fuse (**syngamy)** with the formation of a diploid zygote.

24.4.2   Sex determination
■ The chromosomal sex

The sex of a mammal is determined at fertilisation and depends on the combination of its **sex chromosomes**. While the egg can only carry X chromosomes, spermatozoa, which can carry both X and Y chromosomes, are produced by meiosis from the male germ cells.

Two X chromosomes (XX) lead to the development of ovaries and a female phenotype. The presence of one Y chromosomes (XY) results in the formation of testes and male development. **Sex differentiation** therefore begins with the chromosomal sex at fertilisation and is followed by the development of gonads in the resulting embryo. After this, the secondary sexual characteristics or the sexual phenotype then develop. All three stages of development are interconnected, which was first formulated by Jost in 1953 and this is therefore called the **Jost paradigm**.

> **IN A NUTSHELL**   !
>
> Jost paradigm: chromosomal sex → gonadal sex → sexual phenotype.

The **Y chromosome** is responsible for male development. Even when there are an unusual number of X chromosomes (e.g. XXY, XXXY), the presence of a Y chromosome leads to testis formation, although in these situations the fertility of the eventual male is limited by disruption of spermatogenesis. Whether a testis will develop from the indifferent gonadal plants depends essentially on the presence of a single gene locus on the short arm of the Y chromosome, the **SRY gene (sex-determining region of the Y chromosome**). SRY codes for the **testis-determining factor** (TDF), so its presence determines male development.

> **MORE DETAILS**   TDF stimulates the expression of those genes necessary for testis formation. If SRY is missing on the Y chromosome, the development of an ovary and thus a female appearance will inevitably occur. If the nearby SRY gene is transferred to the X chromosome during the combining of X and Y chromosomes in the course of meiosis, so that there is a crossing over in the pseudoautosomal region, a testis and a male appearance are formed, despite the presence of two X chromosomes (XX males; **Fig. 24.27**).

The presence of germ cells is not essential for the formation of testes. Even after experimental removal or selective destruction of the primordial germ cells the development of the testis is still initiated. TDF is produced for a limited time in the somatic cells of the germ line shortly before differentiation of the gonadal anlage. In pigs, SRY transcripts are only detectable between days 21 and 26 of gestation, and not at day 31, when male development of the gonadal anlage is histologically evident. TDF is probably expressed in the precursors of the Sertoli cells, and induces undifferentiated cells of the gonadal anlage to develop as Sertoli cells..

> **MORE DETAILS**   The SRY gene occurs exclusively in mammals, including marsupials as well as placentals. This shows that the SRY gene acquired the function of a sex-determining factor more than 80–180 million years ago, before marsupials separated from placentals. A functional SRY homologue could not be detected in birds, which have sex chromosomes Z and W and where females represent the heterogamous sex (ZW). In reptiles, where sex is also determined by chromosomes Z and W or where sex determination is also temperature-dependent, and in lower vertebrates, a functional SRY homologue could also not be detected.

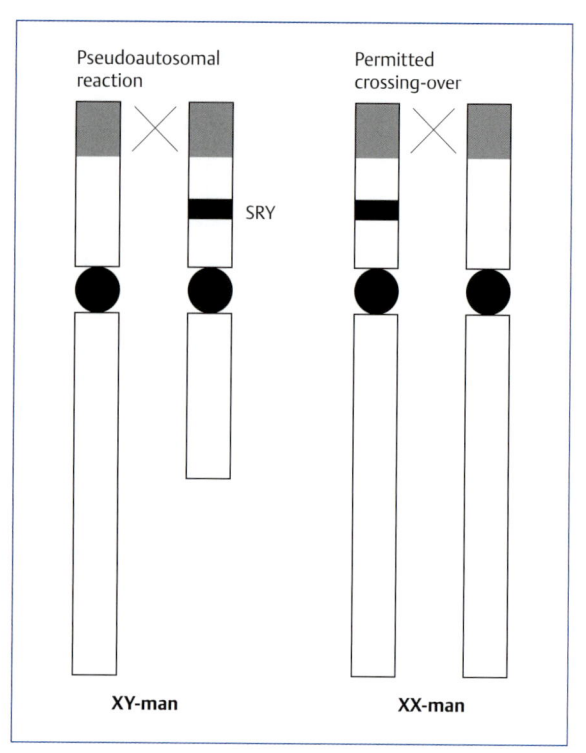

Fig. 24.27 Sex chromosomes in the male with physiological chromosome set (XY) and in the XX male. The SRY gene on the short arm of the Y chromosome is essentially responsible for the development of the **indifferent gonadal plant** to the **testis**. If the SRY gene is transferred to the X chromosome by crossing over, a testis and a male phenotype develop.

◼ The gonadal sex

Differentiation of the **primordial germ cells** begins at a very early stage. In domestic mammals they are detectable in the yolk sac wall during the first weeks of development, in larger domestic mammals after about three weeks, and in mice after seven days. After this they migrate into the germinal ridge by some yet unknown mechanism. They are easily distinguished from somatic cells by their size, round nucleus and histological staining with alkaline phosphatase. During migration in the germ line and in the later gonads, the primordial germ cells divide and multiply to produce several million cells. They settle mainly in the middle of the germ line, from which the undifferentiated gonadal anlage develops. Male germ cells (XY) arrange themselves in the centre and female germ cells (XX) in the periphery. The first sign of the formation of a testis is the development of the foetal Sertoli cells and their aggregation into the primitive spermatic cords in which they enclose the germ cells. In humans and cattle, this step occurs around the sixth week of development. Differentiation into the testis precedes that into the ovary by some days or weeks.

> **IN A NUTSHELL**   !
>
> The Sertoli cells control the development of the undifferentiated gonad system to form the testis.

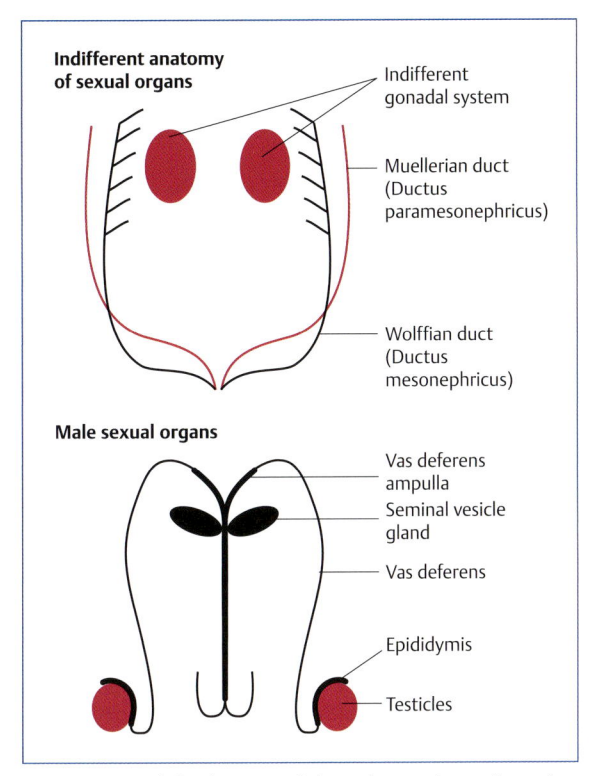

Fig. 24.28 Foetal development of the male sexual tract from the undifferentiated gonad system. Under the influence of AMH (anti-Muellerian hormone), the Muellerian duct regresses. Under the influence of testosterone, the epididymis, the vas deferens and the seminal vesicle develop from the Wolffian duct.

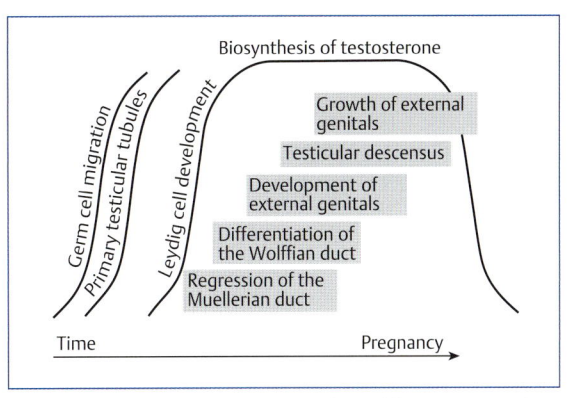

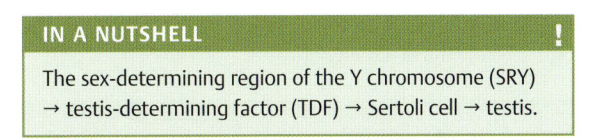

Fig. 24.29 Schematic representation of sex differentiation in the male embryo/foetus during gestation in mammals.

> **IN A NUTSHELL** !
>
> The sex-determining region of the Y chromosome (SRY) → testis-determining factor (TDF) → Sertoli cell → testis.

In addition to their important role in the early development of the testis, foetal Sertoli cells also ensure that the male germ cells can continue to divide mitotically, but unlike the female germ cells in the foetal ovary, they do not enter meiosis. This **meiosis arrest** lasts until the onset of **sexual maturity**. This ensures that spermatozoa are not being produced during foetal and early postnatal development, and that spermatogenesis is only initiated at the onset of puberty.

■ The male phenotype

While the development of the female urogenital tract is largely independent of hormone production by the foetal ovary, development of the male phenotype must be induced by hormones (**Fig. 24.29**). Maturation of the testis and the development of a male appearance can only occur under the influence of **testosterone**.

Under the influence of testosterone, the **Wolffian duct develops** to form the **epididymis** (epididymis), the **vas deferens** (ductus deferens) and the **seminal vesicle gland** (vesicula seminalis). Furthermore, under the influence of testosterone, there is masculinisation of the urogenital germ line and development of the external genitalia. In order to bring about the morphological changes of the external genitalia, testosterone must be converted into dihydrotestosterone in its target cells by the enzyme 5α-reductase. **Dihydrotestosterone** (DHT) has a much higher affinity than testosterone for the androgen receptor, and thus compensates for low androgen concentrations (p.574). A defect in 5α-reductase leads to feminisation of the external genitalia.

Leydig cells appear somewhat later than the Sertoli cells during embryonic development and are located in the interstitium between the primitive tubules of the testis. The conversion of precursor cells into Leydig cells is induced by the expression of testosterone synthesising enzymes and of LH receptors in the cell membrane. The morphological differentiation of Leydig cells correlates with

While the differentiation of Sertoli cells from primitive supporting cells begins under the influence of SRY or its gene product TDF, further testicular development is hormone-dependent. The first biochemical activity of foetal Sertoli cells is the production of anti-Muellerian hormone (AMH), which causes regression of the **Muellerian duct**, a structure which in females would form the female genital tract.

Anti-Muellerian hormone acts locally to suppress development of the Müllerian duct, and also organises Sertoli and germ cells to form the primitive spermatic cords (**Fig. 24.28**). Müller's duct is sensitive to AMH for only a very limited time after the onset of testicular differentiation. In cattle, AMH synthesis begins at about the time when the primitive spermatic cords begin to organise and reaches a maximum when Müller's duct regresses. In cattle, same-sex twin pregnancies cause a species-typical fusion of the placental vessels. AMH in the circulation of a female twin foetus also causes regression of Mueller's duct and a masculinisation of the genital tract. This phenomenon is referred to as **pinch formation** or **freemartinism**. Female calves from male-female twin pregnancies are therefore almost always infertile. However, this phenomenon only occurs in cattle. In other species such as sheep, goats, horses or multiparous species such as dogs, cats and pigs, the sexual development of female foetuses is not affected by their male siblings.

Endocrinology, reproduction

the onset of **testosterone biosynthesis**. It is stimulated either by maternal LH or LH produced by the foetus itself.

In most mammals, there are two phases of Leydig cell growth. Before birth, Leydig cells have the task of producing **testosterone**, necessary for the development and growth of the testes, the internal and external genitalia, and finally for testicular descensus. Another important task of foetal testosterone is the sex-specific imprinting of the brain. Already in the early foetal stage, later male behaviour is determined. It is noteworthy that it is not testosterone itself that exerts this effect on the brain, but its aromatised downstream product (oestradiol), since receptors only exist for oestrogens in the brain. Depending on the species however, the Leydig cells regress before or shortly after birth and for a time cease producing testosterone. They do not resume this until the onset of puberty and then continue to produce testosterone throughout the entire fertile life of a male.

> **IN A NUTSHELL** !
>
> The development of the male **phenotype** only occurs in the presence of testosterone.

24.4.3 Assisted reproduction

Today, **assisted reproduction techniques** are used in animal breeding, both for farm animals and increasingly for individual animals. These offer either the possibility of producing more offspring from animals with above-average **breeding value**, of conserving the genetic potential of such animals, or of producing offspring from animals with **fertility problems**. The methods used today include, **artificial insemination**, **embryo transfer**, in vitro production of embryos, and techniques for sexing offspring. To be successful, these procedures often depend on influencing the female cycle with medication, to optimise the time of insemination, to synchronise oestrus of several females, or to induce multiple follicle ovulation.

■ Oestrus and ovulation synchronisation

The **induction of oestrus** at predetermined times in groups of animals facilitates farm management because the farmer is only concerned with observing and handling the animals during oestrus and parturition within a predictable timeframe. Induction of oestrus can also be useful for individual females, if a sire is only available at a particular time. For embryo transfer, the oestrus cycles of the donor and recipient animals must be synchronised to ensure successful pregnancies.

There are two basic methods of synchronising oestrus and ovulation:
- The administration of **progesterone** or synthetic gestagens is used to prolong the luteal phase and thus postpone oestrus.
- The administration of **PGF$_{2\alpha}$ analogues** is used to cause existing corpora lutea to regress and thus induce oestrus or synchronise a wave of follicle maturation.

There is a wide variety of modifications in the way these methods are applied, depending on the species and the available hormone preparations. Proven treatment protocols have been devised for domestic **cattle, sheep, goats** and **horses**.

In **pigs**, PGF$_{2\alpha}$-induced luteolysis has no practical benefit because the corpus luteum does not respond to PGF$_{2\alpha}$ injection until the 12th day after ovulation. Some protocols have been developed for dogs and cats, but these differ significantly from those for other domestic species, and are often much less successful because of the particular characteristics of dog and cat oestrous cycles.

■ Artificial insemination

In breeding of many species, **instrumental semen transfer** (**"artificial insemination"**) has largely replaced natural mating. For semen transfer, the ejaculate is collected by means of an **artificial vagina** and transferred into the genital tract of the female animal without the two partners coming into physical contact. Apart from hygienic advantages, which avoid transmission of **mating infections** (infectious diseases that can be transmitted during mating and affect fertility or health), there is better use of sires that are in high demand or have valuable genetic potential. The number of **insemination doses** (the amount of sperm required for successful insemination) from one ejaculate, varies from a few in dogs to several hundred in cattle. Storage is possible by adding preservation media and cooling or deep freezing. For short-term preservation, i.e. cooled semen (pig at 15 °C, other species at 5 °C), an ejaculate preparation can be kept for several days. With appropriate addition of **antifreeze agents**, and storage in liquid nitrogen (−196 °C), the fertilising ability can be maintained for decades. Furthermore, storage in liquid nitrogen allows **semen to be transported** in specially designed containers, for worldwide **semen trade**. This trade has become very important in the breeding of species such as cattle, small ruminants, horses and dogs. By creating **frozen semen reserves**, valuable sires can be used for breeding even after their death. "**Semen banks**" of frozen semen are also important in the conservation of endangered breeds or species.

■ Embryo transfer and associated biotechniques

In farm animals and horses, embryos that have not yet implanted can be obtained from the uterus of a **donor animal** and transferred into the uterus of **cycle-synchronised recipient animals**. In so-called in vivo production, late morulae or blastocysts are obtained from the uterus of a donor animal. For **in vitro production**, oocytes are obtained and matured from a donor animal, and then fertilised in vitro, either with appropriately prepared sperm, or by direct injection of sperm into the matured oocytes (**Intracytoplasmic Sperm Injection ICSI**). These can then either be transferred directly to cycle-synchronised recipient animals, or transported under refrigeration to recipient animals in a distant location, or preserved for an indefinite period by deep freezing in liquid nitrogen. By taking biopsies (tissue samples) from the embryos, **genotyping** can also be carried out to determine the sex, colour or genetic defects of the potential offspring. Embryo transfer, like artificial insemination, is now a standard procedure in animal breeding to make better use of the genetic potential of female animals. In cattle and horses, embryo collection can be carried out non-invasively without harmful effects on general health and subsequent fertility of the donors. For small ruminants and pigs, collection is more complex and requires anaesthesia of the donors.

■ Sex determination

In animal breeding, it can be beneficial to increase the proportion of male or female offspring. In dairy breeds, female calves are preferred because they can eventually be milk producers, while male calves are only useful as future potential breeding bulls, and often have poor fattening characteristics. Two methods of sex determination are currently in use. Either **sperm are sorted** into those that carry an X or Y chromosome, so that a decision can be made at the time of artificial insemination as to whether male or female calves are to be preferred. Since the DNA content of the Y-chromosome-bearing sperm is lower, they can be separated from other sperm by a sorting process after vital staining with fluorochromes This procedure is used by breeding organisations for special sires in cattle and pig breeding. In **postconceptional sex determination**, one or more blastomeres are removed from the donor embryos and Y-chromosome-specific DNA sequences are determined using molecular biological techniques. This procedure is routinely used in cattle breeding and is now also routine in horses.

Suggested reading

Bazer FW, Spencer TE, Johnson GA et al. Comparative aspects of implantation. Reproduction 2009; 138:195–209

Ebling FJP, Lincoln GA. Endogenous opioids and the control of seasonal LH secretion in Soay rams. J Endocrinol 1985; 107: 341–353

Fowden AL, Silver M. Comparative development of the pituitary-adrenal axis in the foetal foal and lamb. Reprod Dom Anim 1995; 30: 170–177

Ginther OJ. Reproductive biology of the mare. Basic and applied aspects. 2nd ed. Wisconsin: Equiservices; 1992

Ginther OJ. Selection of the dominant follicle in cattle and horses. Anim Reprod Sci 2000; 60–61: 61–79

Hunter MG, Robinson RS, Mann GE et al. Endocrine and paracrine control of follicular development and ovulation rate in farm species. Anim Reprod Sci 2004; 82–83: 461–477

Rommerts FFG. Testosterone: an overview of biosynthesis, transport, metabolism and action. In: Nieschlag E, Behre HM, eds. Testosterone (action, deficiency, substitution). Berlin, Heidelberg: Springer; 1990: 1–22

Schjenken JE, Robertson SA. The female response to seminal fluid. Physiol Rev 2020; 100: 1077–1117

Senger PL. Pathways to Pregnancy and Parturition. REV. 2011. New York: McGraw-Hill; 2011

Spencer TE, Bazer FW. Biology of progesterone action during pregnancy recognition and maintenance of pregnancy. Front Biosci 2002; 7: 1879–1898

Stormshak F. Biochemical and endocrine aspects of oxytocin production by the mammalian corpus luteum. Reprod Biol Endocrinol 2003; 1: 92

Terasawa E, Guerriero KA, Plant TM. Kisspeptin and puberty in mammals. Adv Exp Med Biol 2013; 784: 253–273

24.5 Reproduction in birds

Almuth Einspanier, Susanne Reitemeier; former collaboration: A. Weißmann

24.5.1 Female reproductive organs

> **ESSENTIALS** ✖
>
> Although the female reproductive organs are laid out in pairs during embryogenesis, for most avian species only the left ovary and oviduct are fully functional. The entire reproductive tract is subject to seasonal influences and the photoperiod is particularly important. When daylight is prolonged, hierarchical functional bodies mature in the ovary in so-called follicle maturation waves. Ovulation of an F1 follicle is followed, independently of any fertilisation, by the process of egg formation in the oviduct.

The female reproductive tract consists of an **ovary** and an **oviduct**. The oviduct in turn is subdivided into **infundibulum, magnum, isthmus, uterus and vagina** (Fig. 24.30). Although in the embryo, the ovary and oviduct are arranged in pairs, the right system regresses to a non-functional tissue strand in the majority of avian species. Only the left gonad and Mueller's duct develop into a functional ovary and oviduct under the influence of oestrogens.

> **MORE DETAILS** Avian exceptions, where paired ovaries are present, include kiwis, some hawk species, vultures and eagles. Outside the laying period or breeding season, the female reproductive organs regress.

The ovary is located caudal to the adrenal gland at the cranial pole of the kidney and is attached to the dorsal wall of the peritoneal cavity by a short **mesovarium**. It is divided into an outer cortex zone (localisation of the follicles) and an inner, well vascularised medullary zone. The process of ovogenesis already begins in the early embryonic stage. In a functional ovary, several mitotic divisions of the migrated **primordial germ cells** produce several million **ovogonia**. However, at the time of hatching, over 90% of these ovogonia regress. At the end of the division phase the remaining ovogonia enter the prophase of meiosis stage 1 and thus become ovocytes. The attachment of follicular epithelial cells around the ovocytes gives rise to the **primordial follicles** about 3–4 days after hatching. This is followed by a phase of slow growth lasting several months to years. The increase in size occurs by the accumulation of yolk proteins produced in the liver and transported via blood to the ovocyte. The follicle wall differentiates into stratum

Endocrinology. reproduction

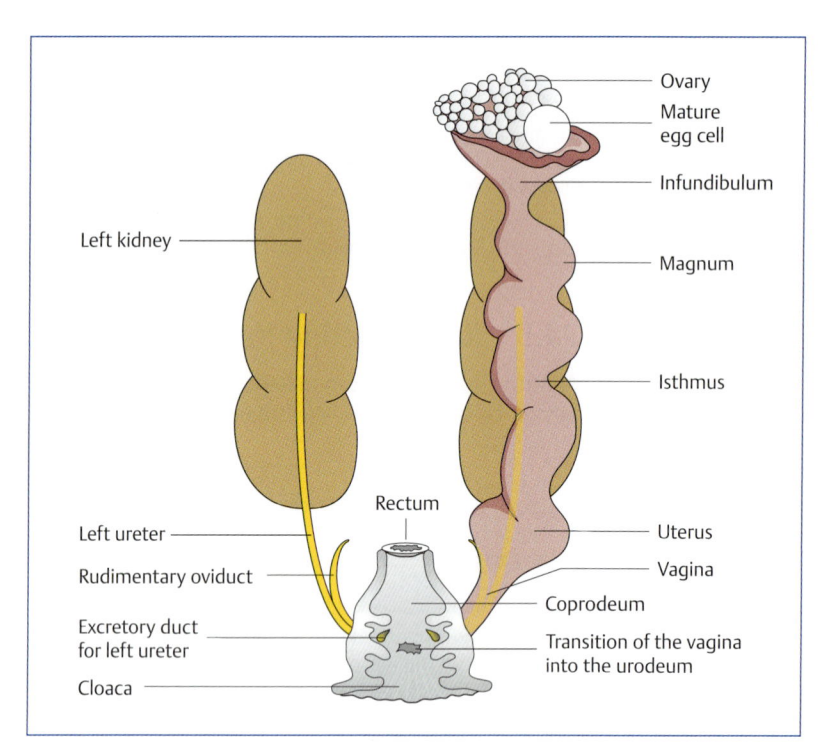

Fig. 24.30 The reproductive tract (ventral view, schematic) of the laying hen (left side only) is composed of ovary, infundibulum, magnum, isthmus, egg-shell gland (uterus) and vagina opening into the cloaca.

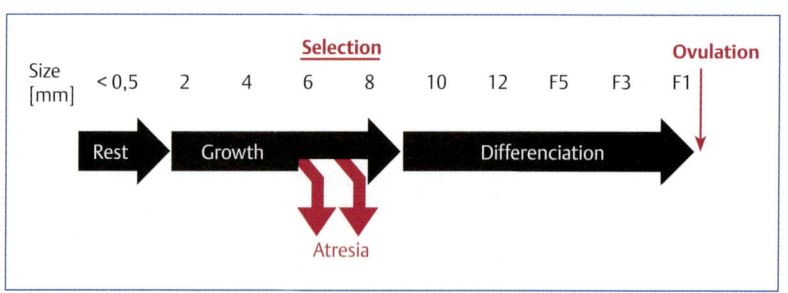

Fig. 24.31 The hierarchy of follicles in a bird ovary ensures the continuity of mature follicles on successive days. As shown in the example of the domestic hen, the follicles grow over a period of 2–3 weeks until ovulation. Of the prehierarchical follicles selected for the slow growth phase, most undergo atresia. Only a few of the 6–8 mm prehierarchical follicles are selected for further differentiation into mature preovulatory follicles.

granulosum, theca interna, theca externa and a final tunica superficialis. During folliculogenesis, the ovocytes remain in the first prophase. Continuation of meiosis stage 1 does not occur until about two hours before ovulation under the influence of luteinising hormone (LH). Physiological atresia can occur in primordial follicles during the active reproductive phase, either through apoptosis of stratum granulosum cells with subsequent resorption of the ovocyte into the vascular system, or through rupture of the follicle wall, so that the ovocyte enters the coelom (abdominal cavity) and is resorbed there.

After reaching **sexual maturity** (in the domestic hen at the age of approx. 150 days), the follicles develop in regular cycles ready for ovulation. At the start there is **follicle selection** approx. every 24 hours from the embryonically created pool of follicles. This then enters a phase of rapid growth as a so-called hierarchical or preovulatory follicle (**Fig. 24.31**). Over a period of 1–2 weeks, a large quantity of yolk lipids and proteins formed in the liver are accumulated. Their hepatic synthesis is regulated by oestrogens produced by the selected follicles. These hormones stimulate the production of the precursor molecule, previtellogenin, in the liver. Subsequently, enzymatically catalysed coupling takes place of this precursor molecule with phosphate, carbohydrate and fatty acid groups. This produces

vitellogenin which is transported in blood to the follicles. While circulating in blood, it assumes an additional function as a transport protein for calcium. Uptake into the ovum occurs by micropinocytosis and is controlled by follicle-stimulating hormone (FSH). In the ovum, vitellogenin is enzymically cleaved into **phosvitin** and **lipovitellin**. The follicular oestrogens also stimulate the synthesis of triacylglycerols in the liver. These enter the bloodstream as "very low density lipoprotein" (VLDL) and travel to the follicles where they are deposited in the yolk (**Fig. 24.32**). The mature follicle is the largest body cell in the animal kingdom and weighs about 20–30 g in the domestic hen. The granulosa cells of the selected follicles are primarily LH-dependent, which induces the formation of progesterone. In contrast, the granulosa cells of non-selected follicles are primarily influenced by FSH.

> **IN A NUTSHELL**   **!**
>
> In the avian ovary, the primordial follicles develop hierarchically into mature follicles. During this phase, in addition to increasing in size, differentiation of the follicle wall into stratum granulosum and theca interna/externa takes place. If follicle selection does not occur, follicular atresia then follows.

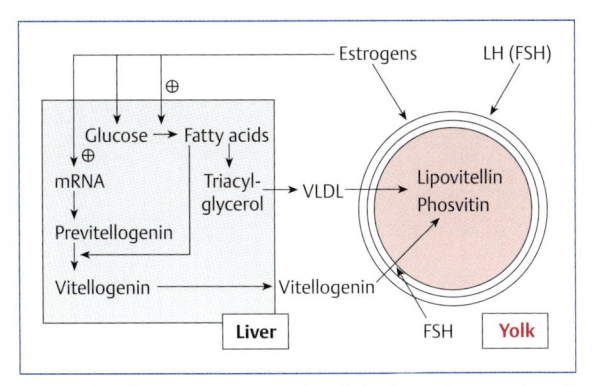

Fig. 24.32 Schematic representation of the formation and deposition of the yolk. Molecular precursors of the yolk substances are synthesised in the liver under the control of ovarian hormones, secreted into the blood and absorbed into the follicular lumen in the ovary.

During the time when eggs are being laid, several follicles in the ovary are present at the same time, each in a different, hierarchically ordered stage of development (**Fig. 24.33**). This is in contrast to the synchronous follicle maturation waves of multiparous mammals (e.g. pigs and dogs, see ch. 24.2.1 (p.560)), in which a different number of growing follicles are in the same stage of maturation. In birds, the selected follicles grow pedunculated and protrude above the surface of the ovary. This gives an active ovary a macroscopically grape-shaped appearance. However, only the largest follicle (the so-called dominant or F1 follicle) proceeds to ovulation; subsequently, the next smaller follicle (F2 follicle) grows into a new F1 follicle. In most species of birds, only one follicle matures in each cycle. In large gull species and penguins, just one follicle ovulates each breeding season.

As in mammals, **ovulation is** induced by an increase in LH (p.565) from the pituitary gland. In birds, this release of LH is in turn coupled to the light regime, related to the time of day. In the domestic hen, the ovulation-inducing LH surge usually occurs about ten hours after the onset of the dark period. Ovarian steroids (p.594) are of great importance in the control of LH secretion.

Approximately 3–6 hours after the LH surge, ovulation occurs with release of the ovum (yolk and germinal disc) at the stigma (for a detailed description of the endocrine control of ovulation in birds, see ch. 24.5.4 (p.594)). After ovulation, the so-called postovulatory follicle, which is endocrinologically active, develops from the former follicle. Prostaglandin $F_{2\alpha}$ produced in the postovulatory follicle influences the transport of the egg in the **oviduct** and then **oviposition**. In birds, no corpus luteum develops from the theca and granulosa cells (p.566), of the type formed in mammals after ovulation, because embryonic development is external to the body of the bird. The ovum enters the oviduct after ovulation, but pathologically, it can also enter the coelom where it is usually reabsorbed within 24 hours. The ovum stays in the infundibulum for approx. 15–30 min in the domestic hen, where the second maturation division of the ovocyte and fertilisation take place. In birds, several sperm penetrate the ovocyte. However, the actual

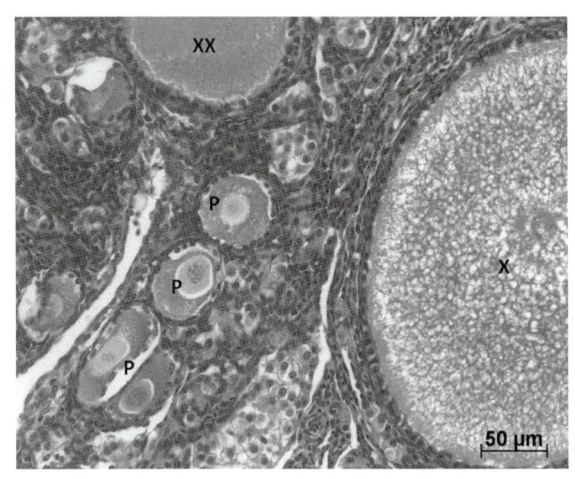

Fig. 24.33 The active ovary of a pigeon with different follicle maturation stages: F1 follicle (X), F2 follicle (XX), non-selected primordial follicle (P). Regardless of size, all follicles have a similar basic morphological structure: Centrally, there is the ovocyte (germ cell and yolk) surrounded by a basement membrane, cells of the stratum granulosum and the theca interna and externa. In contrast to mammals, there is a massive increase in the size of the ovocyte during folliculogenesis in birds. After this the follicle is completely filled and no antrum folliculi is formed. 200x magnification. [Source: Dr. Susanne Reitemeier]

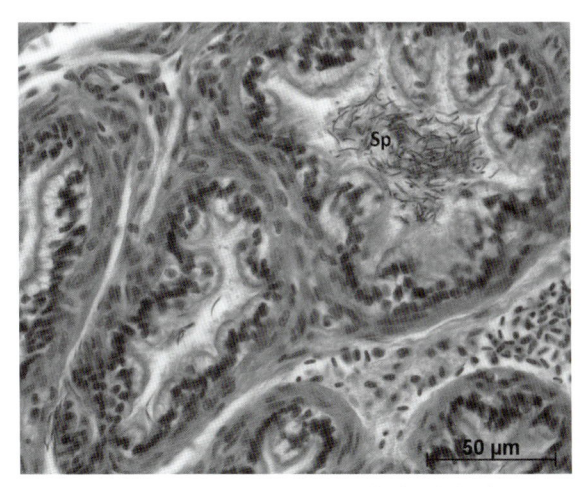

Fig. 24.34 Uterovaginal sperm reservoir of a female budgerigar: spermatozoa (Sp) visible in the lumen. 400x magnification. [Source: Dr. Susanne Reitemeier]

fertilisation is carried out by only one sperm. Female birds have the ability to store sperm in so-called **sperm reservoirs** (**Fig. 24.34**). These consist of gland-like depressions in the mucosa of the infundibulum and at the uterovaginal junction. In the female mammal, sperm storage (p.581) occurs in the folds of the cervix and in the caudal segment of the oviductal isthmus. The duration of sperm storage varies, depending on species, from six days in the red-tailed hawk to 117 days in the turkey.

> ### IN A NUTSHELL   !
>
> Female birds can store sperm in sperm reservoirs for several days without the sperm losing their ability to fertilise.

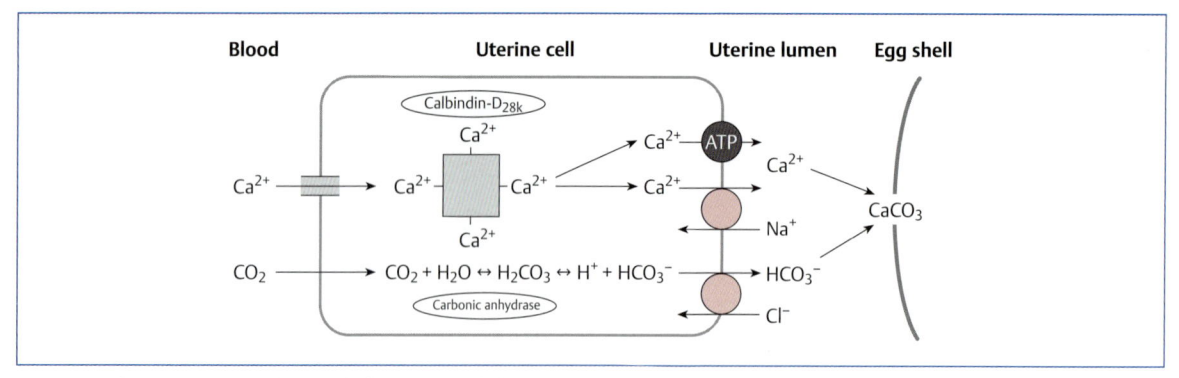

Fig. 24.35 The mineral part of the eggshell is composed of about 98% calcium carbonate ($CaCO_3$). Ionised Ca^{2+}, CO_2 and H_2O are required for eggshell formation. The active, transcellular secretion of Ca^{2+} into the uterine lumen includes influx from the blood through Ca^{2+} channels, intracellular binding to calbindin-D_{28k} and "uphill transport" into the uterine lumen by means of a Ca^{2+}-ATPase and a Na^+/Ca^{2+} exchanger. CO_2 diffuses from the blood into the uterine cells or is produced in these cells from their own metabolic activity. CO_2 and H_2O are first combined as carbonic acid (H_2CO_3) under the influence of carbonic anhydrase in the uterine cells. This then dissociates into bicarbonate (HCO_3^-) and a hydrogen ion (H^+), which is buffered intracellularly. The HCO_3^- then enters the uterine lumen via a Cl^-/HCO_3^- exchanger, followed by Ca^{2+}. These ions are then available to form the $CaCO_3$ for eggshell calcification.

Furthermore, in the **infundibulum**, the **proprioceptive glands** produce the middle and outer yolk membrane as well as the precursors of the chalazae. The ovocyte then enters the magnum, the longest section of the oviduct. During the 2–3 hours that it is retained there, the glandular cells, under the influence of oestrogens, secrete most of the egg white proteins (including **ovalbumin, ovotransferrin, ovomucoid, lysozyme**) along with minerals (e.g. sodium, potassium, magnesium). The formation of the chalazae is also completed. In the following **isthmus** (passage time approx. 75 min), the synthesis of sulphur-containing proteins and collagen fibres takes place, from which the inner and outer shells are formed. The water accompanying these secretions then determines the eventual shape of the egg. As it approaches the terminal end of the isthmus, the organic part of the eggshell, the nipple layer, starts to be laid down. The egg then moves to the uterus, where it remains for the longest time, 18–26 hours. There the calcareous shell is formed with the cuticle secreted by the uterine glands (waxy protective layer on the outside). A schematic illustration of the mineralisation of the eggshell is shown in **Fig. 24.35**. At the junction of the uterus and the vagina is the vaginal sphincter, the most powerful muscle of the oviduct. The vagina serves to transport the egg into the **cloaca**, which is the end of both the gastrointestinal and reproductive tracts. At this point, the egg formation processes are complete. Finally, oviposition occurs, with contraction of the uterus and simultaneous relaxation of the abdominal muscles and the uterovaginal sphincter. This process is controlled by prostaglandins from the postovulatory follicle and the hormones arginine vasotocin and oxytocin produced in the hypothalamus and stored in the neurohypophysis. This causes contraction of the smooth muscles in the uterine wall, while prostaglandin E causes relaxation of the uterovaginal sphincter. The duration of oviposition depends on the bird species and can last from seconds to hours.

> **IN A NUTSHELL** !
>
> Ovulation is triggered by an initial LH surge. During ovogenesis, albumen is added to the ovulated, yolk-rich follicle first in the magnum, and then the calcareous shell is formed in the uterus. The time from ovulation to oviposition is about 24 hours in the domestic hen.

After successful fertilisation, the first cell divisions of the germinal disc take place during passage through the fallopian tube. By the time of oviposition, the germinal disc already consists of 32000–42000 cells. After oviposition, there is a temporary standstill in development because of the lower external temperatures. Embryonic development then continues at temperatures above 21 °C, at the start of either natural or artificial incubation. The physiological arrest of embryonic development immediately after oviposition of each egg serves to synchronise hatching of the entire clutch, when incubated together.

24.5.2 Egg structure

> **ESSENTIALS** ✗
>
> The egg is composed of the following components from the outside to the inside: Cuticle (antimicrobial barrier), calcareous shell (mechanical protection, respiration), shell skin, albumen (albumen; antimicrobial protection as well as nutrition of the embryo) and yolk (nutrition of the embryo).

The exact structure of an egg is shown in **Fig. 24.36**. The germinal disc, which in the case of an unfertilised egg contains the nucleus of the ovum and in the case of successful fertilisation the blastoderm cells of the early germinal bud, lies on the yolk ball. The yolk itself consists of two parts, the yellow and the white yolk. The white yolk is located in the vicinity of the germinal disc. Also the latebra, a bottle-

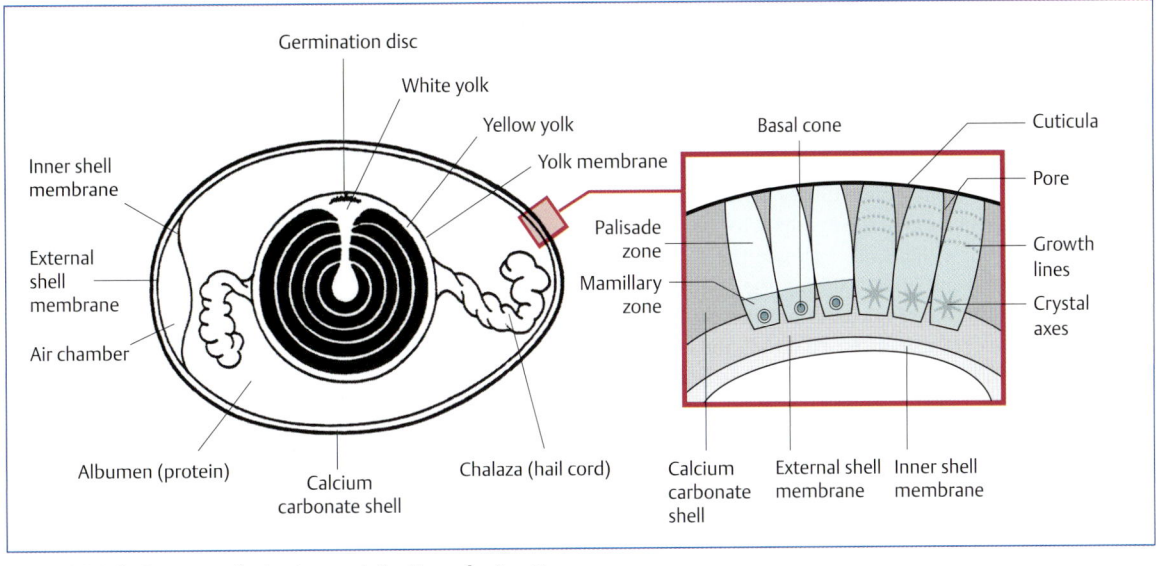

Fig. 24.36 Left: Structure of a hen's egg at the time of oviposition.
Right: Structure of the eggshell. The outermost layer is formed by the cuticle, which has a thickness of 5–12μm and protects the egg from desiccation and microbial invasion. The columnar structure of the palisade zone, which is about 200 μm thick, connects to the inside and merges into the mamillary zone. The mamillary zone is the starting point for the growth and calcification of the eggshell (arrows). In areas without cross-linking of the columnar calcite crystals, pores form in the eggshell (diameter of 0.3–0.9μm). They are important for air and water exchange between the embryo and the environment.

shaped strand that runs from the germinal disc to the centre of the yolk, consists of white yolk. The rest of the yolk is composed of yellow and white yolk, layered concentrically around the latebra. Components of the yolk are predominantly lipids and proteins in an aqueous solution, with white yolk having a greater protein content, while the yellow yolk has a higher lipid content. These nutrients serve as the main source of energy for the embryo throughout its development. Shortly before hatching, the yolk is almost completely absorbed. The remainder is drawn into the abdominal cavity of the embryo via an umbilical cord. Thus, the chick continues to be supplied with energy from the remaining yolk in the first 1–2 days after hatching. The albumen consists of several phases, which are arranged concentrically around the yolk. Directly around the yolk ball is a layer of thin egg white, followed by a middle layer of thick egg white and again an outer layer of thin egg white. Proteins of the albumen also form the **chalazae**. These fibres, stretched along the longitudinal axis, attach to the yolk membrane and hold the yolk ball in position, but allow it to rotate around its own axis. As a result, the germinal disc or embryo always comes to rest on top of the yolk ball due to its lower specific gravity. The albumen consists of about 90% water. The solutes are mainly proteins (ovalbumin, ovotransferrin, ovomucoid), carbohydrates and inorganic ions. The primary function of these proteins is to supply the embryo with amino acids. By the end of embryonic development, the egg white, or albumen, is almost completely absorbed by the embryo via the chorioallantoic circulation and an active protein uptake process. Another function of albumen is inhibition of microbial growth to protect the embryo. This occurs via **enzyme blockade** (ovalbumin, ovomucoid), or binding of substances required for bacterial growth such as iron and biotin (ovotransferrin, avidin), or lysis of bacterial cell walls (lysozyme). Albumen and the **calcareous shell** are separated from each other by the shell skin. This consists of an inner and an outer part, which is supposed to protect the egg against exogenous influences (e.g. germs). Between the outer and inner shells, the **air chamber** develops at the blunt pole of the egg. The size of this chamber increases with longer storage. The thickness, size, shape and pigmentation of the calcareous shell varies with bird species, and to a small extent there may be individual variations within a species. The shell colour is determined by the incorporation of pigments (porphyrin, biliverdin) in the outermost layer of the calcareous shell and is genetically determined. The calcareous shell consists mainly of calcium carbonate, small amounts of organic compounds, and magnesium carbonate. Structurally, it is divided into an inner nipple layer and an outer palisade layer. The nipple layer is the starting point for growth and calcification of the eggshell. It consists of proteinogenic basal cones, which represent crystallisation nuclei for the outward mineralisation process. The columnar crystals of the palisade layer are vertically attached to these nipples. Between the calcified columns are air pores that enable embryonic respiration. The chorioallantoic membrane, formed during embryonic development from the fusion of the allantois and chorion, plays an important role here. The vascular system of the allantois circulation together with the extraembryonic blood vascular system, ensures the gas exchange of CO_2 and O_2 (for a more detailed description of the gas transfer in bird eggs, see ch. 11.12).

The exact composition of the calcified shell and thus its **breaking strength**, is greatly dependent on the maternal mineral supply. Calcium is obtained via absorption from the gastrointestinal tract, and also from the temporary mobilisation of mineral from medullary bone under the regulation of gonadal oestrogens. The uptake of calcium from feed usually occurs during the daylight. However, most of the calcium incorporation during shell formation occurs during the dark period. At that time, mineral supply from the gastrointestinal tract is very low. The temporary mobilisation of Ca^{2+} from the medullary bone thus guarantees adequate calcification of the eggshell. To prevent deficits in calcium supply, hens can increase the enteric absorption of calcium by 70–80% during the laying period. The blood concentration of calcium transport proteins (vitellogenin, albumin) is also increased during the laying period, under the influence of oestrogens. A persistent inadequate supply of calcium results in increasingly poor mineralisation of the long tubular bones (tibia, femur). Furthermore, with inadequate calcium supply, there is a reduction in pituitary FSH secretion, which could ultimately lead to cessation of laying activity. The outermost layer of the egg is the **cuticle**. It is a waxy layer of proteins, polysaccharides and lipids and is secreted by the uterine glands at the end of the egg formation process. The **cuticle** serves as an antimicrobial barrier and as protection against excessive water evaporation.

> ### IN A NUTSHELL !
>
> For the calcification of the eggshell, a sufficient supply of calcium in the hen's diet is important. Medullary bones such as long bones or vertebral bodies serve as temporary Ca^{2+} stores.

The laying performance of the South-East Asian banki chicken (wild predecessor of the domesticated domestic chicken breeds) was 30–40 eggs per year, but by the end of the 1960s, annual production of 220–240 eggs was the norm for laying hybrids. Through intensive crossbreeding, average egg production could be increased enormously as a result of non-additive genetic effects. The hybrid lines used today are selected for low body weight (requiring less space for housing) and high egg production of up to 320 eggs per year.

However, this increasingly affects the behaviour and health of the hens. Hybrid breeds are often less active. They conserve energy for their high egg output (resource allocation theory), and their breeding instinct is markedly decreased. They also show increased aggressiveness, as their high production rate imposes enormous stress with consequent feather pecking and cannibalism. Furthermore, selection for laying performance leads to the loss of genes that are responsible for social interactions.

MORE DETAILS   In high-performance laying hens, a lack of exercise leads to increased demineralisation of the bones. Bone strength decreases and the birds develop cage paralysis (osteoporosis or cage layer fatigue). The hormonal system responsible for calcium metabolism is so stressed that demineralisation is favoured rather than mineralisation. Hens kept in conventional cages (banned in Germany since 2009, EU-wide since 2012) show considerable thinning of bone due to the lack of movement compared to free-range hens. The reduced bone strength results in a higher incidence of fractures.

In addition, diseases of the egg-producing organs increase in permanently laying hybrid breeds. Inflammation of the fallopian tubes, ovary and peritoneum are the most common of these diseases. Tumours of the ovary (especially adenocarcinomas) and prolapsed oviducts are also found in high-performance birds.

> ### IN A NUTSHELL !
>
> The laying performance of hybrid breeds used today is up to 320 eggs per hen per year. This results in an increase in aggressive behaviour, diseases of bone and of the egg producing organs.

24.5.3   Male reproductive organs

> ### ESSENTIALS ✗
>
> With the exception of the cloaca, the male sexual organs in birds are formed in pairs. They consist of paired testicles with little differentiated epididymis and vas deferens (**Fig. 24.37**). In some species the mating organ (phallus) is located in the cloaca. In contrast to mammals, birds lack accessory sex glands. The entire reproductive tract undergoes seasonal changes.

The paired testes are located in the visceral peritoneal sac at the cranial pole of the kidneys and caudal to the adrenal glands. This abdominal location of the testes distinguishes birds from most mammals, where the gonads are displaced into the scrotum due to the lower temperature there, favouring spermatogenesis (p.576) (exceptions: elephants, clipper sheep and whales). The medial boundary is formed by the aorta, caudal vena cava and abdominal air sacs. The gonads are covered by a single layer of serosa (epiorchium) and attached to the dorsal wall of the abdominal cavity by a short serosa double lamella (mesorchium). Their shape, colour and size vary greatly according to age, species, seasonal climatic fluctuations, and the current reproductive stage. Inactive testes are usually small, bean-shaped and yellow-brown in colour. In juveniles they appear rather flattened and pointed. Mature, active gonads enlarge considerably. In wild budgerigars, for example, their weight increases by 30–40 times because of increases in the length and diameter of the seminiferous tubules, and an increased number of Leydig cells. The size of the testes also changes depending on breeding behaviour, mating system, clutch size and geographical location. In the reproductive period, the testes appear rather round and pale white, the vascular markings on the serosa become more intense due to the increased blood supply.

MORE DETAILS   The gonads of some parrot species (e.g. cockatoo species, golden parakeet, yellow-breasted macaw) have a black-brown colouration from melanocytes in the testicular interstitium and capsule. In the active state, however, their colour fades because of expansion of the seminiferous tubules and the lower proportion of melanocytes.

The process of **spermiogenesis** in the seminiferous tubules is divided into spermatogenesis and the transformation of spermatids into sperm (actual spermiogenesis). These

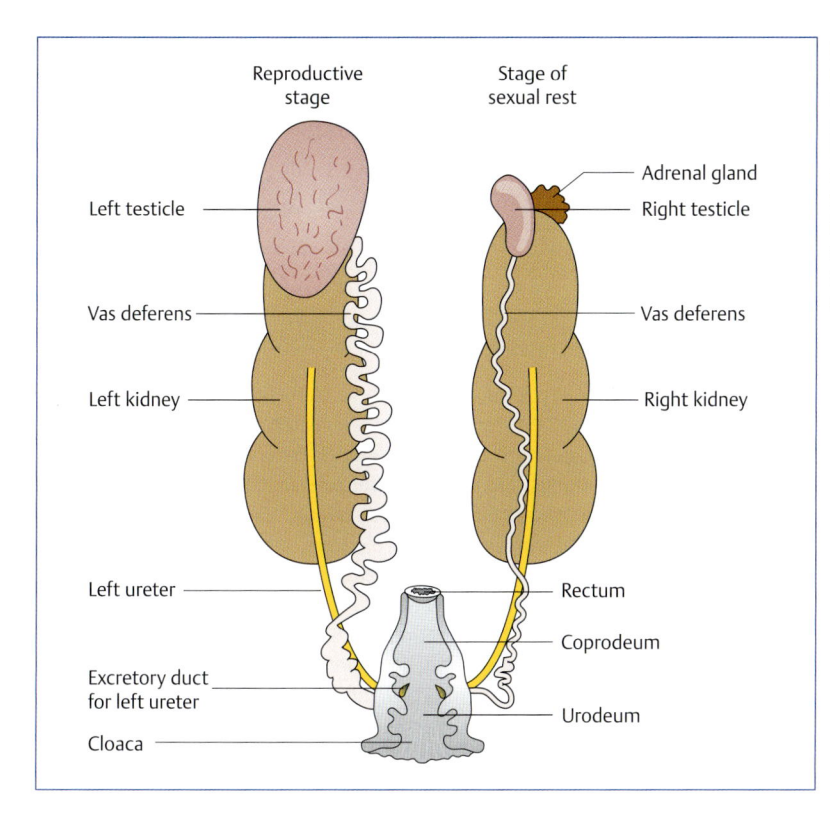

Reproductive stage

Stage of sexual rest

Left testicle

Vas deferens

Left kidney

Left ureter

Excretory duct for left ureter

Cloaca

Adrenal gland

Right testicle

Vas deferens

Right kidney

Rectum

Coprodeum

Urodeum

Fig. 24.37 Schematic ventral view of the urogenital tract of a male bird. In the reproductively active stage the testes are greatly enlarged. The vas deferens also becomes markedly twisted during times of reproductive activity. In the budgerigar, they dilate at the junction with the cloaca to form the so-called seminal glomus. The adrenal glands are only clearly visible in the stage of sexual quiescence, as they are otherwise hidden by the enlarged testicles.

processes are similar to those in mammals (p. 576). However, the spermatozoa of poultry are distinguished by their particular shape and size. The elongated, helical head of the avian sperm carries a dagger-like pointed part (head spine). The latter contains the acrosoma, which is simpler than in mammals. The axial filament, which runs through the entire tail of the sperm, has an identical structure to the mammalian sperm. The short midpiece contains fewer mitochondria in the avian spermatozoon and the segmented columns of the neck as well as the mantle fibres of the midpiece and the main piece of the tail are not present.

The **seminiferous tubules of** the testis open into the testicular meshwork (rete testis), which is connected to the epididymis. The rete testis is not present in all avian species. The epididymis is located dorsomedial to the testis. In some species there is a process that extends cranially to the adrenal gland. Due to its position, the epididymis can hardly be visualised laparoscopically during the reproductive phase, as it is covered by the testis, which has increased considerably in size. There is no division into head, body and tail, as is the case in mammals. In mammals, the individual sections of the epididymis also have specific functions (p. 579), whereas the storage, maturation and nourishment of sperm in the avian epididymis is not assigned to specific compartments. This is where the enrichment of the ejaculate with lipids, proteins and polysaccharides takes place. The epididymis produces secretions that promote maturation of the sperm as well as their motility.

The sperm finally enter the vas deferens, where they mature and are stored. In sexual activity, the vas deferens becomes very tortuous. At the transition of the vas defer-

ens into the middle section of the **cloaca (urodaeum)** is the spermatic duct **papilla**. In passerines, the papilla (promontory) is dilated like a vesicle. It is visible from outside and can therefore be used to identify the sex of a bird. In budgerigars, the spermatic duct (seminal glomus) becomes extended, and has a sperm storage and resorption function. Despite the comparatively high body temperature of 40–42 °C compared to mammals, the sperm of the bird can develop physiologically because the abdominal air sacs provide cooling. In addition, the papilla of passerine birds stores sperm at a constant 4 °C below the internal body temperature.

> ### IN A NUTSHELL !
>
> The sperm formed in the seminiferous tubules of the testis reach the epididymis via the testicular meshwork, from there into the vas deferens, which opens into the middle section of the cloaca as the vas deferens papilla. In passerine birds, this papilla can be used for sex identification.

The **cloaca** forms the common end of the urinary and genital tracts and is divided into three sections (copro-, uro- and proctodaeum). Both ureters and vas deferens open separately into the middle urinary tract. In many birds, the **phallus** is located in the ventral part of the proctodaeum. Basically, a distinction is made between two types of phallus, which function as a seminal duct. Ostriches, geese and breeches have a **protruding phallus**, while the domestic chicken have a **non-protruding, phallus nonprotrudens**. The latter is observed embryonically in pigeons but it later regresses (Phallus types and ejaculation in mammals in **Table 24.8**).

Table 24.9 Ejaculate volume and sperm concentration of selected avian species.

Bird species	Ejaculate volume	Sperm concentration
Domestic fowl	0.5–1 ml	$1.7–3.5 \cdot 10^{12} \cdot ml^{-1}$
Budgie	$3.5–13 \cdot 10^{-3}$ ml	$9.5–11.3 \cdot 10^{12} \cdot ml^{-1}$
Large parrots	$5–10 \cdot 10^{-2}$ ml	$9–10 \cdot 10^{6} \cdot ml^{-1}$
Emu	1.2 ml	$4.4 \cdot 10^{12} \cdot ml^{-1}$
Mallard	$4–8 \cdot 10^{-2}$ ml	$1.3 \cdot 10^{9} \cdot ml^{-1}$
Rockhopper penguin	0.24 ml	$47 \cdot 10^{6} \cdot ml^{-1}$

MORE DETAILS Parrots, sparrows and birds of prey lack a phallus. Here, during copulation, the sperm is transferred via the protruding cloaca into the oviduct of the female.

The erection of the various types of phallus is caused by lymphatic congestion, which at the same time causes mucosal folds in the cloacal wall to swell. As accessory sex glands are absent in birds, the seminal plasma is mainly produced by kinocilia-bearing cells of the epididymis and the seminal ducts (for comparative information on seminal plasma in mammals, see ch. Seminal plasma and ejaculation (p. 580)). In addition, there are transudates from the lymphatic folds and the vascular bodies (corpora vascularia) of the cloaca. The volume of ejaculate in birds is small in comparison to that of mammals (e.g. cock 0.5–1 ml), but it is highly concentrated (**Table 24.9**). The sperm retains fertilising ability in the female sexual tract for several days to weeks.

> **IN A NUTSHELL** !
>
> Depending on the species, male birds have a phallus protrudens (ostriches, geese, breech-hens), a phallus nonprotrudens (domestic chicken) or no phallus (parrots, sparrows and birds of prey). Animals without a phallus transfer their semen via the bulging cloaca into the oviduct of the female.

24.5.4 Endocrine control of reproduction

> **ESSENTIALS** ✘
>
> The endocrine control of reproduction is clearly seasonal in birds. The pineal gland and a pulse generator localised in the anterior hypothalamus are mainly responsible for the translation of external factors into endocrine signals. The hypothalamus-pituitary-gonadal axis is stimulated by the daylight-dependent release of gonadotropin-releasing hormone (GnRH). The resulting release of LH and FSH is responsible, among other things, for follicle maturation, ovulation and proliferation of the oviduct in the female bird. In males, it is responsible for the development and maturation of the seminiferous tubules and vas deferens.

Knowledge of the hormonal regulation of reproduction in both, male and female birds is incomplete. It is known that avian reproduction is clearly subject to seasonal influences (climate, predator presence, social interaction, availability of feed and nesting sites). Gonadal activity is dependent on the interaction of these external factors with internal regulators. Biological clocks control the release of hormones and other messengers that modulate metabolism, reproduction and behaviour. Endogenous circannual rhythms also play a role here, which are genetically preprogrammed and synchronised by seasonally fluctuating environmental factors.

Seasonal variations (p. 557) in gonad size and activity are primarily linked to so-called photoperiods, i.e. the annual variation in daylight duration. Although variations in length of daylight are much less pronounced in the tropics than in temperate latitudes, even tropical birds show seasonal variations in gonadal function depending on photoperiodicity.

Although the **pineal gland** appears to be mainly responsible for photoperiodic control, no light receptors are found there. However, photoreceptor-like cells can be found in the avian pineal gland, and they produce the photopigments **pinopsin** and **melanopsin**. Also, the rhythmic synthesis and release of **melatonin** (p. 553), controlled by the sympathetic nervous system, makes the pineal gland an important component of the circadian pacemaker system. In the domestic chicken (Gallus gallus) and pigeons, the circadian pacemaker system also includes the retina of the eye.

In general, birds register an increase in daylight length by a pulse generator in the anterior hypothalamus (**Fig. 24.38**). Here, extraretinal photoreceptors translate incoming light signals into neuronal impulses and trigger the release of GnRH. The pulse generator is only sensitive to light signals in the phase of increased photosensitivity. During a long light day, this sensitivity coincides with the light period, and gonadal growth is triggered via the hypothalamic-pituitary-gonadal axis (information on its structure and hormones: ch. 24.2.1 (p. 560)). At the time of year of short daylight length, the pulse generator is not stimulated because it is not photosensitive during the short light period. In prolonged periods of long daylight length there is an inhibition of GnRH release, mediated among others by prolactin and the thyroid hormones. In this photorefractory phase, which lasts for different lengths of time depending on species, **gonadal regression** occurs. (compare also **testicular regression** (p. 557) in hamsters and certain breeds of sheep). Thus light influences gonadal function, including spermatogenesis, ovulation and oviposition. For example, germ cell formation in poultry is subject to various lighting regimes. It is known that optimal spermato-

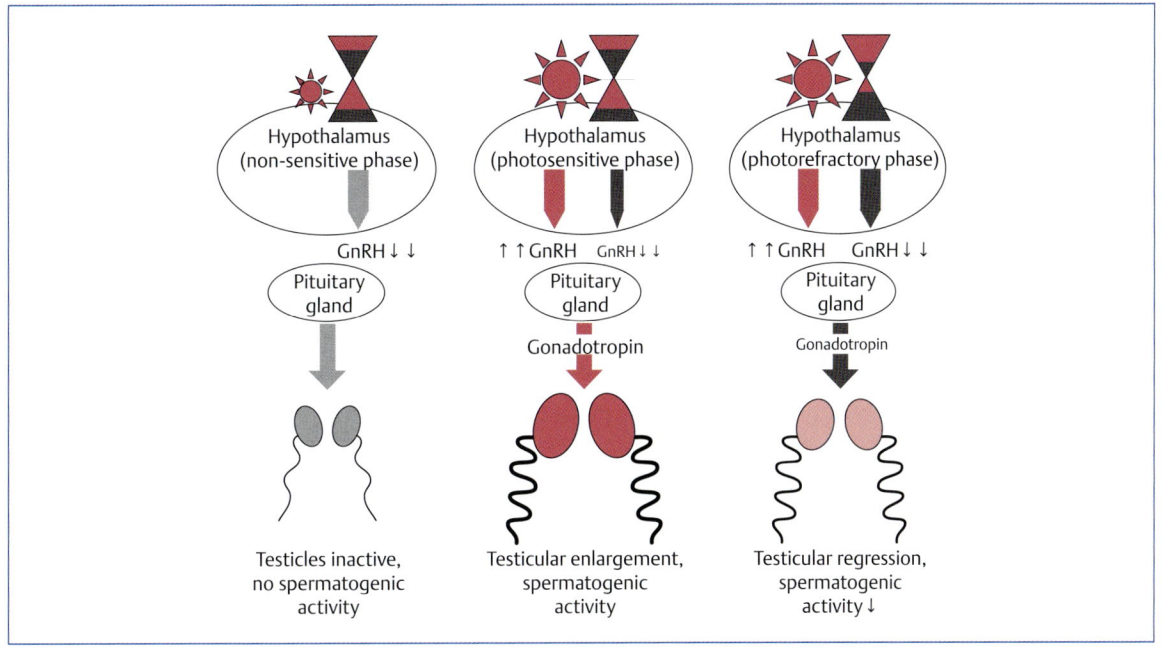

Fig. 24.38 Photoperiodicity of the anterior hypothalamus, and effects on hypothalamic-pituitary-gonadal axis in the male bird: The anterior hypothalamus has a pulse generator by which daylight length (sun) and duration of exposure to a particular length of daylight (hourglass) are recorded, integrated and compared with an endogenous oscillator. When daylight length (short sun) is significantly shortened over a short period of time (full hourglass, short exposure), the short light period falls into the non-sensitive phase of hypothalamic photosensitivity. There are only inhibitory (light grey arrow) but no stimulatory effects on GnRH release. Thus, no gonadotropins are released and the testes remain small and inactive. If the phase of the short light period lasts for a longer period (not shown here), the inhibitory effects on GnRH synthesis also cease and the gonads are again prepared for the start of the new breeding season. Then, as soon as the daylight length increases (long sun), a massive stimulation of GnRH secretion occurs with short exposure (full hourglass), as the phase of increased photosensitivity coincides with the light period. These stimulating effects on the neurosecretory GnRH cells (red arrow) outweigh the inhibitory effects (dark grey arrow) that only set in with a time lag. The consequence is the release of gonadotropins from the pituitary gland, which cause an increase in the size of the testis and maximum sperm production. Prolonged exposure to a long period of light (empty hourglass, long sun) increases the inhibitory influences on GnRH release, causing gonadotropin release to decrease and gonadal regression to occur. The GnRH-producing cells of the hypothalamus become refractory to the long daylight period that still exists.

genesis requires a daily illumination of 12–14 hours, while sperm production decreases significantly with an illumination of less than 9 hours.

GnRH induces, via the pituitary portal system, the secretion of the gonadotropins LH and FSH from the GnRH target cells of the adenohypophysis. As in mammals, the release of GnRH is pulsatile in birds (ch. 24.2.1 (p. 560)). Three isomers of this neurohormone have been isolated from the avian hypothalamus. They differ in structure, distribution and function (general information on peptide hormones in ch. 24.1.1 and ch. 24.3.1). In the hypothalamus of the domestic hen, cGnRH-I and cGnRH-II have been isolated and characterised. Both isomers have been detected in passerine birds, where a third form (ir-lamprey GnRH-III) is also found. The biological activities of GnRH I and II are similar. It is assumed that GnRH I directly stimulates gonadotropin synthesis and secretion.

In female birds, LH is the triggering hormone of ovulation. Its first action on the dominant F1 follicle leads to the formation of the perivitelline cleft, continuation of the first meiotic maturation division, and rupture of the follicular wall at the stigma with subsequent release of the oocyte. In the F2 follicle, it induces the production of androstenedione in theca interna cells. In non-hierarchical follicles, these cells produce progesterone under the influence of

LH, dehydroepiandrostendione and androsterone. From androstenedione, theca-externa cells synthesise oestrogens by the action of aromatase. In birds, as in mammals, androgens are synthesised in the theca cells, but oestrogen synthesis in mammals is localised to the granulosa cells, see ch. 24.2.1 (p. 560). Avian granulosa cells are sensitive to LH only from the time of follicular selection. In hierarchical follicles the synthesis of progesterone is induced by LH.

FSH mainly influences the function of **primordial** and earlier selected follicles, where in theca cells, it increases production of progesterone, androstenedione and oestradiol. Avian granulosa cells mature under the influence of FSH and are thereby sensitised to LH (**Fig. 24.39**). The influence of gonadotropins on follicle maturation and ovulation in mammals is explained in ch. 24.2.1 (p. 560).

> **IN A NUTSHELL** !
>
> In the female bird, LH acts as an ovulation-inducing factor at the dominant F1 follicle, while FSH increases steroid biosynthesis in the theca cells of the primordial follicle.

The oestrogens synthesised in the **theca externa** have multiple functions in avian reproduction. The pituitary gland is sensitised by 17β-oestradiol to hypothalamic

Endocrinology, reproduction

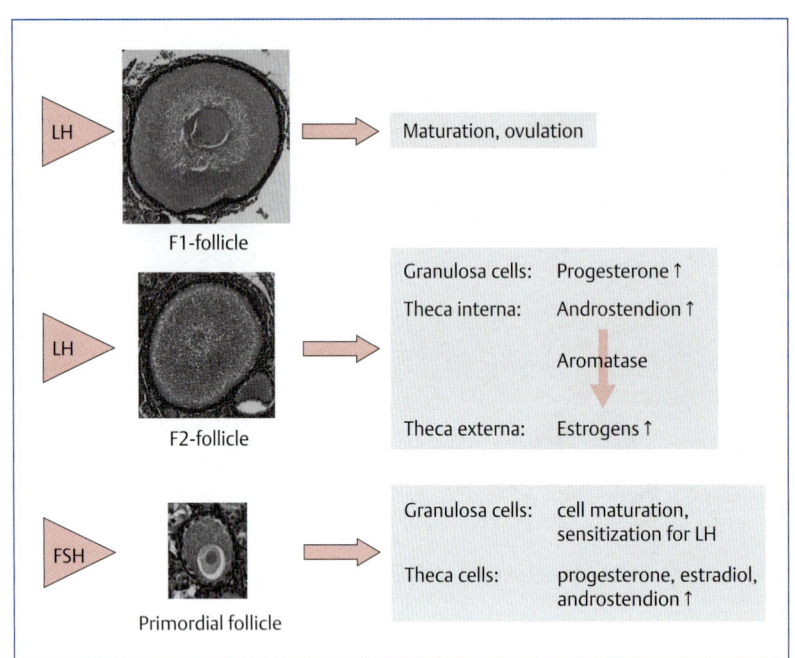

Fig. 24.39 The effect of the gonadotropins LH and FSH on different follicular stages in the avian ovary. LH acts in the dominant F1 follicle to facilitate continuation of the first meiotic maturation division, rupture of the follicular wall at the stigma, and subsequent release of the oocyte. LH also induces cell-specific steroid biosynthesis in the F2 follicle. However, in primordial and earlier selected follicles, hormone production as well as cell maturation is controlled by FSH. Histological representations of the follicles using the example of the pigeon, HE staining, 100x magnification. [Source: Dr. Susanne Reitemeier]

F1-follicle

LH → Maturation, ovulation

F2-follicle

LH →

Granulosa cells:	Progesterone ↑
Theca interna:	Androstendion ↑
	Aromatase
Theca externa:	Estrogens ↑

Primordial follicle

FSH →

| Granulosa cells: | cell maturation, sensitization for LH |
| Theca cells: | progesterone, estradiol, androstendion ↑ |

GnRH. Progesterone receptors in the hypothalamus are also produced in response to 17β-oestradiol. This allows progesterone from the follicular granulosa cells to stimulate the release of GnRH into the pituitary gland, which in turn eenables the piuitary to secrete LH. The embryonic oviduct develops under the influence of gonadal oestrogens. In sexually mature females, oestrogens promote further development of the oviduct and secretory glands. The formation of **egg white proteins** (ovalbumin, ovomucoid, lysozyme) in the glands of the oviduct and the synthesis of yolk proteins in the liver are all mediated by the action of oestrogen. Low oestrogen levels outside the breeding season or the period of egg laying, lead to regression of the oviduct. Regulation of calcium mobilisation for the formation of the calcareous shell, is also under oestrogenic control, see ch. on egg structure (p.590).

The cyclic release of LH causes androgen biosynthesis in the Leydig cells (p.573) of the testis. The androgens **testosterone** and **androstenedione** are responsible for secondary sexual behaviour such as **courtship** and **dominance**, and also for **plumage colour** and male birdsong. Androgens also play an important role in the reproductive tract of male birds and influence the development and maturation of the seminiferous tubules and the vas deferens. Numerous studies on various species of birds have measured plasma testosterone levels in different seasons. In many species, testosterone levels fluctuate depending on the spermatogenic activity of the testis.

MORE DETAILS   In female cockatiels, LH levels rise at the time of nest-building, reach maximum concentrations during the laying period, and then drop again during brooding and hatching. In males, however, LH levels are highest during nest inspection and lowest during the laying period.

FSH (p.573) stimulates **testicular growth** and **spermatogenesis** in male birds by influencing a variety of biosynthetic processes in the Sertoli cells, which consequently undergo hypertrophy. Gonadotropin has the capability of self-potentiation by increasing the number of its receptors on its target cells. There are also synergistic effects of gonadotropin with testosterone which further enhances this mechanism. This may explain the considerable weight gain of the testes during the breeding season. The process of spermatogenesis is thus dependent on the availability of testosterone and FSH, the activity of the Sertoli cells, and the interaction between Sertoli and germ cells.

MORE DETAILS   Other steroid hormones are involved in the control of reproduction in male birds. Oestrogen, for example, influences testicular development in domestic chickens and passerines. Progesterone, on the other hand, stimulates nest care and rearing behaviour in birds of prey and pigeons. It is also involved in the formation of long-term pair bonds, while testosterone plays a subordinate role here.

IN A NUTSHELL   !

In male birds, LH controls androgen synthesis in the Leydig cells, while FSH stimulates testicular growth and spermatogenesis via receptor potentiation on the Sertoli cells. FSH acts synergistically with testosterone to promote sperm production.

Since birds have seasonal reproductive cycles and thus different phases of gonadal activity, it is essential to be able to determine the reproductive status of the gonads, especially for breeding programmes in the conservation of endangered bird species. In male parrots, various methods have been devised to characterise testicular activity from morphological or functional features. Minimally invasive laparoscopy allows a macroscopic assessment of the gonads in terms of size, often in relation to neighbouring organs such as the kidney and adrenal gland, colour and vascular pattern. In active testes, the caudal border of the testis protrudes further into the middle region of the kid-

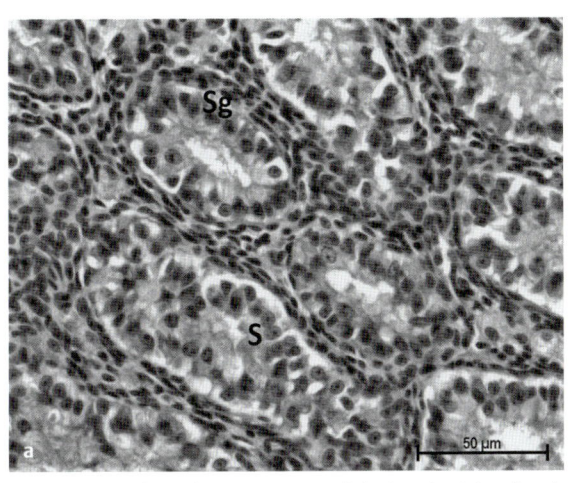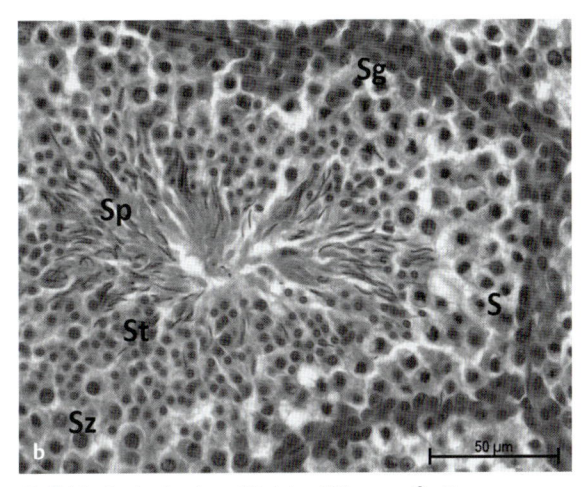

Fig. 24.40 Histological representation of the inactive (**a**) and active testis (**b**) in the budgerigar. HE stain, 400x magnification.
a In the inactive stage, the germinal epithelium of the seminiferous tubules consists only of Sertoli cells (S) and spermatogonia (Sg). [Source: Dr. Susanne Reitemeier]
b In the active stage, other germ cell stages such as spermatocytes (Sz) and spermatids (St) are recognisable. In the centre of the seminiferous tubules there are also the spermatozoa (Sp), the tails of which are arranged in a typical pattern. [Source: Dr. Susanne Reitemeier]

ney, or their length can be up to 4 times that of the adrenal gland. The colour of the testis changes from light brown to yellow in the inactive stage and to yellowish-white in the active stage. Furthermore, a testicular biopsy can be taken during an endoscopic examination. This is followed by cytological, histological or immunocytochemical analysis of the tissue. Cytology gives information on seasonal changes in spermatogenesis in close agreement with histology. The comparison of two tissue sections in **Fig. 24.40** illustrates the differences in the development of the germinal epithelium in the seminiferous tubules of active and inactive testes.

> **MORE DETAILS**   Cytology and histology are important also, for the diagnosis of testicular tumours or orchitis. In parrots, it has been shown that active and inactive stages can be easily distinguished from each other by Sudan black staining of the lipids inside the seminiferous tubules, as inactive testes contain significantly more lipid. Immunocytochemical markers can also be used to distinguish reproductively active gonads from those in sexual quiescence. The steroidogenic enzyme 17β-hydroxysteroid dehydrogenase 2 (17β-HSD-2) is present in the cytoplasm of Sertoli cells of active gonads, but not in inactive gonads. Considerably less invasive tests are the determination of steroid hormone levels (testosterone, oestradiol, corticosterone) in blood and faeces of birds.

24.5.5   Reproduction and breeding

> **ESSENTIALS**   ✖
>
> With over 10000 different species, birds are the most diverse class of terrestrial vertebrates. The variations in body size, feed choice and habitat, as well as in social, reproductive and breeding behaviour, are all correspondingly diverse. However, in reproduction, there are common features across species, such as seasonal reproductive cycles, extramaternal embryonic development in the egg, and progamous sex determination.
>
> In contrast to the mammal (syngamous sex determination female animal = XX, male animal = XY), the female bird has heterogametic (ZW), the male homogametic (ZZ) sex chromosomes. Because of the intraabdominal location of the gonads (primary sex characteristics), only secondary and tertiary characteristics can be used for non-invasive sex identification.

■ Mating and breeding

Mating behaviour in both, female and male birds is influenced by exogenous factors such as daylight length, food supply and temperature. These factors are in turn linked to hormonal regulatory circuits. Steroid-sensitive regions in the brain play an important role in the development of reproductive behaviour patterns such as courtship, birdsong, territorial defence, copulation and the acquiescence reflex. The function of these steroid-sensitive regions is modulated by seasonally variable plasma concentrations, particularly of testosterone.

The endocrine control also influences the mating and breeding behaviour of birds, which varies significantly from species to species.

Monogamous mating patterns develop during the time of breeding (duck), all year round independently of breeding and rearing (cockatoos), and also for life (goose, raven, amazons). In parrots, these pair bonds arise from the attachment to permanent feeding territories. These territories cannot be defended by one bird alone. Pairs therefore function as a social alliance in competition for food sources. In addition, parrots in fixed bonds dominate other unpaired parrots. The monogamous mating system thus has a decisive influence on the dominance behaviour, mainly controlled by androgens. In other species, however, polygamous pair bonding is predominant (domestic chicken, turkey, budgerigar). Colony breeders (budgerigar) show a much stronger competition between individuals for nesting opportunities than single breeders (large parrots). This is associated with higher steroid hormone levels in birds breeding in groups.

Breeding cycles can be distinguished in different bird species by their duration and the time of onset of reproductive activity. Continuous breeders (domestic fowl) are reproductively active throughout the year under optimal conditions. Many wild species in temperate, subarctic and arctic climates show annual cycles, while species in tropical and arid regions have shorter intervals or breed irregularly, depending on favourable environmental conditions. Budgerigars, for example, are such opportunistic breeders and start breeding at the most favourable time for successful reproduction. In arid areas, this is usually when there is an abundant food supply following plentiful rainfall. The start of a breeding season therefore varies with the species.

Egg incubation. The eggs are incubated in a species-specific manner, either by the female (domestic chicken, turkey, duck, budgerigar), the male (ostrich, nandu, Odin's partridge) or alternatively by both parents (stork, cormorant). Further species-related variations in the site of nesting, the length of the breeding period and the number of eggs in a clutch are listed in Table 24.10.

If eggs are destroyed or removed from the clutch in the early breeding phase, non-determinate layers (e.g. domestic fowl, mallards, cockatiels, passerines) produce more eggs until the set point number is reached again. In captive ornamental birds, removing eggs from the cage can give rise to a behavioural disorder of excessive egg laying, which then leads to calcium and protein deficiency. These birds may later show feathering disorders, cramps, prolapse of the oviduct and laying distress. Set point layers (e.g. pigeons), produce a fixed number of eggs, and stop laying as soon as that number is reached.

MORE DETAILS

Progame Sex Determination

In birds, sex is genetically determined by the inheritance of sex chromosomes. In contrast to mammals, however, female birds are heterogamous (sex chromosomes ZW) and males homogamous (sex chromosomes ZZ). Thus, sex is determined by the female producing either "male" or "female" ovocytes (progamous sex determination). The mechanism of sex determination is also different from that of mammals, but has not yet been definitively identified. In mammals, the SRY gene localised on the Y chromosome is crucial for the development of the male sex. The absence of this gene leads to the development of female sex characteristics. The SRY gene is not present on the male sex chromosomes of birds. Here, the DMRT-1 gene located on the Z chromosome is probably the male sex determining factor. In homogamous male birds, the genes are expressed from both Z chromosomes, and the level of expression depends on the number of Z chromosomes. In mammals, on the other hand, only the genes of one X chromosome are expressed in the homogametic female sex (so-called dosage compensation). The influence of the DMRT-1 gene in birds on the development of the embryonic sex characteristics is dependent on dose. When there is a double expression of the gene (ZZ), male sexual characteristics develop. A single expression (ZW) leads to the development of female sexual characteristics.

Table 24.10 Species-dependent variations in the localisation of the nesting site, breeding duration and the number of eggs in an incubated clutch.

Bird species	Brood type	Breeding period	Clutch size
Blackbird	Free brooder	10–19 days	4–5 eggs
Woodpigeon	Predominantly crown breeders, occasionally also ground and niche breeders	16–17 days	2 eggs
Rook	Crown breeders	16–19 days	3–9 eggs
Bankiva chicken	Ground-nesting birds	19–20 days	6–12 eggs
Mallard	Ground-nesting birds	25–28 days	7–16 eggs
Mute Swan	Ground-nesting birds	35–40 days	5–8 eggs
Congo Grey Parrot	Cavity breeders	approx. 28 days	2–5 eggs

Gender identification

In birds, the gonads are located in the abdominal cavity. Non-invasive sex identification from primary sexual characteristics is therefore not possible. However, since **sexual dimorphism** occurs in many bird species, it is possible to distinguish males from females by secondary (morphology) and tertiary (behaviour) characteristics. Testosterone is responsible for the development of these characteristics in both sexes. Morphological characteristics are the colour and size of the comb (domestic chicken) and beak, as well as the colour and structure of the plumage. Courtship, dominance, territorial and breeding behaviour are also under hormonal influence.

MORE DETAILS Some parrot species show sexual dimorphism. Male budgerigars, for example, have a blue coloured waxy skin on the beak, while that of females is brown. However, when a bird has a testicular tumour, the blue colouring of the beak can fade and make it difficult to distinguish between the sexes. The bright green plumage of male noble parrots is clearly distinguishable from the red of females. In some cockatoo species the colouration of the iris can be used for sexing. (e.g. White-crested Cockatoo: male black iris; female reddish-brown iris).

In the majority of parrots, there is no external differentiation between the sexes. These species are called monomorphic, and sex identification is only possible invasively by means of a sexoscopy, or indirectly via DNA analysis or measurement of hormone concentrations.

MORE DETAILS A special feature of avian sexual dimorphism is seen in the Odin's grouse, an Arctic snipe bird. Here, the females have the more colourful plumage and the more conspicuous courtship behaviour. After laying eggs, the females leave the incubation and rearing of the offspring to the males.

In parrots, minimally invasive laparoscopy under inhalation anaesthesia has been used for many years to identify sex and to assess suitability for breeding. The unique structure of the avian respiratory tract, which provides extensive ventilation of the **coelomic cavity**, offers suitable conditions for endoscopy of birds. When the abdominal cavity is explored with an endoscope, the lungs do not collapse.

Routine sexoscopy is performed using rigid endoscopes of 1.9–2.7 mm diameter. Access is from the left side, as only the left ovary is developed in females. The scope is usually inserted caudally of the last rib and cranially of the femur after blunt dissection of the tibialis cranialis muscle. The caudal air sac ruptures spontaneously or must be depressed with the endoscope. The ovary or testis can then be visualised ventrally of the cranial renal pole. Sexoscopy can only be performed after a certain age or at the onset of sexual maturity, as the gonads of juvenile males and females are sometimes very similar. The method requires anaesthesia and thus involves certain risks for the bird, including bleeding and injuries to the kidney or glandular stomach from the endoscope.

In contrast to endoscopic sexing, DNA analysis can be performed on nestlings. The sample material is blood, or quills containing blood (so-called "blood quills"). The DNA is extracted from these and then analysed for sex-specific gene sequences. There are genes that are present on both the W and the Z chromosome, but differ from each other in the length of their introns. The primers used therefore amplify PCR products of different lengths depending on the sex. These can be separated by gel electrophoresis (e.g. CHD-1 gene). There are also sequences that are mainly on the W chromosome (e.g. Xho-1), and can therefore only be detected in female animals.

Another possibility is sex identification by hormone analysis. Sex steroids are produced in the ovaries or testes and secreted into blood. After biotransformation in the liver, the non-water-soluble steroid metabolites are excreted in bile and thus are present in faeces. The sex steroids or their metabolites can be determined in either blood or faeces. The ratio of oestrogens to androgens is particularly important for sex diagnosis. Compared to males, females have higher concentrations of oestrogens and low androgen concentrations. This results in a higher oestrogen/androgen ratio in females, which can be used for sex identification.

> **IN A NUTSHELL** !
>
> In birds, non-invasive sex identification can only be from secondary and tertiary sex characteristics. Options for invasive sex determination are sexoscopy and DNA analysis of blood.

In poultry production, sexing is usually performed on day-old chicks. The methods and criteria are cloacal sexing, the speed of feathering and sex-specific colouring. Cloacal sexing was developed in Japan at the beginning of the 20th century and is mainly used for sex identification of day-old chicks from so-called "pure" lines, as these do not show any other sexual dimorphism characteristics. The technique requires distinguishing the minimal morphological differences of the cloacal opening between male and female day-old chicks. By manually emptying and everting the cloaca, the sex cusp can be assessed, which is formed in all male and about 40% of female chicks. Due to large inter- and intra-sexual variations in size, shape and position in the cloaca, this technique is very difficult to learn.

In the so-called autosexual chicken lines male and female day-old chicks differ in terms of feathering speed or colouration of the down. Genes that influence the phenotype of day-old chicks are located on the sex chromosomes of some chicken breeds. Through selective crossbreeding, some of these traits have also been introduced into the hybrid lines currently used in the poultry industry. In the case of feathering speed, the allele for fast feathering (k) is inherited recessively and the allele for slow feathering (K) is dominant on the Z chromosome. When hybrid lines are produced, K is introduced into the hen line and k into the cock line. As these genes influence the rate of growth of the flight feathers, male birds feather more slowly, and their flight and cover feathers are approximately the same length. Females, on the other hand, feather faster and their wing feathers are always longer than the cover feathers. The colouration of the down can be determined, among other things, by the **silver factor** or the **sparrow hawk** fac-

Endocrinology, reproduction

tor. These are inherited on the Z chromosome and introduced via the hen line. The silver factor, causes silver-coloured (male) or gold-coloured (female) chicks (e.g. brown layer hybrid). The sparrow hawk factor causes sparrow hawk plumage only in adult males. Day-old chicks with the sparrow hawk factor can be distinguished by a white head patch, which is only pronounced in males.

> **MORE DETAILS** Methods for in-ovo sex determination (before hatching) are already being used industrially. Endocrine, molecular biological or hyperspectral methods are used to detect sex-specific differences in embryos. For endocrine analysis, embryonic allantoic fluid is removed from the egg in a minimally invasive procedure and analysed for oestrogen metabolites. Reliable sex identification is possible by this method from the 8th day of embryogenesis in the domestic chicken. The technique is analysis of allantoic fluid for sex-specific gene sequences by PCR on the 9th embryonic day. Hyperspectral analysis detects colour differences in brown-feathered layers on the 13th embryonic day (cocks white, hens brown plumage). Other methods, such as Raman spectroscopy (optical method for displaying sex-specific differences in the circulating blood spectra of extraembryonic vessels) or magnetic resonance imaging, are still being developed for practical application.

■ Breeding and artificial insemination

The number of threatened and endangered bird species, as well as those already extinct in the wild, is very high all over the world. Therefore, in addition to conservation and restoration of their habitats, there are increasing efforts to increase reproduction of threatened species by human intervention. Ideal environmental conditions such as lighting, climate, nutrition and the availability of suitable nesting sites are essential for successful breeding. In addition, diseases of the reproductive tract must be eliminated in the individuals allocated for breeding. Such diseases can occur in birds of both sexes. For example, neoplasia of the testes in male budgerigars or of the ovaries in female budgerigars and cockatiels are common problems. The correct mating of monomorphic species, the onset of sexual maturity and species-specific reproductive behaviour are also important factors to consider. The onset of sexual maturity varies greatly between species. Quails become sexually mature at the age of two months and budgies at six months, while many large parrots do not start reproducing until they are 5–6 years old. Although natural breeding is generally preferable, artificial incubation of eggs may also be necessary to increase the number of offspring. Numerous variables such as temperature, humidity and turning the eggs during incubation must be controlled for successful breeding.

The breeding procedures for parrots are basically the same as for natural reproduction. However, there are also increasing efforts to establish artificial insemination for these species. This would be particularly helpful for endangered species where only a limited number of individuals exist, and mating problems, disease- or behaviour-related impaired fertility, and geographical separation of individuals able to be mated are major challenges. Successful artificial insemination has been reported for the Blue-crowned Amazon, budgerigar, cockatiel, Green-winged Macaw, Red-vented Cockatoo, Scarlet-headed Parrot and various noble parrot species. Artificial insemination has also been successful in chickens and ducks, pigeons, cranes and birds of prey. For many mammals, instrumental sperm transfer has been replacing natural mating (p. 586) for some time.

> **MORE DETAILS** The collection of semen is done by various techniques. Cooperative artificial insemination is performed on birds of prey, which deliver their semen into a receptacle through intensive imprinting on humans. Far more common and less costly is massage of the inner thigh, ventral abdomen, tail, cloaca and synsacrum. Electrostimulation of the cloaca also leads to the release of sperm in pigeons, water fowl, domestic chickens and parrots. It can be used when cooperation or massage techniques do not work. The semen is usually collected in glass capillaries and then examined for sperm density and motility. Contamination from faeces, urine and secretions from the cloaca can interfere with sperm collection and negatively affect sperm longevity. Most favourable is the immediate insemination of the freshly collected sperm into the female. Short-term storage requires temperatures close to freezing point and protection from contamination and desiccation. For storage > 1 hour, diluents must be added. For longer periods, cryopreservation must be used with the addition of cryoprotectants (e.g. glycerol, DMSO). The insemination techniques vary from cooperative methods, massage to stimulate cloacal eversion and deep vaginal insemination. The timing of insemination is crucial for successful fertilisation. Ideally, it should be done daily after the first egg is laid. Egg laying is stimulated by certain behavioural patterns, primarily the presence of the male. In budgies, for example, hens are stimulated to lay eggs by the presence of vasectomised cocks (i.e. non-fertilising males that show normal courtship and copulatory behaviour despite severed spermatic cords). Two hours after oviposition, 5–10 µl of fresh or 40 µl of thawed and processed semen is introduced into the oviduct through a cannula. These volumes are sufficient for the production of fertilised eggs.

Suggested reading

Hummel G. Anatomy and Physiology of Birds. Stuttgart: Ulmer; 2000

Kaleta EF, Krautwald-Junghanns ME, eds. Compendium of Ornamental Bird Diseases: Parrots – pigeons – passerine birds. Hanover: Schlütersche; 2007

Liebich HG. Functional histology of domestic mammals and birds: textbook and colour atlas for study and practice. Stuttgart: Schattauer; 2010

Mehner A, Hartfiel W, eds. Handbuch der Geflügelphysiologie. Jena: Gustav Fischer; 1983

O'Malley B. Clinical anatomy and physiology of exotic species: Structure and function of mammals, birds, reptiles, and amphibians. Edinburgh, New York: Elsevier Saunders; 2005

Ritchie BW, Harrison GJ and LR, ed. Avian medicine: Principles and application. Lake Worth: Wingers; 1994

Rüsse I, Sinowatz F. Lehrbuch der Embryologie der Haustiere. 2nd ed. Berlin: Parey; 1998

Salomon FV. Textbook of poultry anatomy. Jena: Gustav Fischer; 1993

Scholtyssek S. Poultry. Stuttgart: Ulmer; 1987

Whittow GC, ed. Sturkie's avian physiology. 5th ed. San Diego: Academic Press; 2000

25 Lactation

Gerhard Breves; former collaboration: H. Hammon, R. M. Bruckmaier

25.1 The mammary gland

ESSENTIALS ✗

The development of mammary glands and the production of the glandular secretion milk is common to all mammals:
- Milk production represents a decisive evolutionary advantage for care of offspring in mammals, because it provides the newborn with nutrients largely independent of the mother's nutritional supply and status.
- Evolution has produced a great variety of mammary gland characteristics, and also considerable differences in milk composition, which are optimally tailored to meet the needs of offspring of each species.
- In domestic mammals, the first milk (colostrum, beestings) provides the newborn not only with nutrients, but also with immunoglobulins to build up passive immunity. Colostrum also contains other biologically active substances that control ontogenesis of organ functions and support the newborn in adapting to independent life.
- The development of the mammary gland, the synthesis of milk constituents, and control of milk secretion are all regulated by complex endocrine mechanisms.
- Since the nutrient supply of the mammary gland is a high priority, the metabolism of the dam must adapt to that supply. In animal species that have been selected for high milk yield, lactation can affect intermediary metabolism, the immune system and reproduction.

25.2 Importance of lactation for care of offspring

The mammary gland produces a balanced and wholesome food that the newborn eats after switching from parenteral nutrition via the umbilical cord as a foetus to enteral nutrition after birth. The first milk after birth, **colostrum**, contains, in addition to nutrients, essential **immunoglobulins**, to provide **passive immune protection** during the first weeks of life, until the immune system of the newborn becomes fully functional. Colostrum contains other biologically active substances such as growth factors, hormones and cytokines, which are of great importance for early ontogenetic development and especially for the functional development of the gastrointestinal tract. Over the course of lactation the amount and composition of milk changes, depending on the species. With increasing intake of other feed sources, the gastrointestinal tract of the young animal gradually adapts to the digestion and absorption of nutrients typical for each species after the end of lactation.

As well as providing nutrients and other active substances, suckling the young is also crucial for forming and maintaining a close mother-offspring bond, which also improves the young's chances of survival. In many species, lactation inhibits or delays renewed **cyclic ovarian activity** (e.g. in pigs and sporadically in humans), which largely prevents a new pregnancy during lactation and prioritises survival of the current offspring, especially when nutrient supply of the mother is limited. In other species, this suppression of ovarian activity does not occur (e.g. horse) or there is only slight suppression (e.g. cattle), so that lactation and ovarian activity can function simultaneously.

> **IN A NUTSHELL** !
>
> For a newborn animal, lactation provides nutrition, immunisation, postnatal maturation of tissue and organ functions, and mother-offspring bonding.

25.3 Evolutionary development of the mammary gland and milk

Although milk composition varies considerably from one species to another, the basic mechanisms of milk production are similar in all highly developed mammals. Evolution of the mammary gland and milk production began before viviparous (live birth) animals appeared and before diverse families of mammals had evolved. Nutrient-rich milk probably originated from an initial **antimicrobial secretion** which protected the egg in a pouch in the abdomen, as still occurs today in the only remaining family of **Prototheria** subclass, **Monotremata** (echidna, platypus). A sticky secretion from skin glands in the abdominal pocket holds the eggs and keeps them moist, but at the same time creates ideal living conditions for pathogenic microorganisms that can potentially infect the eggs. Antimicrobial components in the secretion can reduce the threat to the eggs from pathogens. **Lysozyme**, an antibacterial enzyme widespread in the animal kingdom, is found in high concentrations in the milk of early mammalian species. It differs structurally from α-lactalbumin in only a few amino acids. In the evolution of milk from an antimicrobial secretion to a liquid nutrient source, protein B of the lactose synthetase system has become more important in supplying lactose as a source of energy for the newborn.

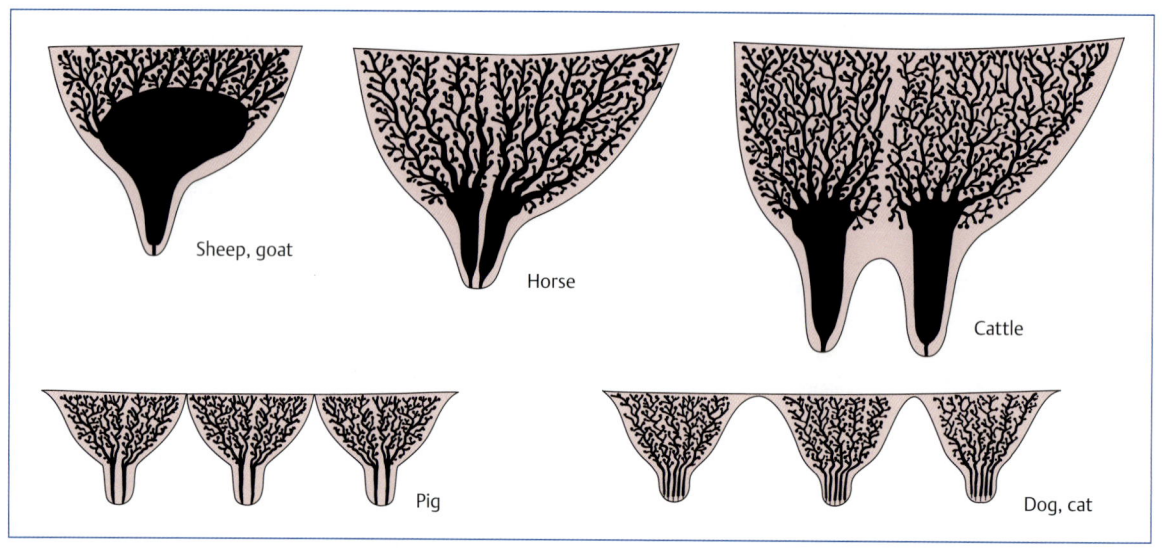

Fig. 25.1 Structure of the mammary glands of different species. Sheep, goat and cattle each have one teat opening per gland complex. Horse and pig have two openings per teat, while dog and cat have several. The mammary glands of sheep and goats have large cistern cavities. In cattle these are much smaller, and are very small in the horse. In pigs, dogs and cats, there are practically no cistern cavities.

> **IN A NUTSHELL** !
>
> The mammary gland evolved before viviparity. The original evolutionary advantage was mainly antimicrobial protection of the offspring.

25.4 Anatomical-histological structure of the mammary gland

The mammary gland is a skin organ and consists of paired gland complexes (mammary complexes). Like sweat or sebaceous glands, it develops from the **ectoderm** of the embryo. The mammary glands are complex structures with different functional components. One of these is the **glandular parenchyma**, which is responsible for milk synthesis, secretion and storage. Other components are the mammary **ducts and cisterns**, through which milk is transported to the teats and stored in a species-specific manner, between suckling and milk synthesis cycles.

> **MORE DETAILS** There are major differences amongst various mammalian species in mammary gland morphology. These differences have important implications for the collection of milk by the suckler or a milking machine. Cattle have two glandular complexes per udder half, each with a teat, whereas horses have two independent secretory units within one glandular complex, which together open into one teat with two orifices. Sheep and goats have one glandular complex and one teat per udder half. The pig's udder consists of 6–8 paired mammary complexes and teats, each with two openings, which discharge the milk from a secretory unit. In dogs and cats there are 4–6 paired glands with one teat each. In dogs there are 7–14 and in cats 4–7 secretory units or openings per teat. There are noticeable species differences in the manner that milk is stored in cistern cavities and in the alveolar tissue (glandular parenchyma). The cistern cavities are particularly large in sheep and goats, somewhat smaller in cattle and water buffalo, and almost absent in pigs, dogs and cats. The arrangement of the secretory units and the cavities of the mammary glands of different species is shown in **Fig. 25.1**. Since alveolar milk is only available after the milk ejection reflex

(p. 612) has been triggered, the location of the stored milk has a great influence on its availability to the suckling infant or for collection by a milking machine.

The **glandular parenchyma** contains a large number of milk-forming cells, the **lactocytes**. They are arranged as a single-layered glandular epithelium on the inner side of the basal membrane of the **alveoli** (< 10 μm), the smallest storage unit for milk in the mammary gland (**Fig. 25.2**). The lactocytes synthesise lactose, lipids and proteins from low-molecular precursors (glucose, volatile fatty acids, amino acids), which they take up from blood. Only some

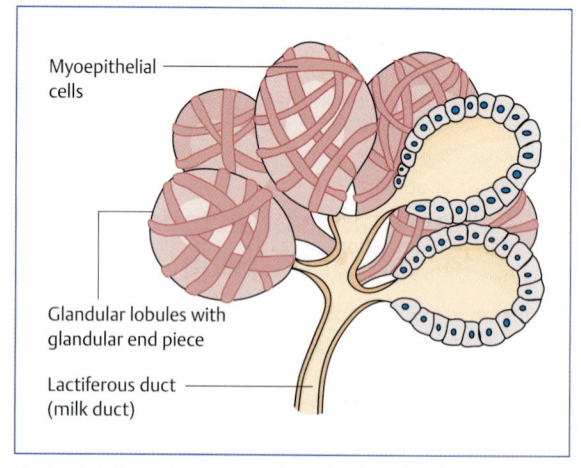

Myoepithelial cells

Glandular lobules with glandular end piece

Lactiferous duct (milk duct)

Fig. 25.2 Schematic structure of an alveolus. The alveolus contains the single-layered glandular epithelium of lactocytes inside the basement membrane. On the outside, the basal membrane is covered with a network of myoepithelial cells (basket cells), which contract under the influence of oxytocin. The myoepithelial cells have the characteristics of smooth muscle cells, but are of ectodermal origin. This distinguishes them from smooth muscle cells of mesodermal origin. A dense network of blood capillaries supplies the lactocytes with precursors for the synthesis of milk and transports oxytocin to the myoepithelial cells. [Source: I care Anatomie, Physiologie. 2nd, updated edition, Stuttgart: Thieme; 2020]

long-chain fatty acids (≥C16) circulating in blood, can be incorporated directly into milk fat.

The cells of the single-layered glandular epithelium are firmly connected to each other by **tight junctions** to form a **blood-milk barrier**.

The glandular parenchyma is exceptionally well supplied with blood. In addition to a dense capillary network, a large number of special muscle cells are present outside the basal membrane, the **myoepithelial cells or basket cells** (**Fig. 25.2**). These have receptors for the peptide hormone **oxytocin**, which is released from the posterior pituitary gland when the mammary gland is stimulated, and thus makes the alveolar milk available for the suckling young animal or for collection by a milking machine.

25.5 Developmental and functional stages of the mammary gland and its endocrine control

The development and function of the mammary gland is divided into various stages, each regulated by different endocrine systems. Depending on the species, these stages may overlap in time. The morphological development and differentiation of the mammary gland, initially with no secretory ability, is called **mammogenesis**. The beginning of milk synthesis and secretion of milk, **lactogenesis**, is specially regulated and is normally activated at the birth of an offspring. The formation of colostrum (**colostrogenesis**) with its special significance for the newborn, is a separate functional component of lactogenesis. The maintenance of lactation, **galactopoiesis**, is in turn controlled by other hormone systems. Again, a separate functional complex during the period of milk secretion is milk ejection (p.612) and milk secretion, which is the prerequisite for the collection of milk both by the infant animal and by mechanical milk extraction. Regular, complete emptying of the mammary gland in turn supports galactopoiesis and has a positive effect on the maintenance of udder health. The end of lactation is characterised by involution of the gland, associated with apoptosis of the lactocytes. In many animal species, this can occur either autonomously due to a steady decline in milk secretion, or it can be induced by external influences with a decreasing demand for milk (weaning of the young, decreasing milking frequency, or suckling with suppressed lactation).

While reproductive hormones are the primary regulators of mammogenesis and lactogenesis, for galactopoiesis and its ultimate involution, it is primarily the hormones that regulate metabolism that mediate those processes.

IN A NUTSHELL   **!**

Mammogenesis, lactogenesis and galactopoiesis are regulated by different hormone complexes. Although these processes run partly in parallel, they are functionally independent.

25.5.1 Mammogenesis

Mammogenesis begins during early embryonic development in utero. At first the mammary gland systems of both sexes develop in the same way. However, with increasing concentrations of foetal male sex steroids (testosterone), mammary gland growth in male foetuses is increasingly suppressed. In cattle, the inhibition of mammogenesis in male foetuses begins around day 65 of gestation. The stimulus for the initial cell division and development of the mammary gland is provided by **oestrogens** and **gestagens**, but also by **prolactin, cortisol**, and **thyroid hormones**. Factors of the **somatotropic axis** (**somatotropin** [STH], **insulin-like growth factor I** [IGF-1]) also play an important role (ch. 24 (p.553) and ch. 25.5.2 (p.604)). **Prenatal mammogenesis** is essentially limited to the formation of the systems for teats, cisternal cavities and milk ducts. The mammary gland grows very little during this phase. During **postnatal mammogenesis** up to the birth of the female's first offspring, mammary growth rate increases, especially influenced by the concentration of ovarian steroids.

Oestrogens are mainly responsible for the growth of the **teats** and the **milk duct system** while the growth of the **alveoli** and the mammary gland epithelial cells, **lactocytes**, are primarily controlled by **progesterone**, but also by oestrogens, prolactin, growth hormone, cortisol and thyroid hormones.

Oestrogens stimulate the secretion of prolactin and somatotropin and at the same time increase the sensitivity of the mammary gland tissue to mammogenic hormones. A massive acceleration of mammary gland growth takes place during puberty due to rising sex steroid levels.

During **pregnancy**, especially in the second half, and thus shortly before milk for the newborn is required, mammary gland development increases rapidly. A proteohormone, **placental lactogenic hormone**, structurally similar to prolactin from the anterior pituitary, also supports mammogenesis during pregnancy. However, this hormone has only been detected in ruminants. Its concentration in blood depends essentially on placental mass, and it acts via receptors for prolactin and somatotropin. In this way, the number of foetuses (e.g. in sheep and goats) or the size of the foetus (e.g. in cattle) indirectly adjusts the intensity of mammary gland development to meet subsequent requirements in the quantity of milk.

Although there is intensive mammogenesis during gestation, there is no requirement for milk production at that time. The high concentrations of progesterone suppress lactation during pregnancy, but these concentrations drop before birth and thus allow lactogenesis to start.

In most mammalian species, mammogenesis is largely completed before the onset of lactation. although in some species, mammogenesis continues during lactation. These are mainly species in which the demand for milk after birth is unpredictable because the number of offspring varies greatly (e.g. mouse and rat), or species in which the demand for milk increases greatly during lactation and the mammary gland develops in parallel with the growth of the offspring (e.g. marsupials).

25.5.2 Colostrogenesis

Some weeks before the onset of lactogenesis, a small amount of glandular secretion has already started, in which, among other things, **immunoglobulins** accumulate. Depending on the animal species, these are either transported **transcellularly** from blood into the glandular secretion through the mammary gland epithelial cells, by means of specific membrane receptors (FcRn) for different immunoglobulin isotypes, or the immunoglobulins are produced by **resident plasma cells in the mammary gland (**IgA, IgM). In cattle, the immunoglobulins in colostrum consist of approx. 70–75% IgG, 15–20% IgA and 5–10% IgM. The FcRn receptor, responsible for IgG_1 transport has been found in many mammalian species, but not in cattle. The storage of immunoglobulins in the glandular secretion before lactogenesis (precolostrum), ensures that their concentration is particularly high in the first milk, the **colostrum**. In the hours after birth, the newborn is able to absorb these immunoglobulins (p. 252) intact (p. 428) in the small intestine. The same receptor type (FcRn) is responsible for the transcellular transport of the immunoglobulins through the intestinal epithelium of the newborn, as for their transcellular transport in the mammary gland epithelium. For the newborn, intake of colostrum within the first hours of neonatal life is crucial. At this time, acid concentration in the stomach and the activity of proteolytic digestive enzymes are still low. The FcRn receptors localised in vacuoles of the newborn's intestinal epithelium also disappear quickly after birth, thus preventing further absorption of immunoglobulins from then on. Thus, effective passive immunisation of the newborn against environmental pathogens is only possible immediately after birth. The absorption of immunoglobulins in the newborn depends on the volume of colostrum ingested and the time after birth. Immunoglobulin absorption is considered optimal if colostrum is ingested up to 6 hours after birth.

Colostrogenesis lasts until birth and then ceases abruptly. However, the exact mechanisms for this are not yet clear. The immunoglobulin content is therefore only particularly high in the **first colostrum**. After colostrum has been drained from the mammary gland, the immunoglobulin content drops rapidly. However, due to incompletely closed alveolar tight junctions during the colostral phase (**Fig. 25.5**), blood components continue to enter the glandular secretion for several days, which clearly distinguishes the composition and appearance of colostrum from mature milk.

The importance of passive immunisation through colostrum depends on the extent of placental transfer of immunoglobulins during pregnancy. The structure of the placenta, and particularly the number of placental tissue layers, determine whether macromolecules can pass from the maternal circulation into foetal blood. In horses, pigs, and ruminants, colostrum is essential and its early and sufficient intake is critical for the newborn's chance of survival. While colostral immunoglobulin transfer is a physiologically desirable mechanism, pathophysiological processes can also be induced by colostrum intake. A disease described as early as the 18th century is the so-called haemolytic syndrome of the foal (neonatal icterus, neonatal isoerythrolysis). In this disease, the foal absorbs maternal antibodies from colostrum, which cause massive haemolysis by binding to surface antigens of the foal's erythrocytes, resulting in a pronounced yellow appearance (jaundice) of mucous membranes. This clinical picture corresponds to the pathophysiological mechanism of rhesus incompatibility in humans.

In dogs, cats, rats, and mice, protective immunisation begins by placental transfer of maternal immunoglobulins and continues postnatally by the intake of colostrum. In rabbits, guinea pigs, and humans, there is efficient placental transfer of macromolecules from the maternal to the foetal circulation, so that in those species, passive immunisation has already been achieved by the time of birth (**Fig. 25.3; Table 16.12**).

MORE DETAILS Besides immunoglobulins the first colostrum also contains a number of other bioactive components such as hormones (insulin, prolactin), growth factors (insulin-like growth factor [IGF]-1 and -2; transforming growth factor [TGF]) and vitamins (vitamin A, C) in particularly high concentrations. It is certain that most hormones and growth factors are not absorbed by the newborn. Therefore, these other colostral components have little systemic effect on the newborn. Nevertheless, they influence the development of the gastrointestinal tract and promote, growth and differentiation of the intestinal epithelium and the mucosal cell villi. By increasing villous growth, colostrum enhances absorptive capacity of the intestinal mucosa and thus contributes to efficient uptake of nutrients.

The enzyme γ-glutamyltransferase is present in high concentrations in colostrum. Its detection in a calf's blood plasma gives evidence of previous colostrum intake, in extensive housing systems.

25.5.3 Lactogenesis

Lactogenesis can be divided into two phases. In the first phase, which partly runs parallel to the formation of the precolostrum, cytological and **enzymatic differentiation** of lactocytes takes place, without any significant secretion by these cells, see ch. 24.1. As a prerequisite for the synthesis of milk constituents, the endoplasmic reticulum and the

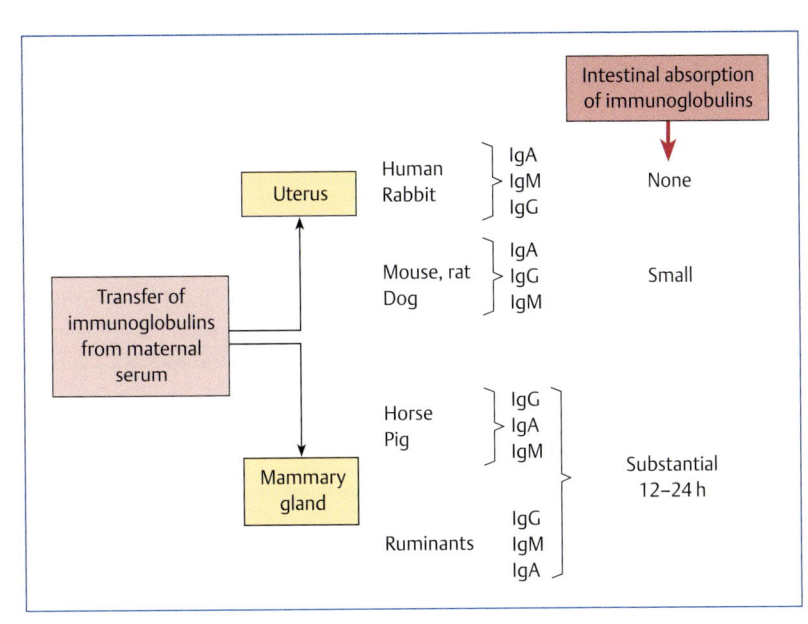

Fig. 25.3 Comparison of the supply of immunoglobulins to the foetus or newborn via the placenta and/or from colostrum in different animal species. Group I: intra-uterine supply of immunoglobulins. Group II: supply of immunoglobulins by intra-uterine transfer and through colostrum; Group III: immunoglobulins almost exclusively supplied by colostrum.

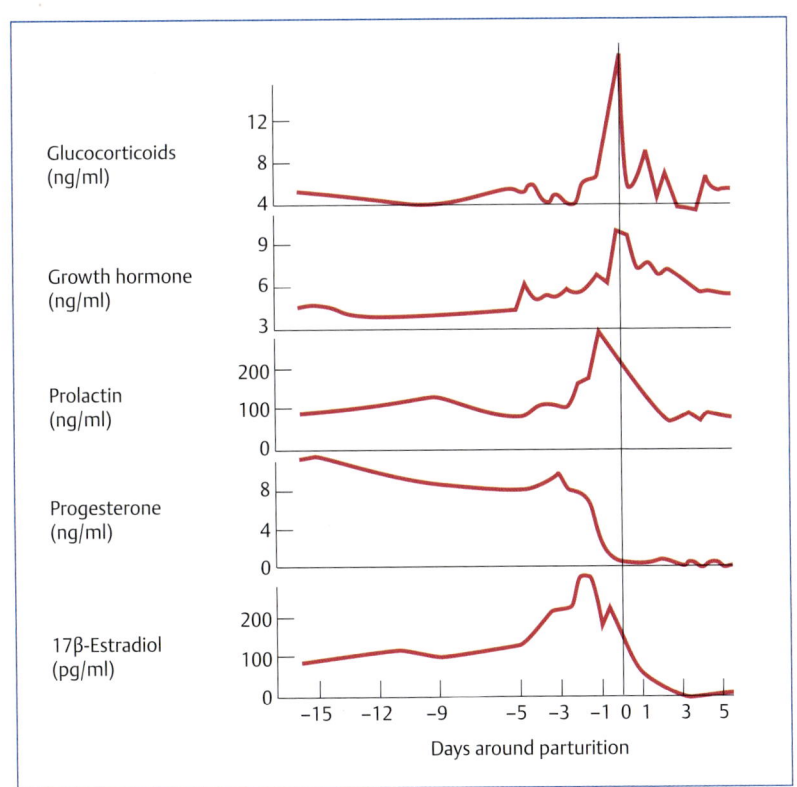

Fig. 25.4 Hormone profiles in maternal plasma in the period close to the time of birth; based on data from Tucker HA. General Endocrine control of Lactation. In: Larson BL, Smith VR (eds.). Lactation: A comprehensive treatise. Vol. 1. New York: Academic Press; 1974: 277–326

Golgi apparatus are further developed. In this phase, the blood plasma concentration of **progesterone** is still **high** and that of **prolactin** is still **low** (Fig. 25.4). The lactogenic effect in this phase is mainly mediated by **glucocorticoids**, a considerable proportion of which is produced by the foetus. At the same time, the concentration of corticoid-binding proteins decreases so that the increased amount of non-protein bound cortisol can exert its full effect. Thus, the foetus influences the development of the mammary gland shortly before birth. In the second phase of lactogenesis, the synthesis of specific milk components begins. The prerequisite for this is a drop in progesterone concentra-

tion in blood, because progesterone suppresses the release of prolactin from the anterior pituitary. In addition, progesterone partially blocks the glucocorticoid receptors of the mammary gland and thus the corticoid-dependent formation of the prolactin receptors. The sharp increase in **prolactin** following the decrease in progesterone is absolutely crucial for the initiation of milk protein and lactose synthesis. In experiments, where prolactin secretion is blocked during lactogenesis, milk secretion is completely suppressed.

Progesterone, a major stimulator of mammogenesis, simultaneously inhibits milk production. Thus, milk is only

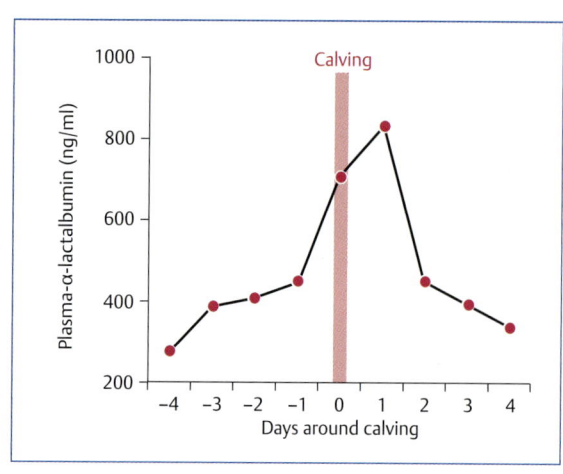

Fig. 25.5 α-Lactalbumin in the blood before and after calving of primiparous cows. There is increasing synthesis of α-lactalbumin at this time, but closure of the tight junctions around birth results in a decrease of α-lactalbumin in blood. [Source: McFadden TB, Akers RM, Kazmer GW. Alpha-lactalbumin in bovine serum: relationships with udder development and function. J Dairy Sci 1987; 71: 826–834]

produced at the time when the newborn is ready to receive it. Differences in the time of onset of lactation come from this effect of progesterone. In ruminants and pigs, progesterone concentration decreases significantly before birth as a result of **luteolysis** induced by prostaglandin F, so that lactation can then begin (**Fig. 25.4**). In contrast, in primates, including humans, progesterone is mainly produced by the placenta shortly before birth. Thus, progesterone levels do not decrease until after the placenta has been ejected, so that milk production does not begin until 1–2 days **after birth**. During lactogenesis, the **tight junctions** of the mammary gland epithelium are close, resulting in a **blood-milk barrier**. (**Fig. 25.5**). This means that the synthesised milk constituents can only enter the glandular secretion and cannot pass into blood. Diffusion of water into the lactocytes, essentially through the osmotic effect of lactose being synthesised, can only function if the blood-milk barrier is intact. Just like the initiation of milk secretion, the **closing** of the **tight junctions** is also inhibited by high concentrations of progesterone. In addition to a **fall in progesterone levels**, **cortisol** and **prolactin are also required** for closure of the tight junctions. At the same time as the histological changes in the mammary gland, **blood flow** more than doubles during lactogenesis, in order to supply the lactocytes with the substrates for synthesis of the milk components.

> **IN A NUTSHELL**   !
>
> Prolactin is essential for the onset of milk production during lactogenesis.

25.5.4 Galactopoiesis

Maintaining milk synthesis and secretion at a high level after the start of lactation is essential during the suckling period for the nutrition of the offspring and also for milk production in dairy farming.

■ Hormonal regulation

Because of the close relationship between nutrient availability, metabolism and milk production it is obvious that **metabolic hormones play a decisive role in** the regulation of galactopoiesis. This is in contrast to the preceding developmental stages of mammogenesis and lactogenesis, where sex hormones are the important regulators. In cattle, the somatotropic axis with **somatotropin** (**STH**), synthesised in the liver, along with the **insulin-like growth factor-1** (**IGF-1**) and the **IGF binding proteins** are needed for efficient **galactopoiesis**. Besides the anabolic effect of IGF-1 in various tissues including the mammary gland, STH also has a direct catabolic, lipolytic effect in adipose tissue.

MORE DETAILS The insulin-like growth factor-1 (IGF-1) stimulates proliferation of lactocytes and simultaneously inhibits their apoptosis. Biotechnologically, increased hepatic production of IGF-1 is achieved by administering **recombinant bovine growth hormone** (rbST). In dairy cows, a significant increase in milk yield (> 20%) can be achieved after administration of rbST. A prerequisite for the stimulation of IGF-1 release after rbST administration is a fully functional somatotropic axis, and also correction of a negative energy balance. When rbST is administered in the last third of lactation, the continued maintenance of good milk production (persistence) is achieved mainly from stimulation of lipolysis and prevention of apoptosis of the lactocytes (which would normally occur at this stage of lactation) (see below). In the USA, the use of growth hormone to increase milk yield in cows has been approved since 1994. In many countries, including the European Union, the use of growth hormone to enhance performance is prohibited.

In **some species**, a significant function of **prolactin** for galactopoiesis has been observed (rabbit, human). By inhibiting prolactin secretion, lactation can be stopped. In ruminants, no increase in milk production can be achieved by the administration of prolactin, and only complete pharmacological inhibition of prolactin secretion by dopamine agonists, will result in a decrease in production or, at the end of lactation, complete cessation of milk secretion (dry lactation).

Thyroid hormones, glucocorticoids as well as **leptin** and a balanced ratio of **insulin** and **glucagon** are also of great importance during galactopoiesis for metabolic regulation in the mammary gland and especially for the necessary metabolic adjustments in the whole animal. The synthesis of milk proteins, especially casein, mobilisation of **calcium** from the bone by **parathyroid hormone-related peptide** (**PTHrP**) and **parathyroid hormone**, as well as the stimulation of gastrointestinal calcium absorption by calcitriol (p. 549), are all of great importance for functioning galactopoiesis. Especially at the beginning of lactation, in high-yielding cows, mobilisation of calcium from bone and gastrointestinal Ca absorption often cannot increase quickly enough to meet the sudden increase in demand for Ca. This can lead to clinical signs of **hypocalcaemia** (parturient paresis, recumbency). As both phosphate and calcium concentration in milk are very high, hypocalcaemia is often associated with hypophosphataemia.

■ Persistence of lactation

Particularly in species where the offspring soon start eating other food, (e.g. in ruminants), milk production peaks not long after birth (in cattle 4–6 weeks) and then declines steadily. For dairy cow production it is therefore important to maintain lactation performance at a high level for a long time (persistence) without, however, imposing too high a yield at peak lactation, which would put excessive strain on the animals' metabolism. In order to achieve persistence at a high level, a high rate of new lactocyte formation, and at the same time, a minimal rate of apoptosis are important.

Effective **control of galactopoiesis** and the time of involution of the mammary gland are determined by the demand for milk and the **frequency** and **completeness of milk withdrawal**. The more completely and the frequency of the mammary gland being emptied, i.e. the higher the demand of the offspring, the longer high level milk secretion would be maintained or even increased. In practical dairy farming. milking frequency can therefore be used to influence performance. If milking is carried out up to 4 times a day, depending on the farm's capability for this, consequent production increases of up to 25% are possible. On the other hand, performance drops very quickly if milkings are cancelled or if milk delivery is disturbed during milking, and large quantities of milk remain in the udder. If regular milk withdrawal is disrupted on several occasions, involution (**apoptosis** of the **lactocytes)** sets in very quickly and milk production ceases. If the performance level is low and lactational persistence of the dairy cows is poor, milk secretion ceases, despite regular milkings.

> **IN A NUTSHELL** !
>
> By increasing milking frequency milk production can be increased.

MORE DETAILS In the past, there have been attempts, especially in organic farming, to milk cows for long periods without a drying off period and without a further pregnancy. Trials have shown that milking in this way did not result in any marked reduction in milk yield. The advantages of this procedure are that the risk periods for animal health around birth could be reduced and the useful life of the animals could be extended. In conventional dairy farming, this procedure is not of practical significance.

> **IN A NUTSHELL** !
>
> The development of the mammary gland (mammogenesis) and the initiation of milk secretion (lactogenesis) are primarily under the control of reproductive hormones and prolactin. In the maintenance of lactation (galactopoiesis), metabolic hormones are primarily involved.

25.6 Synthesis and secretion of milk and its components

Most organic milk constituents are synthesised in the mammary gland. The substrates for this synthesis are mainly β-hydroxybutyrate, glycerol, glucose, amino acids and fatty acids, supplied by blood perfusing the mammary gland. Milk also contains vitamins and smaller organic molecules that are transported from blood into milk unchanged. This also applies to individual proteins such as albumin and immunoglobulins. The number of lactocytes, their substrate uptake capacity, and the rates of synthesis and secretion, define the performance of the mammary gland. There is a close relationship between milk yield and the **number** of **differentiated lactocytes**. Udder size and mass of glandular parenchyma are greater in high yielding cows than in low yielding cows.

The substrate supply for the mammary gland is essentially determined by its **blood supply**. To produce **1 kg of milk**, approx. **500 l of blood** must perfuse the udder of cows and goats. This means that the proportion of cardiac output directed to udder perfusion can be between 20% and 40%, depending on milk yield. During lactation, the lactocytes have a high metabolic rate. This correlates with O_2 uptake from arterial blood, which can be up to approx. 50%.

> **IN A NUTSHELL** !
>
> The synthesis capacity of the mammary gland depends on the genetic characteristics of the animal, the feeding and husbandry conditions, the number of lactocytes and the blood supply to the mammary gland.

Glucose plays a central role in various metabolic pathways for synthesis in the mammary gland. Thus large quantities of **glucose** are used in the synthesis of **lactose**, and also in the **synthesis** of glycerol-3-phosphate (triacylglycerols) for **milk fat** production, where the reducing equivalents of NADPH (**Fig. 25.7**) are also required. Glucose serves to provide NADPH in the cytosol both from the pentose-phosphate cycle and after conversion to citrate in the citrate shuttle. Since carbohydrates can be almost completely degraded to short-chain fatty acids in the forestomachs of ruminants, depending on the composition of the ration, there is little glucose available from the diet for milk production. In ruminants, therefore, glucose (p.469) is an extraordinarily scarce substrate, which must therefore be supplied to a large extent from hepatic (approx. 80%) and kidney (approx. 20%) gluconeogenesis. Because of the limited availability of glucose in the ruminant, the conversion of citrate via isocitrate to alpha-ketoglutarate in the cytosol provides the NADPH required for fatty acid synthesis. NADPH production from conversion of citrate to pyruvate plays no role in the ruminant. As in monogastric animals, glucose is also used in ruminants as a substrate for the pentose phosphate pathway which also is an important source of **NADPH** for fatty acid synthesis, in addition to the isocitrate pathway, described above. The complex functions of glucose in the synthesis of milk constituents result in a very high glucose requirement in high-yielding cows, of approx. 4 kg glucose for a daily milk yield of 55 kg.

In ruminants, the acetate formed in the rumen, along with β-hydroxybutyrate, is the most important substrate for the synthesis of short- and medium-chain fatty acids (up to C16) in the mammary gland (**Fig. 25.8**). Monogastric animals, in contrast to ruminants, have larger amounts of glucose available, so that it is the most important substrate for the formation of short- and medium-chain fatty acids in the mammary gland (**Fig. 25.7**).

The milk-specific proteins (**caseins**, α-lactalbumin, β-lactoglobulin) are synthesised exclusively by the lactocytes The amino acids required for this come from dietary protein and, if the protein supply is insufficient, from the breakdown of body protein. In ruminants, the usable crude protein at the duodenum is composed of the microbial **protein** synthesised in the forestomachs and the forestomach undegraded **feed protein;** see ch. Digestion and absorption in the forestomachs (p. 395).

The **absorption of water** into the mammary gland is mainly determined by the **lactose concentration** in milk, which in cow's milk is therefore largely constant at approx. 4.8–5.0%. Only when the blood-milk barrier is disturbed, as in mastitis, electrolytes can then also become osmotically active and the lactose content of milk can decrease.

IN A NUTSHELL !

The carbohydrate and protein components of milk are completely synthesised in the mammary gland. and are independent of the food consumed. Fluctuations can occur in the concentration of lipids in milk, as the long-chain fatty acids are derived directly from body fat and from dietary fats.

25.6.1 Synthesis of milk fat

In the mammary gland of ruminants, saturated fatty acids can be synthesised up to a chain length of 16 C atoms. Precursors for this are acetate and β-hydroxybutyrate from the microbial fermentation of carbohydrates in the rumen, and the conversion of butyric acid into β-hydroxybutyrate in the rumen mucosa and in the liver (see absorption of short-chain fatty acids (p. 401)). From a chain length of 16 C atoms, the fatty acids originate from food and body fats or from synthesis by rumen microorganisms (p. 404) or the liver. About 50% of palmitic acid (C16) can be synthesised de novo in the udder or absorbed from the blood. Longer-chain fatty acids come exclusively from blood.

Termination of chain elongation in fatty acid synthesis is by special enzymes, the thioesterases. Here there is a clear difference between enzymes in the mammary gland and those in other tissues. **Thioesterase I** (liver, fatty tissue) only stops fatty acid synthesis at a chain length of 16–18 C atoms. **Thioesterase II**, which has so far only been found in the mammary gland, sometimes terminates chain elongation at shorter lengths, but always no longer than 16 C atoms. Therefore, in addition to fatty acids with **14**

and **16 C atoms**, fatty acids with **8, 10** and **12 C atoms** are also synthesised in the mammary gland. The main purpose for this is probably to ensure that milk fat remains as a liquid at 37 °C. Longer fatty acids would increase the melting point of milk fat.

In **monogastric animals, glucose** is the primary substrate in the de novo synthesis of fatty acids. (**Fig. 25.7**). In **ruminants, acetate** from microbial carbohydrate fermentation in the forestomachs, and β-hydroxybutyrate, produced from butyrate in the rumen mucosa or in the liver, are the essential substrates (**Fig. 25.8**).

Because carbohydrates are broken down microbially, mainly to **short-chain fatty acids** in the forestomachs of ruminants, only small amounts of glucose are available for absorption in the intestine. Consequently, ruminants have to expend energy to synthesise glucose. Therefore, since **glucose** is relatively scarce, the short-chain fatty acids, **acetate and β-hydroxybutyrate**, are the preferred substrates for synthesis of long chain **fatty acids**.

About 40–50% of fatty acids (≥ 16 C-atoms) in milk fat of the cow do not originate from de novo synthesis, but come either from **depot fat** (bound to albumin), from the **liver** (very low density lipoproteins, VLDL; in the dairy cow, only very small amounts) or from the **food** (**Fig. 25.8**). In ruminants, however, long-chain unsaturated fatty acids from the food in particular, can only remain unchanged to a limited extent in the forestomach system. They are either saturated microbialogically or converted to cis-trans fatty acids (p. 404). Therefore, milk fat of the cow is normally dominated by saturated palmitic acid (16 C atoms) and monounsaturated oleic acid (18 C atoms). There is a high ATP requirement for de novo synthesis of fatty acids. Thus, 15 moles of ATP are required for the synthesis of 1 mole of palmitate. ATP is required for the transport of acetyl-CoA from mitochondria into the cytosol, and for the synthesis of malonyl-CoA by acetyl-CoA carboxylase.

Despite the transformation of dietary long-chain fatty acids in the forestomach in ruminants, the degree of saturation of long-chain fatty acids in milk fat can still be influenced by feeding. If large amounts of unsaturated fatty acids are ingested (e.g. by feeding fresh grass; grazing), the capacity of the rumen to saturate the long-chain unsaturated fatty acids is exceeded and some of the unsaturated fatty acids are absorbed unchanged in the small intestine. Therefore, the fatty acid composition of the food can influence milk fat composition to a certain extent. In contrast, the carbohydrate and protein composition of milk is not influenced by the food.

MORE DETAILS The fatty acid composition of milk and thus the degree of hardness of butterfat are influenced by feeding. In typical summer feeding with fresh grass, the milk fat (and thus also butter) is relatively soft due to the high proportion of unsaturated fatty acids, whereas in winter feeding with hay, it is typically very hard due to the high proportion of crude fibre. However, by feeding silage and also using special processing techniques, butter that is easier to spread can also be produced in winter.

In ruminants, despite the influence of food composition on the fatty acid pattern described above, it is mainly saturated fatty acids from the food or depot fat that enter the mammary gland. However, the lactocytes have a **micro-**

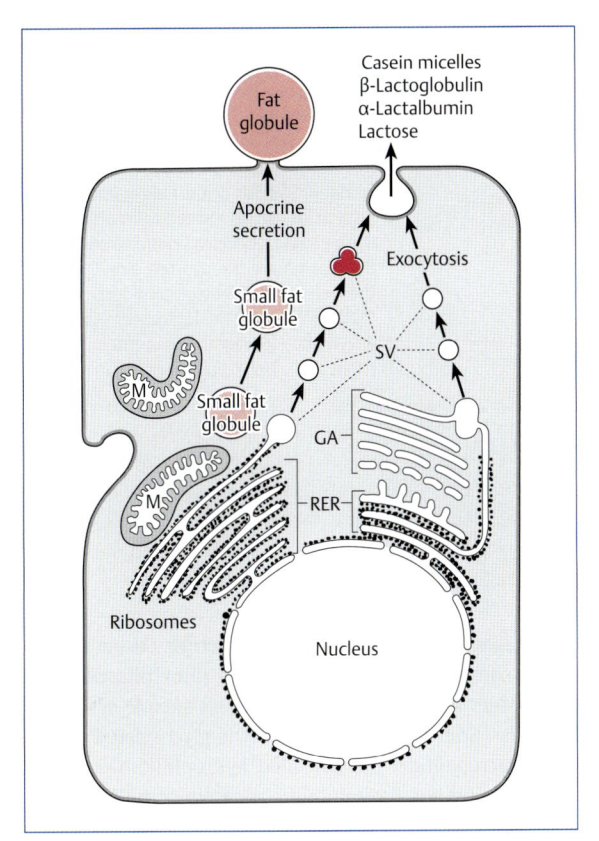

Fat globule

Casein micelles
β-Lactoglobulin
α-Lactalbumin
Lactose

Apocrine secretion

Exocytosis

Small fat globule

SV

Small fat globule

GA

M

RER

Ribosomes

Nucleus

Fig. 25.6 Synthesis and secretion of milk components. Milk proteins including caseins, are synthesised in the rough endoplasmic reticulum (RER). In the Golgi apparatus (GA), casein micelles are formed and together with the other milk proteins and **lactose**, they are packaged into secretory vesicles (VS), which, under the osmotic effect of lactose, absorb water. These vesicles then fuse with the apical cell membrane and the contents enter the alveolar lumen by exocytosis. **Milk fat** is also formed in the RER. Smaller fat globules (FCs) fuse together on their way to the apical cell membrane. There, the enlarged milk fat globules (MFK) are released to the alveolar lumen enclosed in a segment of the apical cell membrane.
M = mitochondrion.

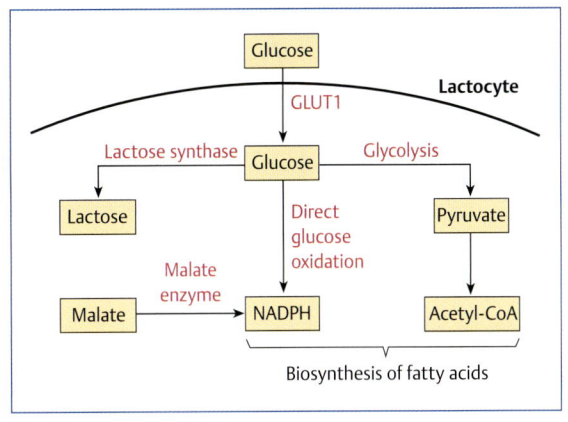

Glucose

Lactocyte

GLUT1

Lactose synthase — Glucose — Glycolysis

Lactose

Malate enzyme

Malate — NADPH

Direct glucose oxidation

Pyruvate

Acetyl-CoA

Biosynthesis of fatty acids

Fig. 25.7 Significance of glucose for milk formation in the lactocytes of the mammary gland. **Glucose** is taken up into the lactocytes by the glucose transporter GLUT1 (facilitated diffusion) and is a substrate for **lactose** synthesis (in all domestic mammals) and, in monogastric animals, also as a substrate for **fatty acid biosynthesis**. Glucose is metabolised in the cytosol to pyruvate (glycolysis), which with oxaloacetate in the mitochondria forms citrate (citrate cycle). Citrate enters the cytosol facilitated by a citrate transporter, where it is cleaved by ATP citrate lyase to acetyl-CoA and oxaloacetate. Acetyl-CoA is a precursor for the synthesis of fatty acids. The conversion of oxaloacetate to malate and then to pyruvate produces **NADPH** (malate enzyme), which is needed for the synthesis of fatty acids. NADPH is also formed directly in glucose oxidation in the pentose phosphate pathway.
GLUT1 = glucose transporter-1; MDH = malate dehydrogenase (cytosolic).

somal desaturase. This can form palmitoleic acid (16:1) from palmitic acid (16:0) and oleic acid (18:1) from stearic acid (18:0), and this in turn lowers the melting temperature of milk fat.

In the uptake of **long-chain fatty acids** into lactocytes, **lipoprotein lipase** (splitting of the triacylglycerole from lipoproteins and chylomicrons into fatty acids and glycerol) and **fatty acid transport proteins** in the plasma membrane, play an important role. Fatty acid transport **proteins** and **acyl-CoA binding** proteins also enable the transport of fatty acids in the cell. For the synthesis of triacylglycerols, the fatty acids are converted into fatty acid acyl-CoAs by means of acyl-CoA synthetase (long-chain form). The glycerol-3-phosphate needed for the synthesis of triacylglycerols comes either from glycolysis or directly by phosphorylation of glycerol obtained from plasma (**Fig. 25.8**).

Most milk fat is therefore in the form of triacylglycerols (triglycerides) and less than 1% is as mono- and diacylglycerols, free fatty acids, phospholipids and steroids. Milk fat also contains fat-soluble vitamins.

Milk fat synthesis takes place in the **endoplasmic reticulum** of **lactocytes**. Initially, small lipovesicles are formed, which fuse together and enlarge on their way to the apical cell membrane. Surrounded by parts of the apical cell membrane, the lipovesicles are released into the alveolar lumen by apocrine secretion (**Fig. 25.6**). These fat droplets can be kept in suspension for a long time as an emulsion in the aqueous milk because they are surrounded by the cell membrane, which is lipophilic on the inside and hydrophilic on the outside. The gradual aggregation of milk fat droplets to form a surface layer of cream on standing, is because of their lower density than water. This effect is not relevant during suckling, as the milk passes directly from the mammary gland into the infant's digestive tract.

MORE DETAILS   A **decrease in milk fat content** occurs when feeding rations that are low in crude fibre and have high contents of starch and unsaturated fatty acids. The high starch content shifts intraruminal conversion of carbohydrates towards more propionic acid and less acetate, and thus less substrate for milk fat synthesis. With a high proportion of unsaturated fatty acids in the ration, unsaturated fatty acids are increasingly transformed by the microorganisms in the rumen into trans fatty acids, of which the trans-10, cis-12 conjugated linoleic acid has a particularly powerful effect in suppressing milk fat synthesis. This effect of suppressing milk fat synthesis can be specifically triggered by the targeted administration of isomers of conjugated linoleic acid (CLA). In experiments where CLA isomers were fed to dairy cows, a reduction in milk fat content of up to 20% was achieved. De novo fatty acid synthesis is also reduced when large amounts of long-chain fatty acids are fed, thereby inhibiting the activity of acetyl-CoA carboxylase, which is essential for the initial step in fatty acid synthesis.

Endocrinology, reproduction

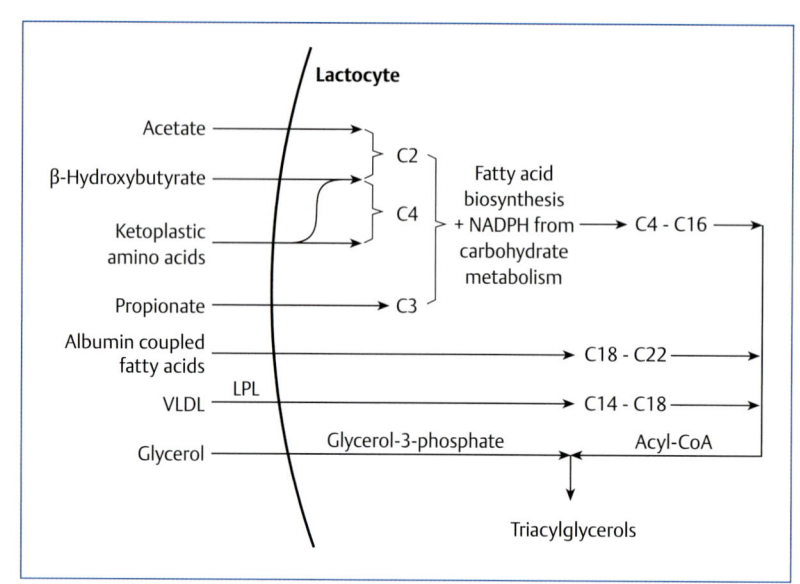

Fig. 25.8 Synthesis of triacylglycerols in ruminants from short and medium chain fatty acids. Acetyl-CoA for **fatty acid biosynthesis** in lactocytes is formed directly from **acetate** and β-hydroxybutyrate in ruminants. Other precursors are the ketogenic amino acids. Odd-numbered fatty acids can be formed from propionate. Long-chain fatty acids bound to albumin in the plasma are transported directly into the lactocytes. Triacylglycerol fatty acids in VLDL, only enter the lactocytes after enzymatic cleavage by lipoprotein lipase (LPL).

25.6.2 Synthesis of milk proteins

The proteins which are specific to milk, caseins and whey proteins, are synthesised de novo in the mammary gland by the lactocytes. Proteins from the plasma are found in milk only during the colostral period (immunoglobulins) and pathologically in mastitis when plasma proteins, such as serum albumin, can diffuse into milk through leaky tight junctions.

The substrates for the de novo synthesis of proteins are amino acids from blood plasma, which are taken up by lactocytes by specific membrane transport. Small peptides can also be taken up by the lactocytes. However, these are largely broken down into the individual amino acids in the lactocytes before they are used for protein synthesis. As described for other tissues (e.g. the small intestine (p. 427)), Na^+ cotransport systems (e.g. transport systems for neutral [alanine, serine leucine], acidic [glutamic acid, aspartic acid] and β-amino acids [taurine]) are available for the uptake of amino acids in the basal membrane of the lactocytes. In addition, there are also Na^+-independent transport systems in the basal membrane which are mainly responsible for the transport of neutral (e.g. essential amino acids such as leucine and methionine) and basic amino acids (lysine, arginine). Peptide transport systems are present for the uptake of small peptides. Since some free amino acids (e.g. glutamic acid, taurine) are present in milk in very high concentrations in some species, specific transport systems are also present in the apical membrane of the lactocytes, which enable these amino acids to pass from the lactocyte into milk.

The most important specific milk proteins are the **caseins** (α-s₁, α-s₂, β-, κ-casein in a ratio of about 3:1:3:1), which are characterised by high contents of proline and glutamic acid and low contents of glycine and asparagine. Milk also contains small amounts of γ-casein, the C-terminal portion of β-casein, which has been cleaved off by the proteinase, plasmin, present in milk. In addition to the proteins, the casein micelles contain large amounts of calcium and phosphorus as well as smaller amounts of citrate

and magnesium in their colloidal structure. Casein submicelles combine through colloidal calcium phosphate to form larger micelles of 10–300 nm. The outside of the micelles is enriched with κ-casein. It is glycosylated with a glycomacropeptide, the so-called hydrophilic hair, which is responsible for the solubility of casein micelles in milk (**Fig. 25.9**).

Chymosin (rennin) in the calf's abomasum splits off the κ-casein glycomacropeptide, which immediately causes casein **coagulation**. The proteins that are not precipitated by chymosin are called **whey proteins**. These include blood serum proteins potentially present in milk, and the specific milk proteins α-lactalbumin and β-lactoglobulin. The **α-lactalbumin**, found in milk of all species, has an important enzyme function in the synthesis of lactose and its expression determines the rate of lactose **synthesis**. **β-Lactoglobulin** is mainly found in the milk of ruminants, and is not present in the milk of humans, rats and guinea pigs. There is no known function of β-lactoglobulin other than as a nutritional protein. In cow's milk it makes up 50 % of the whey protein and binds small hydrophobic ligands such as retinol. It is thought to be responsible for the development of allergies to cow's milk proteins in human nutrition. **Lactoferrin**, another whey protein, is only found in high concentrations during the colostral phase, in mastitis and at the drying off stage of lactation. It is hardly detectable in healthy mature milk.

Milk proteins are synthesised on ribosomes in the endoplasmic reticulum and is similar in principle to protein synthesis in other cell types. The proteins migrate to the Golgi apparatus where they are packaged into secretory vesicles. The aggregation of casein molecules into submicelles and micelles in the presence of calcium also takes place in the Golgi apparatus (**Fig. 25.6, Fig. 25.9**).

Milk protein synthesis is a high **energy-consuming process** and is therefore determined to a large extent by the energy supply. When there is a nutritional energy deficiency, the **protein content** of milk will therefore **decline**. Milk protein synthesis in high-performance cows can also

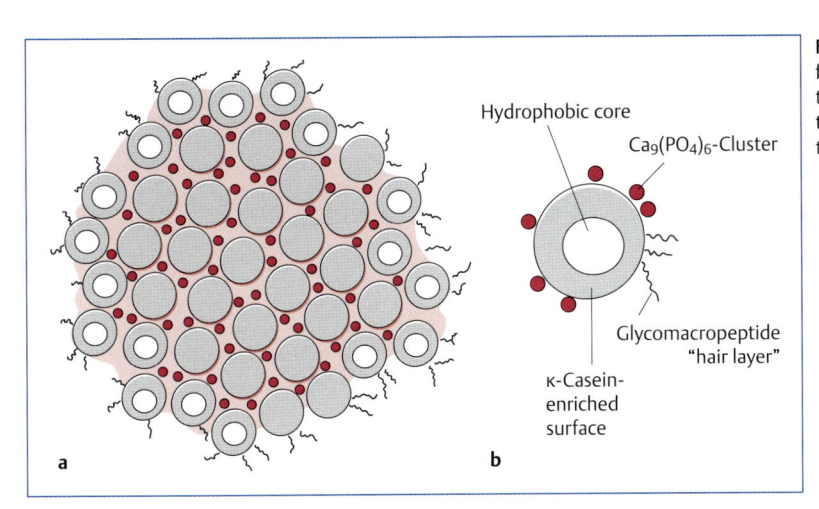

Fig. 25.9 Structure of casein micelles (**a**) from submicelles (**b**). The glycomacropeptide of κ-casein is layered on the surface of the micelles, which prevents further attachment of submicelles.

Hydrophobic core

Ca₉(PO₄)₆-Cluster

Glycomacropeptide "hair layer"

κ-Casein-enriched surface

be impaired by a relative deficiency of essential amino acids (histidine, methionine, phenylalanine, lysine, leucine, isoleucine, valine), when the supply of these amino acids from rumen microbial proteins is not sufficient for milk protein synthesis.

MORE DETAILS Milk urea is used as an indicator of nutritional protein supply. The microbial deamination of amino acids in the rumen produces ammonia, which can be used for microbial protein synthesis. If the protein content of the ration is increased beyond requirement, there is an increased formation of ammonia-N in the rumen fluid. The ammonia-N is absorbed and converted into urea by the urea cycle in the liver. Urea can re-enter the rumen via the ruminohepatic circulation (p. 402) and is broken down by urease into ammonia and CO_2. However, if the protein supply is too high, more urea is excreted in the milk. With a normal milk protein content an increased milk urea indicates an over-supply of protein to dairy cows. A milk urea content that is lower than normal, with a normal milk protein content, indicates a protein undersupply to the dairy cows. A subnormal milk protein content with a milk urea in the normal range indicates that a dairy cow does not have enough energy available for milk protein synthesis.

25.6.3   Synthesis of lactose

Lactose is a **disaccharide** consisting of **galactose and glucose**, linked to each other via a 1,4-β-glycosidic bond. The uptake of glucose into lactocytes, particularly at the beginning of lactation, is through an **insulin-independent** glucose transporter **GLUT1**. In later stages of lactation, glucose transport becomes increasingly insulin-dependent (via GLUT4 and other transporters). Galactose is synthesised from glucose-1-phosphate and UDP-glucose, which is converted to UDP-galactose in the Golgi apparatus under the influence of UDP-galactose-4-epimerase. The combination of UDP-galactose with glucose produces lactose.

In both, monogastric animals and ruminants, lactose is synthesised in cavities of the Golgi apparatus of lactocytes (**Fig. 25.6, Fig. 25.7**).

MORE DETAILS For each mole of lactose synthesised, 3 moles of ATP are required. The enzyme lactose synthase consists of two proteins, galactosyltransferase (protein A) and α-lactalbumin (protein B). While galactosyltransferase is widespread in the animal kingdom and non-specifically links galactose to other sugars, α-lactalbumin is specific for the linkage of galactose and glucose. The quantity of α-lactalbumin determines the rate of lactose formation.

Together with **milk proteins, lactose** is packed into **membrane vesicles** in the **Golgi apparatus** and migrates in vesicles to the apical cell membrane. Lactose cannot pass through the vesicle membrane, so it **osmotically** attracts **water**, which increases the size of the vesicles. The vesicles fuse with the apical cell membrane and their contents are released into the alveolar lumen (**Fig. 25.6**).

25.7   Milk composition in different species

The composition of milk varies considerably not only between animal species, but also during the course of lactation, between individuals of the same species. Table 25.1 gives the average concentrations of the most important constituents and the energy content of milk. For example, the fat content of milk is less than 2% in donkeys and horses, but more than 50% in marine mammals. In the course of evolution, milk composition of each species has adapted to their particular requirements. If the newborns are **nest feeders** the milk must above all be **rich in fat**, since suckling is infrequent, and thus a long-lasting energy supply must be provided.

MORE DETAILS The milk of marine mammals has an extremely high fat content, with very little carbohydrate. One of the most important functions of the milk diet of marine mammals is to supply fat as quickly as possible for the insulating subcutaneous layer, the so-called "blubber". In species such as seals, care of offspring is on land, so the mother is unable to obtain food by hunting. In mother seals, the maternal „blubber" is thus an essential source of nutrients, which are passed on to the newborn in milk.

Table 25.1 Mean concentrations of important milk constituents (g · l^{-1}) and contents of metabolisable energy (MJ/l) in the milk of different animal species.

Animal species	Fat	Casein	Milk serum proteins	Lactose	Calcium	Phosphorus	Energy content
Cow	37	28	6	48	1.2	0.9	3.1
Goat	45	25	4	41	1.2	1.0	3.1
Sheep	74	46	9	48	2.3	1.3	4.7
Pig	68	28	20	55	2.0	1.5	4.7
Horse	19	13	12	62	0.7	0.6	3.2
Human	38	4	6	69	0.3	0.15	3.1
Rat	103	64	20	32	3.2	1.1	n.a.

The course of the **lactation curves** of humans and cattle differ considerably. Since the human infant is nourished exclusively by milk over a long period of time, the demand for milk thus increases as the child grows and the amount of milk produced increases accordingly over the course of lactation. In ruminants, the daily milk yield increases rapidly in early lactation and on average reaches a maximum within the first 6–8 weeks of lactation. In high-yielding dairy cows, daily milk yields can exceed 60 kg during this phase. As lactation progresses, the daily milk yield falls continuously and reaches its minimum at the end of the lactation period, which on average lasts 305 days. The characteristic course of the lactation curve in cows is shown in **Fig. 25.10**. Calves and lambs, under appropriate husbandry conditions, consume fibre-containing food as well as milk in the early period of postnatal life. This additional food source, in association with the establishment of the microbial population, stimulates the development of the forestomach. Thus, milk becomes less important as a source of nutrients.

MORE DETAILS The increases in lactation performance achieved by breeding are usually expressed by increased milk yield at the peak of the lactation curve. The high energy output in milk in the first weeks of lactation cannot be met by the energy intake from food, because compensation for the decreased food **intake** in the last 2–4 weeks of gestation is only achieved after the first weeks of lactation. The imbalance between energy output in milk and energy input in food results in a **negative energy balance**, which can last up to twelve weeks in high-yielding dairy cows. This poses a particular **challenge** to the cow's **intermediary metabolism** and may also be associated with changes in reproductive and immune system functions. These include subclinical and clinical ketosis, ovarian dysfunction and increased susceptibility to infectious diseases, especially of the mammary gland and uterus. It is not yet clear why such changes do not occur in all high-yielding dairy cows. In dairy cattle breeds, yields of more than 10000 kg per lactation and even more are not uncommon today. Outputs of 20000 kg per lactation are possible, and in some cases even higher. In the peak lactation period this can mean a daily milk production of 60–80 kg per day. In addition to high lactation yields, high lifetime yields are aimed for, which require the cows to have a long healthy life. However, dairy cows today often do not live long. On average, dairy cows only complete about 2.8 lactations. Therefore, many cows do not even reach their maximum performance potential, which is only seen in the 3rd–4th lactation.

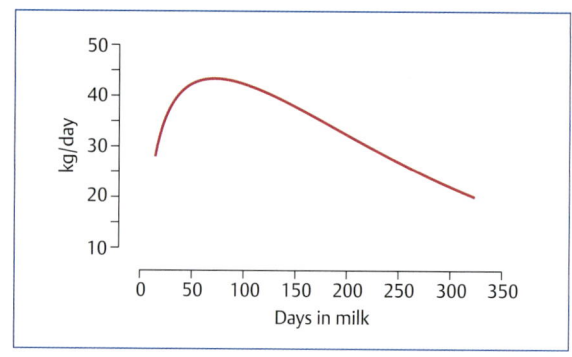

Fig. 25.10 Course of the lactation curve in cows. The maximum daily milk yield is reached on average in the 6th-8th week of lactation. After that, daily milk yield drops continuously.

IN A NUTSHELL   !

The course of the lactation curve depends on the milk requirement relative to the start of the young animal's intake of other food. Milk composition differs greatly between animal species.

25.8   Milk storage and milk ejection

Milk synthesis and milk secretion are continuous, whereas the emptying of the mammary gland is discontinuous during the suckling or milking cycle. In the intervals between emptying, milk accumulates in the alveolar tissue and in the cistern cavities (**Fig. 25.1**). A **negative feedback** on milk secretion is exerted by the presence of **milk** in the **alveoli, but not by milk in the cistern**. Cows with relatively large cisterns therefore react to a decrease in milking frequency with a smaller decrease in milk yield than cows with small cisterns.

Milk in the cistern cavities and large milk ducts (cistern milk) is prevented from flowing out by the milk duct. However, it is immediately available for collection by a suckling offspring or a milking machine. Milk in alveoli and in the small milk ducts (**alveolar milk**), on the other hand, is retained by adhesive friction and capillary forces and must be ejected into the cistern by contraction of the alveoli before it becomes available. This process is called **milk ejection**.

After milk removal, the alveoli then fill because milk is continuously secreted. The cisterns of the mammary gland begin to fill only after a few hours, and after a certain pressure has built up in the alveoli by the accumulating milk secretion. In an average lactation, after an interval of about twelve hours from the previous milking, the **cistern milk content averages** < 10 % in the water buffalo, 20 % in the dairy cow, 50 % in sheep and even up to 80 % of stored milk in goats. In horses, pigs, dogs and cats, on the other hand, milk is almost completely stored in the alveolar tissue. In these latter species, there is therefore no significant cistern milk that would be immediately available (**Fig. 25.1**).

> **IN A NUTSHELL** !
>
> The stored milk can be divided into two fractions in terms of availability. The cistern milk is immediately available, whereas the alveolar milk can only be obtained after milk ejection.

25.8.1 Oxytocin release and milk ejection in the dairy cow

The triggering of oxytocin release and milk ejection differs considerably between the different domestic animal species. First, processes in the dairy cow are considered.

Milk ejection is triggered by mechanical stimulation of the mammary gland (manually, mechanically or by the calf), especially in the teat area, in the form of a **neurohormonal reflex (milk ejection reflex)**.

This mechanical stimulation is converted into afferent action potentials by mechanoreceptors in the teats or in the associated nerves. This neural stimulus reaches the posterior pituitary lobe (PPL) via the spinal cord and the hypothalamus. Oxytocin produced in the hypothalamus and stored in the PPL is released by the neuronal stimulus of the milk ejection reflex and is delivered in blood to the mammary gland (**Fig. 25.11**).

Basal plasma concentrations of oxytocin are in the range of 2–5 pg · ml⁻¹. A small increase in oxytocin concentration above a **threshold value of** approx. 10 pg · ml⁻¹ is sufficient to trigger milk ejection. This increase in blood oxytocin concentration is readily achieved with very **low** intensity **stimulation** (e.g. by a milking cluster hanging on the udder without pulsation). Stimulation by hand or by the normal cycle of a **milking machine** induces oxytocin release to raise blood concentration to usually well above the threshold value. Higher oxytocin releases are achieved when the udder is stimulated by the calf **suckling**. **More oxytocin** is released by **hand milking** than by machine milking. If the applied stimulation persistently raises oxytocin levels in blood above the threshold value, **complete milk ejection** takes place. Occasionally, there may be releases of oxytocin below the threshold that lead to **partial ejections**, i.e. incomplete udder emptying. With excess **oxytocin** secretion, plasma concentrations may temporarily rise significantly above the physiological range. When this happens, additional milk can be obtained. **Residual milk** after the udder has been thoroughly emptied, is about **10 %** of the total milk volume.

The muscle cells that enclose the alveoli like a basket (**basket cells; myoepithelial cells**, **Fig. 25.2**) have receptors for oxytocin. In response to this hormone, the myoepithelial cells contract and alveolar milk is ejected into the cisterns, with a consequent sharp rise in the cistern internal pressure (**Fig. 25.12**). With milk ejection the **cistern cavities enlarge**, while at the same time the emptied glandular tissue is compressed by the pressure in the cistern. Without simultaneous emptying of the udder, however, only some of the milk can be ejected from the alveoli into the cistern (approx. 50 %).

The "**reaction time**" of the udder to the release of oxytocin increases as the **degree of filling** of the udder decreases. The proportion of the udder which is filled depends, in the short term, on the interval since the previous milking, but it also declines in later stages of lactation. If the udder is well **filled**, milk ejection starts after **40–50 seconds**, whereas if the **udder** is only **slightly filled** the first alveolar milk appears in the cistern up to **two minutes** after the start of stimulation.

Endocrinology, reproduction

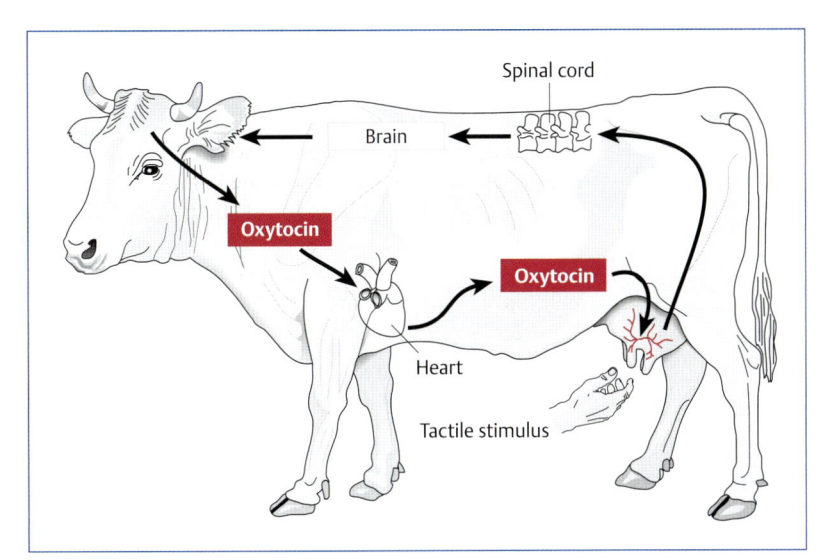

Fig. 25.11 The neuroendocrine reflex arc. Tactile stimulation of the udder results in a neural stimulus via the spinal cord to the hypothalamus and posterior pituitary. There, oxytocin is released into the bloodstream and reaches the udder, where it causes contraction of the myoepithelial cells (basket cells; **Fig. 25.2**) so that milk is expressed into the mammary duct system.

Spinal cord

Brain

Oxytocin

Oxytocin

Heart

Tactile stimulus

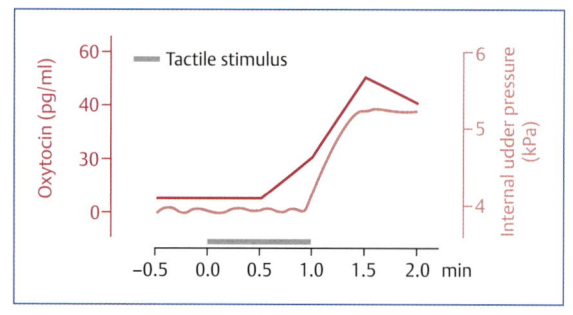

Fig. 25.12 From tactile stimulation, oxytocin is released. This triggers an increase in the udder's internal pressure up to a maximum.

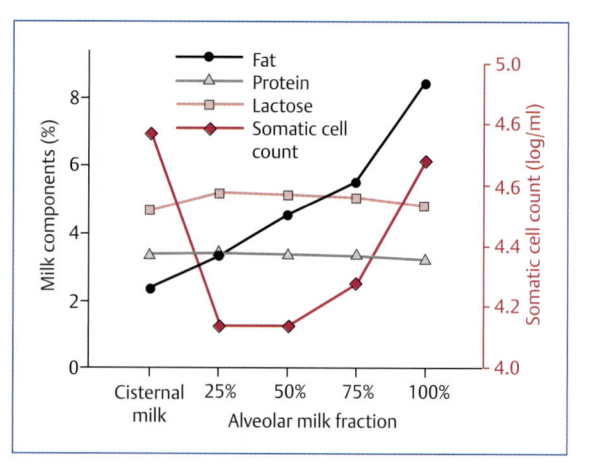

Fig. 25.13 Milk composition and somatic cell count (SCC) in cistern milk and different fractions (25, 50, 75, 100%) of alveolar milk of individual quarters. Fat content is lowest in cistern milk and increases gradually during milking. The somatic cell count is high in cistern milk, reaches its lowest values in the first alveolar milk and then increases steadily to the end of udder emptying. The lactose and protein concentrations hardly change over the course of milk withdrawal.

When machine milking, and the udder fill is low, not only does milk ejection take a particularly long time, but at the same time there is also very little cistern milk available to fill the teats in the relief phases of the milking cycle, until milk ejection begins. In order to avoid the undesirable premature "climbing" of the teat cups in this phase, sufficient udder **preparation (prestimulation) must be done** to trigger milk ejection especially iwhen there is low **udder** filling in late lactation..

> ### IN A NUTSHELL !
>
> If the udder is not very full, the time until milk ejection is prolonged.

MORE DETAILS   The **course of milk flow** during the first few minutes of milking depends on whether milk has already been ejected as a result of udder preparation, or whether ejection is only triggered by stimulation through the application of the milk cup liner during the normal milking cycle. Prestimulation can be carried out manually with the inclusion of premilking and cleaning measures, or mechanically by setting the machine pulsation appropriately, without drawing larger quantities of milk at the same time. If this prestimulation is not carried out, **delayed milk ejection** often takes place after any immediately available cistern milk has already been almost or completely extracted. The consequences are **blind milking phases** at this early stage of milking, which can have a negative effect on further milk ejection. During **prestimulation**, tactile stimulation does **not** necessarily have to be applied **continuously** to the teat. A combination of a short stimulation of at least **15 seconds** followed by a **waiting period of** 45–60 seconds also often leads to even higher milk flow rates than continuous stimulation. However, the waiting time between the end of tactile stimulation and the application of the cluster must not exceed 2 minutes. Otherwise the oxytocin concentration drops and a renewed triggering of milk ejection by stimulation of the cluster leads to a considerable delay in the release of the remaining alveolar milk.

The use of prestimulation is essentially to avoid milking while stimulating the teats. An adequate technical alternative to targeted prestimulation can also be an immediate start of milking with simultaneous lowering of the vacuum and a shortening of the milking phase before milk ejection into the cistern.

As only some of the alveolar milk is transferred into the cistern by milk ejection at the start of milking, it is important that **ejection of alveolar milk** continues during the **entire milking process**. Regardless of the duration of milking, oxytocin concentrations remain elevated. The continuous

stimulating effect of the milking cluster ensures **sustained milk ejection** until the **end of milking**. Because of the short half-life of oxytocin (2–3 minutes), oxytocin secretion must persist during milk withdrawal.

The continuous character of milk ejection during milking also has consequences for the milk **composition** in different milking fractions (**Fig. 25.13**). The **fat content** is lowest in **cistern milk** at the beginning of milking or suckling (in cattle at about 2%), and it increases continuously with the onset of milk ejection until the end of milk withdrawal (in cattle up to 12%). Like milk fat, **the somatic cell count** also **increases** in the different **stages of alveolar milk release**. In contrast to fat, however, the somatic cell count in **cistern milk** is significantly **higher** than in the early alveolar fractions. The concentrations of the electrolytes **Na⁺ and Cl⁻** also change in the course of milking. Like the **cell content**, the electrolyt levels are very high in cistern milk, and lowest in the first alveolar milk, followed by a gradual increase towards the end of milking. The protein and lactose concentrations change little in the course of milking.

> ### IN A NUTSHELL !
>
> Milk ejection is a continuous process throughout the milking cycle. The milk fat content and somatic cell count change significantly during the milking process.

MORE DETAILS   In **mastitis** the somatic cell content (SCC) of milk is increased because gaps in the tight junctions allow cells from blood to pass paracellularly into milk. The changes in tight junctions can also lead to increased electrolytes and other blood plasma components in milk. Indirect measurement of milk electrolyte concentration by electrical conductivity is sometimes used to monitor udder health. A reasonable diagnosis of subclinical mastitis from electrical conductivity of milk only applies to cistern milk because not only the electrolyte content but also the increasing fat content of the milk influences electrical conductivity.

Incontinentia lactis or the "leakage" of milk may be observed, particularly in high-yielding cows. It occurs when the tone of the teat muscles is low, sometimes just before milking, when a kind of "milking readiness" sets in. However, no oxytocin is released in incontinentia lactis without appropriate tactile stimulation. This phenomenon occurs independently of milk ejection and the leaking milk is exclusively cistern milk.

25.8.2 Milk ejection in goat, sheep, pig and horse

In **goats** and **sheep** the proportion of total milk in the cistern is large (**Fig. 25.1**). Prestimulation to trigger milk ejection is unnecessary, as the stimulus of milk withdrawal (suckling or milking,) triggers milk ejection while the cistern milk is being collected. A temporary decrease in milk flow therefore does not occur during machine milking without udder preparation. Some breeds of dairy sheep have a tendency to markedly delay milk ejection, which leads to multi-peak patterns of milk flow. In **pigs**, cistern milk is not present. Therefore, suckling piglets do not receive milk without milk ejection. A characteristic of the lactating sow is that milk ejection is not continuous over the entire suckling period. Only for short periods of 20–30 seconds during suckling is oxytocin released and only during these periods can the piglets obtain milk. The release of oxytocin is accompanied by an increase in grunting sounds from the sow.

Mares have small cistern cavities in their teats. Most of the milk can only be obtained by milk ejection.

> **MORE DETAILS** There are different methods for milking mares. Sometimes the **foal is** allowed to **suckle for a short time** and then the milk is collected by milking. Sometimes manual stimulation is sufficient before the milking cluster is applied. In many farms, however, mares are **milked twice** in succession at intervals of 15–30 minutes, as only about 50% of the milk can be extracted during the first milking period. It has been shown that oxytocin is released by foal suckling or by prestimulation. However, **oxytocin concentrations** drop rapidly **during machine milking**, so that complete udder emptying does not occur.

25.8.3 Disorders of milk ejection in cattle

> **MORE DETAILS** Despite stimulation, **oxytocin release** may be **limited** or may not occur at all. The result is that only **cistern milk** is obtained. These disturbances in oxytocin release often occur in first-lactating cows in the first weeks after calving, or during the peak of oestrus, or when milking is in an unfamiliar environment (e.g. after a change in the milking system, such as when switching from a stall to a milking parlour).
>
> What is certain is that catecholamines cannot trigger such a disorder, as exogenous catecholamines even potentiate the release of oxytocin. In practice, such disorders are often treated by administration of **exogenous oxytocin** which is only effective for one milking. Vaginal stimulation, as an alternative to exogenous oxytocin for milk ejection disorders, has been found to often induce oxytocin release, if this does not happen from udder stimulation.

> **IN A NUTSHELL** !
>
> Milk ejection disorders are caused by failure of oxytocin release.

25.9 Importance of mammary gland milk for postnatal development

Beyond the previously described importance of colostrum, milk is also a complete feed for further postnatal development. Not only the major nutrients, but also trace elements and vitamins are contained in milk to meet the requirements for rapid postnatal growth of musculature and skeleton in the young animal. The calcium and phosphorus content is high, especially in milk caseins, so that an adequate supply of minerals required for ossification and skeletal growth is assured.

> **MORE DETAILS** In species with several newborns, the act of suckling can also be a selection criterion. The stronger offspring win the battle for teats and milk, while underdeveloped young animals do not get access and sooner or later starve to death.
>
> The growth rate during the suckling period differs considerably between species. It is closely correlated with the nutrient or dry matter content of milk of each species. The milk of the rabbit contains 32% dry matter with correspondingly high values of protein and fat, and the birth weight doubles in seven days. Horse milk is very low in nutrient concentration (<10% dry matter) and a doubling of the birth weight is only achieved after 55 days.

25.10 Energy metabolism during lactation

The supply of energy for milk synthesis in the mammary gland is crucial for adequate lactation, and synthesis of milk components, and a lot of ATP is needed. Substrates for the generation of ATP are glucose, acetate and other fatty acids, ketone bodies and amino acids. In **monogastric animals, glucose** is the most important substrate for **ATP formation**. In pigs, more than 50% of the glucose absorbed into the mammary gland is oxidised for energy production. In **ruminants, acetate** is the main substrate for **ATP** production (goat 44%; cow 29%) and little glucose is used (goat 25%, cow 11%).

Especially in the early phase of lactation, the metabolism of the high-performance cow is no longer under the usual **homeostatic regulation**, in which a physiological equilibrium is sought in regulation of energy supply to all organs and tissues. During lactation, **homeostatic** mechanisms faour the mammary gland over the other organs for energy and nutrient distribution, through coordinated changes in metabolism. Because of this, milk yield can increase even further in early lactation despite whole body deficiencies in nutrient and energy supply. The resulting negative energy and nutrient balance requires body reserves to be mobilised from other tissues. The metabolic stress on dairy cows is very high. Significant metabolic consequences are **declining blood glucose levels** and **rising** concentrations of **free (unesterified) fatty acids**. **Propionic acid** produced in the rumen during carbohydrate fermentation is the most important substrate for **gluconeogenesis in the liver**. If the rate of gluconeogensis is at maximum, there is a deficiency of oxaloacetate for the citrate cycle so that oxidation of short-chain fatty acids is limited. An alternative metabolic pathway for these fatty acids is the **synthesis of ketone bodies**. Ketone bodies inhibit gluconeogenesis by suppressing secretion of glucagon. The purpose of this regulatory process is unclear. It possibly increases the availability of oxaloacetate and thus limits the activity of the ketogenic pathway.

> **MORE DETAILS**   An initial slight increase in ketone body concentration is a consequence of a shortfall in energy supply and the simultaneous activation of hepatic gluconeogenesis. A large increase in ketone body production leads to reduced food intake, which further aggrevates the energy deficiency. The **immunosuppressive effect of ketone bodies** then increases the risk of infections, particularly those causing mastitis.
>
> Another special stress on the liver comes from increased **lipolysis** in **adipose tissue** induced by the negative energy balance, which can eventually lead to **fatty liver disease**. Hepatic lipid metabolism is either oxidation of free fatty acids from the circulation in mitochondria, or esterification of these fatty acids in the cytoplasm. In negative energy balance the supply of fatty acids exceeds mitochondrial oxidation capacity so that esterification of the surplus fatty acids produces large quantities of triacylglycerols, which are transported in blood as VLDL to the mammary gland and other tissues, or they are retained in the liver. Since dairy cows have limited capacity for synthesis of VLDL, to remove fatty acids from the liver, thus large quantities of triacylglycerols accumulate, resulting in fatty liver. Because of fat accumulation in the liver, hepatic metabolism can be greatly disturbed in high-yielding cows.

Maximum nutrient flow to the mammary gland is achieved at low ratios of insulin/glucagon and insulin/STH. Even before calving, insulin concentrations begin to fall, which essentially determines the onset of milk production. At the same time as insulin concentration falling, there is decreasing sensitivity of the tissues to insulin (insulin resistance).

Suggested reading

Akers RM. Lactation and the mammary gland. 1st ed. Iowa: Iowa State Press; 2002

Baumann DE, Currie WB. Partitioning of nutrients during pregnancy and lactation: a review of mechanisms involving homeostasis and homeorhesis. J Dairy Sci 1980; 63: 1514–1529

Bauman DE, Perfield JW 2nd, Harvatine KJ, Baumgard LH. Regulation of fat synthesis by conjugated linoleic acid: lactation and the ruminant model. J Nutr 2008; 138: 403–409

Baumrucker CR, Bruckmaier RM. Colostrogenesis: IgG1 transcytosis mechanisms. J Mammary Gland Biol Neoplasia 2014; 19: 103–117

Bruckmaier RM. Normal and disturbed milk ejection in dairy cows. Domest Anim Endocrinol 2005; 29: 268–273

Lacasse P, Ollier S, Lollivier V et al. New insights into the importance of prolactin in dairy ruminants. J Dairy Sci 2015; 99: 864–874

Palmquist DL. Milk Fat: Origin of Fatty Acids and Influence of Nutritional Factors thereon. In: Fox PF, Mc Sweeney PLH (eds.). Advanced Dairy Chemistry, Vol. 2: Lipids. 3rd ed., New York: Springer 2006

Zhao X, Ponchon B, Lanctôt S et al. Invited review: Accelerating mammary gland involution after drying-off in dairy cattle. J Dairy Sci 2019; 102: 6701–6717

Performance physiology

26 Equine exercise physiology as an example for performance physiology

Wolfgang von Engelhardt

26.1 Various performances

ESSENTIALS ✕

Evolution and targeted breeding selection enable horses and some dog breeds to achieve the highest levels of sporting performance. The required performance activities can be very diverse. For example, **quarter horses, thoroughbreds** and **greyhounds** can run very **fast** over short distances. **Sled dogs, draught horses** and **heavy hunters**, on the other hand, are required to run **for long periods of time**. Many animals can run faster (**Fig. 26.5**) and jump higher and further than humans. These very different physical demands require different physiological adaptations.

Here, the physiological reactions to stress in horses are discussed. In order to understand and assess the possibilities, limits and trainability for high performance, it is important to know the different types of stress, especially:

– Energy sources of muscle cells and aerobic and anaerobic processes involved,
– Respiration, oxygen uptake and oxygen transport,
– Adaptations of the cardiovascular system,
– Temperature regulation processes and
– potential influence of training on the complex physiological processes involved.

26.2 The working muscle

26.2.1 Energy metabolism of the working muscle

The working muscle requires energy in the form of adenosine triphosphate (p. 157) (ATP) to enable contractions. In the **muscle cell** only a very **small amount of ATP is stored** and is only sufficient for a few contractions. ATP can then be produced very quickly from the energy stored in **creatine phosphate (CP)**. This energy source is also limited, as CP is only sufficient to meet the energy requirements for the first 20 seconds of muscle contractions (**Fig. 26.1**). For

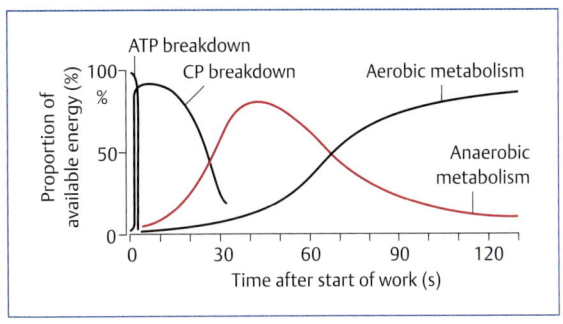

Fig. 26.1 Stored ATP is only sufficient to sustain the first few muscle contractions at the beginning of work. For the following 20 seconds, ATP can then be readily obtained from creatine phosphate (CP) present in muscle. In the next 35–60 seconds, the required ATP must be rapidly produced, mainly by anaerobic metabolism. Only after one minute of work are muscles able to obtain the energy required for contraction, from aerobic metabolism. [Source: Keul J, Doll E, Keppler D. Muskelstoffwechsel: Die Energiebereitstellung im Skelettmuskel als Grundlage seiner Funktion. Munich: J. A. Barth; 1969]

longer periods of work, the energy required for muscle contractions must be obtained from anaerobic and aerobic metabolism in the muscle cells.

For about one minute after the start of work, **ATP is mainly produced** by the **anaerobic breakdown** of glucose via pyruvate to **lactate**. During this process only **2 mol ATP** are produced from **1 mol glucose**. For longer periods of work, the **ATP** required is obtained **aerobically** by oxidation of glucose and free fatty acids (**Fig. 26.2**; **Fig. 6.13**). This aerobic energy production is much more efficient as **aerobic glucose oxidation**, produces **36–38 mol ATP** from **1 mol glucose**. Oxidation of **free fatty acids** produces about **140 mol ATP** per mol of fatty acid, depending on which fatty acids are being oxidised.

IN A NUTSHELL !

During aerobic oxidation of 1 mol glucose, 18–19 times more ATP can be obtained than in anaerobic glucose catabolism.

Performance physiology

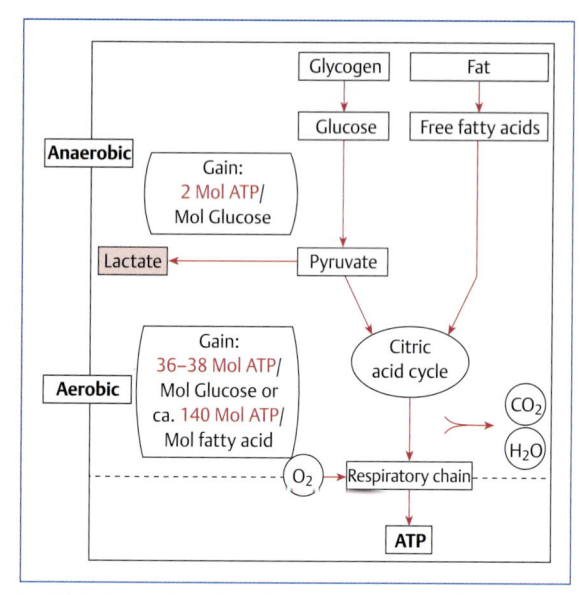

Fig. 26.2 Anaerobic and aerobic energy production during work.

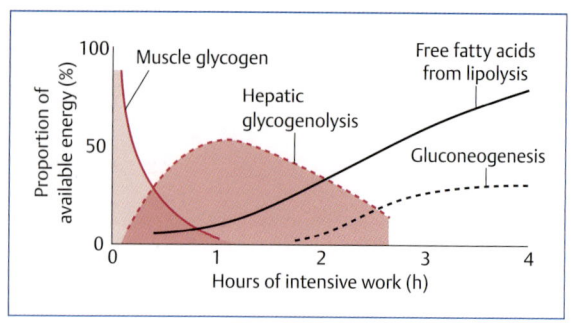

Fig. 26.3 Proportion of available energy during endurance performance lasting several hours, from breakdown of muscle glycogen, from glycogenolysis in the liver, and from the production of free fatty acids (FFA) by lipolysis. Gluconeogenesis maintains the blood glucose concentration.

IN A NUTSHELL !

The level of endurance performance depends on the level of aerobic metabolism.

In this context, it is important that **ATP formation** takes place at **different rates**. **The ATP present in muscle is used up** within the first few seconds after the start of work. ATP is also formed rapidly during the following 10–25 seconds from the breakdown of **creatine phosphate** (**CP**). After 25–60 seconds of starting work, muscle obtains ATP mainly by the **anaerobic** production of **lactate**. Only about 60 seconds after the start of work is ATP increasingly made available from **aerobic metabolism**. The muscle during moderately hard work, is then no longer dependent on the much less efficient anaerobic production of ATP (**Fig. 26.1**).

For **endurance performance**, achieving the greatest level of **aerobic metabolism** is important, while anaerobic metabolism is correspondingly low. With this increasing proportion of anaerobic metabolism (p.627) in prolonged work or in highly intensive work, **blood lactate concentration** increases and muscle fatigue follows.

During **long-term performance** the intracellular energy depots of muscle (mainly **muscle glycogen**) are depleted, and the working muscle is then dependent on glucose or free fatty acids from blood (**Fig. 26.3**). After all intracellular muscle glycogen has been used, there is increased **glycogenolysis** in the **liver**. At the same time, **lipolysis** in the fat depots (p.478) begins slowly at first, and then increases. **Free fatty acids** then become available for energy metabolism. With prolonged exercise, the oxidation of free fatty acids becomes increasingly important. As glycogen levels in the liver and muscles decline, gluconeogenesis must then increase to ensure that blood glucose concentration does not fall below a critical threshold value (gluconeogenesis (p.469); **Fig. 17.5**; **Fig. 26.3**). The substrates for this new formation of glucose after 2½-3 hours of work, come predominantly from glucogenic amino acids released by the degradation of tissue protein (**Fig. 17.5**), and also from glycerol released during lipolysis, and from propionate.

26.2.2 Oxygen deficit at the start of work and oxygen debt at the end

Although at the **start of work**, muscle power increases to the required level within a few seconds, **oxygen supply** ($\dot{V}_{O_2}$) increases only slowly and reaches a steady state after about two minutes of light work. This means that the $\dot{V}_{O_2}$ lags behind the energy demand for aerobic metabolism at the start of work, and thus an **O_2 deficit** develops (**Fig. 26.4**). The increased ATP required immediately after the start of work can be produced without O_2 consumption, by hydrolysis of creatine phosphate and by anaerobic glycolysis producing lactate (**Fig. 26.1**). For the initial aerobic ATP formation, O_2 reserves in myoglobin, haemoglobin and alveolar air (functional residual capacity (p.265)) are available.

In the **steady state** of **light work** the amount of oxygen taken up from inspired air meets the O_2 requirement. However, the O_2 deficit created at the start of work remains, and is not corrected until the recovery phase when the work ends. At that time more oxygen is taken up than needed for the resting state, in order to meet the **O_2 debt**. However, the O_2 debt is usually greater than the O_2 deficit for the following reasons:

- Resynthesis of creatine phosphate
- Glucose formation from lactate (gluconeogenesis) and oxidation of lactate in the citrate cycle
- Energy demand for thermoregulation
- increased heart and respiratory activity

During **heavy** physical **work** oxygen uptake does **not reach a steady state** because the O_2 demand during hard work is greater than the amount of O_2 acquired from inspired air. The ATP formed aerobically is not sufficient to meet the need for muscle contractions, and additional ATP must be obtained during work, from anaerobic metabolism producing lactate (**Fig. 26.2**). The **O_2 debt** at the end of heavy physical work is then **considerably greater** than the O_2 deficit at the start of work, since oxygen is needed for the

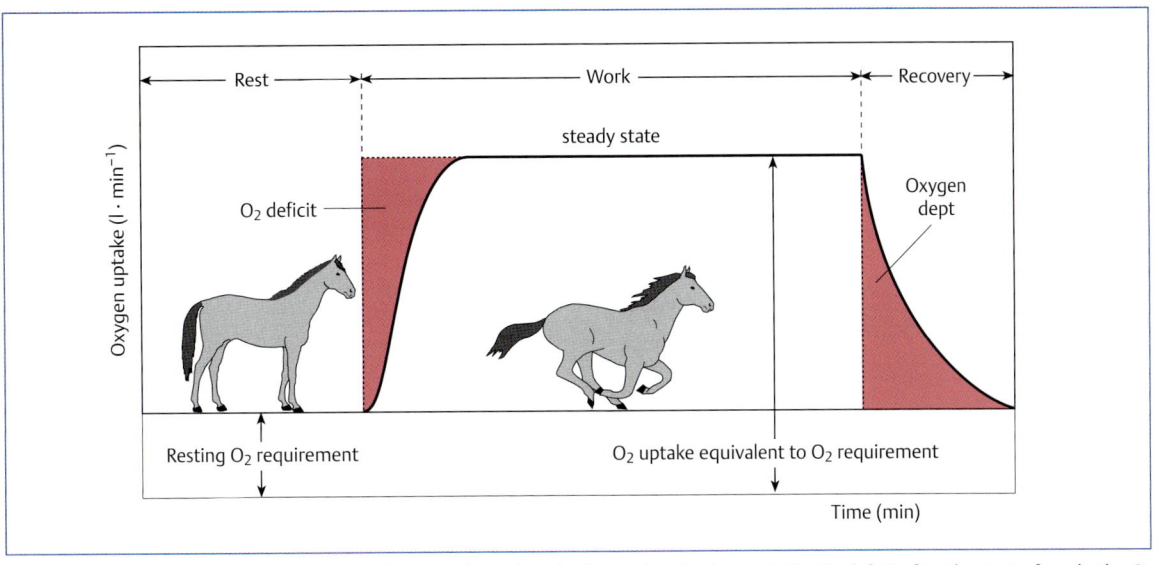

Fig. 26.4 Oxygen uptake during light, short-duration physical work. The resting O_2 demand, the O_2 deficit after the start of work, the O_2 demand during the steady state work, and the O_2 debt after the end of work are shown.

utilisation of lactate being produced and for increased thermoregulation to remove the heat generated by muscle work.

> **IN A NUTSHELL** !
>
> At the start of work, an O_2 deficit is created, which remains during the period of work and is only reduced after the end of work, as a so-called O_2 debt. If ATP formed from aerobic metabolism is not sufficient during heavy work, it must be supplemented from anaerobic metabolism. The O_2 debt at the end of work is then considerably greater than at the beginning.

26.2.3 Where does the required ATP come from for the various types of performance of sport horses?

The **duration** and **intensity** of physical work, determines from where muscles obtain ATP. The **quarter horse** runs a distance of 400 m with a top speed of up to $70\,km \cdot h^{-1}$ in less than 20 seconds, which is twice as fast as a 100 m runner. It can be assumed that 80% of the required ATP comes from creatine phosphate, 18% from anaerobic glycolysis and only 2% from aerobic metabolism (**Table 26.1**).

Thoroughbreds need a little more than two minutes to cover the derby distance of 2400 m. It can be assumed that only about 5% of the required ATP comes from creatine phosphate, while 70% is provided by anaerobic and 25% by aerobic metabolism. During cross-country riding in eventing competitions with alternating loads, the aerobic component is 50%, and in long endurance rides it rises to 94%.

Table 26.1 Estimated proportions of ATP produced from creatine phosphate (CP), from anaerobic and from aerobic metabolism, required for muscle work in different horse performances.

Loads	ATP formation		
	CP	**Anaerobic**	**Aerobic**
Race			
• Quarterhorse (400 m)	80%	18%	2%
• Thoroughbred Derby (2400 m)	5%	70%	25%
Versatility (3.5–7.5 km)	10%	40%	50%
Endurance ride (>60 km)	1%	5%	94%

Source: Snow DH, Vogel CJ. Equine Fitness: The care and training of athletic horse. London: David Charles, Newton Abbot; 1987

26.2.4 Muscle fibre types

MORE DETAILS In the chapter on muscle physiology (p. 156), the three different types of muscle fibres were introduced (**Fig. 6.12**). A distinction is made between **slowly contracting** and **slowly fatiguing** (S or Type I; **red endurance muscles**), the **fast-contracting** and **fast-fatiguing** (FF or type IIB; **white sprinter muscles**), and one or more **transition types** (FR or type IIA) (**Table 26.2**). The oxidative capacity and capillary density are high in type I fibres. In the fast type II fibres, glycogen content is high. Most muscles contain a mosaic of these three muscle fibre types. According to the most important functions of individual muscles, the different fibre types occur with varying frequency. The distribution of muscle fibre types in a muscle seems to a large extent to be genetically determined.

Table 26.2 Muscle fibre types.

Parameter	Type I	Type IIA	Type IIB
	S	FR	FF, Type IIX
Contraction speed	slow	fast	fast
Oxidative capacity	high	medium to high	low
Capillary density	high	medium	low
Glycogen content	medium	high	high
Fatigue	low	medium	high

S = slow; FR = fast, fatigue resistant; FF = fast fatigable

In the **quarter horse**, which specialises in short sprint distances, 93% of muscle fibres are fast contracting and therefore fast fatiguing fibres, and 7% are slow contracting and less susceptible to fatigue. The number of fast-fatiguing fibres is lower in the **Thoroughbred**. In **Heavy Hunters**, which have to gallop long distances as hunting horses, only 69% are fast fibres (**Table 26.3**) and 31% are slow fibres, less susceptible to fatigue. Comparison of the percentages of fast contracting muscle fibres between horse, camel and dog muscles is given in **Table 26.3**. In **dogs**, the distribution of muscle fibre types is comparable to that in horses. In **greyhounds**, a sprinting dog breed, about 97% of the fibres are fast fibres. In contrast, **fox hounds**, which have to perform well in endurance exercise, have only 65% medium to fast fatiguing fibres. In the **camel** and also in **humans**, the low-fatigue slow fibres predominate. Both species run relatively slowly compared to sprinting animals (**Fig. 26.5**), but their endurance is high. For longer lasting work, it is crucial that aerobic ATP production is high. Oxygen uptake is therefore of particular importance for assessing metabolism during endurance exercise.

Table 26.3 Percentages of fast contracting muscle fibres (type II) in the gluteus medius muscle in trained horses, dogs, camels and humans.

Species	Type II fibres
Quarterhorse	93 %
Heavy Hunter	69 %
Greyhound	97 %
Foxhound	65 %
Camel	30 %
Human	25 %

Source: Saltin B, Rose RJ. The Racing Camel – Physiology, metabolic functions, and adaptations. Acta Physiol Scand 1994; 150 (Suppl): 61; Snow DH, Vogel CJ. Equine Fitness: The care and training of athletic horses. London: David Charles, Newton Abbot; 1987

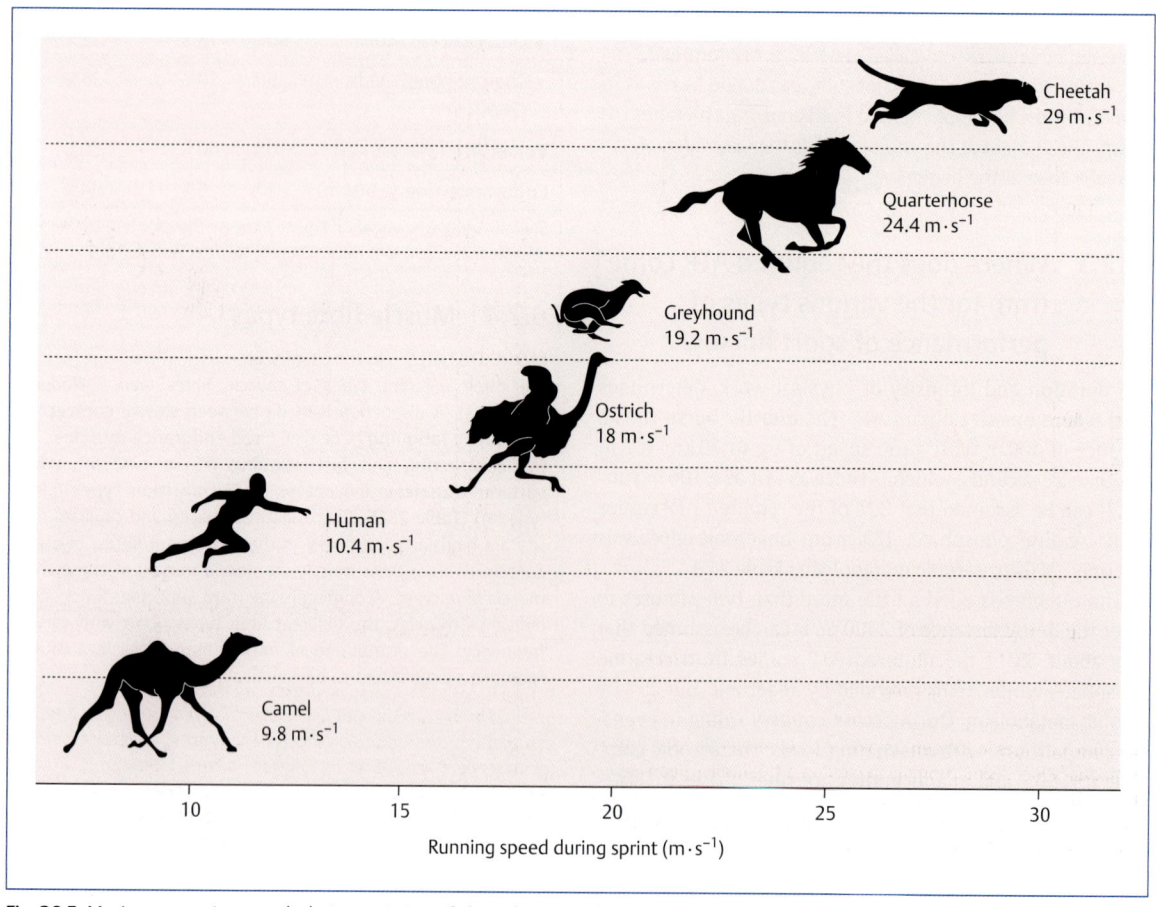

Fig. 26.5 Maximum running speeds during sprinting of cheetah, quarterhorse, greyhound, ostrich, human, dromedary; based on data from Sharp NCC. Animal athletes: A performance review. Vet Rec 2012; 171: 87–94

26.3 Aerobic metabolism and endurance

Numerous functions are involved in high intensity, high capacity aerobic metabolism. These include: respiration, pulmonary gas exchange, O_2 transport in blood, release of O_2 from erythrocytes, diffusion of O_2 through the capillary walls and intracellular O_2 utilisation. **Endurance performance** is the ability to perform work without significant fatigue, over a long period of time. It depends primarily on how much oxygen can be absorbed by the body and brought to the working muscles.

26.3.1 Oxygen uptake, resting metabolic rate and metabolic rate at work

With increasing **running speed** (or other increasing workloads), the **oxygen uptake of** horses ($\dot{V}_{O_2}$) increases linearly (**Fig. 26.6**). From a running speed of about $500\,\text{m} \cdot \text{min}^{-1}$, oxygen uptake reaches a plateau and does not increase any further despite further increases in running speed. This plateau value is the **maximum oxygen uptake** ($\dot{V}_{O_2\text{max}}$) of a horse. In sports medicine, $\dot{V}_{O_2\text{max}}$ is often referred to as **aerobic performance capacity**. Another important characteristic of aerobic performance capacity is the **aerobic threshold**. It is defined as the maximum power performance at a constant lactate concentration (lactate steady-state).

Horses and **camels** during hard work, can **increase their oxygen uptake** by up to **35 times** compared to resting values. A 36-fold increase has also been measured in the South American ratite, the nandu. Smaller animals cannot increase their oxygen uptake per kg of body mass compared to resting values, as much as this capability in large animals (**Fig. 26.7**). The main reason for this is that the **resting metabolic rate** per kg body mass is much **higher in small animals** than in large ones, see ch. Energy metabolism and body size (p.490). The resting metabolic **rate increases** as a function of body mass to the power of **0.75**. The **maximum oxygen uptake** per kg body mass, however, increases to the power of **0.95** (**Fig. 26.7**).

In large animals, the difference between resting and exertion metabolic rates is therefore greater than in small animals. This means that **large animal species** have **more oxygen available** during exercise for working muscles **per kg of body mass** than small animals. Rats can only increase their oxygen consumption per kg of body mass by a factor of 4 compared to resting values, mongrel dogs by a factor of about 10, humans and greyhounds by about

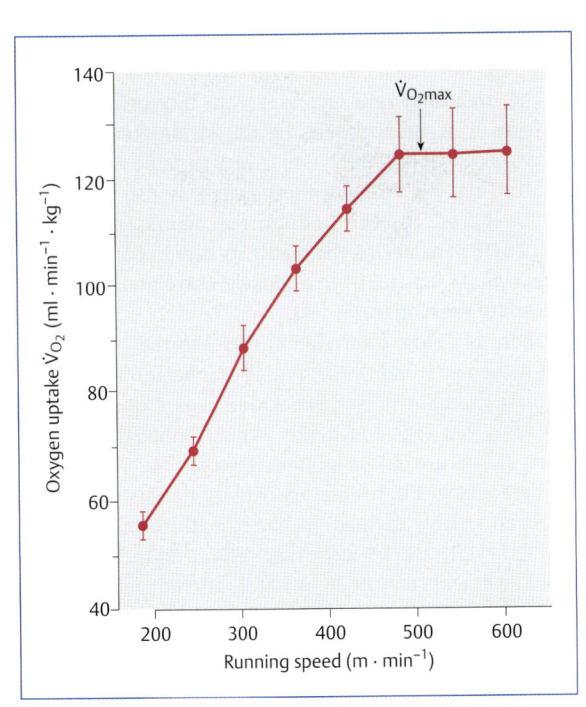

Fig. 26.6 Changes in oxygen uptake ($\dot{V}_{O_2}$) of warm-blooded horses at gradually increasing running speeds on a treadmill (mean values and SEM). Initially the $\dot{V}_{O_2}$ increases linearly with increasing running speed. At about $500\,\text{m} \cdot \text{min}^{-1}$ oxygen uptake no longer increases, so despite further increases in speed, a plateau is reached. This plateau value is the average **maximum oxygen uptake** ($\dot{V}_{O_2\text{max}}$) of horses. [Source: Rose RJ, Evans DL. Cardiovascular and respiratory function in the athletic horse. In: Gillespie JR, Robinson NE (eds). Equine Exercise Physiology 2, Davis: ICEEP Publications; 1987: 1–24]

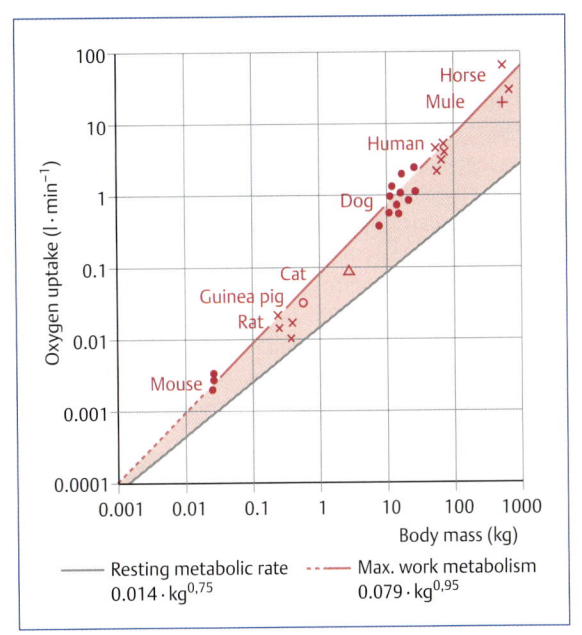

Fig. 26.7 Oxygen uptake at **maximum work rate** as a function of body mass in animals of different weights (**red** regression line). For comparison, the regression line for the **resting metabolic rate** (**grey** straight line). [Source: Regression lines, Hörnicke H. Atmung und Gaswechsel. In: Lenkeit W, Breirem K, Crasemann E (Hrsg.). Handbuch der Tierernährung. Bd. I. Hamburg, Berlin: Paul Parey; 1969: 298–326; the values for the individual animals added by H. Hörnicke]

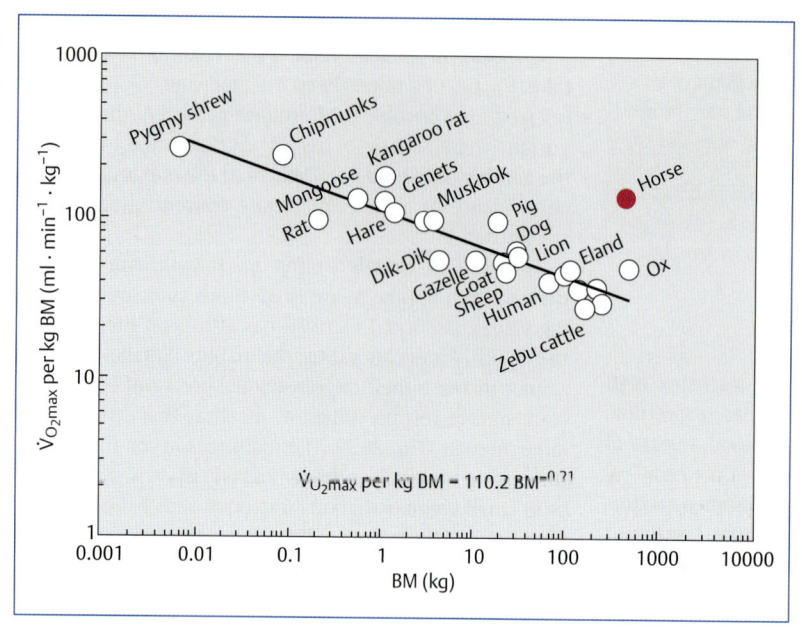

Fig. 26.8 Maximum oxygen uptake ($\dot{V}_{O_2max}$) per kg body mass (BM) in mammals of different weights during heavy muscle work. Small mammals have a greater maximum oxygen uptake in relation to their BM than large animal species. The value for horses (red dot) is 2.5 times higher than for oxen of approximately the same weight. [Source: Lafortuna CL, Saibene F, Albertini M et al. The regulation of respiratory resistance in exercising horses. Eur J Appl Physiol 2003; 90: 396–404]

20 times, and horses and camels by more than 30 times. The high maximum aerobic metabolic activity of the muscle in horses is also expressed in a comparatively **high mitochondrial density** in the muscle cell, which is a measure of oxidative capacity.

The **maximum oxygen uptake** per kg body mass ($\dot{V}_{O_2max}$) decreases with increasing **body mass (BM)** in mammals of different weights during hard work (**Fig. 26.8**). Although large animal species have a lower maximum oxygen uptake per kg BM, they can increase maximum oxygen uptake during hard work significantly more than small animals compared to resting values (**Fig. 26.7**). Small animals, because of their already high resting metabolic rate, have only a comparatively small capability of increasing their maximum work metabolic rate.

Recent studies have also shown that horses are superior to domestic animals of equal weight, such as oxen, in terms of aerobic capacity, because of their comparatively high $\dot{V}_{O_2max}$ per kg BM (**Fig. 26.8**). The $\dot{V}_{O_2max}$ per kg BM is 2.5 times higher in a horse than in a steer. This is probably due to training and genetic factors, and illustrates the special performance characteristics of horses.

> **IN A NUTSHELL**   !
>
> Horses can increase oxygen uptake during exercise much more than most domestic animals of about the same weight that have been studied so far.

26.3.2 Breathing and synchronisation of breathing through the frequency of footfalls at canter

Breathing during work is not only important for O_2 intake and CO_2 release. It also plays a role in the regulation of acid-base balance (p.349) and temperature regulation (p.503). The necessary adaptations of respiration to increasing physical loads are considerably influenced by the galloping movements of horses.

The **breathing rate** increases with increasing load. In humans it is independent of the stride frequency. In horses, also, the breathing rate is very variable while walking, trotting (**Fig. 26.9**). At these gaits it is also influenced by the horse's psyche and by the actions of a rider. (**Fig. 26.9**). In cantering the breathing rate in horses and in **dogs** (ch. 11.8.3 (p.291)) is **closely correlated with the pattern of running (ratio 1:1)**.

There is a close interrelation between the sequence of foot movements and the beginning of inhalation and exhalation in galloping horses. **Exhalation** begins when the first or both front legs touch the ground. **Inhalation** begins when all legs are off the ground. However, the main causes of these changes in respiratory activity in horses have not yet been reliably defined. In horses with respiratory diseases, the 1:1 ratio between inspiration and the pattern of foot movements may be significantly altered.

The synchronisation of breathing and foot movement means that there is some **decoupling** from the usual **regulation of breathing** when **cantering**. When a horse is either trotting or cantering at the same speed, the respiratory minute volume is higher at **cantering** than at trotting due to a higher respiratory frequency. This means that horses **hyperventilate** at low canter speeds compared to the same speed when trotting. Horses galloping fast also have a relatively high respiratory rate compared to humans and other trotting animals, and therefore relatively **shal-**

low breathing. The **dead space ventilation** is therefore relatively high, even when the horse is subjected to higher loads. This is an advantage for **heat dissipation**.

IN A NUTSHELL !

In horses, the breathing rate at a gallop is determined by the pattern of foot movements. The resulting high breathing rate leads to hyperventilation, which facilitates thermoregulation and regulation of acid-base balance.

With increasing hard work, the pH of blood decreases due to lactate accumulation, so that **metabolic acidosis develops**. Humans, dogs and most other animals try to compensate for this acidosis (p.353) by **hyperventilating. Galloping horses hyperventilate** anyway due to the close coupling between foot fall rate and respiratory rate. However, horses **cannot** increase their respiratory rate in a regulated manner while galloping. Also the less sensitive chemosensors in the carotid sinus of the horse may also be partly responsible for a lower ability to regulate ventilation while **trotting**.

Trained **trotters** reach running speeds of up to 800 m · min^{-1}. Trotters also show a 1:1 synchronisation between the pattern of foot movement and breathing at submaximal work. At maximum demand, however, this can change. One inhalation can then be followed by two foot falls in trotters, resulting in a respiration-foot fall ratio of 1:2 (but ratios of 1:1.5; 1:2.5; 1:3 are also possible). This allows trotters to have deep inspirations and a respiratory volume of up to 25 litres at maximum work. At high running speeds, trotters have, due to variable partial synchronisation, a significantly lower respiratory frequency and deeper inspirations than galloping horses.

IN A NUTSHELL !

Trotters only partially synchronise their breathing rate at high running speeds. At a fast trot they have a lower breathing rate and a deeper inspiration than galloping horses.

Since at high running speeds the respiratory rate of horses is largely determined by the stride sequence, changes in **oxygen uptake** are mainly through changes in respiratory **volume**. With increasing running speed, the respiratory frequency increases together with the foot fall frequencies (**Fig. 26.9 a**), but also with the **length** of the **gallop strides**, and thus **respiratory volume increases** linearly (**Fig. 26.9 b**). At the same time, respiratory minute volume and also **alveolar ventilation** increase linearly (**Fig. 26.9 c**). Due to increased **alveolar ventilation**, horses can take in more oxygen. However, this potential capacity of respiratory volume is rarely fully utilised in horses at a fast gallop. Lung ventilation and oxygen uptake of horses during galloping are compared with resting values in **Table 26.4**.

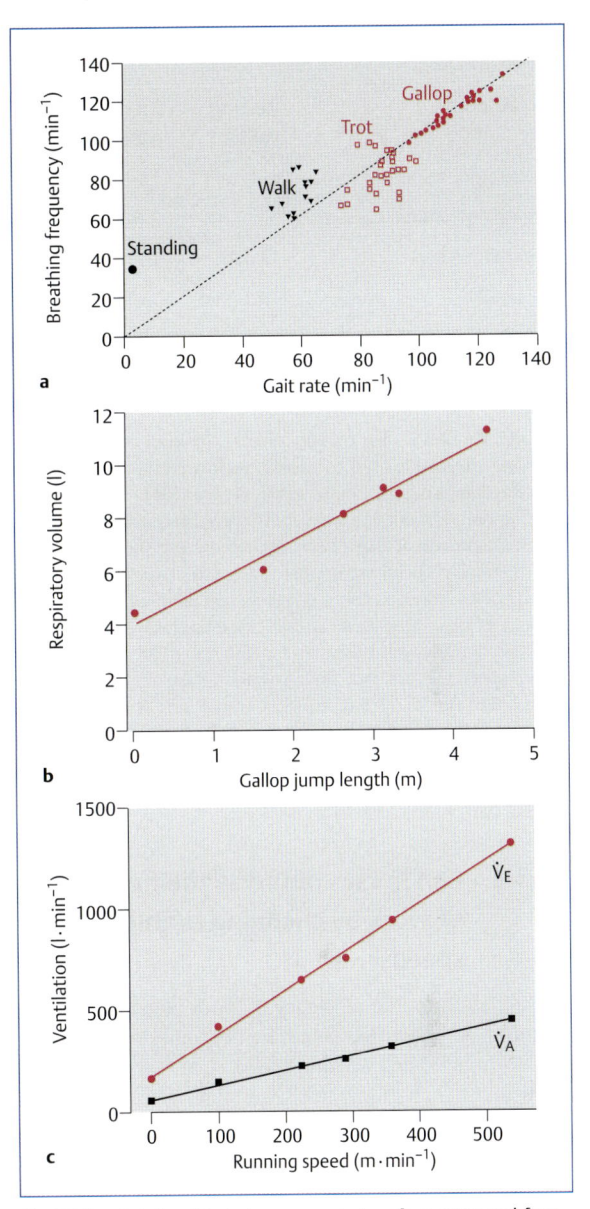

Fig. 26.9 a Relationship between respiratory frequency and foot fall frequency at increasing running speeds of horses. Especially in the galloping horse there is a close 1:1 synchronisation of the two parameters. In trotting horses and in horses at walk, the synchronisation is not so pronounced.
b Linear dependence of the breathing volume of horses on their canter pace length. Furthermore, since breathing rate and canter pace length are largely identical (**a**), there are linear relationships (shown in **c**) between running speed and the respiratory minute volume, and also alveolar ventilation.
$\dot{V}_A$: alveolar ventilation (black); $\dot{V}_E$: respiratory minute volume (red). [Source: (a) Hörnicke H, Meixner R, Pollmann U. Respiration in exercising horses. In: Snow DS, Person SGB, Rose RJ (eds). Equine Exercise Physiology. Cambridge: Granta Editions; 1983: 7–16]

Table 26.4 Respiration and oxygen uptake of horses at rest and at a gallop, mean body weight of horses 550 kg.

Parameter	Resting values	Increase at a fast gallop
Respiratory minute volume	$60 \, l \cdot min^{-1}$	23-fold
Breathing volume	$5 \, l$	2.6-fold
Breathing rate	$12 \, min^{-1}$	10-fold
O_2 uptake	$1.8 \, l \cdot min^{-1}$	33-fold

Source: Hörnicke H, Meixner R, Pollmann U. Respiration in exercising horses. In: Snow DS, Person SGB, Rose RJ, eds. Equine Exercise Physiology. Cambridge: Granta Editions; 1983: 7–16

MORE DETAILS   For human athletes, **oxygen uptake** during defined exercise is used to **assess performance**. Both, oxygen uptake and also load, cannot easily be recorded in sports horses during natural work and training. However, for some years now, such measurements have been made more and more frequently on treadmills. Such measurements are also possible in free-running horses, although this requires quite a lot of equipment. The results of these studies show that oxygen uptake and heart rate increase linearly with increasing running speed. At very high running speeds, heart rate and oxygen uptake reach a plateau (**Fig. 26.6**; **Fig. 26.12**; **Fig. 26.18**). Comparisons of measured parameters show that the **running speed** of **horses** is a useful **reference parameter** to assess endurance performance (ch. 26.7 (p. 630)).

26.3.3   Can horses optimise their efficiency of work by changing running speeds?

At walk and trot, the **efficiency of work** (given as O_2 consumption per 1 metre covered) first becomes more favourable with increasing **walking speed**, then reaches an **optimum**, and then becomes less favourable again (**Fig. 26.10**). If a horse is allowed to independently choose its running speed, it usually prefers a speed at which efficiency is optimal. Both at increasing fast walking and trotting speeds and at very low walking and trotting speeds, the efficiency of work becomes increasingly unfavourable, as more oxygen is required per metre of distance covered. In cantering horses, this relationship with speed is not so apparent. Similarly, trotters with increasing training also run at high trotting speeds with largely constant efficiency – a characteristic which obviously has to be learnt during training.

> **IN A NUTSHELL**   !
>
> For horses that are walking or trotting, the efficiency of work is only optimal in a narrow range of speeds.

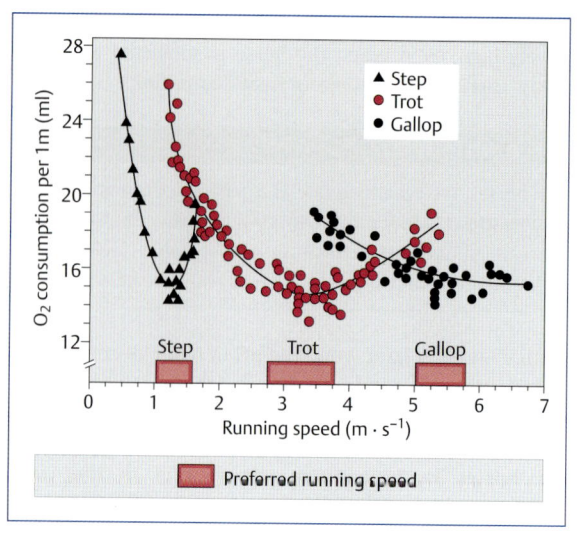

Fig. 26.10 Oxygen consumption of horses at a walk, trot and canter per metre of distance covered, as a function of walking speed. [Source: Hoyt DF, Taylor CR. Gait and energetics of locomotion in horses. Nature 1981; 292: 239–240]

MORE DETAILS

Energy expenditure at high running speeds of camels, horses, and humans

In camels, energy expenditure during races (expressed as oxygen intake per kg body weight for a distance of 1 km) is only half that of horses. In humans, energy expenditure is as much as 2.5 times higher than that of horses (**Fig. 26.11**). This great efficiency of camels is certainly one of their important adaptations to life under desert conditions. The species-specific biomechanics is an important explanation for the different energy consumption during walking. In the camel's pacing gait the body weight has to be lifted only very slightly when walking. In contrast, horses need additional energy for the considerable lifting of body weight required for each canter step. In addition, the length of the legs, their angulations when running, the different anatomy of the feet and the toe, are all important factors affecting energy expenditure. The well-regulated water-saving thermoregulation (p. 503) of camels (p. 629), may also be involved in the economical use of energy. Although they have less favourable efficiency, galloping horses have the advantage of being able to run much faster than camels running at their standard gait (**Fig. 26.5**).

When running fast, humans, just like galloping horses, also have to expend energy to lift their body weight. Another important reason for the higher energy expenditure of humans is that they have a higher resting metabolic rate per kg of body mass than horses and camels, which are about 10 times heavier (see ch. on energy metabolism and body size (p. 490)). Due to the high resting metabolic rate of small mammals, their energy expenditure for locomotion is less efficient than that of large animal species.

26.3.4   Heart rate, cardiac output and arterial blood pressure

The **resting heart rate** of a horse is **30–40 beats** per minute on average, and 120 beats per minute in medium-sized mongrel dogs. At **maximum work, the heart rate** of a **horse** can increase up to **230 beats** per minute, which is almost four heartbeats per second. Up to a running speed of about $650 \, m \cdot min^{-1}$ in trained horses, the heart rate in-

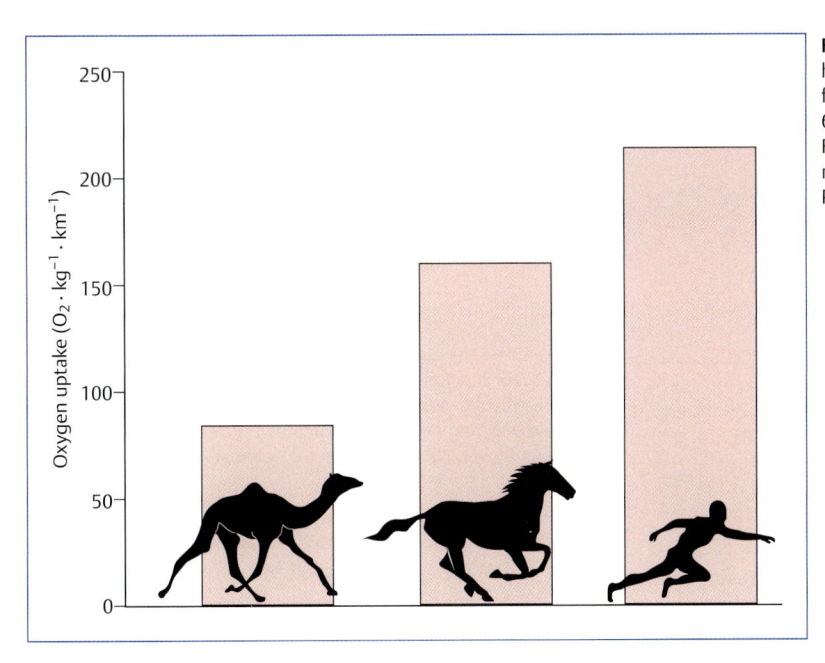

Fig. 26.11 Oxygen uptake of camels, horses, and humans in a race over five kilometres at a running speed of $6–10\,m\cdot s^{-1}$; based on data from Saltin B, Rose RJ. The Racing Camel - Physiological, metabolic functions, and adaptations. Acta Physiol Scand 1994; 150 (Suppl): 61

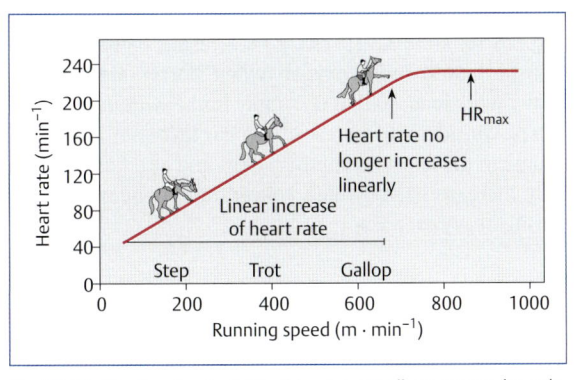

Fig. 26.12 The heart rate (HR) of horses initially increases linearly with increasing running speed. The maximum heart rate (HR_{max}) of about $230\,min^{-1}$ is reached at a running speed of about $700\,m\cdot min^{-1}$.

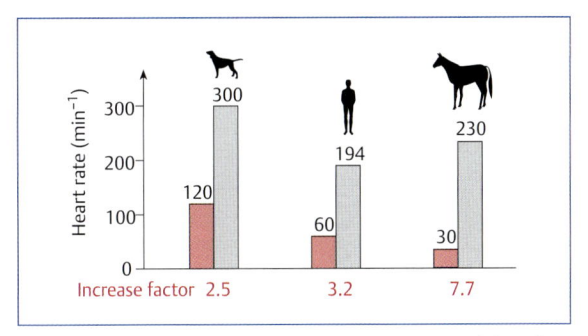

Fig. 26.13 Heart rate in dog, man, and horse at rest (red) and at maximum load (light grey).

creases **linearly** with increasing running speed. At higher running speeds, the heart rate reaches a **plateau**, i.e. when the running speed increases further, the heart rate no longer increases (**Fig. 26.12**; **Fig. 26.18**). This plateau value is the highest possible heart rate of the horse (HR of the horse (HR_{max}).

Although a horse's heart is about 14 times heavier than a human's and 10 times heavier than a greyhound's, the maximum heart rate is as high or even higher than in humans and only slightly lower than in a greyhound. At maximum load, **horses** can increase **heart rate** by **7.7 times**, humans by only 3.2 times and medium-sized dogs by 2.5 times (**Fig. 26.13**).

As the **heart rate** increases, the **diastolic duration** of the horse's heart decreases much more than the **systolic duration**. (**Fig. 26.14**). At a heart rate of 30 beats per minute, diastole, and thus the time during which the myocardium of the left ventricle of the horse's heart is mainly supplied with blood, is 25 times longer than at 230 beats per minute (**Fig. 26.14**), see ch. Current pulse in the arteries (p.201) and energetics of the heart (p.180). At a heart rate of **230 beats** per minute, the **diastolic time is**

only **0.06–0.07 sec**. During this very short time, about 1 l of blood must flow into each ventricle of the horse's heart.

The amount of oxygen that can be supplied to the working muscles of a horse depends mainly on the **pumping capacity of the heart**, the oxygen transport capacity of the blood and the blood flow through the muscles (p.626). The **increase in cardiac output** is mainly due to an increase in **heart rate**. **Cardiac output** increases by about 40% during exercise. Compared to rest, the cardiac output can **increase by a factor of 9.8** when **horses** are working hard (**Fig. 26.16**). This is considerably more than in humans, for whom an increase of only 5–6 times is possible.

The **systolic blood pressure** and, to a lesser extent, the **mean blood pressure** increase exponentially with increasing running speed in horses and other domestic animals (**Fig. 26.15**). These increases are due to the increase in cardiac output. Due to a decrease in total peripheral resistance, **diastolic pressure increases** only slightly or even remains unchanged. With strong vasodilation of the skin blood vessels for thermoregulation, or vasodilation of blood vessels in muscles from severe fatigue, the diastolic pressure may be even lower than the value at rest. **Heart rate increases** linearly with increasing running speed (**Fig. 26.15**).

Performance physiology

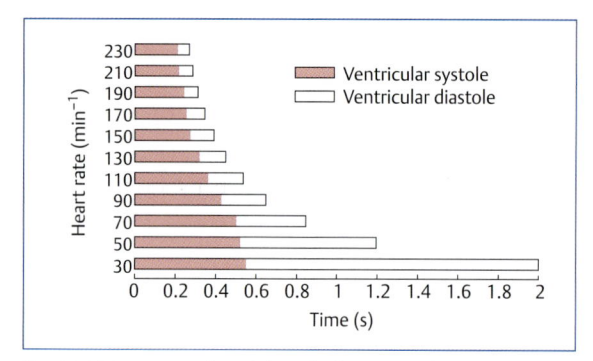

Fig. 26.14 Mean systole and diastole duration with increasing heart rate of horses. [Source: von Engelhardt W. The effect of work and training on the heart and circulation of the horse. Dtsch Tierärztl Wschr 1979; 86: 2–7]

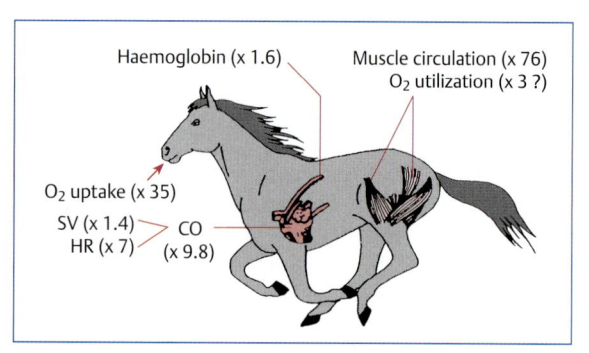

Fig. 26.16 Parameters of heart and circulation involved in the increased oxygen uptake during heavy work in horses. Mean increases during heavy work compared to resting values are given in parentheses. HR = heart rate; CO = cardiac output; SV = stroke volume.

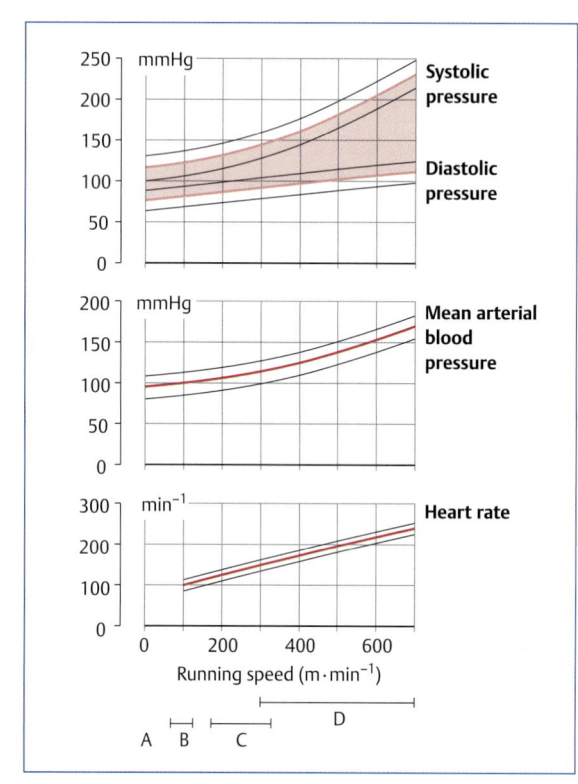

Fig. 26.15 Increase in systolic and diastolic blood pressure, mean arterial blood pressure and heart rate with increasing walking speed of warm-blooded horses. For the regression lines, the standard deviations are drawn as black lines. A=rest; B=stride; C= trot; D=canter. [Source: Hörnicke H, von Engelhardt W, Ehrlein HJ. Effect of exercise on systemic blood pressure in horses. Pfl Arch Physiol 1977; 372: 95–99]

26.3.5   Haemoglobin concentration and oxygen transport capacity of blood

The 35-fold increase in oxygen uptake in horses cannot be explained by the increased cardiac output alone. There is also an increased **oxygen transport capacity of** blood, better **muscle perfusion** and a higher **oxygen utilisation** in the working muscles (Bohr effect (p. 278), **Fig. 11.21 b**). Horses are able to **obtain more oxygen** by **releasing blood stored in their spleen** (ch. 8.3.2 and ch. 9.3.3). The **blood**

haematocrit and thus also the **haemoglobin concentration** in blood can be **increased** by up to 60% compared to resting values (**Fig. 26.16**). The resting haematocrit rises from an average of about $0.40 \, l \cdot l^{-1}$ during workload to $0.65 \, l \cdot l^{-1}$. The blood haemoglobin concentration rises from an average of $150 \, g \cdot l^{-1}$ at rest to $240 \, g \cdot l^{-1}$ at work (**Fig. 26.16**, ch. 8.3.3 (p. 195)). As a result, blood can also transport **60% more oxygen** when horses are under a heavy work **load**, so that O_2 supply to the working muscles can be considerably increased. Similar increases have been shown in the llama. In contrast, dogs and also humans, can only increase haemoglobin concentrations by about 20% during heavy exercise.

26.3.6   Muscle circulation

In horses, it has been shown that in strongly working muscles, blood flow was increased more than 70-fold compared to resting values (**Fig. 26.16**). This great increase in blood flow (p. 208) is due to a marked decrease in peripheral resistance in the working muscles, as a result of low pH-values and increased metabolic products. At the start of work, the O_2 deficit (**Fig. 26.4**) leads to an early increase in muscle blood flow. The low pH values and also the increased temperature in the working muscle increase vasodilation and, through the Bohr effect, facilitate the release of oxygen from haemoglobin. The **Bohr effect** which facilitates O_2 uptake in the lungs and O_2 release in muscle, is more developed in horses than in humans and most small animals (**Fig. 11.21 b**).

The process of **warming up** exercises in horses, improves muscle blood flow and thermoregulation, aerobic energy metabolism, and O_2 release. The O_2 deficit is lower, and return of the heart rate to resting values after exercise is also faster.

IN A NUTSHELL   !

Horses have a high aerobic capacity due to a high oxygen uptake in respiration, a large oxygen transport capacity of blood, a large heart with a large pumping capacity (**Table 26.7**), a high blood flow to working muscles and a well-developed Bohr effect.

26.4 Anaerobic metabolism, fatigue and blood lactate concentration

In many equestrian events, such as short distance races, most show jumping competitions and also in greyhound racing, anaerobic rather than aerobic metabolism is the major mechanism of energy supply (**Table 26.1**). In race-horses and greyhounds, the proportion of **rapidly contracting type II muscle fibres** is high and indicate a **high anaerobic capacity** (**Table 26.3**). The considerable ability of horses and dogs to obtain aerobically the energy required for working muscles, is discussed in the chapter on Aerobic Metabolism and Endurance (p.621). In addition, thoroughbreds and greyhounds can also obtain anaerobically a substantial proportion of their increasing requirement for ATP from the breakdown of pyruvate to lactate. This is seen as high blood lactate concentrations during races (**Table 26.5**). Because there is a high **lactate dehydrogenase activity (LDH)** in **muscle, thoroughbreds** and **greyhounds** can provide ATP quickly by anaerobic metabolism. Thoroughbreds and greyhounds, also have higher LDH activities than humans. LDH catalyses the reduction of pyruvate to lactate, the final reaction of anaerobic glycolysis (**Fig. 26.2**). Rapid muscle contractions and rapid ATP generation are an advantage of type II muscle fibres. However, they have major disadvantages of quickly becoming fatigued, and anaerobic ATP production is energetically much less efficient than that of type I fibres. In racing camels, which have predominantly type I fibres in their muscles, maximum blood lactate concentrations are significantly lower than in thoroughbreds and greyhounds (**Table 26.2**; **Table 26.3**; **Table 26.5**).

Table 26.5 Maximum blood lactate concentrations in racehorses, greyhound dogs, racing camels and trained humans.

Animal species	Maximum blood lactate concentrations (mmol·l^{-1})
Thoroughbreds	30
Greyhound	20
Racing camel	12
Human	15

Source: Values compiled by Derman & Noakes, in: Hodgson DR, Rose RJ. The Athletic Horse. Philadelphia: W. B. Saunders; 1994

In intensive, prolonged work, where sufficient ATP can no longer be provided aerobically, muscle must obtain the required ATP anaerobically. As a result, **lactate is** increasingly produced in the muscle. **Blood lactate concentration** is an indicator for **muscle fatigue** and **general fatigue**.

Fatigue can be defined as the inability to maintain a required force, which results in a drop in performance. Fatigue can be characterised as:

- **general fatigue**, where the whole organism is affected,
- **partial fatigue**, which affects individual muscle groups, or
- **central fatigue**, in which, for example, the sensation of pain is influenced via the CNS.

The following can be involved in **muscle fatigue** above all:

- reduced cross-bridge formation due to intracellular pH drop at increased lactate concentrations, inhibition of ATPase activity, reduced binding of Ca^{2+} to troponin C (**Fig. 6.5**), see ch. on filament sliding and cross-bridge cycle (p.150), disturbances of phosphorylation.
- Disturbances at the cell membranes (e.g. permeability changes) and thus in the excitability of muscle cells.
- Changes in electromechanical coupling (p.149)
- Depletion of glycogen stores in muscle cells
- Tears in the sarcomeres and swollen sarcoplasmic reticulum, see ch. force development and excitation frequency (p.155)

26.5 Thermoregulation and sweat secretion

The considerable increase in metabolic rate during exercise means that the body has to release large amounts of heat. Only 20–25% of the chemical energy can be used by the muscle as mechanical work, 75–80% is released as heat (**Fig. 19.1**); (see ch. on power metabolism (p.490)). A rapid release of heat (p.495) during and **after work** is therefore absolutely essential for the survival of an animal. In the horse, this release takes place mainly through sweating (p.503), and less through respiration than in other domestic animals. During short periods of exertion, heat release is possible without significant difficulties. For longer periods of exertion, such as a long-distance ride of over 80 km, very large amounts of sweat are produced. For a horse weighing 500 kg, a sweat production of 37 litres has been calculated. With longer times of work loads, the evaporation of sweat and thus the effectiveness of cooling, depends on the **air humidity** and the **air movement**. In a dry, warm climate, these conditions for evaporation are favourable. At high humidity and low air movement and also when horses are brought into a stable or into an indoor arena immediately after performing heavy work loads, only ⅓ of the sweat formed may evaporate, while ⅔ flows from the coat without evaporation and thus, without appreciable heat loss for the horse.

Under heavy loads, heat production can be higher than heat release. In thoroughbreds and greyhounds, **core body temperature** will therefore rise accordingly. In horses, blood temperatures of over 42.8 °C have been measured after 8.7 minutes on a treadmill at a running speed of

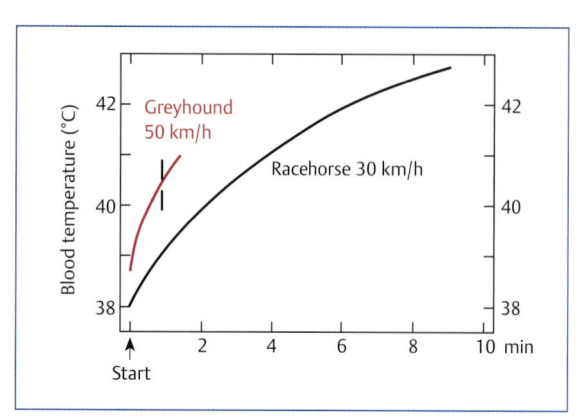

Fig. 26.17 Increase in body temperatures in the pulmonary artery in thoroughbred horses and in greyhounds during running at high running speeds. In horses running 1100 m at a 10% incline on a treadmill at about 90% of maximum oxygen uptake, blood temperature had risen to more than 42 °C at 8.7 minutes after starting. Greyhounds trained for sprinting managed 704 m on the dog track in only 51.2 seconds, and ran much faster than thoroughbred horses. Their weight-related energy expenditure is higher than that of horses. Blood temperature rose much more steeply in dogs (1.82 °C·min⁻¹); Equine progression curves: based on data from Hodgson DR, Rose RJ. The Athletic Horse. Philadelphia: W. B. Saunders; 1994. Curves for the dogs: based on data from Nold JL, Peterson LJ, Fedde MR. Physiological changes in the running greyhoud (Canis domesticus): influence of race length. Comp Biochem Physiol A 1991; 100: 623–627

8.5 m/s (**Fig. 26.17**). In the working muscles average temperatures of even 43.9 °C have been reported. In greyhounds, the body temperature rose very quickly by 1.53 °C within 51.2 seconds at a mean running speed of 13.8 m/s. This is hyperthermia (p. 507) and **not a fever**. If heat dissipation is restricted by high humidity and high ambient temperature during and after heavy exercise, this can quickly lead to **heat exhaustion**.

> **MORE DETAILS   Cloven-hoofed ungulates** and also **cats** can effectively **cool** their brain during exercise hyperthermia through the heat exchanger (p. 497) in the **rete mirabile**. As a result, the regulator in the hypothalamus is not responding to the actual temperature in the rest of the body. The necessary temperature regulation controlled by the regulator, therefore does not occur in these animals as long as their brain is cooled.
> With the help of this brain cooling mechanism, camels can reduce their water losses by very efficient regulation of sweat secretion and impressive water reabsorption in the kidney tubules. This enables them to survive for up to two weeks without drinking during very hot dry periods. Horses and also humans, monkeys, rabbits, guinea pigs, hamsters and rats do not have rete mirabile. In horses, it has been suspected that the air sacs cool the blood flowing to the brain. However, recent studies have shown that this attractive hypothesis is not true. In horses and in zebras, **brain cooling does not** occur during hyperthermia.

IN A NUTSHELL   !

Horses do not have a rete mirabile and cannot cool the hypothalamus region during hyperthermia like cloven-hoofed animals.

Fluid losses from **sweating** can be considerable. During **endurance riding, an** average of 7–8 l of sweat is secreted per hour. After five hours of endurance riding, horses have lost about 8% of their body weight through sweating. At high running speeds in hot climates, sweat secretion rates as high as 15 l per hour can be reached. During prolonged exertion, horses can lose up to 10% of their body weight as a result, and should therefore be given an opportunity to take in water. Since horses usually do not want to take in water spontaneously under such conditions, it is helpful if the animals are already accustomed, by training, to take in water after exertion.

IN A NUTSHELL   !

Due to high energy metabolism, a great deal of heat is generated during hard physical work, which horses mainly release through evaporation of sweat.

The **electrolyte concentrations in sweat** and thus also **electrolyte losses** are much higher in horses than in humans (**Table 26.6**). Whereas human sweat is strongly hypotonic compared to blood, in horses it is isotonic or slightly hypertonic. With heavy sweat secretion, the **osmolarity** of blood in horses, remains largely unchanged, whereas in humans the blood becomes increasingly hypertonic. This constant isotonicity of blood is certainly one of the reasons why horses do not show any clear signs of thirst after prolonged exercise despite a considerable loss of water. With every litre of sweat, horses lose 3 to 4 times more sodium, chloride and potassium than humans. These electrolyte losses can be compensated for by additions to the feed and also by electrolytes in the drinking water.

IN A NUTSHELL   !

The electrolyte concentration in horse sweat is high compared to humans. Horses lose a lot of Na⁺ and Cl⁻ during prolonged sweating.

Table 26.6 Electrolyte concentrations (mmol·l⁻¹) in the sweat of horses and humans.

Species	Sodium	Potassium	Chloride
Horse	130–190	20–50	160–190
Human	40–60	4–5	30–50

Source: Snow DH. Exercise and training. In: Hickman J (ed.). Horse Management. London: Academic Press; 1984: 251–331

> **MORE DETAILS**   The ability to sweat profusely is something that only a few mammals have developed during evolution. Humans, equids, some species of monkeys and also camels, can produce sweat all over their bodies. Sweat glands are also present in large areas of skin of cattle, sheep and goats, as well as in eight African wild ruminants that have been studied. In addition to sweating, these animals can also pant. Very small ruminants in particular, regulate their heat output more through panting than sweating.

In thermoregulation through sweating, there are significant species differences. In **humans**, evaporation can occur directly from hairless skin. **Horses**, on the other hand, have a thick, largely waterproof, **hairy coat**. The secreted sweat must pass through the thick coat, so that evaporation then takes place on the coat surface. In order for this to happen quickly enough, horse sweat contains a very special ingredient, the protein **latherin**. Latherin **reduces** the **water surface tension**. As a result, the sweat is distributed more evenly, the hair is moistened and the sweat can flow more easily through the coat. On the coat, the reduced surface tension causes the **formation of foam**. As a result, the sweat surface is enlarged and a relatively large amount of water can evaporate quickly, reducing the dripping of sweat. In this way, a rapidly running horse can quickly release large amounts of heat over long distances. In addition, the formation of foam results in a shiny sheen on the surface of the hair which improves **reflection** of the **sun's rays**.

Camels can only survive in hot deserts if they can give off enough heat with as little water loss as possible. Camels do not pant and there is no visible sweating. Their coat is always dry. For a long time it was therefore assumed that camels had no sweat glands. However, camels have many sweat glands, distributed over the whole body. However, if camels were to sweat the way horses do, the loss of water in hot desert conditions would be far too high. Camels have therefore developed an interesting, particularly **water-saving method of thermoregulation**. With the help of a cooling system (p.497) in the **rete mirabile** in the brain, they can regulate heat loss only after core body temperature has risen to 41–42 °C. The **sweating that** then follows is extraordinarily **well regulated** and also greatly **reduced**. Only as much sweat is secreted as can completely **evaporate** directly on the **skin surface**. The resulting water vapour passes through the coat to the outside, the coat itself remains dry and remains a very good insulator. With increasing dehydration, camels continue to gradually reduce sweat secretion, so that after 14 days without water, cutaneous water losses are hardly measurable.

26.6 Influence of training on aerobic metabolism, heart and circulation, skeletal muscle and thermoregulation

26.6.1 Haemoglobin concentration and oxygen transport capacity

Training improves the ability of horses to release **erythrocytes** from the **spleen** during exercise and thus increase the **oxygen transport capacity** of blood. However, **blood haemoglobin concentrations** have already reached a **plateau** with moderate training, and **further training** does not cause any further **increase**. This limitation makes sense because a higher increase in erythrocyte concentration and thus also in the **haematocrit**, would increase blood viscosity (p.195) excessively, and thus put a strain on the heart.

26.6.2 Heart size, stroke volume and heart rate

Horses and also other mammals that run longer distances because of the way they live, usually have a **relatively large heart**. In an untrained thoroughbred, the heart weighs, as a proportion of body weight, 0.8–1%, and in warmblood horses 0.6–0.7%. In contrast, rabbits, which only run short distances, have a heart weight of only slightly more than 0.4% of body weight. As an adaptation to training, **hypertrophy** of the **heart muscle** occurs, as it does in human athletes. In trained thoroughbreds, heart muscle weights of 1.04% and in greyhounds of 1.5% of body weight have been measured (**Table 26.7**). Since the heart beat volume increases approximately linearly with heart weight, an **increase** in heart size and thus heart **beat volume** of about 20–25% can be expected after intensive endurance training.

Table 26.7 Heart weights as a percentage of body weight (% bw) in trained racehorses, greyhounds, racing camels and humans.

	Thorough-breds	Grey-hound	Racing camel	Human
Heart weight (% BW)	1.04	1.50	0.60	0.33

Source: Saltin B, Rose RJ. The Racing Camel – Physiology, metabolic functions, and adaptations. Acta Physiol Scand 1994; 150 (Suppl): 61

During a defined, standardised load, the large heart of the trained horse beats more slowly than the smaller heart of the less trained horse. For a given running speed, better trained horses therefore have a lower heart rate than less trained animals. The **dependency** between **heart rate** and **running speed** at defined loads is therefore used as a **parameter** for assessing the **state of training**. A lower slope of the linear dependency between running speed and heart rate (**Fig. 26.18**) is considered an improvement in the endurance performance of a horse. This means that training requires a lower heart rate for a certain running speed, or that a horse can run faster at a defined heart rate than before training. The v_{HR140} is often used as a measurement parameter (running speed of horses in $m \cdot min^{-1}$ at a heart rate of $140\,min^{-1}$). An improved v_{HR140} can also be interpreted as an increase in heart weight and thus as an increased cardiac output.

26.6.3 Oxygen intake

Training can increase maximum oxygen uptake ($\dot{V}_{O_2max}$) (**Fig. 26.6**, **Fig. 26.16**), which improves the **aerobic capacity** of a horse. In trained sport horses, compared to untrained horses, the working muscles are supplied with more blood, O_2 transport capacity of blood is improved and cardiac output is increased. This means that more oxygen is available to the working muscles for ATP production.

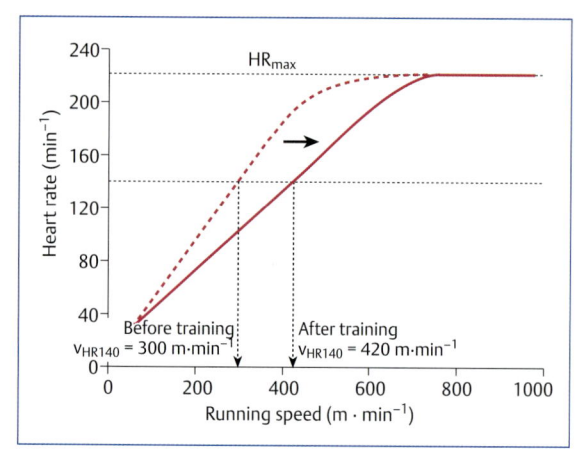

Fig. 26.18 Heart rate (HR) in horses before (dashed red line) and after training (solid red line). In untrained horses the v_{HR140} (running speed at a HR of 140 min⁻¹) was 300 m · min⁻¹, in trained horses 420 m · min⁻¹. The maximum HR (HR$_{max}$) remained unchanged; based on data from Marlin D, Nankervis K. Equine Exercise Physiology. Oxford: Blackwell; 2002

26.6.4 Skeletal muscle

Appropriate **endurance training** of horses can increase maximum oxygen uptake, the pumping capacity of the heart, and blood flow and thus oxygen supply to working muscles. The **oxidative capacity** of the enzymes for the **breakdown of free fatty acids** (Fig. 26.2; Fig. 6.13) can be improved, and the number and size of **mitochondria** can be increased. Training can change the ratio between type I and type II muscle fibres (p.156), although muscle fibres can be changed relatively little. However, type IIB fibres can be converted into type IIA fibres and also somewhat into I fibres (**Table 26.2**). Training can also improve the **glycogen reserve** in muscle cells. However, after complete glycogen depletion during the heaviest work, it takes at least two days for glycogen stores in muscle to be fully replenished. In strong, prolonged exertion, **more ATP** can be made available **aerobically** in the trained horse, so that correspondingly **less** lactate (p.627) is formed (**Fig. 26.19**), and trained horses therefore tire less than untrained horses.

> **IN A NUTSHELL**   !
>
> In trained horses, blood lactate concentrations are lower than in untrained horses at defined standardised loads. Glycogen reserves in muscle cells are improved by training.

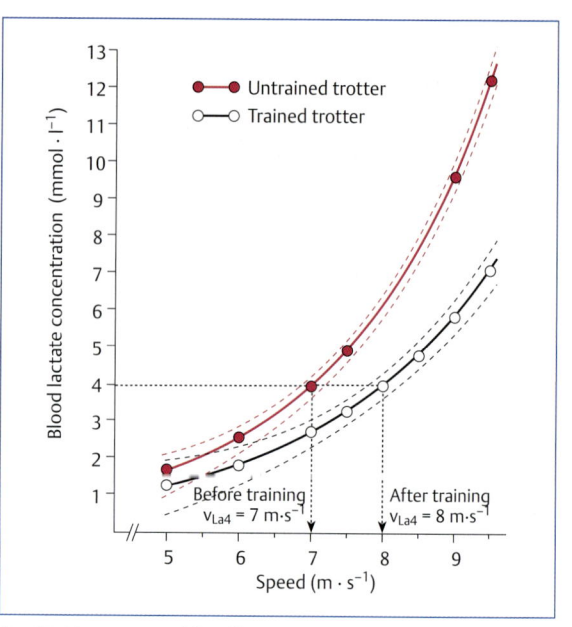

Fig. 26.19 Increase in blood lactate concentrations in venous blood in untrained and trained trotters as a function of running speed. The v_{La4} (running speed at a blood lactate concentration of 4 mmol · l⁻¹) was 7 m · s⁻¹ in the untrained horses and 8 m · s⁻¹ in the trained ones. [Source: Thornton JB, Essén-Gustavsson B, Lindholm A et al. Effects of training and detraining on oxygen uptake, cardiac output, blood gas tensions, pH and lactate concentrations during and after exercise in the horse. In: Snow DH, Person SGB, Rose RJ (eds.). Equine Exercise Physiology. Cambridge: Granta Editions; 1983: 470–486]

26.6.5 Sweat secretion and thermoregulation

Intensive training of horses increases **sweat secretion rates** during standardised exercise. This improves heat release and thus reduces hyperthermia during exercise. In the increased secreted sweat (p.627), the Na⁺ concentration is lower and the concentration of K⁺ higher, while that of Cl⁻ remains unchanged.

26.7 Assessment of the training condition and performance of sport horses

MORE DETAILS Up to now, the available methods have almost exclusively been used to assess only the **aerobic capacity** of horses and thus their **endurance performance**. Endurance plays a decisive role especially in eventing competitions, long races, endurance rides, heavy jumping competitions and also sled dog races.

Measurements of **heart rate** during **standardised exercise tests** and **blood lactate concentrations** immediately afterwards can help to assess an animal's endurance performance. For the assessment of the training condition, the v_{HR140} (running speed at a heart rate of 140 min⁻¹; **Fig. 26.18**) and the v_{La4} (running speed at blood lactate concentrations of 4 mmol · l⁻¹; **Fig. 26.19**) are used. On a treadmill, oxygen uptake (p.621) at **defined loads** can also be recorded as an important parameter (**Fig. 26.6**).

The **maximum oxygen uptake** ($\dot{V}_{O_2 max}$) is a very reliable indicator of the aerobic capacity and thus the endurance performance of a horse. However, such measurements can only be carried out by specialists in this field. Biopsy samples make it possible to assess **glycogen storage** in muscle cells and, to some extent, a transformation towards the slower **muscle fibre types** with more aerobic capacity.

The decrease in heart rate (**recovery pulse sum**) during a forced break in endurance rides, or after the cross-country ride of an eventing competition, is a valuable parameter for assessing the state of exhaustion and thus the condition of horses. However, previous studies on horses show that blood and circulation parameters obtained at rest, do not give any indication of their training condition.

For assessment of **anaerobic performance**, which is so important in many equine **performance** sports, there is no satisfactory test that can be carried out under practical conditions. Investigations of the glycogen stores in muscle cells before and after intensive, very well standardised exertion can provide some indication of anaerobic performance.

Suggested reading

Eaton MD, Evans DL, Hodgson DR et al. Maximal accumulated oxygen deficit in Thoroughbred horses. J Appl Physiol 1995; 78: 1546–1568

Evans DL. Physiology of equine performance and associated tests of function. Equine Vet J 2007; 39: 373–383

Fuller A, Maloney SK, Kamerman PR et al. Absence of brain cooling in free-ranging zebras in their natural habitat. Exp Physiol 2000; 85: 209–217

Hinchcliff KW, Geor RJ, Kaneps AJ. Equine Exercise Physiology. The Science of Exercise in the Athletic Horse. Philadelphia: Saunders, Elsevier; 2008

Hodgson DR, McGowan C, McKeeven K. The athletic horse: Principles and practice of equine sports medicine. St. Louis: Elsevier Saunders; 2013

Hodgson DR, Rose RJ. The athletic horse. Philadelphia: W. B. Saunders; 1994

Lacombe VA, Hinchcliff KW, Geor RJ et al. Muscle glycogen depletion and subsequent replenishment affect anaerobic capacity of horses. J Appl Physiol 2001; 91: 1782–1790

Lafortuna CL, Saibene F, Albertini M et al. The regulation of respiratory resistance in exercising horses. Eur J Appl Physiol 2003; 90: 396–404

Lekeux P. Pulmonary function in healthy, exercising and diseased animals. Flem Vet J, Special Issue; 1993

Marlin D, Nankervis K. Equine exercise physiology. Oxford: Blackwell; 2002

McCutcheon LJ, Geor RJ. Influence of training on sweating responses during submaximal exercise in horses. J Appl Physiol 2000; 89: 2463–2471

McDonald, RE, Fleming RI, Beeley JG et al. Latherin: Surfactant protein of horse sweat and saliva. PLoS ONE 2009; 4: e5726

Mitchell G, Fuller A, Malone SK et al. Guttural pouches, brain temperature and exercise in horses. Biol Lett 2006; 2: 475–477

Padilla DJ, McDonough P, Kindig CA et al. Ventilatory dynamics and control of blood gases after maximal exercise in the thoroughbred horse. J Appl Physiol 2004; 96: 2187–2193

Poole DC, Erickson HH. Highly athletic terrestrial mammals: horses and dogs. Compr Physiol 2011; 1:1–37

Rose RJ, Evans DL. Cardiovascular and respiratory function in the athletic horse. In: Gillespie JR, Robinson NE, eds. Equine exercise physiology 2, Davis: ICEEP Publications; 1987: 1–24.

Saltin B, Rose RJ. The Racing Camel – Physiology, metabolic functions, and adaptations. Acta Physiol Scand 1994; 150 (Suppl): 61

Shave R, Howatson G, Dickson D, Young L. Exercised-induced cardiac remodelling: lessons from humans, horses, and dogs. Vet Sci 2017; 4: 1–16

Sharp NCC. Animal athletes: a performance review. Vet Rec 2012; 171: 87–94

Vance SJ, McDonald RE, Cooper A et al. The structure of latherin, a surfactant allergen protein from horse sweat and saliva. J R Soc Interface 2013: 10(85): 20130453

Appendix

27 Measured quantities and units of measurement

Martin Diener, Gotthold Gäbel, Gerhard Breves, David Fraser

27.1 Greek letters

In the context of physiology, Greek letters are often used and are listed below (**Table 27.1**).

Table 27.1 Greek letters.

Uppercase form	Lowercase form	Name
A	α	alpha
B	β	beta
Γ	γ	gamma
Δ	δ	delta
E	ε	epsilon
H	η	eta
Θ	ϑ	theta
K	κ	kappa
Λ	λ	lambda
M	μ	mu
N	ν	nu
Π	π	pi
P	ρ	rho
Σ	σ	sigma
T	τ	tau
Φ	φ	phi
X	χ	chi
Ψ	ψ	psi
Ω	ω	omega

27.2 Exponentiation and logarithms

Numbers that are much larger or much smaller than 1 are best represented to the base ten (decimal) number system. Numbers greater than 1 have positive exponents in this numbering system (e.g. $10000 = 10^4$), numbers smaller than 1 have negative exponents (e.g. $0.0001 = 10^{-4}$). Frequently used powers of ten have their own names or abbreviations (**Table 27.2**).

Table 27.2 Frequently used powers of ten.

Decimal multiples and parts of units (short scale nomenclature)		Metric prefix	Abbreviation
Quintillionth	10^{-18}	atto	a
Quadrillionth	10^{-15}	femto	f
Trillionth	10^{-12}	pico	p
Billionth	10^{-9}	nano	n
Millionth	10^{-6}	micro	μ
Thousandth	10^{-3}	milli	m
Hundredth	10^{-2}	centi	c
Tenth	10^{-1}	deci	d
Tenfold	10	deca	da
Hundredfold	10^2	hecto	h
Thousandfold	10^3	kilo	k
Millionfold	10^6	mega	M
Billionfold	10^9	giga	G
Trillionfold	10^{12}	tera	T
Quadrillionfold	10^{15}	peta	P

When calculating with the superscripts (exponents), **logarithmic notation is used**. If, for example, 100 is written as a power to the base 10 (10^2), the exponent 2 is called the **decadic logarithm (log$_{10}$)** of 100 ($\log_{10} 100$) ($y = 10^x$ means $x = \log_{10} y$). In physiology, such logarithms are found, for example, in the definition of the pH value, in the Nernst equation or in the specification of the sound pressure level. The **natural logarithm (ln)** is logarithm to the base of the mathematical constant e, where $e = 2.71828$ (Euler's number). Many processes in nature can be described by exponential functions ($y = e^x$ means $x = \ln y$).

Since $\log_{10} x = \ln x \cdot (\ln 10)^{-1}$ and $\ln 10 = 2.3026$, the conversion from ln to $\log_{10}$ and vice versa is done:

$$\log_{10} x = \ln x \cdot 2.3^{-1}$$

$$\ln x \quad = 2.3 \cdot \log_{10} x$$

When comparing very small and very large values, logarithms are often used.

27.3 International System of Units (SI)

In 1960, the 11th "Conférence Générale des Poids et Mesures" (CGPM) recommended the "Système International d'Unités (SI)" as the international system of units (**Table 27.3**).

The units of all measured quantities can be derived from the SI base units. A selection is compiled in **Table 27.4**.

27.4 Older units of measurement

In medical subjects, older units of measurement are often used in addition to the SI units. Often both units are used side by side. In **Table 27.5** some conversions from the older to the SI units are compiled.

Table 27.3 Names and symbols of the 7 SI base units.

Measurand	Basic units	Symbol
Length	metre	m
Mass	kilogram	kg
Amount of substance	mole	mol
Time	second	s
Electric current	ampere	A
Thermodynamic temperature	kelvin	K
Luminous intensity	candela	cd

Table 27.4 Names and symbols of some derived SI units.

Measurand	Definition	SI unit	Abbreviation	Symbol
Force	Mass times acceleration	$kg \cdot m \cdot s^{-2}$	newton	N
Work, energy, heat quantity	Force times distance	$kg \cdot m^2 \cdot s^{-2} = N \cdot m$	joule	J
Power	Work per time	$kg \cdot m^2 \cdot s^{-3} = J \cdot s^{-1}$	watt	W
Pressure	Force per area	$kg \cdot m^{-1} \cdot s^{-2} = N \cdot m^{-2}$	pascal	Pa
Voltage	Power per current	$kg \cdot m^2 \cdot A^{-1} \cdot s^{-3} = W \cdot A^{-1}$	volt	V
Resistance	Voltage per current	$kg \cdot m^2 \cdot A^{-2} \cdot s^{-3} = V \cdot A^{-1}$	ohm	Ω
Electrical conductance	Current per voltage	$A^2 \cdot s^3 \cdot kg^{-1} \cdot m^{-2} = A \cdot V^{-1}$	siemens	S
Electric charge	Current times second	$A \cdot s$	coulomb	C

Table 27.5 Conversion of older units to SI units.

Measurand	Old units	Symbol	Conversion to SI units
Length	Ångström	Å	$1\ \text{Å} = 10^{-10}$ m
Pressure	Mercury column	mmHg	1 mmHg = 1 Torr = 133.3 Pa*
	Water column	cmWC	1 cmWC = 98 Pa
	Bar	bar	1 bar = 100 kPa
	Technical atmosphere	at	1 at = 98.07 kPa
	Standard atmosphere	atm	1 atm = 101.325 kPa
Work	Calorie	cal	1 cal = 4.187 J
	Kilowatt-hour	kWh	1 kWh = 3600 kJ
Thermal energy	Calorie	cal	1 cal = 4.187 J
	Watt-second	Ws	$1\ W \cdot s = 1$ J
Temperature	Degree Celsius	°C	t [°C] = T [K] − 273.15[1]

* In medical textbooks, pressures are usually still given in mmHg or in cmWC (cm water column). Temperatures are only given in degrees Celsius.

Index

Abbreviated terms (cf. list of abbreviations) are usually found with the full form (exception: chemical symbols and chemical ratio formulae).